AF577328

Progress in Pain Research and Management
Volume 24

Proceedings of the 10th World Congress on Pain

Mission Statement of IASP Press®

The International Association for the Study of Pain (IASP) is a nonprofit, interdisciplinary organization devoted to understanding the mechanisms of pain and improving the care of patients with pain through research, education, and communication. The organization includes scientists and health care professionals dedicated to these goals. The IASP sponsors scientific meetings and publishes newsletters, technical bulletins, the journal *Pain,* and books.

The goal of IASP Press is to provide the IASP membership with timely, high-quality, attractive, low-cost publications relevant to the problem of pain. These publications are also intended to appeal to a wider audience of scientists and clinicians interested in the problem of pain.

Progress in Pain Research and Management
Volume 24

Proceedings of the 10th World Congress on Pain

Editors

Jonathan O. Dostrovsky, PhD

Physiology Department,
University of Toronto,
Toronto, Ontario, Canada

Daniel B. Carr, MD

Departments of Anesthesia and Medicine,
Tufts-New England Medical Center,
Boston, Massachusetts, USA

Martin Koltzenburg, MD

Institutes of Child Health and Neurology,
University College London,
London, United Kingdom

IASP PRESS® • SEATTLE

Timely topics in pain research and treatment have been selected for publication, but the information provided and opinions expressed have not involved any verification of the findings, conclusions, and opinions by IASP®. Thus, opinions expressed in *Proceedings of the 10th World Congress on Pain* do not necessarily reflect those of IASP or of the Officers and Councillors.

No responsibility is assumed by IASP for any injury and/or damage to persons or property as a matter of product liability, negligence, or from any use of any methods, products, instruction, or ideas contained in the material herein. Because of the rapid advances in the medical sciences, the publisher recommends that there should be independent verification of diagnoses and drug dosages.

Library of Congress Cataloging-in-Publication Data

World Congress on Pain (10th : 2002 : San Diego, Calif.)
Proceedings of the 10th World Congress on Pain / editors, Jonathan O. Dostrovsky, Daniel B. Carr, Martin Koltzenburg.
p. ; cm. -- (Progress in pain research and management ; v. 24)
Includes bibliographical references and index.
ISBN 0-931092-46-9 (alk. paper)
1. Pain--Congresses. 1. Title: Proceedings of the Tenth World Congress on Pain. II. Dostrovsky, Jonathan O. III. Carr, Daniel B. IV. Koltzenburg, Martin, 1962- V. Title. VI. Series.
[DNLM: 1. Pain--Congresses. WL 704 W927p 2003]
RB127.W67 2002
616'.0472--dc21

2002191922

Published by:

IASP Press
International Association for the Study of Pain
909 NE 43rd Street, Suite 306
Seattle, WA 98105-6020 USA
Fax: 206-547-1703
www.iasp-pain.org
www.painbooks.org

Printed in the United States of America

Contents

Part VII: Clinical Epidemiology

Part VIII: Pain Assessment: Quantitative and Qualitative

Part IX: Specific Clinical Syndromes and Settings

Contributing Authors

Abram, S.E., 739
Africano, J.M., 601
Alcala, R., 601
Amris, K., 791
Andrew, D., 213
Arnold, C., 611
Ashby, M., 803
Aziz, Q., 261

Baba, H., 245
Baccarelli, R., 563
Ballantyne, J., 213
Bär, K.-J., 397
Baron, R., 683
Basbaum, A.I., 19
Beaufour, C., 539
Belzberg, A., 155
Benedetti, F., 315
Bimson, W.E., 295
Binder, A., 683
Bond, M.R., 13
Bradley, L.A., 865
Braz, J., 539
Bridges, D., 437
Brooks, J.C.W., 295
Brooks, J.W., 437
Broom, D.C., 387
Bushnell, M.C., 261

Cairns, B.E., 125
Campbell, J., 155
Cao, C.Q., 89
Carlton, S.M., 125
Carr, D.B., 601
Cepeda, M.S., 601
Cervero, F., 327
Cesselin, F., 539
Chiang, C.Y., 345
Christie, M.J., 481
Chung, J.M., 99

Coggeshall, R.E., 387
Cohen, M.L., 865
Craig, A.D., 197
Crombez, G., 651

Davis, K.D., 261
Devor, M., 305, 725
Diamant, N.E., 261
Dib-Hajj, S.D., 99
Dickenson, A.H., 337
Dionne, R.A., 513
Dostrovsky, J.O., 345
Dray, A., 89
Dubner, R., 355
Duncan, G.H., 261

Ebersberger, A., 397
Eccleston, C., 853
Ekholm, O., 551
Eliav, E., 589
Eriksen, J., 551

Faravelli, L., 115
Fariello, R.G., 115
Farquhar-Smith, W.P., 437
Fitzgerald, M., 185
Flor, H., 725
Fors, E.A., 865
Frank, A.W., 619
Furue, H., 245

Garcia-Larrea, L., 277
Garcia-Nicas, E., 327
Gardner, P., 611
Garland, K., 611
Gibson, S.J., 611, 767

Goldman, D., 513
Gracely, R.H., 589
Gregory, L., 261
Griffin, J.W., 155
Guan, Y., 355

Hamon, M., 539
Handwerker, H.O., 141
Hansson, P., 589
Hart, D.L., 893
Hawkins, R., 839
Heinricher, M.M., 251
Herrington, N., 577
Hill, R.G., 419
Honda, T., 227
Hopf, H.-C., 407
Hu, B., 345
Hu, J.W., 345
Huijer Abu-Saad, H., 705
Hunfeld, J.A.M., 853
Hunt, S.P., 337

Iadarola, M.J., 513
Ito, A., 245

Jadad, A.R., 49
Jennings, E.A., 481
Jensen, M.K., 551
Jensen, T.S., 725
Ji, R.-R., 81
Johnson, L., 577
Jost, 803 T.S.,
Julius, D., 63

Kalso, E., 751
Kawasaki, Y., 245
Kim, H., 513

Preface

It is now almost 30 years since the International Association for the Study of Pain (IASP) was formed. This period has seen considerable growth in pain-related research, in our understanding of the complexity of the pain system, in the diversity and sophistication of approaches to manage of pain, and in the awareness of pain as a major health problem among clinicians, policy makers, and the public. This remarkable progress was evident at the 10th World Congress on Pain, held in San Diego, California, August 17–22, 2002. The scenic coastal location and convenient facilities contributed to a very successful meeting, attracting over 6,000 registrants, the largest number to attend any IASP World Congress. In keeping with the aims of the association and previous congresses, the program and participants included researchers and clinicians covering aspects of pain ranging from cellular and molecular mechanisms to cognitive treatments and ethical issues. This mosaic of basic and clinical science was apparent in all of the plenary sessions, workshops, and poster sessions and even within individual talks and workshops.

The Congress consisted of the usual full day of well-attended refresher courses followed by 5 very full days of scientific sessions. The refresher course syllabus is published separately as *Pain 2002—An Updated Review,* edited by Maria Adele Giamberardino (Seattle: IASP Press, 2002). There were over 1,650 poster presentations, 82 workshops, and 20 plenary talks. Attendance at all of the sessions was very high, and the meeting attracted significant media attention. Notably absent, unfortunately, was Professor Patrick Wall, who passed away on August 8, 2001 (his obituary was published in *Pain* 2001; 94(2):125–129). His always-cheerful and inquisitive presence was much missed. Readers may find Allan Basbaum's description of his encounters with Pat (Chapter 3) of interest. As for the past three congresses, these proceedings of the 10th World Congress are published by IASP Press, marking its 10th anniversary in 2003.

This volume includes in its 10 sections all 20 plenary talks as well as 27 free communications. So much interesting new material was presented at the meeting that only a small fraction could be included in this book. As editors, we aimed to provide a sampling of interesting presentations covering a diverse range of topics. In contrast to previous congress proceedings volumes, this book also includes 22 chapters that summarize findings presented at workshops.

In the first section we include the outgoing and incoming presidents' addresses as well as the John J. Bonica Distinguished Lecture. Also in this section, plenary lectures by Morris and Jadad survey ethical issues and implications of the digital information age for pain management. The second group of chapters highlights recent developments in basic pain research on the properties of nociceptors. This section provides a small sample of the many papers presented on this rapidly progressing field, which has greatly benefited from new molecular biology techniques. The chapters in Part III examine issues related to the central processing of nociceptive signals. They range from studies at the single cell level in the spinal cord, to ascending pathways and descending modulation, and to cortical processing as examined with functional imaging. The fourth section focuses on the important and active area of research on central sensitization. Part V presents some recent pharmacological studies illustrating the rapid progress in our understanding of drugs and receptors involved in mediating and modulating pain. This section covers both animal and human studies, including a chapter on side effects of COX-2 inhibitors and other nonsteroidal anti-inflammatory drugs in humans. Part VI provides a glimpse of the rapidly developing fields of genetic influences on pain and gene therapy.

The remaining sections deal with the epidemiology of pain, pain assessment using multiple approaches, descriptions of specific pain syndromes and settings, and the outcomes of pain treatment by pharmacological and nonpharmacological techniques. The chapters grouped under "Clinical Epidemiology" advance our understanding of the incidence and prevalence of pain of different etiologies in different patient groups and nations. Those in Part VIII describe quantitative and qualitative approaches to exploring nociception and its disorders, as well as more subjective, narrative accounts of pain experiences that form the basis for qualitative research. Included in this eighth section are analyses of patient self-reports, which help us to understand the connections between pain, suffering, negative emotions, and responses to treatment of acute and chronic pain.

Given the complexity of clinical pain and the innumerable individuals and settings in which it occurs worldwide, the chapters in Part IX can only hint at the diversity of reports presented at the World Congress. Those selected for publication span topics of pain in patients with well-characterized medical conditions (such as cancer, phantom limb pain, or complex regional pain syndrome), to groups of patients such as the aged, those at the end of life, or the developmentally impaired whose special needs and characteristics require more focused attention. Ethical and legal issues figure prominently in end of life care and are surveyed from an international perspective in this section as well.

The final section surveys the application of several forms of behavioral pain therapies to diverse populations, concluding with two chapters that deal not only with specific results of rehabilitation programs but also more broadly with the assessment of the outcomes of pain treatment. Because of the great financial and human burden of chronic pain and disability, particularly low back pain, these two chapters emphasize the importance of prompt return of those with industrial injury to the workplace. They also illustrate the key role of evidence-based methods (also emphasized by McQuay and others in prior sections) for the development and appraisal of treatment approaches. In assessing the results of pain therapies, multiple authors in these proceedings emphasize that the goal is not simply to minimize pain intensity but also to maximize quality of life and functionality.

While health care systems are at times accused of indifference to the needs for pain control among those under its care, other governmental entities with growing frequency are engaged in deliberate violation of human rights, i.e., torture. The moving chapter on work with survivors of torture bears witness to the extremes of human behavior—from deliberately harming others to achieve some political or economic objective to caring for these often impoverished and marginalized sufferers. Amidst thousands of pain researchers and clinicians sharing their knowledge with colleagues from around the world, abundant reminders were present that the world is full of discord. Adjacent to a large naval base, the conference center had continuous surveillance aircraft overhead, watching for terrorist infiltrators. Troop ships and battle vessels debarked frequently, a sobering reminder of ongoing military activities. In a world perhaps destined never to be at peace and in which the vulnerable are often overlooked, the decade-long advocacy of pain control as a human right by recent IASP presidents has never seemed more timely. Efforts to advance the study of pain and to translate this new knowledge into improved quality of life for the world's inhabitants have never been more needed.

JONATHAN O. DOSTROVSKY
DANIEL B. CARR
MARTIN KOLTZENBURG

Acknowledgments

The editors of this volume and the officers and members of the Council of the International Association for Study of Pain express their appreciation to the many individuals whose efforts were so important to the success of the 10th World Congress on Pain and of this book.

We first thank our colleagues on the Scientific Program Committee, Allan I. Basbaum, Sandra R. Chaplan, Pongparadee Chaudakshetrin, Sergio H. Ferreira, Herta Flor, Maria Adele Giamberardino, Louisa E. Jones, Robert G. Large, Bernard Laurent, Irena Madjar, Douglas M. Justins, Koichi Noguchi, Barry J. Sessle, Maureen J. Simmonds, Bengt Sjolund, and Amanda C. de C. Williams, upon whom the editorial group depended for the outline planning of the scientific program, which was so well received.

We thank Sandra R. Chaplan, chair of the Local Arrangements Committee in San Diego, and her colleagues Nigel Calcutt, Robert R. Myers, Barry J. Sessle, Linda S. Sorkin, and Victor M. Whizar for their excellent planning of the nonscientific aspects of the Congress. Special thanks are due to Uniglobe Main Events, who took great care in overseeing registration and all on-site details. We are grateful for their hard work on our behalf. We also thank the staff at the San Diego Convention Center for their attentive care to our meeting. We extend special gratitude to Louisa Jones, IASP Executive Officer, and Ellen Wilson, IASP Manager of Meetings and Publications, for their invaluable efforts in organizing the Congress. Thanks also to the other IASP staff members—Kathleen Havers, Karen Lauderback, Susan Couch, Stephanie Munson, Marleda Di Pierri, Roberta Scholz, and Elizabeth Endres—whose hard work before and during the congress was an important contribution to the overall success of the meeting.

The editors express appreciation to the staff of IASP Press, Production Editor Elizabeth Endres, Desktop Technician Dale Schmidt, and Managing Editor Roberta Scholz, for their dedicated work in preparing this book for publication.

On behalf of the Council and member of IASP, the editors acknowledge and express their special appreciation for the financial support given to the 10th World Congress on Pain and related IASP programs by the following companies:

Allergan, Inc. (USA)
AstraZeneca (Sweden)
Eli Lilly and Company (USA)
Endo Pharmaceuticals Inc. (USA)
Grünenthal GmbH (Germany)
Janssen Pharmaceutica N.V. (Belgium)
Ligand Pharmaceuticals (USA)
Pfizer Inc (USA)
Pharmacia Corporation (USA)
Purdue/Mundipharma/Napp Associated Companies (USA)

Part I

IASP, Pain, and the 10th World Congress

Proceedings of the 10th World Congress on Pain, Progress in Pain Research and Management, Vol. 24, edited by Jonathan O. Dostrovsky, Daniel B. Carr, and Martin Koltzenburg, IASP Press, Seattle, © 2003.

1

Outgoing President's Address: Issues and Initiatives in Pain Education, Communication, and Research

Barry J. Sessle

Faculty of Dentistry, University of Toronto, Toronto, Ontario, Canada

The 10th World Congress on Pain has presented topics covering virtually every aspect of acute and chronic pain, from basic science to clinical management. It was complemented by several satellite meetings and by the refresher courses that were capably organized by Maria Adele Giamberardino. This highly successful multidisciplinary congress, with 5,500 scientific delegates and over 6,400 registrants, included 20 plenary lectures and addresses, 81 workshops, 1,686 poster presentations, and 83 exhibitors. I thank Jonathan Dostrovsky and the Scientific Program Committee for organizing such a splendid scientific program. In addition, I am grateful to the Local Arrangements Committee, chaired by Sandra Chaplan, which helped provide a diverse range of optional excursions and activities in the beautiful city of San Diego and its surrounding regions.

When I became president of the International Association for the Study of Pain 3 years ago, I noted several areas in the pain field that warranted increased attention (Sessle 1999). This chapter focuses on three of these areas: education, communication, and research. It describes progress that has been made in these areas and highlights the importance of the efforts of IASP and pain researchers and clinicians in continuing to address them.

EDUCATION

IASP INITIATIVES

One of the guiding principles of IASP is the promotion of pain education and training. I mentioned in my incoming president's address (Sessle

1999) that I believed that IASP needed to increase its efforts to establish processes that will enhance pain education for students and health professionals, as well as for patients, the public, government, and the media. In the case of health professionals and trainees, especially those in the pain field, IASP has continued to generate educational material and other opportunities for knowledge transfer through the World Congresses on Pain and other meetings and symposia, and through publications such as the journal *Pain*, IASP Press books, *Pain: Clinical Updates,* and the *IASP Newsletter. Pain* and IASP Press have benefited greatly from the leadership provided by their respective Editors-in-Chief, Ronald Dubner and Howard Fields, who are stepping down from these positions later this year. I believe that Allan Basbaum and Catherine Bushnell are excellent choices as their respective successors and will maintain the high standards set by their predecessors.

Although these publications are important, additional educational approaches are needed if we are to enhance the understanding of pain and its management. I noted 3 years ago that we must also concentrate on "the front lines" by addressing the education of all health professionals in the formative years of their professional lives, and in particular that of students in the health sciences and allied programs. IASP approached this mission by initiating revisions to the IASP *Core Curriculum* and specialty curricula. These curricula represent an important resource that can help ensure the standardization of pain education worldwide by guiding the content of curricula developed within each country or region, taking into account the unique features and challenges of each geographic area. Consequently, I first surveyed IASP chapters on the value and use of the curricula in each region, and it became clear that although considered useful by most chapters, they needed to be revised. This project has included further wide consultation as part of its development, with input sought from IASP chapters, IASP special interest groups (SIGs), and many other IASP members. The revisions to the IASP *Core Curriculum* should be completed within the next year, and the revised *Core Curriculum* will be available on the IASP Web site.

However, these curricula will be useful and important in enhancing the knowledge base of health professionals only if they are used. In this respect, IASP and the pain field must pay particular attention to three issues. The first is the limited, in some cases almost nonexistent, time devoted to pain in the curricula of students in schools of medicine, dentistry, nursing, and pharmacy. The second issue is that although new and important pain-related knowledge has been gained and validated in recent years, often it is not being applied effectively. The third issue relates to the limited global awareness of pain and its management.

CURRICULAR CONTENT ON PAIN

A concerted effort must be made to increase course content on pain and to present it in a multi- or interdisciplinary manner. For example, in my own professional discipline of dentistry, the diagnosis and management of orofacial pain have been integral components of dental practice since the profession became widely recognized in the 19th century. In addition, epidemiological studies indicate that a large proportion of the population in many countries suffers from temporomandibular disorders, toothache, headache, or other orofacial pain conditions. Moreover, it can be reasonably argued on the basis of demographic research that orofacial pain, and especially chronic pain conditions such as temporomandibular disorders, will become even more of a health problem and socioeconomic burden in these countries as changing demographics result in a higher proportion of the population being middle-aged and elderly, the age cohorts in which many of these pain conditions are especially prevalent. It would therefore seem logical and even essential that the topic of pain should be a significant part of the educational program for dental students, yet in most dental schools around the world, this topic occupies only a minor component of the curriculum (Attanasio 2002). An analogous situation applies to most other health professional programs.

I recognize that local academic constraints and school "politics" make it difficult to increase curricular content on pain in many universities, but it must be done if we are to improve awareness and management of pain. And it can be accomplished, as evidenced by a recent initiative at my own university. At the University of Toronto, we recognized shortcomings in the curricula for medical, dental, nursing, and pharmacy students. Riding on the "coat-tails" of the recent pedagogic emphasis on interdisciplinary education, we have been successful in setting aside a "Pain Week" at the same time in the annual curriculum of each faculty. During Pain Week the many facets of pain, from basic science to clinical management to patient issues, are presented in an integrated, interdisciplinary manner (Watt-Watson et al. 2002). I therefore urge IASP chapters and groups of their members to become more "politically" active and aggressive in their own academic institutions and work together to increase the curricular content devoted to pain for all their health professional students.

KNOWLEDGE TRANSFER AND APPLICATION

The issue of transfer and application of knowledge applies to health professionals as well as to students. IASP has played a leadership role in advocating several pain management strategies (e.g., related to the use of opioid analgesics), in establishing standards and ethical guidelines for pain research in human and experimental animals, and in setting forth recommendations for pain treatment facilities, based on the knowledge that is accepted in our field. Nonetheless, adoption and application of this knowledge are still limited. This continuing gap is well documented in published reports on the undertreatment of pain. For example, several studies (e.g., see Breitbart 1997; Bernabei et al. 1998; Pargeon and Hailey 1999; Watt-Watson et al. 2001) have recently pointed out the unacceptable levels of undermedication still existing for patients with cancer, with HIV/AIDS, or after cardiac surgery.

Clearly, there is great variation around the world in implementing new knowledge and standards of practice and management of acute and chronic pain. Application of new knowledge by health professionals treating patients in pain can be particularly difficult in regions with economic and infrastructure limitations. Information on the utilization of research data to appropriately modify standards of practice in pain management is very limited. We as an association, as scientists, as clinicians, or as educators, must determine the major factors facilitating or impeding the transfer of knowledge into evidence-based practice, and then take appropriate steps to ensure that accepted new knowledge of pain and its management is applied for the benefit of pain patients worldwide. As the changing demographics (see above) increase the demand for appropriate pain management by clinicians knowledgeable about pain, the numbers of such clinicians must increase accordingly (e.g., Gibson, this volume; McQuay and Moore 2002; Sessle 2002).

PAIN AWARENESS

On a broader educational front, greater awareness of pain must be achieved not only by health professionals but also by the public and governments. The World Health Organization (WHO) offers an opportunity for this type of education at the global level, and for several years IASP has been trying to strengthen its interactions with WHO. Progress has been slow, but several new initiatives are being explored to enhance worldwide awareness and dissemination of information about pain and its management. Given the uncertainty of the success of this dialogue, we must ensure that other means for fostering pain education and awareness are being utilized. These would include:

- Updating IASP pain curricula, with broad geographic input in their formulation to ensure widespread applicability.

• Increasing curricular time for pain in all the health science faculties.
• Developing information sheets about pain for distribution to health professionals, patients, and governments.
• Synthesizing the new knowledge that is being gained with existing understanding of pain mechanisms and care in the form of readily understandable review articles published in journals or newsletters widely read by health professionals.
• Ensuring that mechanisms exist, for example within the structure of each IASP chapter, for effective liaisons with government, patient advocacy groups, and the media, in order to increase awareness of the health and socioeconomic impact of pain and of the need to support further pain research and management strategies.

IASP chapters have been taking the lead in some of these approaches, and two such initiatives are worth noting because they may provide some guidance for other chapters and members in enhancing pain education in the broadest sense. First, the 25 chapters affiliated with the European Federation of IASP Chapters (EFIC) promoted a national pain awareness week in each of their countries last year. This "Europe Against Pain" initiative pointed out that pain, especially chronic pain, is a disease or disorder that demands greater public and government awareness. Second, the Canadian chapter, in association with the Canadian Consortium on Pain Mechanisms, Diagnosis and Management, has made considerable progress in involving more patient advocacy groups and industry in support of pain education, communication, and research. The Web sites of these organizations (www.efic.org, www.canadianpainsociety.ca, and www.curepain.ca) provide details of these initiatives.

COMMUNICATION

IASP INITIATIVES

For education to be effective, whether it be targeted at students, clinicians, the public, government, or the media, there must be successful communication. The advent of electronic communication has provided IASP with new opportunities to communicate with its members, chapters, and the public. Therefore, the association has encouraged further development of its Web site. IASP's World Wide Web Task Force, with wide geographic representation, has put considerable effort into developing the site and enhancing its usefulness as an educational and information resource. The site now has several services available that allow the public to access or submit information, including a comprehensive list of IASP publications, articles from

Pain: Clinical Updates and the *IASP Newsletter*'s Technical Corner, information on pain definitions and specialty curricula, and announcements about training opportunities, awards, and meetings. The Web site also featured registration material as well as electronic submission of abstracts for the congress this year, a first for IASP, and soon also will provide a members-only section.

Communication is crucial as IASP continues to grow. The past 3 years have seen the formation of four new chapters as well as three new SIGs (Orofacial Pain, Neuropathic Pain, and Pain and Movement), bringing the total number of chapters to 61 (Fig. 1) and that of SIGs to 12 (Fig. 2). Given the number of SIGs and their importance to many IASP members, the association recently initiated a review of SIG guidelines to ensure that these groups remain effective vehicles for communication with and involvement of IASP members.

Another important matter, which I highlighted 3 years ago, is the need to establish additional mechanisms for enhancing communication, support, and interaction between IASP and its chapters. Therefore, IASP established a Chapter Liaison position on Council. A Subcommittee on Chapter Liaison, chaired by the IASP Chapter Liaison, Michael Bond, has been formed and is taking steps to expand interaction with chapters.

IASP aids the activities of chapters, especially those in less developed or currency-restricted regions, through several processes. These include the provision of IASP Press books and other IASP publications; small grants for specific purposes such as translation of IASP materials, visiting lecturers, and Web site development; and financial assistance to increase member participation in the IASP World Congress on Pain. IASP also donates the journal *Pain* to 100 biomedical libraries. Members have also benefited on the research front with IASP's collaborative research grants and training awards.

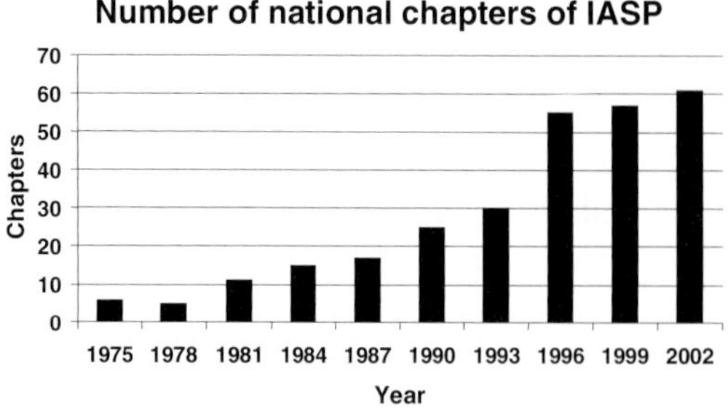

Fig. 1. Growth in number of IASP chapters.

CURRENT IASP SPECIAL INTEREST GROUPS

- Pain in Childhood (1989)
- Pain and the Sympathetic Nervous System (1990)
- Clinical/Legal Issues in Pain (1994)
- Systematic Reviews in Pain Relief (1996)
- Rheumatic Pain (1996)
- Placebo (1997)
- Sex, Gender, and Pain (1997)
- Pain of Urogenital Origin (1998)
- Refractory Angina (1999)
- Orofacial Pain (1999)
- Neuropathic Pain (1999)
- Pain and Movement (2000)

Fig. 2. Growth in number of IASP Special Interest Groups.

These many ongoing activities and new initiatives are funded by approximately $200,000 from IASP's budget. I am pleased to report that, despite the economic instability in the world in recent times, the association has maintained a sound financial state that has allowed this support to continue.

FUTURE CHAPTER ISSUES

The various support mechanisms outlined above are crucial because from a global as well as national or regional perspective, chapters are an extremely important aspect of IASP activities and provide critical links to its nearly 7,000 members. IASP must emphasize communication with its chapters and continue its support of chapter and member activities, especially those based in countries or regions with limited resources. Under the guidance of its new president, Michael Bond, IASP is developing a plan of action that focuses on support for chapters and members in these regions. The new president outlines the major facets of this plan in his incoming president's address (Bond, this volume).

Another chapter-related concern is the limited multidisciplinary nature of the activities and membership of some chapters. These particular chapters must broaden their activities and foster membership from all the professions and disciplines in their region that manage patients in pain or conduct pain-related research. This multidisciplinary growth will not only meet one of the major guiding principles of IASP but also enhance the pain management provided to patients in those regions.

RESEARCH

IASP INITIATIVES

The importance of a multidisciplinary approach also applies to research. One of the major guiding principles of IASP from its inception has been to foster and encourage pain research, and the association has continued to recognize research achievement and foster research training through several awards. In the last few years IASP has also introduced two new programs that fund initiatives emphasizing multi- and interdisciplinary approaches. One is the IASP Research Symposium, which brings together basic scientists, clinical scientists, and clinicians to focus on a specific pain-related research area, and the second is the annual collaborative research grant program, which gives priority to funding international research projects involving basic and clinical scientists.

FUTURE MULTIDISCIPLINARY RESEARCH

Collaborative research initiatives are crucial for the advancement of the pain field. Various chapters in this book attest to the remarkable research advances in this and related fields in the last two decades. The next breakthroughs in understanding and managing pain will most likely come from an even greater emphasis on multidisciplinary and team approaches. For example, we know that the nervous system can undergo neuroplastic changes in the development of chronic or persistent pain, but a combination of experimental approaches (e.g., physiological, anatomical, pharmacological, genetic, and molecular biological) are needed to define the processes underlying neuroplasticity and the factors involved in the transition from acute to chronic pain. A variety of approaches encompassing physiology, pharmacology, molecular biology, and behavioral testing will also expedite the clarification of why inhibitory neural mechanisms in the brain recruited by painful experiences are not always sufficient to prevent the development of chronic pain. Multidisciplinary approaches are also needed to determine the neural substrates underlying the high female predominance in many chronic pain states and those that cause some persons and not others to seek care, and to assess the psychological factors and societal influences involved. These are just some examples of the challenges for the pain field that require an integrated and multidisciplinary attack, and I urge the establishment of research approaches and funding mechanisms that favor multidisciplinary investigations targeting these crucial research issues.

CONCLUDING REMARKS

I am sure that readers will agree that IASP has become the "gold-standard reference" society at the international level, as a result of its exemplary organization, the wide range and impact of its many activities, and the high quality of its publications and meetings. I am confident that it will maintain its well-earned reputation and continue to grow under its new president, Michael Bond, and that its development plan will ensure that IASP maintains its pre-eminence internationally and can successfully address the important matters facing the pain field.

My presidency over the past 3 years has been a wonderful experience, and I have been honored to be in a position to help guide IASP. I owe thanks to many people, including all the IASP officers and members of IASP Council, committees and task forces, as well as Louisa Jones and the IASP office staff, who have provided much assistance and advice. And finally, I send best wishes to all the participants in this enjoyable and informative 10th World Congress on Pain.

ACKNOWLEDGMENTS

The author is Professor, Faculties of Dentistry and Medicine, and member, Centre for the Study of Pain, University of Toronto. He is also Consultant at the Wasser Pain Management Centre, Mount Sinai Hospital, Toronto, and the holder of a Canada Research Chair.

REFERENCES

Attanasio R. The study of temporomandibular disorders and orofacial pain from the perspective of the predoctoral dental curriculum. *J Orofac Pain* 2002; 16:176–180.

Bernabei R, Gambassi G, Lapane K, et al. SAGE Study Group. Management of pain in elderly patients with cancer. Systematic assessment of geriatric drug use via epidemiology. *JAMA* 1998; 279:1877–1882.

Breitbart W. Pain in AIDS. In: Jensen TS, Turner JA, Wiesenfeld-Hallin Z (Eds). *Proceedings of the 8th World Congress on Pain,* Progress in Pain Research and Management, Vol. 8. Seattle: IASP Press, 1997, pp 63–100.

McQuay HJ, Moore RA. Chronic noncancer pain. In: Stevens A, Raftery J (Eds). *Health Care Needs Assessment.* Oxford: Radcliffe Medical Press, 2002, in press.

Pargeon KL, Hailey BJ. Barriers to effective cancer pain management: a review of the literature. *J Pain Symptom Manage* 1999; 18:358–368.

Sessle BJ. Incoming president's address: looking back, looking ahead. In: Devor M, Rowbotham MC, Wiesenfeld-Hallin Z (Eds). *Proceedings of the 9th World Congress on Pain,* Progress in Pain Research and Management, Vol. 16. Seattle: IASP Press, 1999, pp 9–18.

Sessle BJ. Orofacial pain: an educational focus. *J Orofac Pain* 2002; 16:169.
Watt-Watson J, Stevens B, Streiner D, et al. Relationship between pain knowledge and pain management outcomes for their postoperative cardiac patients. *J Adv Nurs* 2001; 36:535–545.
Watt-Watson J, Hunter J, Pennefather P, et al. Integrating IASP curricula: one pain course for six health disciplines. *Abstracts: 10th World Congress on Pain.* Seattle: IASP Press, 2002, p 96.

Correspondence to: Barry J. Sessle, MDS, PhD, Faculty of Dentistry, University of Toronto, 124 Edward Street, Toronto, Ontario, Canada M5G 1G6. Tel: 416-979-4921; Fax: 416-979-4936; email: barry.sessle@utoronto.ca.

Proceedings of the 10th World Congress on Pain,
Progress in Pain Research and Management, Vol. 24,
edited by Jonathan O. Dostrovsky, Daniel B. Carr, and
Martin Koltzenburg, IASP Press, Seattle, © 2003.

2

Incoming President's Address: Planning the Future of IASP

Michael R. Bond

Emeritus Professor of Psychological Medicine, University of Glasgow, Glasgow, United Kingdom

The International Association for the Study of Pain (IASP) was founded in 1973, its purpose being to understand better the nature of pain. This goal was to be achieved by the promotion of scientific research, the improvement of the quality of pain management and standards of care through education, and the dissemination of knowledge. The association hoped to achieve this goal primarily through its publications, its international congresses, and its chapters. IASP has achieved a high level of success and has been the engine of advancement of pain research worldwide. Similarly, it has set world-class standards for improved methods of pain management, including the development and dissemination of a widely accepted terminology for pain conditions.

IASP has enjoyed considerable success scientifically and educationally, but its greatest benefits for the general public have been in the wealthier countries of the world. There remain other areas, poorer in both human and financial resources, that have failed to receive the same benefits for their populations. The association has given aid in various forms to developing countries over many years, but further consideration of their needs is merited. This point was highlighted in recent discussions with the World Health Organization (WHO).

Without detracting from current activities, especially IASP's long-established support for high-quality research and improvement in standards of care, we must explore further how best to improve the management of pain in countries with limited resources.

VISION STATEMENT

Pain relief is a basic duty of all medical and allied professionals dealing with people in pain, and relief from pain is a basic human right. IASP has made significant progress in meeting these ideals through its support for high-quality science and its development and promotion of high standards in methods of care. That work has been supported by a mature administrative structure. Through its leadership as a professional body, its ethos, and its structure, IASP must maintain and, wherever possible, advance its current work. Yet in certain areas of the world there are unmet needs for improvement in treating those in pain so as to meet the high standards of care achieved elsewhere. IASP is in a position to expand its activities on behalf of the basic human right of pain control by applying its existing resources, making greater use of its chapters, collaborating with other non-governmental organizations, and extending its contacts with WHO.

In order to fulfil this vision, flexibility may be required in the structure of IASP, its budgeting system, and the aspirations of its members.

AN ANALYSIS OF STRENGTHS, WEAKNESSES, OPPORTUNITIES, AND THREATS

If IASP is to increase its impact in developing countries, it must augment the stream of activity separate from, but complementary to, the successful work carried out by IASP members and chapters in countries with greater resources. In light of a possible expansion of activity and the additional load that might be borne by the association, I shall review its current strengths and weaknesses, and the threats to and opportunities for its development in the coming years.

STRENGTHS OF IASP

The strengths of IASP include its worldwide reputation for the promotion of high-quality pain research, and its provision of and support for the education of medical and other professionals, including undergraduate students. Its multinational structure and multidisciplinary membership are assets, as are its sound administrative structure and financial base. The association has flexible membership dues linked to members' incomes. It boasts a top-class journal, *Pain,* as well as an 8-year history of well-received books published by IASP Press. Its high-quality triennial congresses feature extensive educational programs, fellowships, scholarships, and prizes. Special interest groups (SIGs) focus upon specific pain problems.

POTENTIAL OR ACTUAL WEAKNESSES OF IASP

With increasing size and autonomy of chapters and professional groups within IASP comes the risk of fragmentation of the association. Should that occur, the global influence of IASP through its chapters, SIGs, and members would decline, as would its income. Its ability to continue its high-quality programs of work in research, education, and other fields could be compromised.

Tensions exist within IASP, in part because of a perception by some clinicians that the association is too strongly oriented toward basic science (as typified by the preponderance of basic science publications in *Pain*). Some members, particularly those in Europe, believe that the association is overly influenced by members in the United States.

Several chapter heads have expressed the opinion that communications between the center and the chapters have been weak, leading to insufficient involvement of the chapters in central decision making. In several countries, chapter members and others who are not members of IASP have formed a national society that takes relatively little account of IASP activities.

THREATS TO IASP'S INTEGRITY

If the weaknesses defined above were to develop into splits within the association, its work would be severely affected. Its ability to speak globally on behalf of pain researchers and clinicians would diminish, and its ability to exert pressure on governments and funding agencies would be lessened. Given a reduced status, its membership might well fall, and its power to attract external funds, and therefore to promote its values and standards, would be reduced.

A second and long-standing threat to the association has been the establishment of rival journals. For example, the American Pain Society's *Journal of Pain* and the *European Journal of Pain* have both appeared in recent years. However, the content and scientific quality of *Pain* have ensured its preeminence in the world of publications on pain and those linked to anesthesiology, neurology, and neuroscience.

The association's Executive Officer, who has played a major role in its development and in the maintenance of its stability throughout its existence, retires in 2006. Her retirement means that its central administration and therefore the association as a whole will undergo a period of adjustment.

Identification of the weaknesses of and threats to IASP provides an opportunity for reviewing existing methods and developing new ones to combat potential problems. The association should develop or recognize new arrangements for chapters that may strengthen their roles. For example,

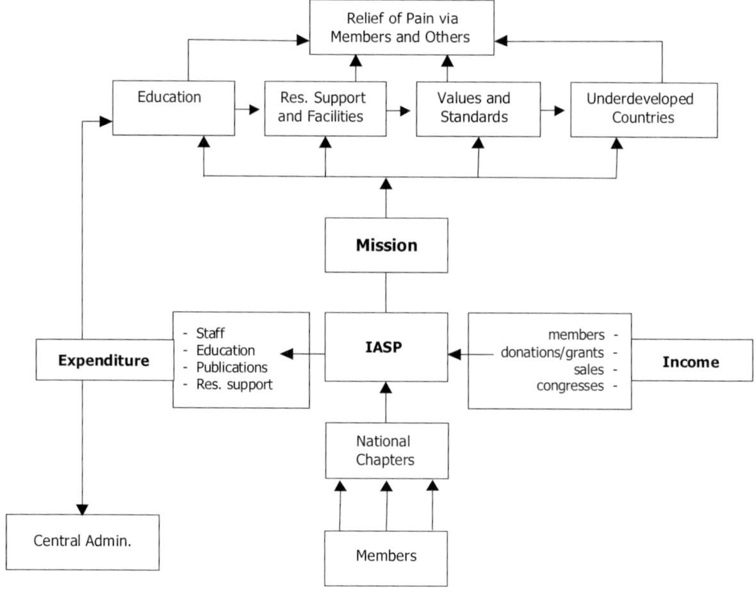

Fig 1. Current structure of IASP.

the formation of the European Federation of IASP Chapters (EFIC) has been accommodated by IASP. The association must also re-assess its administrative needs and define means of meeting them.

The association must extend its work with regard to providing help for countries with lesser resources. To do so offers an opportunity to evaluate their needs and to examine the means whereby the association might address them, alone or in partnership with others. As an aspect of that work, a revision of the funding model of the association should be examined.

SUMMARY

This "SWOT" analysis confirms that the association has a wide range of strengths but also some significant potential and actual areas of weakness. Its future strategies therefore should preserve existing strengths, include plans to deal with threats and to eliminate as far as possible potential or actual weaknesses, and discern and utilize opportunities for further development.

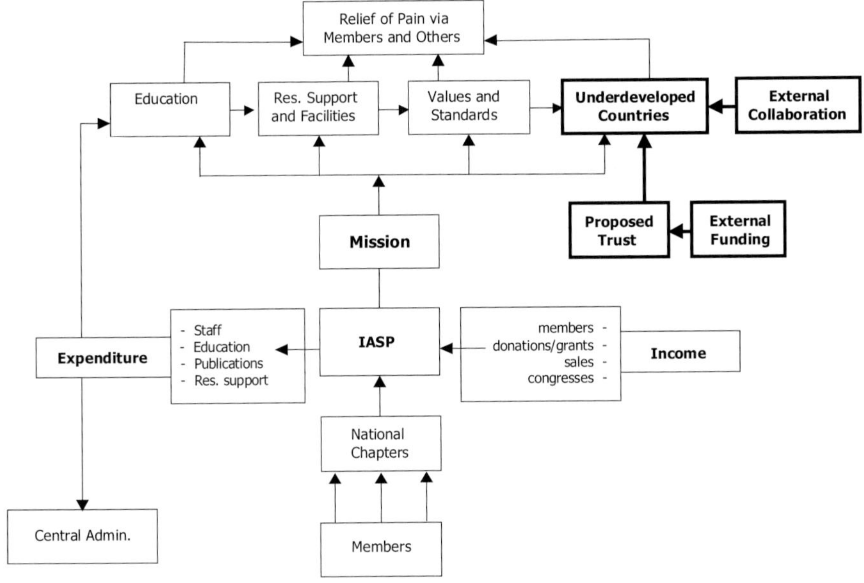

Fig 2. Proposed structure of IASP.

A STRATEGY FOR IASP'S FUTURE

The principles of continuity and development should underpin IASP's strategy for obtaining the following proposed objectives. First, IASP must devise means to maintain and strengthen its structure and function and prevent its fragmentation into competing conglomerates. These conglomerates might comprise professionally based or subject-based groups that no longer feel a need to reside within IASP. Also, chapters and national pain societies may decide to combine their structures and resources and to part from the association.

The second objective is to review the structure and functions of the association's permanent staff and to make changes to be implemented in 2006 or sooner.

The third is to assess basic needs for pain management in developing countries and to examine ways in which IASP may help provide resources to meet these needs. This process should involve IASP chapters, other nongovernmental organizations, and WHO.

Fourth, along with a strengthened agenda to assist developing countries, the association should establish a new income stream directed into a trust fund. This fund would be developed on the basis of an initial donation from the association, augmented by donations from charities and other bodies to support IASP's work in developing countries.

MEETING KEY OBJECTIVES

In order to fulfil this plan, the association will need to establish a working group to assess the risks to its integrity and the means needed to counter them. IASP also must establish a small group to review its current structure and the funding of its central administration and to evaluate its future needs in light of the major staff change in 2006. It also must conduct exploratory meetings with heads of chapters from developing countries to assess "bottom up" needs for improved pain management. Issues to be addressed include the need for professional and public education, and the use of Web-based techniques for educational purposes. Two meetings should be held to pilot the scheme in areas that might include Eastern Europe, South America, Africa, India, and China.

Arrangements should be made to meet with other nongovernmental organizations and WHO to discuss the potential for collaborative work. A Trust Fund to cover work in developing countries should be formed. The development plan proposed will lead to changes in the structure of the Association, as illustrated by comparison of Figs. 1 and 2.

CONCLUSION

IASP is a mature and stable body that has enjoyed steady and fruitful growth over almost 30 years. An appraisal of its current status reveals, however, that certain steps are needed to maintain the staffing of IASP and to permit it to enlarge and extend its current programs. In addition, opportunities exist now for extending its work in developing countries.

Correspondence to: Michael R. Bond, MD, PhD, University of Glasgow, University Avenue, No. 2 The Square, Glasgow G12 8QQ, United Kingdom. Email: m.bond@admin.gla.ac.uk.

Proceedings of the 10th World Congress on Pain,
Progress in Pain Research and Management, Vol. 24,
edited by Jonathan O. Dostrovsky, Daniel B. Carr, and
Martin Koltzenburg, IASP Press, Seattle, © 2003.

3

Learning about Pain from the Friendly Giants[1]

Allan I. Basbaum

Departments of Anatomy and Physiology and W.M. Keck Foundation Center for Integrative Neuroscience, University of California San Francisco, San Francisco, California, USA

There are several approaches to presenting a lecture in the name of John Bonica. One possibility is to discuss the latest news from the laboratory. An alternative is to take a retrospective look at the work that is presumably being recognized by the incredible honor that comes with being asked to present this lecture. When asked to submit an abstract of my talk (months before the 10th World Congress on Pain), I had no idea what it should include and therefore did not submit one. Louisa Jones, Executive Officer of the International Association for the Study of Pain (IASP) asked that at the minimum I submit a title that could be included in the program. Faced with that request, I decided that the lecture would indeed look back, but that it would highlight what to me has been one of the most gratifying and rewarding parts of my pain research studies, namely the opportunity to have worked with many of the real giants in the field. I titled the talk "Learning about pain from the friendly giants" because it has also been my good fortune to have worked with brilliant and genuinely warm people. Of course, some had their tough sides, as do most people who spend much of their life defending scientific ideas, but they were always supportive and had an enormous impact on my career. Without these teachers and colleagues, I would not be writing this chapter.

[1]The John J. Bonica Lecture.

THE FRIENDLY GIANTS OF PAIN RESEARCH

My mentors included clinicians and basic scientists, a combination that I believe is essential for a researcher working in a field that is so directly affected by, and relevant to, the condition of the patient. Although I did not work directly with John Bonica, I was strongly influenced by him. His emphasis on treating the whole patient and his recognition of the importance of a multidisciplinary approach to the treatment of the pain patient are principles to which I can readily relate. Although my research focus is on the transmission side of the nociceptive pathway, my longstanding interest is in how this information is translated into a pain perception and, more importantly perhaps, how treatment can be enhanced. Because of the remarkable contribution that John made to the field of pain research and therapy, and the great respect that I have for him and for his contributions, I am honored to have presented the lecture on which this chapter is based in his name.

I probably should have subtitled my lecture: "With some important incidences of good luck along the way." In fact, the reason that I began doing pain research can be attributed to good luck. It was the summer of 1967, and I had just completed my second (sophomore) year at McGill University in Montreal. The world's fair was about to open and I, like many of my student friends, sought a summer job there, attracted by the exciting surroundings and the opportunity to earn money. Unfortunately, or perhaps very fortunately, I did not receive an offer and had to find another way to earn money during the summer. Ron Melzack, in the Psychology Department at McGill University, had placed an advertisement for a research technician to help run animal behavior experiments. Having just completed his highly regarded course called "Motivation," I applied for the position and was hired. That was my entrance into the world of pain research. I continued working with Ron for the next 2 years, completed an honor's thesis project (which had nothing to do with pain), and then developed an interest in spinal cord mechanisms, an interest that has lasted until this day.

We were trying to test an hypothesis that was articulated in Melzack and Wall's recently published "Gate Control Theory of Pain" (1965), namely that the dorsal column pathway is the route through which descending cortical "pain" control mechanisms are activated. This was the "Central Control Trigger" outlined in the model. I performed a series of studies that evaluated the effects of dorsal column lesions on pain responsiveness under conditions in which a Pavlovian conditioning paradigm was used to inhibit the withdrawal response to a noxious stimulus (by temporally linking a food reward to the presentation of the stimulus). Unfortunately, for time reasons, and because I was on my way to graduate school, these studies were never completed. I regret that Ron and I never published a paper together, but it is because of him that I am this field. And more importantly, despite my intense interest in the spinal cord circuitry that underlies nociceptive processing, it is because of Ron's teaching that I am acutely aware of the difference between nociception and pain and of the importance of supraspinal/cortical regulation of nociceptive processing. There is no question that my subsequent interest in the pathways that contribute to the descending control of "pain" transmission at the level of the spinal cord reflect the initiation into pain research that began under Ron's tutelage.

Ron encouraged me to apply to the University of Pennsylvania, where I could continue my studies into spinal cord mechanisms. I began working with Mel Levitt, an expert in primate somatosensory mechanisms, but he left the university before I graduated. That proved important because I ended up having the opportunity to work with several remarkable scientists at Penn. Most importantly, Eliot Stellar became my thesis advisor. His incredible understanding of animal behavior had a lasting influence on the types of studies that I subsequently designed. And of particular importance were my day-to-day interactions with a remarkable scientific duo, William Chambers and John Liu. Liu and Chambers (1958) were the first to discover the phenomenon of collateral sprouting. They showed that when a single dorsal root is isolated, by deafferenting roots rostral and caudal to it, there is collateral growth from the intact spinal terminals into denervated regions of the cord. These observations were strongly questioned when first published, in part because they relied on silver degeneration methods, which were novel, but considered insensitive. It took many years before the phenomenon was widely accepted.

Among the many things that I learned from Chambers and Liu were a variety of neuroanatomical approaches, tract tracing, lesion reconstruction, and the appreciation of neuroanatomy as both an art and a science. John Liu also taught me how to perform spinal cord surgery in the rat: "Don't make lesions with scissors," he said. "It will only promote bleeding. Use jeweler's forceps and squeeze the axon bundles that you want to transect." That advice, as described below, proved to be among the most important contributors to the success of my subsequent studies into the analysis of descending control pathways.

My lecture at the IASP meeting did not provide enough time to include all of the friendly giants, but I would be remiss if I failed to mention the impact that Fred Kerr had on my research. As part of my graduate thesis, which examined the contribution of short-fiber multisynaptic systems in the spinal cord to the flow of nociceptive information, I began a study of the central projection of primary afferents in the rat. In these studies, which were performed in collaboration with Peter Hand, I used the latest silver degeneration methods, which had just been developed by Bob Fink, who was working at Penn at the time. In the course of these studies, I deafferented the spinal cord by multiple dorsal rhizotomy and observed that the rats often attacked the denervated limb, in a behavior subsequently termed *autotomy*. It seemed to me that this behavior could represent biting of an insensate limb, but I wanted to test the possibility that it represented an attempt on the part of the animal to eliminate abnormal, unpleasant, dysesthetic sensations. In a series of studies designed to test this hypothesis, I concurrently made a variety of spinal cord lesions and found that subtotal lesions prevented the behavior, but importantly, the lesions did not result in paralysis of the limb. Based on the elimination of the abnormal behavior, I concluded that the biting must have arisen because the animal was experiencing something unpleasant, which was eliminated by the superimposed spinal cord lesions. I presented the results at a meeting of the American Association of Anatomists (in some respects the precursor of the Society for Neurosciences meeting). The title of the talk was "Experimental central pain in rats." At the meeting Fred Kerr introduced himself and quickly gave me a lesson in how to talk to clinicians. He suggested that some neurosurgeons might find the suggestion that this was a model of central pain somewhat hard to accept and encouraged me to temper my claims about the clinical relevance of the model.

This brief interchange led to several long discussions with Fred about basic science and its intersection with clinical medicine, gaining a new understanding that has stayed with me since. These discussions continued at every subsequent meeting that we attended. Fred's input has strongly influenced my interest in translating basic laboratory findings to the patient, in seeing patients, and in trying to learn more about the similarities and differences between animal and human pain conditions. My friendship with Fred continued until his premature death. He epitomized the physician-scientist we are trying to train today; if today's upcoming scientists emulate him they will be incredibly successful. As an aside, the title of the paper in which the "preautotomy" data were published was "Effects of central lesions on disorders produced by multiple dorsal rhizotomy in the rat"; only in the discussion is the possible relationship of this model to central pain raised (Basbaum 1974). I took Fred's suggestion of caution to heart.

After completing my PhD I moved to London to do postdoctoral research with Pat Wall. Interestingly, when Pat found out that I came from Montreal, he said that had he known that, he probably would have rejected my application to work with him—Ron Melzack and Lorne Mendell were enough Canadian colleagues for a lifetime. Working with Pat was a remarkable experience. I had never met a scientist like him, nor have I met anyone like him since. He loved his work and was the most imaginative and creative person with whom I have ever collaborated. In many respects he was a phenomenologist; he derived insights from snippets of data that others took years to recognize. He often got bored with the niggling details of experiments and would leave the details to others. It was the big picture that intrigued him. Often the direction that an experiment was going turned in midstream because of the unusual firing of a single cell in response to a novel stimulus. Pat never ignored the unexpected, but rather sought to understand it.

It is of interest that my work with Pat focused less on issues relating to pain than on the problem of injury-induced plasticity, an area of study that Pat had pioneered a few years earlier in his groundbreaking studies with David Egger (Wall and Egger 1971). Together they demonstrated the remarkable plasticity of the somatosensory map in the thalamus after lesions to the input to the thalamus. In many respects this finding was the electrophysiological correlate of the Liu and Chambers collateral sprouting story, and it was criticized almost as harshly when it was first published. Some said that the changes were too small to be believable; others said that the nervous system is hard-wired. The critics were all wrong, as many subsequent studies have shown, not the least of which are the remarkable cortical reorganization studies of Michael Merzenich and his colleagues (Recanzone et al. 1992). Having been steeped in Liu and Chambers tradition, Pat and I decided to look at the spinal cord for reorganization after multiple dorsal rhizotomy. We showed that the plasticity in the spinal cord was even more dramatic than the situation Pat and David had described in the thalamus. Not only was there extensive topographic reorganization of the somatotopic map in the cord, but single cells often developed split receptive fields, spontaneous activity was altered, and the changes could be manifest over large segments of the cord. Those studies emphasized to me how plastic the nervous system is, and more importantly, that tissue or nerve injury can induce dramatic changes that we must take into account when trying to explain the phenomena now referred to as allodynia and hyperalgesia. The nervous system is not hard-wired, but undergoes dramatic reorganization, both during development and after injury. Of course, it is now commonplace to attribute many chronic pain syndromes to injury-induced changes in the central nervous system, rather than to the magnitude of the injury. Pat's studies laid the groundwork for all that has come since.

Of course, if basic scientists interested in nociceptive mechanisms revered Pat, many pain clinicians idolized him. He spoke their language and could offer important explanations for the problems that their patients experienced. He understood that there were limitations to what could be inferred about clinical pain conditions from studies in the laboratory. And most importantly, he encouraged me to learn about patients. In fact, he allowed me to take off one half-day a week to go to the National Hospital at Queen's Square, to see patients with his good friend Peter Nathan, a neurologist who treated many patients with difficult pain problems.

Peter had an enormous influence on my career. It is difficult to summarize how much I learned from him about the incredible heterogeneity of pain problems, about pharmacological approaches to treatment (which unfortunately, have not changed much since the early 1970s), and about the importance of psychology in a patient's pain. Interestingly, it was while I was seeing patients with Peter that tricyclic antidepressants were introduced for the treatment of postherpetic neuralgia. Of course, new drugs are now available (better anticonvulsants, etc.), but we are still awaiting the promised revolution in the treatment of chronic pain. I hope that soon we will treat persistent pain with drugs whose actions differ mechanistically from those that have been used for many years.

Because Peter's patients returned regularly for follow-up, I also had the opportunity to assess the short- and long-term efficacy of different approaches to treatment. I cannot recall how many patients tried complementary approaches (from acupuncture to faith healing) to deal with their pain, but I do recall that such methods rarely worked. Peter also taught me about the importance of peripheral nerve activity to the persistence of peripheral-nerve-injury-induced pain conditions. He showed me how successful peripheral nerve block can be for postherpetic neuralgia and demonstrated that injection of local anesthetics not only could eliminate stump pain in an amputee, but also could abolish the phantom pain, not to mention the phantom. He argued, and I now concur, that there is a critical peripheral nerve activity component to all peripheral-nerve-injury-induced pain conditions. This activity is clearly exacerbated by its interaction with an altered nervous system, but the importance of the peripheral component should never be overlooked. Remarkably, and for reasons that are still not understood, local anesthetic block of peripheral nerves can, in some patients, relieve pain for up to 3 weeks. The pain always comes back, but the fact that it can be eliminated for a time that far exceeds the duration of anesthetic block is dramatic. Whether this is a Livingston type of reverberatory circuit that is being quieted temporarily by the anesthetic is not clear.

Pat also introduced me to William (Bill) Noordenbos, a superb neurosurgeon and neuroscientist from Amsterdam. The introduction came after Pat gave me a copy of Bill's textbook (his thesis), which was published in the mid-1950s (Noordenbos 1959). This book is a gem, and in many respects, it was the precursor to the gate control theory. The book emphasized the importance of activity in multiple types of primary afferent fiber, and espoused the pattern theory over specificity theory, which was popular at the time. Among the book's most remarkable features are its exquisitely detailed descriptions of the neurological examination of patients with neuropathic pain. Bill's descriptions of hyperesthesia and hyperpathia (terms that are largely unused today) are incomparable and provide an invaluable tool to the basic scientist who wants to understand what the clinical problem of pain really is. I have urged my students and postdoctoral fellows to observe, listen to, and talk to patients, so that they can better understand what clinical pain is all about. If they do not have that opportunity I urge them to obtain a copy of Bill's remarkable book.

I also had the wonderful opportunity of meeting the Noordenbos family, under somewhat unusual circumstances. My wife Carol, who was also doing postdoctoral work in London, and I visited the Noordenbos home during the Middle East War of 1973, when gasoline was not available. Because of this we toured Amsterdam by bicycle, a memorable experience. Bill is the honorary godfather of our daughter, who was born in London a month before Carol and I returned to the United States.

In addition to supporting my interest in the pain patient, Pat always encouraged being independent in science. If you had an idea for an experiment that was a bit out of the ordinary he urged you to carry it out. This ability to go off and do one's own experiment, regardless of its relationship to what we were working on together, had a critical impact on my career. In the middle of my postdoctoral fellowship, John Liebeskind and his colleagues published their seminal studies that demonstrated that electrical stimulation in the midbrain periaqueductal grey (PAG) induced a profound antinociception in rats (Mayer et al. 1971). I was fascinated by those studies and particularly intrigued by the fact that not only did the rats not respond to a noxious stimulus by trying to remove it (i.e., they seem to be truly analgesic), but the reflex responses to these stimuli were also suppressed. Because the reflexes were organized at the spinal cord level I hypothesized that the antinociception must involve activation of descending inhibitory controls. It was not a big leap, therefore, to ask whether selective lesions of spinal cord pathways could interrupt the analgesia produced by PAG stimulation.

I wrote to John Liebeskind for advice on targeting the electrodes, as it seemed that putting an electrode through the sagittal sinus was not the best surgical approach to the PAG and the dorsal raphe, which lies right on the midline. John quickly replied that there was no problem putting the electrode through the midline and wished me good luck. The results were clear.

A midthoracic lesion of the dorsolateral funiculus (DLF), bilateral because the stimulation evoked bilateral control, completely abolished the analgesia produced by electrical stimulation of the PAG. Because the lesion was performed at the thoracic level, it is significant that the loss of analgesia occurred only in the hindlimb; a noxious stimulus to the forelimbs still failed to evoke a nocifensive response. That result also firmly dissociated the antinociception from the strong rewarding effects of stimulating the dorsal raphe.

It was around this time that I finished up my postdoctoral work with Pat and moved to San Francisco. Carol was offered a terrific fellowship with John Heuser at the University of California at San Francisco (UCSF). Pat suggested that I contact Howard Fields at UCSF to see if there was an opportunity for me in his laboratory. Howard offered me a position and in November of 1974, my wife and I moved to San Francisco. We have had the good fortune to remain there ever since.

Soon after moving to San Francisco, a very important event occurred, namely the first IASP meeting in Florence, Italy, not a bad place for a young postdoctoral fellow to present what seemed like interesting data. This proved to be a memorable meeting. I learned that how you present your data could make a big difference in how it is perceived. My talk was scheduled on the last day of the meeting. It seemed pretty straightforward; certainly the data were pretty clear, at least to me. Unfortunately for me, a rather senior and respected scientist got up after my talk and, based on his experience, suggested to the audience that it was impossible to perform selective lesions of the DLF without paralyzing the animal. Not unreasonably, he asked where the histology was. The point was well taken. I had shown schematic reconstructions of the lesions, but no histology.

I tried to convince him, and the rest of the now skeptical audience, that such lesions could indeed be performed (having learned them from Chambers and Liu). I reminded the questioner that the corticospinal tract in rodents is uniquely located in the base of the dorsal columns, and thus is not severed when a DLF lesion is performed. I doubt, however, that my discussion of the course of the corticospinal tract helped convince anyone in the audience that such lesions could indeed be performed. Perhaps to boost my spirits, Ron Dubner, whom I had met a couple of times during my postdoctoral work with Pat Wall, invited me to come to his laboratory at the National Institutes of Health (NIH) to present the data. After we spent an enjoyable few hours discussing science, Ron asked whether I could demonstrate the surgery to his laboratory. I have joked with Ron since then about his ulterior motive for inviting me to the NIH, but it proved a useful experience. I did teach the laboratory how to do the surgery, and Ron was sufficiently convinced to spread the word. And when I finally published the data in *Pain*

(Basbaum et al. 1977), I included the histology of the lesions. Ron and I have been great friends ever since. The trauma of that first IASP meeting was a great learning experience; never assume that your audience believes what you say just because you say it. Make sure that you can substantiate the claims—and show the histology!

EVOLUTION OF A MODEL OF DESCENDING ANTINOCICEPTIVE CONTROLS

The demonstration that electrical brain stimulation can support a profound antinociception was revolutionary, but the observation that naloxone can reverse this effect was even more dramatic (Akil et al. 1976). Taken together with the discovery of the endogenous opioid peptides (Lord et al. 1977), these observations led to the suggestion that brain stimulation produces analgesia by activating an endorphin-mediated pain control system. With these ideas and observations as a framework, Howard Fields and I decided to extend the analysis of descending control to the effects of opiates, in particular morphine. It had previously been reported that spinal cord transection significantly reduces the effect of systemic morphine. Our studies established that a pathway in the DLF was critical. Specifically, we showed that bilateral lesions of the DLF almost completely blocked the analgesia produced by systemic morphine. Only very large doses could reinstate pain control.

Based on these results and because of concurrently published studies of the effects of microinjection of opiates into the brain (Pert and Yaksh 1974), Howard and I postulated that systemic morphine exerts its analgesic effects by binding to opiate receptors in the PAG and thus activating a powerful descending inhibitory control system. The output of the descending control, we hypothesized, traveled to the spinal cord via a pathway in the DLF, presumably to regulate the firing of spinal cord "pain" transmission neurons. The problem with that formulation, at least at the time, was that evidence was lacking for direct projections from the PAG to the spinal cord (tracing methods were still rather primitive). Most tracing studies were based on cellular chromatolytic changes after injury to the axons, or else used silver degeneration methods, which were notorious for missing the projections that arise from small-diameter axons.

A clue to the puzzle came from an important series of studies that appeared from the laboratory of my good friend Jean-Marie Besson in Paris (Oliveras et al. 1975). His group demonstrated that electrical stimulation of the nucleus raphe magnus (NRM) of the medulla (called the inferior central nucleus at the time) also generated profound antinociception. That result was of interest for two important reasons. First, it suggested a possible link from the PAG to the spinal cord. And second, because the NRM was known to be rich in serotonin-containing neurons, these studies provided an important anatomical correlate to the growing evidence that serotonin was a major contributor to the inhibitory controls that were exerted. Thus, for example, depleting animals of serotonin reduced stimulation-produced analgesia (Akil and Mayer 1972).

With a view to studying the projections of the NRM and the adjacent reticular formation, Howard and I initiated a long and difficult study using newly developed tracing methods that employed tritiated amino acid injections. The tritiated amino acid (usually leucine) is incorporated into protein at the level of the cell body and transported anterogradely by the axons to the their synaptic terminals, where it can be detected using autoradiographic techniques. The procedures were incredibly cumbersome and time-consuming (because of the long exposures that were required), but they were far more sensitive than the degeneration methods that they eventually replaced. The results from our studies could not have been more exciting. We found that injections into the midline raphe revealed a major pathway that travels to the spinal cord in the DLF (bilaterally, of course, as the raphe is a midline structure). Most importantly, the terminals of these axons were concentrated in laminae I, II and V, precisely where electrophysiological studies had revealed the presence of "pain"-responsive neurons (Basbaum et al. 1978; Basbaum and Fields 1979). The literature up to that time argued strongly that there was no supraspinal projection to the superficial dorsal horn, a conclusion that clearly derived from the poor sensitivity of silver degeneration methods. It is of interest that when we first reported these results at a meeting, the word was that we were looking at an artifact of the autoradiography method. Faith in the dogma based on the silver methods made it difficult for others to accept what was considered a radical observation. Subsequent studies from other laboratories, however, have confirmed the observations, including my own memorable collaboration in primate experiments with Peter and Diane Ralston (Basbaum et al. 1986).

Given that NRM stimulation induced a profound analgesia, and that NRM axons project directly to the spinal cord via the DLF, it was natural to wish to determine the effect of NRM stimulation on the firing of dorsal horn neurons. The results were precisely as predicted (Fields et al. 1977). Only those neurons with nociceptive inputs were inhibited by NRM stimulation. Neurons that only responded to low-intensity stimulation (and which were concentrated in lamina IV) were not affected. Furthermore, a lesion of the DLF completely blocked the inhibitory controls generated by NRM stimulation.

With these different pieces of the puzzle creating an ever clearer picture, Howard and I, with Charles Clanton, published a paper in the *Proceedings of the National Academy of Sciences* that summarized all of these data (Basbaum et al. 1976). The paper described the behavioral effects of DLF lesions, the anatomical pathways that arise from the NRM, and the effects of NRM stimulation on the firing of dorsal horn neurons. The story would probably have ended there if not for a wonderful adjunct to hard work in the laboratory, namely serendipity. Soon after the paper was published I received a call from John Liebeskind. He had agreed to be part of a symposium at the Winter Conference on Brain Research (WCBR) meeting but was unable to attend. He asked whether I could fill in for him. I agreed immediately, even though I had never heard of the WCBR meetings. As an avid skier I let my imagination fill in the blanks as to what went on at the meeting, besides good science.

I went to the meeting and presented the work that had just appeared in the *Proceedings.* It was well received, no doubt because I included the histology. But the morning after the talk proved to be most significant. While waiting in line for the ski lift (after the 2-hour morning session), Fred Plum, the then Editor-in-Chief of *Annals of Neurology,* introduced himself and asked whether I would like to write a review on the data for his journal. To be honest, I did not know Fred Plum and had never heard of the *Annals of Neurology* (Howard is the neurologist), but he convinced me that it was a major journal in that field. I returned to San Francisco and persuaded Howard, who of course knew the *Annals,* to join me in writing the review.

Howard and I decided that we should include a diagram that illustrates the connections that these studies had identified. We are indebted to Stu Anderson, a postdoctoral fellow in the laboratory, who was the artist behind the model. In its simplest form, the model includes a circuit from the PAG to the NRM to the spinal cord dorsal horn (Basbaum and Fields 1978). That is the part that most people remember. But the paper and the model went into much more detail. In particular, around the time that the model was being developed, immunocytochemical studies were beginning to reveal the incredible neurochemical complexity of the dorsal horn. Also, the Jessell and Iversen (1977) model of opioid regulation of substance P release from small-diameter primary afferent nociceptors had just been published. We decided to incorporate many of their ideas into the model. We also emphasized the fact that there were probably multiple opioid receptor links at brainstem and spinal cord levels, all of which almost certainly are concurrently activated by systemic injection of morphine. In addition, we included the hypothesis that what activates this endogenous pain control system is pain itself, i.e., that the system functions in a negative feedback way, limiting the magnitude of pain that is normally experienced in the presence of a noxious stimulus.

In part, these hypotheses derived from the plethora of studies that were examining the effects of injecting naloxone into normal animals and humans, or in the setting of pain. In a subsequent version of the model, published 6 years later, we expanded on the contribution of the enkephalins and emphasized the interesting complexity presented by the fact that GABAergic mechanisms seem to intervene between the enkephalin-containing neurons and the output neurons of the PAG (Basbaum and Fields 1984). Based on these anatomical circuits, we hypothesized that opioids initiate PAG descending inhibitory control by a process of disinhibition, i.e., by blocking a tonic GABAergic inhibitory control. Many subsequent anatomical, pharmacological, and even neurochemical studies have provided considerable support for our hypothesis.

UNRAVELING DORSAL HORN NEUROCHEMISTRY

With the publication of the descending control model, my interest turned more and more to the complexity of the circuitry in the different components of the system. In fact, during the last 20 years, through a thoroughly enjoyable collaboration with many brilliant graduate students, postdoctoral fellows, and research technicians, our laboratory has published a series of papers on the neurochemistry and circuitry in the PAG, the NRM, and especially, the spinal cord. The latter region, of course, is proving ever more complicated. I would, however, like to make specific reference to the work that resulted from a wonderful collaboration with two close friends and colleagues, Jon Levine and Patrick Mantyh. Soon after I began to study the contribution of neuropeptides in the dorsal horn, Jon and I began a series of studies that examined the other end of the primary afferent nociceptor, namely its peripheral end. The nociceptor, of course, branches, and when we began these studies, the contribution of the peripheral release of substance P to the phenomenon of neurogenic inflammation had been well established (Lembeck et al. 1982). These were, however, still relatively early days in the neuropeptide field; calcitonin-gene related peptide, the primary afferent neuropeptide that induces the vasodilatation component of the neurogenic inflammatory response, had not yet been discovered. Jon is a rheumatologist and neurobiologist, an unusual combination that explains his keen interest in the contribution of the nervous system to inflammatory disease. Our studies asked whether manipulations that reduce the innervation of joints alter the severity of joint destruction (i.e., disease) in an experimental model of rheumatoid arthritis in the rat. We showed that this is indeed the case and, more importantly, that the concentration of substance P in the affected joint is critical (Levine et al. 1984).

The studies with Pat Mantyh came several years later and were, in some respects, another example of serendipity in the course of science. At the time, neuroanatomical studies of the circuitry through which neuropeptides act relied almost exclusively on studies that used antisera directed against the neuropeptides. Although there were light microscopic studies of the distribution of neuropeptide receptors, these involved binding of radioactive ligand. Because fixation adversely affected binding, it was not possible to use electron microscopy to identify the synaptic architecture of the neuropeptide and its receptor. Very fortunately for my laboratory, a colleague at UCSF received an aliquot of an antibody from Steve Vigna at Duke University. The antibody was generated against the receptor to which substance P binds, namely the neurokinin-1 (NK-1) receptor (Vigna et al. 1994). The serendipity resulted from the fact that the colleague at UCSF who gave the antisera to our laboratory did so because his team was unable to get the antibody to work well, and asked for our help. It turned out that this group had made the classic mistake with antibodies. Because they had trouble pulling the signal out from the background noise, they mistakenly increased the concentration of antibody that they used in the immunohistochemical reaction, hoping to increase the signal-to-noise ratio. Of course, all that increasing primary antibody concentration does is further increase the background noise; the signal is already saturated.

We "played" with the antibody concentrations and ended up using dilutions that were literally three orders of magnitude higher. The results could not have been more spectacular. Our findings led to a new "view" as to how neuropeptides and receptors are organized in the central nervous system. The long-hypothesized mismatch between peptide and receptor was immediately apparent. More important, perhaps, was the demonstration not only that the NK-1 receptor is not located exclusively at synaptic sites, but also that neurons that express the receptor do so over their entire somatic and dendritic surface (Liu et al. 1994; Brown et al. 1995). Having seen the remarkable results with this antibody, we obviously wanted to pursue the studies and thus asked Steve Vigna if he could send us more antibody so that we could do a complete light and electron microscopic analysis of the NK-1 receptors in the spinal cord. To my surprise, he said that Pat Mantyh had the antibody and that we should contact him. (I learned later that Steve and Pat were colleagues at the Center for Ulcer Research at UCLA).

Pat said that of course he would send us antibody, but understandably he told us that he was also using the antibody in the spinal cord and had observed a labeling pattern comparable to what we had just observed. Some individuals would use such an opportunity to refuse their help, but Pat quickly asked whether we would like to collaborate, and I immediately agreed. This decision led to a long series of studies that took advantage of the "Golgi"-like labeling of NK-1-receptor-positive neurons to study the functional effects of substance P release in the dorsal horn. Because G-protein-linked receptors are internalized after binding ligand, and because the antibody permitted us to identify neurons that "responded" to substance P stimulation, we were able to identify neurons that were activated by different modalities of noxious stimulation (Mantyh et al. 1995). Our studies also showed that the numbers and distribution of activated neurons are significantly increased when the same stimulus is applied in the setting of inflammation (Abbadie et al. 1997). This result, of course, is relevant to the hypothesis that long-term changes that occur in the setting of injury alter nociceptive processing. Subsequently our two laboratories published several studies that examined the regulation of NK-1-receptor internalization by a variety of pharmacological agents, including morphine and baclofen (Trafton et al. 1999; Riley et al. 2001). Those studies provided a new perspective on the pre- and postsynaptic mechanisms through which these drugs function. Pat has since gone on to publish his incredibly exciting work on the selective targeting of NK-1-receptor-expressing neurons using a substance P–saporin conjugate (Mantyh et al. 1997; see Mantyh et al., this volume). It has been a thoroughly wonderful collaboration, intellectually stimulating, highly productive, and absolutely critical to my understanding of the complexity of nociceptive processing in the dorsal horn.

Of course, substance P is but one of the many players in the dorsal horn. From a rather limited number of neurotransmitter and neuromodulator candidates that had been characterized in the mid-1970s, we now have an enormous list of molecules that have been implicated in nociceptive processing (Snider and McMahon 1998; Julius and Basbaum 2001). The identity of many of these molecules arose from the remarkable contribution that molecular biological analysis has brought to the field of pain. Of particular interest is that many of the molecules recently identified appear to be uniquely expressed in primary afferent nociceptors. These include the vanilloid receptor (Caterina et al. 1997), which was cloned in the laboratory of my good friend and colleague, David Julius, a class of tetrodotoxin (TTX)-resistant Na channels, the P2X3 subtype of purinergic receptor (Chen et al. 1995; Cook et al. 1997), and a recently described subclass of G-protein-linked receptors (Dong et al. 2001; Lembo et al. 2002).

The complexity of the neurochemistry of the primary afferent nociceptor is matched by the large number of downstream molecules that have been identified in the dorsal horn (Basbaum and Woolf 1999; Woolf and Salter 2000). Of particular importance are the many second-messenger molecules that have been implicated in the development of central sensitization. Among these are a variety of protein kinases and other enzymes, such as nitric oxide synthase and the gamma isoform of protein kinase, which our laboratory has implicated in the development of neuropathic pain (Malmberg et al. 1997).

My perspective on the diversity of these molecules is that they constitute the biochemical basis for development of memories of noxious stimuli (Basbaum 1996). Presumably, the memories are initially established to sensitize dorsal horn neurons so that allodynia develops as a protective mechanism following injury. Unfortunately, there appear to be far too many situations in which the memory is maladaptive, resulting in long-term allodynia and hyperalgesia, which are the major features of many persistent pain conditions, whether they arise following tissue or nerve injury. Of course, to the extent that these molecules are targets for therapy, their elucidation is of particular clinical importance. The problem, of course, is to fit such a large number of molecules into a comprehensive and meaningful circuit that is relevant to nociceptive processing so that new therapeutic targets can be identified. The London subway map, which I showed during the lecture, is in fact, much less complicated than the neurochemistry of the circuitry of the dorsal horn.

Yet another important question is posed by the complexity of the neurochemistry of nociceptive processing. This question harkens back to the Cartesian view of the transmission of "pain" messages that Melzack and Wall continually criticized. As I continually tell my students, "The bane of pain is plainly in the brain." Nociceptive messages may be transmitted to the brain by labeled lines, but whether or not they produce pain and the magnitude and emotional content of the pain experience cannot be solely predicted by the pathway through which the inputs are transmitted. On the other hand, given the molecular heterogeneity of the nociceptors, it is of interest to ask whether they engage different or identical circuits in the brain. For example, does a C fiber that expresses the P2X3 receptor, but not substance P, activate central circuits that are different from those that are substance P positive, but P2X3 negative? And if separate circuits are activated, what is their functional correlate?

In some respects this question is very similar to the types of questions posed by imagers, who ask whether different patterns of activity across different regions of the cortex, thalamus, and brainstem are activated by different types of noxious stimuli. Our approach to answering the anatomical question has evolved from the tools offered by molecular biology. Specifically, we have recently developed a transgenic mouse that allows us to trace circuits in the brain by inducing the expression of a lectin, wheat germ agglutinin, which has the remarkable capacity to be transported across synapses, so as to reveal the connections made by subsets of neurons (Braz et al. 2002). All neurons in the brain of this transgenic mouse have the capacity to synthesize the tracer, but we can control which neurons do so and when (i.e., during development or in the adult). Thus it is possible, for example, to turn the tracer on in subsets of dorsal root ganglion cells, so as to selectively study their central connections. Modifications in the development of future transgenic mouse lines will allow us to more selectively study the connections made by C-fiber nociceptors that uniquely express a particular molecule.

Needless to say, because we can control the time when the gene that encodes the tracer is activated, it may also be possible to ask questions about the circuits that are newly created after injury. For example, although considerable evidence indicates that Aβ mechanoreceptive afferents sprout into the superficial dorsal horn after peripheral nerve injury (Woolf et al. 1992), we have little information about the neurons that are contacted by these sprouted afferents, and know nothing about the neurons that lie further downstream. We are optimistic that we will soon be able to answer such questions. Our hope is that we will eventually be able to trace the connections from the nociceptor to the cortex, and to identify the many collateral systems that are likely to be engaged. Ultimately we may be able to correlate these patterns of connections with the results from imaging studies. This line of study will not, of course, tell us where pain is processed in the cortex, but it will provide important insights into the complex pathways through which different types of injury inputs are transmitted to higher brain centers and how these circuits are altered in the setting of tissue or nerve injury. This information also promises to provide insights into new therapeutic approaches to the management of pain. That is a goal that I am sure John Bonica would have enthusiastically endorsed.

ACKNOWLEDGMENTS

This work was supported over many years by generous research grants from the NIH.

REFERENCES

Abbadie C, Trafton J, Liu H, Mantyh PW, Basbaum AI. Inflammation increases the distribution of dorsal horn neurons that internalize the neurokinin-1 receptor in response to noxious and non-noxious stimulation. *J Neurosci* 1997; 17:8049–8060.

Akil H, Mayer DJ. Antagonism of stimulation-produced analgesia by p-CPA, a serotonin synthesis inhibitor. *Brain Res* 1972; 44:692–697.

Akil H, Mayer DJ, Liebeskind JC. Antagonism of stimulation-produced analgesia by naloxone, a narcotic antagonist. *Science* 1976; 191:961–962.

Basbaum AI. Effects of central lesions on disorders produced by multiple dorsal rhizotomy in rats. *Exp Neurol* 1974; 42:490–501.

Basbaum AI. Memories of pain. *Science Med* 1996; 3:22–31.

Basbaum AI, Fields HL. Endogenous pain control mechanisms: review and hypothesis. *Ann Neurol* 1978; 4:451–462.

Basbaum AI, Fields HL. The origin of descending pathways in the dorsolateral funiculus of the spinal cord of the cat and rat: further studies on the anatomy of pain modulation. *J Comp Neurol* 1979; 187:513–532.

Basbaum AI, Fields HL. Endogenous pain control systems: brainstem spinal pathways and endorphin circuitry. *Ann Rev Neurosci* 1984; 7:309–338.

Basbaum AI, Woolf CJ. Pain. *Curr Biol* 1999; 9:R429–431.

Basbaum AI, Clanton CH, Fields HL. Opiate and stimulus-produced analgesia: Functional anatomy of a medullo-spinal pathway. *Proc Natl Acad Sci USA* 1976; 73:465–468.

Basbaum AI, Marley NJ, O'Keefe J, Clanton CH. Reversal of morphine and stimulus-produced analgesia by subtotal spinal cord lesions. *Pain* 1977; 3:43–56.

Basbaum AI, Clanton CH, Fields HL. Three bulbospinal pathways from the rostral medulla of the cat. An autoradiographic study of pain modulating systems. *J Comp Neurol* 1978; 178:209–224.

Basbaum AI, Ralston DD, Ralston III HJ. Bulbospinal projections in the primate: a light and electron microscopic study of a pain modulating system. *J Comp Neurol* 1986; 250:311–323.

Braz JM, Rico B, Basbaum AI. Transneuronal tracing of diverse CNS circuits by Cre-mediated inductin of wheat germ agglutinin in transgenic mice. *Proc Natl Acad Sci USA* 2002; in press.

Brown JL, Liu H, Maggio JE, et al. Morphological characterization of substance P receptor-immunoreactive neurons in the rat spinal cord and trigeminal nucleus caudalis. *J Comp Neurol* 1995; 356:327–344.

Caterina MJ, Schumacher MA, Tominaga M, et al. The capsaicin receptor: a heat-activated ion channel in the pain pathway. *Nature (Lond)* 1997; 389:816–824.

Chen CC, Akopian AN, Sivilotti L, et al. A P2X purinoceptor expressed by a subset of sensory neurons. *Nature (Lond)* 1995;377:428–431.

Cook SP, Vulchanova L, Hargreaves KM, Elde R, McCleskey EW. Distinct ATP receptors on pain-sensing and stretch-sensing neurons. *Nature (Lond)* 1997; 387:505–508.

Dong X, Han S, Zylka MJ, Simon MI, Anderson DJ. A diverse family of GPCRs expressed in specific subsets of nociceptive sensory neurons. *Cell* 2001; 106:619–632.

Fields HL, Basbaum AI, Clanton CH, Anderson SD. Nucleus raphe magnus inhibition of spinal cord dorsal horn neurons. *Brain Res* 1977; 126:441–453.

Jessell TM, Iversen LL. Opiate analgesics inhibit substance P release from rat trigeminal nucleus. *Nature (Lond)* 1977; 268:549–551.

Julius D, Basbaum AI. Molecular mechanisms of nociception. *Nature (Lond)* 2001; 413:203–210.

Lembeck F, Donnerer J, Bartho L. Inhibition of neurogenic vasodilatation and plasma extravasation by substance P antagonists, somatostatin and (D-Met^2,Pro^5) enkephalinamide. *Eur J Pharm* 1982; 85:171–176.

Lembo PM, Grazzini E, Groblewski T, et al. Proenkephalin A gene products activate a new family of sensory neuron–specific GPCRs. *Nat Neurosci* 2002; 5:201–209.

Levine JD, Clark R, Devor M, et al. Intraneuronal substance P contributes to the severity of experimental arthritis. *Science* 1984; 226:547–549.

Liu C-N, Chambers WW. Intraspinal sprouting of dorsal root axons. *Arch Neurol Psychiat* 1958; 79.
Liu H, Brown JL, Jasmin L, et al. Synaptic relationship between substance P and the substance P receptor: light and electron microscopic characterization of the mismatch between neuropeptides and their receptors. *Proc Natl Acad Sci USA* 1994; 91:1009–1013.
Lord JAH, Waterfield AA, Hughes J, Kosterlitz HW. Endogenous opioid peptides: multiple agonists and receptors. *Nature (Lond)* 1977; 267:495–499.
Malmberg AB, Chen C, Tonegawa S, Basbaum AI. Preserved acute pain and reduced neuropathic pain in mice lacking PKCγ. *Science* 1997; 278:279–283.
Mantyh PW, DeMaster E, Malhotra A, et al. Receptor endocytosis and dendrite reshaping in spinal neurons after somatosensory stimulation. *Science* 1995; 268:1629–1632.
Mantyh PW, Rogers SD, Honoré P. Inhibition of hyperalgesia by ablation of lamina I spinal neurons expressing the substance P receptor. *Science* 1997; 278:275–279.
Mayer DJ, Wolfle TL, Akil H, Carder B, Liebeskind JC. Analgesia from electrical stimulation in the brainstem of the rat. *Science* 1971; 174:1351–1354.
Melzack R, Wall PD Pain mechanisms: a new theory. *Science* 1965; 150:971–979.
Noordenbos W. *Pain: Problems Pertaining to the Transmission of Nerve Impulses Which Give Rise to Pain.* Amsterdam: Elsevier, 1959, pp 182.
Oliveras JL, Redjemi F, Guilbaud G, Besson JM. Analgesia induced by electrical stimulation of the inferior centralis nucleus of the raphe in the cat. *Pain* 1975; 1:139–145.
Pert A, Yaksh T. Sites of morphine induced analgesia in the primate brain: relation to pain pathways. *Brain Res* 1974; 80:135–140.
Recanzone GH, Merzenich MM, Jenkins WM, Grajski KA, Dinse HR. Topographic reorganization of the hand representation in cortical area 3b of owl monkeys trained in a frequency-discrimination task. *J Neurophysiol* 1992; 67:1031–1056.
Riley RC, Trafton JA, Chi SI, Basbaum AI. Presynaptic regulation of spinal cord tachykinin signaling via GABA(B) but not GABA(A) receptor activation. *Neuroscience* 2001; 103:725–737.
Snider WD, McMahon SB. Tackling pain at the source: new ideas about nociceptors. *Neuron* 1998; 20:629–632.
Trafton JA, Abbadie C, Marchand S, Mantyh PW, Basbaum AI. Spinal opioid analgesia: how critical is the regulation of substance P signaling? *J Neurosci* 1999; 19:9642–9653.
Vigna SR, Bowden JJ, McDonald DM, et al. Characterization of antibodies to the rat substance P (NK-1) receptor and to a chimeric substance P receptor expressed in mammalian cells. *J Neurosci* 1994; 14:834–845.
Wall PD, Egger MD. Formation of new connexions in adult rat brains after partial deafferentation. *Nature (Lond)* 1971; 232:542–545.
Woolf CJ, Salter MW. Neuronal plasticity: increasing the gain in pain. *Science* 2000; 288:1765–1769.
Woolf CJ, Shortland P, Coggeshall RE. Peripheral nerve injury triggers central sprouting of myelinated afferents. *Nature (Lond)* 1992; 355:75–78.

Correspondence to: Allan Basbaum, PhD, Department of Anatomy, University of California San Francisco, 513 Parnassus Avenue, Box 0452, San Francisco, CA 94143, USA. Tel: 415-476-5270; Fax: 415-476-4845; email: aib@ phy.ucsf.edu.

Proceedings of the 10th World Congress on Pain,
Progress in Pain Research and Management, Vol. 24,
edited by Jonathan O. Dostrovsky, Daniel B. Carr, and
Martin Koltzenburg, IASP Press, Seattle, © 2003.

4

Ethics beyond Guidelines: Culture, Pain, and Conflict

David B. Morris

*University Professor, University of Virginia,
Charlottesville, Virginia, USA*

Ethics is an enterprise in which pain and culture clearly overlap. Surprisingly, there is at present no good book—or any book—on the ethics of pain. This lack is not restricted to whole books. Although specialists in pain medicine have devoted relatively little attention to ethics, bioethicists in turn have more or less ignored pain (Rich 1997). This mutual inattention is no doubt normal in professional worlds where few specialists are expert in both the intricacies of ethical thought and the complexities of pain medicine. This division of labor, however, is not ultimately beneficial either for patients or for providers.

There are exceptions that signal important changes ahead. Pain specialist Mark Sullivan (2000) expertly describes and critiques various major philosophical positions in ethics. The International Association for the Study of Pain (IASP)'s *Core Curriculum for Professional Education in Pain* (Fields 1995) includes material on ethical standards in pain management and research. From the perspective of nursing, Swenson (2002) has recently called attention to ethical issues in pain management. Scattered articles have begun to discuss pain-related ethical dilemmas in particular specialties and conditions, such as the treatment of infants and children (Walco et al. 1994; Kenny 2001), end-of-life care (Pellegrino 1998), and sickle cell disease (Ballas 2001). In 1998 the American Pain Society and the American Academy of Pain Medicine formed a joint multidisciplinary task force to examine ethical issues in pain management (Dubois 1999). Their initial conclusions, published in *The Journal of Pain,* say that ethical dilemmas are common in pain management practice and that their resolution requires commitment both by individual professionals and by health systems (Ferrell et al. 2001). This chapter is meant as a contribution to this newly emerging interest in an ethics of pain, and my central purpose is to encourage formal, official, and ongoing discussion of ethical issues related to pain.

Despite promising exceptions and recent signs of change, guidelines represent the major public occasion on which pain specialists have focused on ethics, especially the indispensable 1983 and 1995 ethical guidelines written by the Committee on Ethical Issues of IASP. The value of these guidelines is obvious. Yet, once in place, guidelines may also tend to deflect ethical discussion, as if vital matters have been settled once and for all. As a prelude to a movement beyond guidelines, this chapter will examine several specific provisions of the IASP guidelines and then discuss two general shifts in focus that suggest supplemental approaches to an ethics of pain: a shift from principles to values and a shift toward understanding pain as interpersonal. Both shifts find productive support in the work of philosopher Emmanuel Levinas, discussed briefly later in this chapter, where brevity (in its failure to engage complexities and nuances) at least dramatizes the need for regular, extended ongoing discussion of ethics at professional meetings devoted to the study of pain.

The need for a continuing discussion of pain ethics is easy to demonstrate. A sample consisting of 229 oncology nurses in the United States concluded that the most frequently cited ethical dilemma involves the management of pain (Raines 2000). Edmund Pellegrino, a pioneer of modern bioethics, asserts in a discussion of palliative care ethics that failure to relieve pain optimally is "tantamount to moral and legal malpractice" (1998, p. 1521). Moral malpractice is a significant concept, because the well-known problem of undertreatment for pain is usually treated as an issue demanding reform in medical education, in professional training, and in drug regulation. As a result, its ethical dimensions have gone mostly unaddressed. In the United States, even a welcome recent Joint Commission on Accreditation of Health Care Organizations directive linking adequate pain management to institutional certification, while based in a firm assertion about patients' rights, has the practical effect of obscuring ethical questions in favor of regulations whose force is ultimately financial (Joint Commission on Accreditation of Healthcare Organizations 2002). Financial incentives as a basis for improved pain treatment may, however, prove less than dependable in times of economic downturn. What finance gives, finance may take away. Ethics offers a more durable and, arguably, a more appropriate standard for adequate professional pain management.

Ongoing discussion of ethical questions is necessary especially because pain and its dilemmas cannot be fully subsumed under the general principles of bioethics. It is important to recognize limitations in the familiar four-principle approach to bioethics advocated in the widely influential textbook by Beauchamp and Childress (1994). For instance, what should we do when (as often happens) two principles clash? Are principles necessarily self-explanatory or self-evident? Different social groups may interpret a specific principle quite differently, basing their interpretation on distinctive cultural traditions, much as the principle of patient autonomy draws upon Western traditions sometimes quite foreign to immigrant families where medical decisions rest with a patriarch or matriarch or eldest son (Blackhall et al. 1995). Even the Enlightenment assumption that reason constitutes a universal basis for moral judgment is no longer universally shared in a postcolonial, postmodern world that regularly tests the limits of what people regard as reasonable and ethical (MacIntyre 1988; Bauman 1993). Englehardt in *The Foundations of Bioethics* (1996) observed the impossibility, given cultural differences, of affirming any universalist "appeal to general rational justifications" (p. 14). The ethical doctrine known as "principlism" has come under significant criticism recently (Clouser and Gert 1990). More important, what constitutes right action in any specific case is often a matter of debate among reasonable people, so that principles alone will never avert or resolve all ethical conflict concerning pain.

Conflict is the native ground of ethics. Although it sometimes appears that ethical positions are the product of pure reason, timeless and transcendent, they also express and embody the particular conflicts of specific historical eras, even if they sometimes address such historical conflicts through an appeal to divinely bestowed principles or through the procedures of detached rational calculation. Conflict is inherent in ethical matters; there is no evading the ultimate need to acknowledge and confront debate. An ethics of pain thus has no valid alternative to ongoing discussion that moves beyond the calm high ground of principle. Evidence suggests that guidelines alone are insufficient to alter physician behavior (Lomas et al. 1989). A down-to-earth ethics of pain committed to ongoing, regular, official discussion of medical conflict offers a supplement to guidelines that is not only useful but also, in the long run or the short run, indispensable.

The earliest IASP guideline ("Ethical guidelines for investigations of experimental pain in conscious animals") was published in the association's journal *Pain* in 1983, and it offers a useful starting point from which to examine the limits of guidelines. Limits, of course, are not identical with defects. Limitations rather are inherent in the nature of guidelines, and discussion is often necessary in order to make such limits visible. For example, the IASP guidelines open with an assertion that research involving experimental pain in conscious animals is "essential" for producing clinically relevant new knowledge. Most IASP members surely agree. Yet the assertion acknowledges no room for significant difference of opinion, for debate, or for changing cultural standards. By contrast, the *Journal of the American Society of Veterinary Medicine* recently devoted a long discussion to pain in animals, and its article on ethics by Livingston (2002) is remarkable chiefly for its open acknowledgment that questions of animal pain evoke serious conflict.

After 20 years it is time to revisit the 1983 IASP guidelines on animal research and to ask some hard (but not ungenerous) questions. Some provisions in the 1983 guidelines sound as if they are calculated to defuse rather than to acknowledge conflict. Conflict, indeed, is implicit in the 1983 guidelines, which addressed the mostly unregulated experimental practices common in the 1970s. Such historical practices, combined with the emergence of new fields soon called pain medicine and bioethics, made guidelines seem urgently needed. The committee deliberations that produce consensus guidelines usually require members to hammer out compromise positions. Compromise often appears to erase all traces of the conflict in which it originated. How should we understand, for example, the guideline provision stating that researchers should "accept a general attitude in which the animal is regarded not as an object for exploitation, but as a living individual"? A sudden shift from the regulation of practices to the stipulation of mental attitudes manages to bury in high-mindedness any serious engagement with the conflict implicit in opposing answers to the question of exactly what it is that *constitutes* scientific exploitation or objectification of an animal.

Unacknowledged conflict may account for another provision in the 1983 guidelines that today sounds decidedly odd. It states that researchers should if "possible" try out the pain stimulus on themselves. Yet, what beyond public relations is the point of this gesture? How many researchers really manage to calibrate the body-weight ratios, interspecies differences, and gender distinctions necessary in order to assure that they experience a one-time stimulus genuinely equivalent with what they administer, repeatedly, to a laboratory rodent? Questions might even be asked about the very sensible provision stating that researchers treat animals ethically when the experiment undergoes prior review and when researchers give "reasonable assurance" that animals are exposed to "the minimal pain necessary for the purposes of the experiment." However, does the language here obscure recognition that the purposes of any experiment are human purposes, not qualities objectively present in a piece of research? It is open to debate whether judgments concerning what measures count as "reasonable" are based on universal standards of rationality, or on current cultural beliefs, including beliefs in the culture of biomedical science. A provision that researchers inflict only "minimal pain necessary" in effect can be employed to justify whatever pain a researcher claims is needed, so long as a review panel—in practice often configured to reduce diversity and dissent (Hurst 2001)—certifies the study. Peer review, while clearly valuable, covers a multitude of sins and fails to ensure that actions are ethical. It only guarantees, at a bare minimum, that they are approved by a small group of more or less like-minded colleagues.

The questions raised here about the 1983 guidelines are meant not as objections but as probes that honor the IASP committee's invitation to ongoing dialogue: "It is expected that responses from readers will help to improve these guidelines." Continuing ethical discussion is especially important today when researchers must explain their work to a new, curious, and sometimes skeptical public that extends far beyond the circles of scientific research. This new public just might include your vegetarian children or grandchildren, and it certainly includes such post-1980s figures as the distinguished animal rights philosopher Tom Regan, who argues that humans have no right to inflict pain on animals, no matter what the justification. As he writes: "The best we can do when it comes to using animals in science is—not to use them. That is where our duty lies, according to the rights view" (1989, p. 113). Although most biomedical researchers completely disagree with Regan, his arguments cannot be fairly described or wisely dismissed as irrational. An appeal to current scientific consensus offers one sound response to his conflicting arguments and principles. Conflict, in this case, is better acknowledged than ignored. Even if, as seems likely, ongoing discussion will not significantly alter the substance of the 1983 guidelines, renewed and vigorous deliberation can improve its assumptions, logic, point, persuasiveness, and language.

Human pain, with the more complicated questions it evokes, did not receive published IASP guidelines until 1995. Also published in the journal *Pain*, "Ethical guidelines for pain research in humans" is described, like its predecessor, as "intended to stimulate debate among members." The principles it articulates, however, are consistent with established and very noncontroversial guidelines involving research with human subjects, including stipulations regarding informed consent and peer review. It seems such a successful guide—so consonant with current thinking—that it leaves little to debate. The particularity of research involving pain does receive specific attention, as in guideline number seven: "[S]ubjects should be able to escape or terminate a painful stimulus at will." Animals were offered no such escape clause, so that the right to terminate a painful stimulus at will seems a privilege granted by humans to humans as a perquisite of being human, which is fair enough: we grant ourselves all kinds of species-specific privileges, and human pain is in many ways unique. Beyond the safeguards it extends, however, the most important thing about the 1995 guide may be what it does *not* cover. Research involving human subjects is merely a small, if crucial, subclass of ethical questions raised by pain. We also need serious supplemental ongoing discussion that extends to the daily practice of pain management and to the difficult region that lies, thus far, beyond even the best pain guidelines.

The region beyond guidelines seems difficult in part because ethics has a reputation as a specialized subfield of philosophy already staked out with major and mutually incompatible theoretical approaches from Kantianism and utilitarianism to various rights-based theories, all open to critique (Sullivan 2000). In these technical versions, ethics at times resembles an abstract hyperlogic, unintelligible to all but philosophers. Meanwhile, health care professionals in their everyday practice are left to muddle through the social, familial, and personal dilemmas of treatment with the sole guidance of an equally abstract four-principle bioethics that so far has failed to wrestle with such urgent problems as adequate pain treatment for infants, children, dying patients, the elderly, women, ethnic minorities, the poor, people with AIDS, the uninsured, and the entire developing world. (Justice as a principle in bioethics has clearly received many conflicting interpretations—and mere disregard.) This expanded, even global, context creates a space for two shifts in focus that promise to move discussion ahead: a focus on values as distinct from principles and a focus on pain as interpersonal.

An ethics of pain that shifts focus from principles to values cannot offer rock-solid rules for conduct such as guidelines propose. Yet, whereas guidelines often submerge or conceal conflict, one major contribution of a values-based ethics is its promise to clarify the concealed or evaded disagreements that often underlie and perpetuate conflict. Such disagreements and misunderstandings are a regular outcome of exchanges among patients, providers, institutions, third-party insurers, regulatory agencies, and even governments. It is hard to imagine how parties with such different interests and agendas could possibly avoid regular conflict. What often goes unappreciated in partisan clashes, however, is the extent to which disagreements and misunderstandings are rooted in conflicting values. Values differ not only among individuals but also across ethnicities and cultures. The corporate values of health care systems, organizations, and governments may conflict openly or covertly with the values of people whom they serve or employ, from patients to physicians. Such conflicts in values, especially when ignored, create a simmering potential for dispute. One productive role for an ethics of pain is thus to identify the open or unacknowledged conflicting values that often underlie and perpetuate specific disputes.

Here is one example of a situation where the source of conflict lies less in principles than in values. When Pellegrino asserted that suboptimal treatment for pain is tantamount to moral malpractice, he presumably based his assertion on the four-principle standard of nonmalificence. However, also writing in the context of palliative care, Cahana (2002) pertinently asks whether optimal pain relief is always optimal. Relief that seems optimal to a physician who is concerned with reducing pain or to a health care organization that is concerned with certification may not coincide with values that matter deeply to a specific patient. For a dying patient who values mental clarity far above technically optimal pain relief, a specific treatment may cause more distress than the pain it relieves. Knotty disputes over pain management at the end of life regularly expose deep differences in values that separate patients not only from caregivers but also at times from children, spouses, ex-spouses, and assorted in-laws. An ethics focused on values promises to untangle or at least to clarify some of the intractable conflicts over pain.

A values-based ethics is implicitly, although not exclusively, patient-centered. It cannot, of course, always resolve conflict—some disagreements follow us to the grave—but paying attention to values helps shift the focus away from abstract principles and toward whatever it is that matters deeply to each patient. The effect of such a shift toward a patient-centered, value-based ethics is quite visible when we look again at the 1995 IASP guidelines on human subject research. Significantly, this document identifies its primary aim as benefit for "patients in general": "the individual patient," it acknowledges, "may or may not benefit directly." A values-based ethics of pain requires that caregivers attend less to abstract "patients in general" than to a specific patient. In this sense, a focus on values will directly benefit the individual. The values of an individual patient will not always prevail in the circumstantial give-and-take of ethical deliberation, but at least they cannot be ignored or assigned to secondary importance in favor of abstract principles or general patienthood.

A values-based, patient-centered ethics of pain need not be invented from the ground up. In fact, a useful model for values-based ethical thinking is available in the 1996 book by Fiona Randall and R.S. Downie entitled *Palliative Care Ethics: A Good Companion.* In contrast to an ethics focused on narrow codes of conduct, they argue for understanding ethics in a broad sense as including "the whole area of value judgments about good and harm." They argue: "It is because many health care professionals take ethics or morality in the narrow sense that they are unaware of the extent to which they are continually making moral or value judgements in the broad sense" (p. 2). Oddly, the index to *Palliative Care Ethics* includes only one reference to pain, although palliative care specialists have long been among the vanguard in a concern for pain ethics. What matters is the opportunity that pain specialists might seize to extend values-based ethical thinking beyond questions especially appropriate to end-of-life care. Such an extension needs to acknowledge and investigate how far the individual values of caregivers (or their shared corporate values) affect their own medical or research decisions. In settings from the emergency department to obstetrics, it has been repeatedly demonstrated that ethnicity and its associated cultural values correlate directly with medical judgments about pain (Morris 2002a).

A values-based, patient-centered approach to ethics raises the fascinating possibility that pain specialists need to focus on how their own daily practice reflects the impact of innumerable, all-pervasive judgments of value. There is thus good reason why pain medicine might explore what Komesaroff (1995) calls a "microethics" attentive to the subtle ways in which value judgments continually influence medical research and treatment (Frank 1998). Microethics does not focus on headline issues like abortion or cloning but on the nuances of everyday conduct. It works at a level of magnification that helps to reveal the values implicit in even the most casual operations of medical judgment and ordinary practice. Moreover, the model or approach that Randall and Downie represent is attractive especially because it seems consistent with a related conceptual change that merits more extended discussion among pain specialists. This conceptual change, which introduces the second shift in focus beyond guidelines and principles, understands pain (like ethics and dying) as basically interpersonal.

The concept of pain as interpersonal at first seems wholly counterintuitive. Common sense says that pain resides within the confines of an individual nervous system. But perhaps common sense does not tell the whole story. Quantum physics is also counterintuitive, but not therefore wrong. Sullivan (2001) has discussed at length a second-person view of chronic pain that he calls fundamentally "inter-subjective." Subjectivity as it relates to pain may build upon a basic recognition that we are in the proximity of fellow creatures: in certain strains of laboratory rats, the identity of cagemates can largely override genetic predispositions to pain behavior (Raber and Devor 2002). An argument that human pain is interpersonal and intersubjective requires more discussion than is possible here. As a provisional view, however, an interpersonal and intersubjective approach to pain finds important support in the work of the late French philosopher Emmanuel Levinas, professor of philosophy at the Sorbonne, who bases ethics on a recognition of the intrinsic, permanent, interpersonal human differences that he calls "otherness."

An accessible introduction to the thought of Levinas—who has influenced fellow philosophers from Sartre to Derrida—is readily available in the published collection of interviews he gave on French radio entitled *Ethics and Infinity* (1985). Whereas Randall and Downie represent a plain-speaking, pragmatic style in Anglo-American ethical and philosophical thought, Levinas represents continental philosophy in a style of writing and thinking that poses a basic challenge to Anglo-American traditions. It forces us to reexamine assumptions—which must give productive pause to the study of values—that we can ever fully understand another person's words or actions. It urges an attention to the complex interweaving of textual strands that makes any statement or action an instance of potentially endless indeterminacy. Values, statements, and behaviors, according to this continental perspective, are best understood not as well-defined, nugget-like packets of information, cleanly extractable from their surroundings. Instead, embedded in their human context, they possess an indefinite, indeterminate, dialogical quality resistant to any final, fully authoritative summation. This way of thinking, needless to say, drives certain practical, no-nonsense, get-to-the-point people right up the wall!

Ethics for Levinas begins with recognition of the infinitude of each person, as the title *Ethics and Infinity* suggests. This human infinitude—one synonym for otherness—refers to the inherent, inexhaustible differences that make each person more than simply unique, as the cliché tells us. Our otherness for Levinas makes us also irreducible to an objective knowledge that can summarize or "contain" us. One of the repeated words he employs to describe human otherness translates as "uncontainable." Pain, too, has an intrinsic dimension of uncontainable otherness.

It is the uncontainable otherness of each individual that for Levinas gives rise to an ethics of everyday practice. Levinas is distinctive among philosophers in viewing ethics not as a rationalist enterprise deduced from higher abstract philosophical principles, but as social and personal action implicit in a recognition of the otherness of another person. The repeated image that he uses to represent the uncontainable otherness of all human beings is prosaically nonabstract: the face. The face, as Levinas employs it figuratively, evokes the mysterious presence of another person: a presence that he regards as making an immediate ethical claim upon us. As he writes: "The epiphany of the face is ethical" (1969, p. 199). The face, whose radiance we miss or conveniently manage to forget, evokes a bond that precedes reason or principle, an ethics born of immediate contact, as if we stood face-to-face with a revelation of the mundane infinitude of another person—an otherness we can never fully comprehend or overcome. Husbands, Levinas observes, never fully understand wives, nor do wives fully understand husbands. Empathy, no matter how desirable, cannot allow us to know or feel another person's pain. (Whatever distress you may feel if I cut my finger, it is your distress you are feeling, not my pain.) For Levinas, ethics has nothing to do with empathetic self-projection. It begins in acknowledgment of the radical otherness of each person that moves beyond abstract principles and beyond generous illusions about feeling someone else's pain into the demanding daily care for a human being whom we will never fully know or understand.

One major challenge that Levinas poses to traditional ethics is the importance he assigns to emotion. The face for Levinas is not fully knowable as an object of thought. (As he employs it metaphorically, the face is not identical with our physical features and is not even primarily a visual object.) The face for Levinas represents the implicit ethical bond created in the contact between two people that always contains at least a flicker of emotion. He describes the impact of the face as an "obsession" or "shuddering" (*frémissement*), as if to indicate how far this direct, personal encounter taps into emotional strata more primal than language, reason, logic, principle, or philosophy. As he puts it: "The neighbor assigns me before I designate him. This is a modality not of a knowing, but of an obsession, a shuddering of the human quite different from cognition" (1981, p. 87). Levinas explains that the word "shuddering" (*frémissement*) translates a term from Plato's *Phaedrus*, the dialogue in which Socrates calls love a divine madness that lifts the soul toward truth.

It is important to emphasize that Levinas does not regard ethical action as the product of pure reason but as embedded within interpersonal relations that include an emotional component so intense that a rationalist might dismiss it as madness. Neurophysiology and functional brain imaging show that pain emerges from activity not only in the somatosensory cortex but also in affect-related limbic areas of the cortex (Chapman et al. 2001). Emotion is as central to moral choice—brain-damaged patients without affect can reason but not choose—as it is to the human experience of pain (Morris 2002b). With or without Levinas, emotion cannot be wholly foreign to the everyday work of pain ethics. One practical problem that his work poses is how, short of the impossible claims sometimes made for empathy, ethicists should allow for the presence of emotion in human affairs.

The practical ethics that concerns Levinas is, in contrast to standard biomedical emphasis upon patient rights, an ethics of responsibility. It arises from and demands a specific concern for the dialogical and interpersonal nature of human speech. In effect, the prerational, impassioned, obsessive relation to the face—to the "call" of the other—initiates a move into language that for Levinas is implicitly (or, as he likes to say, "straightaway") ethical. "Face and discourse are tied," he explains. "The face speaks. It speaks, it is in this that it renders possible and begins all discourse" (1985, p. 87). Verbal response—to cite a Levinasian pun—is a sign and source of ethical responsibility. Responsibility implies a relation to the other person that reaches beyond the codified layers of professional duty. As he insists: "The face opens the primordial discourse whose first word is obligation" (1961, p. 201).

Significantly, pain too for Levinas shares in the primordial power to call forth an implicit ethical response. Pain and suffering reach beyond an individual nervous system into interpersonal relations where the primary, overriding ethical obligation is our responsibility to relieve the pain of the other. Unlike many religious traditions, Levinas in his essay "Useless suffering" (1988) finds no redeeming or transcendent value in pain. He allows, however, that another person's pain takes on a limited but crucial purpose when it calls forth, in us, the same ethical response implicit in the face. Pain in effect initiates an ethical movement where otherness entails an overriding obligation to the other person. Hostage, stranger, exile: these three repeated images take their significance for Levinas in an embodiment of the vulnerability always present within otherness. Pain specialists might want to add to this emblematic trio, which calls forth an implicit ethical response, another vulnerable and often neglected figure: the patient. Admittedly, Levinas offers an unconventional approach to ethics. Like any philosopher, he has intellectual opponents, in addition to his unique buildup of cult followers. More conventional approaches, however, have failed to move discussion of pain ethics into questions beyond principles. In the challenge of its otherness, the work of Levinas suggests why professional associations concerned with pain might consider creating an official, regular, ongoing forum for extended discussion of the difficult ethical conflicts that lead into—not away from—the vital terrain beyond guidelines.

REFERENCES

Ballas SK. Ethical issues in the management of sickle cell pain. *Am J Hematol* 2001; 68:127–132.

Bauman Z. *Postmodern Ethics*. Oxford: Blackwell, 1993.

Beauchamp TL, Childress JF. *Principles of Biomedical Ethics*, 4th ed. New York: Oxford University Press, 1994.

Blackhall LJ, Murphy ST, Frank G, Michel V, Azen S. Ethnicity and attitudes toward patient autonomy. *JAMA* 1995; 274:820–825.

Cahana A. Is optimal pain relief always optimal? Bioethical considerations of interventional pain management at the end of life. *APS Bulletin* 2002; 12(5):1,4.

Chapman CR, Nakamura Y, Donaldson GW, et al. Sensory and affective dimensions of phasic pain are indistinguishable in the self-report and psychophysiology of normal laboratory subjects. *J Pain* 2001; 2:279–294.

Clouser KD, Gert B. A critique of principlism. *J Med Philos* 1990; 15:219–236.

Committee on Ethical Issues of the International Association for the Study of Pain. Ethical guidelines for investigations of experimental pain in conscious animals. *Pain* 1983; 16:109–110.

Committee on Ethical Issues of the International Association for the Study of Pain. Ethical guidelines for pain research in humans. *Pain* 1995; 63:277–278.

DuBois MY. Ethics in pain management. *APS Bulletin* 1999; 9:1.

Englehardt HT, Jr. *The Foundations of Bioethics*, 2nd ed. New York: Oxford University Press, 1996.

Ferrell BR, Novy D, Sullivan MD, et al. Ethical dilemmas in pain management. *J Pain* 2001; 2:171–180.

Fields HL (Ed). *Core Curriculum for Professional Education in Pain*. Seattle: IASP Press, 1995, pp 117–123.

Frank AW. First-person microethics: deriving principles from below. *Hastings Cent Rep* 1998; 28(4):37–42.

Hurst M. The value of difference: nonaffiliates on IRBs provide alternative views. *Protecting Human Subjects* 2001; 5:1–3.

Joint Commission on Accreditation of Healthcare Organizations. *2002 Comprehensive Accreditation Manual for Hospitals: The Official Handbook*. Oakbrook Terrace, IL: Joint Commission Resources, Inc., 2002.

Kenny NP. The politics of pediatric pain. In: Finley GA, McGrath PJ (Eds). *Acute and Procedure Pain in Infants and Children,* Progress in Pain Research and Management, Vol. 20. Seattle: IASP Press, 2001, pp 147–158.

Komesaroff PA. From bioethics to microethics: ethical debate and clinical medicine. In: Komesaroff PA (Ed). *Troubled Bodies: Critical Perspectives on Postmodernism, Medical Ethics, and the Body*. Durham, NC: Duke University Press, 1995, pp 62–86.

Levinas E. *Ethics and Infinity: Conversations with Philippe Nemo*. Cohen RA (Trans). Pittsburgh: Duquesne University Press, 1985.

Levinas E. *Otherwise Than Being or Beyond Essence*. Lingis A (Trans). Pittsburgh: Duquesne University Press, 1981.

Levinas E. *Totality and Infinity: An Essay on Exteriority*. Lingis A (Trans). Pittsburgh: Duquesne University Press, 1969.

Levinas E. Useless suffering. In: Cohen R (Trans). *The Provocation of Levinas*. London: Routledge, 1988, pp 156–167.

Livingston AL. Ethical issues regarding pain in animals. *J Am Soc Vet Med* 2002; 221:229–233.

Lomas J, Anderson GM, Dominick-Pierre K, et al. Do practice guidelines guide practice? The effect of a consensus statement on the practice of physicians. *N Engl J Med* 1989; 321:1306–1311.

MacIntyre A. *Whose Justice? Which Rationality?* Notre Dame, IN: University of Notre Dame Press, 1988.

Morris DB. Ethnicity and pain. *Pain: Clin Updates* 2002a; 9(4):1–4.

Morris DB. Narrative, ethics, and pain: thinking with stories. In: Montello M, Charon R (Eds). *Stories Matter: The Role of Narrative in Medical Ethics*. New York: Routledge, 2002b, pp 196–218.

Pellegrino ED. Emerging ethical issues in palliative care. *JAMA* 1998; 279:1521–1522.

Raber P, Devor M. Social variables affect phenotype in the neuroma model of neuropathic pain. *Pain* 2002; 97:139–150.

Raines ML. Ethical decision making in nurses: relationships among moral reasoning, coping style, and ethics stress. *JONA's Healthcare Law, Ethics, and Regulation* 2000; 2(1):29–41.

Randall F, Downie RS. *Palliative Care Ethics: A Good Companion*. New York: Oxford University Press, 1996.

Regan T. The case for animal rights. In: Regan T, Singer P (Eds). *Animal Rights and Human Obligations*, 2nd ed. Englewood Cliffs, NJ: Prentice Hall, 1989, pp 105–114.

Rich BA. A legacy of silence: bioethics and the culture of pain. *J Med Humanit* 1997; 18:233–259.

Sullivan M. Ethical principles in pain management. *Pain Med* 2000; 1:274–279.

Sullivan MD. Finding pain between minds and bodies. *Clin J Pain* 2001; 17:146–156.

Swenson CJ. Ethical issues in pain management. *Semin Oncol Nurs* 2002; 18:135–142.

Walco GA, Cassidy RC, Schechter NL. Pain, hurt, and harm: the ethics of pain control in infants and children. *N Engl J Med* 1994; 331:541–544.

Correspondence to: David B. Morris, PhD, 138 Bryan Hall, University of Virginia, Charlottesville, VA 22904-1478, USA. Email: dbm6e@virginia.edu.

Proceedings of the 10th World Congress on Pain,
Progress in Pain Research and Management, Vol. 24,
edited by Jonathan O. Dostrovsky, Daniel B. Carr, and
Martin Koltzenburg, IASP Press, Seattle, © 2003.

5

Pain Relief in the Information Age: Let's Meet Our Children's Expectations

Alejandro R. Jadad

Centre for Global eHealth Innovation, Rose Family Chair in Supportive Care, Canada Research Chair in eHealth Innovation, and Departments of Health Policy, Management and Evaluation, and Anesthesia, University Health Network, University of Toronto, Toronto, Canada

A PERSONAL INTRODUCTION

On May 13, 2002, my father died of lung cancer. He was a family physician who cared deeply about his patients. He was fully aware of his bad prognosis but was not afraid of death. He wanted to maintain the highest possible quality of life for as long as possible and to die with dignity. The 2 years between his diagnosis and his death taught me a lot about the health system we could have in the information age.

During this time, I had more conversations with my father than in the previous 20 years. We used the telephone and email often. His oncologists in South America sent me copies of his records and tests over the Internet. I was then able to share this information with my colleagues in Canada. I conducted literature searches over the Internet trying to find answers to their questions. When successful, the searches were followed by long telephone or email sessions, led by my father, to discuss the findings. Rapidly, thanks to the Internet and the telephone, we developed a strong international team focused on my father's needs. Knowledge continued to flow well, through the Internet, between South America and Canada. My father received several rounds of chemotherapy followed by radiotherapy that kept him functional. He received his treatments late in the week, so as to be able to see patients on Monday. When he developed pain, it was moderate and could be relieved completely by carefully titrated doses of opioids. He kept working and driving until the very end. We had long sessions on the Internet or the telephone, discussing his concerns, fears, and satisfactions. At the end of such conversations, he would tell me that they made him feel better than anything else. Thanks to technology, we were closer than ever.

His last day was a good reflection of his life and caring nature. He had breakfast with his family. Eight patients came to his house in the morning, seeking his advice. Although he was in worse shape than those patients, he saw them all, taking some oxygen in between consultations. According to his records of that day, six of the patients could not pay. As always, lack of money did not make any difference in how he treated them. After having lunch with his family and some close friends, he hugged his wife and daughter, then took a nap. Two hours later, he woke up, had an episode of coughing that triggered bleeding from an artery in his lungs, and died in a few minutes. Although a year earlier than he had hoped, his wishes had been granted: he died at home, with his family, close to his friends, active professionally, pain-free, and with dignity.

Soon after my father's death, I was fascinated to reflect that what had happened did not appear to surprise my children. They are growing up in an open, respectful family environment, in which death can be discussed frankly and the Internet and other information and communications technologies are a normal part of life. They attend a school in which Internet use is encouraged to support their projects and to promote good communication among peers, parents, and teachers. For these children, now just 8 and 10 years of age, the flow of information across the world and the attention that we paid to my father's needs seemed perfectly appropriate. How disappointed they would feel if they knew that they are part of a small minority and that no health system, even in the most "developed" countries, is currently using the Internet or paying attention to patients at the level to which they have grown accustomed, both at home and at school.

With positions in Supportive Care, eHealth Innovation, and Health Policy, I now find myself leading several initiatives that hope to bridge "high-tech" with "high-touch" approaches, globally. With increasing frequency, I reflect on the risk we face of limiting experiences such as my father's or my children's to the benefit of the well-connected, affluent, and highly educated. In a world in which more than 100 years after the invention of the telephone fewer than 50% of the world's inhabitants have used it, and in which less than 1% of the population owns a computer, we will need to be very creative, persistent, resilient, and committed if we are to ensure that the information age promotes equity, not more disparity.

THE VISION

Regardless of who or where we are, we all feel strongly about our health care system. We want a system that is trustworthy, understandable, accountable, responsive, and efficient. We want a system that answers our questions and provides support. We want responsible care in our homes as well as in the hospital. We want a system that does not only focus on treating disease, but promotes the highest possible level of health for each person throughout life, regardless of location or circumstance. We want care that is responsive to our culture and sensitive to our unique individual needs. We want the best care to be available to us and to everyone else (Jadad 1999).

In sum, we want a health care system that behaves like a good companion, not like the franchise of inefficient repair shops we have now. Transforming the health system into a good companion will not be easy, but it is possible.

Can the use of information and communications technologies help us realize this vision with regard to pain relief and research? Of course it can. Rapid developments in information technology are creating new ways for people to communicate with each other, to interact with machines, and to access and exchange information. Thanks to those developments, and particularly the Internet, for the first time in history we have the tools needed to ensure that all human beings have the same opportunity to share information, regardless of who or where they are (Jadad and Enkin 2000). But we need much more than technological power. Solutions are starting to emerge through a creative blend of technological innovation, effective knowledge management, balanced partnerships among the government, academic institutions, the public, and industry, rigorous interdisciplinary research and development, increasing public participation, strong input from social scientists, and political will (Jadad et al. 2001).

To realize this vision, however, we will need to overcome many significant barriers. Rapid developments in information technology not only have outpaced the ability of the health care system to keep up and adapt, but are also creating a widening gap between those who have and those who lack efficient access to technology and knowledge. This disparity can be seen both within and across countries, and across all groups of decision makers. This is a scenario common to many technologies in the world and one that we cannot afford to ignore within the context of health systems.

WILL WE BE ABLE TO MEET OUR CHILDREN'S EXPECTATIONS?

The rest of this chapter will compare the expectations of children like mine with the current status of the health system. My hope is to highlight the challenges we must meet to ensure that patients and health professionals in the near future find the health system that they need, expect, and deserve. Obviously, all the issues described below will apply first to high-income countries with a high level of Internet usage. It is my expectation, although this may not be feasible in the short term, that low-income countries will see the use of technology as a means by which to improve the efficiency of their health systems and will make doing so a priority, while exploring and adopting strategies to become active and respected participants in a truly global community.

OUR CHILDREN EXPECT US TO BE TRUSTWORTHY

A vast amount of information about pain is already available on the Internet and in the peer-reviewed literature. A search of the Internet on September 15, 2002, using Google and the term "pain," yielded over 13 million sites in 0.15 seconds! A search of MEDLINE the same day and with the same term yielded over 240,000 citations. My children, however, would not be surprised by these figures, as they, too, experience information overload almost every day.

What would shock them is the wide gap that still exists between what we could know and what we do know, between what we think we should do and what we really do (Jadad and Enkin 2000). My question, then, is: How can we ensure that our decisions are based on the best available knowledge, when we have so much information and not enough time or skills to handle it?

During the past decade, proponents of evidence-based decision-making have created several "information distilleries," a series of efforts that use information and communication technologies to help us handle information overload. The following are some examples of these efforts, with an emphasis on those that are available free online and are relevant to the study and management of pain.

"New breed journals" or secondary publications. Secondary publications result from scanning and filtering the contents of a large number of journals using explicit methods to identify valid and clinically useful articles. They provide concise informative titles, abstracts, and commentaries that help readers discern whether the information applies to their own decisions. These publications are typically thin and relatively infrequent, reflecting the fact that a very small proportion of the literature is really worth reading.

Bandolier is perhaps the most important member of this group of tools to those interested in the study and management of pain. This publication is produced monthly by the Oxford Anglia National Health Service Region in the United Kingdom. It lists useful "bullet points of evidence-based medicine" on the Internet, free of charge (www.jr2.ox.ac.uk/bandolier/). Bandolier supports the Oxford Pain Internet Site (www.jr2.ox.ac.uk/bandolier/booth/painpag/), a free online publication that provides access to systematic reviews of randomized controlled trials (RCTs) on all aspects of pain.

Specialized compendia of evidence. Two superb examples are the Cochrane Library and the National Guideline Clearinghouse.

The Cochrane Library is the main product of The Cochrane Collaboration (www.cochrane.org), an international organization that aims to help people make informed decisions about health by preparing, maintaining, and ensuring the accessibility of rigorous, systematic, and up-to-date reviews (and where possible, meta-analyses) of the benefits and risks of health care interventions. The rapid growth and recognition of the Cochrane Collaboration has been due, to a great extent, to its extensive use of the Internet to provide interested individuals with access to manuals, tools, and training materials to facilitate the design and conduct of reviews, easy access to them, and continuous open peer-review.

The regularly updated electronic Cochrane Library was designed to give decision makers the evidence they need to make informed health care decisions, with special emphasis on data from RCTs. It is issued quarterly and provides two databases online that could be particularly valuable to people interested in the management of pain.

The Cochrane Database of Systematic Reviews (CDSR) is a rapidly growing collection of regularly updated systematic reviews of the effects of health care prepared by members of collaborative review groups affiliated with the Cochrane Collaboration. It also includes protocols of reviews in progress. One of the groups, known as the Cochrane Pain, Palliative and Supportive Care (PaPaS) Collaborative Review Group (www.jr2.ox.ac.uk/Cochrane), focuses on reviews on the prevention and treatment of pain, in addition to reviews of supportive care and interventions for symptoms at the end of life.

The Database of Abstracts of Reviews of Effectiveness (DARE) contains structured abstracts of thousands of systematic reviews from around the world, all of which have been completed independently of the Cochrane Collaboration. These reviews have been approved by reviewers at the National Health Service Centre for Reviews and Dissemination at the University of York, England. DARE also includes brief records of reviews that may be useful for background information, abstracts of reports of health technology agencies worldwide, and abstracts of reviews in selected secondary publications. In September 2002, DARE included information from over 700 reviews related to pain.

The National Guideline Clearinghouse (NGC; www.guidelines.gov) is an Internet-based public resource that enables access to clinical practice guidelines and allows comparisons of recommendations produced by different organizations in North America. It includes a comprehensive database of evidence-based clinical practice guidelines and related documents produced by the Agency for Healthcare Research and Quality (AHRQ) (formerly the Agency for Health Care Policy and Research, AHCPR), in partnership with the American Medical Association (AMA) and the American Association of Health Plans (AAHP).

Its mission is to provide physicians, nurses, other health professionals, health plans, integrated delivery systems, health care purchasers, and others an accessible mechanism for obtaining objective, detailed information on clinical practice guidelines and to further their dissemination and implementation. Key components of NGC include: (1) Structured abstracts (summaries) about the guidelines included and their development; (2) a tool for comparing two or more guidelines side by side; (3) syntheses of guidelines covering similar topics, highlighting areas of similarity and difference; (4) links to full-text guidelines, where available, and information on how to order printed copies; (5) an electronic forum, NGC-L, for exchanging information on clinical practice guidelines and their development and use; and (6) annotated bibliographies on guideline development methodology and implementation of guidelines. In September 2002, the database included almost 400 guidelines on pain-related issues.

Other compendia of distilled knowledge are evolving rapidly. Examples include *Clinical Evidence* (www.clinicalevidence.com), *UpToDate* (www.uptodate.com), and *Scientific American Medicine* (www.samed.com).

Although most of these efforts focus on evidence from research, they illustrate how technology could be used to produce, organize, and distribute health-related information, of any kind, globally.

OUR CHILDREN EXPECT US TO EMBRACE ELEARNING

It would be difficult for children in developed nations today to understand that most of the sources of high-quality evidence available on the Internet, like the ones mentioned above, remain unknown to most health professionals and patients (Sigouin and Jadad 2002), and that we continue to rely on ineffective, inefficient, and passive modes of education (Davis et al. 1999).

These children would expect us to adopt, with enthusiasm, strategies and devices that could help us optimize our levels of competence, performance, and behavior. Some simple interventions have been shown to be surprisingly effective. A recent study, for instance, suggests that closed, moderated discussion groups can help patients with chronic back pain improve their function, reduce their level of pain and distress, and seek fewer physician visits (Lorig et al. 2002). New technologies such as hand-held devices, Internet-based telephone- and videoconferencing, wireless networks with high-speed data transmission, and multimedia applications are already making possible "just in time" learning at the point of care (www.pdamd.com/vertical/home.xml; www.zdnet.com/special/filters/sc/pda/). Wearable computers and virtual reality, although still in their infancy, promise yet another convenient way to access, generate, and exchange information easily, cheaply, and quickly (Mann et al. 2001). Pain relief provides an ideal model for the development, refinement, and use of these technologies, and to help us understand and minimize potential harmful effects.

OUR CHILDREN EXPECT STRONG PARTNERSHIPS BETWEEN PATIENTS AND HEALTH PROFESSIONALS

Most children in industrialized countries now have access to the Internet and are encouraged to use it as a source of information to enrich their school projects and homework. Because of this unprecedented access to information, the main role of parents and teachers has shifted now to one of support and guidance, rather than one of control. How could we explain to modern children that most of the interactions between health professionals and patients follow a paternalistic model of care and that use of the Internet by patients is still viewed by many health professionals as threatening? Instead, these children would expect patients to participate in interactions with their health professionals as respected and welcome partners, being able to ask questions of interest to them and to obtain answers in a timely and honest fashion. Research, in fact, suggests that such an approach could lead to improved health outcomes with no associated increase in consultation time. Studies have shown, consistently, that patients feel more satisfied and obtain better health outcomes when they are able to identify and discuss the issues that are of greatest importance to them, obtain information on available treatments, and ask pertinent questions of health professionals involved in their care (Jadad 1995; Stewart 1995; Oliver et al. 2001).

Based on this literature, we have developed an evidence-based, patient-centered guide for the treatment of cancer pain. Prepared with input from patients, family members and health professionals, this guideline includes strategies to improve patient participation in treatment decisions and also stresses the uncertainty surrounding most decisions on the treatment of cancer pain. Each component of the guide, known as *A Team Approach to Pain Relief,* was developed following research evidence on how to improve health outcomes through increased patient participation in decisions. The contents of the guide that relate to the management of pain were based on the best available evidence from systematic reviews and guidelines. Decisions on the language, format, and graphics of the guide were made by a group of patients and family members, with support from health professionals. A refined version of the guide (with four different formats) was presented separately to 113 patients, 100 family members or close friends, and 25 health professionals, who were selected randomly at a major cancer center in Ontario. Of the 238 individuals approached, 227 (95%) agreed to participate. Of the participating patients, 46.4% had reported pain over the previous week. Overall, 98% of the participants (including health professionals) said that the guide was easy to understand, 88% found it of adequate length, 93% agreed with the order of the ideas presented, 72% reported that it improved their understanding of pain and its treatment (including 41% of the health professionals!), and 79% said that it could help them communicate better about pain and its treatment. Eighty-three percent said that it would help them ask questions about cancer pain, and 70% that it would help improve the treatment of cancer pain (26% of the participants were unsure and 4% said it would not help at all). Seventy-six percent expressed interest in using the guide during the treatment of cancer pain, and 77% reported interest in the use of similar guides for the treatment of other conditions in patients with cancer. Further evaluation, using experimental methods, will determine the impact of such a partnership-based intervention on pain outcomes, process of care, and resource utilization.

With input from patients and health professionals working in partnership, we are also developing and evaluating a "Virtual Coach" to train patients on how to identify and ask questions of importance to them, and how to seek answers from Web sites and health professionals. Intelligent tools of this kind will become increasingly frequent and could help us ensure that computers take care of the repetitive tasks that currently hinder the patient-health professional relationship, leaving more time for in-person encounters (Jadad 1999).

OUR CHILDREN EXPECT ONLINE COMMUNICATION WITHIN AN INTEGRATED HEALTH INFORMATION SYSTEM

Most children in industrialized countries, either through their own experience or that of a family member, have seen how bank cards provide access to financial records in seconds, regardless of their location. Increasingly, they are being exposed to online systems to order movie tickets, rent cars, make flight reservations, and book hotel rooms. It would be difficult to explain to them that in most of the world, hospitals and community-based organizations have poor information infrastructure, that even in industrialized countries it is rare to find integration of information systems across institutions, and that most patients do not have access to their health records over the Internet.

Recent surveys of over 2,000 patients attending the University Health Network in Toronto have revealed that more than half have access to the Internet, and more than two-thirds with such access use it as a source of health information and are willing to use it to communicate with health professionals. Other studies have shown that patients would be willing to use computers to support activities such as renewal of prescriptions, scheduling of appointments, and accessing of health records (Balas et al. 1997). Based on this research, a team of researchers at the Centre for Global eHealth Innovation has developed and is currently evaluating an "Internet Clinical Communication Centre," also known as iC3. This application creates continuous channels of communication between patients and health professionals, supporting all types of communication through the Internet, from simple email to instant messaging systems with video and audio functions that will allow patients and health professionals to see and be seen by each other. When fully developed, the iC3 will allow patients and health professionals to renew prescriptions online, to access clinic schedules and summaries of health records remotely, and to communicate about non-urgent matters. It will also provide patients with tools to record information on quality of life and symptoms between consultations, to create summaries of those assessments and share them with health professionals, to create their own health information portal, and to communicate with other patients.

The iC3 will have one set of resources for patients and one for health professionals. One of the main aims of the project is to create a friendly interface in the major languages spoken in the world (e.g., English, Spanish, and Mandarin). The project will allow easy navigation for people of various ages, health conditions, cultural background, literacy levels, and socioeconomic status. The iC3 is also being used to evaluate the impact of Internet-based communication on waiting times, on patient and health professional satisfaction with care, on resource utilization, on the organization of health services, and on health outcomes.

Many barriers must still be overcome if we are to reach the full potential for Internet-mediated communication between the public and health professionals. For health professionals, the most important include fear of liability, lack of appropriate reimbursement mechanisms, and concerns about work overload and interference with their lives outside work. For the public, the main barriers are lack of open communication channels with most health professionals, the lack of clear guidelines on how to communicate with them, and still, for about half the population in North America and a much greater proportion in most other regions of the world, lack of easy access to the Internet.

OUR CHILDREN EXPECT US TO COLLABORATE EFFECTIVELY

Our children would be shocked to learn how little collaboration exists across sectors, groups, and institutions. They would expect us to use technology to eliminate geographic, cultural, and institutional barriers, and to share resources, experiences, and ideas across remote locations. They also would expect us to build strong relationships with others interested in conducting, supporting, and participating in pain relief research; to adopt common methods to capture data from research studies (e.g., forms to capture core data from studies over the Internet); and to use tools for group-to-group online interactions.

In 2002, federal and provincial agencies in Canada funded the creation of the Centre for Global eHealth Innovation, at the University Health Network and University of Toronto (www.uhnres.utoronto.ca/ehealth). This center was conceived as a resource to study and promote Internet-based innovations that help people, regardless of who or where they are, maintain the highest levels of health, while making efficient use of health resources. The center is becoming the hub for the Global eHealth Innovation Network, a rapidly growing group of individuals, research settings, and tools that provides unique conditions to support, worldwide, the study of how technology may accelerate the reconceptualization and transformation of the study of pain and the health system at large in the information age (Jadad et al. 2001).

During the 10th World Congress on Pain, the Secretariat and the World Wide Web Task Force of the International Association for the Study of Pain, together with the Centre for Global eHealth Innovation, conducted a survey of participants to assess their patterns of use of the Internet and their interest in participating in a global collaborative community of people involved in studying and managing pain. This survey will provide the basis for a strategic effort to integrate the existing fragmented efforts throughout the world to study pain, and foster the development and implementation of creative solutions to current problems.

CONCLUSION

The Internet and other information and communication technologies are transforming all aspects of human life. They are also creating radically new approaches to promote efficient interactions among scientists, clinicians, regulatory agencies, and members of the public, in order to accelerate the transformation of ideas into successful ways to control pain.

However, it is naive to think that fancy gadgets will lead, on their own, to more efficient and successful studies and better management of pain. Many barriers, mostly political, financial, and cognitive rather than technological, prevent us from having a health system that acts as a lifelong companion for people.

Many of us are now in a privileged position to make a contribution, albeit small, to meeting these challenges. Perhaps for the first time in history, thanks to the Internet, we have a real opportunity to achieve equitable and efficient access to information, honest and balanced communication, and groundbreaking research, with a global reach. Because of the high prevalence and global extent of pain, its study and management provide ideal models to understand how to improve the system at large. We cannot afford to miss this opportunity. If we take it and succeed, we will provide future generations with the health system they expect and deserve. If we fail, they will know that we tried, and will try again (Jadad 2001).

REFERENCES

Balas EA, Jaffrey F, Kuperman GJ, et al. Electronic communication with patients. Evaluation of distance medicine technology. *JAMA* 1997; 278:152–159.

Davis D, Thomson MA, Freemantle N, et al. Impact of formal continuing medical education: do conferences, workshops, rounds and other traditional continuing education activities change behavior or health care outcomes? *JAMA* 1999; 282:867–874.

Jadad AR. Asking patients to write lists—randomised controlled trials support it. *BMJ* 1995; 311:746.

Jadad AR. Promoting partnerships: challenges for the Internet age. *BMJ* 1999; 319:761–764.

Jadad AR. Quo vadis health system? On wishes, magic and the power of eHealth. *Healthcare Information Management & Communications* 2001; 25:8.

Jadad AR, Enkin M. The new alchemy: transmuting information to knowledge in the electronic age. *CMAJ* 2000; 162(13):1826–1828.

Jadad AR, Goel V, Rizo C, Hohenadel J, Cortinois A. The Global eHealth Innovation Network: building a vehicle for the transformation of the health system in the information age. Business briefing—next generation healthcare. *World Medical Association* 2001; 48–50.

Lorig K, Laurent DD, Deyo RA, et al. Can a back pain e-mail discussion group improve health status and lower health care costs? A randomized study. *Arch Intern Med* 2002; 162:792–796.

Mann S, Niedzviecki, H. *Cyborg: Digital Destiny and Human Possibility in the Age of the Wearable Computer*. Canada: Doubleday, 2001.

Oliver JW, Kravitz RL, Kaplan SH, Meyers FJ. Individualized patient education and coaching to improve pain control among cancer outpatients. *J Clin Oncol* 2001; 19(7):2206–2212.

Sigouin C, Jadad AR. Awareness of sources of peer-reviewed research evidence on the internet. *JAMA* 2002; 287:2867–2869.

Stewart MA. Effective physician-patient communication and health outcomes: a review. *CMAJ* 1995; 152:1423–1433.

Correspondence to: Alejandro R. Jadad, MD, DPhil, FRCPC, Centre for Global eHealth Innovation, R. Fraser Elliot Building, 4th Floor, Elizabeth Street, Toronto, ON, Canada M5G 2C4. Email: ajadad@uhnres.utoronto.ca.

Part II

Nociceptors: Membrane Receptors, Channels, and Types

Proceedings of the 10th World Congress on Pain,
Progress in Pain Research and Management, Vol. 24,
edited by Jonathan O. Dostrovsky, Daniel B. Carr, and
Martin Koltzenburg, IASP Press, Seattle, © 2003.

6

The Molecular Biology of Thermosensation

David Julius

Department of Cellular and Molecular Pharmacology, University of California San Francisco, San Francisco, California, USA

NATURAL PRODUCTS AS PROBES OF THE PAIN PATHWAY

Pain-producing stimuli are detected by a subset of primary afferent neurons that have the remarkable ability to recognize a range of physical and chemical stimuli and transduce this information into electrochemical signals called action potentials (Fields 1987). As suggested by Sherrington (1906) and later validated by Burgess and Perl (1967), these neurons, called nociceptors, can be distinguished from other sensory nerve fibers by their relatively high thresholds for activation; that is, they can be excited by intense (noxious) chemical, thermal, or mechanical stimuli, but not by innocuous stimuli, such as warming or light touch. The concept of the nociceptor presents a challenge for the molecular biologist: to identify molecules that define the nociceptor and account for the unusual and specific functional properties of these cells, most notably, their high threshold sensitivity to noxious physical and chemical stimuli. We would therefore like to obtain answers to the following questions: (1) how are noxious stimuli detected? (2) how do these molecular detectors transduce noxious stimuli into action potentials? (3) how are sensitivity thresholds determined by the biophysical and biochemical properties of these signal detectors? and (4) how are thresholds reset following injury (at least with regard to peripherally mediated events)?

Molecular studies of visual transduction were facilitated by the fact that the machinery governing phototransduction is concentrated in one easily obtainable structure, namely the eye, making biochemical, physiological, and ultimately molecular genetic studies possible (Nathans 1987). In the case of olfaction, physiological experiments suggested that signal transduction occurs through the activation of G-protein-coupled receptors, providing the essential clue for genomics-based cloning strategies that led to the eventual identification of a family of odorant receptors (Buck and Axel 1991). In contrast to these examples, the somatosensory system has not been very amenable to biochemical analysis, nor have physiological studies pointed the way to any particular class or family of molecules as being especially important in signal detection and transduction. For these reasons, we have taken a pharmacological approach to gaining insight into the molecular mechanisms underlying somatosensation and nociception in the vertebrate nervous system. In particular, we have exploited natural products as powerful tools with which to identify cellular targets that mediate their often potent and selective physiological and psychophysical effects. Indeed, the pain pathway has provided some of the best examples of this approach, as illustrated by morphine and aspirin, two plant-derived analgesic agents whose use in the laboratory led to the discovery of endogenous opioid and cyclooxygenase signaling pathways, respectively. We have used products of the chili pepper and mint leaf to determine how primary afferent neurons detect hot and cold.

THE CAPSAICIN RECEPTOR IS A DETECTOR OF NOXIOUS HEAT

Capsaicin is the pungent ingredient in chili peppers that elicits the familiar tingling and burning sensation associated with spicy foods (Jancso et al. 1977; Szolcsanyi 1993). As has been appreciated for many years, capsaicin produces its psychophysical sensations by serving as a selective excitatory agent for a subset of primary afferent neurons that detect painful (noxious) stimuli; indeed, capsaicin sensitivity has been widely used as one functional hallmark of nociceptors (Jancso et al. 1977). Moreover, cellular studies have shown that capsaicin elicits nonselective cationic currents in a subset of cultured dorsal root ganglion neurons, thereby promoting influx of both sodium and calcium ions into these cells (Bevan and Docherty 1993). We took advantage of this response to identify a capsaicin receptor from rat dorsal root ganglia using expression cloning methods, in conjunction with a sensitive calcium imaging-based screen (Caterina 1997). Gene sequence and functional analyses of this cDNA (vanilloid receptor subtype 1, or VR1, now termed TRPV1) showed that the expressed protein is, indeed, a nonselective cation channel with relatively high permeability to calcium ions (being approximately nine times more permeable to Ca^{2+} than to Na^{+}). Moreover, in situ hybridization and immunohistochemistry studies have clearly shown that TRPV1 is expressed by a subpopulation of dorsal root and trigeminal neurons with the small- to medium-diameter soma (~19 μm in diameter), most of which probably correspond to unmyelinated C-fiber nociceptors. TRPV1-positive cells include both peptidergic neurons (expressing substance P and calcitonin gene-related peptide) and nonpeptidergic (IB4- and P2X3-positive) neurons (Tominaga et al. 1998; Guo et al. 1999; Michael and Priestly 1999).

One of the most important discoveries that we have made regarding TRPV1 function is to show that this channel can be activated by heat (Caterina 1997). Salient characteristics of this response include a thermal activation threshold of ~43°C; a rather steep temperature dependence (Q_{10} >20), suggesting a highly cooperative or allosteric mechanism of activation; and nonselective permeability to cations, including calcium (Caterina 1997; Tominaga et al. 1998; Welch et al. 2000). These properties resemble those of native heat-evoked currents in cultured sensory neurons or single nerve fibers (Treede et al. 1995; Cesare and McNaughton 1996; Vyklicky et al. 1999). While there are certainly many similarities between native heat-evoked currents and those mediated by heterologously expressed TRPV1 channels, not all characteristics reported for these responses are believed to be identical (Nagy and Rang 1999). We and others have therefore used genetic methods to test the roles of TRPV1 in thermo- and chemonociception (Caterina et al. 2000; Davis et al. 2000). Mice bearing targeted deletions within the TRPV1 gene were examined for thermal sensitivity at numerous levels of the pain pathway, including cultured sensory neurons, primary afferent nerve fibers (skin-nerve preparation), spinal cord dorsal horn neurons, and animal behavior. At each level, significant deficits were observed in heat sensitivity. At the same time, it is clear (especially from results of the single-fiber recording and behavioral response data) that TRPV1 knockout mice are not thermally analgesic, suggesting that this channel underlies some, but not all, aspects of acute heat sensitivity. We have hypothesized that this residual heat sensitivity is mediated by other, structurally related ion channels belonging to the greater family of mammalian transient receptor potential (TRP) channels (Caterina et al. 1999). Indeed, a number of such candidates have been cloned and shown to respond to heat or cold, at least when expressed in heterologous systems (see below).

Another robust and important phenotype observed in these genetic experiments was an almost complete lack of thermal hypersensitivity among TRPV1-deficient mice in the setting of inflammation; importantly, these animals showed normal hypersensitivity to mechanical stimuli (Caterina et al. 2000; Davis et al. 2000). Thus, TRPV1 is an essential component of the signal transduction pathway that produces thermal hyperalgesia following tissue injury, consistent with the idea that TRPV1 is a polymodal signal detector whose thermal activation threshold can be dramatically influenced by a variety of factors that make up the "inflammatory soup," including protons, bioactive lipids, peptides, and neurotrophic factors (Tominaga et al. 1998; Zygmunt et al. 1999; Chuang et al. 2001).

THE MENTHOL RECEPTOR IS A DETECTOR OF COLD

Compared to our understanding of noxious heat sensation, less is known about how we detect cold. Depending on the study and experimental system, approximately 10–15% of C and Aδ fibers respond to application of a cold stimulus (Hensel and Zotterman 1951; Bessou and Perl 1969; Kress et al. 1992). Importantly, many of these fibers show increased sensitivity to cold in the presence of menthol (Hensel and Zotterman 1951). Studies of cold or menthol responses in nerve fibers or cultured sensory neurons have produced several models to explain how these stimuli promote neuronal depolarization, including inhibition of background potassium channels, inhibition of Na^+/K^+ ATPases, activation of Na^+-selective epithelial sodium channel/degenerin channels, and activation of Ca^{2+}-permeable channels (Pierau et al. 1974; Braun et al. 1980; Suto and Gotoh 1999; Askwith et al. 2001; Reid and Flonta 2001a,b). Thus, there has been some debate as to whether cold excites sensory neurons by activating a specific "cold receptor," or by simultaneously modulating a variety of excitatory and inhibitory channels that, together, determine the electrical status of the cell.

To address this question, we and others have used calcium imaging methods to identify cold- and/or menthol-sensitive cells among cultured neurons from dorsal root or trigeminal ganglia, where they represent ~15% of the population. These responses were then examined in greater physiological detail using whole-cell patch-clamp recording methods. Our results and those from Reid's group indicate that cold activates a nonselective cation current that can be significantly potentiated by menthol (Reid and Flonta 2001b; McKemy et al. 2002), reminiscent of seminal studies by Hensel and Zotterman (1951) on trigeminal fibers of the cat. Moreover, we found that menthol or cold produced currents in cultured sensory neurons with biophysical properties similar to those exhibited by the cloned capsaicin receptor, most notably a pronounced outward rectification (McKemy et al. 2002). This finding differs from contemporaneous studies of Viana and colleagues (2002), who propose that cold depolarizes sensory neurons through differential effects on potassium conductances.

Based on our physiological results, we decided to clone a menthol receptor using the same calcium imaging-based cloning strategy that enabled us to identify the TRPV1 cDNA. In this manner, we identified a single clone that, when expressed in transfected mammalian cells or frog oocytes, rendered them sensitive to menthol (McKemy et al. 2002). Moreover, menthol elicited membrane currents in these cells that were virtually identical to those observed in cultured sensory neurons. Amazingly, expression of this same cDNA rendered cells sensitive to cold thermal stimuli such that application of cold perfusate produced outwardly rectifying, nonselective cation currents that were, again, indistinguishable from native cold-evoked responses in cultured sensory neurons. We have therefore named this cold- and menthol-sensitive receptor CMR1.

It has been argued that the sensation of cold is based on a mechanism that detects a temperature differential or rate of cooling, rather than a specific temperature threshold. However, CMR1 is activated with a characteristic thermal threshold of ~26°C, independent of the rate or direction of temperature change, suggesting that, as in the case of noxious heat, our sensation of cold is defined by a specific thermal threshold for channel activation (McKemy et al. 2002). This specific threshold can be altered by menthol, which shifts the activation threshold of CMR1 to warmer temperatures, accounting for its ability to produce cooling sensations at normal body temperature. Taken together, our findings show that cooling compounds and cold are detected by one and the same receptor on sensory nerve endings, providing a molecular explanation for the common psychophysical experience evoked by these chemical and physical stimuli. While our findings strongly support the idea that cold and menthol depolarize sensory neurons by activating CMR1, we must ask how the observations of Viana and colleagues relate to this model. Perhaps the most parsimonious explanation would be if other channels, such as cold-sensitive potassium channels, contribute to this process by altering the kinetics or magnitude of cold-evoked action potentials in cells expressing CMR1 or functionally related excitatory channels.

TRP CHANNELS MEDIATE THERMOSENSATION FROM HOT TO COLD

We cloned CMR1 based solely on its ability to respond to menthol. However, the deduced amino acid sequence of this receptor showed that it is also a member of the TRP ion channel family, making CMR1 (also called

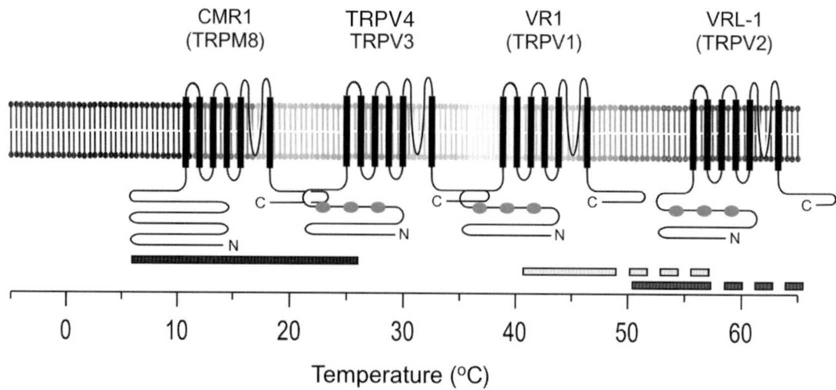

Fig. 1. Proposed range of thermosensitivity for members of the transient receptor potential (TRP) channel family. A number of TRP channels have been proposed to function as thermosensors in the vertebrate peripheral nervous system. Approximate range of temperature sensitivity for each channel (based on in vitro electrophysiological studies) is indicated on the temperature scale below the structure. Thus, TRPV1 and TRPV2 are proposed to detect noxious heat, TRPV3 and TRPV4 are proposed to detect warm stimuli, and TRPM8 is proposed to detect stimuli in the cool to noxious cold range (see text for relevant references).

TRPM8) a close molecular cousin of TRPV1 (McKemy et al. 2002). This exciting discovery bolsters our hypothesis that TRP channels function as primary detectors of temperature in the mammalian peripheral nervous system. Moreover, these findings support the idea that primary afferent neurons can detect temperature over a remarkably wide dynamic range because they express a number of different TRP channel subtypes, each of which is tuned to respond to temperature over a discrete window of stimulus intensities (Caterina et al. 1999). Indeed, several groups have now screened the mouse and human genome for TRP-like channels and have examined several of these novel channels for cold or heat sensitivity using heterologous expression systems. In this manner, new candidate thermosensors have been identified, including the contemporaneous cloning and characterization of CMR1/TRPM8 (Peier et al. 2002), as well as putative warm receptors, TRPV3 and TRPV4 (Guler et al. 2002; Peier et al. 2002; Smith et al. 2002; Xu et al. 2002). The proposed range of temperature sensitivity for each of these channels is summarized in Fig. 1.

REFERENCES

Askwith CC, Benson CJ, Welsh MJ, Snyder PM. DEG/ENaC ion channels involved in sensory transduction are modulated by cold temperature. *Proc Natl Acad Sci USA* 2001; 98:6459–6463.

Bessou P, Perl ER. Response of cutaneous sensory units with unmyelinated fibers to noxious stimuli. *J Neurophysiol* 1969; 32:1025–1043.

Bevan SJ, Docherty RJ. Cellular mechanisms of the action of capsaicin. In: Wood J (Ed). *Capsaicin in the Study of Pain.* London: Academic Press, 1993, pp 27–44.

Braun HA, Bade H, Hensel H. Static and dynamic discharge patterns of bursting cold fibers related to hypothetical receptor mechanisms. *Pflugers Arch* 1980; 386:1–9.

Buck L, Axel R. A novel multigene family may encode odorant receptors: a molecular basis for odor recognition. *Cell* 1991; 65:175–187.

Burgess, Perl ER. Myelinated afferents fibres responding specifically to noxious stimulation of the skin. *J Physiol* 1967; 190:541–562.

Caterina MJ, Schumacher MA, Tominaga M, et al. The capsaicin receptor: a heat-activated ion channel in the pain pathway. *Nature* 1997; 389:816–824.

Caterina MJ, Leffler A, Malmberg AB, et al. Impaired nociception and pain sensation in mice lacking the capsaicin receptor. *Science* 2000; 288:306–313.

Caterina MJ, Rosen TA, Tominaga M, Brake AJ, Julius D. A capsaicin-receptor homologue with a high threshold for noxious heat. *Nature* 1999; 398:436–441.

Cesare P, McNaughton P. A novel heat-activated current in nociceptive neurons and its sensitization by bradykinin. *Proc Natl Acad Sci USA* 1996; 93:15435–15439.

Chuang HH, Prescott ED, Kong H, et al. Bradykinin and nerve growth factor release the capsaicin receptor from PtdIns(4,5)P2-mediated inhibition. *Nature* 2001; 411:957–962.

Davis JB, Gray J, Gunthorpe MJ, et al. Vanilloid receptor-1 is essential for inflammatory thermal hyperalgesia. *Nature* 2000; 405:183–187.

Fields HL. *Pain.* New York: McGraw-Hill, 1987.

Guler AD, Lee H, Iida T, et al. Heat-evoked activation of the ion channel, TRPV4. *J Neurosci* 2002; 22:6408–6414.

Guo A, Vulchanova L, Wang J, Li X, Elde R. Immunocytochemical localization of vanilloid receptor 1 (TRPV1): relationship to neuropeptides, the P2X3 purinoceptor and IB4 binding sites. *Eur J Neurosci* 1999; 11:946–958.

Hensel H, Zotterman Y. The effect of menthol on the thermoreceptors. *Acta Physiol Scand* 1951; 24:27–34.

Jancso G, Kiraly E, Jancso-Gabor A. Pharmacologically induced selective degeneration of chemosensitive primary sensory neurons. *Nature* 1977; 270:741–743.

Kress M, Koltzenburg M, Reeh PW, Handwerker HO. Responsiveness and functional attributes of electrically localized terminals of cutaneous C-fibers in vivo and in vitro. *J Neurophysiol* 1992; 68:581–595.

McKemy DD, Neuhausser WM, Julius D. Identification of a cold receptor reveals a general role for TRP channels in thermosensation. *Nature* 2002; 416:52–58.

Michael GJ, Priestly JV. Differential expression of the mRNA for the vanilloid receptor subtype 1 in cells of the adult rat dorsal root and nodose ganglia and its downregulation by axotomy. *J Neurosci* 1999; 19:1844–1854.

Nagy I, Rang HP. Similarities and differences between the responses of rat sensory neurons to noxious heat and capsaicin. *J Neurosci* 1999; 19:10647–10655.

Nathans J. Molecular biology of visual pigments. *Ann Rev Neurosci* 1987; 10:163–194.

Peier AM, Reeve AJ, Andersson DA, et al. A heat-sensitive TRP channel expressed in keratinocytes. *Science* 2002; 296:2046–2049.

Peier AM, Moqrich A, Hergarden AC, et al. A TRP channel that senses cold stimuli and menthol. *Cell* 2002; 108:705–715.

Pierau FK, Torrey P, Carpenter DO. Mammalian cold receptor afferents: role of an electrogenic sodium pump in sensory transduction. *Brain Res* 1974; 73:156–160.

Reid G, Flonta M. Cold transduction by inhibition of a background potassium conductance in rat primary sensory neurones. *Neurosci Lett* 2001a; 297:171–174.

Reid G, Flonta ML. Cold current in thermoreceptive neurons. *Nature* 2001b; 413:480.

Sherrington C. *The Integrative Action of the Nervous System*. New York: Scribner, 1906.

Smith GD, Gunthorpe MJ, Kelsell RE, et al. TRPV3 is a temperature-sensitive vanilloid receptor-like protein. *Nature* 2002; 418:186–190.

Suto K, Gotoh H. Calcium signaling in cold cells studied in cultured dorsal root ganglion neurons. *Neuroscience* 1999; 92:1131–1135.

Szolcsanyi J. In: Wood J (Ed). *Capsaicin in the Study of Pain*. London: Academic Press, 1993, pp 1–26.

Tominaga M, et al. The cloned capsaicin receptor integrates multiple pain-producing stimuli. *Neuron* 1998; 21:1–20.

Treede R, Meyer RA, Srinivasa RN, Campbell JN. Evidence for two different heat transduction mechanisms in nociceptive primary afferents innervating monkey skin. *J Physiol* 1995; 483:747–758.

Viana F, de la Pena E, Belmonte C. Specificity of cold thermotransduction is determined by differential ionic channel expression. *Nat Neurosci* 2002; 5:254–260.

Vyklicky L, Vlachova V, Vitaskova Z, et al. Temperature coefficient of membrane currents induced by noxious heat in sensory neurones in the rat. *J Physiol (Lond)* 1999; 517:181–192.

Welch JM, Simon SA, Reinhart PH. The activation mechanism of rat vanilloid receptor 1 by capsaicin involves the pore domain and differs from the activation by either acid or heat. *Proc Natl Acad Sci USA* 2000; 97:13889–13894.

Xu H, Ramsey IS, Kotecha SA, et al. TRPV3 is a calcium-permeable temperature-sensitive cation channel. *Nature* 2002; 418:181–186.

Zygmunt PM, Petersson J, Andersson DA, et al. Vanilloid receptors on sensory nerves mediate the vasodilator action of anandamide. *Nature* 1999; 400:452–457.

Correspondence to: David Julius, PhD, Department of Cellular and Molecular Pharmacology, University of California San Francisco, San Francisco, CA 94143-0450, USA. Email: julius@cmp.ucsf.edu.

Proceedings of the 10th World Congress on Pain,
Progress in Pain Research and Management, Vol. 24,
edited by Jonathan O. Dostrovsky, Daniel B. Carr, and
Martin Koltzenburg, IASP Press, Seattle, © 2003.

7

ASIC3, but Not ASIC1, Channels Are Involved in the Development of Chronic Muscle Pain

Kathleen A. Sluka,[a,b] Margaret P. Price,[c]
John A. Wemmie,[b,d,e] and Michael J. Welsh[b,c]

[a]*Physical Therapy and Rehabilitation Science Graduate Program,* [b]*Neuroscience Graduate Program, and Departments of* [c]*Internal Medicine and* [d]*Psychiatry, University of Iowa, Iowa City, Iowa, USA;* [e]*Department of Veterans Affairs Medical Center, Iowa City, Iowa, USA*

Chronic musculoskeletal pain syndromes, such as fibromyalgia and myofascial pain syndrome, are associated with significant disability and high medical costs and can be difficult to treat (McCain 1994; Yelin and Callahan 1995). Patients with chronic muscle pain show decreases in mechanical pain thresholds not only at the site of pain but also in areas remote from it (Berglund et al. 2002; Leffler et al. 2002). For this reason, our laboratory developed a new animal model of chronic muscle-induced pain to examine mechanisms of chronic pain development and maintenance (Sluka et al. 2001). In the mouse, injections of acidic saline into one gastrocnemius muscle 2–5 days apart produce a long-lasting bilateral hyperalgesia with no associated tissue damage. The hyperalgesia seems to be maintained without continued primary afferent input because lidocaine injected into the muscle or unilateral dorsal rhizotomy after the development of hyperalgesia has no effect (Sluka et al. 2001). This bilateral mechanical hyperalgesia is reversed by blockade of spinal *N*-methyl D-aspartate (NMDA) or non-NMDA glutamate receptors (Skyba et al. 2002) and by activation of spinal μ- or δ-opioid receptors (Sluka et al. 2002). This model thus produces a secondary mechanical hyperalgesia maintained by changes in the central nervous system.

The induction of the long-lasting bilateral hyperalgesia only occurs after a second intramuscular injection of pH 4 saline. This finding suggests that induction involves activation of acid-sensing ion channels (ASICs) in the muscle. These channels include ASIC3, also referred to as dorsal root acid-sensing ion channel (DRASIC), ASIC2a and ASIC2b, and ASIC1. Both ASIC1 and ASIC3 are activated by low pH and are found on primary afferent neurons (Waldmann and Lazdunski 1998). ASIC1s are found predominantly on small to medium-sized primary afferent fibers, and in terminals in the superficial dorsal horn, laminae I and II (Olson et al. 1998). ASIC1 colocalizes with calcitonin gene-related peptide in the superficial dorsal horn, and neonatal capsaicin treatment eliminates ASIC1 immunoreactivity in the dorsal horn (Olson et al. 1998), suggesting that ASIC1 channels are located on capsaicin-sensitive primary afferent fibers. ASIC3s have been cloned from dorsal root ganglia, are found in large- and small-diameter primary afferents, and have a biphasic component with a fast inward current followed by a sustained current (Price et al. 2001;Waldmann et al. 1997). Thus, decreasing pH may result in activation of ASIC1s and/or ASIC3s on primary afferent fibers, which in turn could produce mechanical hyperalgesia.

METHODS

All experiments were approved by the Animal Care and Use Committee at the University of Iowa and are in accordance with the guidelines of the International Association for the Study of Pain and the National Institutes of Health. Experiments were performed in mice, either ASIC1 or ASIC3 knockouts and their wild-type littermates, or the C57BL6 strain. The ASIC1 and ASIC3 knockouts have been previously described (Price et al. 2001; Wemmie et al. 2002).

Mice were injected with 20 μL of pH 4 sterile saline into one gastrocnemius muscle 5 days apart. This treatment results in a bilateral mechanical hyperalgesia that lasts for 4 weeks, does not depend on continued primary afferent input, and does not damage the injected muscle (Sluka et al. 2001).

Mechanical hyperalgesia was measured as the number of responses (average of 10 trials) out of 5 repeated applications of a von Frey filament (0.4 mN bending force) to the plantar surface of both the ipsilateral and contralateral hindpaws. Because we measured responses outside the site of injection, we interpreted the responses as secondary hyperalgesia.

In C57BL6 mice, amiloride was injected either intramuscularly at doses of 0.15 (n = 9) and 0.5 (n = 6) mg/20 μL in 25% dimethyl sulfoxide (DMSO), or intrathecally at 11.3 (n = 14), 37.6 (n = 6), 113 (n = 6) and 376 (n = 10) nmol/5 μL in separate animals. A vehicle control consisted of 25% DMSO for intramuscular injections (n = 8) or saline (n = 13) for intrathecal injections.

Extracellular recordings of wide-dynamic-range (WDR) neurons were made in ASIC3 knockouts (n = 10) and compared to those of wild-type littermates (n = 9) before and for up to 4 hours after the second injection of pH 4 saline. Animals were anesthetized intraperitoneally with 50 mg/kg sodium pentobarbital and given supplemental anesthesia as necessary. A laminectomy was performed, and animals were placed in a stereotactic frame. A recording electrode was inserted into the ipsilateral dorsal horn, and a single cell was isolated. Cells were classified as WDR neurons if they responded to both brushing and pinching of the skin. We mapped the receptive field size in response to brushing or pinching the skin before and after injection of pH 4 saline. We also examined the number of responses to a 10-second application of brush or pinch to the ipsilateral skin of the calf and paw, and the comparable site on the contralateral skin of the calf and paw. The activity of single units was collected and stored for later analysis using Spike 2 software. Background activity was subtracted, and changes in evoked responses were calculated.

RESULTS

Initially, to test for a role for ASICs, we administered the nonselective channel blocker, amiloride, intramuscularly (i.m.) prior to the second injection of pH 4 saline and examined the effects on mechanical hyperalgesia. I.m. injection of amiloride (0.5 mg/20 μL, in 25% DMSO) prevented the development of bilateral mechanical hyperalgesia that normally occurs after the second injection of pH 4 saline (Fig. 1B) when compared to vehicle injection. To determine whether there was involvement of ASICs in the spinal cord, we administered amiloride (11.3–376 nmol/5 μL) intrathecally (i.t.) just prior to the second injection of pH 4 saline in C57BL6 mice. Similar to the i.m. injection, i.t. injection of amiloride dose-dependently prevented the bilateral mechanical hyperalgesia that normally occurs after the second i.m. injection of pH 4 saline (Fig. 1A). The highest dose of amiloride tested, 376 nmol, produced agitation in the mice and had no effect on the hyperalgesia, and thus the drug probably has nonspecific actions at this dose.

To assess which ASICs were involved in the development of mechanical hyperalgesia, we utilized animals with a null mutation of either ASIC1 (Wemmie et al. 2002) or ASIC3 (Price et al. 2001). In ASIC1 knockout animals, the hyperalgesia was similar to that of their wild-type littermates (Fig. 2A,B) at all time points tested. There was an initial increase 4 hours after the first injection of pH 4 saline that returned to baseline responses 24 hours after the first injection. On day 5, a second injection of pH 4 saline

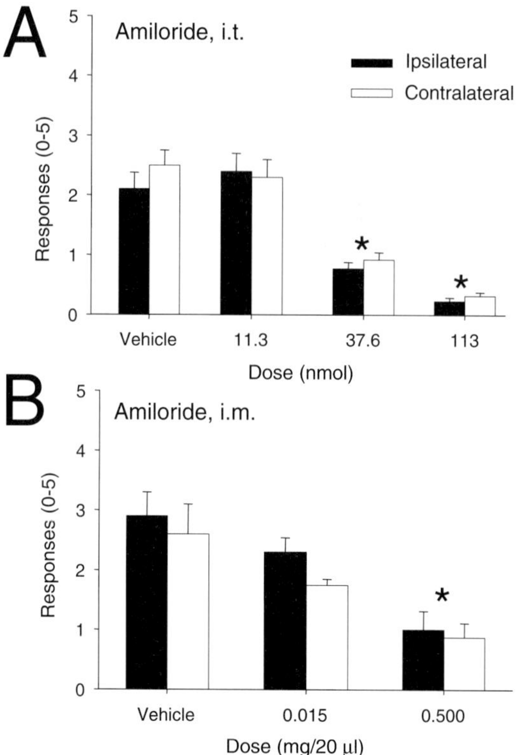

Fig. 1. Responses to von Frey filaments in animals administered amiloride either (A) intrathecally (i.t.) or (B) intramuscularly (i.m.) just prior to the second injection of pH 4 saline on day 5. Significant differences from vehicle control occurred for the mice injected with 37.6 or 113 nmol i.t. or with 0.5 mg/20 μL i.m. Asterisks (*) denote results significantly different from vehicle.

produced a bilateral increase in the number of responses to the 0.4 mN force in both the ASIC1 knockouts and their wild-type littermates that lasted for 1 week after the second injection. However, in ASIC3 knockouts, the hyperalgesia was significantly less severe when compared to that of the wild-type littermates (Fig. 2C,D). The number of responses to repeated application of a von Frey filament was significantly decreased 4 hours after the first injection of pH 4 saline, and again 4 hours, 24 hours, and 1 week after the second injection of pH 4 saline.

To assess the effects of repeated acid injection on spinal dorsal horn neurons, we examined the receptive field size and the responses of WDR dorsal horn neurons to innocuous (brush) and noxious (pinch) stimuli of the ipsilateral and contralateral paw and calf. In wild-type littermates of the ASIC3 knockouts, isolated dorsal horn neurons demonstrated an expansion

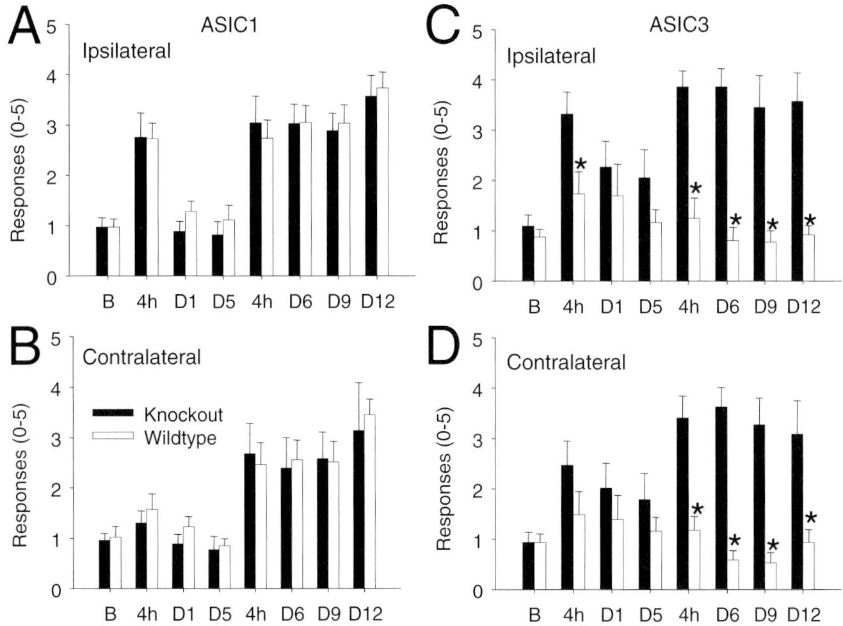

Fig. 2. Responses to 0.4 mN bending force for wild-type (solid bars) and knockout animals (open bars) of ASIC1 (A,B) or ASIC3 (C,D) for the ipsilateral (top panels) or contralateral hindpaws (bottom panels). Injections of pH 4 saline were given i.m. after baseline testing on day 0 (B) and again after testing on day 5 (D5). In wild-type animals, increased responses occurred for the ipsilateral paw 4 hours after the first i.m. injection and through 1 week after the second i.m. injection (4 hours, D6, D9, and D12). Contralateral increases occurred after the second intramuscular injection of pH 4 saline through 1 week (4 hours, D6, D9, D12). Similar responses to wild-type littermates occurred in ASIC1 knockouts. On the other hand, ASIC3 knockouts showed significantly weaker responses to mechanical stimuli when compared to their wild-type littermates both ipsilaterally and contralaterally. Asterisks (*) denote results significantly different from wild-type littermates.

of the receptive field to include the contralateral limb, in response to both innocuous and noxious stimuli within 4 hours after the second injection of pH 4 saline. This expanded receptive field did not spread to the contralateral side in DRASIC knockout animals. A representative example of the expanded receptive field for wild-type littermates is shown in Fig. 3, and the receptive field from an ASIC3 knockout is also shown in Fig. 3.

Further, the responses on the contralateral side to brushing and pinching were increased in wild-type littermates within 3–4 hours after the second injection of pH 4 saline. Contralaterally, the response to brushing increased from –0.12 ± 0.09 and 0.03 ± 0.19 spikes/second from the paw and calf, respectively, before the second i.m. injection of pH 4 saline to 0.15 ± 0.10 and 0.27 ± 0.19 spikes/second after injection. The responses to pinching

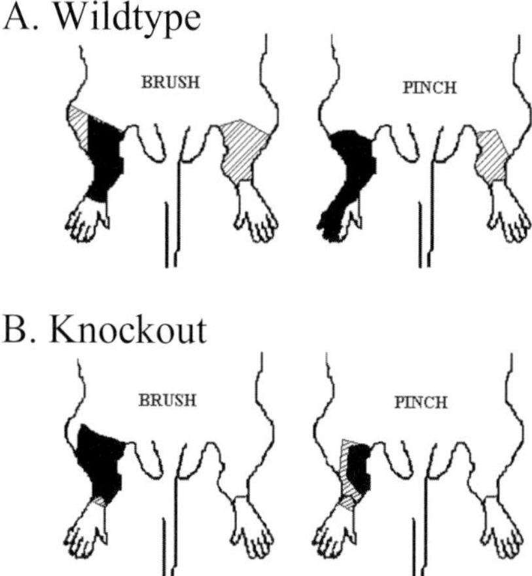

Fig. 3. Representative maps of receptive fields of wide-dynamic-range dorsal horn neurons recorded from wild-type and ASIC3 knockout mice before (filled area) and 4 hours after (diagonal filled area) the second intramuscular injection of pH 4 saline for responses to brushing the skin (BRUSH) or pinching the skin (PINCH).

increased from –0.19 ± 0.11 and –0.12 ± 0.16 spikes/second from the paw and calf, respectively, before the second i.m. injection of pH 4 saline to 0.52 ± 0.3 and 0.75 ± 0.37 spikes/second after injection. These increases did not occur in the ASIC3 knockouts. Responses to brushing were –0.006 ± 0.003 and –0.005 ± 0.003 spikes/second from the paw and calf, respectively, before the second i.m. injection of pH 4 saline and 0.06 ± 0.06 and 0.001 ± 0.01 spikes/second after injection. The responses to pinching were 0.01 ± 0.01 and 0.03 ± 0.03 spikes/second for the paw and calf, respectively, before the second intramuscular injection of pH 4 saline and 0.1 ± 0.1 and 0.09 ± 0.09 spikes/second after injection. No changes were observed for responses to brushing and pinching the skin of the calf or the paw ipsilateral to the site of injection.

DISCUSSION

These experiments show that mice lacking the ASIC3 channel do not develop mechanical hyperalgesia and that spinal WDR neurons do not show an expansion of the receptive field to the contralateral side in these mice. The mechanical hyperalgesia induced by acid in C57BL6 mice is prevented by amiloride applied to the muscle. In contrast, ASIC1 animals develop a bilateral mechanical hyperalgesia similar to that of wild-type littermates. These data suggest that ASIC3 (but not ASIC1), in the muscle, is essential for the development of bilateral mechanical hyperalgesia associated with repeated injection of pH 4 saline into the gastrocnemius muscle. Our findings further suggest that contralateral hyperalgesia may be mediated by a spread of the receptive field of WDR neurons to the contralateral limb and that the initial input from ASIC3 channels in the muscle may result in the contralateral spread.

Low pH activates nociceptors in rats and produces pain in humans (Reeh and Steen 1996; Steen and Reeh 1993). Low pH also activates ASIC1 and ASIC3, with ASIC3 being most sensitive to smaller changes in pH (Benson et al. 2002). The lack of effect in ASIC1 knockouts is surprising because these channels are located in dorsal root ganglion (DRG) neurons that contain capsaicin and thus presumably nociceptors (Olson et al. 1998). Interestingly, in DRG cells from ASIC1 knockouts, the overall amplitude of the pH current is significantly reduced but the pH response is not eliminated (Benson et al. 2002). Further, there is a decreased rate of desensitization and an increased rate of recovery from desensitization when compared to DRG cells from wild-type littermates (Benson et al. 2002). Thus, ASIC1 channels would be expected to be involved in sensing acid changes in peripheral tissue. However, because these channels form heteromultimers (Benson et al. 2002), elimination of ASIC1 may not be sufficient to produce a behavioral effect but may still show differences in recording single channels in DRG neurons.

Previously, we demonstrated that ASIC3 was necessary for the mechanical hyperalgesia that occurs after the first i.m. injection of pH 4 saline (Price et al. 2001). In contrast, carrageenan injection into the paw elicits an enhanced response to mechanical stimulation of the paw when compared to wild-type littermates but no difference in response to radiant heat of the paw (Price et al. 2001). Similarly, Chen et al. (2002) show a reduced mechanical threshold (i.e., hyperalgesia) in the paw-pressure test after carrageenan paw inflammation. However, in the hot-plate test at temperatures of 52.5° or 55°C, ASIC3 knockout mice showed a reduced latency to paw withdrawal (i.e., heat hyperalgesia) when compared to wild-type littermates. This finding did not occur at temperatures of 50°C. Further high doses of intraperitoneal acetic acid resulted in an increased number of writhes and a shorter duration to onset. These data suggest that a null mutation of ASIC3 results in increased hyperalgesia in response to high-intensity stimulation. Our results, in contrast, suggest that acid-induced muscle hyperalgesia is dependent on activation of muscle ASIC3s to initiate the hyperalgesia. Further, Price et al. (2001) found increased responses of rapidly adapting mechanoreceptors and decreased responses of A-fiber mechanonociceptors utilizing the skin nerve preparation. Thus, the response may be complex, with some aspects of mechanical and nociceptive responses increased and others decreased. The response and its direction may depend on the composition of the subunits that form channels at a specific site and on the specific stimulus used.

Loss of ASIC3 does not eliminate acid-evoked currents (Price et al. 2001). Loss of ASIC3, however, alters acid-evoked currents in DRG neurons such that ASIC3s are less sensitive to pH 6.5 than are neurons from wild-type littermates (Price et al. 2001). In the skin nerve preparation, cutaneous Aδ mechanoreceptors showed a decreased number of action potentials to displacement of the skin and decreased responsiveness to von Frey filaments (Price et al. 2001). However, there were no differences in C fibers (Price et al. 2001). Thus, different fiber types (Aδ versus C), different tissues (cutaneous versus muscle), different stimuli (carrageenan, pH), or different tests (von Frey filaments, hot-plate, radiant heat test) could be critical to the involvement of different ASIC channels in the transmission of painful stimuli. In summary, ASIC3, but not ASIC1, channels are important in the development of acid-induced chronic muscle pain including behavioral and dorsal horn neuron responses.

ACKNOWLEDGMENTS

These experiments were funded by National Institutes of Health grants R01 NS39734 and K02 AR 02201 to K.A. Sluka, and by a Department of Veterans Affairs Research Career Development Award to J.A. Wemmie. M.J. Welsh is an Investigator of the Howard Hughes Medical Institute. We thank Tammy Lisi, Ellen King, and Brooke Bond for excellent technical assistance.

REFERENCES

Benson CJ, Xie J, Wemmie JA, et al. Heteromultimers of DEG/ENaC subunits form H+-gated channels in mouse sensory neurons. *Proc Natl Acad Sci USA* 2002; 99:2338–2343.

Berglund B, Harju EL, Kosek E, et al. Quantitative and qualitative perceptual analysis of cold dysesthesia and hyperalgesia in fibromyalgia. *Pain* 2002; 96:177–187.

Chen CC, Zimmer A, Sun WH, et al. A role for ASIC3 in the modulation of high-intensity pain stimuli. *Proc Natl Acad Sci USA* 2002; 99:8992–8997.

Leffler AS, Hansson P, Kosek E. Somatosensory perception in a remote pain-free area and function of diffuse noxious inhibitory controls (DNIC) in patients suffering from long-term trapezius myalgia. *Eur J Pain* 2002; 6:149–159.

McCain GA. Fibromyalgia and myofacial pain syndromes. In: Wall PD, Melzack R (Eds). *Textbook of Pain.* New York: Churchill Livingstone, 1994, pp 475–493.

Olson TH, Riedl MS, Vulchanova L, et. al. An acid sensing ion channel (ASIC) localizes to small primary afferent neurons in rats. *Neuroreport* 1998; 9:1109–1113.

Price MP, McIlwrath SL, Xie J, et al. Channel contributes to the detection of cutaneous touch and acid stimuli in mice. *Neuron* 2001; 32:1071–1083.
Reeh PW, Steen KH. Tissue acidosis in nociception and pain. *Prog Brain Res* 1996; 113:143–151.
Skyba DA, King EW, Sluka KA. Effects of NMDA and non-NMDA ionotropic glutamate receptor antagonists on the development and maintenance of hyperalgesia induced by repeated intramuscular injection of acidic saline. *Pain* 2002; 98:69–78.
Sluka KA, Kalra A, Moore SA. Unilateral intramuscular injections of acidic saline produce a bilateral, long-lasting hyperalgesia. *Muscle Nerve* 2001; 24:37–46.
Sluka KA, Rohlwing JJ, Bussey RA, et al. Chronic muscle pain induced by repeated acid injection is reversed by spinally administered μ-, and δ-, but not κ-, opioid receptor agonists. *J Pharmacol Exp Ther* 2002; 302:1146–1150.
Steen KH, Reeh PW. Sustained graded pain and hyperalgesia from harmless experimental tissue acidosis in human skin. *Neurosci Lett* 1993; 154:113–116.
Waldmann R, Champigny G, Bassilana F, et al. A proton-gated cation channel involved in acid-sensing. *Nature* 1997; 386:173–177.
Waldmann R, Lazdunski M. H(+)-gated cation channels: neuronal acid sensors in the NaC/DEG family of ion channels. *Curr Opin Neurobiol* 1998; 8:418–424.
Wemmie JA, Chen J, Askwith CC, et al. The acid-activated ion channel ASIC contributes to synaptic plasticity, learning, and memory. *Neuron* 2002; 34:463–477.
Yelin E, Callahan LF. The economic costs and social and psychological impact of musculoskeletal conditions. *Arthritis Rheum* 1995; 38:1351–1362.

Correspondence to: Kathleen A. Sluka, PT, PhD, Physical Therapy and Rehabilitation Science Graduate Program, Medical Education Building, 1-242, University of Iowa, Iowa City, IA 52242, USA. Tel: 319-335-9791; Fax: 319-335-9707; email: kathleen-sluka@uiowa.edu.

Proceedings of the 10th World Congress on Pain,
Progress in Pain Research and Management, Vol. 24,
edited by Jonathan O. Dostrovsky, Daniel B. Carr, and
Martin Koltzenburg, IASP Press, Seattle, © 2003.

8

Activation of MAP Kinases in Primary Sensory Neurons

Ru-Rong Ji

Neural Plasticity Research Group, Department of Anesthesia and Critical Care, Massachusetts General Hospital and Harvard Medical School, Boston, Massachusetts, USA

MAP KINASE FAMILY

Mitogen-activated protein kinases (MAPK) transduce a broad range of extracellular stimuli into diverse intracellular responses by transcriptional and translational regulation, as well as by post-translational modification (Widmann et al. 1999; Ji et al. 2001). Early studies indicate a critical role of MAPK in regulating mitosis, proliferation, differentiation, and survival of mammalian cells during development. Recently, accumulating evidence has implicated the MAPK cascade in neuronal plasticity in the adult. ERK (extracellular signal-regulated kinase, including ERK1 and ERK2) is the best-studied member of the MAPK family, especially with regard to its activity-dependent activation and its regulation of neuronal plasticity, such as learning and memory, as well as its involvement in generating pain hypersensitivity (Ji and Woolf 2001; Sweatt 2001). Another two MAPK family members, p38 and c-Jun-N-terminal protein kinase (JNK), originally identified as stress-activated protein kinase (SAPK), are activated in many cells by cellular stress and cytokines. ERK5 is the least well-known member of the MAPK family (Widmann et al. 1999).

Intense noxious stimuli and tissue inflammation produce pain hypersensitivity that results both from peripheral sensitization (an increased responsiveness of the peripheral terminals of nociceptor primary sensory neurons) and from central sensitization (an increased excitability of dorsal horn neurons) (Woolf and Salter 2000). ERK activation in dorsal horn neurons is involved in generating central sensitization. It induces upregulation of prodynorphin and NK-1 in dorsal horn neurons and maintains inflammatory pain (Ji et al. 1999a, 2002a; Karim et al. 2001). ERK activation in peripheral terminals of primary sensory neurons contributes to peripheral sensitization (Aley et al. 2001; Dai et al. 2002). Recently we have found that p38 is activated in primary nociceptive neurons in the dorsal root ganglia (DRG) after inflammation and participates in inflammatory pain (Ji et al. 2002b). In this chapter, I first review several major findings about p38 activation in DRG neurons, and then report some new data about ERK activation in the cell body, as well as in the terminals of DRG neurons.

ACTIVATION OF p38 MAPK IN DRG NEURONS BY INFLAMMATION

Immunohistochemistry using a phospho-specific p38 antibody shows that activated (phosphorylated) p38 (p-p38), is normally present in 15% of DRG neurons. The p-p38 is located in the nucleus and cytoplasm of these neurons, as well as in some surrounding non-neuronal cells. Intraplantar injection of complete Freund's adjuvant (CFA) produces inflammation and slowly increases the percentage of p-p38-immunoreactive DRG neurons. This increase reaches significance at 24 hours and reaches its peak at 48 hours, with high levels persisting at 7 days. However, total levels of p38 (nonphosphorylated and phosphorylated) do not increase after inflammation, indicating that the increase in p-p38 after inflammation is caused by increased phosphorylation, rather than by elevated substrate. Furthermore, p-p38 is present mainly in small DRG neurons (cross-sectional area <600 μm^2) in both control and inflamed animals. Because p-p38 rarely colocalizes with neurofilament-200, a marker for myelinated A fibers, in either control or inflamed conditions, it seems to be predominantly expressed in neurons with unmyelinated axons, the C fibers. However, p-p38 heavily colocalizes with trkA and TRPV1, formerly known as capsaicin receptor vanilloid receptor-1 (VR1) (Ji et al. 2002b).

To examine whether p38 activation in the DRG is involved in producing inflammatory pain hypersensitivity, we administered a specific p38 inhibitor, SB203580, into the intrathecal space via a catheter. The tip of the catheter was positioned close to the L4 DRG in order to target p38 activity in the DRG. The drug was delivered by an osmotic pump (0.5 μg/μL/h) connected to the catheter. The catheter was implanted at least 6 hours prior to injection of CFA. Neither heat nor mechanical basal sensitivity is affected by SB203580 administration in noninflamed rats. The inhibitor does, however, reduce inflammation-induced heat hyperalgesia 24 and 48 hours after CFA injection. Intrathecal SB 203085 infusion does not reduce CFA-induced inflammatory swelling, as measured by paw thickness. Post-treatment with SB203580 (1 μg), 48 hours after CFA injection, also decreases heat hyperalgesia at 3 and 24 hours (Ji et al. 2002b).

TRPV1 is expressed in nociceptors and plays an important role in inflammatory heat hyperalgesia (Caterina et al. 2000; Davis et al. 2000). To test whether p38 mediates heat hyperalgesia by regulating TRPV1 expression, we examined TRPV1 expression in the DRG after inflammation. Peripheral inflammation induces a sustained increase in TRPV1 protein levels in the DRG, as detected by both Western blot and immunohistochemistry, reaching a peak at 2 days, as does p-p38. Intrathecal infusion of SB203580 via an osmotic pump reverses the increase in the percentage of TRPV1-immunoreactive neurons after inflammation. Moreover, SB203580 (1 μg, administered intrathecally twice a day for 2 days, with the first injection given 30 min prior to CFA injection) decreases inflammatory heat hyperalgesia as effectively as does osmotic pump administration of the drug. This treatment also blocks the CFA-induced upregulation of the total level of TRPV1 at 2 days, as measured by Western blot analysis (Ji et al. 2002b).

ACTIVATION OF ERK/MAPK IN DRG NEURONS BY ACTIVITY AND GROWTH FACTORS

In order to test whether there is an activity-dependent activation of ERK in primary sensory neurons, as is the case in dorsal horn neurons (Ji et al. 1999a,b), we depolarized adult DRG neuronal cultures with 50 mM KCl. Western blot analysis shows that KCl induces a very rapid and transient ERK phosphorylation, reaching peak levels at 1 minute (Fig. 1a). This very transient pERK induction is also observed in vivo following peripheral noxious stimuli, reaching its peak at 2 minutes and returning to nearly baseline levels after 10 minutes (Dai et al. 2002). Comparatively, pERK induction in postsynaptic dorsal horn neurons after painful stimuli is more sustained, lasting for more than an hour (Ji et al. 1999a). Moreover, the percentage of pERK-positive neurons is much lower than that of p-p38 in either normal or stimulated conditions.

In addition to activity, target-derived growth factors can influence intracellular signaling. Growth factors can be retrogradely transported from the periphery to neuronal cell bodies in the DRG, where they can activate intracellular signaling pathways. Nerve growth factor (NGF) and glial-derived neurotrophic factor (GDNF) are two of the most important signaling molecules for DRG neurons. Bath application of either NGF or GDNF to adult DRG cultures strongly activates ERK at 10 minutes (Fig. 1b). Furthermore,

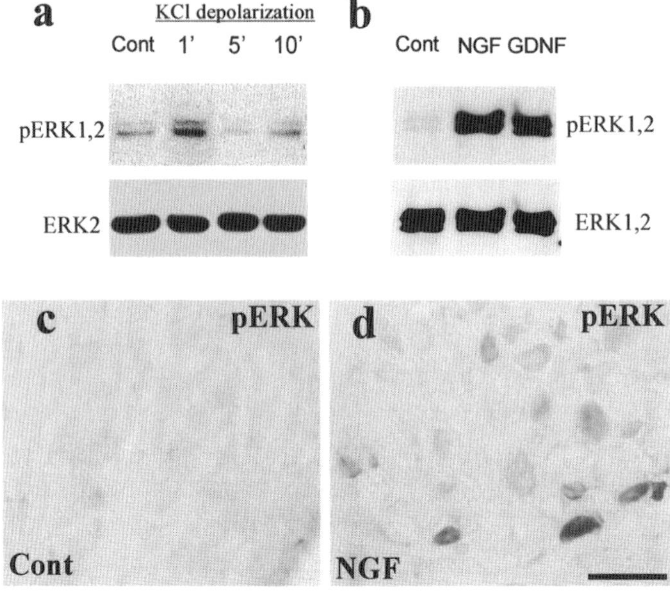

Fig. 1. (a,b) Western blot analysis showing pERK induction in day 5 adult DRG cultures following (a) 50 mM KCl depolarization and (b) addition of NGF (100 ng/ml) and GDNF (20 ng/ml) for 10 minutes. The blots were first probed with pERK antibody, then stripped and reprobed with anti-ERK1/2 or ERK2 antibody as a total ERK control. Both ERK isoforms, ERK1 (p44 MAPK) and ERK2 (p42 MAPK), are present in the DRG and are activated by these reagents. (c,d) Immunostaining indicates pERK induction in many DRG neurons 10 minutes after intrathecal injection of NGF (d, 2 μg), as compared to control (c). Scale, 50 μm.

intrathecal injection of NGF (2 μg) induces a rapid pERK induction, within 10 minutes, in many DRG neurons (Fig. 1c,d), as does GDNF (0.5 μg) (data not shown). This rapid ERK activation is very likely to be mediated by a direct effect of NGF or GDNF on the DRG neuronal cell body via the intrathecal route, because axonal terminal uptake and retrograde transport take much longer. NGF appears to induce sustained ERK activation because many pERK-labeled neurons are found in the DRG 24 hours after systematic NGF administration (Averill et al. 2001).

ERK is induced not only in the soma of DRG neurons, but also in their peripheral axons. Intraplantar injection of formalin increases pERK labeled nerve fibers in the epidermis within 2 minutes (Fig. 2a,b), suggesting a possible role of pERK in peripheral sensitization. ERK contributes to epinephrine-induced mechanical hyperalgesia (Aley et al. 2001) and to capsaicin-induced heat hyperalgesia (Dai et al. 2002). pERK is also found in nerve

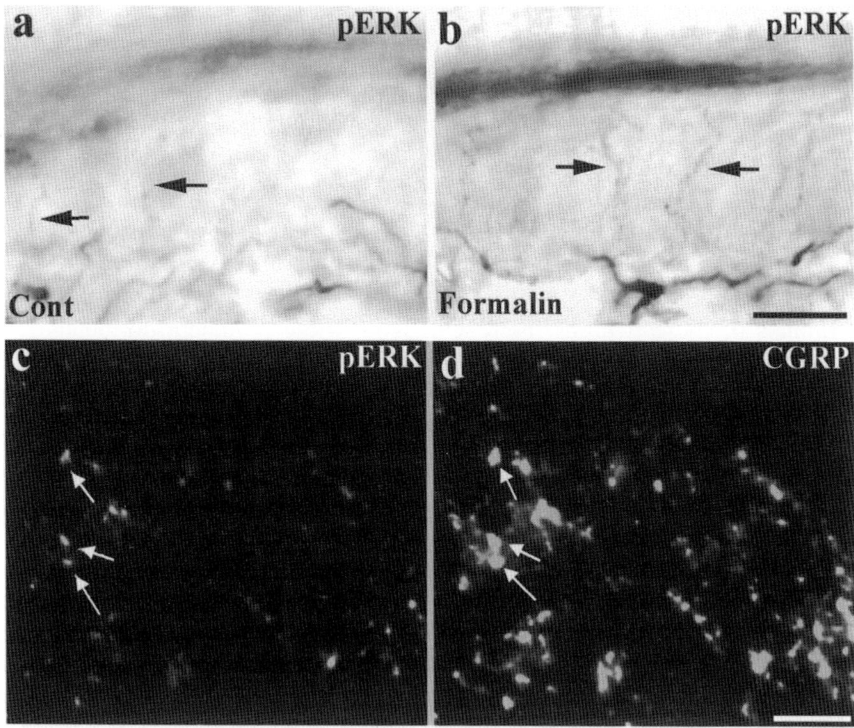

Fig 2. (a,b) pERK immunoreactivity in control and formalin-stimulated skin. More pERK-labeled nerve fibers are found in the epidermis after formalin stimulation. Arrows indicate labeled epidermal nerve fibers. Two minutes after intraplantar formalin injection (5%, 50 μL), the plantar hindpaw skin was fixed with 4% paraformaldehyde for 16 hours. Scale, 50 μm. (c,d) Double immunostaining showing colocalization of pERK and CGRP in presynaptic terminals in the superficial dorsal horn. Naive rats were perfused with 4% paraformaldehyde, and spinal cord sections were incubated with monoclonal anti-pERK and polyclonal anti-CGRP antibodies. Arrows indicate double-labeled axonal terminals. Scale, 10 μm.

fibers of the sciatic nerve (Averill et al. 2001). Furthermore, pERK appears to be present in the central axonal terminals of DRG neurons in the superficial dorsal horn. Double-labeled staining shows that pERK is almost totally colocalized in presynaptic terminals with calcitonin gene-related peptide (CGRP), a neuropeptide that originates exclusively from primary afferents (Fig. 2c,d). In addition to a dramatic ERK activation in postsynaptic dorsal horn neurons, pERK seems to increase in presynaptic terminals in the superficial dorsal horn following noxious stimulation (data not shown).

CONCLUSION

Both p38 and ERK are specifically activated in response to nociceptive stimuli in nociceptors of primary sensory neurons in the DRG, and are involved in pain hypersensitivity. However, these members of the MAPK family are differentially activated in DRG neurons. First, p-p38 is expressed by more DRG neurons than pERK in both control and stimulated conditions. Second, p38 is activated in the cell body of DRG neurons, whereas ERK is activated not only in the cell body but also in the peripheral and central terminals of these neurons. ERK activation in the peripheral terminals results in peripheral sensitization, possibly due to post-translational regulation, by phosphorylation of key receptors and channels in nociceptor terminals. ERK activation in the central terminals may be involved in neurotransmitter release in the dorsal horn. Third, nociceptive input (activity) induces a very transient ERK activation (less than 10 minutes), whereas growth factors such as NGF and GDNF are likely to induce more persistent ERK activation in the DRG. Therefore, neuronal activity and growth factors produce transient and sustained pERK induction in the DRG, respectively, differentially regulating neuronal plasticity. Inflammation produces a delayed but sustained p38 activation (more than 1 week) via a retrograde signal, such as NGF (Ji et al. 2002b).

In summary, activation of p38 and ERK MAPK in primary sensory neurons by nociceptive activity and/or inflammatory mediators is likely to play an important role in regulating the plasticity of these neurons via transcriptional, translational, and posttranslation modification, contributing to the development and maintenance of pathological pain following tissue injury.

ACKNOWLEDGMENT

This work was supported by NIH RO1 NS40698 to the author.

REFERENCES

Aley KO, Martin A, McMahon T, et al. Nociceptor sensitization by extracellular signal-regulated kinases. *J Neurosci* 2001; 21:6933–6939.

Averill S, Delcroix JD, Michael GJ, et al. Nerve growth factor modulates the activation status and fast axonal transport of ERK 1/2 in adult nociceptive neurons. *Mol Cell Neurosci* 2001; 18:183–196.

Caterina MJ, Leffler A, Malmberg AB, et al. Impaired nociception and pain sensation in mice lacking the capsaicin receptor. *Science* 2000; 288:306–313.

Dai Y, Iwata K, Fukuoka T, et al. Phosphorylation of extracellular signal-regulated kinase in primary afferent neurons by noxious stimuli and its involvement in peripheral sensitization. *J Neurosci* 2002; 22:7737–7745.

Davis JB, Gray J, Gunthorpe MJ, et al. Vanilloid receptor-1 is essential for inflammatory thermal hyperalgesia. *Nature* 2000; 405:183–187.

Ji RR, Woolf CJ. Neuronal plasticity and signal transduction in nociceptive neurons: implications for the initiation and maintenance of pathological pain. *Neurobiol Dis* 2001; 8:1–10.

Ji RR, Baba H, Brenner GJ, Woolf CJ. Nociceptive-specific activation of ERK in spinal neurons contributes to pain hypersensitivity. *Nat Neurosci* 1999a; 2:1114–1119.

Ji RR, Brenner GJ, Schmoll R, Baba H, Woolf CJ. Phosphorylation of ERK and CREB in nociceptive neurons after noxious stimulation. In: Devor M, Rowbotham MC, Wiesenfeld-Hallin Z (Eds). *Proceedings of the 9th World Congress on Pain*. Progress in Pain Research Management, Vol 16. Seattle: IASP Press, 1999b, pp 191–198.

Ji RR, Befort K, Brenner GJ, Woolf CJ. ERK MAP kinase activation in superficial spinal cord neurons induces prodynorphin and NK-1 upregulation and contributes to persistent inflammatory pain hypersensitivity. *J Neurosci* 2002a; 22:478–485.

Ji RR, Samad TA, Jin SX, Schmoll R, Woolf CJ. p38 MAPK activation by NGF in primary sensory neurons after inflammation increases TRPV1 expression and maintains heat hyperalgesia. *Neuron* 2002b; 36:57–68.

Karim F, Wang CC, Gereau RW. Metabotropic glutamate receptor subtypes 1 and 5 are activators of extracellular signal-regulated kinase signaling required for inflammatory pain in mice. *J Neurosci* 2001; 21:3771–3779.

Sweatt JD. The neuronal MAP kinase cascade: a biochemical signal integration system subserving synaptic plasticity and memory. *J Neurochem* 2001; 76:1–10.

Widmann C, Gibson S, Jarpe MB, Johnson GL. Mitogen-activated protein kinase: conservation of a three-kinase module from yeast to human. *Physiol Rev* 1999; 79:143–180.

Woolf CJ, Salter MW. Neuronal plasticity: increasing the gain in pain. *Science* 2000; 288:1765–1769.

Correspondence to: Ru-Rong Ji, PhD, Neural Plasticity Research Group, Department of Anesthesia, Massachusetts General Hospital, 149 13th Street, Room 4309, Charlestown, MA 02129, USA. Tel: 617-724-3302; Fax: 617-724-3632; email: ji@helix.mgh.harvard.edu.

Proceedings of the 10th World Congress on Pain,
Progress in Pain Research and Management, Vol. 24,
edited by Jonathan O. Dostrovsky, Daniel B. Carr, and
Martin Koltzenburg, IASP Press, Seattle, © 2003.

9

Tonic Effects of BAM8-22, an Agonist at the Novel Sensory Neuron Specific Receptor, on the Nociceptive Flexor Reflex in Rats

Chang Qing Cao, Andy Dray, and Martin N. Perkins

AstraZeneca R&D Montreal, St-Laurent, Montreal, Quebec, Canada

A novel family of G-protein-coupled receptors named sensory neuron specific receptors (SNSRs) has recently been identified (Lembo et al. 2002). The receptors show a unique expression pattern restricted to dorsal root and trigeminal ganglia in rat and human studies. Double-labeling studies have shown that SNSRs are expressed predominantly in isolectin B4 (IB4)-positive, small-diameter nociceptors (Lembo et al. 2002), one of two major classes of unmyelinated fibers conducting noxious stimuli (Snider and McMahon 1998; Vulchanova et al. 2001; Simonin and Kieffer 2002). No other G-protein-coupled receptors (GPCRs) except SNSRs and Mas-related genes (MRGs) (Dong et al. 2001) demonstrate such a localized and colocalized distribution exclusive to the sensory ganglia. Given that small-diameter sensory neurons are believed to mediate nociceptive transmission in both acute and chronic pain states (Snider and McMahon 1997), SNSRs are probably involved in nociception.

SNSRs are a non-opioid class of receptors and BAM8-22, a C-terminal fragment of bovine adrenal medulla peptide 22 (BAM22), is a selective endogenous agonist at SNSRs (Lembo et al. 2002). However, the function of the SNSRs/BAM8-22 system is unknown; for example, it is not known whether SNSR activation by BAM8-22 is pro- or antinociceptive. Our study was designed to answer this question by measuring the excitability of a spinal nociceptive flexor reflex (Woolf 1983; Cao et al. 2001; Skljarevski and Ramadan 2002) following the application of BAM8-22.

METHODS

The experiments used male Sprague-Dawley rats (260–350 g). All animal procedures adhered to the guidelines of *Guide to the Care and Use of Experimental Animals* (Olfert et al. 1993). In addition, the local Animal Care Committee examined and approved all animal protocols.

ANIMAL PREPARATION

Rats were anesthetized with halothane in NO_2/O_2, and the jugular vein was cannulated. A laminectomy was performed at the T3–T4 level to expose the spinal cord, and an intrathecal (i.t.) catheter was implanted with its tip at the L4–L5 level of the lumbar spinal cord for drug administration. Animals were decerebrated by aspiration of all the cranial contents rostral to the mesencephalon. The trachea was then cannulated, anesthetic was discontinued, and the rat was placed in an experimental frame with its lower limbs immobilized in an extended position. Animals were paralyzed with gallamine, artificially ventilated, and then spinalized at the T3–T4 level. Rectal temperature was maintained at 35.8°–36.2°C.

An incision in the popliteal fossa on one side of the lower left leg exposed the nerves to the principal head of posterior biceps femoris/semitendinosus (PBF/ST) muscles. The nerve was cut distally and covered with paraffin. Its proximal end was placed on a silver wire recording electrode.

EXPERIMENTAL PROCEDURES

Extracellular recordings of flexor α-motoneuron activity were made from the nerve to the PBF/ST muscles, which responded to mechanical simulation of the ipsilateral hindlimb. Recordings were started no earlier than 1 hour after spinalization, to allow for recovery from the anesthetic and stabilization of the preparation.

To determine the excitability of flexor reflex, we measured the following: (1) spontaneous activity for 10 seconds; (2) the total discharges elicited by eight standard touch stimuli (light touches applied with the flat surface of an experimenter's thumb to the plantar surface of the foot, each lasting 2 seconds and moving from the middle position of the foot to the distal foot pads, applied every 4 seconds); (3) the total discharges elicited by a standard test pinch applied with a clip (sprung at 200 g) on the three middle toes of the ipsilateral hindpaw for 2 seconds; and (4) the total discharges evoked by heat stimuli applied by immersing the hindpaw into hot water (52ºC) for 8 seconds. The above test protocol was applied at 5-minute intervals.

Prior to drug administration, we obtained baseline values by repeating the protocol at 5-minute intervals for at least 30 minutes until a stable reflex level (defined as less than 25% variation for the evoked responses) was established. All individual results for a particular animal were calculated as a percentage of the mean baseline discharge value.

Drugs were administrated by the spinal route in four doses (0.1, 0.5, 1.0, and 5.0 nmol/10 µL/rat, i.t.), either cumulatively or as a single dose given to different animals. The effect of each dose was measured for at least 30 minutes. BAM8-22 was dissolved in Hank's buffered saline solution (HBSS) and administered by slow infusion followed by flushing with 10 µL of saline. All solutions were prepared immediately prior to an experiment.

DATA ANALYSIS

Touch, pinch, and heat responses were analyzed as the total number of spikes recorded, minus the extrapolated spontaneous activity in the same period. Data, expressed as percentages of the baseline calculated from the first three readings, were tested with one-way analysis of variance (ANOVA) followed by Tukey's test for multiple comparisons, or nonparametric ANOVA followed by Dunnett's multiple comparison tests in case of unequal standard deviations (SDs).

RESULTS

BAM8-22 ENHANCED TOUCH, PINCH, AND HEAT RESPONSES

Touch-evoked responses showed a dose-dependent increase following the administration of BAM8-22 (0.1–5.0 nmol, i.t.) (Fig. 1A,B). At a dose of 5 nmol/10 µL/rat, BAM8-22 enhanced the touch response by 719 ± 125%, ($P < 0.005$, $n = 15$). BAM8-22 also enhanced noxious pinch-evoked responses (Fig. 2). At 5 nmol, BAM8-22 enhanced the pinch response by 225 ± 62% ($P < 0.005$, $n = 16$) with a latency of 5–10 minutes and a duration of more than 40 minutes.

Finally, BAM8-22 enhanced thermal responses in a dose-dependent manner (Fig. 3). At 5 nmol, BAM8-22 increased the thermal response by 742 ± 200% ($P < 0.005$, $n = 15$), which is about threefold higher than the increase in the pinch response.

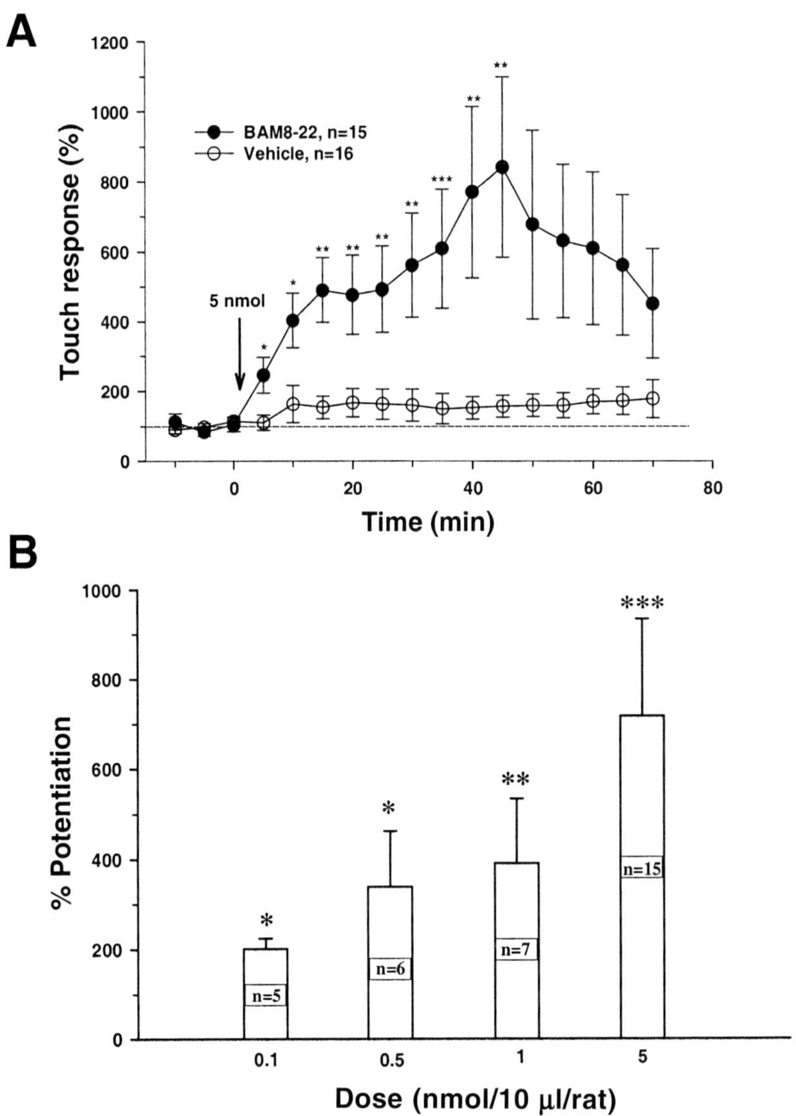

Fig. 1. Enhancement of touch response by BAM8-22. (A) BAM8-22 potentiated the touch response of flexor α-motoneurons. Excitability is expressed as the percentage deviation from the baseline value taken as an average of the last three tests before drug application. The first three measurements were averaged and constitute the baseline. The subsequent data have been normalized and are illustrated as mean ± SEM. BAM8-22 (5 nmol, i.t.) was administered at the time indicated by the arrow. The open circle in all plots represents vehicle control (HBSS) and the filled circle BAM8-22. (B) Pooled data taken 30 minutes after drug delivery from all neurons tested in the dose range of 0.1, 0.5, 1.0, and 5.0 nmol. Potentiation is expressed as the percentage increase in touch response over the baseline control. *$P < 0.05$, **$P < 0.01$, ***$P < 0.005$ compared with predrug control.

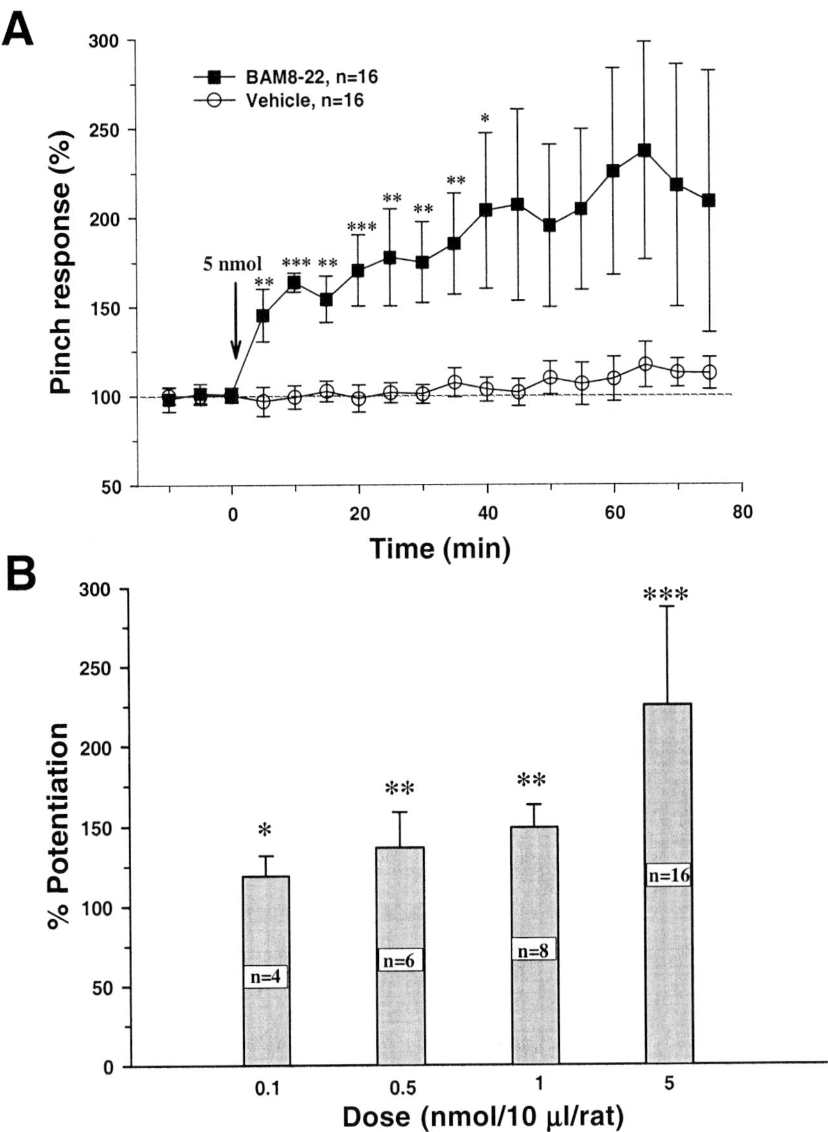

Fig. 2. Enhancement of the noxious pinch response by BAM8-22. (A) BAM8-22 potentiated the noxious pinch response of flexor α-motoneurons. Other details are as for Fig. 1, except that the noxious pinch stimulus was used to evoke a nociceptive response. (B) Pooled dose-response data taken 30 minutes after drug delivery from all neurons tested.

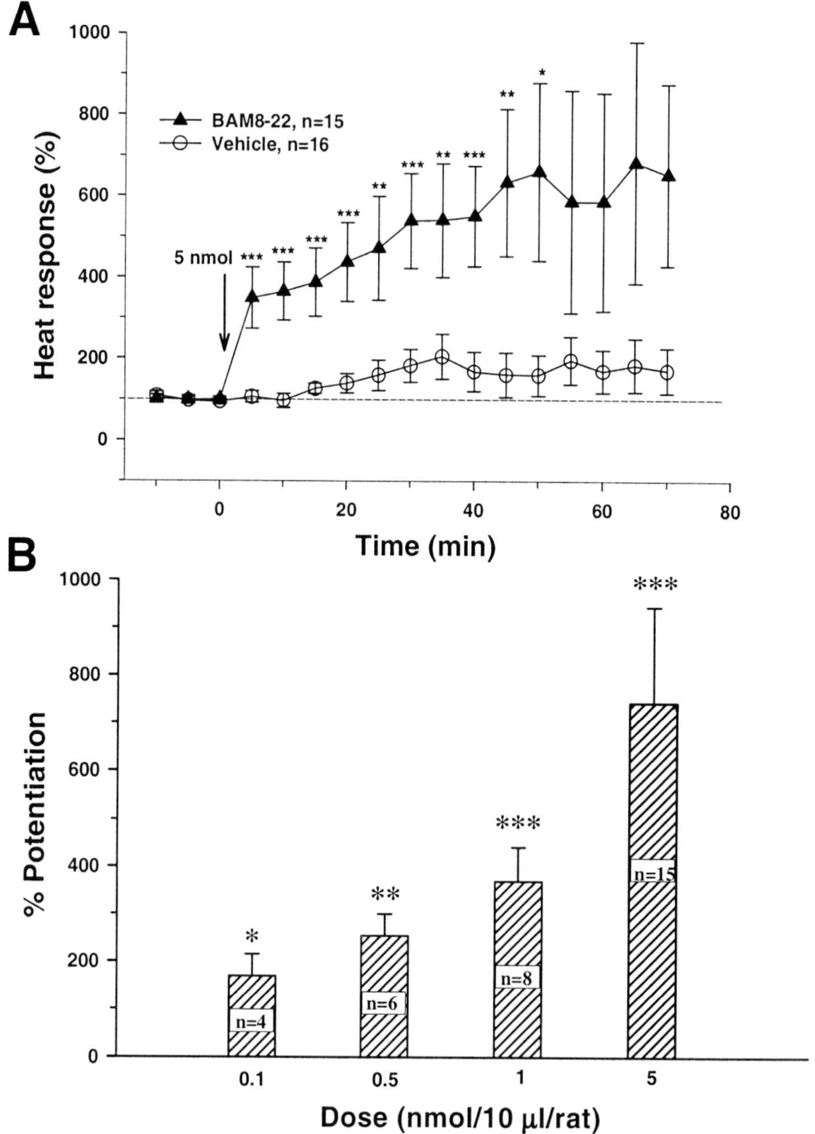

Fig. 3. Potentiation of the heat response by BAM8-22. (A) BAM8-22 potentiated the noxious heat responses of spinal flexor α-motoneurons. Other details are as for Fig. 1, except that the noxious heat stimulus (hot water at 52°C) was used to evoke thermal nociceptive response. (B) Pooled dose-response data taken 30 minutes after drug delivery from all neurons tested.

BAM8-22 POTENTIATED SPONTANEOUS ACTIVITY OF FLEXOR α-MOTONEURONS

Apart from the changes in evoked responses, BAM8-22 also dose-dependently increased spontaneous activity in all preparations (data not shown). At 5 nmol, BAM8-22 increased the background activity of the flexor α-motoneurons from 1.5 ± 0.4 Hz to 11.4 ± 4.4 Hz ($P < 0.01$, $n = 16$).

DEGRADATION ANALYSIS OF BAM8-22

To determine whether degradation of the peptide or any of its metabolites might be responsible for its effects, we used liquid chromatography mass spectrometry to analyze samples of preperfusion, 20-, 40-, and 60-minute recycled perfusion of 1 μM BAM8-22 in L1 to S1 of the spinal cord. We saw no evidence of degradation or metabolism of BAM8-22 after perfusion, as all samples showed the characteristic mass spectrometry peaks of the peptide; m/z 662 ($[M + 4H]^{4+}$), 882 ($[M + 3H]^{3+}$), and 1322 ($[M + 2H]^{2+}$).

DISCUSSION

The recent discovery of the SNSR and its endogenous ligand has stimulated the exploration of this novel family of GPCRs as a potential target for analgesics. Our study provides the first electrophysiological characterization of the action of SNSR/BAM8-22 in the spinal cord.

BAM22, one of the preproenkephalin A products (Dores et al. 1990), binds to all three subtypes of opioid receptors with high affinity. BAM22 also activates SNSRs in a naloxone-insensitive manner (Lembo et al. 2002), which suggests a non-opioid mechanism. BAM22 may therefore have dual opioid and non-opioid or dual pro- and antinociceptive activities at the spinal level. The tonic effect of BAM8-22 in our study may represent a non-opioid effect of BAM22; this C-terminal fragment bound to and activated SNSRs but lacked activity at opioid receptors (Lembo et al. 2002). Interestingly, BAM8-22 occurs endogenously as a peptidase cleavage product of proenkephalin A-derived peptide E (Zhang et al. 1999). It is unlikely that a metabolite of BAM8-22 was responsible for these effects because this peptide did not degrade after 20, 40 and 60 minutes of recycled perfusion in the rat spinal cord. Further characterization of BAM8-22 in broad receptor screen has not revealed binding affinity and activity at receptors other than SNSRs. Thus, the increased excitability and potentiation of the nociceptive flexor reflex could be attributed to specific interaction with SNSRs.

The BAM8-22-induced thermal hypersensitivity was about three-fold higher than the mechanical hypersensitivity. This result is consistent with the morphological finding that mRNA expression of SNSR is preferentially colocalized with heat-responsive vanilloid receptor TRPV1, formerly known as VR1 (~56%), and IB4 (~80%) positive dorsal root ganglion (DRG) neurons (Lembo et al. 2002). The colocalization with TRPV1 indicates that SNSR-positive receptors may differ in their sensitivity to thermal stimuli. IB4-deficient rats showed a markedly elevated thermal nociceptive threshold (Vulchanova et al. 2001), indicating a pronociceptive role of the IB4 class of nociceptors. In cultured sensory neurons, a subset of IB4-positive cells responded to noxious heat stimuli in the mouse (Stucky and Lewin 1999). The preferential enhancement of thermal nociception by BAM8-22 in our study may reflect a functional correlation of these colocalizations.

Because SNSR mRNA is solely expressed in small DRG neurons, the SNSR protein presumably would be located at the presynaptic site of its primary afferent terminals in the superficial layer of the dorsal horn. It is therefore unlikely that the increases in spontaneous activity and the evoked responses are direct actions of BAM8-22 on the flexor α-motoneuron. It is tempting to speculate that an increased excitability along the central pathway of the flexor reflex arc induced by excitatory neurotransmitters might be responsible. Activation of SNSRs by BAM8-22, for example, might induce release of a nonpeptidergic transmitter such as glutamate from IB4-positive primary afferent terminals (Malmberg et al. 1997; Mantyh et al. 1997; Nichols et al. 1999). However, the mechanisms and site of this tonic action remain to be determined.

In conclusion, BAM8-22 enhanced the nociceptive flexor reflex, indicating that SNSRs have a role in modulating spinal nociceptive transmission. The highly restricted distribution of SNSRs in peripheral tissue may be of great advantage in developing analgesics with limited central nervous system side effects.

ACKNOWLEDGMENTS

We wish to thank Dr. Angelo Filosa for the mass spectrometer analysis of BAM8-22.

REFERENCES

Cao CQ, Hong Y, Dray A, Perkins MN. Spinal delta opioid receptors mediate suppression of systemic SNC80 on excitability of the flexor reflex in normal and inflamed rat. *Eur J Pharmacol* 2001; 418:79–87.

Dong X, Han S, Zylka MJ, Simon MI, Anderson DJ. A diverse family of GPCRs expressed in specific subsets of nociceptive sensory neurons. *Cell* 2001; 106:619–632.

Dores RM, McDonald LK, Steveson TC, Sei CA. The molecular evolution of neuropeptides: prospects for the '90s. *Brain Behav Evol* 1990; 36:80–99.

Lembo PM, Grazzini E, Groblewski T, et al. Proenkephalin A gene products activate a new family of sensory neuron-specific GPCRs. *Nat Neurosci* 2002; 5:201–209.

Malmberg AB, Chen C, Tonegawa S, Basbaum AI. Preserved acute pain and reduced neuropathic pain in mice lacking PKC gamma. *Science* 1997; 278:279–283.

Mantyh PW, Rogers SD, Honore P, et al. Inhibition of hyperalgesia by ablation of lamina I spinal neurons expressing the substance P receptor. *Science* 1997, 278:275–279.

Nichols ML, Allen BJ, Rogers SD, et al. Transmission of chronic nociception by spinal neurons expressing the substance P receptor. *Science* 1999; 286:1558–1561.

Olfert D, et al. (Eds). *Guide to the Care and Use of Experimental Animals,* Vol. 2. Canadian Council of Animal Care, 1993.

Simonin F, Kieffer BL. Two faces for an opioid peptide—and more receptors for pain research. *Nat Neurosci* 2002; 5:185–186.

Skljarevski V, Ramadan NM. The nociceptive flexion reflex in humans. *Pain* 2002; 96:3–8.

Snider WD, McMahon SB. Tackling pain at the source: new ideas about nociceptors. *Neuron* 1998; 20:629–632.

Stucky CL, Lewin GR. Isolectin B (4)-positive and -negative nociceptors are functionally distinct. *J Neurosci* 1999; 19:6497–6505.

Vulchanova L, Olson TH, Stone LS, et al. Cytotoxic targeting of isolectin IB4-binding sensory neurons. *Neuroscience* 2001; 108:143–155.

Woolf CJ. Evidence for a central component of post-injury pain hypersensitivity. *Nature* 1983; 306:686–688.

Zhang H, Stoeckli M, Andren PE, Caprioli RM. Combining solid-phase preconcentration, capillary electrophoresis and off-line matrix-assisted laser desorption/ionization mass spectrometry: intracerebral metabolic processing of peptide E in vivo. *J Mass Spectrom* 1999; 34:377–383.

Correspondence to: Chang Qing Cao, PhD, AstraZeneca R&D Montreal, 7171 Frederick Banting, St. Laurent, PQ, Canada H4S 1Z9. Tel: 514-832-3200; Fax: 514-832-3232; email: changqing.cao@astrazeneca.com.

Proceedings of the 10th World Congress on Pain,
Progress in Pain Research and Management, Vol. 24,
edited by Jonathan O. Dostrovsky, Daniel B. Carr, and
Martin Koltzenburg, IASP Press, Seattle, © 2003.

10

Sodium Channel Subtypes and Neuropathic Pain[1]

Jin Mo Chung,[a] Sulayman D. Dib-Hajj,[b] and Sally N. Lawson[c]

[a]Department of Anatomy and Neurosciences, University of Texas Medical Branch, Galveston, Texas, USA; [b]Department of Neurology and PVA/EPVA Neuroscience Research Center, Yale Medical School and Rehabilitation Center, VA Connecticut Healthcare System, West Haven, Connecticut, USA; [c]Department of Physiology, Medical School, University of Bristol, Bristol, United Kingdom

Peripheral nerve injury can result in chronic neuropathic pain, in which normally painful peripheral stimuli produce severe pain (hyperalgesia), and normally nonpainful stimuli produce pain (allodynia). This state involves abnormal central processing that is initiated and maintained by abnormal peripheral input (Gracely et al. 1992). Peripheral nerve injuries are likely to include mechanical damage and local inflammation, both of which lead to development of pathological afferent activity, including ectopic discharges from axotomized afferents and spontaneous activity of sensitized nociceptors. Dynamic changes in Na^+ channels after nerve injury may play an important role in generating these abnormal activities, thus contributing to neuropathic pain. Many of the recently cloned subtypes of Na^+ channels are localized in dorsal root ganglion (DRG) neurons. This chapter discusses the evidence linking certain Na^+ channel subtypes to the generation and maintenance of neuropathic pain.

---

[1] Based on a Congress workshop.

NOCICEPTIVE DRG NEURONS

Nociceptive neurons as well as low-threshold mechanoreceptive (LTM) neurons have fibers that conduct in all three conduction velocity (CV) ranges: C, Aδ, and Aα/β (Lawson 2002). A high proportion of somatic C-fiber neurons are nociceptive, and a high proportion of Aα/β-fiber neurons are LTM units. DRG neurons with small somata may have fibers in any of the three CV groups (Harper and Lawson 1985). Thus many, but not all, small to medium-sized neurons are nociceptive, and many, but not all, large neurons are LTM units. The membrane properties of nociceptive DRG neurons, however, differ from those of LTM neurons in the following respects: they have broader and/or inflected action potentials (APs) and longer afterhyperpolarizations, higher electrical thresholds, and larger AP overshoots in all CV groups (Ritter and Mendell 1992; Djouhri et al. 1998; for review, see Lawson 2002). These properties, many of which depend on a mixture of distinct Na^+ currents, appear to limit the information carried along nociceptive pathways. In nociceptors and possibly also in LTM neurons, changes in Na^+ currents that result in altered membrane properties such as those described above probably contribute to chronic neuropathic pain.

DYNAMIC EXPRESSION OF MULTIPLE Na^+ CHANNELS IN SENSORY NEURONS

CHANNEL STRUCTURE AND TYPES OF Na^+ CURRENTS

Voltage-gated Na^+ channels underlie the unique ability of excitable cells to generate and transmit electrical activity. Ten distinct pore-forming α-subunits have been identified in vertebrates and have been classified into two subfamilies under a unified nomenclature, Na_v1 and Na_x (Goldin et al. 2000). The α-subunit of Na^+ channels consists of four domains (D1–D4) connected by intracellular loops, and each domain contains six transmembrane segments (S1–S6) (Catterall 2000); the extracellular S5–S6 linker of each domain contributes pore-lining residues with one residue from each linker constituting the selectivity filter. The amino acids serine (S), as in $Na_v1.8$ and $Na_v1.9$, or cysteine (C), as in $Na_v1.5$, in the pore-lining segment from D1 causes the channel to be resistant to tetrodotoxin (TTX) as follows: S: IC_{50} ~40–60 μM (Akopian et al. 1996; Cummins et al. 1999); C: IC_{50} ~1–2 μM (Satin et al. 1992). A residue with an aromatic side chain causes the channel to be sensitive to TTX (IC_{50} <10 nM; Satin et al. 1992). Based on the kinetics of activation, inactivation, and sensitivity to TTX, Na^+ currents have been classified into four types (Fig. 1): fast-inactivating TTX-sensitive

(TTX-s_F), fast-inactivating TTX-resistant (TTX-r_F), slow-inactivating TTX-r (TTX-r_S), and persistent TTX-r (TTX-r_P) currents.

EXPRESSION PATTERN OF Na^+ CHANNELS IN SENSORY NEURONS

Rat sensory neurons in DRG and trigeminal ganglia display the four types of Na^+ currents described above (Kostyuk et al. 1981; Caffrey et al. 1992; Roy and Narahashi 1992; Elliott and Elliott 1993; Akopian et al. 1996; Cummins et al. 1999). The complexity of the Na^+ currents in adult rat DRG neurons is paralleled by the presence of multiple Na^+ channel transcripts. A multiplex reverse transcription polymerase chain reaction (RT-PCR) and subsequent restriction enzyme mapping of amplicons (the RT-PCR/REP assay) was used to determine the expression pattern of Na^+ channel genes (Dib-Hajj et al. 1998b). The combination of length and restriction enzyme polymorphism identifies individual Na^+ channels. Transcripts for six Na^+ channels ($Na_v1.1$, $Na_v1.6$, $Na_v1.7$, $Na_v1.8$, $Na_v1.9$, and Na_x) account for most of the signal in adult rat DRG neurons, while transcripts of $Na_v1.2$ and $Na_v1.3$ are also detected but at much reduced levels (Waxman et al. 1994; Black et al. 1996; Dib-Hajj et al. 1998b; Kim et al. 2001). Immunocytochemical analysis confirms the presence of individual channels in DRG neurons (Toledo-Aral et al. 1997; Caldwell et al. 2000; Sleeper et al. 2000; Benn et al. 2001).

The expression of the TTX-r channels and some of the TTX-s channels is developmentally regulated. The levels of the TTX-s_F channels $Na_v1.1$, $Na_v1.2$, and $Na_v1.3$ change during development while levels of $Na_v1.6$, $Na_v1.7$, and Na_x remain steady (Fig. 2). $Na_v1.2$ and $Na_v1.3$ amplicons are still detectable at postnatal day 0 but are significantly attenuated by postnatal day 7, while $Na_v1.1$ signal increases during the same period. The TTX-r_F current produced by $Na_v1.5$ (Satin et al. 1992) is recorded from most embryonic DRG neurons at embryonic day 18 but is detectable in only ~5% of small DRG neurons of adult rats, consistent with the results of the RT-PCR/REP assay (Renganathan et al. 2002). Transcripts of $Na_v1.8$ and $Na_v1.9$ are first detected around embryonic day 15 and remain at abundant levels through adulthood (Fig. 2 and Benn et al. 2001). The TTX-r_S current produced by $Na_v1.8$ (Akopian et al. 1996) is in both small and some large DRG neurons (Black et al. 1996; Fjell et al. 1999), while the TTX-r_P current produced by $Na_v1.9$ (Cummins et al. 1999) is only in small DRG neurons (Tate et al. 1998; Dib-Hajj et al. 1998b). Both TTX-r_S and TTX-r_P currents increase in density during development until birth, and sustain that level thereafter (Renganathan et al. 2002).

Na^+ CHANNEL SUBTYPES IN SMALL DRG NEURONS

Of the Na^+ channel subtypes expressed in DRG neurons, only three ($Na_v1.7$, 1.8, and 1.9) are normally preferentially expressed in smaller DRG neurons, indicating possible involvement in determining nociceptive properties. $Na_v1.8$ and $Na_v1.9$ subtypes are expressed only in primary afferent neurons and not in the central nervous system (CNS), thus future novel analgesic drugs that target them may have few or no CNS side effects. The TTX-r_S current associated with $Na_v1.8$ has slow kinetics and a high activation threshold (~–30 to –35 mV) and is thought to contribute to the AP inward current (Akopian et al. 1996). $Na_v1.8$ therefore may be largely responsible for the TTX-r broad APs in nociceptive neurons (Waddell and Lawson 1990; Ritter and Mendell 1992; Djouhri et al. 1998). This quality of $Na_v1.8$, and its expression (mRNA and protein) in small and medium-sized DRG neurons, has suggested an important role in nociceptors (Akopian et al. 1996; Novakovic et al. 1998). $Na_v1.9$ is expressed only in small DRG neurons. The hyperpolarized (low-threshold) voltage dependence of activation, and the ultra-slowly inactivating and therefore, persistent nature of the $Na_v1.9$ current (Cummins et al. 1999), may influence membrane potential in small DRG neurons (Herzog et al. 2001). The TTX-s_F $Na_v1.7$ channel appears to be more abundant in neurons in the peripheral nervous system, for example in DRG and sympathetic ganglia, than in the CNS (Sangameswaran et al. 1997; Toledo-Aral et al. 1997). Although $Na_v1.7$ mRNA is present in DRG neurons of all sizes (Black et al. 1996), more immunoreactivity (protein) is found in small than in large DRG neurons in adult rats and guinea pigs (Gould et al. 2000; Djouhri et al. 2003), but not in fetal rats (Toledo-Aral et al. 1997).

EXPRESSION OF Na^+ CHANNEL SUBTYPES IN IDENTIFIED NOCICEPTIVE AND NON-NOCICEPTIVE NEURONS

Electrophysiological recordings from DRG neurons in vivo were combined with subsequent immunohistochemical analysis to determine the presence of $Na_v1.7$, 1.8, and 1.9 in nociceptive and non-nociceptive neurons. Intracellular voltage recordings were made in L4 and L5 DRG in deeply anesthetized female Wistar rats ($Na_v1.8$ and $Na_v1.9$) and in L5 and L6 DRG in deeply anesthetized young female guinea pigs ($Na_v1.7$). Dorsal roots were electrically stimulated, the shapes of evoked intracellular APs were analyzed, and the CV was classified as C, Aδ or Aα/β. Each individual unit was classified as nociceptive, LTM, thermoreceptive, or unresponsive based on responses to mechanical and thermal stimulation applied to the hindlimb and flank. Because C-fiber unresponsive neurons had membrane properties similar to

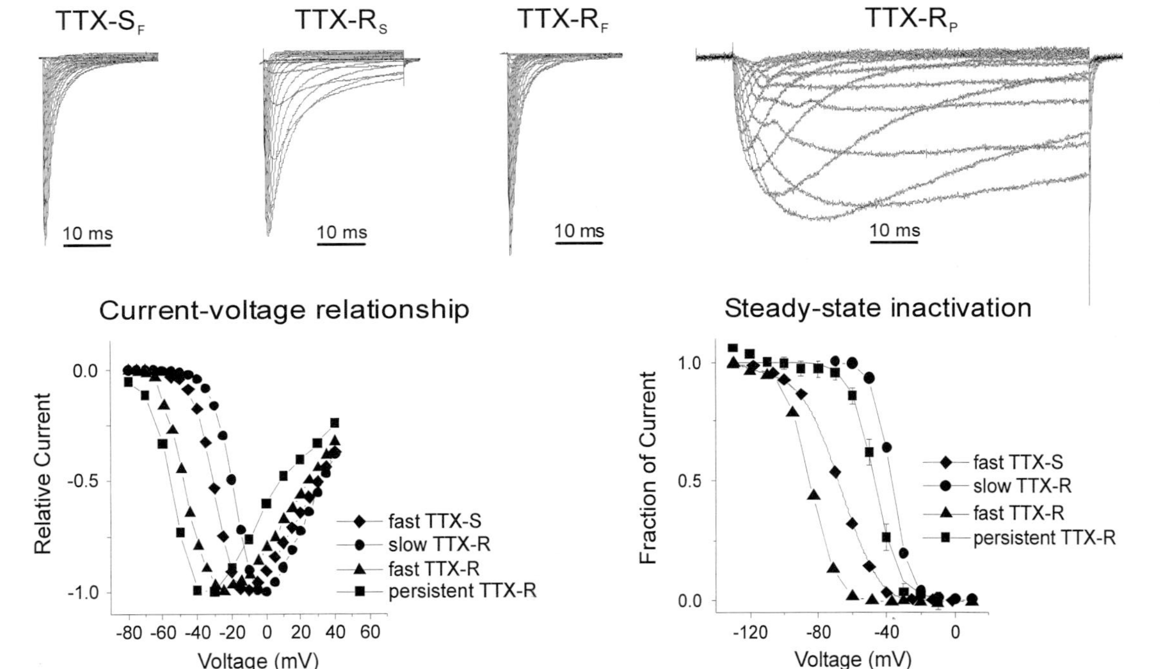

Fig. 1. Types of Na^+ currents in dorsal root ganglion (DRG) neurons. Top panel shows the four major types of Na^+ currents from DRG neurons. TTX-s_F: fast-inactivating TTX-s Na^+ current, produced by multiple channels; TTX-r_F: fast-inactivating TTX-r Na^+ current, produced by $Na_v1.5$; TTX-r_S: slow-inactivating TTX-r Na^+ current, produced by $Na_v1.8$; TTX-r_P: persistent TTX-r Na^+ current, produced by $Na_v1.9$. The TTX-r_S and TTX-r_F were recorded from DRG neurons in the presence of 250 nM TTX. The TTX-r_P was recorded from DRG neurons of $Na_v1.8$ null mice in the presence of 250 nM TTX. Left and right lower panels show current-voltage relationships and voltage-dependence of inactivation, respectively, for TTX-s_F (diamond), TTX-r_F (triangle), TTX-r_S (circle), and TTX-r_P (square).

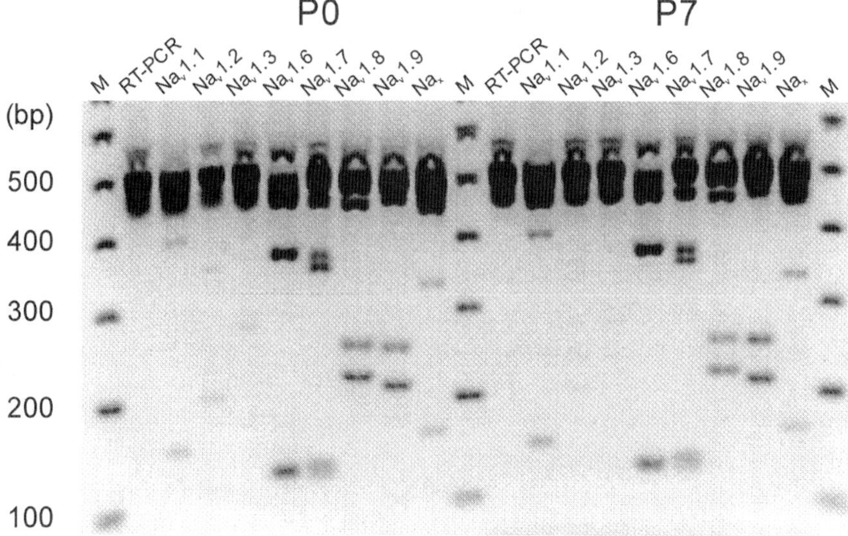

Fig. 2. Restriction enzyme mapping of RT-PCR products from rat DRG. "M" lanes contain 100 bp ladder marker; RT-PCR lane contains uncut products. Equal aliquots were digested by the restriction enzymes *EcoR V*, *EcoN I*, *Ava I*, *Sph I*, *Bam H I*, *Afl II*, *Eco R I*, and *Xba I*, which are specific to subunits $Na_v1.1$, $Na_v1.2$, $Na_v1.3$, $Na_v1.6$, $Na_v1.7$, $Na_v1.8$, $Na_v1.9$, and Na_x channels, respectively. The predicted length of amplicons and digestion products are: $Na_v1.1$ (558 bp, 152 and 406 bp); $Na_v1.2$ (561 bp, 204, 357 bp); $Na_v1.3$ (561 bp, 279, 282 bp); $Na_v1.6$ (507 bp, 126, 381 bp); $Na_v1.7$ (501 bp, 134, 367 bp); $Na_v1.8$ (479 bp, 224, 255 bp); $Na_v1.9$ (468 bp, 185, 283 bp); and Na_x (501 bp, 165, 336 bp). $Na_v1.7$ and $Na_v1.8$ amplicons contain *Bam H1* site. The two amplicons, however, differ in length and in *Bam H1* digestion products, thus it is feasible to demonstrate the presence of either amplicon or both in the pool.

those of C-nociceptive neurons, they probably included very high-threshold (sometimes called "silent") nociceptors. Both nociceptive and C-unresponsive neurons are thus included in the term "nociceptor-type" neurons. Intracellular dye injection enabled subsequent immunocytochemical identification of individual Na^+ channels. The cross-sectional area of the largest 8-μm section through the neuron was an indication of soma size.

$Na_v1.9$-like immunoreactivity (LI) was seen only in nociceptive neurons, but it was not found in all of them. It was detected in 64%, 54%, and 31% of C-, Aδ-, and Aα/β-fiber nociceptive units, respectively, and in 90% of C-unresponsive units; it was absent from all LTM units examined (Fang et al. 2002). $Na_v1.8$-LI was detected in most nociceptive neurons, but in contrast to $Na_v1.9$-LI, moderate immunoreactivity was also seen in some LTMs in all CV groups (Fang et al. 2001). $Na_v1.7$-LI was detected in most C- and Aδ-fiber nociceptive units, and in less than half the Aα/β nociceptive units; however, it was also present in Aδ LTMs and in about half the cutaneous afferent Aα/β LTMs, but not in muscle spindle afferents (Djouhri et al. 2003). Thus, all these three subunits are present in a substantial proportion of nociceptive neurons, but with varying selectivity for nociceptive units. The relative intensities of the immunoreactivity for all three subunits were negatively correlated with soma size and CV in all neurons and were positively correlated (especially $Na_v1.7$) with AP duration; that is, intense immunolabeling was detected in smaller, slowly conducting neurons that tended to have broader spikes (Fang et al. 2001, 2002; Djouhri et al. 2003).

ABNORMAL AFFERENT ACTIVITY AND Na^+ CHANNELS

ECTOPIC DISCHARGES AND NEUROPATHIC PAIN

Neuropathic pain behaviors are reversed by approximately 50% by removing ectopic discharge input to the spinal cord, suggesting that at least part of the pain behaviors are maintained by ectopic discharges from injured primary afferent neurons (Chung and Chung 2002). Primary afferent neurons manifest altered membrane properties in animal models of chronic pain that involve inflammation and/or peripheral nerve injury. For instance, injured neurons become hyperexcitable and produce exaggerated responses to suprathreshold stimuli. It is therefore important to establish which ion channels are responsible for any alterations in membrane properties that contribute to increased information traffic to the CNS. For example, after axotomy the changes that occur in DRG neurons include broadening of APs and increased spontaneous activity at least in A-fiber neurons (Kim et al. 1998; Stebbing et al. 1998; Liu et al. 2001). Whether these changes occur only in neurons that prior to axotomy were nociceptive is unknown.

Na^+ CHANNELS AND ECTOPIC DISCHARGES IN AXOTOMIZED AFFERENTS

Because Na^+ channels are critical for the initiation and propagation of APs, injury-induced changes to the expression of these channels have been extensively investigated. The view that Na^+ channels may be important for the generation of ectopic discharges is supported by the accumulation of Na^+ channels at the neuroma of a cut sensory nerve where some ectopic discharges may arise (Devor et al. 1989) and by the ability of Na^+ channel blockers to silence these discharges (Devor et al. 1992; Matzner and Devor 1994). Furthermore, application of Na^+ channel blockers reduces neuropathic pain in humans (Chabal et al. 1992) and diminishes pain behaviors in animal models of neuropathic pain (Abram and Yaksh 1994).

TTX SENSITIVITY OF ECTOPIC DISCHARGES AND NEUROPATHIC PAIN

Ectopic discharges are sensitive to TTX applied topically to the neuroma (Matzner and Devor 1994), but because the effective dose in vivo is hard to determine, it is difficult to ascertain the role of TTX-s_F, TTX-r_S, and TTX-r_P currents. To determine TTX sensitivity of ectopic discharges more accurately, TTX was applied to injured DRGs in vitro (Liu et al. 2001). The L5 spinal nerve of the rat was ligated and, at various times after L5 spinal nerve ligation (SNL), the ipsilateral L5 DRG and its connected dorsal root and ligated spinal nerve were placed in a recording chamber, each in a separately perfused compartment. Single-unit ectopic discharges were recorded from teased proximal dorsal root filaments. Following peripheral nerve injury, ectopic discharges are known to arise from both the injury site and the DRG. After SNL, however, ectopic discharges arose in the DRG in 98% of tested units (Liu et al. 1999, 2001); the rate of this discharge was significantly reduced after the application of ~20 nM TTX to the DRG (Liu et al. 2001). This reduction was not due to conduction block, which required ~400 nM of TTX. TTX-s_F subtypes must, therefore, play an important role in generating ectopic discharges in the DRG, because the doses of TTX required to block these discharges were about two orders of magnitude lower than those needed to block TTX-r Na^+ channels. This finding suggests that TTX-s_F subtypes of Na^+ channels may be important in generating neuropathic pain. TTX sensitivity of animal behavior in models of neuropathic pain was therefore examined by applying TTX topically onto the L5 DRG in the SNL model using a chronically implanted catheter (Lyu et al. 2000). Neuropathic pain behavior is indeed significantly reduced by doses of TTX (12.5–50 nM) but not of vehicle (saline); these doses are too low to involve any TTX-r subtype and are indicative of a role for TTX-s channels in this behavior.

UPREGULATION OF TTX-S SODIUM CHANNEL SUBTYPES AFTER NERVE INJURY

The preceding section suggests that TTX-s_F Na^+ channels are important in ectopic discharges as well as in generation of neuropathic pain behavior after nerve injury. Molecular and electrophysiological approaches were used to investigate changes in the expression of the TTX-s_F channels ($Na_v1.1$, $Na_v1.2$, $Na_v1.3$, $Na_v1.6$, $Na_v1.7$, and Na_x). An upregulation of one or more subtype in synchrony with the development of ectopic discharge would suggest a role in neuropathic pain.

Molecular studies have demonstrated that $Na_v1.3$ mRNA is upregulated in adult rat DRG neurons following axotomy (Waxman et al. 1994; Dib-Hajj et al. 1996), chronic constriction injury (CCI) (Dib-Hajj et al. 1999), and SNL (Kim et al. 2001), but not after dorsal rhizotomy (Black et al. 1999). Immunocytochemical studies have demonstrated the accumulation of $Na_v1.3$ protein in the somata of axotomized small-diameter DRG neurons and in the transected fibers at the site of ligation (Black et al. 1999). The increase of $Na_v1.3$ mRNA is evident 16 hours after injury (Kim et al. 2001) and is maintained for several weeks (Dib-Hajj et al. 1996). Transcripts of Na_x, a putative TTX-s channel, are upregulated at 5 days but not 1 day after SNL (Fig. 3). In contrast, transcript levels of $Na_v1.1$, $Na_v1.2$, $Na_v1.6$, and $Na_v1.7$ declined after nerve injury (Kim et al. 2001, 2002). Increased levels of $Na_v1.3$ mRNA and protein following injury are paralleled by the emergence of a rapidly repriming TTX-s_F Na^+ current in small-diameter DRG neurons (Cummins and Waxman 1997). The hypothesis that the rapidly repriming TTX-s_F is produced by $Na_v1.3$ (Cummins and Waxman 1997) is supported by the production of a similar current in HEK293 cells expressing recombinant $Na_v1.3$ (Cummins et al. 2001; Leffler et al. 2002). Furthermore, upregulation of $Na_v1.3$ is in synchrony with ectopic discharge development in DRG neurons, which begins 13 hours after SNL and continues for weeks (Liu et al. 1999), while upregulation of Na_x occurs at a later time point (Fig. 3). Together, all these data point to a central role for $Na_v1.3$, although a possible contribution by Na_x at a later postoperative period cannot be ruled out.

INJURY-INDUCED CHANGES IN THE EXPRESSION OF $Na_v1.8$ AND $Na_v1.9$ CHANNELS AND TTX-R CURRENTS

Transcripts and proteins of the TTX-r channels $Na_v1.8$ and $Na_v1.9$ are significantly reduced following axotomy, CCI, and SNL (Dib-Hajj et al. 1996, 1999; Okuse et al. 1997), but not after dorsal rhizotomy (Sleeper et al. 2000). $Na_v1.8$ transcript levels were slightly attenuated after establishment of diabetic neuropathy (Okuse et al. 1997). The TTX-r_S and TTX-r_P currents that are produced by $Na_v1.8$ and $Na_v1.9$, respectively, are also attenuated following axotomy, but not rhizotomy (Sleeper et al. 2000). The loss of TTX-r_S in axotomized small DRG neurons persists for several weeks following injury (Cummins and Waxman 1997).

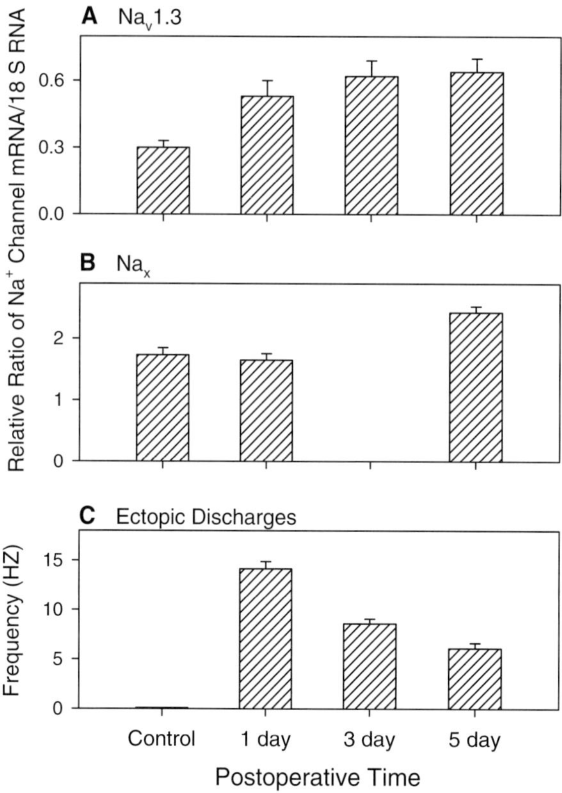

Fig. 3. Comparison of upregulation of mRNAs for TTX-sensitive (TTX-s) Na^+ channel subtypes and the development of ectopic discharges. mRNAs for 6 TTX-s Na^+ channel subtypes ($Na_v1.1$, $Na_v1.2$, $Na_v1.3$, $Na_v1.6$, $Na_v1.7$, and Na_x) were measured in the DRG by RNAse protection assay at different times after spinal nerve ligation. Four channels were found to be downregulated. Data for the remaining two that were upregulated are shown here in panels A and B. In panel B, no measurement was made at postoperative day 3. Panel C shows the rate of ectopic discharges recorded (n = 128–211) using an in vitro set-up during the same time periods. Upregulation of Na_x was not evident at postoperative day 1, while that of $Na_v1.3$ was obvious from postoperative day 1. On the other hand, ectopic discharges developed quickly (maximum at postoperative day 1) and gradually declined in frequency. The data in panels A and B are adapted from Kim et al. (2001, 2002); those in panel C are unpublished data from J.M. Chung's laboratory.

EFFECT OF NEUROTROPHIC FACTORS ON THE EXPRESSION OF Na CHANNELS

Changes to the expression of $Na_v1.3$, $Na_v1.7$, $Na_v1.8$, and $Na_v1.9$ following injury might be explained in part by the action or loss of target-derived neurotrophic factors. For example, axotomy reduces the amount of peripherally derived nerve growth factor (NGF) reaching the DRG cell body

(Lee et al. 1998), while inflammation increases it (see below). The hypothesis that growth factors may be involved in Na^+ channel plasticity is further supported by experiments that provide exogenous NGF and glial-derived neurotrophic factor (GDNF) to DRG neurons in culture (Fjell et al. 1999; Sleeper et al. 2000), and in vivo via an osmotic pump (Dib-Hajj et al. 1998a; Cummins et al. 2000; Leffler et al. 2002). NGF restored primarily the expression of $Na_v1.8$ and TTX-r_S (Dib-Hajj et al. 1998; Fjell et al. 1999), while GDNF restored both $Na_v1.8$ and $Na_v1.9$ channels and the currents that they produce (Fjell et al. 1999; Cummins et al. 2000). In addition, $Na_v1.8$ is upregulated by exogenous NGF (Gould et al. 2000). In contrast both NGF and GDNF downregulate $Na_v1.3$ expression and the rapidly repriming TTX-s_F current that emerges following axotomy (Leffler et al. 2002). Intrathecal administration of GDNF produces analgesic effects in a model of neuropathic pain, perhaps due to its effects on the expression of Na^+ channels (Boucher et al. 2000).

INFLAMMATION

During inflammation of tissues, such as that induced by complete Freund's adjuvant (CFA), NGF is upregulated in the tissues, is transported to the DRG, and leads to hyperalgesia (Woolf et al. 1994). Thus, in contrast to axotomy, there is an increased availability of NGF in DRG somata. NGF-dependent changes that occur in nociceptive neurons include decreased AP duration, a threefold increase in maximum rate of firing along the fibers, and increased spontaneous activity, especially in C-fiber nociceptors, more than half of which fire spontaneously 4 days after CFA application (Djouhri and Lawson 1999; Djouhri et al. 2001). These changes would considerably increase the numbers of APs reaching the spinal cord along the nociceptive pathway. The slow time scale of these changes (>1 day) is consistent with changes in gene expression, perhaps induced (see above) by altered growth factor availability. The changes may result, at least in part, from the increased levels of $Na_v1.8$ and $Na_v1.9$ transcripts (Tanaka et al. 1998; Tate et al. 1998), of increased TTX-r_S current (Tanaka et al. 1998) in small DRG neurons, and of greater $Na_v1.7$ protein accumulation (Gould et al. 2000) resulting from chronic inflammation of the rat hindpaw. If the changes in AP duration were simply due to increased expression of $Na_v1.7$, $Na_v1.8$, and $Na_v1.9$, then increased rather than decreased AP durations might be expected. That this appears not to be the case may indicate the importance of altered properties of these Na^+ channels under the influence of molecules such as β subunits, other accessory proteins, inflammatory mediators, or growth factors. For instance, the inflammatory mediators prostaglandin E_2

(PGE_2) and serotonin acutely increase the amplitude of the TTX-r_S current in DRG neurons in culture (England et al. 1996; Gold et al. 1996). Acute PGE_2-mediated hyperalgesia was ameliorated by treatment with $Na_v1.8$ antisense oligonucleotides (Khasar et al. 1998). However, a study using $Na_v1.8$ null mutant mice (Kerr et al. 2001) did not support a role of $Na_v1.8$ channel in PGE_2-mediated hypersensitivity or neuropathic pain, but did suggest a role in NGF-induced thermal hyperalgesia. Overall, it is clear that patterns of change in Na^+ channel expression or properties may be quite different, even opposite, during inflammation and following peripheral axotomy. Nonetheless in both cases they appear to contribute to increased excitability of DRG neurons and to the generation of chronic pain states. Indeed, depending on the injury, both axotomy- and inflammation-induced changes are likely to contribute in differing degrees to neuropathic pain.

CONCLUSIONS

Recent cloning and characterization of various Na^+ channel subtypes have triggered many studies on the role of individual channels in pain mechanisms. Several Na^+ channel subtypes appear to play unique roles in different aspects of nociceptive function or in the generation of abnormal activity in models of chronic pain. The accumulation of $Na_v1.3$ channels in the injured DRG somata and at neuromas may play a significant role in the development and maintenance of ectopic discharges. In contrast, the loss of the TTX-r_P currents in injured DRG neurons may contribute to the hyperexcitability of these neurons by allowing the resting membrane to hyperpolarize, thus reducing resting inhibition of the TTX-s channels (Cummins and Waxman 1997; Herzog et al. 2001). Genetic manipulation of expression of individual channel subunits both in vitro and in vivo will help to elucidate more precisely the roles of each Na^+ channel subtype in different types of sensory neurons in inflammatory and neuropathic pain.

ACKNOWLEDGMENTS

J.M. Chung was supported by NIH grants NS 31680 and NS 11255. S. Dib-Hajj was supported in part by grants from the National Multiple Sclerosis Society and from the Rehabilitation Research and Development Service and Medical Research Services, Department of Veterans Affairs, and by gifts from the Paralyzed Veterans of America and Eastern Paralyzed Veterans Association. S.N. Lawson was supported by Wellcome Trust UK grants.

REFERENCES

Abram SE, Yaksh TL. Systemic lidocaine blocks nerve injury-induced hyperalgesia and nociceptor-driven spinal sensitization in the rat. *Anesthesiology* 1994; 80:383–391.

Akopian AN, Sivilotti L, Wood JN. A tetrodotoxin-resistant voltage-gated sodium channel expressed by sensory neurons. *Nature* 1996; 379:257–262.

Benn SC, Costigan M, Tate S, Fitzgerald M, Woolf CJ. Developmental expression of the TTX-resistant voltage-gated sodium channels Nav1.8 (SNS) and Nav1.9 (SNS2) in primary sensory neurons. *J Neurosci* 2001; 21:6077–6085.

Black JA, Dib-Hajj S, McNabola K, et al. Spinal sensory neurons express multiple sodium channel alpha-subunit mRNAs. *Mol Brain Res* 1996; 43:117–131.

Black JA, Cummins TR, Plumpton C, et al. Upregulation of a silent sodium channel after peripheral, but not central, nerve injury in DRG neurons. *J Neurophysiol* 1999; 82:2776–2785.

Boucher TJ, Okuse K, Bennett DL, et al. Potent analgesic effects of GDNF in neuropathic pain states. *Science* 2000; 290:124–127.

Caffrey JM, Eng DL, Black JA, Waxman SG, Kocsis JD. Three types of sodium channels in adult rat dorsal root ganglion neurons. *Brain Res* 1992; 592:283–297.

Caldwell JH, Schaller KL, Lasher RS, Peles E, Levinson SR. Sodium channel Na(v)1.6 is localized at nodes of Ranvier, dendrites, and synapses. *Proc Natl Acad Sci USA* 2000; 97:5616–5620.

Catterall WA. From ionic currents to molecular mechanisms: the structure and function of voltage-gated sodium channels. *Neuron* 2000; 26:13–25.

Chabal C, Jacobson L, Mariano A, Chaney E, Britell CW. The use of oral mexiletine for the treatment of pain after peripheral nerve injury. *Anesthesiology* 1992; 76:513–517.

Chung JM, Chung K. Importance of hyperexcitability of DRG neurons in neuropathic pain. *Pain Practice* 2002; 2:87–97.

Cummins TR, Waxman SG. Downregulation of tetrodotoxin-resistant sodium currents and upregulation of a rapidly repriming tetrodotoxin-sensitive sodium current in small spinal sensory neurons after nerve injury. *J Neurosci* 1997; 17:3503–3514.

Cummins TR, Dib-Hajj SD, Black JA, et al. A novel persistent tetrodotoxin-resistant sodium current In SNS-null and wild-type small primary sensory neurons. *J Neurosci* 1999; 19:RC43-1–RC43-6.

Cummins TR, Black JA, Dib-Hajj SD, Waxman SG. Glial-derived neurotrophic factor upregulates expression of functional SNS and NaN sodium channels and their currents in axotomized dorsal root ganglion neurons. *J Neurosci* 2000; 20:8754–8761.

Cummins TR, Aglieco F, Renganathan M, et al. Nav1.3 sodium channels: rapid repriming and slow closed-state inactivation display quantitative differences after expression in a mammalian cell line and in spinal sensory neurons. *J Neurosci* 2001; 21:5952–5961.

Devor M, Keller CH, Deerinck TJ, Levinson SR, Ellisman MH. Na^+ channel accumulation on axolemma of afferent endings in nerve end neuromas in *Apteronotus. Neurosci Lett* 1989; 102:149–154.

Devor M, Wall PD, Catalan N. Systemic lidocaine silences ectopic neuroma and DRG discharge without blocking nerve conduction. *Pain* 1992; 48:261–268.

Dib-Hajj S, Black JA, Felts P, Waxman SG. Down-regulation of transcripts for Na channel alpha-SNS in spinal sensory neurons following axotomy. *Proc Natl Acad Sci USA* 1996; 93:14950–14954.

Dib-Hajj SD, Black JA, Cummins TR, et al. Rescue of alpha-SNS sodium channel expression in small dorsal root ganglion neurons following axotomy by in vivo administration of nerve growth factor. *J Neurophysiol* 1998a; 79:2668–2676.

Dib-Hajj SD, Tyrrell L, Black JA, Waxman SG. NaN, a novel voltage-gated Na channel, is expressed preferentially in peripheral sensory neurons and down-regulated after axotomy. *Proc Natl Acad Sci USA* 1998b; 95:8963–8968.

Dib-Hajj SD, Fjell J, Cummins TR, et al. Plasticity of sodium channel expression in DRG neurons in the chronic constriction injury model of neuropathic pain. *Pain* 1999; 83:591–600.

Djouhri L, Lawson SN. Changes in somatic action potential shape in guinea pig nociceptive primary afferent neurons during inflammation *in vivo*. *J Physiol* 1999; 520:565–576.

Djouhri L, Bleazard L, Lawson SN. Association of somatic action potential shape with sensory receptive properties in guinea pig dorsal root ganglion neurons. *J Physiol* 1998; 513:857–872.

Djouhri L, Dawbarn D, Robertson A, Newton R, Lawson SN. Time course and nerve growth factor dependence of inflammation-induced alterations in electrophysiological membrane properties in nociceptive primary afferent neurons. *J Neurosci* 2001; 21:8722–8733.

Djouhri L, Newton R, Levinson SR, Lawson SN. Sensory and electrophysiological properties of guinea-pig sensory neurons expressing Na_v1.7 (PN1) Na^+ channel α subunit protein. *J Physiol* 2003; 546:565–576.

Elliott AA, Elliott JR. Characterization of TTX-sensitive and TTX-resistant sodium currents in small cells from adult rat dorsal root ganglia. *J Physiol* 1993; 463:39–56.

England S, Bevan S, Docherty RJ. PGE2 modulates the tetrodotoxin-resistant sodium current in neonatal rat dorsal root ganglion neurones via the cyclic AMP-protein kinase A cascade. *J Physiol* 1996; 495:429–440.

Fang X, Djouhri L, Okuse K, Wood JN, Lawson SN. Sensory and electrophysiological properties of DRG neurones with SNS-like immunoreactivity (SNS-LI) in rats. *Soc Neurosci Abstr* 2001; 27:819.5.

Fang X, Djouhri L, Black JA, et al. The presence and role of the TTX resistant sodium channel Nav1.9 (NaN) in nociceptive primary afferent neurons. *J Neurosci* 2002; 22:7425–7433.

Fjell J, Cummins TR, Dib-Hajj SD, et al. Differential role of GDNF and NGF in the maintenance of two TTX-resistant sodium channels in adult DRG neurons. *Mol Brain Res* 1999; 67:267–282.

Gold MS, Reichling DB, Shuster MJ, Levine JD. Hyperalgesic agents increase a tetrodotoxin-resistant Na^+ current in nociceptors. *Proc Natl Acad Sci USA* 1996; 93:1108–1112.

Goldin AL, Barchi RL, Caldwell JH, et al. Nomenclature of voltage-gated sodium channels. *Neuron* 2000; 28:365–368.

Gould HJ, III, Gould TN, England JD, et al. A possible role for nerve growth factor in the augmentation of sodium channels in models of chronic pain. *Brain Res* 2000; 854:19–29.

Gracely RH, Lynch SA, Bennett GJ. Painful neuropathy: altered central processing maintained dynamically by peripheral input. *Pain* 1992; 51:175–194.

Harper AA, Lawson SN. Conduction velocity is related to morphological cell type in rat dorsal root ganglia. *J Physiol* 1985; 359:31–46.

Herzog RI, Cummins TR, Waxman SG. Persistent TTX-resistant Na^+ current affects resting potential and response to depolarization in simulated spinal sensory neurons. *J Neurophysiol* 2001; 86:1351–1364.

Kerr BJ, Souslova V, McMahon SB, Wood JN. A role for the TTX-resistant sodium channel Nav1.8 in NGF-induced hyperalgesia, but not neuropathic pain. *Neuroreport* 2001; 3077–3080.

Khasar SG, Gold MS, Levine JD. A tetrodotoxin-resistant sodium current mediates inflammatory pain in the rat. *Neurosci Lett* 1998; 256:17–20.

Kim CH, Oh Y, Chung JM, Chung K. The changes in expression of three subtypes of TTX sensitive sodium channels in sensory neurons after spinal nerve ligation. *Mol Brain Res* 2001; 95:153–161.

Kim CH, Oh Y, Chung JM, Chung K. Changes in three subtypes of tetrodotoxin sensitive sodium channel expression in the axotomized dorsal root ganglion in the rat. *Neurosci Lett* 2002; 323:125–128.

Kim YI, Na HS, Kim SH, et al. Cell type-specific changes of the membrane properties of peripherally-axotomized dorsal root ganglion neurons in a rat model of neuropathic pain. *Neuroscience* 1998; 86:301–309.

Kostyuk PG, Veselovsky NS, Tsyndrenko AY. Ionic currents in the somatic membrane of rat dorsal root ganglion neurons. I. Sodium currents. *Neuroscience* 1981; 6:2423–2430.

Lawson SN. Phenotype and function of somatic primary afferent nociceptive neurones with C, A delta or A alpha/beta-fibres. *J Exp Physiol* 2002; 87:239–244.

Lee SE, Shen H, Taglialatela G, Chung JM, Chung K. Expression of nerve growth factor in the dorsal root ganglion after peripheral nerve injury. *Brain Res* 1998; 796:99–106.

Leffler A, Cummins TR, Dib-Hajj SD, et al. GDNF and NGF reverse changes in repriming of TTX-sensitive Na^+ currents following axotomy of dorsal root ganglion neurons. *J Neurophysiol* 2002, 88:650–658.

Liu X, Chung K, Chung JM. Ectopic discharges and adrenergic sensitivity of sensory neurons after spinal nerve injury. *Brain Res* 1999; 849:244–247.

Liu X, Zhou J-L, Chung K, Chung JM. Ion channels associated with the ectopic discharges generated after segmental spinal nerve injury in the rat. *Brain Res* 2001; 900:119–127.

Lyu YS, Park SK, Chung K, Chung JM. Low dose of tetrodotoxin reduces neuropathic pain behaviors in an animal model. *Brain Res* 2000; 871:98–103.

Matzner O, Devor M. Hyperexcitability at sites of nerve injury depends on voltage-sensitive Na^+ channels. *J Neurophysiol* 1994; 72:349–359.

Novakovic SD, Tzoumaka E, McGivern JG, et al. Distribution of the tetrodotoxin-resistant sodium channel PN3 in rat sensory neurons in normal and neuropathic conditions. *J Neurosci* 1998; 18:2174–2187.

Okuse K, Chaplan SR, McMahon SB, et al. Regulation of expression of the sensory neuron-specific sodium channel SNS in inflammatory and neuropathic pain. *Mol Cell Neurosci* 1997; 10:196–207.

Renganathan M, Dib-Hajj SD, Waxman SG. Nav1.5 underlies the "third TTX-R sodium current" in rat small DRG neurons. *Mol Brain Res* 2002; 106:70–82.

Ritter AM, Mendell LM. Somal membrane properties of physiologically identified sensory neurons in the rat: effects of nerve growth factor. *J Neurophysiol* 1992; 68:2033–2041.

Roy ML, Narahashi T. Differential properties of tetrodotoxin-sensitive and tetrodotoxin-resistant sodium channels in rat dorsal root ganglion neurons. *J Neurosci* 1992; 12:2104–2111.

Sangameswaran L, Fish LM, Koch BD, et al. A novel tetrodotoxin-sensitive, voltage-gated sodium channel expressed in rat and human dorsal root ganglia. *J Biol Chem* 1997; 272:14805–14809.

Satin J, Kyle JW, Chen M, et al. A mutant of TTX-resistant cardiac sodium channels with TTX-sensitive properties. *Science* 1992; 256:1202–1205.

Sleeper AA, Cummins TR, Dib-Hajj SD, et al. Changes in expression of two tetrodotoxin-resistant sodium channels and their currents in dorsal root ganglion neurons after sciatic nerve injury but not rhizotomy. *J Neurosci* 2000; 20:7279–7289.

Stebbing MJ, McLachlan EM, Sah P. Are there functional P2X receptors on cell bodies in intact dorsal root ganglia of rats? *Neuroscience* 1998; 86:1235–1244.

Tanaka M, Cummins TR, Ishikawa K, et al. SNS Na+ channel expression increases in dorsal root ganglion neurons in the carrageenan inflammatory pain model. *Neuroreport* 1998; 9:967–972.

Tate S, Benn S, Hick C, et al. Two sodium channels contribute to the TTX-R sodium current in primary sensory neurons. *Nature Neurosci* 1998; 1:653–655.

Toledo-Aral JJ, Moss BL, He ZJ, et al. Identification of PN1, a predominant voltage-dependent sodium channel expressed principally in peripheral neurons. *Proc Natl Acad Sci USA* 1997; 94:1527–1532.

Waddell PJ, Lawson SN. Electrophysiological properties of subpopulations of rat dorsal root ganglion neurons *in vitro*. *Neuroscience* 1990; 36:811–822.

Waxman SG, Kocsis JD, Black JA. Type III sodium channel mRNA is expressed in embryonic but not adult spinal sensory neurons, and is reexpressed following axotomy. *J Neurophysiol* 1994; 72:466–470.

Woolf CJ, Safieh Garabedian B, Ma QP, Crilly P, Winters J. Nerve growth factor contributes to the generation of inflammatory sensory hypersensitivity. *Neuroscience* 1994; 62:327–331.

Correspondence to: Jin Mo Chung, PhD, Department of Anatomy and Neurosciences, University of Texas Medical Branch, 301 University Boulevard, Route 1069, Galveston, TX 77555-1069, USA. Email: jmchung@utmb.edu.

Proceedings of the 10th World Congress on Pain,
Progress in Pain Research and Management, Vol. 24,
edited by Jonathan O. Dostrovsky, Daniel B. Carr, and
Martin Koltzenburg, IASP Press, Seattle, © 2003.

11

Inhibition of TTX-r Na^+ Currents in Rat Sensory Neurons by NW-1029, a New Antihyperalgesic Agent

Laura Faravelli, Ruggero G. Fariello, and Patricia Salvati

Newron Pharmaceuticals Research and Development, Gerenzano, Varese, Italy

After peripheral nerve injury, ectopic generation of action potentials can occur along the damaged axons or in their cell bodies within the dorsal root ganglion (DRG). This hyperexcitability and increased baseline sensitivity leads to abnormal spontaneous bursting and can cause chronic pain (Waxman et al. 1999). Based on their differential sensitivity to tetrodotoxin (TTX) and on their kinetic properties, Na^+ currents in the DRG have been classified into three subgroups: fast TTX-sensitive (TTX-s) currents are mediated by multiple Na^+ channel α subunits (Goldin 2001), slow TTX-resistant (TTX-r) currents have a high-voltage-dependent activation and inactivation, and persistent TTX-r currents have a much lower activation threshold (Cummins et al. 1999; Dib-Hajj et al. 2002). The different TTX-r currents are thought to be mediated by two sensory-specific Na^+ channels named Na_v 1.8 and Na_v 1.9, respectively, according to the new standardized nomenclature (Goldin et al. 2000).

Numerous studies have associated TTX-s and TTX-r Na^+ currents with chronic pain pathologies of both inflammatory and neuropathic types. Because of their selective expression in small-diameter DRG neurons, the channels encoding TTX-r currents are of particular interest because they may make important contributions to the membrane properties of nociceptors. Indeed, because of their different voltage sensitivities of activation and inactivation, TTX-r channels are still capable of generating impulses at depolarized potentials (which characterize the chronically damaged nerve fibers), whereas TTX-s channels are inactivated and cannot contribute to excitability (Elliott and Elliott 1993).

Furthermore, the dynamic relocalization of TTX-r Na^+ channels along the axonal membrane following nerve injury and their accumulation at the injury site represent the main mechanisms underlying the ectopic discharges responsible for both inducing and maintaining pain (Novakovic et al. 1998, 2001; Coward et al. 2000). Antisense studies using in vivo pain models (Porreca et al. 1999; Laj et al. 2002) have given further support to the hypothesis of a key role of TTX-r channels in the pathobiology of chronic pain, with a particular involvement of the Na_v 1.8 channel subtype.

Although no known drug exhibits selectivity toward Na^+ channel subtypes underlying TTX-r currents, over the past few years it has become increasingly apparent that Na^+-channel-blocking agents such as anticonvulsants (lamotrigine, topiramate, and carbamazepine), and local anesthetics and antiarrhythmics (lidocaine and mexiletine) offer benefit in neuropathic pain (Clare et al. 2000; Anger 2001).

NW-1029 is a new drug developed to treat chronic pain conditions by the oral route. Selected from several α-amino-amide derivatives, a novel chemical class of Na^+ channel blockers (Pevarello et al. 1999), it has demonstrated antinociceptive properties in animal models of inflammatory and chronic pain (Faravelli et al. 2000; Veneroni et al., in press).

This chapter describes a study that investigates the electrophysiological effects of NW-1029 on TTX-r Na^+ currents of acutely dissociated DRG neurons from adult rats. This study aimed to elucidate the mechanism of action of NW-1029 and explain its marked antihyperalgesic effect in animal models.

MATERIALS AND METHODS

CELL PREPARATION

Acutely isolated DRG neurons were prepared from adult Wistar rats (150–200 g). Animals were anesthetized and sacrificed by decapitation in accordance with the Guide for the Care and Use of Laboratory Animals (Clark et al. 1997). The spinal cord was exposed and removed. L4 and L5 DRG were plucked from their recesses and after the connective tissue had been removed they were enzymatically digested at 37°C for 30 minutes with collagenase/dispase (3 mg/mL) in Ca^{2+} free solution and for an additional 30 minutes with collagenase II-S (1 mg/mL). Ganglia were then mechanically dissociated using fire-polished Pasteur pipettes. Neurons were centrifuged and resuspended for plating on poly-L-lysine-coated Petri dishes in medium containing nerve growth factor (NGF) at 75 ng/mL. Cells were used for patch-clamp experiments after 1–24 hours.

PATCH-CLAMP RECORDINGS AND SOLUTIONS

Experiments were conducted on isolated cells using standard whole-cell patch-clamp methods. Membrane currents were recorded with an EPC7 patch-clamp amplifier. Data were digitized with a Digidata 1200 instrument. Voltage steps and data acquisition were controlled online using pClamp6 software. Access resistance ranged from 5 to 10 MΩ. Linear leakage and capacitative currents were eliminated using the P/4 subtraction protocol; the membrane currents were filtered at 10 kHz. Drug or control solutions were locally delivered by means of a rapid solution changer.

The external bath solution consisted of 60 mM NaCl, 60 mM choline Cl, 1.3 mM $CaCl_2$, 2 mM $MgCl_2$, 0.4 mM $CdCl_2$, 0.3 mM $NiCl_2$, 20 mM TEA Cl, 10 mM HEPES, and 10 mM glucose. TTX-r Na^+ currents were studied in the presence of 0.25 μM TTX. The patch electrode solution contained 65 mM CsCl, 65 mM CsF, 10 mM NaCl, 1.3 mM $CaCl_2$, 2 mM $MgCl_2$, 10 mM HEPES, 10 mM EGTA, and 1 mM Mg ATP. Stock solution of NW-1029 was made in distilled water at a concentration of 10 mM. It was diluted in the external bath solution to the desired final concentrations just before experiments.

STATISTICS

Drug concentration/inhibition curves were constructed according to the logistic equation $y = A2 + (A1 - A2)/[1 + (x/IC_{50})^p]$, where $A1$ and $A2$ are fixed values for 0% and 100% of current inhibition, respectively, x is the drug concentration, and IC_{50} is the drug concentration required to produce 50% current inhibition; p is the slope. For construction of steady-state inactivation curves, the peak current (I) was normalized relative to the maximal value (I_{max}) obtained at a holding potential (V_h) of –90 mV and plotted against the conditioning pulse potentials. Data were fitted by a Boltzman function according to the following equation: $I/I_{max} = 1/\{1 + \exp[(V - V_{1/2})/kh]\}$, where V is the membrane potential during prepulses, $V_{1/2}$ is the potential at which the half-maximal channel inactivation occurs, and kh is the slope of the line. Data points indicate means ± SEM; n refers to the number of cells in each experimental group. IC_{50} and $V_{1/2}$ are fitted values ± SE, where the latter represents the 95% confidence interval for the estimated parameter.

RESULTS

Cells used in this study had an average cell-body capacitance of 30.3 ± 1.1 pF (n = 33). Two Na^+ current phenotypes could be identified on the basis of their kinetics and their relative sensitivity to TTX in DRG sensory neurons, the fast TTX-s and the slow TTX-r currents. TTX-s Na^+ currents were completely blocked by 0.25 μM TTX, which was added to the external solution during the experiments in order to isolate and study the TTX-r currents. Current amplitudes ranged from 200 pA to 10 nA under the condition of reduced extracellular Na^+ concentrations.

NW-1029 (3–200 μM) reversibly reduced the amplitude of the peak Na^+ currents (tonic block) in a concentration-dependent manner. The effect was strictly dependent on the membrane potential. TTX-r Na^+ currents evoked from a resting membrane potential (V_h = –90 mV) were inhibited by NW-1029 with a mean IC_{50} of 130.7 ± 6.4 μM (n = 13). A voltage-dependent increase of the sensitivity to the drug was obtained when depolarized/inactivating preconditioning membrane potentials (V_h = –60 mV, V_h = –40 mV) were used, yielding lower IC_{50} values of 50.9 ± 7.1 μM (n = 13) and 11.9 ± 1.4 μM (n = 4), respectively (Fig. 1).

Repeated activation of TTX-r currents by trains of 50 depolarizing pulses at a frequency of 10 Hz further enhanced the inhibitory effects of NW-1029, due to the development of a use-dependent drug action (phasic block) (Fig. 2A,B). To quantify the use-dependent blocking potencies, concentration-inhibition curves were constructed from fractional block of the peak current during the 50th pulse. From a holding potential of –90 mV, the IC_{50} for the phasic block was 55.0 ± 3.3 (n = 8) (Fig. 2C; see the comparison with the tonic-block curve at the same V_h, –90 mV). Lowering the holding potential to –60 mV strongly enhanced the phasic block, yielding an IC_{50} of 10.0 ± 1.0 μM (n = 7) (Fig. 2D; see the comparison with the tonic-block curve at the same V_h, –60 mV).

Na^+ channel blockers acting in a use-dependent fashion are known to shift the availability curve of Na^+ currents depending on voltage in the hyperpolarizing direction. This mechanism of action was confirmed for NW-1029 by measuring the leftward displacement of the steady-state inactivation curves of TTX-r in the presence of the drug (50 μM). In control conditions, inactivation curves of TTX-r currents were characterized by $V_{1/2}$ values of –43.3 ± 0.4 mV (n = 7). NW-1029 shifted the inactivation curve by about 10 mV in the hyperpolarizing direction ($V_{1/2}$ = –52.5 ± 0.6 mV, n = 4) (Fig. 3A).

The influence of NW-1029 on the rate of recovery from inactivation also confirmed the preferential binding of the drug to the inactivated state of

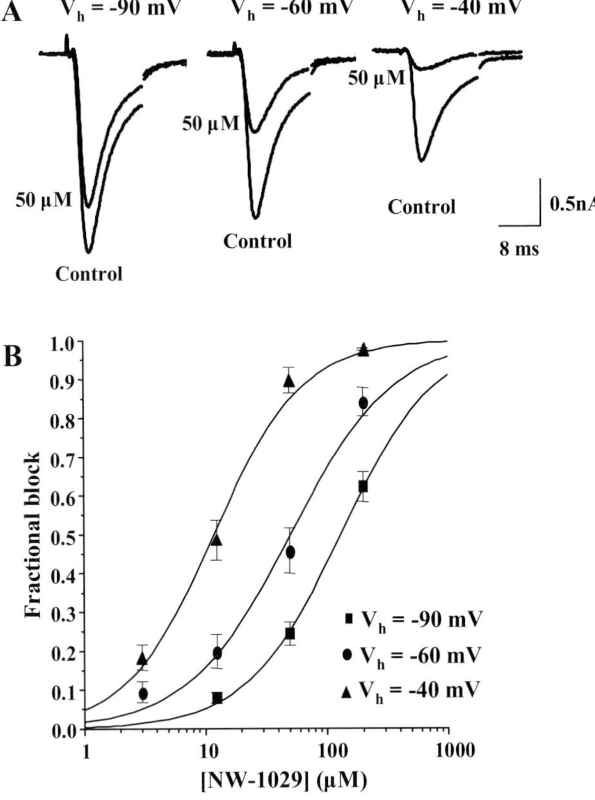

Fig. 1. Effect of holding potential on tonic block by NW-1029. (A) Representative recordings of whole-cell TTX-r Na^+ currents are evoked by a single depolarizing step to + 10 mV from different holding potentials in the absence and in the presence of NW-1029. (B) The amount of block, calculated in the condition of a single depolarizing step from the holding potentials indicated above, is plotted against blocker concentration. The half-maximal blocking concentrations for the best fits of NW-1029-induced tonic block are 130.7 ± 6.4 µM (*n* = 13) from –90 mV, 50.9 ± 7.1 µM (*n* = 13) from –60 mV, and 11.9 ± 1.4 µM (*n* = 4) from –40 mV.

the channels. Indeed, NW-1029 (50 µM) stabilizes the inactivated state by delaying the recovery from fast inactivation (Fig. 3B).

DISCUSSION

In a previous study that compared the electrophysiological effect of NW-1029 on TTX-r and TTX-s currents in cultured rat sensory neurons, we demonstrated that NW-1029's affinity for both types of Na^+ currents is almost

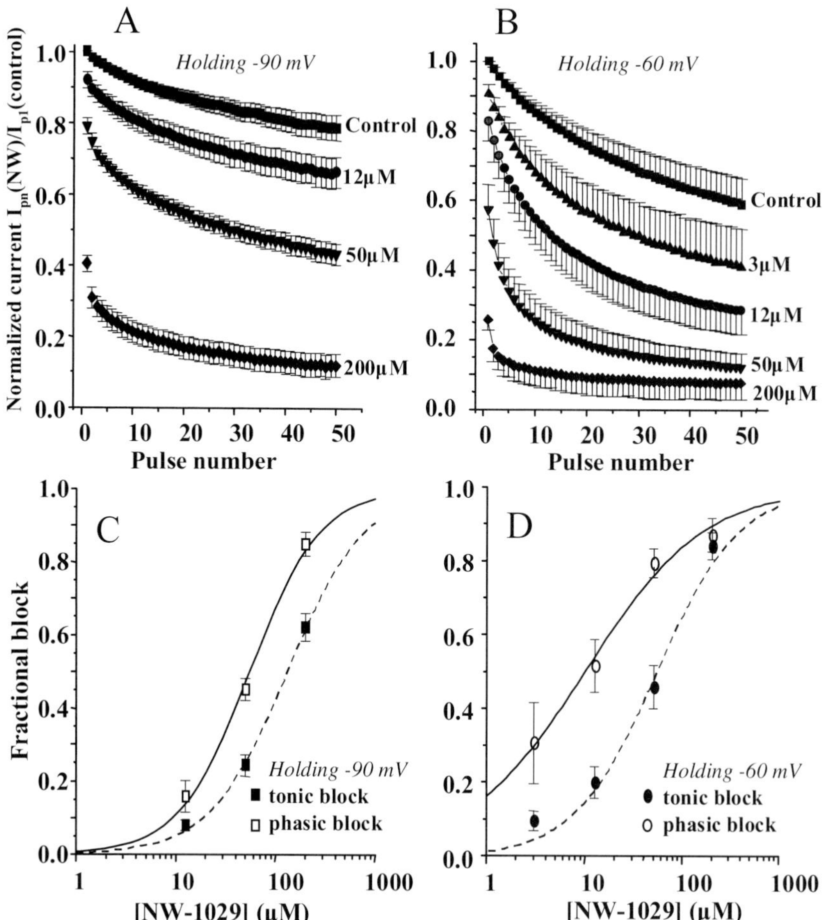

Fig. 2. Use-dependent block of TTX-r Na^+ currents by NW-1029. Upper panels: 50 consecutive pulses to 0 mV for 10 ms were delivered at 10 Hz from holding potentials of –90 mV (A) and –60 mV (B). Current amplitudes were normalized to the first amplitude evoked in the control condition and plotted as a function of the pulse number. Lower panels: concentration-inhibition curves for 10-Hz use-dependent block, from holding potentials of –90 (C) and –60 (D). Each phasic-block curve is compared to its relative tonic block. The potency of the drug for blocking the TTX-r channels under the condition of high-frequency stimulation was calculated using the value of the current at the 50th pulse in the presence of different concentrations of NW-1029 normalized with respect to the 50th episode in the absence of the drug. The resulting IC_{50}s for phasic block are 55.0 ± 3.3 (n = 8) from –90 mV and 10.0 ± 1.0 μM (n = 7) from –60 mV.

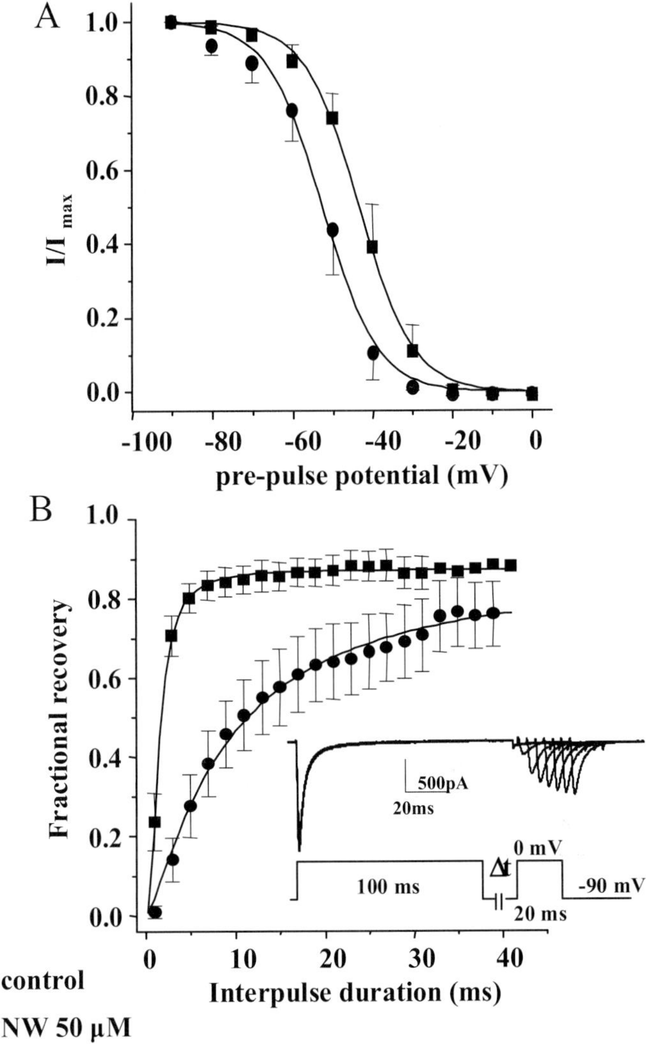

Fig. 3. Effects of NW-1029 on the inactivation properties of TTX-r Na^+ currents. (A) NW-1029-induced shift of the steady-state inactivation curve. The preconditioning potential was held at various levels for 1.8 seconds and was immediately followed by a 15-ms step depolarization to 0 mV. Na^+ current was normalized to its respective maximum value obtained from –90 mV and was plotted as a function of the pre-pulse potential. Half-maximal inactivating potentials in the absence and in the presence of NW-1029 are –43.3 ± 0.4 mV (n = 7) and –52.5 ± 0.6 mV (n = 4), respectively. (B) Effect of NW-1029 on the recovery from inactivation. A double-pulse protocol was used to determine the rate of recovery for TTX-r. Fractional recovery (peak current evoked with test pulse divided by peak current evoked during conditioning pulse) is plotted as a function of interpulse duration. The lines of best fit are a double exponential function with t values of 1.1 and 7.9 ms in the control condition and a single exponential with a t value of 9.5 in the presence of NW-1029.

the same when the channels are free of inactivation. However, a significant threefold higher selectivity for the TTX-r channels compared to TTX-s channels becomes apparent when depolarizing conditions lead the channels to the same level of inactivation (Faravelli et al. 2000).

The persistent low-threshold TTX-r current described by Cummins et al. (1999) and mediated by Na_v 1.9 channels activates so slowly and inactivates at such negative membrane potentials that they could not be detected with the voltage clamp protocols used in the present study. Thus, the TTX-r current recorded may reflect the activation of Na_v 1.8. Furthermore, in wild-type neurons, the only way to obtain Na_v 1.9 current is by a double-pulse protocol (Cummins et al. 1999). We believe that the attempt to separate them by subtraction of the biophysical properties of Na_v 1.9 current from the total TTX-r currents and to study their voltage and use-dependent modulation by drug application would lead to many interpretative errors.

In the present study we better characterized the functional effects of NW-1029 on the TTX-r Na^+ currents in acutely isolated sensory neurons from adult rats. In particular, the dependence of NW-1029-blocking properties on membrane potential and repetitive activation may be of relevance for the successful use of the drug in pain management. In peripheral fibers both TTX-r and TTX-s currents are expressed, but because of their biophysical properties, TTX-r currents are the best candidate for impulse generation under the pathological conditions found in the ectopic sites. Indeed, the voltage dependence of activation and inactivation of TTX-r currents lies in a more depolarized range of potentials compared to the TTX-s currents (Elliott and Elliott 1993). Thus TTX-r channels are available for generating spontaneous activity in the condition of sustained depolarized potentials that is characteristic of damaged peripheral fibers, while a much higher proportion of TTX-s channels have become inactivated. Our results lend support to this interpretation. In fact, in absence of the blocker the TTX-r current is only slightly reduced by depolarization, being the half-maximal steady state inactivation potential at –43 mV.

The inhibition of TTX-r currents was strictly voltage-dependent, characterized by a strong gain in the potency at depolarizing/inactivated conditions. Moreover, during high-frequency repetitive stimulations (10 Hz), NW-1029 produced a further decrease in the amplitude of Na^+ currents owing to the development of a use-dependent (phasic) block. Our data show that the depolarized membrane potential combined with repetitive firing has a strong impact on the NW-1029-induced blockage. Indeed, the half-maximal blocking concentration decreases more than 10-fold from 130 μM at –90 mV for tonic block to 10 μM at –60 mV for use-dependent block when stimulated at 10 Hz.

In terms of antihyperalgesic profile, this mechanism abolishes bursting activity in the damaged peripheral fibers, where TTX-r channels provide the basis for spontaneous firing of action potentials. On the other hand, healthy cells are less susceptible to the drug because of the intact negative membrane potential, so that physiological excitability is not affected.

The voltage- and use-dependent block can be rationalized in terms of preferential binding of the drug to the inactivated state of the channels. This interpretation is supported by the evidence that in the presence of NW-1029, a much higher proportion of Na^+ channels is kept in the inactivated state (as demonstrated by the NW-1029-induced hyperpolarizing shift of the steady-state inactivation curve), and the channels are prevented from becoming activated (shown as the NW-1029-induced delay in the recovery from inactivation).

In summary, our findings provide strong support for the hypothesis that NW-1029 blockade of Na^+ currents in sensory neurons and in particular the preferential drug activity against the TTX-r current in the condition of depolarized membrane are functionally important mechanisms underlying the antinociceptive effects observed in animal models of neuropathic and inflammatory pain (Faravelli et al. 2000, Veneroni et al., in press). Thus this drug may prove to be effective for the treatment of some types of chronic pain and is being prepared for phase I clinical trials.

REFERENCES

Anger T, Madge DJ, Mulla M, Riddall D. Medicinal chemistry of neuronal voltage-gated sodium channel blockers. *J Med Chem* 2001; 44(2):115–137.

Clare JJ, Tate SN, Nobbs M, Romanos MA. Voltage-gated sodium channels as therapeutic targets. *Drug Discovery Today* 2000; 5(11):506–520.

Clark JD, Gebhart GF, Gonder JC, Keeling ME, Kohn DF. Special report: the 1996 guide for the care and the use of laboratory animals. *ILAR J* 1997; 38(1):41–48.

Coward K, Plumpton C, Facer P, et al. Immunolocalization of SNS/PN3 and NaN/SNS2 sodium channels in human pain states. *Pain* 2000 85(1–2):41–50.

Cummins TR, Dib-Hajj SD, Black JA, et al. A novel persistent tetrodotoxin-resistant sodium current in SNS-null and wild-type small primary sensory neurons. *J Neurosci* 1999; 19(RC43):1–6.

Dib-Hajj S, Black JA, Cummins TR, Waxman SG. NaN/Nav1.9: a sodium channel with unique properties. *Trends Neurosci* 2002 May; 25(5):253–259.

Elliott AA, Elliott JR. Characterization of TTX-sensitive and TTX-resistant Na^+ currents in small cells from adult rat dorsal root ganglia. *J Physiol* 1993; 463:39–56.

Faravelli L, Maj R, Veneroni O, Fariello RG, Benatti L, Salvati P. NW-1029 is a novel Na^+ channel blocker with analgesic activity in animal models. *Soc Neurosci* 2000; 26(1):1218 (454.9).

Goldin AL. Resurgence of sodium channel research. *Annu Rev Physiol* 2001; 63:871–894.

Goldin AL, Barchi RL, Caldwell JH, et al. Nomenclature of voltage-gated sodium channels. *Neuron* 2000; 28(2):365–368.

Laj J, Gold MS, Kim C-S, Bian D, et al. Inhibition of neuropathic pain by decreased expression of the tetrodotoxin-resistant sodium channel, NaV1.8. *Pain* 2002; 95(1–2):143–152.

Novakovic SD, Tzoumaka E, McGivern JG, et al. Distribution of the tetrodotoxin-resistant sodium channel PN3 in rat sensory neurons in normal and neuropathic conditions. *J Neurosci* 1998; 18:2174–2187.

Novakovic SD, Eglen MR, Hunter JC. Regulation of Na^+ channel distribution in the nervous system. *Trends Neurosci* 2001; 24(8):473–478.

Pevarello P, Bonsignori A, Caccia C, et al. Sodium channel activity and sigma binding of 2-aminopropanime anticonvulsants. *Bioorgan Med Chem Lett* 9; 1999:2521–2524.

Porreca F, Lai J, Bian D, et al. A comparison of the potential role of the tetrodotoxin-insensitive sodium channels, PN3/SNS and NaN/SNS2, in rat models of chronic pain. *Proc Natl Acad Sci USA* 1999; 96:7640–7644.

Veneroni O, Maj R, Calabresi M, et al. Antiallodynic effect of NW-1029, a novel Na^+ channel blocker, in experimental animal models of inflammatory and neuropathic pain. *Pain;* in press.

Waxman SG, Dib-Hajj S, Cummins TR, Black JA. Sodium channels and pain. *Proc Natl Acad Sci USA* 1999; 96:7635–7639.

Correspondence to: Laura Faravelli, PhD, Electrophysiology Unit, Newron Pharmaceuticals, via Lepetit 34, 21040 Gerenzano, Varese, Italy. Email: laura.faravelli@newron.it.

Proceedings of the 10th World Congress on Pain,
Progress in Pain Research and Management, Vol. 24,
edited by Jonathan O. Dostrovsky, Daniel B. Carr, and
Martin Koltzenburg, IASP Press, Seattle, © 2003.

12

Peripheral Glutamate Receptors: Novel Targets for Analgesics?[1]

Susan M. Carlton,[a] Terry A. McNearney,[b] and Brian E. Cairns[c,d]

[a]*Department of Anatomy and Neurosciences, Marine Biomedical Institute, and* [b]*Department of Internal Medicine and Microbiology and Immunology, and Anatomy and Neurosciences, University of Texas Medical Branch, Galveston, Texas, USA;* [c]*Department of Anesthesia, Harvard Medical School, Boston, Massachusetts, USA;* [d]*Children's Hospital, Boston, Massachusetts, USA*

It has been over 15 years since the first experiments confirmed the presence of glutamate receptors on primary afferent neurons (Agrawal and Evans 1986; Evans et al. 1987; Lewis et al. 1987; Lovinger and Weight 1988). Since then animal and human studies have confirmed that glutamate and its receptors contribute to nociceptive processing and thus offer novel targets for treatment of pain of peripheral origin.

A ROLE FOR PERIPHERAL GLUTAMATE RECEPTORS IN ACUTE AND INFLAMMATORY PAIN

Several lines of evidence indicate that glutamate receptors in the skin contribute to normal nociception and to the persistent pain of inflammation. Anatomical studies confirm that dorsal root ganglion (DRG) neurons express the ionotropic glutamate receptors. Virtually all DRG cells have *N*-methyl-D-aspartate (NMDA) receptors, but only subpopulations of neurons express kainate and α-amino-3-hydroxy-5-methyl-4-isoxazole propionate (AMPA) receptors (Sato et al. 1993). Immunohistochemistry at the electron microscopic level demonstrates that 48 ± 18% of unmyelinated axons in the rat digital nerve are positively labeled for the R1 subunit of the NMDA

[1] Based on a Congress workshop.

receptor, while 27 ± 3% and 23 ± 8% are labeled for subunits of the kainate and AMPA receptors, respectively (Coggeshall and Carlton 1998). Activation of these receptors following intraplantar injection of glutamate or specific glutamate receptor ligands results in increased mechanical and thermal sensitivity (Fig. 1A) (Carlton et al. 1995, 1998; Zhou et al. 1996). Recording from identified nociceptors using an in vitro skin-nerve preparation demonstrates that nociceptors are excited and sensitized by application of glutamate (Du et al. 2000) or NMDA (Fig. 1B) (Du et al. 2003) and that glutamate will sensitize nociceptors to heat.

We used the complete Freund's adjuvant (CFA) model of inflammation to demonstrate that 48 hours after application of CFA, the number of digital

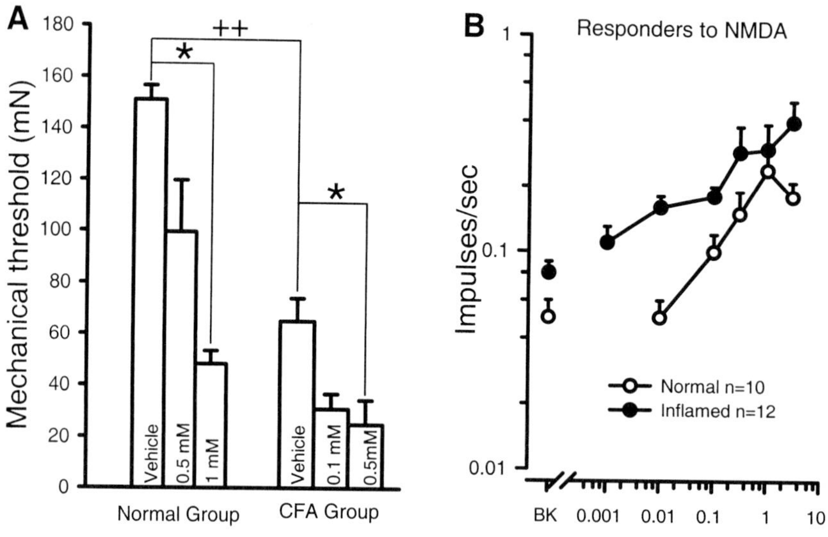

Fig. 1. (A) Behavioral responses to intraplantar NMDA. Subcutaneous injection of NMDA in normal and 5-day CFA-inflamed hindpaws results in a significant decrease in the von Frey threshold. Injection of 1 mM NMDA in normal animals can induce an enhanced mechanical sensitivity equivalent to that seen in the inflamed state; 0.5 mM NMDA in normal animals has no significant effect but produces a significant decrease in threshold in CFA-injected animals ($n = 6$ animals for each concentration except for CFA vehicle where $n = 12$; $*P < 0.05$, $++P < 0.01$, Kruskal-Wallis followed by Dunn's test). (B) Dose-response curves of nociceptor responses to NMDA. The curves illustrate the discharge rate of NMDA "responders" in normal (10/21) and inflamed (12/15) skin. Responders are units in which NMDA-generated activity is greater than the mean + 2 SD of mean background (BK) activity. Note the shift to the left in the dose-response curve for NMDA-induced excitation of nociceptors in inflamed compared to normal skin. An asterisk (*) indicates a significant increase compared to the background (Friedman's ANOVA followed by Dunnett's post hoc test, $P < 0.05$).

axons expressing the ionotropic glutamate receptors significantly increases (Carlton and Coggeshall 1999). These results suggest an increased potential for activation of glutamate receptors in the inflamed state. Intraplantar injection of NMDA results in enhanced mechanical sensitivity as previously reported (Zhou et al. 1996), and 1 mM NMDA in normal animals produces a change in mechanical sensitivity that is equivalent to that seen 48 hours post-CFA injection (Fig. 1A). Furthermore, concentrations of NMDA that have no effect in normal animals significantly reduce mechanical thresholds in the inflamed hindpaw (Fig. 1A). These data suggest that subthreshold concentrations of glutamate activate glutamate receptors in the inflamed hindpaw. In the skin-nerve preparation, a slight shift to the left in the dose-response curve for NMDA-induced activation of nociceptors indicates that NMDA induces activity in nociceptors in both normal and inflamed skin. The amount of NMDA required to induce activation is reduced in inflamed skin (Fig. 1B). Furthermore, NMDA lowers thresholds and increases nociceptor activity to heat in normal and inflamed skin. The percentage of NMDA-activated nociceptors is significantly increased in inflamed compared to normal skin, and this activity can be blocked by coapplication of the NMDA antagonist MK-801 (Du et al. 2003).

Primary afferents may be a source of ligand for activation of peripheral glutamate receptors because DRG cells contain glutamate at concentrations considered to be higher than that representing metabolic stores (Battaglia and Rustioni 1988). Stimulation of primary afferent fibers in the non-noxious or noxious range results in release of glutamate from peripheral primary afferent terminals (deGroot et al. 2000). Given that glutamate receptors are localized on peripheral nociceptors and primary afferents contain and release glutamate, it is probable that through autocrine or paracrine regulation, glutamate can initiate or enhance the activity of nociceptors.

Several lines of evidence suggest that glutamate content increases in inflamed tissue in animal and human studies. Nerves innervating inflamed knee joints show an increase in glutamate immunoreactivity, suggesting enhanced glutamate content (Westlund et al. 1992). Glutamate content increases in inflamed hindpaws (Omote et al. 1998). Macrophages (Piani et al. 1991) and sera (McAdoo et al. 1997) that infiltrate inflamed regions will contribute to the glutamate content. In human studies, glutamate content increases in the synovial fluid of arthritic patients (McNearney et al. 2000) and glutamate immunoreactivity increases in inflamed human skin (Nordlind et al. 1993). Thus, inflamed regions offer a ready source of ligand for glutamate receptors. Glutamate receptors are present on unmyelinated axons in human skin (Kinkelin et al. 2000), and local treatment of the skin with ketamine, an NMDA antagonist, reduces hyperalgesia associated with experimental burn injuries (Warncke et al. 1997).

These recent findings indicate that modulation of peripheral glutamate receptors may provide a non-opioid approach to pain control. Formulation of glutamate receptor antagonists that do not cross the blood-brain barrier may reduce peripheral nociceptor activity while avoiding central side effects. Glutamate antagonists could be used in the periphery in combination with drugs that target the central nervous system. This approach would be more efficacious in relieving pain of peripheral origin because it would target nociceptors to reduce peripheral sensitization and also target dorsal horn neurons to reduce central sensitization.

THE EXCITATORY AMINO ACIDS IN ARTHRITIS

Over 90% of the population will suffer from arthritis at some point in life. The present treatment regimens for arthritis cannot completely stop arthritis inflammation and pain. The cost of arthritis to the United States in medicines, disability, and lost wages is estimated at $60 billion dollars per year. The involvement of neurogenic mediators in human arthritis has been clinically observed for many years. Several case reports and case series (usually in stroke) document the sparing of arthritis on the paralyzed side, compared to the contralateral, neurologically intact side in rheumatoid arthritis, gout, and osteoarthritis (Winter 1952; Thomason and Bywater 1962; Glyn and Clayton 1976). One case report describes the reversal of established joint damage after a stroke, with improvement of erosions and partial reversal of the ulnar deviation (Velayos and Cohen 1972). These reports encouraged studies to determine whether neurotransmitter substances might be released into the joint and contribute to arthritis.

The Westlund laboratory has published a substantial body of work, first characterizing the neurotransmitter changes in the spinal cord and later describing glutamate receptor activation in the periphery with initiation of experimental arthritis (Sluka and Westlund 1993b; Sluka et al. 1995; Lawand et al. 1997b, 2000). Reports from experimental models suggest that several neurogenic mediators of inflammation and pain affect the course of arthritis. These mediators include substance P, calcitonin gene-related peptide (CGRP), and excitatory amino acids (EAAs) such as glutamate. Substance P causes plasma extravasation and vasodilatation (Sluka and Westlund 1993b). CGRP also causes vasodilatation (Schwab et al. 1997). Moreover, hyperalgesia does not develop in CGRP knockout animals (Zhang et al. 2001). Glutamate is involved in joint swelling and increased nociception (Chapman and Dickenson 1992; Sluka and Westlund 1993a).

Elucidation of the dorsal root reflexes has greatly improved our understanding of neurogenic contributions to peripheral inflammation. Pathological events in the periphery cause the central terminals of the primary afferent fibers to initiate action potentials back out to the periphery that probably release peptides, EAAs such as glutamate, aspartate, and inflammatory mediators from nociceptive terminals into the joints (Sluka et al. 1995).

Previous studies have demonstrated that intra-articular kaolin and carrageenan-induced arthritic measures in rats could be significantly reduced by pre-administration of lidocaine (Lawand et al. 2000) (Fig. 2A), a glutamate receptor antagonist (Sluka et al. 1994a), or by previous dorsal rhizotomy (Sluka et al. 1994b). Blood flow measured by Doppler markedly increases following release of glutamate into the joint (Fig. 2B; N.B. Lawand, K.N. Westlund, and W.D. Willis, unpublished data). Behavioral responses have also been characterized in the context of neurogenic inflammation. Intra-articular injections of EAA reduce paw withdrawal latency to heat and withdrawal threshold to mechanical stimuli that last for 4–8 hours (Fig. 3) (Lawand et al. 1997b).

To characterize the role of EAA in human arthritis, we analyzed synovial fluid (SF) from 144 patients with active arthritis and found a mean 4.61-fold increase in glutamate and 2.15-fold increase in aspartate, compared to metabolic control amino acids (Fig. 4A) (McNearney et al. 2000). Levels of glutamate and aspartate in SF were independent of SF cell counts and can be independent of other body compartments, such as plasma and SF simultaneously harvested from other joints, and reflect local pathology (McNearney et al. 1999). In cadavers, we noted marked mean plasma/SF EAA ratios for samples harvested <24 hours after witnessed death, and compared them to 10 additional amino acid ratios studied. Results provided further support that EAA concentrations in body compartments can be independent and may reflect the presence of glutamate transporter mechanisms previously described in neuronal tissue (Sonnewald et al. 2002).

Neurogenic and inflammatory mediators also contribute to pain states. Increasing numbers of studies are characterizing neurotransmitter-immune interactions and their consequences. In our comparison of mean SF EAA levels to SF inflammatory mediators tumor necrosis factor α (TNF-α), RANTES, MIP-1α, and interleukin-8 (IL-8), we noted a significant correlation (T.A. McNearney, unpublished data). Evidence suggests that cytokine antagonists or immunosuppression diminish hyperalgesia and allodynia in animal models (Lawand et al. 1997a; Hashizume et al. 2000; Sweitzer et al.

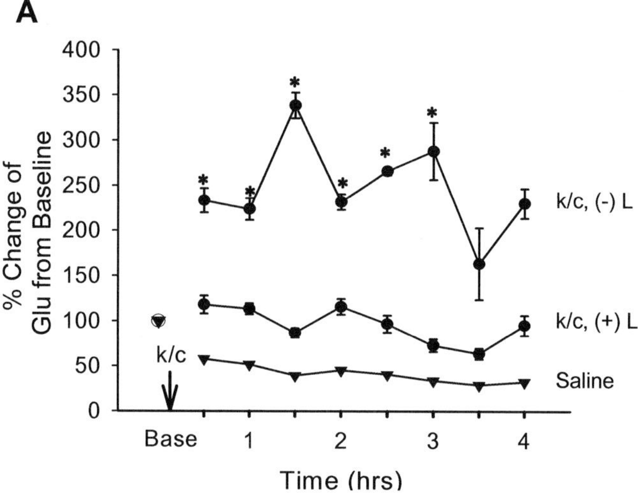

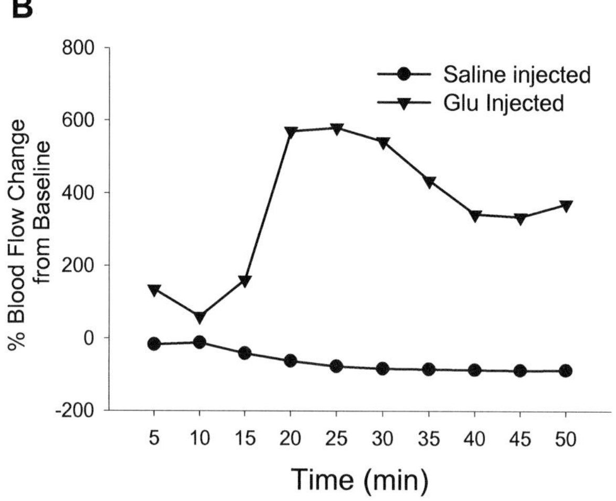

Fig. 2. (A) Pretreatment of rats with intra-articular lidocaine (L) abrogates the increased glutamate (Glu) levels in the synovial fluid (SF) due to arthritis induced by kaolin and carrageenan (k/c). Intra-articular injection of saline does not affect SF glutamate levels. $N = 6$. Reprinted from Lawand et al. (2000), with permission. (B) Intra-articular glutamate injection increases blood flow to the rat joint. Injection of intra-articular glutamate increased blood flow to the joint to six-fold over intra-articular saline controls by Doppler measurements. The effect was sustained for over 50 minutes. $N = 4$.

Fig. 3. Intra-articular injections of the excitatory amino acids glutamate and/or aspartate result in decreased paw-withdrawal latency to radiant heat (A) and withdrawal thresholds to innocuous mechanical stimuli (B), compared to phosphate buffer (PB) controls. The effects lasted 4 hours in rats and could be abrogated by glutamate receptor antagonists. Reprinted from Lawand et al. (1997b), with permission. →

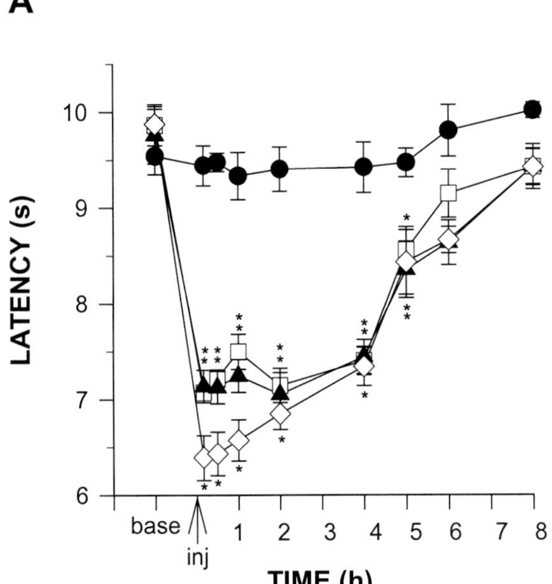
A
LATENCY (s)
10
9
8
7
6
base
inj
1 2 3 4 5 6 7 8
TIME (h)
PB
ASP/GLU
ASP/ARG
ASP/GLU/ARG

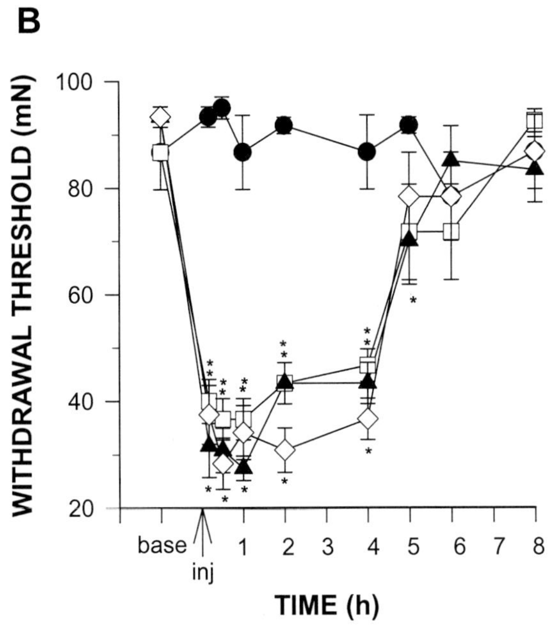
B
WITHDRAWAL THRESHOLD (mN)
100
80
60
40
20
base
inj
1 2 3 4 5 6 7 8
TIME (h)

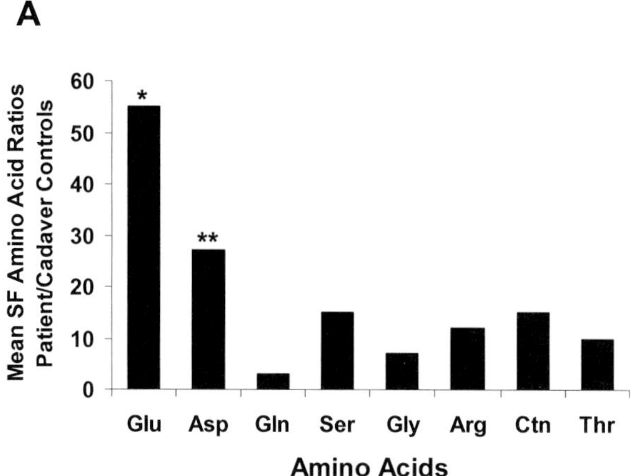

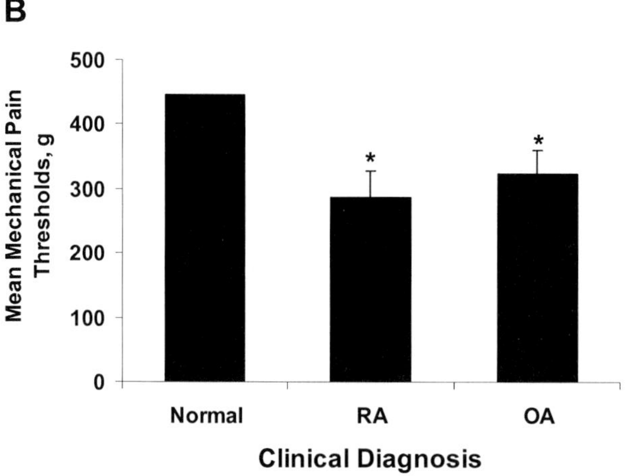

Fig. 4. (A) Mean synovial fluid (SF) glutamate (Glu) and aspartate (Asp) levels are elevated in patients with arthritis, compared to amino acids assessed as metabolic controls. * $P < 0.05$ compared to other amino acids; ** $P < 0.05$ compared to Gln, Gly, Arg, and Thr. (B) Mean total mechanical pain thresholds (measured in grams) are decreased in rheumatoid arthritis (RA) and osteoarthritis (OA) patients, compared to normal controls. * $P < 0.05$ compared to normal controls. Average of both knees of each patient or control. Mechanical pain thresholds were measured by von Frey monofilaments. Reprinted from McNearney et al. (2000), with permission.

2001). Evidence also indicates that glutamate receptor antagonists, or neural interruption, diminishes hyperalgesia and allodynia in animal models (Sluka et al. 1994a; Willis 2001). Patients having active arthritis (rheumatoid arthritis or osteoarthritis) longer than 3 months were assessed for mechanical sensation and pain thresholds related to reported pain, surface joint temperature, and joint circumference. They demonstrated significantly decreased mechanical pain thresholds (Fig. 4B) and significantly increased mechanical sensation thresholds compared to normal subjects with no arthritis or reported pain. The mechanical pain thresholds significantly correlate to surface joint temperature (Hendiani et al. 2003).

In summary, appreciation is growing for the role of neurotransmitters in human arthritic states, particularly that of glutamate in peripheral inflammation. Increasing evidence suggests that the animal models will correlate to the arthritic indices in humans. Characterization of the abnormal pain states will enhance the search for novel and synergistic therapies to more effectively manage the pain and inflammation of human arthritis.

PERIPHERAL GLUTAMATE RECEPTORS IN DEEP CRANIOFACIAL TISSUE

The demonstration of an association between peripheral glutamate receptor activation and craniofacial pain could lead to the development of novel analgesics for the treatment of craniofacial pain conditions. Both NMDA and non-NMDA receptors are found on trigeminal ganglion neurons and can be activated by glutamate to depolarize both large- and small-diameter trigeminal ganglion neurons in vitro (Puil and Spigelman 1988; Sahara et al. 1997; Pelkey and Marshall 1998). In an acute rat model of inflammatory temporomandibular joint (TMJ) injury, the inflammatory irritant and algogenic compound mustard oil is injected into the TMJ to evoke prolonged jaw muscle reflex responses. Preinjection of the noncompetitive NMDA-receptor antagonist MK801 into the TMJ attenuates this activity (Yu et al. 1996). Similar jaw muscle reflexes can be evoked in a concentration-related manner by injection of glutamate (50–1000 mM), or of the selective glutamate receptor agonists NMDA, AMPA, and kainate, into the TMJ (Cairns et al. 1998). Jaw muscle reflex responses evoked by injection of glutamate can be significantly attenuated by injection of the competitive NMDA receptor antagonist DL-2-amino-5-phosphonovalerate (APV) or the non-NMDA-receptor antagonist 6-cyano-7-nitroquinoxaline-2,3-dione (CNQX). Taken together, these results suggest that peripheral NMDA and non-NMDA receptors are present in deep craniofacial tissues and can be activated to evoke reflex jaw muscle responses that are similar to those evoked by an algogenic compound.

To investigate the effect of glutamate on deep craniofacial afferent fibers, we developed an acute in vivo rat model that enabled simultaneous recording of the activity of trigeminal ganglion neurons and the jaw muscles in response to injection of glutamate into these tissues (Cairns et al. 2001b). A unique feature of this model is that it identifies TMJ and masseter muscle afferent fibers that project to the caudal brainstem, a principal projection target for small-diameter putative nociceptive afferent fibers from these tissues (Fig. 5) (Nishimori et al. 1986; Capra 1987; Arvidsson and Raappana 1989). Recent findings indicated that TMJ and masseter muscle afferent fibers that project to the caudal brainstem have conduction velocities under 25 m/s (Cairns et al. 2001b, 2002a). Most of these afferent fibers are excited by injection of 500 mM glutamate into their receptive fields, although glutamate evokes the largest responses in afferent fibers with conduction velocities of less than 5 m/s (Fig. 5) (Cairns et al. 2001a,b). As with glutamate-evoked reflex responses, glutamate-evoked afferent fiber discharge appears to be due, in part, to peripheral NMDA-receptor activation because it can also be attenuated by APV (Cairns and Berde 2002). However, the duration of glutamate-evoked TMJ afferent discharge is shorter than that of reflex jaw muscle activity evoked by the injection of glutamate into the TMJ, which may indicate that the afferent barrage from these tissues is amplified by the central nervous system.

Injection of 1000 mM, but not 100 mM, glutamate into the rat masseter muscle also results in a prolonged (>30-minute) decrease in the mechanical threshold of the muscle afferent fibers (Cairns et al. 2002a). The extent of glutamate-induced afferent mechanical sensitization is not dependent on conduction velocity, initial mechanical threshold, or the sex of the rat. Despite the high concentration of glutamate required, osmosis-induced changes to the muscle tissue do not appear to play a role in glutamate-induced mechanical sensitization (Gambarota et al. 2001). Indeed, activation of peripheral NMDA and non-NMDA receptors underlies glutamate-induced mechanical sensitization of masseter muscle afferent fibers, given that co-injection of the NMDA and non-NMDA receptor antagonist kynurenate with glutamate into the masseter muscle significantly attenuates development of mechanical sensitization (Cairns et al. 2002a).

Prevalence of TMJ disorders and related craniofacial pain conditions is much greater among women of reproductive age, which suggests that sex-related factors may play a role in the pathogenesis of these conditions (Dao and Leresche 2000). Injection of glutamate into deep craniofacial tissues can be used as a tool to investigate the possible role of physiological mechanisms in these sex-related differences. In rats, injection of glutamate into the TMJ produces a concentration-dependent increase in reflex jaw muscle activity in both sexes. It evokes greater jaw muscle activity in females than in males when injected glutamate concentrations exceed 100 mM (Cairns et al. 2001b, 2002b). This sex-related difference disappears if female rats are gonadectomized and reappears if gonadectomized female rats are given estrogen replacement therapy. Further, glutamate-evoked TMJ and masseter

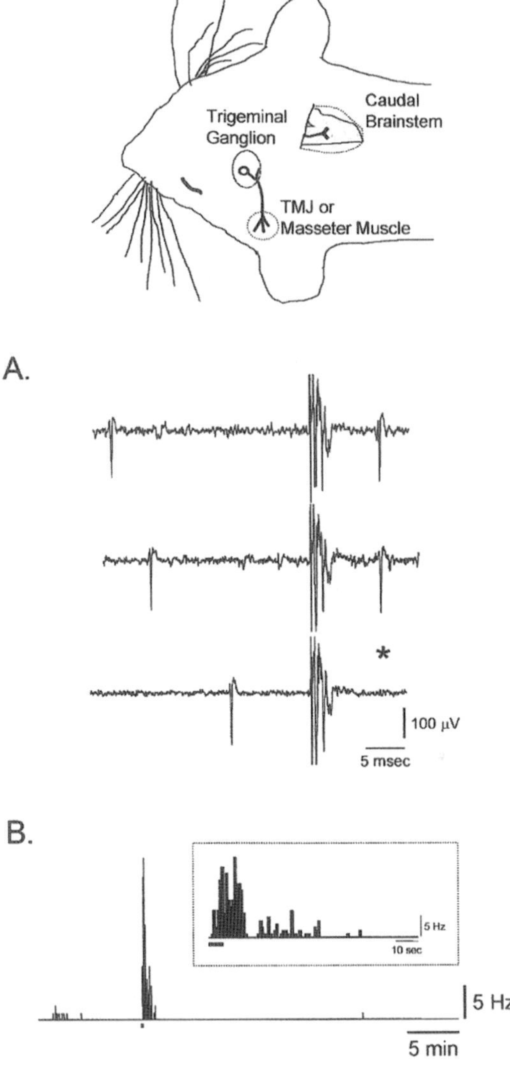

Fig. 5. The line drawing illustrates the projection pathway of putative nociceptive TMJ and masseter muscle afferent fibers through the trigeminal ganglion to the trigeminal subnucleus caudalis in the caudal brainstem. (A) The projection of this fiber from the masseter muscle to the caudal brainstem was demonstrated by a collision (*) of the orthodromic action potential evoked by mechanical stimulation of the masseter muscle with the antidromic action potential evoked by electrical stimulation (indicated by the stimulus artifact) of the caudal brainstem. In addition to its projection to the caudal brainstem, the conduction velocity of this C fiber (1.4 m/s) and its high mechanical threshold (600 kPa) identify it as a putative muscle nociceptor. (B) Injection of glutamate (500 mM, 10 μL, black bar) into the receptive field of this afferent fiber evoked a brief afferent discharge. The inset box reveals in more detail the burst-pause nature of this glutamate-evoked C-fiber discharge.

muscle afferent fiber discharge is also significantly greater in female than in male rats, which suggests that a peripheral mechanism contributes to the observation of enhanced glutamate-evoked jaw muscle responses in female rats (Cairns et al. 2001a,b, 2002a). In contrast, injection of glutamate into the rat masseter muscle does not induce a sex-related difference in afferent sensitization (Cairns et al. 2002a).

Parallel experiments in human subjects can explore the relevance of animal findings to sex-related differences in deep craniofacial pain. Both sexes perceive injection of 500 or 1000 mM glutamate into the human masseter muscle as significantly more painful than injection of isotonic saline; however, the intensity of glutamate-evoked muscle pain is significantly greater in women than in men (Cairns et al. 2001a). Further, injection of 1000 mM, but not 100 mM, glutamate into the human masseter muscle results in a prolonged (>25-minute) period of mechanical sensitization that is similar in men and women (Svensson et al. 2003). Thus, injection of glutamate into deep craniofacial tissues evokes pain in human subjects and activates putative nociceptive afferent fibers and jaw muscle reflex responses in anesthetized rats that differ in a sex-related manner.

Relatively high concentrations of glutamate are required to evoke pain and afferent fiber discharge and it is not yet clear under what natural conditions tissue glutamate levels could be sufficiently elevated to cause masseter muscle or TMJ pain. Therefore, the development of clinically useful analgesic drugs that target peripheral glutamate receptors to treat craniofacial pain awaits experimental verification of a link between elevated craniofacial tissue glutamate levels, activation of peripheral glutamate receptors, and pain from deep craniofacial tissues.

ACKNOWLEDGMENTS

Work described in this chapter was supported by NIH grants NS27910 and NS40700 to S.M. Carlton; by grant PO1-NS11255 and funding from the Charles A. Dana Foundation to T.A. McNearney; and by grants from the Medical Research Council of Canada, the Canadian Arthritis Society, the Danish National Research Foundation, the National Institutes of Health, and the Boston Children's Hospital Pain Research Endowment Fund to B.E. Cairns. Special thanks to Dr. Karin N. Westlund for valuable comments and critical review of sections of this chapter.

REFERENCES

Agrawal SG, Evans RH. The primary afferent depolarizing action of kainate in the rat. *Br J Pharmacol* 1986; 87:345–355.

Arvidsson J, Raappana P. An HRP study of the central projections from primary sensory neurons innervating the rat masseter muscle. *Brain Res* 1989; 480:111–118.

Battaglia G, Rustioni A. Coexistence of glutamate and substance P in dorsal root ganglion neurons of the rat and monkey. *J Comp Neurol* 1988; 277:302–312.

Cairns BE, Berde CB. Glutamate excites muscle afferent fibers via activation of peripheral NMDA receptors. *Abstracts: 10th World Congress on Pain.* Seattle: IASP Press, 2002, p 156.

Cairns BE, Sessle BJ, Hu JW. Evidence that excitatory amino acid receptors within the temporomandibular joint region are involved in the reflex activation of the jaw muscles. *J Neurosci* 1998; 18:8056–8064.

Cairns BE, Hu JW, Arendt-Nielsen L, Sessle BJ, Svensson P. Sex-related differences in human pain and rat afferent discharge evoked by injection of glutamate into the masseter muscle. *J Neurophysiol* 2001a; 86:782–791.

Cairns BE, Sessle BJ, Hu JW. Characteristics of glutamate-evoked temporomandibular joint afferent activity in the rat. *J Neurophysiol* 2001b; 85:2446–2454.

Cairns BE, Gambarota G, Svensson P, Arendt-Nielsen L, Berde CB. Glutamate-induced sensitization of rat masseter muscle fibers. *Neuroscience* 2002a; 109:389–399.

Cairns BE, Sim Y-L, Bereiter DA, et al. Influence of sex on reflex jaw muscle activity evoked from the rat temporomandibular joint. *Brain Res* 2002b; 957:338–344.

Capra NF. Localization and central projections of primary afferent neurons that innervate the temporomandibular joint in cats. *Somatosens Res* 1987; 4:201–213.

Carlton SM, Coggeshall RE. Inflammation-induced changes in peripheral glutamate receptor populations. *Brain Res* 1999; 820:63–70.

Carlton SM, Hargett GL, Coggeshall RE. Localization and activation of glutamate receptors in unmyelinated axons of rat glabrous skin. *Neurosci Lett* 1995; 197:25–28.

Carlton SM, Zhou S, Coggeshall RE. Evidence for the interaction of glutamate and NK1 receptors in the periphery. *Brain Res* 1998; 790:160–169.

Chapman V, Dickenson AH. The combination of NMDA antagonism and morphine produces profound antinociception in the rat dorsal horn. *Brain Res* 1992; 573:321–323.

Coggeshall RE, Carlton SM. Ultrastructural analysis of NMDA, AMPA and kainate receptors on unmyelinated and myelinated axons in the periphery. *J Comp Neurol* 1998; 391:78–86.

Dao TTT, LeResche L. Gender differences in pain. *J Orofac Pain* 2000; 14:169–184.

deGroot JF, Zhou S, Carlton SM. Peripheral glutamate release in the hindpaw following low and high intensity sciatic stimulation. *Neuroreport* 2000; 11:497–502.

Du J, Koltzenburg M, Carlton SM. Glutamate-induced excitation and sensitization of nociceptors in rat glabrous skin. *Pain* 2000; 89:187–198.

Du J, Coggeshall RE, Carlton SM. N-methyl-D-aspartate (NMDA)-induced excitation and sensitization of normal and inflamed nociceptors. *Neuroscience* 2003; in press.

Evans RH, Evans SJ, Pook PC, Sunter DC. A comparison of excitatory amino acid antagonists acting as primary afferent C fibres and motoneurones of the isolated spinal cord of the rat. *Br J Pharmacol* 1987; 91:531–537.

Gambarota G, Cairns BE, Berde CB, Mulkern RV. Osmotic effects on the T2 relaxation decay of in vivo muscle. *Magn Reson Med* 2001; 46:592–599.

Glyn J, Clayton M. Sparing effect of hemiplegia on tophaceous gout. *Ann Rheum Dis* 1976; 35:534–535.

Hashizume H, Rutkowski MD, Weinstein JN, DeLeo JA. Central administration of methotrexate reduces mechanical allodynia in an animal model of radiculopathy/sciatica. *Pain* 2000; 87:159–169.

Hendiani JA, Westlund KN, Lawand N, et al. Mechanical sensation and pain thresholds in patients with chronic arthropathies. *J Pain* 2003; in press.

Kinkelin I, Brocker E-B, Koltzenburg M, Carlton SM. Localization of ionotropic glutamate receptors in peripheral axons of human skin. *Neurosci Lett* 2000; 283:149–152.

Lawand NB, Willis WD, Westlund KN. Blockade of joint inflammation and secondary hyperalgesia by L-NAME, a nitric oxide synthase inhibitor. *Neuroreport* 1997a; 8:895–899.

Lawand NB, Willis WD, Westlund KN. Excitatory amino acid receptor involvement in peripheral nociceptive transmission in rats. *Eur J Pharmacol* 1997b; 324:169–177.

Lawand NB, McNearney T, Westlund KN. Amino acid release into the knee joint: key role in nociception and inflammation. *Pain* 2000; 86:69–74.

Lewis SJ, Cincotta M, Verberne AJM, et al. Receptor autoradiography with [^{3}H]L-glutamate reveals the presence and axonal transport of glutamate receptors in vagal afferent neurones of the rat. *Eur J Pharmacol* 1987; 144:413–415.

Lovinger DM, Weight FF. Glutamate induces a depolarization of adult rat dorsal root ganglion neurons that is mediated predominantly by NMDA receptors. *Neurosci Lett* 1988; 94:314–320.

McAdoo DJ, Hughes M, Xu G-Y, Robak G, DeCastro R. Microdialysis studies of the role of chemical agents in secondary damage upon spinal cord injury. *J Neurotrauma* 1997; 14:507–515.

McNearney TA, Goel N, Lisse J, et al. Temporal fluctuations in excitatory and inhibitory amino acid profiles of synovial fluids derived from patients with arthropathies. *J Investig Med* 1999; 47:109A.

McNearney T, Speegle D, Lawand NB, Lisse J, Westlund KN. Excitatory amino acid profiles of synovial fluid from patients with arthritis. *J Rheumatol* 2000; 27:739–745.

Nishimori T, Sera M, Suemune S, et al. The distribution of muscle primary afferents from the masseter nerve to the trigeminal sensory nuclei. *Brain Res* 1986; 372:375–381.

Nordlind K, Johansson O, Liden S, Hökfelt T. Glutamate- and aspartate-like immunoreactivities in human normal and inflamed skin. *Cell Path Mol Path* 1993; 64:75–82.

Omote K, Kawamata T, Kawamata M, Namiki A. Formalin-induced release of excitatory amino acids in the skin of the rat hindpaw. *Brain Res* 1998; 787:161–164.

Pelkey KA, Marshall KC. Actions of excitatory amino acids on mesencephalic trigeminal neurons. *Can J Physiol Pharmacol* 1998; 76:900–908.

Piani D, Frei K, Do KQ, Cuénod M, Fontana A. Murine brain macrophages induce NMDA receptor mediated neurotoxicity *in vitro* by secreting glutamate. *Neurosci Lett* 1991; 133:159–162.

Puil E, Spigelman I. Electrophysiological responses of trigeminal root ganglion neurons in vitro. *Neuroscience* 1988; 24:635–646.

Sahara Y, Noro N, Iida Y, Soma K, Nakamura Y. Glutamate receptor subunits GluR5 and KA-2 are coexpressed in rat trigeminal ganglion neurons. *J Neurosci* 1997; 17:6611–6620.

Sato K, Kiyama H, Park HT, Tohyama M. AMPA, KA and NMDA receptors are expressed in the rat DRG neurones. *Neuroreport* 1993; 4:1263–1265.

Schwab W, Bilgicyildirim A, Funk RH. Microtopography of the autonomic nerves in the rat knee: a fluorescence microscopic study. *Anat Rec* 1997; 247:109–118.

Sluka KA, Westlund KN. Behavioral and immunohistochemical changes in an experimental arthritis model in rats. *Pain* 1993a; 55:367–377.

Sluka KA, Westlund KN. Spinal cord amino acid release and content in an arthritis model: the effects of pretreatment with non-NMDA, NMDA, and NK1 receptor antagonists. *Brain Res* 1993b; 627:89–103.

Sluka KA, Jordan HH, Westlund KN. Reduction in joint swelling and hyperalgesia following post-treatment with a non-NMDA glutamate receptor antagonist. *Pain* 1994a; 59:95–100.

Sluka KA, Lawand NB, Westlund KN. Joint inflammation is reduced by dorsal rhizotomy and not by sympathectomy or spinal cord transection. *Ann Rheum Dis* 1994b; 53:309–314.

Sluka K, Willis W, Westlund K. The role of dorsal root reflexes in neurogenic inflammation. *Pain Forum* 1995; 4:141–149.

Sonnewald U, Qu H, Aschner M. Pharmacology and toxicology of astrocyte-neurons glutamate transport and cycling. *J Pharmacol Exp Ther* 2002; 301:1–6.

Svensson P, Cairns BE, Wang K, et al. Glutamate-evoked pain and mechanical allodynia in the human masseter muscle. *Pain* 2003; 101:221–227.

Sweitzer S, Martin D, DeLeo J. Intrathecal interleukin-1 receptor antagonist in combination with soluble TNF-α receptor exhibits an anti-allodynic action in the rat model of neuropathic pain. *Neurosci* 2001; 103:529–539.

Thomason M, Bywater E. Unilateral rheumatoid arthritis following hemiplegia. *Ann Rheum Dis* 1962; 21:370–377.

Velayos E, Cohen D. The effect of stroke on well established rheumatoid arthritis. *Md State Med J* 1972; 21:38–42.

Warncke T, Jorum E, Stubhaug A. Local treatment with the *N*-methyl-D-aspartate receptor antagonist ketamine, inhibits development of secondary hyperalgesia in man by a peripheral action. *Neurosci Lett* 1997; 227:1–4.

Westlund KN, Sun YC, Sluka KA, et al. Neural changes in acute arthritis in monkeys. II. Increased glutamate immunoreactivity in the medial articular nerve. *Brain Res Rev* 1992; 17:15–27.

Willis W. Role of neurotransmitters in sensitization of pain responses. *Ann NY Acad Sci* 2001; 933:142–156.

Winter S. Unilateral Heberden's nodes in a case of hemiplegia. *NY State J Med* 1952; 52:349–350.

Yu X-M, Sessle BJ, Haas DA, et al. Involvement of NMDA receptor mechanisms in jaw electromyographic activity and plasma extravasation induced by inflammatory irritant application to temporomandibular joint region of rats. *Pain* 1996; 68:169–178.

Zhang L, Hoff AO, Wimalawansa SJ, et al. Arthritic calcitonin/alpha calcitonin gene-related peptide knockout mice have reduced nociceptive hypersensitivity. *Pain* 2001; 89:265–273.

Zhou Z, Bonasera L, Carlton SM. Peripheral administration of NMDA, AMPA or KA results in pain behaviors in rats. *Neuroreport* 1996; 7:1–6.

Correspondence to: Susan M. Carlton, PhD, Department of Anatomy and Neurosciences, University of Texas Medical Branch, MRB 2.138, 301 University Boulevard, Galveston, TX 77555-1069, USA. Tel: 409-772-2124; Fax: 409-772-2789; email: smcarlto@utmb.edu.

Proceedings of the 10th World Congress on Pain,
Progress in Pain Research and Management, Vol. 24,
edited by Jonathan O. Dostrovsky, Daniel B. Carr, and
Martin Koltzenburg, IASP Press, Seattle, © 2003.

13

The Differential Effect of Nociceptor Subtypes for Generating Chronic Pain[1]

Martin Koltzenburg,[a] Hermann O. Handwerker,[b] and H. Richard Koerber[c]

[a]*Institute of Child Health and Institute of Neurology, University College London, London, United Kingdom;* [b]*Institute of Physiology and Pathophysiology, University of Erlangen-Nuremberg, Erlangen, Germany;* [c]*Department of Neurobiology, School of Medicine, University of Pittsburgh, Pittsburgh, Pennsylvania, USA*

Unmyelinated afferent neurons are considerably heterogenous. These neurons differ in their neurotransmitter phenotype, their biophysical and receptive properties, and their central termination patterns. While psychophysical experiments in conjunction with differential nerve blocks and reaction time measurements have shown that unmyelinated nociceptive afferent fibers signal pain in humans, our understanding of the relative contribution of the different subtypes of C-fiber nociceptors for pain perception and hyperalgesia is incomplete. However, recent research has begun to indicate that the different subtypes of nociceptors contribute differentially to the generation of pain and hyperalgesia.

DIFFERENTIAL CONTRIBUTIONS TO HYPERALGESIAS BY DIFFERENT CLASSES OF NOCICEPTORS IN HUMAN SKIN

The technique of microneurography, the percutaneous recording of single nerve fibers, was first adapted to recordings of human afferent C fibers by Torebjörk and Hallin (1970) more than three decades ago. Since then this technique has been used extensively to study the discharge patterns of human cutaneous and muscle C-fiber nociceptors (Marchettini et al. 1996). The

[1] Based on a Congress workshop.

development of a refined "marking technique" that employs the postexcitatory slowing of unmyelinated axons for identification and characterization has made it possible to study for many hours responses from single C-fiber units in healthy subjects and in patients suffering from neuropathies (Schmidt et al. 1995; Campero et al. 1998; Orstavik et al. 2003).

On the basis of their postexcitatory subnormal and supernormal conduction, three classes of afferent C fibers have been distinguished in human skin nerves: *cold fibers,* which show very little postexcitatory slowing (Serra et al. 1999); *mechano-heat-sensitive nociceptors* (CMH, also named "polymodal," nociceptors), which have an intermediate level of slowing; and *mechano-insensitive* C fibers (CMi), which exhibit the most pronounced slowing upon repetitive stimulation (Weidner et al. 1999) (Fig. 1). CMi fibers also show a pronounced supernormal conduction when a conditioning spike precedes a test stimulus at short intervals (e.g., 20–50 ms), leading to higher conduction velocities within burst discharges (Weidner et al. 2002).

The discovery of CMi nociceptors, also known as "sleeping" or "silent" nociceptors, in human nerves has greatly changed our concepts of peripheral nociceptor mechanisms in humans (Schmidt et al. 1995; Torebjörk et al. 1996). This class comprises about 20% of the cutaneous nociceptors in the peroneal nerve. These fibers are insensitive even to destructive mechanical stimuli such as pricking with a hypodermic needle. However, a subgroup of these units is responsive to heating, with thresholds slightly above those of the CMH units. Most of the mechano-insensitive nociceptors are responsive to chemical irritants, in particular to capsaicin. Therefore, these fibers are "chemonociceptors" or "heat-chemonociceptors." A subgroup of the CMi units is highly sensitive to histamine and probably mediates itch sensations (Schmelz et al. 1997).

Under the influence of inflammatory mediators, CMi units regularly become responsive to mechanical stimuli, and start to respond to von Frey hair stimuli in the threshold range of CMH units of normal skin (around 30 mN). They are thus likely to contribute to inflammatory pain and hyperalgesias.

PRIMARY HYPERALGESIAS

Ample evidence indicates that the hyperalgesia to heating induced following a mild burn or injection of capsaicin is largely due to the sensitization of CMH units (LaMotte et al. 1982, 1992; Torebjörk et al. 1984). However, the concomitant primary mechanical hyperalgesia to blunt pressure that is mediated by C fibers (Kilo et al. 1994) cannot be due to CMH activity because these units often are desensitized after noxious heating or

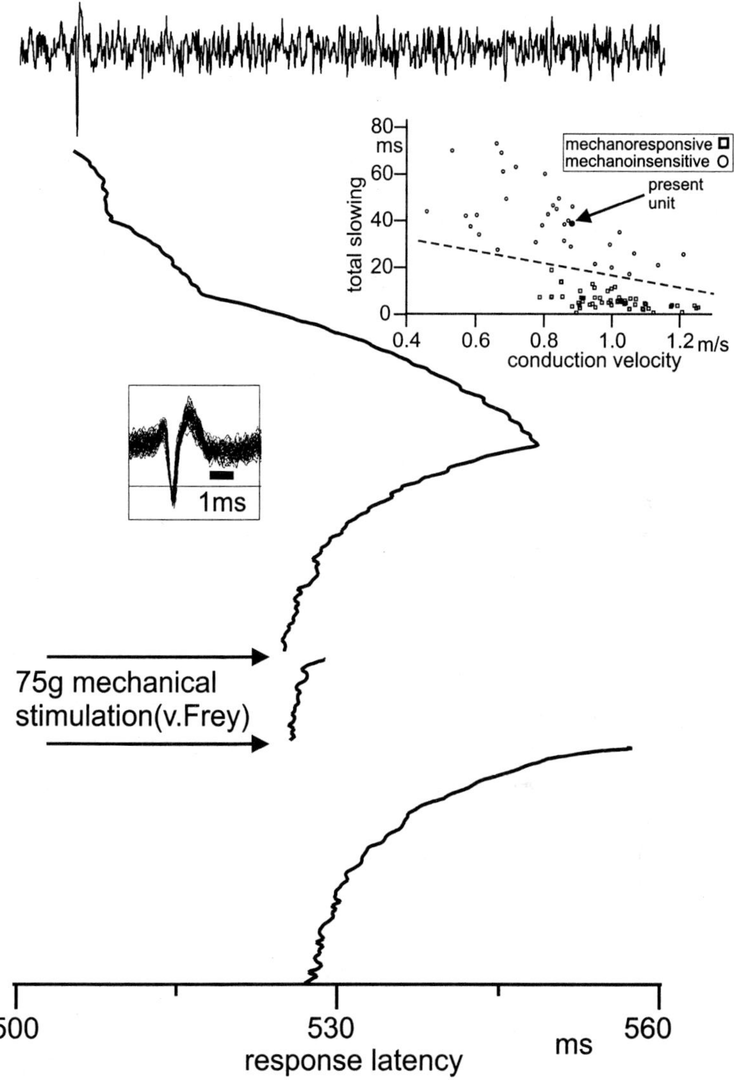

Fig. 1. Microneurography recordings from a C fiber in the superficial peroneal nerve of a patient suffering from erythromelalgia. The upper trace represents the recordings of a spike response following electrical stimulation of the nerve endings in the receptive skin field with a latency of about 500 ms. The trace running down from the spike shows the changes in conduction delay upon increasing stimulus frequency. According to its pronounced poststimulatory slowing and its slow conduction velocity this unit belongs to the class of "mechano-insensitive nociceptors" (see small scatter diagram; for details see Weidner et al. 1999). The small spike inset demonstrates the unitary spike form throughout the recording time of more than 2 hours. This unit was responsive to mechanical probing in the receptive field with a bristle of 750 mN bending force and is therefore a sensitized CMi unit. (Data from Orstavik et al. 2003.)

capsaicin application. In particular, intracutaneous capsaicin injection regularly leads to a rapid discharge in CMH fibers followed by desensitization after less than a minute. In contrast, after capsaicin injection CMi units show long-lasting discharges that after subsiding can be rekindled by warming the skin, which also elicits a burning pain sensation. Furthermore, these units become mechanically responsive after capsaicin treatment. This finding suggests that CMi, but not CMH, units mediate hyperalgesia to blunt pressure, besides mediating most of the input for the ongoing burning pain sensation after capsaicin.

SECONDARY HYPERALGESIAS

Secondary hyperalgesia to gentle stroking (also known as brush-evoked pain) is present in a wide area around a capsaicin injection site (LaMotte et al. 1991). Experiments with selective nerve blocks reveal that this kind of hyperalgesia is only detectable when conduction in large myelinated fibers is intact, and can be mimicked by intraneural electrical microstimulation of low-threshold mechanoreceptive afferents that normally signal nonpainful touch (Torebjörk et al. 1992). Brush-evoked pain disappears when the ongoing activity in the sensitized nociceptors is reduced. The close correlation between the nociceptor-mediated background pain and touch-evoked pain has also been observed in patients with neuralgia (Koltzenburg et al. 1994). Thus, it appears that this particular form of secondary hyperalgesia represents an altered response of the central nervous system to mechanoreceptor input and is a consequence of an ongoing nociceptor barrage. At least in the case of capsaicin-induced secondary hyperalgesia, the main sensitizing input is probably provided by CMi units that become tonically active.

Another form of secondary mechanical hyperalgesia, pinprick hyperalgesia, is largely independent of ongoing nociceptor barrage from the traumatized region. It has recently been shown to be related to altered central nervous responsiveness to the impulses of Aδ units (Magerl et al. 2002). Although not maintained by a peripheral input, this type of hyperalgesia is initiated by nociceptor firing, although it is unclear which nociceptor subtype is involved.

From the described model experiments with capsaicin injections or burn lesions it is obvious that CMi units play a crucial role in several forms of primary and secondary mechanical hyperalgesias, namely in primary hyperalgesia to blunt pressure and in secondary hyperalgesia to gentle touch. To what extent CMi units are involved in clinically important forms of more chronic hyperalgesias due to tissue damage or nerve lesions is currently under investigation.

We have recently studied patients suffering from long-standing erythromelalgia, a chronic painful condition that most often affects one foot or leg (Orstavik et al. 2003). In these experiments we have encountered units with the conduction-slowing characteristics of CMi units that were responsive to mechanical probings and hence presumably were chronically sensitized (see Fig. 1). In addition, spontaneous activity was observed in CMi units, which may explain the ongoing pain and hyperalgesia to gentle touch regularly encountered in this chronic pain condition.

IDENTIFICATION OF A SUBPOPULATION OF NOCICEPTORS IN VITRO

Activity-dependent slowing of C-fiber conduction velocity can also be demonstrated in rodents in vivo (Gee et al. 1996) and in vitro. We used a skin-nerve in vitro preparation of the mouse to record from functionally identified neurons innervating the hairy skin (Beggs et al. 2002). Following functional characterization the neurons were subjected to repetitive stimulation. When the neurons were stimulated every 3 seconds the latency of the electrically evoked response was stable. However, short periods of excitation of a unit interspersed between such low-frequency stimulation often resulted in strong latency shifts (Fig. 2). This activity-dependent slowing varied between different units and was correlated with the thermal sensitivity of the fibers. In the mouse the degree of activity-dependent slowing appears to correlate best with the heat sensitivity of nociceptors. Heat-sensitive fibers show a profound increase in latency on repetitive electrical stimulation, whereas heat-insensitive units show only a modest change of conduction velocity (Fig. 2A,B). This phenomenon is best illustrated by units that are both heat- and cold-sensitive in comparison to units that are sensitive to only one thermal modality. This finding indicates that the cellular mechanisms conferring thermal sensitivity are correlated with those that regulate activity-dependent slowing. Moreover, the pattern of activity-dependent slowing in rodents closely resembles that observed in human microneurography experiments, suggesting that the mechanisms underling activity-dependent latency slowing arc similar, if not identical, in rodents and humans.

The mechanisms for this activity-dependent slowing are not fully understood. It is minimal, if not absent, in myelinated nerve fibers. This finding could mean that activity-dependent slowing is caused by a differential recovery from the inactivation of sodium currents and that blockade of voltage-gated sodium channels can produce increases in conduction velocity. Another possibility is that the different activity profiles of the sodium pump

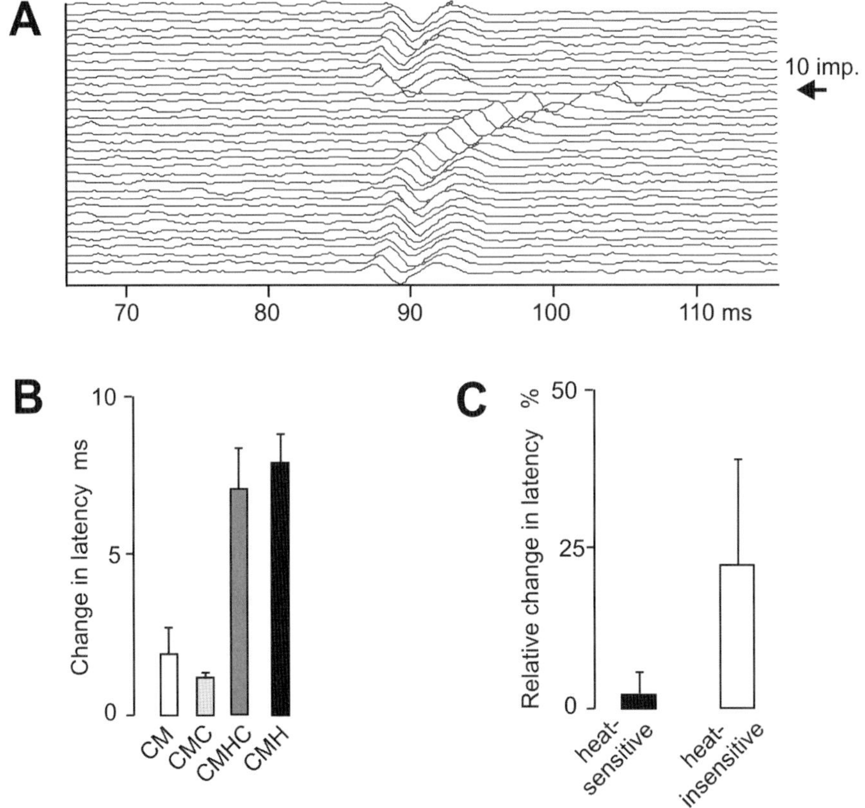

Fig. 2. Latency changes of mouse C fibers. (A) Response of a mechano-heat-sensitive C fiber to electrical stimulation at a regular interstimulus interval of 3 seconds. A short train of impulses (10 impulses at 10 Hz) during the interstimulus interval results in a significant delay in the latency. (B) Mean (± SEM) latency changes differ between different subtypes of C fibers. CM, mechanosensitive, CMC, mechano-cold-sensitive, CMHC, mechano-cold- and heat-sensitive, CMH, mechano-heat-sensitive. (C) Mean (± SEM) relative changes of the activity-dependent latency increases induced by 10 stimuli during the application of 10 μM of ZD7228. (Based on F. Pracher, S. Beggs, and M. Koltzenburg, unpublished data.)

could lead to this effect. Currently, the contribution of these two alternatives for the activity-dependent slowing is incompletely understood, but recent studies have implicated other voltage-gated cation channels.

THE PACEMAKER CURRENT Ih IS DIFFERENTIALLY EXPRESSED IN A SUBPOPULATION OF NOCICEPTORS

Studies using compound action potential recordings indicate that some of the activity-dependent slowing is related to a hyperpolarization-activated cation current (Ih) because blockers of this current such as cesium ions or the compound ZD7228 enhance the slowing (Takigawa et al. 1998). Hyperpolarization-activated currents are found in many excitable cells including central and peripheral neurons. Their best understood function is the pacemaker current in the sinoatrial node providing the inward current that slowly depolarizes the cells during diastole when the membrane is hyperpolarized after an action potential (Accili et al. 2002). Ih is encoded by four members of a gene family of hyperpolarization-activated, cyclic nucleotide-gated channels (HCN1–4), a branch of the superfamily of voltage-gated cation channels (Biel et al. 1999). HCN isoforms have been found in the dorsal root ganglion (DRG) using in situ hybridization (Moosmang et al. 2001), reverse transcription polymerase chain reaction, Western blotting, and immunohistochemistry (Huerta and Koltzenburg 2002). HCN1–3 channels are abundant in the DRG of mice, whereas HCN4, the isoform strongly expressed in cardiac tissue, appears to be absent. Interestingly, HCN isoforms are more strongly expressed in large cells than in small cells. Using capsaicin-induced cobalt uptake or calcium imaging in combination with immunohistochemistry, it is possible to correlate the functional properties of DRG neurons with the expression of various HCN isoforms and other neuronal markers. As expected from the preponderance of HCN in large cells, many neurons containing heavy chain neurofilament are capsaicin insensitive and strongly stain for HCN1 and 2. Amongst the small-diameter neurons, HCN1 and 2 can be found in both the peptidergic neurons, where it can be identified by staining for CGRP, and in the nonpeptidergic neurons, where it can be labeled with IB4. However, HCN staining is absent or of low intensity in cells that are capsaicin sensitive (Huerta and Koltzenburg 2002). By contrast, many cells that are cold or menthol sensitive show strong staining for HCN1 and HCN2. This expression pattern is consistent with the view that heat- and capsaicin-sensitive DRG neurons show absent or low levels of Ih and hence have marked activity-dependent slowing, whereas many cold-sensitive neurons express high levels of HCN and Ih and therefore display less slowing.

To test the functional importance of Ih in a subpopulation of sensory neurons, we recorded from identified cutaneous sensory afferents in vitro and tested the effect of blockers of Ih during electrical stimulation of the terminals. In the presence of cesium ions, many C fibers show a conduction block without significant prior slowing. It is presently unclear whether this effect of cesium can be attributed to blockade of Ih in this preparation. However, application of the more selective blocker of Ih, ZD7228, increases the activity-dependent slowing of heat-insensitive units more strongly than those of heat-sensitive fibers (Fig. 2C). This finding indicates that the presence of Ih normally prevents activity-dependent slowing in heat-insensitive units, whereas its relative lack of effect in heat-sensitive units is in agreement with the view that Ih is normally absent or weakly expressed in such units.

It is currently not established how the differential expression of Ih influences its receptive properties. In analogy to the pacemaker currents of the heart where blockade of Ih produces bradycardia, blockade of Ih in nociceptive neurons could dampen excitability and may therefore be a target for analgesic drugs. Conversely, increases in HCN expression could lead to an increase in excitability. Thus, knowledge of the factors that control HCN expression or modulate Ih currents would be important for our understanding of the excitability of nociceptors. The identification of subpopulations of nociceptors on the basis of their activity-dependent slowing may also be an important tool to identify the functional properties of C fibers, whose receptive properties cannot be studied after axotomy. Given that microneurographic studies in humans have shown that subpopulations of nociceptors contribute differentially to pain and hyperalgesia, it would be of importance to identify differences in their central connectivity. Detailed knowledge of the differential expression of Ih and the corresponding isoforms 1–3 of HCN may facilitate immunohistochemical investigations of the central projections and connections to second-order neurons that underlie the differential central effects of C fibers for generating pain and hyperalgesia.

CUTANEOUS NOCICEPTORS DURING DEVELOPMENT AND FOLLOWING NERVE INJURY

It is widely thought that following peripheral nerve injury, some large-diameter (Aβ) low-threshold mechanoreceptors produce collateral sprouts from the deep dorsal horn that ascend dorsally to provide novel input into laminae I and II (Woolf et al. 1992; Shortland et al. 1993; Koerber et al. 1989, 1994, 1999; Woolf et al. 1995). Sprouting of large-diameter, low-threshold fibers into nociceptive spinal regions following peripheral nerve injury provides an obvious potential substrate for resulting neuropathic pain syndromes such as mechanical hyperalgesia. Interestingly, during the first several weeks after birth, it is also thought that large-diameter (Aβ) low-threshold mechanoreceptors ignore the usual boundary separating them from C-fiber projections and project extensively in laminae I–II (Fitzgerald et al. 1994; Coggeshall et al. 1996). Similarly, the existence of low-threshold mechanoreceptive fibers projecting into the nociceptive regions of the spinal cord during development provides an attractive model to explain the phenomenon of neonatal hypersensitivity, whereby innocuous mechanical stimuli evoke a range of responses normally associated with noxious stimuli in adults.

Apart from its obvious implication for the generation of chronic pain, the transient presence of tactile inputs into spinal regions involved in nociception raises several interesting neurobiological questions, including the nature of the factors regulating the growth, retraction, and subsequent regrowth of these ectopic projections. In order to begin to answer these questions we decided to determine the identity of those myelinated fibers capable of supporting projections in laminae I–II during these states of altered central morphology. We used an ex vivo preparation of skin, nerve, and spinal cord that allowed us to evaluate the phenotypic characteristics of sensory neurons in a comprehensive fashion (Ritter et al. 2000; Woodbury et al. 2001). In these studies sensory neurons are impaled in DRG, and their somal membrane properties and peripheral response properties are characterized. The tracer neurobiotin is then injected to permit histological visualization of the cells and their peripheral and central projections.

Myelinated cutaneous sensory neurons exhibit diverse morphological and functional properties. Large and small myelinated fibers innervating cutaneous low-threshold mechanoreceptors have narrow uninflected somal spikes, rarely contain peptides, and have central projections confined primarily to laminae III–V. Large and small myelinated cutaneous nociceptive fibers have broad somal spikes with inflections on the falling phase of the spike, occasionally contain peptides, and are generally thought to have central projections primarily confined to laminae I and II_o or I, II_o, and V.

PROJECTIONS OF MYELINATED FIBERS DURING POSTNATAL DEVELOPMENT

We have used this ex vivo preparation to evaluate cutaneous sensory neurons during the first postnatal week. We have characterized, stained, and recovered the central projections of over 60 cutaneous sensory neurons. These fibers include all different fiber types ranging from large-diameter, low-threshold mechanoreceptors to nociceptive C fibers. We have analyzed the somal action potentials and central projections of 19 well-characterized and labeled low-threshold (mean 0.6 ± 1.3 mN) rapidly adapting afferents. These were a mixture of large-diameter fibers innervating guard-hair follicles and small-diameter fibers normally associated with down-hair follicles. An additional seven slowly adapting low-threshold (mean 0.2 ± 0.4 mN) mechanoreceptors were also characterized and stained. All of these low threshold cutaneous fibers had narrow uninflected somal action potentials, as seen in adult mice. In addition, these 26 fibers gave rise to 240 central collaterals that were indistinguishable from those seen in adult mice. That is, they had projections confined to laminae II_i–V and did not overlap with C-fiber projections in lamina II_o (Woodbury et al. 2001).

An additional 28 slowly adapting fibers with broad inflected somal spikes were also analyzed. These fibers had a wide range of peripheral thresholds (0.3–7.8 mN) and could be separated into two groups based on central morphology. The first group consisted of large- and medium-diameter fibers with relatively high mechanical thresholds (mean 3.2 ± 2.6 mN) that gave rise to projections ramifying in laminae I–II. The second group were of similar diameter but had somewhat lower mechanical thresholds (mean 1.5 ± 1.4 mN) and central projections traversing the entire dorsal horn (laminae I–V) (Woodbury and Koerber 1993).

In summary, the only myelinated cutaneous fibers that maintained projections that overlapped with C-fiber terminals were those with broad inflected somal action potentials and relatively elevated peripheral thresholds and response properties indicative of myelinated nociceptors.

PROJECTIONS OF MYELINATED FIBERS FOLLOWING PERIPHERAL NERVE INJURY

We have used the same preparation in adult animals to determine the identity of cutaneous fibers capable of supporting ectopic projections into the superficial dorsal horn following peripheral injury. The somas of peripherally regenerated fibers were impaled in thoracic DRG 2–7 weeks following transection of 7–9 consecutive dorsal cutaneous nerves. Each fiber's peripheral response properties (if any) were determined, its somal spike was recorded, and the cell was stained with neurobiotin. Using this approach we were able to examine the cell's central projections, somal morphology, and immunohistochemistry and investigate the peripheral morphology of individual regenerated fibers.

We have examined the central projections of 36 peripherally regenerated myelinated fibers. Of these, 25 fibers had conduction velocities in the Aδ–Aβ conduction velocity range and had brief uninflected somal spikes. Those that had successfully reinnervated the skin could be easily characterized as slowly adapting type I or rapidly adapting fibers innervating hair follicles. Analysis of the central projections of these fibers revealed morphological changes consistent with possible retraction and new growth. However, the projections were confined to the same spinal laminae as seen in intact preparations. That is, they did not give rise to ectopic projections in the superficial laminae.

In addition, 11 fibers in the same conduction velocity ranges had broad inflected somal spikes, and those that successfully reinnervated the skin had response properties indicative of myelinated nociceptors. Analysis of the central projections of these fibers revealed extensive collateralization throughout laminae I and II. Fibers giving rise to these projections were morphologically very similar to those seen during postnatal development. Some fibers had projections primarily in laminae I–II, while others projected across all dorsal horn laminae (I–V). These results suggest that following transection of cutaneous nerves, it is myelinated nociceptors, and not low-threshold mechanoreceptors, that are supplying direct inputs into the superficial dorsal horn.

PROJECTIONS OF MYELINATED NOCICEPTORS IN NAIVE ADULTS

There are two possible explanations for these observations. The first hypothesis is that put forth for low-threshold mechanoreceptors. At birth cutaneous myelinated nociceptors give rise to extensive projections throughout the superficial laminae (I–II), and during maturation most of the projections in lamina II are retracted and replaced by C-fiber inputs. Subsequent peripheral injury induces collateral sprouting of these fibers that reinstates their neonatal morphology. The second hypothesis is that the central projections of myelinated nociceptors have not been adequately studied in the past and that the neonatal projections are retained throughout life.

In order to determine which of these possible explanations was correct, we conducted more experiments in intact animals focusing specifically on this population of myelinated nociceptive fibers. Recently, we have examined six myelinated nociceptors (both Aβ and Aδ) in naive adult control preparations. All six gave rise to extensive projections throughout the superficial dorsal horn. The basic central morphology and peripheral response properties, including mechanical thresholds, of these fibers were indistinguishable from those seen for myelinated nociceptors observed in the neonatal preparations.

In conclusion, shortly after birth cutaneous myelinated nociceptors and low-threshold mechanoreceptors are essentially miniature replicas of those found in adults. Given the locations of their central terminations in the superficial dorsal horn, myelinated nociceptors are positioned to provide direct inputs to the superficial layers during development and following injury. These inputs previously were thought to be provided by ectopic sprouts of low threshold mechanoreceptors.

REFERENCES

Accili EA, Proenza C, Baruscotti M, DiFrancesco D. From funny current to HCN channels: 20 years of excitation. *News Physiol Sci* 2002; 17:32–37.

Beggs S, Pracher F, Koltzenburg M. Heat sensitivity of mouse C-fibre afferents as a predictor of use-dependent slowing. *Abstracts: 10th World Congress on Pain.* Seattle: IASP Press, 2002, p 465.

Biel M, Ludwig A, Zong X, Hofmann F. Hyperpolarization-activated cation channels: a multi-gene family. *Rev Physiol Biochem Pharmacol* 1999; 136:165–181.

Campero M, Serra J, Marchettini P, Ochoa JL. Ectopic impulse generation and auto excitation in single myelinated afferent fibers in patients with peripheral neuropathy and positive sensory symptoms. *Muscle Nerve* 1998; 21:1661–1667.

Coggeshall RE, Jennings EA, Fitzgerald M. Evidence that large myelinated primary afferent fibers make synaptic contacts in lamina II of neonatal rats. *Dev Brain Res* 1996; 92:81–92.

Fitzgerald M, Butcher T, Shortland P. Developmental changes in the laminar termination of A-fiber cutaneous sensory afferents in the rat spinal cord dorsal horn. *J Comp Neurol* 1994; 348:225–233.

Gee MD, Lynn B, Cotsell B. Activity-dependent slowing of conduction velocity provides a method for identifying different functional classes of C-fibre in the rat saphenous nerve. *Neuroscience* 1996; 73:667–675.

Huerta JJ, Koltzenburg M. HCN channel distribution in mouse DRG sensory neurons. *Abstracts: 10th World Congress on Pain.* Seattle: IASP Press, 2002, p 485.

Koerber HR, Seymour AW, Mendell LM. Mismatches between peripheral receptor type and central projection after peripheral nerve regeneration. *Neurosci Lett* 1989; 99:67–72.

Koerber HR, Mirnics K, Brown PB, Mendell LM. Central sprouting and functional plasticity of regenerated primary afferents. *J Neurosci* 1994; 14(6):3655–3671.

Koerber HR, Mirnics K, Kavookjian AM, Light AR. Ultrastructural analysis of ectopic synaptic boutons arising from peripherally regenerated primary afferent fibers. *J Neurophysiol* 1999; 81:1636–1644.

Kilo S, Schmelz M, Koltzenburg M, Handwerker HO. Different patterns of hyperalgesia induced by experimental inflammation in human skin. *Brain* 1994; 117:385–396.

Koltzenburg M, Torebjörk HE, Wahren LK. Nociceptor modulated central sensitisation causes mechanical hyperalgesia in acute chemogenic and chronic neuropathic pain. *Brain* 1994; 117:579–591.

LaMotte RH, Thalhammer JG, Torebjörk HE, Robinson CJ. Peripheral neural mechanisms of cutaneous hyperalgesia following mild injury by heat. *J Neurosci* 1982; 2:765–781.

LaMotte RH, Shain CN, Simone DA, Tsai EF. Neurogenic hyperalgesia: psychophysical studies of underlying mechanisms. *J Neurophysiol* 1991; 66:190–211.

LaMotte RH, Lundberg LER, Torebjörk HE. Pain, hyperalgesia and activity in nociceptive-C units in humans after intradermal injection of capsaicin. *J Physiol* 1992; 448:749–764.

Magerl W, Fuchs P, Meyer RA, Treede RD. Roles of capsaicin-insensitive nociceptors in cutaneous pain and secondary hyperalgesia. *Brain* 2002; 124:1754–1764.

Marchettini P, Simone DA, Caputi G, Ochoa JL. Pain from excitation of identified muscle nociceptors in humans. *Brain Res* 1996; 740:109–116.

Moosmang S, Stieber J, Zong X, et al. Cellular expression and functional characterization of four hyperpolarization-activated pacemaker channels in cardiac and neuronal tissues. *Eur J Biochem* 2001; 268:1646–1652.

Orstavik K, Weidner C, Schmidt R, et al. Pathological C-fibres in patients with a chronic painful condition. *Brain* 2003; 126:567–578.

Ritter AM, Woodbury CJ, Mirnics K, et al. Maturation of cutaneous sensory neurons from normal and NGF overexpressing mice. *J Neurophysiol* 2000; 83:1722–1732.

Schmelz M, Schmidt R, Bickel A, Handwerker HO, Torebjörk HE. Specific C-receptors for itch in human skin. *J Neurosci* 1997; 17:8003–8008.

Schmidt R, Schmelz M, Forster C. Novel classes of responsive and unresponsive C nociceptors in human skin. *J Neurosci* 1995; 15:333–341.

Serra J, Campero M, Ochoa J, Bostock H. Activity-dependent slowing of conduction differentiates functional subtypes of C fibres innervating human skin. *J Physiol (Lond)* 1999; 515:799–811.

Shortland P, Woolf CJ. Chronic peripheral nerve section results in a rearrangement of the central axonal arborizations of axotomized A beta primary afferent neurons in the rat spinal cord. *J Comp Neurol* 1993; 330:65–82.

Takigawa T, Alzheimer C, Quasthoff S, Grafe P. A specific blocker reveals the presence and function of the hyperpolarization-activated cation current I-H in peripheral mammalian nerve fibres. *Neuroscience* 1998; 82:631–634.

Torebjörk HE, Hallin RG. C-fibre units recorded from human sensory nerve fascicles in situ: a preliminary report. *Acta Soc Med Upsal* 1970; 75:81–84.

Torebjörk HE, LaMotte RH, Robinson CJ. Peripheral neural correlates of magnitude of cutaneous pain and hyperalgesia: simultaneous recordings in humans of sensory judgments of pain and evoked responses in nociceptors with C-fibers. *J Neurophysiol* 1984; 51:325–339.

Torebjörk HE, Lundberg LER, LaMotte RH. Central changes in processing of mechanoreceptive input in capsaicin-induced secondary hyperalgesia in humans. *J Physiol* 1992; 448:765–780.

Torebjörk HE, Schmelz M, Handwerker HO. Functional properties of human cutaneous nociceptors and their role in pain and hyperalgesia. In: Belmonte C, Cervero F (Eds). *Neurobiology of Nociceptors.* Oxford: Oxford University Press, 1996, pp 349–369.

Weidner C, Schmelz M, Schmidt R, et al. Functional attributes discriminating mechano-insensitive and mechano-responsive C nociceptors in human skin. *J Neurosci* 1999; 19:10184–10190.

Weidner C, Schmelz M, Schmidt R, et al. Neural signal processing: the underestimated contribution of peripheral human C-fibers. *J Neurosci* 2002; 22:6704–6712.

Woodbury CJ, Koerber HR. Widespread projections from myelinated nociceptors throughout the substantia gelatinosa provide novel insights into neonatal hypersensitivity. *J Neurosci* 2003; 23:601–610.

Woodbury CJ, Ritter AM, Koerber HR. Central anatomy of individual rapidly adapting low-threshold mechanoreceptors innervating the hairy skin of newborn mice: early maturation of hair follicle afferents. *J Comp Neurol* 2001; 436:304–323.

Woolf CJ, Shortland P, Coggeshall RE. Peripheral nerve injury triggers central sprouting of myelinated afferents. *Nature* 1992; 355:75–78.

Woolf CJ, Shortland P, Reynolds ML, et al. Central regenerative sprouting: the reorganization of the central terminals of myelinated primary afferents in the rat dorsal horn following peripheral nerve section or crush. *J Comp Neurol* 1995; 360:121–134.

Correspondence to: Martin Koltzenburg, MD, Institute of Child Health, University College London, 30 Guilford Street, London WC1N 1EH, United Kingdom. Email: m.koltzenburg@ich.ucl.ac.uk.

Proceedings of the 10th World Congress on Pain,
Progress in Pain Research and Management, Vol. 24,
edited by Jonathan O. Dostrovsky, Daniel B. Carr, and
Martin Koltzenburg, IASP Press, Seattle, © 2003.

14

Painful Peripheral Neuropathies and C-Fiber Nociceptors

John W. Griffin,[a,b,c] Justin C. McArthur,[b] Michael Polydefkis,[a,b,c] Beth B. Murinson,[a,c] Alan Belzberg,[d] James Campbell,[d] Matthias Ringkamp,[d] and Richard A. Meyer[d]

[a]Peripheral Nerve Laboratories, [b]Cutaneous Neurology Laboratory, and [c]Daniel B. Drachman Neuromuscular Service, Department of Neurology; [d]Pain Physiology Laboratory, Department of Neurosurgery, Johns Hopkins University School of Medicine, Baltimore, Maryland, USA

Peripheral neuropathies are among the most prevalent disorders that cause neuropathic pain. An indication of the magnitude of the problem is seen in the number of individuals with either the painful neuropathy of diabetes or that associated with HIV/AIDS. This chapter focuses on a series of studies relevant to painful neuropathies that were performed in laboratories at Johns Hopkins University. The Hopkins studies were motivated by clinicopathological experience with painful "small-fiber" neuropathies (Holland et al. 1997, 1998; Periquet et al. 1999; Polydefkis et al. 2000), and by experimental investigations that were triggered by recent reports (Sato and Perl 1991; Koltzenburg et al. 1994; Myers et al. 1996; Wagner and Myers 1996; Ramer et al. 1997; Sorkin et al. 1997) suggesting that Wallerian degeneration might contribute to neuropathic pain.

The four laboratories that joined in these studies are the cutaneous neurology laboratory, the neuromuscular service, and the peripheral nerve laboratories in the Department of Neurology, and the pain physiology laboratories in the Department of Neurosurgery. Encapsulating in a few sentences a single distinctive hypothesis from these studies is neither possible nor appropriate, given the relevant data that derive from many other laboratories, as well as the diversity of favored hypotheses and of interpretations of data among the Hopkins investigators. However, both our clinical and experimental studies share several perspectives. First, we are interested in the possibility that "spared," uninjured peripheral nerve fibers, as well as injured fibers, might contribute to the development of neuropathic pain. Second, we are asking to what extent physiological and structural changes in C-fiber nociceptors might contribute to neuropathic pain. Third, we are investigating to what extent Wallerian degeneration of neighboring nerve fibers might influence uninjured nociceptors in a fashion that favors development of neuropathic pain.

Some basic terms are used in different ways among different disciplines. Table I presents a glossary of operational definitions used in this chapter. In the first section of this chapter we address the clinical features of the painful neuropathies, particularly the small-fiber sensory neuropathies, and review recent data on the underlying pathological changes in the peripheral nerves. We then summarize recent observations on the biology of small sensory fibers, of Remak bundles, and of the C-fiber nociceptor terminals within the epidermis. New models of experimental degeneration and regeneration of C-fiber nociceptors in humans are presented. The final section turns to experimental models of partial nerve injury and consequent hyperalgesia in the rat. In particular, we summarize the responses of Remak bundles and C fibers to injury of neighboring nerve fibers, and review the current status of the controversy about whether neuropathic pain is driven by injured afferents, spared afferents, or both.

Table I
Definitions of terminology

Nerve fiber: an axon and the Schwann cell that ensheaths it
Peripheral neuropathy*: a length-dependent symmetrical polyneuropathy, not a mechanical nerve injury
Unmyelinated fiber: one or more unmyelinated axons ensheathed by a single Schwann cell (i.e., a Remak bundle)
Small-fiber neuropathy: a neuropathy in which C and Aδ fibers are prominently or predominantly affected
Small sensory fiber: a C or Aδ (small myelinated) fiber. C-fiber nociceptors can be recognized physiologically. Some have TRPV1 (VR1) receptors and are sensitive to capsaicin

*The term "peripheral neuropathy" could arguably be used to describe any nerve injury or disease, include nerve root compression, carpal tunnel syndrome, or causalgia. Here we will use it in the restricted sense usually understood by neurologists. Because we will not discuss multiple mononeuropathies, in this chapter it can be thought of as a shorthand for what might more properly be termed a length-dependent symmetrical polyneuropathy.

PAINFUL SENSORY NEUROPATHIES

CLINICAL FEATURES

Many neuropathies produce neuropathic pain, including toxic neuropathies induced by drugs such as vincristine, nutritional and alcoholic neuropathies, and angiopathic neuropathies such as those due to vasculitis. In these disorders, large and small nerve fibers are lost. A group of painful neuropathies are characterized by preferential loss of small nerve fibers. Some of the disorders most frequently associated with painful "small-fiber" sensory neuropathies are listed in Table II.

The symptoms in most of these neuropathies are dominated by pain beginning in the toes and feet. While affected individuals use a number of descriptors, "burning" is the term most frequently used. The pain is often described as "always present" and is usually largely stimulus-independent, although it may be aggravated by activity, and the amplified symptoms may last for several hours. Conversely, some patients feel that activity improves their symptoms. For many patients nighttime is worst, perhaps because of the absence of distracting stimuli. A subgroup of patients fidget their feet or develop frank "restless legs." Polydefkis and colleagues (2000) identified a group of older individuals with restless leg syndrome who lacked family histories of the disorder. Electrodiagnostic studies or skin biopsy provided

Table II
Disorders associated with painful "small-fiber" neuropathies

Diabetes
Impaired glucose tolerance
HIV/AIDS
Distal sensory polyneuropathy
Antiretroviral toxic neuropathy (neurotoxic dideoxynucleoside antiretrovirals)
Amyloidosis
Acquired
Familial
Some heritable sensory neuropathies
Fabry's disease
Idiopathic small-fiber sensory neuropathy (tabes dorsalis due to syphilis*)

* Tabes dorsalis, a late complication of syphilitic infection, is now uncommon and therefore often ignored. Although tabes is best known for the occurrence of painless injuries to the extremities, it also produces neuropathic pain, often with typical lightning pains. This is instructive, because tabes pathologically appears to be a virtually pure dorsal radiculopathy, with preservation of dorsal root ganglion cells and peripheral sensory fibers, but degeneration of both large and small fibers in the dorsal roots. Theories of neuropathic pain need to take into account the occurrence of pain in tabes.

evidence of peripheral neuropathy in over 50% of these individuals. This finding contrasts with a group of individuals with onset before 45 years of age, most of whom had family histories of the disorder. In this group, peripheral neuropathy is uncommon.

A frequent feature of painful neuropathies is the development of "lightning pains" (Holland et al. 1998; Periquet et al. 1999)—sudden stabbing or electrical sensations that may occur in one portion of one foot or leg and then reoccur later elsewhere. Typically these pains last for only seconds, but they are sufficiently severe that they can interrupt ongoing activities and divert the patient's attention.

Hyperalgesia induced by light stroking is present in some patients with painful neuropathies. Punctate hyperalgesia is less frequent. Often the rubbing of the bed sheets at night is uncomfortable, and such patients may sleep with their feet uncovered. Many wear socks to bed, in part to reduce stroking hyperalgesia. Many patients say that they benefit from cooling of the feet, and some plunge their feet into cold water or even ice water for relief. This remedy is not invariable, and many prefer to warm their feet.

Some patients with ongoing spontaneous pain in sensory neuropathies also have a potential for painless injuries due to hypesthesia in the feet. This problem can apply even to individuals with striking tactile hyperalgesia. Painless injuries can, of course, develop in patients without neuropathic pain. Plantar ulcers and Charcot joints in the feet and ankles are the most frequent painless injuries. The development of painless injuries is a contributing factor in the development of osteomyelitis and soft tissue infections in the legs in diabetes, and thus may indirectly lead to the need for amputation.

ETIOLOGIES

The frequency and prevalence of painful neuropathies are not known with precision, but an approximation of the magnitude of the problem derives from estimates of their prevalence in diabetes and in HIV/AIDS infection. The most prevalent neuropathy, diabetic polyneuropathy, is frequently complicated by painful neuropathy. Data from the National Health and Nutrition Examination Survey indicate that 5.1% of U.S. adults have diagnosed diabetes, 2.7% have undiagnosed diabetes, and another 6.9% have impaired fasting glucose, cumulating to a total of 12.3% of the population (Harris et al. 1998). Similarly, HIV/AIDS, affecting over one million individuals in the United States, can produce painful neuropathic symptoms in up to 30% of infected individuals (Schifitto et al. 2002), and the highly active antiretroviral therapies frequently involve use of dideoxynucleosides like DDC, ddI, and D4T that can in themselves produce and amplify painful neuropathies.

It used to be argued that only patients with severe, longstanding hyperglycemia and frank diabetes develop diabetic polyneuropathy and neuropathic pain. The status of painful neuropathy associated with diabetes has recently become more complex. Recent studies found that that a population of individuals with impaired glucose tolerance as determined by glucose tolerance testing, but lacking frank diabetes, developed burning feet (Novella et al. 2001; Singleton et al. 2001a,b; Smith et al. 2001). Polydefkis and colleagues (Sumner et al. 2002) have provided presumptive evidence that in such patients there is a progression from a predominant involvement of small sensory fibers to involvement of both small and large sensory fibers, and that in more advanced stages of diabetic neuropathy there is involvement of motor fibers as well. Why some individuals with prediabetes develop painful neuropathies and others remain asymptomatic is unknown. The development of neuropathic pain can provide a useful "warning" of impending diabetes, allowing the opportunity to alter the course of the disease. A rigorous diet and exercise program can prevent or delay the subsequent development of diabetes in individuals with impaired glucose tolerance (Tuomilehto et al. 2001). The implications of such regimens for the development of diabetes-associated neuropathic disease are unexplored.

C-FIBER NOCICEPTORS

NORMAL ANATOMY OF C-FIBER NOCICEPTORS

C-fiber nociceptors are by definition unmyelinated nerve fibers. In their course from the primary sensory neurons to their target in, for example, the skin, they are organized into Remak bundles. The Remak bundle is the basic axon/Schwann unit in which one or more unmyelinated axons are ensheathed by a Schwann cell process. Normally each unmyelinated axon in a Remak bundle is separately ensheathed, and a tightly applied basal lamina lies over the whole bundle. Histograms of axons in Remak bundles in the rat sciatic nerve show that the median number of axons per Remak bundle is between six and seven (B.B. Murinson, unpublished data). Nociceptors may be mixed with postganglionic sympathetic axons in the same Remak bundle. Similarly, in the rat sciatic nerve, fibers from both L4 and L5 may share the same bundle (Murinson, unpublished data). Tracing studies have shown that individual axons exchange from one Remak bundle to another frequently.

C-fiber nociceptor neurons respond to either nerve growth factor (NGF) or glial-derived neurotrophic factor (GDNF), reflecting the presence on the neuron of high-affinity receptors for these growth factors (Molliver et al. 1997). The GDNF-responsive neurons tend to bear a number of other markers, including P2X3 receptors, fluoride-resistant alkaline phosphatase (FRAP), and carbohydrates that bind the lectin, isolectin B4 (IB4). In contrast to C fibers, Aδ nociceptors are small-caliber myelinated axons. In general, these categories are considered immutable in adult animals, and correlate with different response properties and physiologies. However, Höke and colleagues (2003) have recently shown that very high doses of GDNF can drive a population of C fibers to myelinate. The physiological correlates of this induced myelination have not been studied. Murinson (unpublished data) has found that NGF- and GDNF-responsive axons can share the same Remak Schwann cell.

Cutaneous C-fiber nociceptors pass through an extensive subepidermal plexus, then ascend vertically through the dermal-epidermal junction and the epidermis. Most reach the stratum corneum at the surface of the epidermis (Hsieh et al. 1996). These axons lose their Schwann cell ensheathment at the dermal-epidermal junction, and ascend as true "free nerve endings," running between adjacent keratinocytes (Hsieh et al. 1996).

The advent of skin biopsies has substantially changed researchers' ability to assess small fibers in humans. The procedure can be done as punch biopsies (Holland et al. 1997, 1998; Periquet et al. 1999; Polydefkis et al. 2000) or as epidermal blisters (Kennedy et al. 1999). Both procedures are well tolerated by patients and can be repeated as needed over time. It is also possible to assess multiple samples from different anatomical areas. The technical capacity to successfully stain epidermal nerve fibers was markedly advanced by the development of panaxonal markers, such as PGP 9.5, that "see" C fibers. Most previous markers had been directed toward antigens of proteins relatively low in abundance in small fibers, such as the neurofilament proteins and peptide transmitters. The advent of immunostaining with PGP 9.5 provided a robust panaxonal marker that allowed identification and enumeration of small fibers in the epidermis. In glabrous skin of the rat hindpaw virtually all of these fibers are sensory, as reflected by their degeneration following dorsal root ganglionectomy (Li et al. 1997). Rice has found evidence that in hairy skin a population of postganglionic sympathetics reaches into the epidermis as well (Davis et al. 1997; Fundin et al. 1997).

The sites that are biopsied can be determined by the experimental questions of interest. In the cutaneous neurology laboratory at Johns Hopkins our standard diagnostic series is a 3-mm punch biopsy performed at the distal leg above the ankle, the distal thigh above the knee, and the proximal thigh below the hip (Holland et al. 1998).

PATHOLOGY OF C-FIBER NOCICEPTORS IN PAINFUL NEUROPATHIES

Because a wide variety of neuropathic disorders can produce pain, there can be a wide variety of underlying pathologies. Dyck and colleagues (1976) identified active Wallerian degeneration within cutaneous nerves as a correlate of neuropathic pain. In their study there was no predilection for the type of sensory fibers—small or large—that were affected, but other studies have identified the prominence of small sensory fiber involvement in painful neuropathies. In general, one lesson of the last few years has been that in regions of spontaneous burning pain the density of C-fiber nociceptors in the skin is reduced or virtually absent (Holland et al. 1997, 1998; Herrmann et al. 1999; Periquet et al. 1999; Polydefkis et al. 2000). This loss of C fibers may be accompanied by loss of other classes of sensory fibers.

Several studies have examined epidermal innervation in patients with peripheral nerve disease (Holland et al. 1997, 1998; Herrmann et al. 1999; Periquet et al. 1999; Polydefkis et al. 2000) (Fig. 1). Correlative studies of sural nerve biopsy and electrophysiology (Holland et al. 1998; Herrmann et al. 1999) confirmed the expected close relationship between abnormalities

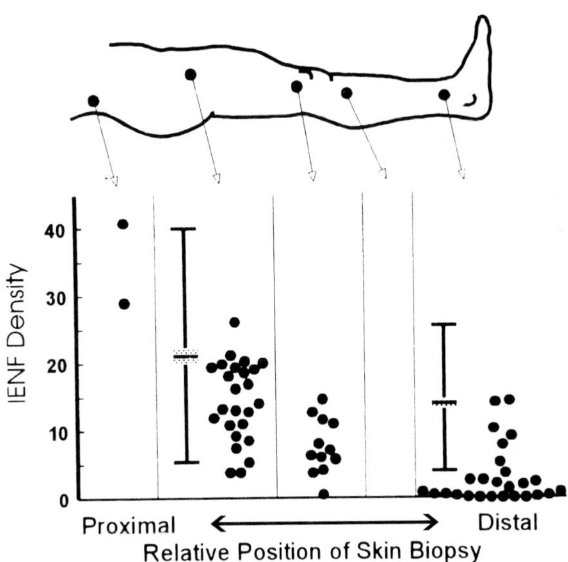

Fig. 1. Intraepidermal nerve fiber (IENF) densities in skin sampled at various levels from the patients with chronic progressive idiopathic small-fiber sensory neuropathies (SFSN) (filled circles) compared with the 5th to 95th percentile range for normal controls (bars), demonstrating length-dependent cutaneous denervation. Reprinted from Holland et al. (1998), with permission.

of electrophysiology—particularly action potential amplitudes of sensory nerves—and preservation of large fibers in sural nerve biopsies (Fig. 2). In general, there was little correlation between electrophysiology and numbers of Aδ and C fibers in sural nerves. Again, this finding was not unexpected, because large fibers are the predominant determinants of action potential amplitudes of sensory nerves. In contrast, there was an excellent correlation between the density of Aδ fibers and the epidermal innervation in the distal leg by skin biopsy. Similarly, there was a correlation with C fibers in the sural nerve. This relationship was less tight than with Aδ fibers (Herrmann et al. 1999). Because most of the epidermal fibers represent C-fiber terminals, this relationship should be the closest biologically, but two factors confound it. First, quantitation of unmyelinated fibers in the sural nerve has inherent technical limitations and variability (Herrmann et al. 1999), and second, there is a population of patients with small-fiber sensory neuropathies in whom fibers are lost from the skin but remain intact at the level of the sural nerve. This finding presumably means that the fibers degenerated between the distal sural nerve and their normal termination in the epidermis over the ankle. Holland and colleagues (1998) pointed out that such patients may be particularly valuable subjects in future studies of nerve fiber regeneration, because if an agent were found to promote regrowth of C fibers, the nerve fibers in such patients would have the shortest distance to regenerate in order to reinnervate the skin of the distal leg and foot.

EXPERIMENTAL ASSESSMENT OF C-FIBER REGENERATION IN HUMANS

The foregoing discussion indicates that in many patients with painful neuropathies, C-fiber nociceptors degenerate and are lost from the skin, and that the loss occurs first in the most distal regions, innervated by the longest fibers. If the longest C-fiber nociceptors are unable to be maintained, and thus degenerate, might shorter ones that are still present have difficulty regenerating after an injury? In other words, might the ability of C-fiber nociceptors to regenerate after an experimental injury be altered in some neuropathies? The ability to assess C-fiber regeneration is also important because several approaches proposed to promote nerve fiber regeneration could augment C-fiber regeneration in humans. These approaches include the administration of growth factors (NGF, GDNF, and insulin-like growth factor-1), administration of neuroimmunophilins, and electrical stimulation of nerve fibers. Models are needed to determine their efficacy.

Three models have been recently used to study regeneration of sensory C fibers in humans (Table II). In the first model, termed the *excision model*

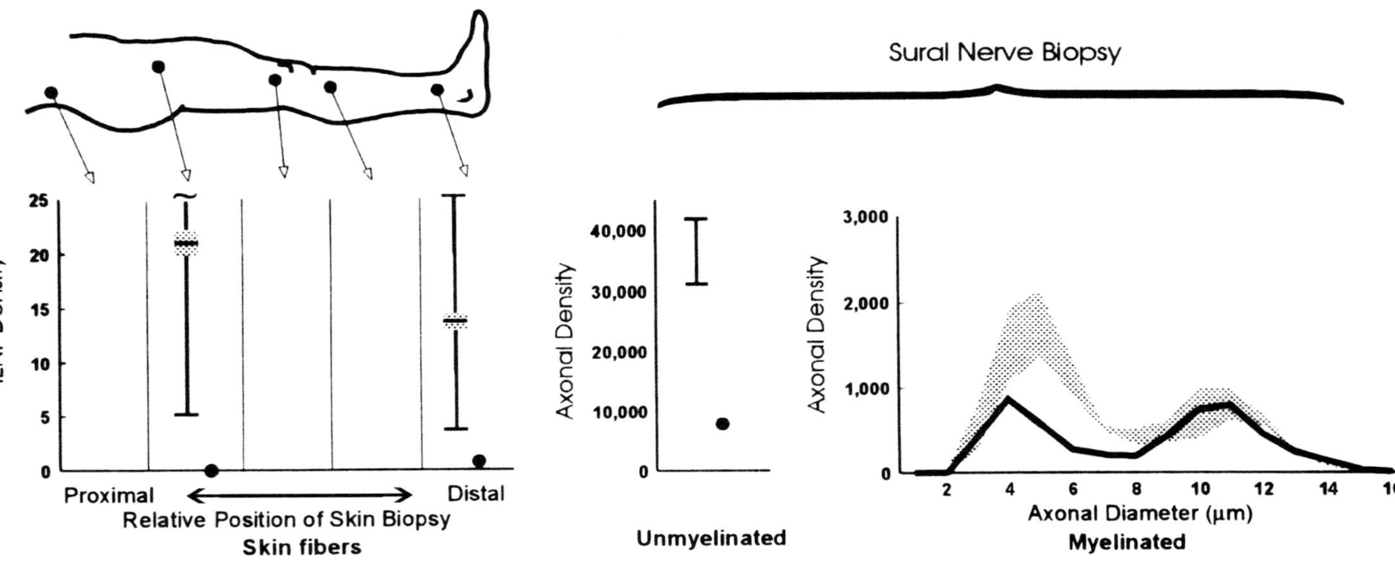

Fig. 2. Sural nerve morphometry and IENF densities from a patient with severe SFSN. The density of small-diameter myelinated and unmyelinated axons is reduced in the sural nerve biopsy specimen. There is marked cutaneous denervation in skin from both proximal and distal sites. See Fig 1. legend for further details. Shaded area in graph on right represents the range of values in normal subjects. Reprinted from Holland et al. (1998), with permission.

(Fig. 3), Rajan and colleagues (in press) inserted a 3-mm diameter circular knife vertically into the skin and removed the resulting cylinder to perform a 3-mm skin excision. In this model, both the epidermis and the dermis were removed, and collagen bundles promptly grew into the dermis. Within 3 days a thin layer of epidermis covered most of the excised region. There were no Schwann cell bands within this new dermis. Probably for this reason, regeneration occurred almost entirely by sprouting from the epidermal

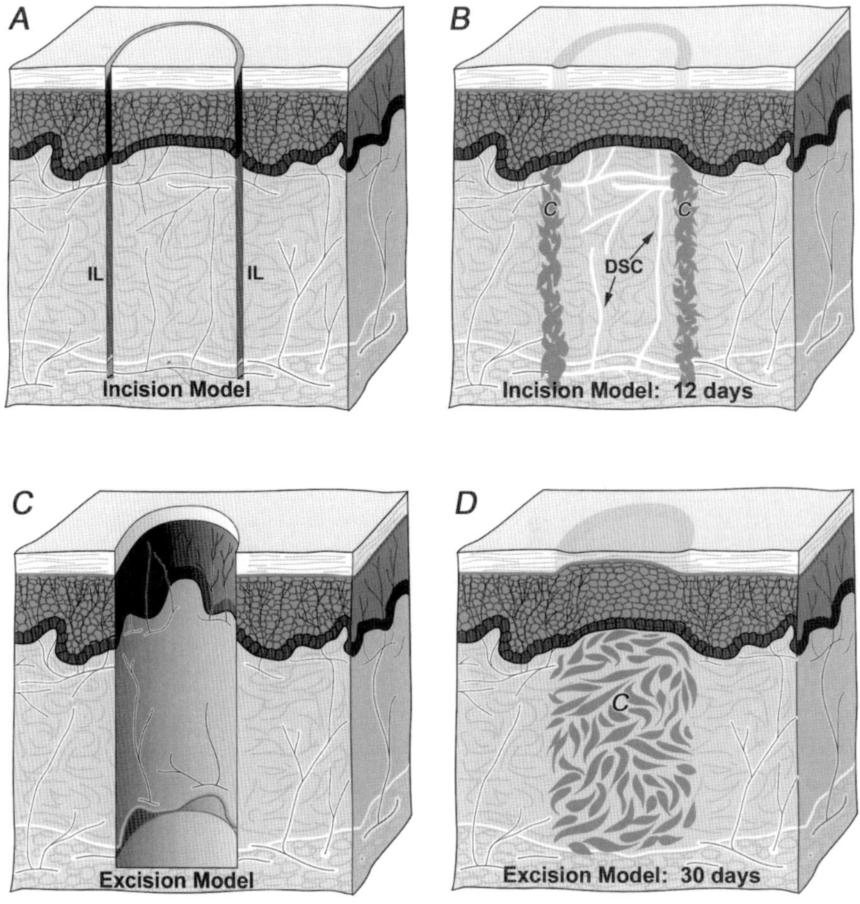

Fig. 3. (A,B) Schematic of the incision model: the vertical incision (IL) is shown immediately after lesioning (A), and after 12 days (B). Nerve fibers are indicated by black lines with white margins. The collagen (*C*) bands at the incision lines are shown, along with the denervated Schwann cell bundles (DSC, white lines). (C,D) Schematic of the excision model: a cylinder of skin is removed at the time of the lesioning (C); after 30 days (D) collagen (*C*) completely fills the lesion, and there are no remaining Schwann cell bands. Reprinted from Rajan et al. (in press), with permission.

nerve fibers at the cut margins. These fibers provided reinnervation in two fashions. First, they bent and grew horizontally into the suprabasal regions of the epidermis in a pattern termed *ultraterminal sprouting* (Fig. 4). Second, collaterals from these fibers grew down to the epidermal side of the

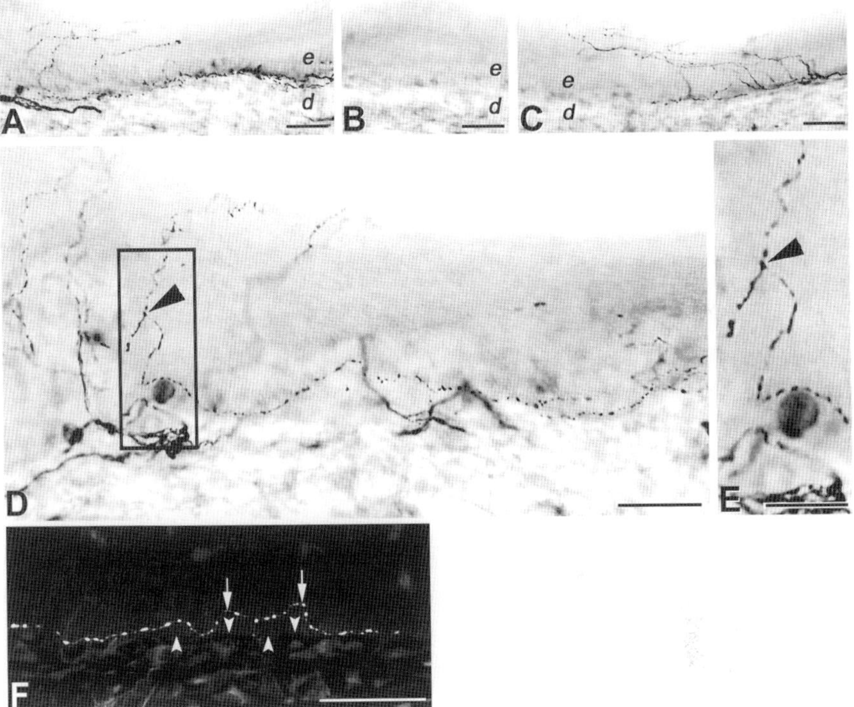

Fig. 4. (A–C) A 50-μm thick frozen vertical section of a skin biopsy taken from an experimental subject 30 days after excision of a smaller skin punch biopsy. The biopsy is immunostained for PGP9.5. The cut margins (A and C) have suprabasal axons that are elongated and leaning into the denervated zone. In addition, there are abundant axons growing down the dermal-epidermal junction. In contrast, the central region (B) of the denervated zone has no axons. Scale marker 50 μm. (D) A 50-μm frozen vertical section taken 30 days after excision, immunostained for PGP9.5. The incision passed just to the right of the boxed region. Scale marker 50 μm. In the boxed region an intraepidermal axon gives rise to a branch (seen at higher magnification in panel E) that drops down to the dermal-epidermal junction and then extends into the denervated zone. The branch is identified by arrowheads. Scale marker 25 μm. (F) Confocal microscopy of a 50-μm frozen section 30 days after excision, immunostained for PGP9.5 using Texas red. This section follows a single fluorescent axon, using a total confocal depth of 30 μm. Note that the axon is on the epidermal side of the dermal-epidermal junction (arrowheads), as seen unequivocally (arrows) where it rises above the junction, presumably to pass over a basal keratinocytes. Scale marker 50 μm. Reprinted from Rajan et al. (in press), with permission.

basal lamina at the dermal-epidermal junction, and then grew toward the center of the denervated region (Fig. 4). Whole mounts of the epidermis, obtained by taking 5-mm biopsies at intervals after the initial 3-mm biopsies, demonstrated that these collateral branches tended to grow relatively straight toward the center of the denervated area. Their rate of growth was slow, and as they reached the center of the denervated disks, they began to arborize.

A second model, termed the *incision model,* involved a similar incision of the skin in which the skin plug was not removed (Fig. 3). This lesion interrupted the subepidermal fibers, but left the dermal Schwann cell bands in place, resulting in Wallerian degeneration of subepidermal and epidermal fibers. In the incision model, similar behavior to the excision model was seen at the cut margin, indicating that a collateral reinnervation process as well as ultraterminal sprouting began in this setting as well. However, this process competed with regenerating axons growing up from the denervated Schwann cell bands in the dermis. As these regenerating sprouts reached the epidermis, the ultraterminal sprouts and the collateral sprouts regressed. Recovery thus occurred primarily by regeneration from the site of transection in the dermis up the denervated Schwann cell bands, a form of regrowth that can be termed *regenerative regeneration.*

These behaviors strongly suggest that growth-stimulating molecules are produced within the denervated epidermis, and that they exist in gradients, so that reinnervation reduces their abundance. Such gradients could occur by regulation of the production of molecules such as NGF or GDNF, or it could result from the accumulation of such proteins due to the absence of nerve terminals to take them up and remove them from the epidermis. In either event, a gradient could be established.

The third model, initially developed by Simone and coworkers (1998) and Nolano and coworkers (1999), uses capsaicin to produce degeneration of the C-fiber nociceptors within the epidermis. Polydefkis and colleagues (Sumner et al. 2002) have shown that application of an occlusion patch containing 0.075% capsaicin produces a predictable loss of all epidermal fibers and degeneration of subepidermal fibers as well. As might be expected, innervation of sweat glands and around blood vessels remained intact. Polydefkis' team used this approach to examine subsequent reinnervation. Fibers grew back toward the epidermis from deep dermal sites along the denervated Schwann cell bands. Successive biopsies performed within the first 100 days after denervation showed that epidermal denervation was complete, and that epidermal nerve fiber density subsequently gradually increased back toward normal through regenerative regrowth. This technique offers a potential means of assessing the rate of regeneration in individuals with neuropathy, and of assessing the effects of agents intended to promote regeneration and reinnervation.

LESSONS FROM EXPERIMENTAL STUDIES IN RODENTS

Several well-known animal models have been used to study experimental neuropathic pain. All are based on partial injuries to the peripheral nervous system (Bennett and Xie 1988; Seltzer et al. 1990; Kim and Chung 1992; Decosterd and Woolf 2000). A widely studied rat model is ligation of the L5 and L6 mixed spinal roots distal to the dorsal root ganglion, developed by Kim and Chung (1992). At the outset it is important to acknowledge the limitations of these models for studies of pain in neuropathies. Partial nerve injuries have many pathophysiological differences from the slowly progressing "dying back" neuropathies we have been describing in humans. There have been few models of neuropathic pain in experimental peripheral neuropathies. The recent advent of painful neuropathic models due to vincristine (Nozaki-Taguchi et al. 2001) and paclitaxel (Polomano et al. 2001) may help alleviate this problem. A second barrier to investigation is that, as noted above, most patients with painful neuropathies have stimulus-independent, ongoing pain; only a minority have hyperalgesia. Yet in most experimental studies the "readout" is based on detection of hyperalgesia. The extent to which these models produce ongoing pain is unknown.

In any event, in all of the models it is presumed that abnormal electrical activity in the peripheral nervous system leads to changes in the segmental spinal cord that result in hyperexcitability or central sensitization (Campbell et al. 1988). Abnormal electrical activity can be generated at the cut end of the injured nerve fibers within neuromas. It is now clear that an important component of spontaneous electrical activity arises at the level of the nerve cell bodies of the axotomized fibers (Coggeshall et al. 1993; Michaelis et al. 2000). This activity in turn is likely to represent altered gene expression in the axotomized neurons; changes in sodium channels, including Na_v 1.3 (type III) and Na_v 1.8 (sensory neuron specific), may be especially relevant. Axotomy has long been known to induce changes in synthesis of proteins within the perikaryon, including increased message for tubulins and reduced message for neurofilament proteins, induction of regeneration-associated proteins such as growth-associated protein 43 (GAP43), and changes in transmission-relevant products, including reduced substance P and calcitonin gene-related peptide in nociceptor neurons and increased galanin in A fibers. Production of brain-derived neurotrophic factor (BDNF) is reduced. A unifying hypothesis is that all of these genetic changes may reflect the consequences of an axotomy-induced reduction in delivery of neurotrophic agents such as NGF and GDNF from the periphery. NGF can reverse the changes in cytoskeletal protein synthesis and GAP43, and GDNF can prevent or reverse the expression of the Na_v 1.3 Na^+ channel (Boucher et al. 2000).

While these changes are well established, there is currently interest in the possibility that changes in the uninjured sensory afferents may contribute to development or maintenance of neuropathic pain in these models. Studies conducted by Myers and colleagues (Myers et al. 1996; Wagner and Myers 1996; Sorkin et al. 1997) and by Ramer and colleagues (1997) demonstrated that mice with slow Wallerian degeneration on a genetic basis develop hyperalgesia later than animals with normal brisk Wallerian degeneration. This observation raised the possibility that degenerating fibers distal to the site of the lesion might in some fashion alter neighboring intact fibers, so that they could drive central sensitization.

We have undertaken a series of studies to evaluate this possibility. In a modified Chung lesion in which the L5 mixed spinal root only was ligated and cut, the Hopkins group found that hyperalgesia was unchanged when the L5 dorsal root was cut (Li et al. 2000). However, transection of the neighboring L4 dorsal root eliminated hyperalgesia, as would be expected, because the combined lesions virtually eliminated the afferent innervation of the hindpaw. Further, the Hopkins group found that a dorsal root ganglionectomy was sufficient to produce hyperalgesia. In this setting, all of the L5 sensory fibers were degenerated, so that the process would by necessity be driven by fibers passing through the L4 dorsal root (Li et al. 2000). In these models the hyperalgesia was greater when the stimulus was applied in the lateral aspect of the paw, its most extensively denervated aspect.

If degeneration of neighboring fibers were sufficient to induce properties in neighboring intact fibers that result in central sensitization, then it was reasoned that injury to the ventral root could be sufficient. Studies at Hopkins (Sheth et al. 2002) demonstrated that this was indeed the case. L5 ventral rhizotomy stimulated development of hyperalgesia in the hindpaw of rats. In this model no afferents were injured, and the degenerating fibers were myelinated motor fibers almost exclusively; there are very few C fibers within the L5 ventral root (Coggeshall et al. 1977).

The development of hyperalgesia is thought to be driven by central sensitization in response to spontaneous peripheral electrical activity. We asked whether there was spontaneous electrical activity in the spared sensory afferents, particularly in C-fiber nociceptors. Low-level spontaneous activity was found in C-fiber nociceptors of the L4 dorsal root in the modified Chung model, in which the L5 mixed spinal nerve was transected (Wu et al. 2001). These data confirmed and extended previous data from Koltzenburg et al. (1994) and Ali et al. (1999). Strikingly, similar activity was present after selective L5 ventral rhizotomy (Wu et al. 2002). That the activity took place in intact C-fiber nociceptors was shown by identifying the receptive field for several of the spontaneously active fibers (Wu et al. 2001). The spontaneous activity in these models is likely to be induced by diffusible factors released into the endoneurial space or at the nerve terminals during the process of Wallerian degeneration of neighboring fibers. These factors could be derived from macrophages or from Schwann cells and could affect the L4 axons or nociceptor cell bodies, or possibly the Remak Schwann cells ensheathing the intact L4 nociceptors.

The last possibility is suggested because a series of structural changes occurs in the Remak bundles after these lesions. In the modified Chung lesion, the number of axons in the Remak bundles decreases and the degree of ensheathment is changed. Remak Schwann cells enter the cell cycle, with consequent proliferation (B.B. Murinson, unpublished manuscript).

Recent data from other laboratories have shown a series of changes in the dorsal root L4 ganglia in this model that largely reciprocate those in the L5 ganglia. Substance P in C fibers is abundant, and levels of BDNF are increased. These changes raise the possibility that these ganglia may be receiving increased levels of growth factors because of increased growth factor production by denervated Schwann cells of the degenerating fibers.

CONCLUSIONS

The experimental studies summarized above suggest the following hypothesis: Degeneration of myelinated nerve fibers releases into the endoneurial space factors that affect neighboring uninjured Remak bundles to produce spontaneous electrical activity within C-fiber nociceptors. This activity originates in the skin. In addition, there is structural remodeling of Remak bundles, including stimulation of Remak Schwann cell proliferation. This spontaneous electrical activity might in turn contribute to central sensitization and thereby to spontaneous neuropathic pain and/or hyperalgesia. Such a hypothesis generates a series of questions: What factors might be generated by degeneration of neighboring fibers? Are they derived from axonal breakdown per se, by new synthesis by denervated Schwann cells, or from invading macrophages? Candidate molecules might include cytokines such as tumor necrosis factor α, chemokines that can influence C-fiber nociceptors through axonal chemokine receptors, nitrous oxide, or growth factors such as NGF.

The studies of patients with painful "small-fiber" neuropathies also direct attention to the small sensory fibers, but there are important differences from the experimental models. First, we emphasized the prominence of loss of C-fiber nociceptors from the epidermis, but in the experimental models the fibers generating spontaneous activity are intact. It is possible that degenerating C-fiber nociceptors might also generate spontaneous activity, or at least respond to neighboring degenerating fibers with spontaneous activity similar to or greater than that of intact C fibers. Second, most patients with painful neuropathies complain of spontaneous ongoing pain without hyperalgesia, whereas in the experimental model only hyperalgesia can be detected. The underlying mechanisms need not be the same. The value of the data available to this point will be in their capacity to suggest studies that will dissect the contributions of the various components of these hypothesized mechanisms.

REFERENCES

Ali Z, Ringkamp M, Hartke TV, et al. Uninjured cutaneous C-fiber nociceptors develop spontaneous activity and alpha adrenergic sensitivity following L6 spinal nerve ligation in the monkey. *J Neurophysiol* 1999; 81:455–466.

Bennett GJ, Xie YK. A peripheral mononeuropathy in rat that produces disorders of pain sensation like those seen in man. *Pain* 1988; 33:87–107.

Boucher TJ, Okuse K, Bennett DL, et al. Potent analgesic effects of GDNF in neuropathic pain states. *Science* 2000; 290:124–127.

Campbell JN, Raja SN, Meyer RA, MacKinnon SE. Myelinated afferents signal the hyperalgesia associated with nerve injury. *Pain* 1988; 32:89–94.

Coggeshall RE, Emery DG, Haruhide I, Maynard CW. Unmyelinated and small myelinated axons in rat ventral roots. *J Comp Neurol* 1977; 173:175–184.

Coggeshall RE, Dougherty PM, Pover CM, Carlton SM. Is large myelinated fiber loss associated with hyperalgesia in a model of experimental peripheral neuropathy in the rat? *Pain* 1993; 52:233–242.

Davis BM, Fundin BT, Albers KM, et al. Overexpression of nerve growth factor in skin causes preferential increases among innervation to specific sensory targets. *J Comp Neurol* 1997; 387:489–506.

Decosterd I, Woolf CJ. Spared nerve injury: an animal model of persistent peripheral neuropathic pain. *Pain* 2000; 87:149–158.

Dyck PJ, Lambert EH, O'Brien PC. Pain in peripheral neuropathy related to rate and kind of fiber degeneration. *Neurology* 1976; 26:466–477.

Fundin BT, Silos-Santiago I, Ernfors P, et al. Differential dependency of cutaneous mechanoreceptors on neurotrophins, trk receptors, and P75 LNGFR. *Dev Biol* 1997; 190:94–116.

Harris MI, Flegal KM, Cowie CC, et al. Prevalence of diabetes, impaired fasting glucose, and impaired glucose tolerance in U.S. adults. The Third National Health and Nutrition Examination Survey, 1988–1994. *Diabetes Care* 1998; 21:518–524.

Herrmann DN, Griffin JW, Hauer P, Cornblath DR, McArthur JC. Epidermal nerve fiber density and sural nerve morphometry in peripheral neuropathies. *Neurology* 1999; 53:1634–1640.

Höke A, Ho H, Crawford TO, et al. Glial cell-line derived neurotrophic factor alters axon-Schwann cell units and promotes myelination in unmyelinated nerve fibers. *J Neurosci* 2003; 23:561–567.

Holland NR, Stocks EA, Hauer P, et al. Intraepidermal nerve fiber density in patients with painful sensory neuropathy. *Neurology* 1997; 48:708–711.

Holland NR, Crawford TO, Hauer P, et al. Small-fiber sensory neuropathies: clinical course and neuropathology of idiopathic cases. *Ann Neurol* 1998; 44:47.

Hsieh S-T, Choi S, Lin W-M, McArthur JC, Griffin JW. Epidermal denervation and its effects on keratinocytes and Langerhans cells. *J Neurocytol* 1996; 25:513–524.

Kennedy WR, Nolano M, Wendelschafer-Crabb G, Johnson TL, Tamura E. A skin blister method to study epidermal nerves in peripheral nerve disease. *Muscle Nerve* 1999; 22:360–371.

Kim S-H, Chung JM. An experimental model for peripheral neuropathy produced by segmental spinal nerve ligation in the rat. *Pain* 1992; 50:355–363.

Koltzenburg M, Kees S, Budweiser S, Ochs G, Toyka KV. The properties of unmyelinated nociceptive afferents change in a painful chronic constriction neuropathy. In: Gebhart GF, Hammond DL, Jensen TS (Eds). *Proceedings of the 7th World Congress on Pain,* Progress in Pain Research and Management, Vol. 2. Seattle: IASP Press, 1994, pp 511–522.

Li Y, Hsieh S-T, Chien H-F, et al. Sensory and motor denervation influence epidermal thickness in rat foot glabrous skin. *Exp Neurol* 1997; 147:452–462.

Li Y, Dorsi MJ, Meyer RA, Belzberg AJ. Mechanical hyperalgesia after an L5 spinal nerve lesion in the rat is not dependent on input from injured nerve fibers. *Pain* 2000; 85:493–502.

Michaelis M, Liu X, Jänig W. Axotomized and intact muscle afferents but no skin afferents develop ongoing discharges of dorsal root ganglion origin after peripheral nerve lesion. *J Neurosci* 2000; 20:2742–2748.

Molliver DC, Wright DE, Leitner ML, et al. IB4-binding DRG neurons switch from NGF to GDNF dependence in early postnatal life. *Neuron* 1997; 19:849–861.

Myers RR, Heckman HM, Rodriguez M. Reduced hyperalgesia in nerve-injured WLD mice: relationship to nerve fiber phagocytosis, axonal degeneration, and regeneration in normal mice. *Exp Neurol* 1996; 141:94–101.

Nolano M, Simone DA, Wendelschafer-Crabb G, et al. Topical capsaicin in humans: parallel loss of epidermal nerve and pain sensation. *Pain* 1999; 81:135–145.

Novella SP, Inzucchi SE, Goldstein JM. The frequency of undiagnosed diabetes and impaired glucose tolerance in patients with idiopathic sensory neuropathy. *Muscle Nerve* 2001; 24:1229–1231.

Nozaki-Taguchi N, Chaplan SR, Higuera ES, Ajakwe RC, Yaksh TL. Vincristine-induced allodynia in the rat. *Pain* 2001; 93:69–76.

Periquet MI, Novak V, Collins MP, et al. Painful sensory neuropathy: prospective evaluation using skin biopsy. *Neurology* 1999; 53:1641–1647.

Polomano RC, Mannes AJ, Clark US, Bennett GJ. A painful peripheral neuropathy in the rat produced by the chemotherapeutic drug, paclitaxel. *Pain* 2001; 94:293–304.

Polydefkis M, Allen RP, Hauer P, et al. Subclinical sensory neuropathy in late-onset restless legs syndrome. *Neurology* 2000; 55:1115–1121.

Rajan B, Polydefkis M, Hauer P, Griffin JW, McArthur JC. Epidermal innervation after intracutaneous axotomy in man. *J Comp Neurol,* in press.

Ramer MS, French GD, Bisby MA. Wallerian degeneration is required for both neuropathic pain and sympathetic sprouting into the DRG. *Pain* 1997; 72:71–78.

Sato J, Perl ER. Adrenergic excitation of cutaneous pain receptors induced by peripheral nerve injury. *Science* 1991; 251:1608-1610.

Schifitto G, McDermott MP, McArthur JC, et al. Incidence of and risk factors for HIV-associated distal sensory polyneuropathy. *Neurology* 2002; 58:1764-1768.

Seltzer Z, Dubner R, Shir Y. A novel behavioral model of neuropathic pain disorders produced in rats by partial sciatic nerve injury. *Pain* 1990; 43:205–218.

Sheth RN, Dorsi MJ, Li Y, et al. Mechanical hyperalgesia after an L5 ventral rhizotomy or an L5 ganglionectomy in the rat. *Pain* 2002; 96:63–72.

Simone DA, Nolano M, Johnson T, Wendelschafer-Crabb G, Kennedy W. Intradermal injection of capsaicin in humans produces degeneration and subsequent reinnervation of epidermal nerve fibers: correlation with sensory function. *J Neurosci* 1998; 18:8947–8959.

Singleton JR, Smith AG, Bromberg MB. Increased prevalence of impaired glucose tolerance in patients with painful sensory neuropathy. *Diabetes Care* 2001a, 24:1448–1453.

Singleton JR, Smith AG, Bromberg MB. Painful sensory polyneuropathy associated with impaired glucose tolerance. *Muscle Nerve* 2001b; 24:1225–1228.

Smith AG, Ramachandran P, Tripp S, Singleton JR. Epidermal nerve innervation in impaired glucose tolerance and diabetes-associated neuropathy. *Neurology* 2001; 57:1701–1704.

Sorkin LS, Xiao WH, Wagner R, Myers RR. Tumour necrosis factor-alpha induces ectopic activity in nociceptive primary afferent fibers. *Neuroscience* 1997; 81:255–262.

Sumner CJ, Sheth S, Griffin JW, Cornblath DR, Polydefkis M. The spectrum of neuropathy in diabetes and impaired glucose tolerance. *Neurology* 2003; in press.

Tuomilehto J, Lindstrom J, Eriksson JG, et al. Prevention of type 2 diabetes mellitus by changes in lifestyle among subjects with impaired glucose tolerance. *N Engl J Med* 2001; 344:1343–1350.

Wagner R, Myers RR. Endoneurial injection of TNF-alpha produces neuropathic pain behaviors. *Neuroreport* 1996; 7:2897–2901.

Wu G, Ringkamp M, Hartke TV, et al. Early onset of spontaneous activity in uninjured C-fiber nociceptors after injury to neighboring nerve fibers. *J Neurosci* 2001; 21:RC140.

Wu G, Ringkamp M, Murinson BB, et al. Degeneration of myelinated efferent fibers induces spontaneous activity in uninjured C-fiber afferents. *J Neurosci* 2002; 22:7746–7753.

Correspondence to: John W. Griffin, MD, Johns Hopkins University School of Medicine, Department of Neurology, 600 N. Wolfe Street, Meyer 6-113, Baltimore, MD 21287-7613, USA. Tel: 410-955-5103; Fax: 410-955-0672; email: jgriffi@jhmi.edu.

Proceedings of the 10th World Congress on Pain,
Progress in Pain Research and Management, Vol. 24,
edited by Jonathan O. Dostrovsky, Daniel B. Carr, and
Martin Koltzenburg, IASP Press, Seattle, © 2003.

15

Potential Anatomical and Neurochemical Substrates of Cutaneous Pain: A Role for Meissner's Corpuscles

Michel Paré,[a] Karin L. Petersen,[b] and Frank L. Rice[c]

[a]Department of Pharmacology and Therapeutics, McGill University, Montreal, Quebec, Canada; [b]UCSF Pain Clinical Research Center, University of California San Francisco, San Francisco, California, USA; [c]Center for Neuropharmacology and Neuroscience, Albany Medical College, Albany, New York, USA

Most research on primary sensory neurons pertaining to nociception and pain perception has focused on smaller neurons with thin-caliber axons that are either unmyelinated C fibers or lightly myelinated Aδ fibers. A wide variety of C fibers and Aδ fibers collectively have preferred stimuli that cover a range of temperatures (thermoreceptors), a variety of exogenous and endogenous molecules (chemoreceptors), intense mechanical impact (high-threshold mechanoreceptors), or some polymodal combination of such stimuli (Burgess and Perl 1973; Fields 1987; Birder and Perl 1994). Extremes in such stimuli are perceived as pain. In general, C-fiber-mediated nociception has been implicated in slow, burning pain, whereas Aδ-fiber nociception has been implicated in sharp, pricking pain. Under a variety of pathological conditions, pain perception increases acutely or chronically due to reduced thresholds to normally noxious stimuli (hyperalgesia) or to changes that result in normally non-noxious stimuli becoming noxious (allodynia).

Larger primary sensory neurons give rise to the larger caliber, heavily myelinated Aβ fibers that are exceptionally sensitive to mild mechanical stimuli (low-threshold mechanoreceptors) (Burgess and Perl 1973; Darian-Smith 1984; Birder and Perl 1994). Each axon terminates peripherally as one of many varieties of morphologically distinct end organs, such as Merkel disks or Pacinian corpuscles, that, respectively, have slowly or rapidly adapting responses preferential to particular mechanical submodalities such as compression or high-frequency vibration. However, selective loss of Aβ-fiber activity results in a reduction of more discriminative aspects of pain perception above and beyond that of sensations mediated by C fibers and Aδ fibers. Moreover, tactile allodynia can also be mediated by a contingent of fibers having fast conduction velocities in the Aβ-fiber range. Research has not yet identified the types of Aβ fibers that may contribute to normal pain perception and abnormal tactile allodynia.

Recent advances in molecular biology have begun to unravel molecular mechanisms in primary sensory neurons that are consistent with thermal, mechanical, and chemical stimuli that induce or modulate pain sensation (Julius and Basbaum 2001). These mechanisms include a variety of receptors and ion channels that respond to opioids, purines, catecholamines, agents such as capsaicin and menthol, and neuropeptides such as substance P (SP) and calcitonin gene-related peptide (CGRP). Some ion channels respond to extreme hot and cold temperatures and changes in pH. Of particular interest are receptors that have multimodal properties such as the vanilloid receptor-1 (TRPV1, also known as VR1), which responds to capsaicin, high temperatures, and low pH (Caterina and Julius 2001). Immunochemical and in situ hybridization studies have shown that these receptors and ion channels, and also peptides such as SP and CGRP that are implicated in nociception, have an especially concentrated expression, mostly among the smaller primary sensory neurons and thin-caliber axons. Changes in sensory neuron response characteristics associated with hyperalgesia or allodynia may be due to changes in neuronal molecular expression. For example, under inflammatory conditions, an increase reportedly occurs in the number of primary sensory neurons that have detectable immunoreactivity (IR) for SP and CGRP (Neumann et al. 1996).

As part of ongoing studies of peripheral neuropathies related to naturally occurring type II diabetes in aging monkeys (Paré et al. 2001b, 2002a), we recently investigated the immunochemical characteristics of glabrous skin innervation in the fingers of normal young-adult old-world monkeys, *Macaca mulatta* and *M. fascicularis* (Paré et al. 2001a). The dermal papillae in digital glabrous skin of the monkey and also the human hand contain numerous Meissner's corpuscles that receive Aβ-fiber innervation that most likely responds to low-frequency, flutter vibration (Cauna 1956; Paré et al. 2001a, 2002c). However, we discovered that two types of C fibers also innervate the Meissner's corpuscles in monkey digital glabrous skin (Fig. 1). One type expresses CGRP-IR and SP-IR and the other type expresses IR for TRPV1. The peptidergic C fibers had also been seen in structurally similar human Meissner's corpuscles (Johansson et al. 1999). As we have consistently observed in a variety of species (Fundin et al. 1997a,b; Rice et al. 1997; Rice and Rasmusson 2001; Paré et al. 2001a,b,c), Aβ fibers and nonpeptidergic

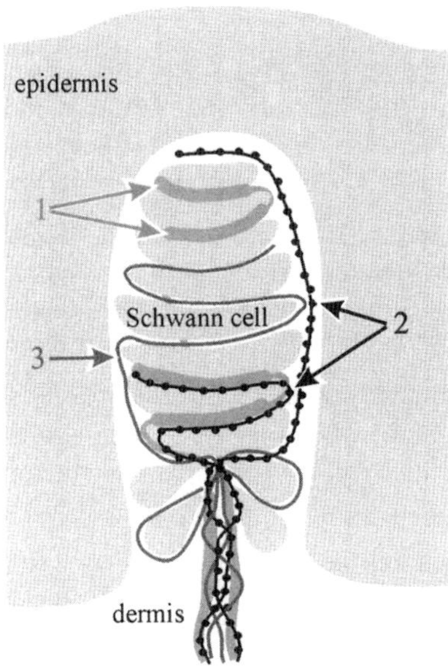

Fig. 1. Schematic drawing of a Meissner's corpuscle shown in a plane perpendicular to the skin surface and illustrating three different types of innervation (from Paré et al. 2001): (1) neurofilament protein (NF)-positive Aβ-fiber innervation, (2) varicose CGRP-positive C-fiber innervation, and (3) nonpeptidergic TRPV1-positive C-fiber innervation. The Meissner's corpuscles are located in dermal papillae that protrude into the epidermis. The CGRP-positive C-fiber innervation is closely affiliated with the Aβ-fiber endings, although some distributes independently around the contour of the Meissner's corpuscle. The nonpeptidergic TRPV1 innervation is segregated to zones interdigitated between the intertwined Aβ-fiber and CGRP-positive C-fiber innervation. Schwann cells are distributed between the innervation and at the base and apex of each Meissner's corpuscle. The most likely additional immunochemical characteristics for each type of innervation are as follows: (1) NF 200, myelin basic protein, CGRP, SP, NK1, δ-opioid receptor, α_{2A} and α_{2C} adrenergic receptors, P2X2, P2X3, TRPV2; (2) CGRP, SP, μ-opioid receptor, δ-opioid receptor, α_{2A} adrenergic receptor, P2X1, P2X3, nociceptin; (3) TRPV1, P2X1, nociceptin, possibly μ- and δ-opioid receptors.

Aδ fibers have intense IR for 200-kD neurofilament protein (NF), which is lacking in C fibers and is weak in peptidergic Aδ fibers.

Within the monkey Meissner's corpuscles, the endings of the TRPV1-positive C fibers formed alternating layers with the NF-positive Aβ-fiber endings (Fig. 1). In contrast, the CGRP/SP-positive C-fiber endings were closely intertwined with the Aβ-fiber endings. In addition, our analysis revealed that the Aβ-fiber innervation also contained CGRP/SP-IR, but at a lower intensity than on the intertwined peptidergic C fibers. This finding suggested that the Meissner's Aβ-fiber innervation may have neuropeptide properties that have been associated with some types of nociceptors. The Aβ fibers and endings also were immunoreactive for the neurokinin-1 (NK1) receptor for SP, which suggests that the peptidergic C-fiber endings may interact functionally with the Aβ-fiber endings.

The presence of relatively low levels of CGRP/SP-IR in the Aβ-fiber Meissner's endings raises the question of whether these neuropeptides are normally endogenous to this large-caliber innervation. Although the presence of CGRP and SP is commonly associated with small sensory neurons and their C fibers, in which immunolabeling for these peptides is relatively intense, lower levels of CGRP and SP-IR have been consistently observed among many medium to large sensory neurons (Lawson 1992, 1995). Conceivably, these larger neurons could be producing just as much CGRP and SP as are the smaller neurons, and the weaker immunoreactivity in both the larger cell bodies and thicker axons (and weaker message as seen by in situ hybridization) could merely be due to greater volumetric dilution. Such a dilution might also explain why many other biochemical components commonly associated with nociception typically have more intense expression in or on relatively small neurons and thin axons, whereas less intense expression is also commonly evident on larger neurons. Therefore, we may generally be underestimating the contribution of Aβ-fiber innervation to normal nociception.

The predictable anatomical relationships of the three types of innervation within the Meissner's corpuscles of the monkey provided an opportunity to compile additional immunochemical characteristics of each type of ending, especially because antibodies raised in different species were available for NF (rabbit and mouse), TRPV1 (rabbit and guinea pig), and CGRP (rabbit and sheep). Therefore, a wide variety of double-label combinations could be run with other antibodies for purinergic receptors, opioid receptors, adrenergic receptors, other vanilloid-related receptors, acid-sensing ion channels, and enzymes (Paré et al. 2001a). As shown schematically in Fig. 1, each type of Meissner's innervation has a complex biochemistry consisting of several combinations of properties implicated in nociceptive mechanisms. Importantly, multiple nociceptive-implicated properties—in addition to CGRP and SP—were present on the Aβ-fiber and on the C-fiber innervation. Interestingly, only the Aβ fibers expressed the vanilloid-like receptor (TRPV2, also known as VRL1), whose only known stimulus is high temperature that results in pain perception under sustained exposure.

An important control is that other Aβ-fiber innervation terminating on Merkel cells, within the same tissue sections, lacked most of the putative nociceptive immunochemical characteristics seen on the Aβ fibers terminating in the Meissner's corpuscles. Also, most of the antibodies labeled overlapping subsets of C-fiber and Aδ-fiber endings in the epidermis. Due to the lack of predictable anatomical arrangement of epidermal endings, the comparable full range of immunochemical characteristics has not yet been unraveled for specific endings within the epidermis. However, these epidermal endings include sets that have detectable IR either for CGRP and SP or for TRPV1, or that lack IR for neuropeptides or TRPV1.

Our results indicate that the Aβ-fiber Meissner's innervation has immunochemical properties consistent with the possibility that they may contribute to normal pain perception or may be involved in Aβ-fiber-mediated allodynia. By analogy, the Aβ-fiber lanceolate endings that terminate around hair follicles may perform a similar role in hairy skin. The lanceolate endings also express detectable SP and CGRP-IR and are intimately associated with C-fiber endings (Fundin et al. 1997a; Rice et al. 1997). Like the Aβ-fiber Meissner's endings, the lanceolate endings are considered to be rapidly adapting, low-threshold mechanoreceptors. Such an Aβ-fiber contribution to pain perception may be mediated by collaterals to the dorsal horn that terminate on presumptive wide-dynamic-range neurons located deep to laminae I and II.

The functional significance of the close anatomical affiliation of the C- and Aβ-fiber endings in the Meissner's corpuscles and around the hair follicles remain to be determined. As noted above, the peptidergic C-fiber endings in the monkey Meissner's corpuscles may exert a trophic effect on, or modulate the physiological activity of, the Aβ-fibers that express the NK1 receptor. Likewise, the TRPV1 C fibers presumably are functionally related to the other types of endings within the Meissner's corpuscle. We hypothesize that these peptidergic and vanilloid C fibers, and also the Aβ fibers, are each monitoring and integrating different complementary aspects of stimuli that affect the Meissner's corpuscle. Although peptidergic and vanilloid endings also terminate in the epidermis, we hypothesize that they are performing other, perhaps similar, functional roles specific to the epidermis.

For example, Meissner's corpuscles are purportedly stimulated by low-frequency vibrations such as those generated from the friction encountered when stroking an object. Such vibrations would also be generated if an object is slipping due to insufficient force exerted during a prehensile grasping task. In contrast, excessive force would generate heat-producing shear forces within the skin that could cause a blister injury. Therefore, the mix of endings with the Meissner's corpuscle may provide a means for calculating the necessary force to grasp an object while minimizing the mechanical impact on the structure of the skin. As such, heat generated within the skin may activate the potential thermal properties of the various types of Meissner's innervation. In contrast, endings with potential thermal properties in the epidermis may be more involved in detecting exogenous thermal stimuli applied to the skin. Importantly, our preliminary analyses indicate that Meissner's corpuscles in the rat and mouse lack the complexity of those seen in the monkey, and only occasionally do they contain some C-fiber innervation in addition to Aβ-fiber innervation. The reason may be that rodents do not engage in powerful, prehensile grasping tasks common to primates. Consequently, peripheral neuropathies generating chronic pain in the glabrous hand skin of primates may involve a different mix of innervation than that in comparable rodent skin used in experimental models of chronic pain.

Based on the preceding observations, we hypothesize that biochemically different types of endings to the same target are likely to be more functionally related than are biochemically similar endings that terminate in different targets. While this premise logically seems evident in relation to such extremely different targets like viscera and skin, we hypothesize that such functional divisions also occur among different types of targets within the skin. Consistent with this hypothesis, a previous study used unique anatomical features of the whisker pad innervation to assess the brainstem connections via transganglionic transport of horseradish peroxidase (HRP) (Arvidsson and Rice 1991). In one type of experiment, HRP was applied to single nerves that supply a mix of several hundred Aβ, Aδ, and C fibers that collectively terminate only in the deeper two-thirds of whisker follicles. All of the innervation, including that from numerous peptidergic and nonpeptidergic C fibers, terminated in a dense, consolidated column with lamina IV of the trigeminal nucleus caudalis and in a less dense site within lamina V. No labeling was found in laminae I and II, which are generally regarded as the principal sites of Aδ- and C-fiber terminations (Fields 1987). However, labeling of laminae I and II was obtained from the application of HRP to the whisker pad epidermis, which is a different site of Aδ and C-fiber terminations. We hypothesize that both the Aβ and C fibers innervating the monkey Meissner's corpuscles would also have a common central projection that may be deep to laminae I and II, whereas projections from the epidermis would be in laminae I and II. Consequently, inflammatory conditions involving innervation to both the Meissner's corpuscles and the epidermis would more extensively affect dorsal horn neurons than would acute conditions that only affect the epidermis or the Meissner's corpuscles.

Importantly, our observations indicate that individual cutaneous sensory endings from Aβ and C fibers can normally have a highly complex chemistry that would enable them to respond to a variety of stimuli implicated in nociception. However, the response properties of these fibers under normal conditions are partially dictated by the composition of the site where the endings terminate and the types of stimuli that can normally impact those sites. The normal perception of the inputs from a given peripheral target in turn depends upon their central terminations. As such, hyperalgesia and allodynia may result not only from a change in the molecular properties of a sensory ending, but also from a change in where they terminate in the skin. Some types of postherpetic neuralgia (PHN) may be an example of such a combination of problems.

We recently analyzed the cutaneous innervation in a patient with severe intractable PHN persisting 6 years after an acute herpes zoster attack (Petersen et al. 2002). His right T6 distribution had persistent, daily, deep pain, shooting pain, and severe allodynia. Brief trials of capsaicin at 0.025% and 0.075% produced intense burning pain. Various treatments including nortriptyline, methadone, lidocaine patches, and gabapentin provided only partial relief. At the patient's insistence, the painful area of skin was excised. A 3-mm punch biopsy was also taken from an unafflicted mirror image site. This treatment reduced the patient's pain symptoms, suggesting that activity of the primary afferent neurons contributed to ongoing pain and allodynia.

Immunofluorescence assessments revealed that the PHN skin had a substantial reduction in innervation density, in accordance with the findings of other studies. However, double-label assessments with various antibody combinations revealed several structural and chemical changes among the remaining endings and the skin, as summarized in Fig. 2. Among the changes was the absence of most of the epidermal innervation that normally lacks either CGRP or TRPV1. Virtually all the remaining epidermis endings had detectable IR for CGRP or TRPV1, or both. In contrast, TRPV1-positive fibers were only observed subepidermally in the biopsy from the unafflicted contralateral site and did not colabel with CGRP. These results indicated either that TRPV1-positive innervation had sprouted into the epidermis, or that some epidermal endings had upregulated TRPV1. Moreover, remaining endings in the epidermis of the PHN skin were longer, more tortuous, and more branched, and extended more superficially than in the epidermis of the contralateral biopsy. These observations indicate that the remaining epidermal endings were in a more exposed location, had more surface area, and had a higher concentration of TRPV1 receptors. Collectively, these changes indicate that these endings would have lower thresholds to potentially noxious stimuli such as capsaicin.

Relatively large-caliber, NF-positive fibers—presumably indicative of Aβ fibers—in the contralateral biopsy only ended as small tangles within dermal papillae. This location indicates that these endings may be the thoracic skin equivalent of Meissner's corpuscles, although they are smaller and less elaborate than in the glabrous skin of the hand. NF-IR was not present on epidermal endings in the contralateral biopsy. In contrast, dermal

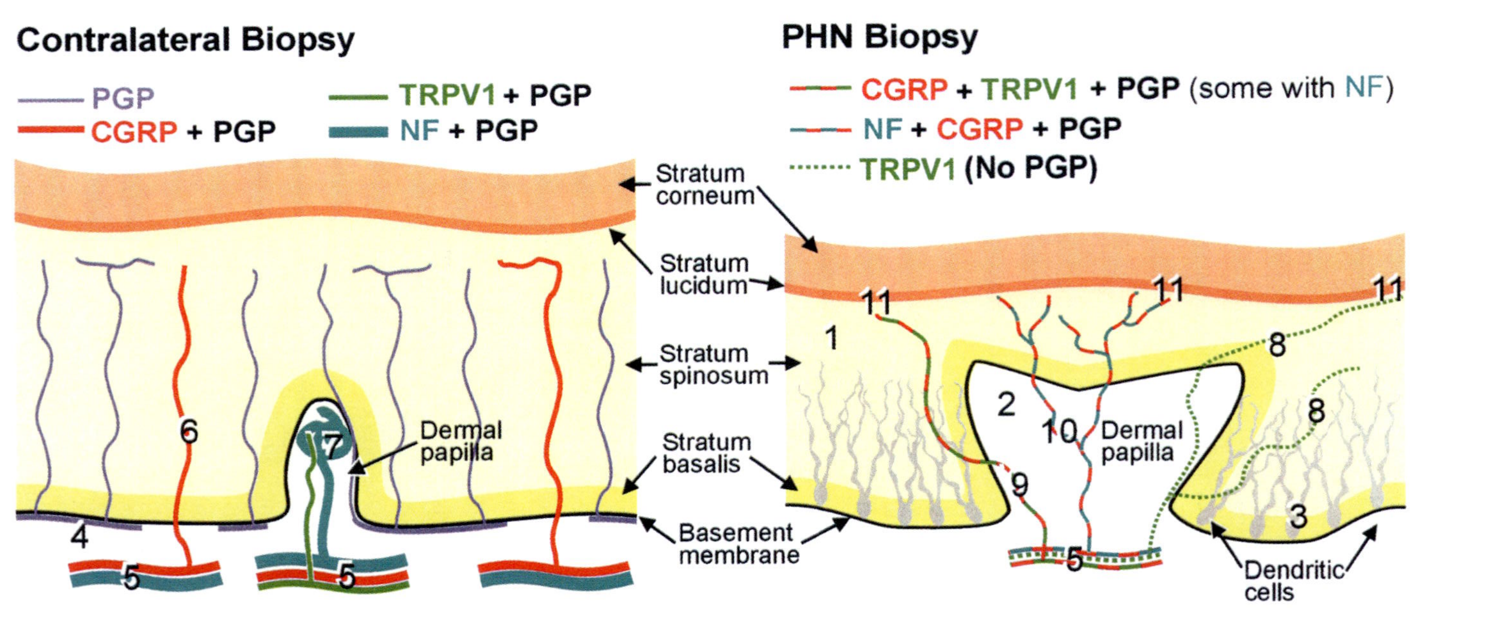

Contralateral Biopsy
PGP
CGRP + PGP
TRPV1 + PGP
NF + PGP
PHN Biopsy
CGRP + TRPV1 + PGP (some with NF)
NF + CGRP + PGP
TRPV1 (No PGP)
Stratum corneum
Stratum lucidum
Stratum spinosum
Stratum basalis
Basement membrane
Dermal papilla
Dermal papilla
Dendritic cells
1
2
3
4
5
5
5
5
6
7
8
8
9
10
11
11
11

← **Fig. 2.** Schematic summary of differences between skin affected by postherpetic neuralgia (PHN) and unaffected skin (from Petersen et al. 2002, reprinted with permission). Numbering refers to numbers on the figure. (1) The epidermis was thinner in the PHN skin. (2) The dermal papillae were larger and more irregularly shaped in PHN skin. Virtually all of the innervation to the epidermis entered via the dermal papillae, whereas most fibers in the contralateral skin entered the epidermis between the dermal papillae (see 4, 5). (3) Only the PHN skin contained numerous anti-protein gene product 9.5 (PGP9.5)-labeled presumptive dendritic cells concentrated primarily in lamina basalis between the dermal papillae. (4) Innervation that only labels with anti-PGP 9.5 is virtually absent in the epidermis of PHN skin. In the contralateral skin, this innervation consisted of axons located immediately subjacent to the basement membrane that terminate as very thin, fairly simple, predominantly radially oriented endings. At least some endings had short T-shaped terminal branches. (5) PHN skin lacked most of the small nerves in the upper dermis that were not in contact with the basement membrane. The remaining nerves were small, with fewer and thinner axons. (6) PHN skin lacked CGRP-positive endings that were supplied directly from the small nerves in the upper dermis and penetrated the epidermis between the dermal papillae. (7) PHN skin lacked axons that terminated like a knot in the dermal papillae. In contralateral skin, this was the only upper dermal and epidermal innervation that labeled with anti-NF, and it may be myelinated. (8) TRPV1-positive profiles in PHN skin were present in virtually all dermal papillae, often had several branches, and often had long oblique trajectories into the epidermis. About half had little or no detectable anti-PGP 9.5 immunoreactivity (IR). In contralateral skin, TRPV1-positive profiles were restricted to only a few dermal papillae, had simple profiles, and also had PGP IR. (9,10) Virtually all the innervation to PHN epidermis that labeled with anti-PGP 9.5 also labeled with anti-CGRP. This innervation had a more oblique instead of radial orientation, could be highly branched, and may also express TRPV1 and/ or NF IR.

papillae in the PHN skin lacked NF-positive terminals, but NF-IR was present on many endings in the epidermis. Many of these aberrant NF-positive epidermal endings also had detectable CGRP-IR. These observations indicate that NF was either upregulated in some types of epidermal innervation that normally lack detectable NF, or that the Aβ-fiber innervation may have sprouted into the epidermis where the fibers would be exposed to stimuli that may not normally contribute to their activation. Conceivably, these aberrant endings may contribute to the tactile allodynia experienced by the patient.

REFERENCES

Arvidsson J, Rice FL. Central projections of primary sensory neurons innervating different parts of the vibrissae follicles and intervibrissal skin on the mystacial pad of the rat. *J Comp Neurol* 1991; 309:1–16.

Birder J, Perl ER. Cutaneous sensory receptors. *Clin Neurophysiol* 1994; 11:534–552.

Burgess PR, Perl ER. Cutaneous mechanoreceptors and nociceptors. In: Iggo A (Ed). *Handbook of Sensory Physiology: Somatosensory System.* Heidelberg: Springer-Verlag, 1973, pp 29–78.

Caterina MJ, Julius D. The vanilloid receptor: a molecular gateway to the pain pathway. *Annu Rev Neurosci* 2001; 24:487–517.

Cauna N. Nerve supply and nerve endings in Meissner's corpuscles. *Am J Anat* 1956; 99:315–327.

Darian-Smith I. The sense of touch: performance and peripheral neural processes. In: Brookhart JM, Mountcastle VB (Eds). *Sensory Processes,* The Nervous System, Vol. III, Part 2. Bethesda, MD: American Physiological Association, 1984, pp 739–788.

Fields HL. *Pain.* New York: McGraw-Hill, 1987.

Fundin BT, Arvidsson J, Aldskogius H, et al. A comprehensive immunofluorescence and lectin binding analysis of intervibrissal fur innervation in the mystacial pad of the rat. *J Comp Neurol* 1997a; 385:185–206.

Fundin BT, Silos-Santiago I, Ernfors PJ, et al. Differential dependency of developing mechanoreceptors on neurotrophins, trk receptors and p75 LNGFR. *Develop Biol* 1997b; 190:94–116.

Johansson O, Fantini F, Hu H. Neuronal structural proteins, transmitters, transmitters enzymes and neuropeptides in humans Meissner's corpuscles: a reappraisal using immunohistochemistry. *Arch Dermatol Res* 1999; 291:419–424.

Julius D, Basbaum AI. Molecular mechanisms of nociception. *Nature* 2001; 413:203–210.

Lawson SN. Morphological and biochemical cell types of sensory neurons. In: Scott SA (Ed). *Sensory Neurons, Diversity, Development and Plasticity.* New York: Oxford University Press, 1992, pp 27–59.

Lawson SN. Neuropeptides in morphologically and functionally identified primary afferent neurons in dorsal root ganglia: substance P, CGRP and somatostatin. *Prog Brain Res* 1995; 104:161–173.

Neumann S, Doubell TP, Leslie T, Woolf CJ. Inflammatory pain hypersensitivity mediated by phenotypic switch in myelinated primary sensory neurons. *Nature* 1996; 384:360–364.

Paré M, Elde R, Mazurkiewicz JE, Smith AM, Rice FL. The Meissner corpuscle revised: multi-afferented mechanoreceptor with nociceptor immunochemical properties. *J Neurosci* 2001a; 21:7236–7246.

Paré M, Rice FL, Bodkin NL, Hansen BC. Aging and diabetes related changes in the innervation to glabrous skin in rhesus monkeys. *Soc Neurosci Abstr* 2001b; 31:282.1.

Paré M, Bodkin NL, Schreyer DJ, Rice FL. Transient increase and subsequent loss of cutaneous innervation in the glabrous skin of diabetic monkeys. *Soc Neurosci Abstr* 2002a; 32:757.1.

Paré M, Schreyer DJ, Rice FL. Selective expression of GAP-43 in C-fiber, δ-fiber and sympathetic innervation in glabrous skin of rats and monkeys. *Abstracts: 10th World Congress on Pain.* Seattle: IASP Press, 2002b, pp 159–160.

Paré M, Smith AM, Rice FL. Distribution of skin mechanoreceptors in the thumb and index fingerpads of the monkey determined by fluorescence microscopy. *J Comp Neurol* 2002c; 445:347–359.

Petersen KL, Rice FL, Suess F, Berro M, Rowbotham MC. Relief of post-herpetic neuralgia by surgical removal of painful skin. *Pain* 2002; 98:119–126.

Rice FL, Fundin BT, Arvidsson J, Aldskogius H, Johansson O. A comprehensive immunofluorescence and lectin binding analysis of vibrissal follicle sinus complex innervation in the mystacial pad of the rat. *J Comp Neurol* 1997; 385:149–184.

Rice FL, Rasmusson DD. Innervation of the digit on the forepaw of the raccoon. *J Comp Neurol* 2000; 417:467–490.

Correspondence to: Frank L. Rice, PhD, Center for Neuropharmacology and Neuroscience, Albany Medical College, 47 New Scotland Avenue, Albany, NY 12208, USA. Email: ricef@mail.amc.edu.

Part III

Nociceptive Pathways, Central Processing, and Imaging

Proceedings of the 10th World Congress on Pain,
Progress in Pain Research and Management, Vol. 24,
edited by Jonathan O. Dostrovsky, Daniel B. Carr, and
Martin Koltzenburg, IASP Press, Seattle, © 2003.

16

The Role of Activity in Developing Pain Pathways

Maria Fitzgerald and Suellen Walker

Department of Anatomy and Developmental Biology,
University College London, London, United Kingdom

The postnatal period is a critical time in the development of spinal sensory systems. It is a time of structural and functional reorganization of sensory connections accompanied by marked changes in expression of molecules, receptors, and channels associated with sensory transmission (Alvares and Fitzgerald 1999; Fitzgerald and Jennings 1999). In addition, it is becoming increasingly evident that these postnatal events are dependent upon neural activity and that synaptic development requires defined patterns of afferent input (Ben-Ari 2002; Debski and Kline 2002; Fox 2002). Abnormal or excessive activity related to pain and injury in early life may therefore change the course of development and cause long-term changes in somatosensory and pain processing (Alvares et al. 2000; Anand 2000). Clinical studies suggest that early pain related to surgical and procedural interventions during intensive care management of premature neonates can have long-term consequences upon pain behavior and perception in later life (Porter et al. 1999; Grunau 2000). This chapter discusses clinical and laboratory evidence for these changes and outlines possible underlying mechanisms.

EVIDENCE THAT EARLY PAIN EXPERIENCE ALTERS FUTURE SOMATOSENSORY PROCESSING: HUMAN STUDIES

Preterm infants in intensive care can receive many invasive procedures, and adequate levels of analgesia are frequently hard to gauge (Anand and Porter 1998). Even the youngest preterm infant will display clear responses to noxious stimuli and tissue injury (Johnston et al. 1995; Fitzgerald and DeLima 2000). Several studies have addressed whether such early pain experience, if excessive or repeated, may alter future pain responses. These responses have been divided here into shorter-term changes (days and weeks) and longer-term changes (months and years).

SHORTER-TERM EFFECTS

Several studies have investigated lasting pain and sensitivity in and around an area of injury in infants. They have shown that even very young preterm babies are capable of displaying a prolonged cutaneous sensitization or hyperalgesia for days and weeks, when exposed to repeated painful stimulation such as heel lances (Fitzgerald et al. 1989). In addition, secondary hyperalgesia can be observed, for instance in the contralateral limb following local ischemic injury (Andrews and Fitzgerald 1994). The area around an abdominal surgical wound shows a similar enhanced cutaneous sensitivity in the postoperative period (Andrews and Fitzgerald 2002). A recent study shows that reactions (evidenced by grimacing or crying) to the pain caused by venipuncture on the forearm are also increased in full-term infants who have undergone repeated heel lances in the previous 24–36 hours, compared to control infants (Taddio et al. 2002). This effect, which extends to increased grimacing even during non-noxious skin cleansing, suggests a spread of central sensitization well outside the area of direct injury.

Other studies have asked a rather different question: Does the overall experience of several weeks of intensive care alter pain responsiveness? These studies do not demonstrate an enhanced response. In fact, facial expression and autonomic and other biobehavioral measures show that pain responses in infants of 32 weeks postconceptional age who have undergone 4 weeks of repeated invasive procedures can be blunted compared to those of age-matched controls (Johnston and Stevens 1996, Grunau et al. 2001).

The debate on how best to measure pain responses in such studies continues (Stevens and Franck 2001), and it is clear that there is great individuality of response, even at very young ages (Franck et al. 2000; Morison et al. 2001). One advantage of measuring cutaneous sensitization and hyperalgesia is that they are relatively simple spinally mediated responses with direct parallels with laboratory studies (Fitzgerald and De Lima 2001). Interestingly, it appears that below 32 weeks, grimacing (facial action coding) and autonomic measures may also be mediated subcortically, because there is no difference in these responses to heel lance in intact and severely brain-injured infants (Oberlander et al. 2002).

LONGER-TERM EFFECTS

While understanding the persistent effects of early pain over days and weeks is extremely important for adequate pain management and recovery, our interest here really lies in the potential for such stimuli to cause changes in responses lasting into childhood, adolescence, or adulthood. Very few data are available in this area, and what little information we have is hard to interpret. Grunau (2000) emphasized the complexity of such studies and the need for careful design and interpretation. As yet no studies have been directed toward sensitivity in and around the site of injury itself as the child matures.

One important study shows that boys who have been circumcised at birth show increased pain responses to vaccinations at 4–6 months compared to those who have not (Taddio et al. 1995). In a follow-up, prospective study on 87 infant boys, uncircumcised infants were found to have the lowest pain scores at vaccination 4–6 months later, followed by those circumcised after treatment with lidocaine-prilocaine cream (EMLA), while those circumcised after placebo cream showed the greatest responses (Taddio et al. 1997).

There is also evidence of persistent hypersensitivity following infant surgery. A follow-up study of infants 3 months after corrective surgery for unilateral hydronephrosis showed that the majority still displayed increased abdominal sensitivity compared to control infants of the same age (Andrews et al. 2003).

Again, the situation is somewhat different when examining former preterm infants and the effects of multiple invasive procedures in intensive care. The blunting of pain responses after several weeks of intensive care, as described above, appears to have disappeared by the time the infants are 4 months old. Biobehavioral pain responses to blood collection by finger lance at 4 months were similar overall between former extremely low birth weight infants and term-born controls (Oberlander et al. 2002). This finding appears inconsistent with the pioneering study of 195 toddlers at 18 months of varying birth weights from 480 g to over 2500 g, in which parents perceived the lowest birth weight groups to have the lowest pain responsiveness and where, unlike the case for toddlers of greater birth weight, there was no relationship between temperament and pain perception (Grunau et al. 1994a). Also, in older children of 4.5 years, "somatization," the occurrence of numerous pains that cannot be accounted for medically, was significantly greater in the lowest birth weight children (Grunau et al. 1994b), although this finding was not observed at age 8–10 years (Grunau et al. 1998). Interestingly, these older children do rate pictures of painful events as more painful than do their peers of normal birth weight (Grunau et al. 1998).

All these longer-term studies are hard to design due to confounding factors such as gestational age at birth (Grunau 1994a), length of intensive care stay (Johnston and Stevens 1996), intensity of the stimulus (Porter et al. 1999a), therapeutic management (Grunau et al. 2001), and parenting style (Grunau 1994b). In addition, children born preterm can have reduced cortical growth (Ajayi-Obe et al. 2000), reduced cognitive test scores, and increased incidence of attention deficit and hyperactivity disorder and other behaviors (Bhutta et al. 2002). The older the child gets, the harder the studies are to conduct because learned patterns of behavior within families are a major determinant of perceived sensitivity to pain (MacGregor et al. 1997).

Changes, if they occur, may be hard to detect in human subjects because the very plasticity that we are investigating may act elsewhere in the nervous system to compensate for the adverse effects of altered or excessive inputs. For instance, in contrast to the intense pain that occurs in adults, no chronic long-term pain follows brachial plexus avulsion at birth, and there is excellent restoration of sensory function and localization of restored sensation in avulsed spinal root dermatomes following surgical repair (Anand and Birch 2002). This finding is consistent with the observation in rat pups that despite profound alterations of plantar hindpaw innervation induced by early nerve transection, cutaneous nociceptive reflexes maintain an essentially normal spatial organization (Holmberg and Schouenborg 1996). In these cases of early nerve damage, an impressive reorganization must have taken place in the nervous system to limit the sensory deficit.

EVIDENCE THAT EARLY PAIN EXPERIENCE ALTERS FUTURE SOMATOSENSORY PROCESSING: ANIMAL STUDIES

BEHAVIORAL STUDIES

A key step toward evaluating the impact of early pain upon future somatosensory processing is to establish animal models where tissue injury or repeated noxious stimuli applied at infancy lead to changes in adult sensory behavior. Such models have been reported, but the effects depend critically upon the nature of the injury.

Exposure to repetitive needle pricks to the paw four times a day in rat pups from postnatal (P) days P0 to P7 produces hyperalgesia, in the form of reduced hot-plate latencies, at day P16, but this does not last into adulthood (Anand et al. 1999). The neonatally injured animals do, however, show an increased preference for alcohol and also manifest other behavioral changes as adults. On the other hand, a more severe injury of repeated 10% formalin injections into paws from P1 to P7 leads to hypoalgesia in adulthood, in the form of increased hot-plate and tail-flick latency. Preemptive morphine treatment before the first injection of formalin ameliorates the effects in males only, but the situation is complicated by the fact that morphine alone at birth increases adult tail-flick latencies more severely than does an injury. In this model, neonatal pain and morphine decrease alcohol preference (Bhutta et al. 2001). The differences in these results may be explained by the fact that formalin is a more damaging stimulus that may lead to some sensory neuron death (Tsujino et al. 2000), whereas repeated needle prick will presumably only produce local inflammation.

The long-term effects of an injection of inflammatory agents at birth is a subject of some controversy and clearly depends on the agent and dose used. Nociceptive thresholds fall in neonatal animals within a few hours of an inflammatory lesion (Jiang and Gebhart 1998; Marsh et al. 1999), but the question here is whether the effects last beyond the resolution of the peripheral damage. One report describes neonatal hindpaw injection of 0.25% carrageenan in newborn rat pups causing mechanical and heat hypoalgesia in 60-day-old adults while increasing the hyperalgesia produced by an injection of complete Freund's adjuvant (CFA) (Lidow et al. 2001). These effects were reversed if the neonatal inflammation was accompanied by four injections of sciatic bupivacaine nerve block, lasting up to 9 hours after the inflammation. However, in two other separate, blinded studies, no changes in mechanical or heat responses were observed in adults following neonatal carrageenan injection (Alvares et al. 2000; Walker and Fitzgerald 2002). Despite the profound and long-lasting inflammation (14 days) produced by a single injection of 10 μL 2% carrageenan in the neonatal hindpaw, no difference was found in the three groups (neonatal carrageenan, saline, and anesthetic only) in mechanical or heat thresholds (either between left and right paws or between inflamed and control groups) at any stage tested. In addition, the reapplication of 2% carrageenan or CFA in these rats, when they had reached maturity, caused normal inflammatory, hyperalgesic, and allodynic responses that did not differ from those of controls. A stronger inflammatory agent (25 μL CFA) injected into the hindpaw at birth also leaves adult baseline thermal withdrawal latencies unchanged, but following a second challenge with CFA, hyperalgesia increases very slightly and the time course, but not the magnitude, of the formalin response is altered (Ruda et al. 2000). The volumes and doses of inflammatory agents used in infant rats for such studies must be considered with care. Injection of 25 μL CFA in a newborn rat leaves the paw swollen into adulthood (Walker and Fitzgerald 2001) and thus is clearly not an injury that resolves itself in the neonatal period.

Another type of injury that has been investigated is a full-thickness skin wound in the hindpaw of the newborn rat pup, which heals rapidly. A long-lasting hypersensitivity, in the form of lowered von Frey mechanical threshold, persists in the previously injured region (Reynolds and Fitzgerald 1995; DeLima et al. 1999). The effect is apparent after 1 week and lasts for at least 6 weeks (DeLima et al. 1999); it only occurs if the wound is made in the postnatal period (Reynolds et al. 1997). In this case, local sciatic nerve block with bupivacaine for the first 24 hours after wounding did not affect the onset or magnitude of mechanical hypersensitivity.

NEUROBIOLOGICAL STUDIES

While changes in animal behavior are important, they are prey to almost as many confounding factors as human studies. There is considerable advantage in looking for direct effects of early injury upon the development of neural connections. Analysis at the cellular level can reveal changes in sensory connections that are not evident in behavioral tests.

Early peripheral inflammation has a transient influence on the postnatal development of rat primary sensory neuron subtypes (Beland and Fitzgerald 2001). This phenomenon has been studied using calcitonin gene-related peptide (CGRP) to label peptide-containing and IB4 to label nonpeptide-containing nociceptive neurons and using NF200 to label larger non-nociceptive neurons. Following carrageenan inflammation in rats on day P1, the normal rise in IB4-positive binding in the dorsal root ganglion occurs earlier but is the same as that in controls by day P21. The CGRP-positive population increases at 2 and 6 days after carrageenan, because of an increase in both small CGRP/IB4 and larger CGRP/NF200 double-labeled cells, but again, is normal by 3 weeks. The effects are different from adult inflammation, where carrageenan causes a transient increase in CGRP/IB4 cells only (Beland and Fitzgerald 2001).

There is also a clear acute effect (within 2–5 hours) of carrageenan inflammation upon the properties of dorsal horn cells, including increased spontaneous activity, evoked responses, and A-fiber sensitization, although the pattern of effects is age dependent (Torsney and Fitzgerald 2002). These short-term effects do not last beyond the acute inflammation, however, and in parallel with the behavioral results described above, the dorsal horn cell properties 6 weeks later do not differ from controls (C. Torsney and M. Fitzgerald, unpublished manuscript).

CFA injections in the neonate, on the other hand, do cause long-lasting changes in spinal circuitry that can be observed in the adult. These consist of expanded central C-fiber terminal fields and CGRP expression and increased fos-like immunoreactivity, a measure of neuronal activity in dorsal horn neurons (Ruda et al. 2000; Tachibana et al. 2001). These central changes must be viewed in the context of very severe tissue damage caused by large volumes of inflammatory agents that may have neuropathic and systemic consequences and that produce an inflammatory response that lasts into adulthood (Walker and Fitzgerald 2002).

Of all the early models of pain, skin wounding at birth has some of the longest-lasting peripheral and central consequences upon sensory connections. The wound heals rapidly, but the sensory nerve terminals in the area show a profound sprouting response, which long outlasts the injury (at least 12 weeks in the rat) (Reynolds and Fitzgerald 1995; De Lima et al. 1999; Alvares et al. 2000). The effect is most dramatic when wounds are performed at birth and decreases progressively with age at wounding. This is a sensory A- and C-fiber nerve response with no sympathetic involvement (Reynolds and Fitzgerald 1995). In addition, skin wounding at birth leads to a long-lasting expansion of dorsal horn cell receptive fields, which is clearly observed at 6 weeks (C. Torsney and M. Fitzgerald, unpublished observations).

The only other infant model that leads to central changes of this kind is neonatal colonic distension or irritation with mustard oil between postnatal days 8 and 21, which leads to sensitization of the abdominal withdrawal reflex and heightens the responses of viscerosensitive neurons during colon distension in adult rats. This model appears to lead to chronic visceral hypersensitivity in the adult in the absence of identifiable peripheral pathology and only occurs if the colon is distended in young animals (Al-Chaer et al. 2000).

MECHANISMS UNDERLYING THE EFFECTS OF EARLY PAIN EXPERIENCE UPON FUTURE SOMATOSENSORY PROCESSING

The mechanisms by which early experience alters somatosensory processing are likely to involve activity-dependent changes in the developing nervous system. The influence of sensory experience upon the formation of somatosensory synaptic connections is well established in the rodent trigeminal system, where alterations in whisker stimulation during a critical period of postnatal development result in receptive field reorganization in the brainstem, thalamus, and cortex (O'Leary et al. 1994; Fox 2002; Kaas and Catania 2002). This period of plasticity is transitory, usually encompassing only a short time soon after the onset of the sensory stimulus, which is immediately postnatal for whisker barrel formation (Fox 1992), and after eye opening in relation to the visual cortex (Berardi et al. 2000). If the source of activity is altered during this critical period, normal patterns of connectivity are disrupted. A common mechanism has been proposed whereby synaptic connections are strengthened when pre- and postsynaptic activity is correlated, with those connections that are uncorrelated being weakened and eliminated (Feldman et al. 1999; Sanes and Yamagata 1999). The molecular basis of this mechanism is thought to involve the induction of *N*-methyl D-aspartate (NMDA)-dependent long-term potentiation and depression (Fox 2002). In support of this theory, normal sensory connectivity patterns are disrupted in NMDA-R1-receptor knockout mice (Iwasato et al. 1997). While the limits of sensory connections are dependent upon afferent terminal patterns, functional somatotopic maps are determined by the size and pattern of receptive fields of individual target neurons, and the construction of these receptive fields in the developing visual system is also NMDA-dependent (Huang and Pallas 2001).

EVIDENCE FOR ACTIVITY-DEPENDENT DEVELOPMENT OF SPINAL SENSORY PATHWAYS

Spinal cord dorsal horn somatosensory maps also undergo postnatal refinement over a critical postnatal period. Primary afferent A fibers extend more superficially to laminae I and II of the dorsal horn at early postnatal stages, with a subsequent gradual withdrawal down to lamina III and below over the first three postnatal weeks (Fitzgerald et al. 1994; Beggs et al. 2002). This withdrawal is accompanied by a progressive reduction in A-fiber input to the substantia gelatinosa (Park et al. 1999; Nakatsuka et al. 2000) and a gradual reduction in the cutaneous receptive field size of dorsal horn cells (Fitzgerald and Jennings 1999; Torsney and Fitzgerald 2002). The postnatal refinement of sensory inputs in the spinal dorsal horn is likely to contribute to sensory processing in the postnatal period and may underlie the increase in cutaneous mechanical reflex thresholds that occurs between birth and adulthood (Fitzgerald 1999; Fitzgerald and Jennings 1999).

The postnatal withdrawal of A-fiber terminals from the substantia gelatinosa may be the result of a competitive process because neonatal destruction of C fibers with capsaicin prevents the effect (Torsney et al. 2000). Recently we have shown that chronic, local exposure of the dorsal horn of the lumbar spinal cord to the NMDA antagonist MK801 from birth prevents the normal functional and structural reorganization of A-fiber connections (Beggs et al. 2002). Dorsal horn cells in spinal MK801-treated animals, investigated at 8 weeks of age by "in vivo" electrophysiological recording, had significantly larger cutaneous mechanoreceptive fields and greater A-fiber-evoked responses than did vehicle-treated controls. C-fiber-evoked responses were unaffected. Chronic application of MK801 also prevented the normal structural reorganization of A-fiber terminals in the spinal cord. The postnatal withdrawal of superficially projecting A-fiber primary afferents to deeper laminae did not occur in treated animals, although C-fiber afferent terminals and cell density in the dorsal horn were apparently unaffected. Spinal MK801-treated animals also had significantly reduced behavioral reflex thresholds to mechanical stimulation of the hindpaw compared to naive and vehicle-treated animals, whereas noxious heat thresholds remained unaffected. The results indicate that the normal postnatal structural and functional development of A-fiber sensory connectivity within the spinal cord is an activity-dependent process requiring NMDA-receptor activation (Beggs et al. 2002).

The finding that blockade of NMDA activation of dorsal horn neurons during a critical period of development selectively alters the normal development of spinal sensory connections demonstrates the plasticity and vulnerability of this system. It seems likely, therefore, that altered patterns of C-fiber excitation resulting from local injury in neonates will modify synaptic connectivity within the central nervous system via an NMDA-dependent mechanism and so alter the normal maturation of sensory pathways.

CONCLUSION

In common with other areas of the central nervous system, synaptic development of spinal sensory connections is experience or activity dependent. Evidence from both animal and human studies shows that alterations in the pattern of sensory activity that can arise from tissue injury and pain in early life may disrupt normal synaptic organization within the somatosensory system. While these studies are incomplete and more investigation is needed in this area, the potential clinical importance of neonatal plasticity in pain development is clear.

ACKNOWLEDGMENTS

Suellen Walker was an IASP John J. Bonica Fellow. Support from the Medical Research Council and Children Nationwide is gratefully acknowledged.

REFERENCES

Ajayi-Obe M, Saeed N, Cowan FM, Rutherford MA, Edwards AD. Reduced development of cerebral cortex in extremely preterm infants. *Lancet* 2000; 356:1162–1163.

Al-Chaer ED, Kawasaki M, Pasricha PJ. A new model of chronic visceral hypersensitivity in adult rats induced by colon irritation during postnatal development. *Gastroenterology* 2000; 119:1276–1285.

Alvares D, Fitzgerald M. Building blocks of pain: the regulation of key molecules in spinal sensory neurones during development and following peripheral axotomy. *Pain* 1999; 6(Suppl):S71–S85.

Alvares D, Torsney C, Beland B, Reynolds M, Fitzgerald M. Modelling the prolonged effects of neonatal pain. *Prog Brain Res* 2000; 129:365–373.

Anand KJS. Pain, plasticity and premature birth: a prescription for permanent suffering? *Nat Med* 2000; 6:971–973.

Anand KJS, Porter FL. Epidemiology of pain in neonates. *Res Clin Forums* 1998; 20(4)9–18.

Anand KJS, Coskun V, Thrivikraman KV, Nemeroff CB, Plotsky PM. Long-term behavioural effects of repetitive pain in neonatal rat pups. *Physiol Behav* 1999; 66:627–637.

Anand P, Birch R. Restoration of sensory function and lack of long-term chronic pain syndromes after brachial plexus injury in human neonates. *Brain* 2002; 125:113–122.

Andrews KA, Fitzgerald M. The cutaneous withdrawal reflex in human neonates: sensitization, receptive fields and the effects of contralateral stimulation. *Pain* 1994; 56:95–101.

Andrews KA, Fitzgerald M. Wound sensitivity as a measure of analgesic effects following surgery in human neonates and infants. *Pain* 2002; in press.

Andrews KA, Desai D, Dhillon K, Wilcox T, Fitzgerald M. Abdominal sensitivity in the first year of life: comparison of infants with and without prenatally-diagnosed unilateral hydronephrosis. *Pain* 2003; in press.

Beggs S, Torsney C, Drew L, Fitzgerald M. The postnatal reorganisation of primary afferent input and dorsal horn cell receptive fields in the rat spinal cord is an activity-dependent process. *Eur J Neurosci* 2002; 16:1249–1258.

Beland B, Fitzgerald M. Influence of peripheral inflammation on the postnatal maturation of primary sensory neuron phenotype in rats. *J Pain* 2001; 2:36–45.

Ben-Ari Y. Excitatory actions of GABA during development: the nature of the nurture. *Nat Rev Neurosci* 2002; 3:728–7239.

Berardi N, Pizzorusso T, Maffei L. Critical periods during sensory development. *Curr Opin Neurobiol* 2000; 10:138–145.

Bhutta AT, Rovnaghi C, Simpson PM, et al. Interactions of inflammatory pain and morphine in infant rats. Long term behavioural effects. *Physiol Behav* 2001; 73:51–58.

Bhutta AT, Cleves MA, Casey PH, Cradock MM, Anand KJS. Cognitive and behavioural outcomes of school aged children who were born preterm. *JAMA* 2002; 288:728–737.

Debski EA, Cline HT. Activity-dependent mapping in the retinotectal projection. *Curr Opin Neurobiol* 2002; 12:93–99.

De Lima J, Alvares D, Hatch DJ, Fitzgerald M. Sensory hyperinnervation after neonatal skin wounding: effect of bupivacaine sciatic nerve block. *Br J Anaesth* 1999; 83:662–664.

Feldman DE, Nicoll RA, Malenka RC. Synaptic plasticity at thalamocortical synapses in developing rat somatosensory cortex: LTP, LTD, and silent synapses. *J Neurobiol* 1999; 41:92–101.

Fitzgerald M. The developmental neurobiology of pain. In: *Textbook of Pain*, 4th ed. Wall PD, Melzack R (Eds). Edinburgh: Churchill Livingstone, 1999, pp 235–252.

Fitzgerald M, De Lima J. Hyperalgesia and allodynia in infants. In: Finley A, McGrath PJ (Eds). *Acute and Procedure Pain in Infants and Children*, Progress in Pain Research and Management, Vol. 20. Seattle: IASP Press, 2001, pp 1–12.

Fitzgerald M, Jennings E. The postnatal development of spinal sensory processing. *Proc Natl Acad Sci USA* 1999; 96:7719–7722.

Fitzgerald M, Millard C, Macintosh N. Cutaneous hypersensitivity following peripheral tissue. *Pain* 1989; 39:31–36.

Fitzgerald M, Butcher T, Shortland P. Developmental changes in the laminar termination of A-fibre cutaneous sensory afferents in the rat spinal cord dorsal horn. *J Comp Neurol* 1994; 348:225–233.

Fox K. A critical period for experience-dependent synaptic plasticity in rat barrel cortex. *J Neurosci* 1992; 12(5):1826–1838.

Fox K. Anatomical pathways and molecular mechanisms for plasticity in the barrel cortex. *Neuroscience* 2002; 111:799–814.

Franck LS, Boyce WT, Gregory GA, et al. Plasma norepinephrine levels, vagal tone index, and flexor reflex threshold in premature neonates receiving intravenous morphine during the postoperative period: a pilot study. *Clin J Pain* 2000; 16:95–104.

Grunau RE. Long-term consequences of pain in human neonates. In: Anand KJS, Stevens BJ, McGrath PJ (Eds). *Pain in Neonates,* 2nd ed. Pain Research and Clinical Management, Vol. 10. Amsterdam: Elsevier, 2000.

Grunau RE, Whitfield MF, Petrie JH. Pain sensitivity and temperament in extremely low birth weight premature toddlers and preterm and fullterm controls. *Pain* 1994a; 58:341–346.

Grunau RE, Whitfield MF, Petrie JH, Fryer EL. Early pain experience, child and family factors, as precursors of somatization: a prospective study of extremely premature and fullterm children. *Pain* 1994b; 56:353–359.

Grunau RE, Whitfield MF, Petrie J. Children's judgements about pain at age 8–10 years: do extremely low birthweight (<=1000 g) children differ from full birthweight peers? *J Child Psychol Psychiatry* 1998; 39:587–594.

Grunau RE, Oberlander TF, Whitfield MF, Fitzgerald C, Lee SK. Demographic and therapeutic determinants of pain reactivity in very low birth weight neonates at 32 weeks' postconceptional age. *Pediatrics* 2001; 107:105–112.

Holmberg H, Schouenborg J. Developmental adaptation of withdrawal reflexes to early alteration of peripheral innervation in the rat. *J Physiol* 1996; 495:399–409.

Huang L, Pallas SL. NMDA antagonists in the superior colliculus prevent developmental plasticity but not visual transmission or map compression. *J Neurophysiol* 2001; 86:1179–1194.

Iwasato T, Erzurumlu RS, Huerta PT, et al. NMDA receptor-dependent refinement of somatotopic maps. *Neuron* 1997; 19:1201–1210.

Jiang MC, Gebhart GF. Development of mustard oil–induced hyperalgesia in rats. *Pain* 1998; 77:305–313.

Johnston CC, Stevens BJ. Experience in a neonatal intensive care unit affects pain response. *Pediatrics* 1996; 98:925–930.

Johnston CC, Stevens BJ, Yang F, Horton L. Differential response to pain by very premature neonates. *Pain* 1995; 61:471–479.

Kaas JH, Catania KC. How do features of sensory representations develop? *Bioessays* 2002; 24:334–343.

Lidow MS, Song Z-M, Ren K. Long-term effects of short lasting early local inflammatory insult. *Neuroreport* 2001; 12:399–403.

Marsh D, Dickenson A, Hatch D, Fitzgerald M. Epidural opioid analgesia in infant rats II: responses to carrageenan and capsaicin. *Pain* 1999; 82:33–38.

McGregor AJ, Griffiths GO, Baker J, Spector TD. Determinants of pressure pain threshold in adult twins: evidence that shared environmental influences predominate. *Pain* 1997; 73:253–257.

Morison SJ, Grunau RE, Oberlander TF, Whitfield MF. Relations between behavioral and cardiac autonomic reactivity to acute pain in preterm neonates. *Clin J Pain* 2001; 17:350–358.

Nakatsuka T, Ataka T, Kumamoto E, Tamaki T, Yoshimura M. Alteration in synaptic inputs through C-afferent fibres to substantia gelatinosa neurons of the rat spinal dorsal horn during postnatal development. *Neuroscience* 2000; 99:549–556.

O'Leary D, Ruff NL, Dyck RH. Development, critical period plasticity, and adult reorganizations of mammalian somatosensory systems. *Curr Opin Neurobiol* 1994; 4:535–544.

Oberlander TF, Grunau RE, Whitfield MF, et al. Biobehavioral pain responses in former extremely low birth weight infants at four months' corrected age. *Pediatrics* 2000; 105:e6.

Oberlander TF, Grunau RE, Fitzgerald C, Whitfield MF. Does parenchymal brain injury affect biobehavioral pain responses in very low birth weight infants at 32 weeks' postconceptional age? *Pediatrics* 2002; 110:570–576.

Park JS, Nakatsuka T, Nagata K, Higashi H, Yoshimura M. Reorganization of the primary afferent termination in the rat spinal dorsal horn during post-natal development. *Brain Res Dev Brain Res* 1999; 113:29–36.

Porter FL, Grunau RE, Anand KJ. Long-term effects of pain in infants. *J Dev Behav Pediatr* 1999; 20:253–261.

Reynolds M, Fitzgerald M. Long-term sensory hyperinnervation following neonatal skin wounds. *J Comp Neurol* 1995; 358:487–498.

Reynolds ML, Alvares D, Middleton J, Fitzgerald M. Neonatally wounded skin induces NGF-independent sensory neurite outgrowth in vitro. *Dev Brain Res* 1997; 102:275–283.

Ruda MA, Ling Q-D, Hohmann AG, Peng YB, Tachibana T. Altered nociceptive neuronal circuits after neonatal peripheral inflammation. *Science* 2000; 289:628–630.

Sanes JR, Yamagata M. Formation of lamina-specific synaptic connections. *Curr Opin Neurobiol* 1999; 9:79–87.

Stevens BJ, Franck LS. Assessment and management of pain in neonates. *Paediatr Drugs* 2001; 3:539–358.

Tachibana T, Ling QD, Ruda MA. Increased fos induction in adult rats that experienced neonatal peripheral inflammation. *Neuroreport* 2001; 12:925–927.

Taddio A, Goldbach M, Ipp M, Stevens B, Koren G. Effect of neonatal circumcision on pain responses during vaccination in boys. *Lancet* 1995; 345:291–292.

Taddio A, Shah V, Gilbert-MacLeod C, Katz J. Conditioning and hyperalgesia in newborns exposed to repeated heel lances. *JAMA* 2002; 288:857–861.

Tsujino H, Kondo E, Fukuoka T, et al. Activating Transcription Factor 3 (ATF3) induction by axotomy in sensory and motoneurons: a novel neuronal marker of nerve injury. *Mol Cell Neurosci* 2000; 15:170–182.

Torsney C, Fitzgerald M. Age-dependent effects of peripheral inflammation on the electrophysiological properties of neonatal rat dorsal horn neurons. *J Neurophysiol* 2002 87:1311–1317.

Torsney C, Meredith-Middleton J, Fitzgerald M. Neonatal capsaicin treatment prevents the normal postnatal withdrawal of A fibres from lamina II without affecting fos responses to innocuous peripheral stimulation. *Brain Res Dev Brain Res* 2000; 121:55–65.

Walker SM, Fitzgerald M. Acute and chronic inflammatory pain models in infant rats: effects of volume and inflammatory mediator. *Soc Neurosci Abstracts* 2001; 27:159.8.

Walker SM, Fitzgerald M. Long-term plasticity of primary afferent terminal fields following neonatal inflammation is maintained by prolonged injury. *Abstracts: 10th World Congress on Pain.* Seattle: IASP Press, 2002, pp 272–273.

Correspondence to: Maria Fitzgerald, PhD, Department of Anatomy and Developmental Biology, University College London, Gower Street, London WC1E 6BT, United Kingdom. Email: m.fitzgerald@ucl.ac.uk.

Proceedings of the 10th World Congress on Pain,
Progress in Pain Research and Management, Vol. 24,
edited by Jonathan O. Dostrovsky, Daniel B. Carr, and
Martin Koltzenburg, IASP Press, Seattle, © 2003.

17

Specificity and Integration in Central Pain Pathways

A.D. Craig

Atkinson Pain Research Laboratory, Division of Neurosurgery, Barrow Neurological Institute, Phoenix, Arizona, USA

As a functional neuroanatomist, I believe it is axiomatic that the nervous system is well-organized. Approximately 65 million years of mammalian evolution have generated neural pathways, reproduced in each individual, that reliably maintain the health of the body—in other words, autonomic, neuroendocrine, immune, and behavioral systems that efficiently maintain homeostasis and promote survival. I also believe, in agreement with Darwin's thesis, that whereas only humans have both the self-awareness and the language required to describe it explicitly, pain is a basic mammalian emotion involving these inherent systems that serves to protect the individual. Like other basic emotions (e.g., fear, anger, disgust, sadness, or happiness), pain generates both a distinct feeling (sensation) that can be introspectively evaluated and a behavioral motivation (affect) that can overwhelm one's attention completely. Similarly, temperature, itch, sensual touch, hunger, thirst, and all other aspects of homeostatic afferent activity have the same characteristics—they generate both a distinct feeling and a graded motivation. As a neuroanatomist, I know that by dissecting the nervous system according to its natural divisions—reading the data rather than imposing preconceptions—we will discover that it is organized in distinct, specific neural pathways that correlate with, and engender, the different aspects of the emotion of pain that can be distinguished psychophysically. As Sherrington taught, the organization of the nervous system is based on the integration of specific components.

Most current investigators and clinicians have learned a model of the central neural pathways underlying pain based on the gate control theory (Melzack and Wall 1965), which denied a role for specificity in pain. In this model, pain is not represented by specific or well-organized elements in the brain, but by patterns of activity within the somatosensory system (Price and Dubner 1977; Price 1988; Bonica 1990; Willis and Westlund 1997). Clinicians in particular appreciate this view because they recognize that pain is more than just a specific sensation. In this model, activity carried by "pain transmission neurons" ascends in the crossed spinothalamic tract (STT) to the ventral posterior (VP) nucleus of the thalamus and thence to the main somatosensory cortex in the postcentral gyrus. The "pain transmission neurons" in this model are convergent, multireceptive pain-and-touch neurons, the so-called "wide dynamic range" or WDR neurons, which have been studied extensively in the deep dorsal horn (lamina V), in the VP, and in the somatosensory cortex (Casey 1966; Willis 1985; Kenshalo et al. 1988; Bushnell et al. 1993). Nonspecific WDR neurons are thought to be essential for pain because they seem to provide a ready basis for the allodynia and referred pain encountered in patients (Wall 1973; Price and Dubner 1977). Imaging, evoked potential, and lesion studies in humans from some laboratories are interpreted as supportive of a role for the first and second (S1 and S2) parietal somatosensory cortices in pain, consistent with this model (e.g., Ploner et al. 1999; Treede et al. 2000; Chen et al. 2002).

This model has several fundamental shortcomings. First, it has been known for at least a century that lesions of parietal somatosensory cortices almost never affect pain sensation, and pain is almost never caused by stimulation there. On the contrary, stimulation in VP, the lemniscal relay to S1, is often used to alleviate chronic pain. Second, the convergent WDR cells are inherently modality-ambiguous; the data indicate that the activity of individual WDR neurons does not distinguish innocuous brushing from noxious pinch, or pinch from heat, or cutaneous stimuli from muscle or visceral input, or histamine from mustard oil, even though all of these cause very different sensations that are easily distinguishable (Surmeier et al. 1988; Carstens 1997). Third, this model of pain includes at best a minor role for well-documented STT neurons that are specifically sensitive to stimuli that cause painful sensations, even though such neurons must be involved in pain processing. Fourth, this model ignores the classic evidence (the Brown-Sequard syndrome) that the pathways in the central nervous system underlying pain, temperature, itch, and sensual touch are distinguished from those associated with discriminative touch and positional senses by their immediate segregation at the spinal level into the contralateral STT and the ipsilateral lemniscal pathway, respectively. The functional significance of this separation is supported by the observation that all of the feelings associated with the STT generate autonomic (i.e., homeostatic) reflexes and behavioral motivation (affect), whereas fine touch and positional senses do not and instead are intimately associated with motor control. (Recall that a primary symptom of a dorsal column lesion is loss of fine dexterity [Nathan 1986].)

The essential conceptual difference between the convergent model and the new view described in this chapter stems from the fundamental recognition that the feelings from the body represented in the STT are all aspects of the sense of the body's physiological condition, referred to as interoception, whereas the discriminative touch and positional senses provide information about the relationship between the body and the external environment, that is, exteroception. In this view, pain is distinct from touch, and it is a feeling and a motivation related to the physiological condition of the material body, like temperature, itch, and hunger.

This chapter presents an overview of recent functional, anatomical, and imaging findings indicating that pain is represented in a well-organized system that conveys homeostatic afferent activity, including an interoceptive spinothalamocortical pathway that is visible only in primates and is well-developed only in humans. However, this model incorporates both spinal neurons that represent specific aspects of the condition of the body's tissues and convergent neurons that represent the cumulative sum of all afferent activity. The specific neurons are associated with distinct sensations, including first ("sharp") pain and second ("burning") pain, whereas the convergent neurons modify integration in forebrain systems and could be involved in neuropathic dysfunction. Thus, the neural substrates underlying pain sensation in this model include both specific sensory channels (virtual "labeled lines") and integrative pathways, and integration of these ascending pathways in the forebrain engenders perceived sensation. Further details, numerous illustrations, and complete references can be found in recent reviews (Craig and Dostrovsky 1999; Craig 2000, 2002a,b).

TWO PAIN-RELATED COMPONENTS OF THE STT

Small-diameter (Aδ and C) primary afferents from all tissues of the body terminate in lamina I of the superficial spinal dorsal horn. (The adjacent lamina II [substantia gelatinosa] contains only local interneurons in cats and monkeys and essentially receives C fibers only from skin. In rodents, lamina II is less distinct from lamina I.) Cells in the deep dorsal horn receive direct Aδ-nociceptor input and polysynaptic C-fiber input. Lamina I is the source of output from the superficial dorsal horn and contributes half of the STT; the second component originates in laminae IV–VII.

The small-diameter afferents and lamina I neurons are developmentally associated and are differentiated from the large-diameter exteroceptive and proprioceptive afferents that project to the deep dorsal horn (Altman and

Bayer 1984). The fine afferents originate from small (B) dorsal root ganglion cells and enter the spinal cord in a second wave, subsequent to the larger fibers that issue from the A cells. Their arrival in the dorsal horn is genetically coordinated to coincide with the arrival of lamina I neurons. The lamina I cells originate from the progenitors of autonomic interneurons in the lateral horn and migrate to their superficial dorsal position during a ventromedial rotation of the entire dorsal horn that occurs simultaneously with the arrival of the small-diameter afferents. (This also results in the recurrent trajectory of the large-diameter fibers, which do not contact lamina I neurons.) This phenomenon supports the view that small-diameter afferents and lamina I neurons constitute a cohesive homeostatic afferent system distinct from the exteroceptive/proprioceptive system.

The Aδ and C afferent fibers that monosynaptically activate lamina I neurons relate homeostatic information from all tissues—not only painful mechanical stress and noxious heat and cold, but also innocuous temperature, local metabolism (e.g., acidic pH, hypoxia, hypo-osmolarity, lactic acid), cell rupture (ATP, glutamate), parasite penetration (histamine), mast cell activation (serotonin, eicosanoids), and immune and hormonal activity (cytokines, somatostatin) (for references, see Craig 2002b). Microneurographic data indicate that only the summated activation of "C-nociceptors" causes a conscious perception of "pain" in humans (Gybels et al. 1979), and C fibers often have slow ongoing discharge without provocation that is not perceived (Mense and Stahnke 1983; Schaible and Schmidt 1996; Adreani and Kaufman 1998) and that is most likely related to current tissue metabolic status. In addition, many cutaneous C fibers are selectively sensitive to weak mechanical stimuli that evoke sensual ("limbic") touch (Vallbo et al. 1999), as are certain neurons in lamina I (Light and Willcockson 1999).

The ascending projections of lamina I neurons in cats and monkeys directly indicate their role in homeostasis (Craig 1995). They project strongly to the sympathetic cell columns of the thoracolumbar spinal cord and to the major homeostatic integration sites in the brainstem. The latter include regions that also receive parasympathetic afferent activity (by way of the solitary nucleus) and are heavily interconnected with the hypothalamus and amygdala (e.g., ventrolateral medulla, catecholamine cell groups A1–2 and A5–7, parabrachial nucleus [PB]). These lamina I projections substantialize the hierarchical somato-autonomic reflexes activated by small-diameter afferents that are critical for homeostatic functions (Sato and Schmidt 1973). In turn, lamina I receives descending modulation directly from brainstem pre-autonomic sources, and most strikingly, directly from the hypothalamus.

Lamina I neurons comprise several distinct, modality-selective classes that receive input from particular subsets of small-diameter fibers and relate the ongoing physiological status of the tissues of the body. These classes of neurons can be termed "labeled lines," because they differ morphologically, physiologically, and biochemically, and because their activity corresponds with distinct sensations (Han et al. 1998; Craig et al. 2001), although they must be integrated in the forebrain (see below). Based on cutaneous stimulation, two classes of nociceptive lamina I STT neurons that receive predominantly Aδ-nociceptor and polymodal C-nociceptor inputs correlate with sharp ("first") pain and burning ("second") pain, respectively (Andrew and Craig 2002; Craig and Andrew 2002). These have been distinguished by using a maintained mechanical stimulus paradigm with a graded series of fine probes that produces a selective sensation of first pain and a repeated brief contact heat stimulus paradigm that produces a selective sensation of augmenting second pain. Only the responses of the first class of lamina I STT neurons (nociceptive-specific, or NS fusiform cells) closely parallel the psychophysics of first pain, and only those of the other class (polymodal nociceptive multipolar cells, or HPC for heat, pinch, and cold) parallel the sensation of second pain produced by the latter paradigm. The activity of HPC neurons also can explain the burning sensation elicited by noxious cold or by the thermal grill illusion of pain.

In addition, there are two types of thermoreceptive lamina I cells that respond selectively to cooling (pyramidal cells) or to warming, distinct types of chemoreceptive cells that respond selectively to histamine or to noxious chemicals, and other classes that respond selectively to muscle or joint afferents or to mechanical "slow brush" (tickle). The role of lamina I neurons is dramatically highlighted by the characteristics of the histamine-responsive cells that constitute a specific pathway for the sensation of itch (Andrew and Craig 2001) and by the characteristics of thermoreceptive lamina I neurons that correspond precisely with thermal sensation (Craig et al. 2001). We also recently identified lamina I neurons that are selectively responsive to metaboreceptive input caused by muscle contraction (Wilson et al. 2002). It is important to recognize that muscles normally produce ongoing homeostatic adjustments without the behaviorally motivating signal of pain, yet large increases in such activity causes the familiar aching or burning sensation from muscles, and synchronous activation causes a painful cramping sensation (Simone et al. 1994). It is similarly important to recognize that the threshold of the "noxious cold" sensitivity of HPC neurons is ~24°C, i.e., just below the level of a comfortable ambient temperature for homeothermic mammals. Lamina I cells that receive visceral input generally have convergent cutaneous input, although specific cells must also exist.

The STT cells in the deep dorsal horn are large neurons with dendrites that extend across much of the dorsal horn. They receive mainly large-diameter (myelinated) primary afferent input from cutaneous and deep sources, as well as direct Aδ-nociceptor input and polysynaptic C-fiber input. Thus, they provide a modality-ambiguous representation of most primary afferent input to the spinal cord, including mechanoreceptive and proprioceptive as well as nociceptive activity (Milne et al. 1982; Surmeier et al. 1988; Carstens 1997). Almost all are WDR cells, some of which respond better to innocuous stimulation, others better to noxious stimulation. They generally have large receptive fields and high ongoing discharge (related to limb position). Their responses do not differentiate any particular modality of noxious stimulation. As first suggested by Wall (1967), they represent as a population the integrated sum of all afferent activity that arrives in the dorsal horn, or an "intensive trajectory" (Surmeier et al 1988). In contrast to lamina I neurons, they are not somatotopically organized, and recent evidence indicates that their complex excitatory and inhibitory receptive fields can be regarded as musculotopically organized (Schouenborg et al. 1995; McGaraughty et al. 1997). This finding is consistent with the proposal that they have a fundamental role in flexor withdrawal mechanisms and somatomotor integration (Lundberg 1971; Perl 1984; Levinsson 2000). The deep laminae contain many premotor interneurons, and they have extensive propriospinal connections and strong projections to the brainstem reticular formation.

An essential role in pain sensation for WDR lamina V STT neurons was imputed based on their sensitization and extensive segmental radiation in response to strong noxious stimulation or spinal cord injury; this response parallels neuropathic pain but also hyperexcitability of flexor reflexes (Wall et al. 1988; Palecek et al. 1992; Coghill et al. 1993). One key study claimed to have shown that only electrical stimulation of WDR STT axons in awake humans caused well-localized burning pain (Price and Mayer 1975), but the hypothesized pattern of multi-unit WDR activation required for spatial localization could not have been created by the synchronous electrical stimuli; furthermore, the responses were elicited at sites where thermal sensations (cool, warm) were evoked at lower currents, so the observations can be easily explained by activation of HPC lamina I STT axons, which were unrecognized at the time of the study, coursing in the lateral STT. The involvement of WDR STT cells in pain sensation was also inferred from correlations between their discharge activity and simultaneous operant responses of well-trained monkeys to noxious heat stimuli (Dubner et al. 1989), but a role in somatomotor integration can also explain such observations.

In contrast, in recent studies of rat models of pain, abolition of lamina I cells bearing NK-1 (substance P) receptors caused behavioral hypalgesia (Mantyh et al. 1997; De Felipe et al. 1998), mechanical allodynia after nerve injury was associated with c-fos activation of lamina I projection neurons (Bester et al. 2000), and allodynic behavior indicative of spinal cord injury pain appeared only after chemical lesions of the deep dorsal horn that spared lamina I (Gorman et al. 2001).

The lamina I and lamina V components of the STT are differentiated by their ascending locations. Anatomical data indicate that lamina I STT axons course in the middle of the lateral funiculus, the classical "lateral STT," whereas the STT axons of laminae V–VII are concentrated in the ventral (anterior) funiculus in the "anterior STT." These bundles are also distinguished by their immunoreactivity for calbindin and parvalbumin, respectively (Craig et al. 2002). Cordotomy lesions that reduce pain, temperature, itch, and sensual touch involve the lateral STT, whereas lesions of the anterior STT reportedly affect "crude touch and movement" (May 1906; Kuru 1949).

Thus, the available evidence is consistent with the view that lamina I is an integral component of the central representation of pain, temperature, and itch sensibilities, that subclasses of lamina I STT neurons can be directly associated with distinct aspects of these sensations, and that the population of deep STT cells carries intensity-related activity in its integrated output.

THALAMIC SUBSTRATES

In primates, lamina I STT neurons project heavily to a dedicated thalamocortical relay nucleus in the posterolateral thalamus, the posterior part of the ventral medial nucleus, or VMpo (Craig et al. 1994). Whereas the VMpo is diminutive in the macaque monkey thalamus and only primordially represented in subprimates, it is proportionately very large in the human thalamus (Blomqvist et al. 2000). Its anatomical characteristics are those of a thalamic relay nucleus; dense clusters of large, glutamatergic lamina I boutons are organized topographically (in the rostrocaudal direction) within cytoarchitectonically distinguishable cell nests and terminate in triadic arrangements with GABAergic presynaptic dendrites and proximal relay cell dendrites. There is also weak lamina I input to VP that is morphologically different (boutons of passage), and some input to the ventral posterior inferior nucleus (VPI) and the ventral caudal portion of the medial dorsal nucleus (MDvc).

The VMpo forms a cohesive structure with the basal part of the ventral medial nucleus, or VMb (which is denoted by some as the parvicellular part of the ventral posterior medial nucleus, or VPMpc, though it does not project to somatosensory cortex like VPM proper does), which in primates receives direct input from the nucleus of the solitary tract (NTS) that conveys visceral and gustatory afferent activity (Beckstead et al. 1980). Together, VMpo and VMb represent all homeostatic afferent inflow (i.e., both sympathetic and parasympathetic) and form a rostrocaudally organized column that is orthogonal to the mediolateral orientation of the exteroceptive/proprioceptive representation in VP, to which they are connected at the representation of the mouth. The direct lamina I pathway to VMpo and the direct NTS pathway to VMb are visible only in primates; in subprimates, homeostatic afferent activity reaches the forebrain after integration in the brainstem parabrachial nucleus (Cechetto and Saper 1990) or by spinohypothalamic projections (in rats) (Burstein 1996).

Specifically nociceptive and thermoreceptive neurons with properties similar to lamina I neurons have been identified in VMpo in macaque and owl monkeys, and similar neurons have also been recorded in the region of VMpo in awake humans (Lenz et al. 1993a; Davis et al. 1999). Significantly, microstimulation within this region of the thalamus in awake humans elicits discrete pain or cooling or visceral sensations (Dostrovsky et al. 1992; Lenz et al. 1993a,b; Davis et al. 1999).

Anatomical data indicate that VMpo and VMb project topographically to the middle layers of a cytoarchitectonically distinct field at the dorsal margin of insular cortex (see Craig 2002a). A corollary projection from each terminates in area 3a near the central sulcus. The MDvc projects to area 24c in the cingulate sulcus.

Lamina V STT axons terminate in VP, VPI, the ventral lateral nucleus (VL, or motor thalamus), and the intralaminar nuclei (which project to the basal ganglia). Their terminations in VP occur in separate bursts predominantly along the borders of the lemniscal VP subnuclei, where WDR neurons have been recorded. The available evidence suggests that such neurons are immunohistochemically distinct within VP and project to areas 3b and 1—the S1 cortical region—though to the superficial layers rather than the middle layers, suggesting a modulatory role (Rausell and Jones 1992; Shi et al. 1993). Similar nociceptive neurons have been reported in these areas (Kenshalo et al. 1988; Treede et al. 2000). Lamina V and lamina I STT terminations converge in VPI, where clusters of WDR neurons are found and where projections originate to the parietal opercular (S2/PV) region.

Thus, lamina I STT projections reach a specific pain and temperature relay nucleus, VMpo, that projects to the dorsal insula and area 3a, and also a medial thalamic nucleus that projects to anterior cingulate cortex. Lamina V STT projections reach cells that are interspersed within the lemniscal (touch) relay VP and project to superficial layers of S1. Both STT components converge in VPI, which projects to S2.

CORTICAL SUBSTRATES

Functional imaging results verify that dorsal insular cortex is activated by temperature, pain, and numerous interoceptive modalities that cause feelings from the body, consistent with the functional anatomical data. It is the only site activated by graded thermal stimuli (Craig et al. 2000). It is activated in every study using noxious heat (e.g., Hofbauer et al. 2001; Brooks et al. 2002). It is active in chronic pain patients (Kupers et al. 2000) and in neuropathic pain patients during allodynia (Peyron et al. 2000). Consistent with the broader role of this region in interoception, it is also activated during itch, isometric and dynamic exercise, blood pressure manipulations, air hunger, hypoglycemia (hunger), and hyperosmolarity (thirst) (for references see Craig 2002b). Consistent with the tracing studies, the dorsal insular cortex more rostrally is activated by gustatory stimuli. In addition, slow tactile stimulation that evoked an indistinct pleasant sensation in a polyneuropathy patient who has only peripheral nerve C-fiber conduction caused activation of interoceptive cortex, consistent with the essential role of lamina I and the lateral STT in sensual (limbic) touch (Olausson et al 2002).

In human atlases, this dorsal insular site has been included with the parietal operculum as part of S2, based on a mistake in the anatomy literature prior to the recognition of VMpo. However, this site is distinct from S2. The S2 has a topography aligned from lateral to medial face to foot (Disbrow et al. 2000), orthogonal to the rostrocaudal topography in the interoceptive VMpo cortical field; thus, tactile stimulation of the hand activates a region in S2 much closer to the lip of the lateral sulcus, >16 mm lateral to the site in the dorsal posterior insula activated by thermal, noxious, pruritic, or other interoceptive stimuli. This site also coincides with the location of cortical lesions that produce thermanesthesia and hypalgesia (Schmahmann and Leifer 1992; Greenspan et al. 1999).

Thus, the evidence indicates that in primates the dorsal insular cortex contains a primary sensory representation of the small-diameter afferent activity carried in the lamina I spinothalamocortical pathway that relates the physiological condition of the entire body. This area constitutes an interoceptive image of homeostatic afferents. It provides the cortical representations of several highly resolved, distinct sensations, including temperature, pain, itch, muscular and visceral sensations, sensual touch and other feelings from the body. The importance of this cortex for homeostasis is underscored by its delimitation by labeling for receptors for corticotropin-releasing factor, thought by many to be a definitive indicator of an association with homeostatic stress (Sanchez et al. 1999). In humans, successive re-representations of interoceptive cortex in the right (nondominant) anterior insula seem to provide the basis for subjective awareness of the material self as a feeling (sentient) entity, consistent with the "somatic marker" hypothesis of consciousness (Damasio 1993; Craig 2002b).

The medial lamina I spinothalamocortical pathway by way of MDvc activates area 24c in anterior cingulate cortex (ACC), and imaging data in humans consistently show activation in this region during pain. In particular, results obtained with the thermal grill illusion of pain indicate that ACC activation is selectively associated with thermal distress (Craig et al. 1996), and hypnotic modulation of unpleasantness is selectively associated with graded activation in ACC (Rainville et al. 1997). This indication fits with the idea that the ACC is involved in behavioral motivation associated with homeostatic distress. Many recent functional imaging studies have documented the role of the ACC in behavioral drive and volition (for references, see Craig 2002b). Like the lamina I pathway to the VMpo, the direct medial lamina I pathway to the ACC does not exist in subprimates, in which a phylogenetically older lamina I projection is relayed by the thalamic submedial nucleus to the orbitofrontal cortex. Despite this underlying anatomical difference, data from studies in rats substantiate a primordial role of the ACC in behavioral motivation by homeostatic distress, probably due to parabrachial and other brainstem inputs to the medial thalamus and ACC (Vogt 1987; Gabriel et al. 1991; Krout and Loewy 2000; Johansen et al. 2001). Thus, activation of ACC is associated with motivation, and activation of the insula is associated with sensation, which together form an emotion, and like all feelings from the body and other emotions, pain consists of both a sensation and a motivation. The role of the ACC in the inhibition of pain by cooling, indicated by analysis of the thermal grill illusion, may be of particular importance clinically (Craig 2002b), and preliminary data indicate that this begins in the MDvc (Craig 1997).

Notably, the absence of the direct cortical interoceptive representation in subprimates implies that they cannot experience feelings from the body in the same way that humans do. The available data indicate that emotional behavior in subprimates reflects motivational signals from homeostatic integration centers in the brainstem and hypothalamus. A new, anatomically concrete proposal suggests that such brainstem activity may underlie central pain in humans (Craig 2002b). The occurrence of central pain after lesions that disrupt evoked temperature and pain sensibility was a key argument made against the existence of a specific neural representation of pain (Melzack and Wall 1965). However, this new proposal suggests that central pain can be regarded as thermoregulatory distress due to the loss of descending control of brainstem integration by thermosensory cortex. This idea is consistent with the recognition that pain is both an aspect of interoception and a behavioral drive caused by a physiological imbalance that homeostatic systems alone cannot rectify. It is also consistent with the heuristic model of central pain originally proposed by Head and Holmes (1911).

About half of all imaging studies of cutaneous pain do not show activation in the parietal somatosensory cortices, like studies of visceral and deep pain, but the other half do. These studies have been interpreted to support a role for S1 and S2 in pain. Attempts have been made to reconcile these different findings by direct comparisons with low-threshold activation or by modulation of attention to discriminative features (Ploner et al. 2000; Hofbauer et al. 2001; Chen et al. 2002). An alternative interpretation is that the activation near the central sulcus actually occurs in area 3a, where VMpo projects, rather than in areas 3b and 1, where VP projects. Because area 3b contains the primary representation of low-threshold mechanoreception, it is considered to be S1 proper. Imaging data in the monkey support this interpretation, because repeated noxious heat evokes infrared optical activity in area 3a and suppresses activity in area 3b (Tommerdahl et al. 1996); multi-unit recordings were also obtained in that study that corroborated this finding (which have been confirmed in my laboratory; A.D. Craig, unpublished data). In addition, these findings indicate that the supragranular lamina V WDR input to areas 3b and 1 is not sufficient to cause macroscopic activation observable with optical imaging. Furthermore, fMRI activation by noxious cold in the anesthetized monkey has been observed only in the dorsal insula, anterior cingulate, and area 3a (See Fig. 1). The simplest explanation is that nociceptive activation in the region of the central sulcus in humans occurs similarly in area 3a, but that its localization in human PET and fMRI studies is still below the obtainable level of resolution.

CONCLUSIONS

The data available indicate that distinguishable types of pain (first and second pain, muscle pain, and allodynic pain) are represented together with other interoceptive feelings in a primary sensory cortex in the dorsal posterior insula that receives direct input from the lamina I–lateral STT–VMpo spinothalamocortical pathway. An ancillary projection from VMpo to area 3a in the fundus of the central sulcus may be responsible for activation that is misinterpreted as occurring in S1 in the imaging literature; this component fits with a prior interpretation of clinical literature (Perl 1984), but its role in sensation remains to be clarified. Confusion over the anatomical region designated as S2 may be responsible for a misinterpretation that interoceptive insular activation occurs in S2, or there may be a separate

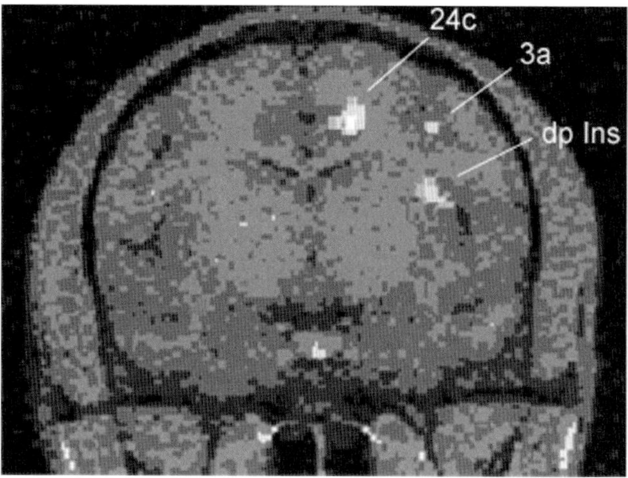

Fig. 1. A preliminary fMRI image of activation produced by noxious cold stimulation in an anesthetized monkey, localized in area 24c (MDvc target), area 3a (VMpo target), and the dorsal posterior insula (VMpo target). The latter two sites are probably interpreted as "S1" and "S2," respectively, in human imaging studies.

activation of S2 by way of input from laminae I and V to VPI that has not yet been distinguished. There is also a direct lamina I STT activation of ACC by way of MDvc that is associated with the motivation (affect) of pain, and this component may be important for the inhibition of pain by cold and for the disinhibited pain in the central pain syndrome. Modulation of activity in the cortex and in the striatum by the integrated signals arriving by way of the lamina V–anterior STT–VP/VL and intralaminar nuclei does not encode distinguishable aspects of pain but could have great importance for forebrain integration of the various sites activated by these two STT components, for example in neuropathic pain. This new view makes explicit anatomical and functional predictions, and it is my hope that these will be tested in the near future.

ACKNOWLEDGMENTS

I thank M. Castro and A. Godinez for technical assistance. The work in this laboratory is supported by grants from the NIH (NS40413 and 41287) and funding from the Barrow Neurological Foundation.

REFERENCES

Adreani CM, Kaufman MP. Effect of arterial occlusion on responses of group III and IV afferents to dynamic exercise. *J Appl Physiol* 1998; 84:1827–1833.

Altman J, Bayer SA. The development of the rat spinal cord. *Adv Anat Embryol Cell Biol* 1984; 85:1–164.

Andrew D, Craig AD. Spinothalamic lamina I neurons selectively sensitive to histamine: a central neural pathway for itch. *Nat Neurosci* 2001; 4:72–77.

Andrew D, Craig AD. Responses of spinothalamic lamina I neurons to maintained noxious mechanical stimulation in the cat. *J Neurophysiol* 2002; 87:1889–1901.

Beckstead RM, Morse JR, Norgren R. The nucleus of the solitary tract in the monkey: projections to the thalamus and brain stem nuclei. *J Comp Neurol* 1980; 190:259–282.

Bester H, Beggs S, Woolf CJ. Changes in tactile stimuli-induced behavior and c-Fos expression in the superficial dorsal horn and in parabrachial nuclei after sciatic nerve crush. *J Comp Neurol* 2000; 428:45–61.

Blomqvist A, Zhang ET, Craig AD. Cytoarchitectonic and immunohistochemical characterization of a specific pain and temperature relay, the posterior portion of the ventral medial nucleus, in the human thalamus. *Brain* 2000; 123:601–619.

Bonica JJ. Anatomic and physiologic basis of nociception and pain. In: Bonica JJ (Ed). *The Management of Pain*, Vol. 1. Philadelphia: Lea & Febiger, 1990, pp 28–95.

Brooks JC, Nurmikko TJ, Bimson WE, Singh KD, Roberts N. fMRI of thermal pain: effects of stimulus laterality and attention. *Neuroimage* 2002; 15:293–301.

Burstein R. Somatosensory and visceral input to the hypothalamus and limbic system. *Prog Brain Res* 1996; 107:257–267.

Bushnell MC, Duncan GH, Tremblay N. Thalamic VPM nucleus in the behaving monkey. I. Multimodal and discriminative properties of thermosensitive neurons. *J Neurophysiol* 1993; 69:739–752.

Carstens E. Responses of rat spinal dorsal horn neurons to intracutaneous microinjection of histamine, capsaicin, and other irritants. *J Neurophysiol* 1997; 77:2499–2514.

Casey KL. Unit analysis of nociceptive mechanisms in the thalamus of the awake squirrel monkey. *J Neurophysiol* 1966; 29:727–750.

Cechetto DF, Saper CB. Role of the cerebral cortex in autonomic function. In: Loewy AD, Spyer KM (Eds). *Central Regulation of Autonomic Function*. New York: Oxford University Press, 1990, pp 208–223.

Chen JI, Ha B, Bushnell MC, Pike B, Duncan GH. Differentiating noxious- and innocuous-related activation of human somatosensory cortices using temporal analysis of fMRI. *J Neurophysiol* 2002; 88:464–474.

Coghill RC, Mayer DJ, Price DD. The roles of spatial recruitment and discharge frequency in spinal cord coding of pain: a combined electrophysiological and imaging investigation. *Pain* 1993; 53:295–309.

Craig AD. Distribution of brainstem projections from spinal lamina I neurons in the cat and the monkey. *J Comp Neurol* 1995; 361:225–248.

Craig AD. The primate MDvc contains nociceptive neurons. *Soc Neurosci Abstr* 1997; 23:1012.

Craig AD. The functional anatomy of lamina I and its role in post-stroke central pain. In: Sandkühler J, Bromm B, Gebhart GF (Eds). *Nervous System Plasticity and Chronic Pain*, Vol. 129. Elsevier: Amsterdam, 2000, pp 137–151.

Craig AD. New and old thoughts on the mechanisms of spinal cord injury pain. In: Yezierski RP, Burchiel KJ (Eds). *Spinal Cord Injury Pain: Assessment, Mechanisms, Management*, Progress in Pain Research and Management, Vol. 23. Seattle: IASP Press, 2002a, pp 237–264.

Craig AD. Opinion: How do you feel? Interoception: the sense of the physiological condition of the body. *Nat Rev Neurosci* 2002b; 3:655–666.

Craig AD, Dostrovsky JO. Medulla to thalamus. In: Wall PD, Melzack R (Eds). *Textbook of Pain.* Edinburgh: Churchill Livingstone, 1999, pp 183–214.

Craig AD, Andrew D. Responses of spinothalamic lamina I neurons to repeated brief contact heat stimulation in the cat. *J Neurophysiol* 2002; 87:1902–1914.

Craig AD, Bushnell MC, Zhang E-T, Blomqvist A. A thalamic nucleus specific for pain and temperature sensation. *Nature* 1994; 372:770–773.

Craig AD, Reiman EM, Evans A, Bushnell MC. Functional imaging of an illusion of pain. *Nature* 1996; 384:258–260.

Craig AD, Chen K, Bandy D, Reiman EM. Thermosensory activation of insular cortex. *Nat Neurosci* 2000; 3:184–190.

Craig AD, Krout K, Andrew D. Quantitative response characteristics of thermoreceptive and nociceptive lamina I spinothalamic neurons in the cat. *J Neurophysiol* 2001; 86:1459–1480.

Craig AD, Zhang ET, Blomqvist A. Association of spinothalamic lamina I neurons and their ascending axons with calbindin-immunoreactivity in monkey and human. *Pain* 2002; 97:105–115.

Damasio AR. *Descartes' Error: Emotion, Reason, and the Human Brain.* New York: Putnam, 1993.

Davis KD, Lozano AM, Manduch M, et al. Thalamic relay site for cold perception in humans. *J Neurophysiol* 1999; 81:1970–1973.

De Felipe C, Herrero JF, O'Brien JA, et al. Altered nociception, analgesia and aggression in mice lacking the receptor for substance P. *Nature* 1998; 392:394–397.

Disbrow E, Roberts T, Krubitzer L. Somatotopic organization of cortical fields in the lateral sulcus of *Homo sapiens*: evidence for SII and PV. *J Comp Neurol* 2000; 418:1–21.

Dostrovsky JO, Wells FEB, Tasker RR. Pain sensations evoked by stimulation in human thalamus. In: Inoka R, Shigenaga Y, Tohyama M (Eds). *Processing and Inhibition of Nociceptive Information,* International Congress Series 989. Amsterdam: Excerpta Medica, 1992, pp 115–120.

Dubner R, Kenshalo DR Jr, Maixner W, Bushnell MC, Oliveras J-L. The correlation of monkey medullary dorsal horn neuronal activity and the perceived intensity of noxious heat stimuli. *J Neurophysiol* 1989; 62:450–457.

Gabriel M, Kubota Y, Sparenborg S, Straube K, Vogt BA. Effects of cingulate cortical lesions on avoidance learning and training-induced unit activity in rabbits. *Exp Brain Res* 1991; 86:585–600.

Gorman AL, Yu CG, Ruenes GR, Daniels L, Yezierski RP. Conditions affecting the onset, severity and progression of a spontaneous pain-like behavior following excitotoxic spinal cord injury. *J Pain* 2001; 2:229–240.

Greenspan JD, Lee RR, Lenz FA. Pain sensitivity alterations as a function of lesion location in the parasylvian cortex. *Pain* 1999; 81:273–282.

Gybels J, Handwerker HO, VanHees J. A comparison between the discharges of human nociceptive nerve fibres and the subject's ratings of his sensations. *J Physiol (Lond)* 1979; 292:193–206.

Han Z-S, Zhang E-T, Craig AD. Nociceptive and thermoreceptive lamina I neurons are anatomically distinct. *Nat Neurosci* 1998; 1:218–225.

Head H, Holmes G. Sensory disturbances from cerebral lesions. *Brain* 1911; 34:102–254.

Hofbauer RK, Rainville P, Duncan GH, Bushnell MC. Cortical representation of the sensory dimension of pain. *J Neurophysiol* 2001; 86:402–411.

Johansen JP, Fields HL, Manning BH. The affective component of pain in rodents: direct evidence for a contribution of the anterior cingulate cortex. *Proc Natl Acad Sci USA* 2001; 98:8077–8082.

Kenshalo DR Jr, Chudler EH, Anton F, Dubner R. SI nociceptive neurons participate in the encoding process by which monkeys perceive the intensity of noxious thermal stimulation. *Brain Res* 1988; 454:378–382.

Krout KE, Loewy AD. Parabrachial nucleus projections to midline and intralaminar thalamic nuclei of the rat. *J Comp Neurol* 2000; 428:475–494.

Kupers RC, Gybels JM, Gjedde A. Positron emission tomography study of a chronic pain patient successfully treated with somatosensory thalamic stimulation. *Pain* 2000; 87:295–302.

Kuru M. *The Sensory Paths in the Spinal Cord and Brain Stem of Man.* Tokyo: Sogensya, 1949, p 675.

Lenz FA, Seike M, Richardson RT, Lin YC, et al. Thermal and pain sensations evoked by microstimulation in the area of human ventrocaudal nucleus. *J Neurophysiol* 1993a; 70:200–212.

Lenz FA, Seike M, Lin YC, Baker FH, et al. Neurons in the area of human thalamic nucleus ventralis caudalis respond to painful heat stimuli. *Brain Res* 1993b; 623:235–240.

Levinsson A. Spinal cord processing of sensory information: spatial organization and adaptive mechanisms. PhD Thesis, Dept. of Physiological Sciences, Lund University, Sweden, 2000.

Light AR, Willcockson HH. Spinal laminae I–II neurons in rat recorded in vivo in whole cell, tight seal configuration: properties and opioid responses. *J Neurophysiol* 1999; 82:3316–3326.

Lundberg A. Function of the ventral spinocerebellar tract: a new hypothesis. *Exp Brain Res* 1971; 12:317–330.

Mantyh PW, Rogers SD, Honore P, et al. Inhibition of hyperalgesia by ablation of lamina I spinal neurons expressing the substance P receptor. *Science* 1997; 278:275–279.

May WP. The afferent path. *Brain* 1906; 29:742–803.

McGaraughty S, Henry JL. Relationship between mechano-receptive fields of dorsal horn convergent neurons and the response to noxious immersion of the ipsilateral hindpaw in rats. *Pain* 1997; 70:133–140.

Mense S, Stahnke M. Responses in muscle afferent fibres of slow conduction velocity to contractions and ischaemia in the cat. *J Physiol* 1983; 342:383–397.

Melzack R, Wall PD. Pain mechanisms: a new theory. *Science* 1965; 150:971–979.

Milne RJ, Foreman RD, Willis WD. Responses of primate spinothalamic neurons located in the sacral intermediomedial gray (Stilling's nucleus) to proprioceptive input from the tail. *Brain Res* 1982; 234:227–236.

Nathan PW, Smith MC, Cook AW. Sensory effects in man of lesions of the posterior columns and of some other afferent pathways. *Brain* 1986; 109:1003–1041.

Palecek J, Dougherty PM, Kim SH, et al. Responses of spinothalamic tract neurons to mechanical and thermal stimuli in an experimental model of peripheral neuropathy in primates. *J Neurophysiol* 1992; 68:1951–1966.

Perl ER. Pain and nociception. In: Darian-Smith I (Ed). *Sensory Processes,* Handbook of Physiology, Section 1, The Nervous System, Vol. III. Bethesda: American Physiological Society, 1984, pp 915–975.

Peyron R, Garcia-Larrea L, Gregoire MC, et al. Parietal and cingulate processes in central pain. A combined positron emission tomography (PET) and functional magnetic resonance imaging (fMRI) study of an unusual case. *Pain* 2000; 84:77–87.

Ploner M, Freund HJ, Schnitzler A. Pain affect without pain sensation in a patient with a postcentral lesion. *Pain* 1999; 81:211–214.

Ploner M, Schmitz F, Freund HJ, Schnitzler A. Differential organization of touch and pain in human primary somatosensory cortex. *J Neurophysiol* 2000; 83:1770–1776.

Price DD. *Psychological and Neural Mechanisms of Pain.* New York: Raven Press, 1988.

Price DD, Dubner R. Neurons that subserve the sensory-discriminative aspects of pain. *Pain* 1977; 3:307–338.

Price DD, Mayer DJ. Neurophysiological characterization of the anterolateral quadrant neurons subserving pain in *M. mulatta. Pain* 1975; 1:59–72.

Rainville P, Duncan GH, Price DD, Carrier B, Bushnell MC. Pain affect encoded in human anterior cingulate but not somatosensory cortex. *Science* 1997; 277:968–971.

Rausell E, Bae CS, Viñuela A, Huntley GW, Jones EG. Calbindin and parvalbumin cells in monkey VPL thalamic nucleus: distribution, laminar cortical projections, and relations to spinothalamic terminations. *J Neurosci* 1992; 12:4088–4111.

Sanchez MM, Young LJ, Plotsky PM, Insel TR. Autoradiographic and in situ hybridization localization of corticotropin-releasing factor 1 and 2 receptors in nonhuman primate brain. *J Comp Neurol* 1999; 408:365–377.

Sato A, Schmidt RF. Somatosympathetic reflexes: afferent fibers, central pathways, discharge characteristics. *Physiol Rev* 1973; 53:916–947.

Schaible H-G, Schmidt RF. Neurobiology of articular nociceptors. In: Belmonte C, Cervero F (Eds). *Neurobiology of Nociceptors.* Oxford: Oxford University Press, 1996, pp 202–220.

Schmahmann JD, Leifer D. Parietal pseudothalamic pain syndrome: clinical features and anatomic correlates. *Arch Neurol* 1992; 49:1032–1037.

Schouenborg J, Weng HR, Kalliomäki J, Holmberg H. A survey of spinal dorsal horn neurones encoding the spatial organization of withdrawal reflexes in the rat. *Exp Brain Res* 1995; 106:19–27.

Sherrington CS. Cutaneous sensations. In: Schäfer EA (Ed). *Text-book of Physiology*. Edinburgh: Pentland, 1900, pp 920–1001.

Shi T, Stevens RT, Tessier J, Apkarian AV. Spinothalamocortical inputs nonpreferentially innervate the superficial and deep cortical layers of SI. *Neurosci Lett* 1993; 160:209–213.

Simone DA, Marchettini P, Caputi G, Ochoa JL. Identification of muscle afferents subserving sensation of deep pain in humans. *J Neurophysiol* 1994; 72:883–889.

Surmeier J, Honda CN, Willis WD Jr. Natural groupings of primate spinothalamic neurons based on cutaneous stimulation: physiological and anatomical features. *J Neurophysiol* 1988; 59:833–860.

Tommerdahl M, Delemos KA, Vierck CJ Jr, Favorov OV, Whitsel BL. Anterior parietal cortical response to tactile and skin-heating stimuli applied to the same skin site. *J Neurophysiol* 1996; 75:2662–2670.

Treede RD, Apkarian AV, Bromm B, Greenspan JD, Lenz FA. Cortical representation of pain: functional characterization of nociceptive areas near the lateral sulcus. *Pain* 2000; 87:113–119.

Vogt BA, Pandya DN, Rosene DL. Cingulate cortex of the rhesus monkey: I. Cytoarchitecture and thalamic afferents. *J Comp Neurol* 1987; 262:256–270.

Wall PD. The laminar organization of the dorsal horn and effects of descending impulses. *J Physiol (Lond)* 1967; 188:403–424.

Wall PD. Dorsal horn electrophysiology. In: Zotterman Y (Ed). *Handbook of Sensory Physiology—Somatosensory System.* Berlin: Springer-Verlag, 1973.

Wall PD, Coderre TJ, Stern Y, Wiesenfeld-Hallin Z. Slow changes in the flexion reflex of the rat following arthritis or tenotomy. *Brain Res* 1988; 447:215–222.

Willis WD. *The Pain System.* Basel: Karger, 1985.

Willis WD, Westlund KN. Neuroanatomy of the pain system and of the pathways that modulate pain. *J Clin Neurophysiol* 1997; 14:2–31.

Wilson LB, Andrew D, Craig AD. Activation of spinobulbar lamina I neurons by static muscle contraction. *J Neurophysiol* 2002; 87:1641–1645.

Correspondence to: A.D. Craig, PhD, Atkinson Pain Research Laboratory, Barrow Neurological Institute, 350 West Thomas Rd., Phoenix, AZ 85013, USA. Tel: 602-406-3385; Fax: 602-406-4121; email: bcraig@chw.edu.

Proceedings of the 10th World Congress on Pain,
Progress in Pain Research and Management, Vol. 24,
edited by Jonathan O. Dostrovsky, Daniel B. Carr, and
Martin Koltzenburg, IASP Press, Seattle, © 2003.

18

Itch: Mechanisms and Mediators[1]

David Andrew,[a,b] Martin Schmelz,[c]
and Jane Ballantyne[d]

[a]Atkinson Pain Research Laboratory, Division of Neurosurgery, Barrow Neurological Institute, Phoenix, Arizona, USA; [b]Spinal Cord Research Group, Institute of Biomedical and Life Sciences, University of Glasgow, Glasgow, United Kingdom; [c]Department of Anesthesiology Mannheim, University of Heidelberg, Mannheim, Germany; [d]Department of Anesthesiology, Harvard Medical School, Boston, Massachusetts, USA

ITCH MECHANISMS

Several competing theories of the mechanisms that produce itch sensations have been developed over the years. In broad terms, these theories suggest either that specific elements, both peripherally and centrally, respond only to itch-inducing agents (*specificity theory*), or that a subset of nociceptive neurons that encode "itch" at low firing frequencies also evoke the sensation of pain at higher frequencies (*intensity theory*). There is evidence to support both of these mechanisms. The results of microstimulation studies (Torebjörk and Ochoa 1981) and clinical observations on the effects of spinal opioids (Hales 1980; Duffy 1981) support the specificity theory, whereas psychophysical (Graham et al. 1951) and human and animal single-fiber recording studies (Tuckett and Wei 1987; Handwerker et al. 1991) support the intensity theory, albeit indirectly. However, analysis of the histamine-evoked discharge patterns of the most common type of C-fiber nociceptor (mechano-heat [CMH] or "polymodal nociceptors"), which have been extensively studied in animal (Bessou and Perl 1969) and human (Torebjörk 1974) skin, indicates that such units are either insensitive to histamine or only weakly activated. Thus, they are unlikely to account for the lasting itch

[1] Based on a Congress workshop.

sensation observed, for example, following histamine application to the skin.

C fibers recently discovered within the class of mechano-insensitive C nociceptors (Schmelz et al. 1997) respond to histamine iontophoresis in parallel to the itch ratings of the subjects (Fig. 1), as postulated previously (LaMotte et al. 1988). These peripheral "itch" fibers have low conduction velocities and large innervation territories, and show mechanical unresponsiveness and high thresholds to transcutaneous electrical stimulation. These characteristics identify the histamine-sensitive fibers as a distinct subset of units that differ both from conventional "polymodal" C-fiber nociceptors (Perl 1996) and from the "silent" or "sleeping" nociceptors (Meyer and Campbell 1988; Schmidt et al. 1994) that are also mechanically insensitive

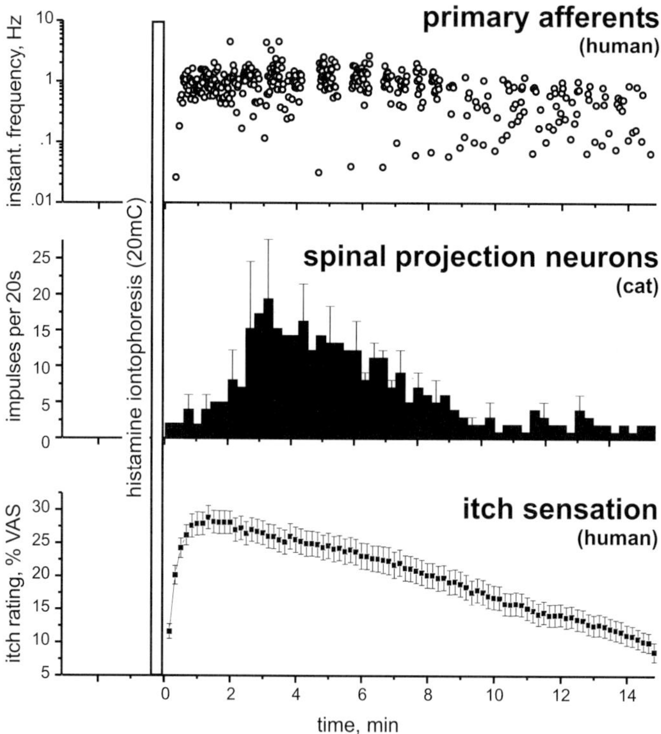

Fig. 1. The upper panel shows instantaneous discharge frequency of a mechano- and heat-insensitive C fiber in the superficial peroneal nerve following histamine iontophoresis (20 mC; marked as open box in the diagram). The unit was not spontaneously active before histamine application. The middle panel depicts neuronal activity of a spinothalamic projection neuron following histamine iontophoresis in the periphery. The lower panel shows average itch magnitude ratings of a group of 21 healthy volunteers after an identical histamine stimulus. Ratings at 10-s intervals on a visual analogue scale with the end points "no itch" and "unbearable itch." Bars: standard error of means (modified from Schmelz et. al. 1997 and Andrew and Craig 2001).

but are activated by algogenic chemicals (Schmelz et al. 2000). Units with a strong and sustained histamine response are found only in the group of mechano-insensitive nociceptors, and they comprise about 20% of this group.

A "LABELED LINE" FOR ITCH

Early lesion studies (Bickford 1938) identified the lateral spinothalamic tract as being crucial to itch sensibility. Neurophysiological studies of spinal neurons in cats have clarified the critical link between the spinothalamic tract and itch sensation. Specifically, a subset of spinothalamic neurons in lamina I of the spinal dorsal horn that respond selectively to histamine iontophoretically administered to the skin have recently been identified (Andrew and Craig 2001). The time course of their responses was similar to that of itch sensation in humans, and it also matched the responses of the peripheral C fibers that respond to histamine (Schmelz et al. 1997) (Fig. 1). Like the histamine-sensitive C fibers, the histamine-sensitive spinothalamic neurons were also mechanically insensitive. The histamine-sensitive spinothalamic neurons were considered a distinct subset of cells because they differed from nociceptive and thermoreceptive spinothalamic neurons by their slower central conduction velocities, their level of background activity, and their pattern of projection to the thalamus (Andrew and Craig 2001). Thus, the combination of dedicated peripheral and central neurons with a unique response pattern to pruritic mediators and anatomically distinct projections to the thalamus provides the basis for a specific neuronal pathway for itch.

CORTICAL REGIONS ACTIVATED DURING ITCHING

Recent studies using functional brain imaging have investigated the supraspinal processing of itch and its corresponding scratch response in humans. Although itch was induced by injecting histamine into the skin (which also can produce pain; Keele and Armstrong 1964), rather than by iontophoresis (Magerl et al. 1990), itching evoked activity in the anterior cingulate cortex, supplementary motor area, and inferior parietal lobe with a contralateral predominance (Hsieh et al. 1994; Darsow et al. 2000; Drzezga et al. 2001). The anterior cingulate cortex was the most strongly activated cortical area, and this was interpreted as representing the "urge to scratch" (Hsieh et al. 1994). In addition to finding activation of the same motor-related cortical areas during itching, Drzezga and colleagues (2001) also described correlations between itch unpleasantness and intensity and activation in the contralateral insula, primary somatosensory cortex, and supplemental motor areas bilaterally. The multiple activation sites in the brain during itching argue against the existence of a single itch center and reflect the multidimensionality of the itch sensation.

D. ANDREW

PRURITIC MEDIATORS

Only a few mediators can induce histamine-independent pruritus. Prostaglandins enhance histamine-induced itch in the skin (Hägermark and Strandberg 1977), but also act directly as pruritogens in the conjunctiva (Woodward et al. 1995) and in human skin when applied via microdialysis fibers (Neisius et al. 2002). Intradermal injection of serotonin elicits pain and a weak itch sensation (Hägermark 1992). Recent results suggest that the peripheral effect of serotonin may be partly due to release of histamine from mast cells (Weisshaar et al. 1999). Acetylcholine is a pruritic in atopic dermatitis, but induces pain in normal subjects (Vogelsang et al. 1995). This mechanism could easily explain the itch that many patients with atopic dermatitis experience when sweating. The role of serotonin in the pathogenesis of itch is unclear. It might be involved in pruritus seen in polycythemia vera.

The potency of the main known pruritics can be defined as histamine >> prostaglandin E_2 (PGE_2) > acetylcholine > serotonin; in contrast, bradykinin and capsaicin application basically induces a pure pain sensation. Neurons responsible for the itch sensation would thus be expected to exhibit a graded response according to the pruritic potency of the mediators. Fig. 2 depicts responses of different types of C nociceptors to stimulation with histamine, PGE_2, acetylcholine, and capsaicin. Only the units showing lasting activation following histamine application were also excited by PGE_2. In contrast, we did not observe any lasting activation of mechanoresponsive nociceptors by histamine or by PGE_2. Similarly, none of the mechano-insensitive fibers that were unresponsive to histamine were activated by PGE_2 application. Thus, the response pattern of the histamine-responsive "itch" units corresponds to the psychophysically observed pruritic effect of PGE_2.

HISTAMINE AND NEUROPEPTIDES

Histamine has been a widely used pruritic in experimental settings (Magerl et al. 1990). Most experimental itch stimuli act indirectly via histamine release from skin mast cells. Upon activation by histamine, nociceptors release vasodilatory neuropeptides such as substance P (SP) and calcitonin gene-related peptide (CGRP), which, via axon reflexes, induce an erythema surrounding the application site. In turn, intradermal injection of high

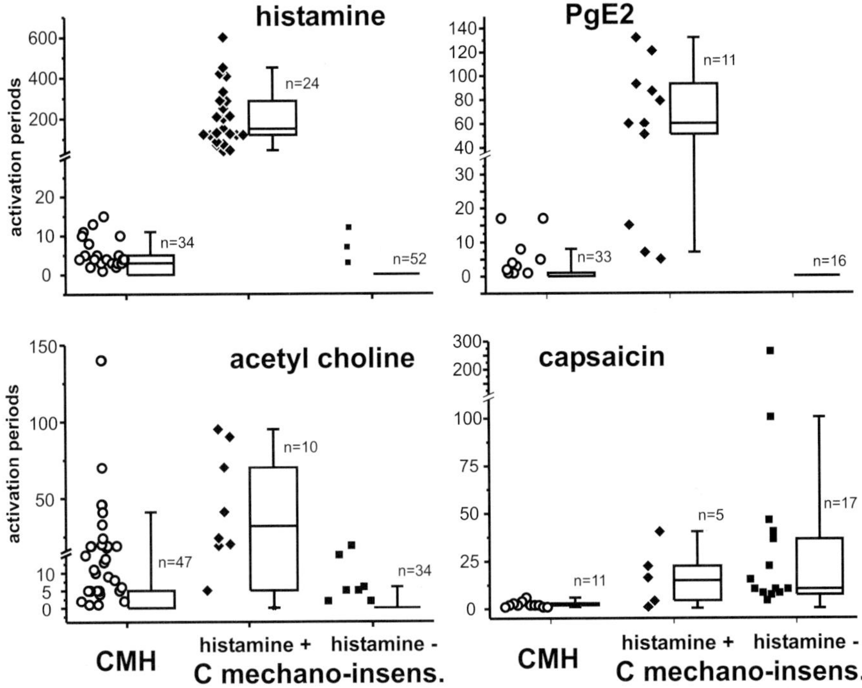

Fig. 2. Intensity of chemically induced activation of different classes of C nociceptors, namely mechano-heat-positive fibers (CMH), which are polymodal nociceptors, histamine-positive ("histamine +") and histamine-negative ("histamine –"); and mechano-insensitive fibers (C mechano-insens.). The units were stimulated with histamine (iontophoresis; 20 mC), prostaglandin E_2 (PGE_2; 10^{-5} M, 20 μL injection), acetylcholine (iontophoresis; 60 mC), or capsaicin (0.1%, 20 μL injection).

concentrations of exogenous SP degranulates mast cells and provokes an itch sensation (Hägermark et al. 1978). However, under physiological conditions the concentrations of endogenous neuropeptides released upon nociceptor activation are too low to degranulate mast cells (Schmelz et al. 1999). Although direct excitatory effect of SP may explain itch in humans, no experimental evidence implicates histamine-independent SP-induced itch in humans (Weidner et al. 2000; Schmelz and Petersen 2001) or SP-induced excitation of nociceptors (Kessler et al. 1992). The concentration of intradermal SP injections used to elicit itch in animals is unphysiologically high (2 mM) (Andoh et al. 1998), especially if compared to the half-maximal concentration needed to elicit inward currents in the cell bodies of primary afferent neurons (6 nM) (Akasu et al. 1996) or to the half-maximal concentration needed to produce protein extravasation in human skin (0.1 μM). Thus, reduction of itch behavior seen in SP receptor (NK1) knockout mice

(Akasu et al. 1996) can most probably be attributed to inhibition of the spinal transmission directly via the NK1 receptor or indirectly via presynaptic $GABA_A$ receptors (Yamada and Akasu 1996).

PROTEINASES

While previous research has mainly focused on histamine as the main pruritic mediator in itch, microdialysis has also provided evidence for a histamine-independent mechanism by which mast cells can induce itch. In patients with atopic dermatitis, mast cell degranulation by compound 48/80 provokes itch, which is not suppressed by antihistamines (Rukwied et al. 2000). One hypothesis suggests that tryptase derived from mast cells is a possible candidate for this effect, as it specifically activates proteinase receptors (PAR-2). While proteinases such as papain were identified several decades ago as histamine-independent itch mediators (Rajka 1969; Hägermark 1973), they have received little recent attention. However, the identification of specific proteinase-activated receptors on afferent nerve fibers (Steinhoff et al. 2000) has initiated various successful studies investigating the role of PAR-2 in the pain pathway (Vergnolle et al. 2001a,b; Fiorucci and Distrutti 2002). Meanwhile, convincing evidence points to an involvement of PAR-2 for activation and sensitization of both somatic (Steinhoff et al. 2000; Kawabata et al. 2001) and visceral afferent nerve fibers (Corvera et al. 1999; Hoogerwerf et al. 2001; Coelho et al. 2002). Apart from the involvement in the pain pathway, recent results from PAR-2 knockout mice also indicate a role of PAR-2 in itchy skin diseases including atopic dermatitis (Kawagoe et al. 2002). The latest microdialysis results suggest that tryptase concentration is elevated in patients with atopic dermatitis, as could be expected from the higher percentage of tryptase-positive mast cells (Jarvikallio et al. 1997), and indicate that activation of PAR-2 receptors may induce itch in these patients (Steinhoff and Schmelz, ongoing work).

PERIPHERAL SENSITIZATION FOR PAIN AND ITCH

Classical inflammatory mediators such as bradykinin, serotonin, prostanoids, and low pH sensitize nociceptors. Regulation of gene expression induced by trophic factors such as nerve growth factor (NGF) play a major role in prolonged increases in neuronal sensitivity (Shu and Mendell 1999). Trophic factors also initiate sprouting of nerve fibers and thus change their morphology. Sprouting of epidermal nerve fibers in combination with localized pain and hypersensitivity has been reported (Bohm-Starke et al. 1998, 2001).

Similarly, increased intradermal nerve fiber density occurs in patients with chronic pruritus (Sugiura et al. 1997; Urashima and Mihara 1998). Also, patients with atopic dermatitis have increased epidermal levels of neurotrophin 4 (NT4) (Grewe et al. 2000) and massively increased serum levels of NGF and SP that are correlated to the severity of the disease (Toyoda et al. 2002). It is well known that NGF (Shu and Mendell 1999; Romero et al. 2000) and NT4 (Shu et al. 1999) can sensitize nociceptors. These findings suggest an apparent match of mechanisms by which peripheral nociceptors proliferate and are sensitized in patients with chronic itch and those with chronic pain. However, these similarities do not explain the fundamental difference between chronic itch and chronic pain sensation observed in these patients. We have no way to morphologically differentiate between neurons responding to pruritogens and to algogens and no evidence for a specific peripheral sensitization of pruriceptive neurons that would spare the noceptive neurons. Thus, peripheral mechanisms alone can not account for the obvious differences between patients with chronic itch and those with chronic pain.

M. Schmelz

INTERACTION OF PAIN AND ITCH

ITCH MODULATION BY PAINFUL AND NONPAINFUL STIMULI

It is common experience that pain induced by scratching lessens the itch sensation. Studies using various painful thermal, mechanical, and chemical stimuli confirm that painful stimuli inhibit itch. Electrical stimulation via an array of pointed electrodes, known as "cutaneous field stimulation," has been successfully used to inhibit itch for several hours in an area of more than 10 cm around the stimulated site, and suggests a central mode of action (Nilsson et al. 1997). In line with these results, itch is suppressed inside the secondary zone of capsaicin-induced mechanical hyperalgesia (Brull et al. 1999). This central effect of capsaicin should be clearly separated from the neurotoxic effect it exerts locally on the nerve fibers (Simone et al. 1998), with both mechanisms inhibiting itch.

The inhibition of itch by pain is not relevant just in the situation of enhanced painful input. The converse mechanism also has significant implications: inhibition of pain processing may reduce its inhibitory effect and thus enhance itch (Atanassoff et al. 1999).

OPIOIDS

Endogenous and exogenous opioids are capable of inducing itch, a phenomenon widely observed both experimentally and clinically. Opioid-induced pruritus became a greater clinical problem after the use of neuraxial opioids was popularized in the 1980s. Clinicians observed a greater incidence than that associated with systemic use, and it became clear that a central mechanism of opioid-induced itch was occurring via the μ-opioid receptor (Ballantyne et al. 1988). The concept of an endogenous opioid role in the pruritus of systemic diseases such as cholestasis and uremia has been evolving over the past two decades (Bernstein and Swift 1979; Summerfield 1980; Thornton and Losowsky 1988; Bergasa and Jones 1995). Opioid antagonists can reverse experimental itch (Heyer et al. 1997), and are successful in the treatment of opioid-induced itch and itch associated with systemic disease (Peer et al. 1996; Wolfhagen et al. 1997; Slappendel et al. 2000). More recent studies have recognized a potential clinical role for κ-opioid receptor agonists in the treatment of pruritus (Karnei and Nagase 2001; Togashi et al. 2002), secondary to the recognition that the κ-opioid receptor has μ-opioid-receptor opposing actions (Pan 1998). Conversely, in animal experiments κ-opioid antagonists enhanced itch (Kamei and Nagase 2001). A recent meta-analysis found that the κ-opioid agonist nalbuphine reduced μ-opioid-induced pruritus (Kjellberg and Tramer 2001). Studies using a newly developed κ-opioid agonist have successfully tested this new therapeutic concept in patients with chronic itch (Kumagai 2001).

The exact mechanism of μ-opioid-induced itch is unclear. While the analgesic effects per se may play a role, an excitatory effect is another possibility. The hyperalgesic effects of opioids are now well established (Mao 2002), and pruritus may be one manifestation of the spectrum of central excitatory or disinhibitory events that are induced by endogenous or exogenous opioids (see Fig. 3). Some opioids, morphine in particular, induce pruritus through histamine activity in the periphery, although this effect is usually transient and clinically unimportant.

CENTRAL SENSITIZATION FOR PAIN AND ITCH

Beyond the direct interaction of pain and itch is a remarkable homology of central sensitization phenomena for the two perceptions. Activity in chemonociceptors subserving the pain sensation will not only lead to an acute pain sensation, but in addition can sensitize second-order neurons in the dorsal horn and lead to increased pain sensitivity (hyperalgesia). Two different types of hyperalgesia can be differentiated. First, normally painless touch sensations in the uninjured surroundings of the trauma can be felt as

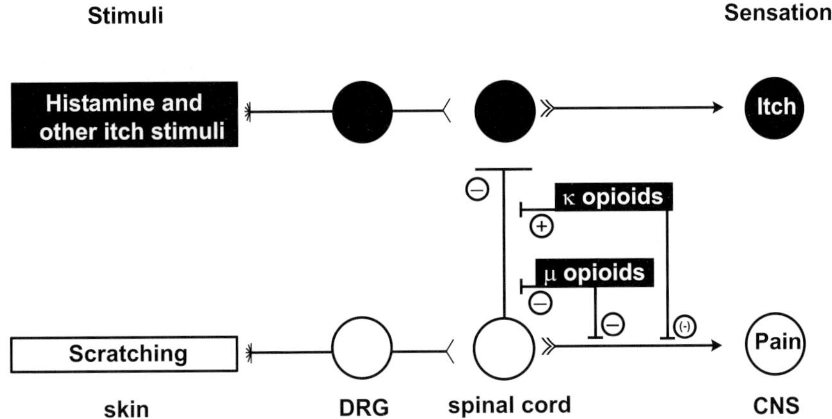

Fig. 3. Simplified schematic view of the central interaction between pain and itch under physiological conditions. CNS = central nervous system; DRG = dorsal root ganglion. While having a similar inhibitory effect on pain processing, μ and κ opioids differentially modify spinal itch processing.

painful "stroke-evoked allodynia." This type of sensitization requires ongoing activity of primary afferent nociceptors. Second, slightly painful pinprick-like stimulation is felt as more painful in the secondary zone of "punctate hyperalgesia." Punctate hyperalgesia does not require ongoing activity in primary nociceptors, but can persist for hours following a trauma (LaMotte 1986).

Similar phenomena occur in itch processing: touch-evoked pruritus around an itching site has been termed "itchy skin" or alloknesis (Bickford 1938; Simone et al. 1991; Heyer et al. 1995). Like allodynia it requires ongoing activity in primary afferents and is elicited by low-threshold mechanoreceptors (Aβ fibers). Also, more intense prick-induced itch sensations, or "hyperknesis," have been reported following histamine iontophoresis in healthy volunteers (Atanassoff et al. 1999). Fig. 4 summarizes the similar central sensitization phenomena.

While a major role for central sensitization in chronic pain is well established, the exact mechanism and role of central sensitization for itch in clinical circumstances still require exploration. Evidence is emerging for a clinical interaction between chronic pain and chronic itch, in parallel with the similarities between experimentally induced pain and itch secondary to sensitization phenomena. Recently, Baron and colleagues (2001) found that histamine iontophoresis, which provokes a pure itch sensation in normal patients, is felt as burning pain by neuropathic pain patients. Conversely, cutaneous stimulation with an acidified solution, which provokes a purely

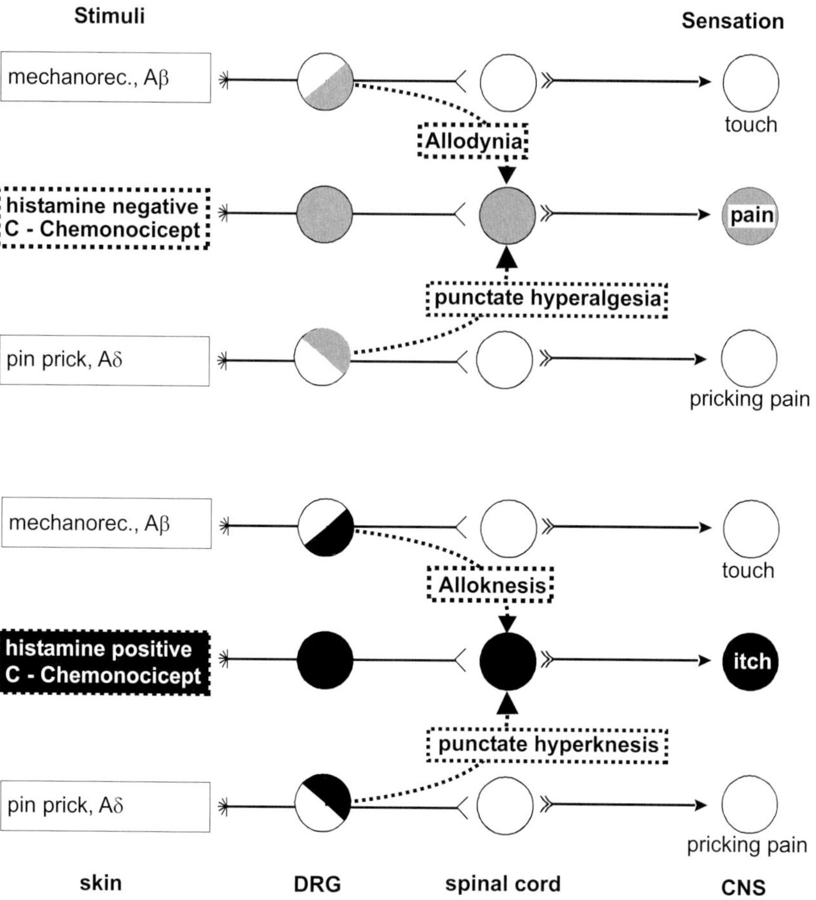

Fig. 4. Similarities between central sensitization phenomena for pain and itch.

painful sensation in normal subjects, is felt as itching by patients with atopic dermatitis when applied in or close to their eczematous skin (A. Ikoma, personal communication). Mechanisms of peripheral sensitization of nociceptors could be identical for painful and pruritic diseases. Therefore, therapeutic approaches for pain treatment may also be beneficial for antipruritic therapy, at least in the case of peripheral events, including peripheral sensitization. However, the question why certain inflammatory processes lead to a painful condition, whereas others provoke itch, is unsolved and the clinically relevant pruritic mediator(s) still have to be identified.

J. Ballantyne

ACKNOWLEDGMENTS

This work was supported by the Deutsche Forschungsgemeinschaft (SFB 353) and by the Royal Society of Edinburgh.

REFERENCES

Akasu T, Ishimatsu M, Yamada K. Tachykinins cause inward current through NK1 receptors in bullfrog sensory neurons. *Brain Res* 1996; 713:160–167.

Andoh T, Nagasawa T, Satoh M, Kuraishi Y. Substance P induction of itch-associated response mediated by cutaneous NK1 tachykinin receptors in mice. *J Pharmacol Exp Ther* 1998; 286:1140–1145.

Andrew D, Craig AD. Spinothalamic lamina 1 neurons selectively sensitive to histamine: a central neural pathway for itch. *Nat Neurosci* 2001; 4:72–77.

Atanassoff PG, Brull SJ, Zhang J, et al. Enhancement of experimental pruritus and mechanically evoked dysesthesiae with local anesthesia. *Somatosens Mot Res* 1999; 16:291–298.

Bar-Shavit R, Maoz M, Yongjun Y, et al. Signalling pathways induced by protease-activated receptors and integrins in T cells. *Immunology* 2002; 105:35–46.

Baron R, Schwarz K, Kleinert A, Schattschneider J, Wasner G. Histamine-induced itch converts into pain in neuropathic hyperalgesia. *Neuroreport* 2001; 12:3475–3478.

Bennett DL. Neurotrophic factors: important regulators of nociceptive function. *Neuroscientist* 2001; 7:13–17.

Bessou P, Perl ER. Responses of cutaneous sensory units with unmyelinated fibers to noxious stimuli. *J Neurophysiol* 1969; 32:1025–1043.

Bickford RGL. Experiments relating to itch sensation, its peripheral mechanism and central pathways. *Clin Sci* 1938; 3:377–386.

Bohm-Starke N, Hilliges M, Falconer C, Rylander E. Increased intraepithelial innervation in women with vulvar vestibulitis syndrome. *Gynecol Obstet Invest* 1998; 46:256–260.

Bohm-Starke N, Hilliges M, Brodda-Jansen G, Rylander E, Torebjork E. Psychophysical evidence of nociceptor sensitization in vulvar vestibulitis syndrome. *Pain* 2001; 94:177–183.

Brull SJ, Atanassoff PG, Silverman DG, Zhang J, LaMotte RH. Attenuation of experimental pruritus and mechanically evoked dysesthesiae in an area of cutaneous allodynia. *Somatosens Mot Res* 1999; 16:299–303.

Coelho AM, Vergnolle N, Guiard B, Fioramonti J, Bueno L. Proteinases and proteinase-activated receptor 2: a possible role to promote visceral hyperalgesia in rats. *Gastroenterology* 2002; 122:1035–1047.

Corvera CU, Dery O, McConalogue K, et al. Thrombin and mast cell tryptase regulate guinea-pig myenteric neurons through proteinase-activated receptors-1 and -2. *J Physiol (Lond)* 1999; 517:741–756.

D'Andrea MR, Rogahn CJ, Andrade-Gordon P. Localization of protease-activated receptors-1 and -2 in human mast cells: indications for an amplified mast cell degranulation cascade. *Biotech Histochem* 2000; 75:85–90.

Darsow U, Drzezga A, Frisch M, et al. Processing of histamine-induced itch in the human cerebral cortex: a correlation analysis with dermal reactions. *J Invest Dermatol* 2000; 115:1029–1033.

Drzezga A, Darsow U, Treede R, et al. Central activation by histamine-induced itch: analogies to pain processing: a correlational analysis of O-15 H_2O positron emission tomography studies. *Pain* 2001; 92:295–305.

Fiorucci S, Distrutti E. Role of PAR2 in pain and inflammation. *Trends Pharmacol Sci* 2002; 23:153–155.

Grewe M, Vogelsang K, Ruzicka T, Stege H, Krutmann J. Neurotrophin-4 production by human epidermal keratinocytes: increased expression in atopic dermatitis. *J Invest Dermatol* 2000; 114:1108–1112.

Hägermark O. Influence of antihistamines, sedatives, and aspirin on experimental itch. *Acta Derm Venereol* 1973; 53:363–368.

Hägermark O. Peripheral and central mediators of itch. *Skin Pharmacol* 1992; 5:1–8.

Hägermark O, Strandberg K. Pruritogenic activity of prostaglandin E2. *Acta Derm Venereol* 1977; 57:37–43.

Hägermark O, Hokfelt T, Pernow B. Flare and itch induced by substance P in human skin. *J Invest Dermatol* 1978; 71:233–235.

Heyer G, Ulmer FJ, Schmitz J, Handwerker HO. Histamine-induced itch and alloknesis (itchy skin) in atopic eczema patients and controls. *Acta Derm Venereol (Stockh)* 1995; 75:348–352.

Heyer G, Dotzer M, Diepgen TL, Handwerker HO. Opiate and H1 antagonist effects on histamine induced pruritus and alloknesis. *Pain* 1997; 73:239–243.

Hoogerwerf WA, Zou L, Shenoy M, et al. The proteinase-activated receptor 2 is involved in nociception. *J Neurosci* 2001; 21:9036–9042.

Hsieh JC, Hägermark O, Stahle Backdahl M, et al. Urge to scratch represented in the human cerebral cortex during itch. *J Neurophysiol* 1994; 72:3004–3008.

Jarvikallio A, Naukkarinen A, Harvima IT, Aalto ML, Horsmanheimo M. Quantitative analysis of tryptase- and chymase-containing mast cells in atopic dermatitis and nummular eczema. *Br J Dermatol* 1997; 136:871–877.

Kamei J, Nagase H. Norbinaltorphimine, a selective kappa-opioid receptor antagonist, induces an itch-associated response in mice. *Eur J Pharmacol* 2001; 418:141–145.

Kawabata A, Kawao N, Kuroda R, et al. Peripheral PAR-2 triggers thermal hyperalgesia and nociceptive responses in rats. *Neuroreport* 2001; 12:715–719.

Kawagoe J, Takizawa T, Matsumoto J, et al. Effect of protease-activated receptor-2 deficiency on allergic dermatitis in the mouse ear. *Jpn J Pharmacol* 2002; 88:77–84.

Kessler W, Kirchhoff C, Reeh PW, Handwerker HO. Excitation of cutaneous afferent nerve endings in vitro by a combination of inflammatory mediators and conditioning effect of substance P. *Exp Brain Res* 1992; 91:467–476.

Kidd BL, Urban LA. Mechanisms of inflammatory pain. *Br J Anaesth* 2001; 87:3–11.

Kingston WP, Greaves MW. Actions of prostaglandin E2 metabolites on skin microcirculation. *Agents Actions* 1985; 16:13–14.

Kjellberg F, Tramer MR. Pharmacological control of opioid-induced pruritus: a quantitative systematic review of randomized trials. *Eur J Anaesthesiol* 2001; 18:346–357.

Kumagai H. Prospects for a novel opioid kappa receptor agonist Trk-820 in uremic pruritus. Hiroo Kumagai, Japan: International Workshop on Itch, 2001.

Lambert RW, Granstein RD. Neuropeptides and Langerhans cells. *Exp Dermatol* 1998; 7:73–80.

LaMotte RH. James Daniel Hardy (1904–1985). Tribute to a pioneer in pain psychophysics. *Pain* 1986; 27:127–130.

LaMotte RH, Simone DA, Baumann TK, Shain CN, Alreja M. Hypothesis for novel classes of chemoreceptors mediating chemogenic pain and itch. In: Dubner R, Gebhart GF, Bond MR (Eds). *Proceedings of the Vth World Congress on Pain,* Pain Research and Clinical Management, Vol. 3. Amsterdam: Elsevier, 1988, pp 529–535.

Magerl W, Westerman RA, Mohner B, Handwerker HO. Properties of transdermal histamine iontophoresis: differential effects of season, gender, and body region. *J Invest Dermatol* 1990; 94:347–352.

Meyer RA, Campbell JN. A Novel electrophysiological technique for locating cutaneous nociceptive and chemospecific receptors. *Brain Res* 1988; 441:81–86.

Neisius U, Olsson R, Rukwied R, Lischetzki G, Schmelz M. Prostaglandin E2 induces vasodilation and pruritus, but no protein extravasation in atopic dermatitis and controls. *J Am Acad Dermatol* 2002; 47:28–32.

Nilsson HJ, Levinsson A, Schouenborg J. Cutaneous field stimulation (CFS): a new powerful method to combat itch. *Pain* 1997; 71:49–55.

Perl ER. Cutaneous polymodal receptors: characteristics and plasticity. *Prog Brain Res* 1996; 113:21–37.

Rajka G. Latency and duration of pruritus elicited by trypsin in aged patients with itching eczema and psoriasis. *Acta Derm Venereol* 1969; 49:401–403.

Romero MI, Rangappa N, Li L, et al. Extensive sprouting of sensory afferents and hyperalgesia induced by conditional expression of nerve growth factor in the adult spinal cord. *J Neurosci* 2000; 20:4435–4445.

Rukwied R, Lischetzki G, McGlone F, Heyer G, Schmelz M. Mast cell mediators other than histamine induce pruritus in atopic dermatitis patients: a dermal microdialysis study. *Br J Dermatol* 2000; 142:1114–1120.

Schmelz M, Petersen LJ. Neurogenic inflammation in human and rodent skin. *News Physiol Sci* 2001; 16:33–37.

Schmelz M, Schmidt R, Bickel A, Handwerker HO, Torebjörk HE. Specific C-receptors for itch in human skin. *J Neurosci* 1997; 17:8003–8008.

Schmelz M, Zeck S, Raithel M, Rukwied R. Mast cell tryptase in dermal neurogenic inflammation. *Clin Exp Allergy* 1999; 29:652–659.

Schmelz M, Schmidt R, Handwerker HO, Torebjörk HE. Encoding of burning pain from capsaicin-treated human skin in two categories of unmyelinated nerve fibres. *Brain* 2000; 123:560–571.

Schmidt RF, Schaible HG, Messlinger K, Hanesch U, Pawlak M. Silent and active nociceptors: structure, functions, and clinical implications. In: Gebhart GF, Hammond DL, Jensen TS (Eds). *Proceedings of the 7th World Congress on Pain,* Progress in Pain Research and Management, Vol. 2. Seattle: IASP Press, 1994, pp 213–250.

Schmidt R, Schmelz M, Forster C, et al. Novel classes of responsive and unresponsive C nociceptors in human skin. *J Neurosci* 1995; 15:333–341.

Sciberras DG, Goldenberg MM, Bolognese JA, James I, Baber NS. Inflammatory responses to intradermal injection of platelet activating factor, histamine and prostaglandin E2 in healthy volunteers: a double blind investigation. *Br J Clin Pharmacol* 1987; 24:753–761.

Shu XQ, Llinas A, Mendell LM. Effects of trkB and trkC neurotrophin receptor agonists on thermal nociception: a behavioral and electrophysiological study. *Pain* 1999; 80:463–470.

Shu XQ, Mendell LM. Neurotrophins and hyperalgesia. *Proc Natl Acad Sci USA* 1999; 96:7693–7696.

Simone DA, Alreja M, LaMotte RH. Psychophysical studies of the itch sensation and itchy skin ("alloknesis") produced by intracutaneous injection of histamine. *Somatosens Mot Res* 1991; 8:271–279.

Simone DA, Nolano M, Johnson T, Wendelschafer-Crabb G, Kennedy WR. Intradermal injection of capsaicin in humans produces degeneration and subsequent reinnervation of epidermal nerve fibers: correlation with sensory function. *J Neurosci* 1998; 18:8947–8954.

Steinhoff M, Vergnolle N, Young SH, et al. Agonists of proteinase-activated receptor 2 induce inflammation by a neurogenic mechanism. *Nat Med* 2000; 6:151–158.

Sugiura H, Omoto M, Hirota Y, Danno K, Uehara M. Density and fine structure of peripheral nerves in various skin lesions of atopic dermatitis. *Arch Dermatol Res* 1997; 289:125–131.

Torebjörk HE. Afferent C units responding to mechanical, thermal and chemical stimuli in human non-glabrous skin. *Acta Physiol Scand* 1974; 92:374–390.

Toyoda M, Nakamura M, Makino T, et al. Nerve growth factor and substance P are useful plasma markers of disease activity in atopic dermatitis. *Br J Dermatol* 2002; 147:71–79.

Urashima R, Mihara M. Cutaneous nerves in atopic dermatitis—a histological, immunohistochemical and electron microscopic study. *Virchows Arch Int J Pathol* 1998; 432:363–370.

Vergnolle N, Bunnett NW, Sharkey KA, et al. Proteinase-activated receptor-2 and hyperalgesia: a novel pain pathway. *Nat Med* 2001a; 7:821–826.

Vergnolle N, Wallace JL, Bunnett NW, Hollenberg MD. Protease-activated receptors in inflammation, neuronal signaling and pain. *Trends Pharmacol Sci* 2001b; 22:146–152.

Vogelsang M, Heyer G, Hornstein OP. Acetylcholine induces different cutaneous sensations in atopic and non-atopic subjects. *Acta Derm Venereol* 1995; 75:434–436.

Weber M, Birklein F, Neundorfer B, Schmelz M. Facilitated neurogenic inflammation in complex regional pain syndrome. *Pain* 2001; 91:251–257.

Weidner C, Klede M, Rukwied R, et al. Acute effects of substance P and calcitonin gene-related peptide in human skin—a microdialysis study. *J Invest Dermatol* 2000; 115:1015–1020.

Weisshaar E, Ziethen B, Rohl FW, Gollnick H. The antipruritic effect of a 5-HT3 receptor antagonist (tropisetron) is dependent on mast cell depletion—an experimental study. *Exp Dermatol* 1999; 8:254–260.

Wolfhagen FH, Sternieri E, Hop WC, et al. Oral naltrexone treatment for cholestatic pruritus: a double-blind, placebo-controlled study. *Gastroenterology* 1997; 113:1264–1269.

Woodward DF, Nieves AL, Hawley SB, et al. The pruritogenic and inflammatory effects of prostanoids in the conjunctiva. *J Ocul Pharmacol Ther* 1995; 11:339–347.

Yamada K, Akasu T. Substance P suppresses GABA-A receptor function via protein kinase C in primary sensory neurones of bullfrogs. *J Physiol* 1996; 496(Pt 2):439–449.

Correspondence to: Martin Schmelz, Dr med, Department of Anesthesiology and Intensive Care Medicine, Faculty of Clinical Medicine Mannheim, University of Heidelberg, Theodor-Kutzer Ufer 1-3, 68167 Mannheim, Germany. Tel: 49-6121-383-5616; email: martin.schmelz@anaes.ma.uni-heidelberg.de.

Proceedings of the 10th World Congress on Pain, Progress in Pain Research and Management, Vol. 24, edited by Jonathan O. Dostrovsky, Daniel B. Carr, and Martin Koltzenburg, IASP Press, Seattle, © 2003.

19

The Central Projection of Unmyelinated (C) Primary Afferent Fibers from Gastrocnemius Muscle in the Guinea Pig

Li Jun Ling,[a,b] Takashi Honda,[c] Noriyuki Ozaki,[a] Yasuhiro Shimada,[b] and Yasuo Sugiura[a]

Departments of [a]Functional Anatomy and Neuroscience and [b]Anesthesiology, Nagoya University Graduate School of Medicine, Nagoya, Japan; [c]Department of Anatomy, Fukushima Medical College, Fukushima, Japan

Spinal termination of fine afferent fibers from muscle mediates mechanical sensation, including local pressure and pain sensation. Thinly myelinated (group III) and unmyelinated (C or group IV) fibers are known to be a major component of muscle afferent fibers (Mense 1993). A few reports have dealt with central terminals of C-afferent fibers from muscles, but information in this regard is still fragmentary (Hirakawa et al. 1992; Torre et al. 1995).

Neck and forelimb muscle afferents terminate in laminae I and V (Abraham and Swett 1986), while dense projections from the gastrocnemius and soleus muscle are reported to terminate in the substantia gelatinosa (Brushart et al. 1981) or diffusely terminate in laminae I–V (Kalia et al. 1981). Other studies report that muscle afferents terminate clearly in laminae I and V, but not in lamina II (Mense and Craig 1988).

Intra-axonal labeling with horseradish peroxidase (HRP) of group III afferents from muscle or deep tissues demonstrates that the axons terminate in lamina I only or in laminae I, IV, and V (Hoheisel et al. 1989). By contrast, unmyelinated (C) afferent fibers from the skin terminate mainly in laminae I and II of the spinal cord of guinea pigs (Sugiura et al. 1986, 1989) and monkeys (Alvarez et al. 1993). On the other hand, visceral C-afferent axons terminate in laminae I, V, and X (Sugiura et al. 1989, 1993).

However, complete trajectories in the spinal cord of C or group IV afferent fibers from muscle have not been demonstrated. This chapter describes a study designed to elucidate the central terminals of unmyelinated C fibers from the lateral gastrocnemius (LGC) muscle in guinea pigs.

MATERIALS AND METHODS

ANIMALS AND SURGICAL TECHNIQUES

The experiments were conducted under the control of the local animal ethics committee in accordance with the Guidelines for Animal Experiments of Nagoya University Graduate School of Medicine , and with the guidelines of International Association for the Study of Pain (Zimmerman 1983).

The experiments were performed on 40 female guinea pigs weighing 200–300 g. Under deep anesthesia with sodium pentobarbital (50 mg/kg i.p.), respiration was maintained by a positive pressure pump, and additional doses of anesthesia were given as necessary. The L5 dorsal root ganglion (DRG), LGC muscle, and muscular branches of the tibial nerve were exposed for recording and stimulation (Fig. 1a). Fine glass micropipettes filled with a solution of 2.5% *Phaseolus vulgaris* leucoagglutinin (PHA-L) dissolved in 0.1 M KCl were used to record the neuronal activity from DRG cell bodies.

Recordings were made from the L5 DRG cell bodies of responses to electrical stimulation (6–10 V or 5 mA) of the tibial nerve branch to the LGC muscle above the C-fiber threshold (Fig. 1b). Conduction velocity was calculated from the response latency recorded and the conduction distance (40–50 mm) between the stimulation electrode and the L5 DRG cell. After C-fiber latency had been confirmed, PHA-L was applied intracellularly by positive current (5×10^{-9} A) for 5 minutes. After the experiment, animals recovered and were kept for 3 to 5 days. Animals were perfused transcardially with a fixative containing 2% paraformaldehyde and 10% saturated picric acid under deep anesthesia. Tissue of the L1–L6 spinal cord and L5 DRG was removed and kept in the same fixative overnight. All tissue blocks were processed using 20% sucrose and embedded into a freezing compound.

IMMUNOHISTOCHEMISTRY

L1 to L6 spinal segments were sectioned serially at 50 μm in the parasagittal plane on a freezing microtome. All tissue sections were processed for PHA-L immunohistochemistry. Tissue sections were immersed in goat anti-PHA-L solution (×1,000) for 3 days. Sections were immersed in a biotinylated rabbit anti-goat-immunoglobulin solution (×200) for 2 hours,

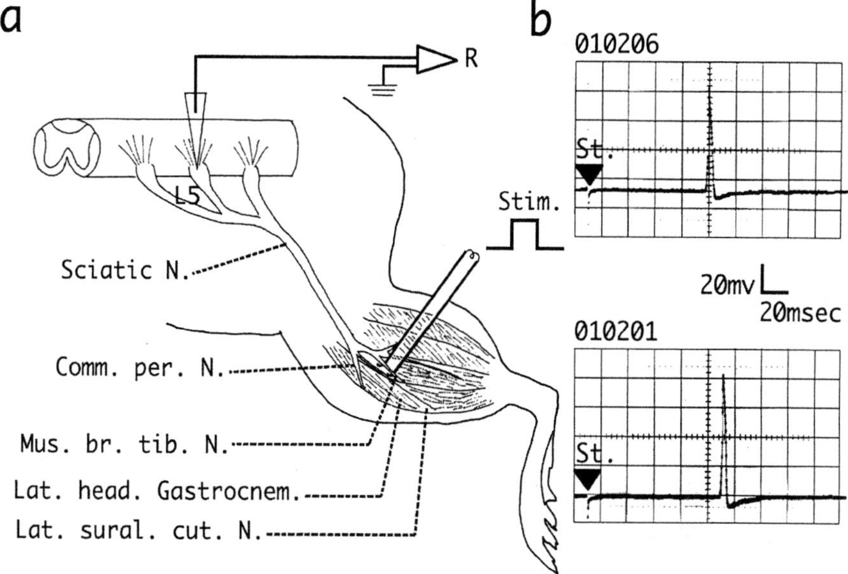

Fig. 1. (a) Diagram of the experimental design of the intracellular recording. A micropipette was inserted in an L5 DRG cell for intracellular recording and iontophoretic injection with the PHA-L solution. Stim, electric stimulation; Comm. per N., common peroneal nerve; Mus. br. tib. N., muscle branch of tibial nerve; Lat, lateral; Gastrocnem, gastrocnemius; cut, cutaneous. (b) Intracellular recordings in L5 DRG cells. Stimulation at 5 mA evoked an action potentials of approximately 80 mV with a 100 ms latency (in fiber 010201) at –60 mV resting potential and an action potential with a 90 ms latency (in fiber 010206) at –50 mV resting potential. St indicates the time of electrical stimulation.

incubated in an avidin, biotin-peroxidase complex (1:200) solution at room temperature for 90 minutes, and immersed in 0.1% 3-3' diaminobenzidine tetrahydrochloride containing 0.023% H_2O_2. Composite camera lucida drawings were made of arbors of the labeled central processes in the spinal cord as found in consecutive parasagittal sections.

RESULTS

Muscle C fibers (group IV fibers) were identified in 40 female guinea pigs by the latency of the unitary response after electrical stimulation (Fig. 1a). In the present study, the unitary responses of all the C fibers had an 80–100 ms latency (Fig. 1b). We could not find any responses elicited by natural stimuli (touch or pinch by forceps) from the skin, muscle, tendon, or deep connective tissues, or any spontaneous activity relating to muscle tone. In previous studies on cutaneous C fibers (Sugiura et al. 1986, 1993), receptive fields in the skin or toe were identified in almost half of the neurons. Central terminal projections of six C fibers were recovered in the 40 labeled C-afferent neurons. The mean conduction velocity of these afferents was approximately 0.5 m/second. In two recordings of 40 neurons the excitable membrane did not repolarize immediately after depolarization, and the potential remained on a plateau near the peak of the spike for several milliseconds before repolarization began.

The central collaterals and branches of the LGC muscle C fibers were very thin in the superficial dorsal horn of the lumbar cord. The arbors of well-labeled fibers could generally be traced up to terminal enlargements in the entry segment of the root, and some fiber terminals were traced in several segments regardless of faint staining or interruption of fiber trajectories in the dorsal funiculus (DF).

SPINAL DISTRIBUTION OF CENTRAL TERMINALS OF C MUSCLE AFFERENT FIBERS

We noted three representative fiber terminals in the six recovered fibers. The axon of the reconstructed fiber (numbered 010327) issued collaterals to make a few small circumscribed distributions of terminals in laminae I and II and in the DF, and some terminal collaterals extended to the border of lamina III, whose terminal areas extended 100–200 μm rostrocaudally.

C fiber 010403 showed terminal areas, forming a nest-like terminal field in the DF, at the border of laminae I and II and in the middle of lamina II. Two major terminal plexuses were connected with the very fine fibers and had thin, small terminals extending about 700 μm rostrocaudally. Total terminal areas in this case extended 1 mm (about one-quarter segment) in the spinal cord.

In the case of fiber 010201, the axon ran along the surface of the DF, then issued collaterals to laminae I and II and the DF. This C-afferent fiber extended almost 1 cm rostrocaudally in the spinal segment and gave off several collaterals from the main branches running along the DF to terminate in laminae I and II and form three terminal areas; some collaterals also terminated in the DF.

In summary, the LGC muscle C afferents, which were not identified as to their receptor modality, projected to the dorsal spinal cord and extended rostrocaudally over several segments and ran along the surface of the DF, giving off collaterals to laminae I and II and to the border of lamina III. Terminal branches of C fibers were found not only in the gray matter in the superficial dorsal horn, but also in the DF around the dorsal horn. A muscle C-afferent fiber typically had a few (two or three) terminal regions distributed over the rostrocaudal length of two or three spinal segments.

DISCUSSION

This study is, to our knowledge, the first report to demonstrate the central projection of unmyelinated C or group IV muscle afferent fibers. In this study about 15% of the unmyelinated muscle fibers could be recovered and their terminals traced almost to their full extent..

DIFFERENTIAL TERMINATION OF MUSCLE AFFERENT FIBERS

Several investigators have described central projections of myelinated muscle afferent fibers . Large-diameter afferent fibers terminate in laminae IV, V, VI, VII, and IX (Brown and Fyffe 1979; Ishizuka et al. 1979). Thinly myelinated afferent and small-diameter fibers from muscle send terminals to laminae I and V (Craig and Mense 1983; Nyberg and Blomqvist 1984; Mense and Craig 1988).

Early studies have partially clarified the terminal areas of unmyelinated muscle afferent fibers in the dorsal horn by using electrophysiological recording (MacMahon and Wall 1985; Hoheisel and Mense 1990). Studies using application of HRP or cholera toxin B subunit to the muscle have labeled the superficial dorsal horn and lamina II including central terminals of C-muscle afferent fibers (Hirakawa et al. 1992). Capsaicin-sensitive muscle afferent fibers, which are C fibers, terminate in laminae I and II (Torre et al. 1995). Our observations in this study modified and detailed morphological and electrophysiological findings.

In Fig. 2, comparative distributions of various C-afferent fibers are schematically drawn. Cutaneous C fibers terminate principally in laminae I and II of the dorsal horn in a circumscribed and concentrated zone containing many enlargements and synaptic boutons (Sugiura et al. 1986, 1989). The visceral afferent C fibers, on the other hand, typically have only one or two terminal branches at each terminal locus, unlike the somatic fibers that have a concentrated terminal focus. C fibers of visceral origin terminate ipsilaterally in laminae I, II, V, and X, and some fibers project contralaterally to laminae V and X (Sugiura et al. 1989) (Fig. 2).

The LGC muscle C afferents projected rostrocaudally over several segments running on the surface of the DF and giving off collaterals ipsilaterally to laminae I and II, and partly to lamina III. Most of the terminal arbors and boutons were localized in laminae I and II and the DF (Fig. 2). The terminal locations of the unmyelinated muscle afferents are similar to those of the cutaneous C-afferents, but the distribution of the terminals in the plexus is different from that of cutaneous and visceral C-afferent fibers. Our observations demonstrate that the central projections of muscle C-afferent

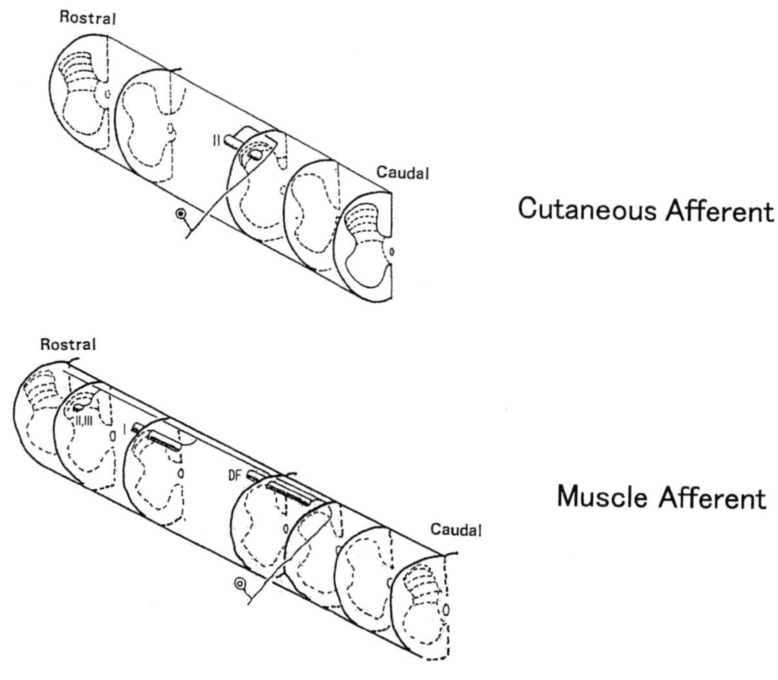
Rostral
II
Caudal
Cutaneous Afferent
Rostral
II,III
I
DF
Caudal
Muscle Afferent

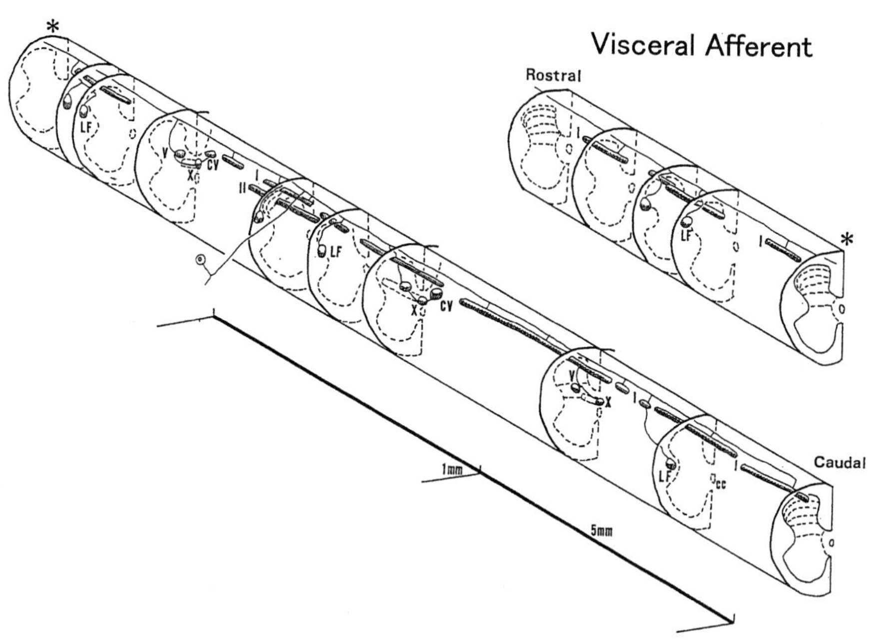
*
LF
V
X
CV
I
II
LF
X
CV
V
X
I
LF
cc
I
Caudal
1mm
5mm
Visceral Afferent
Rostral
I
LF
I
*

← **Fig. 2.** Schematic three-dimensional drawings of the central collateral distribution of single unmyelinated (C) afferent fibers. The cutaneous afferent illustrated shows the typical central terminals labeled in a T13 DRG cell. Central terminals are located in the lamina I or II in the superficial dorsal horn within a circumscribed and dense concentrated zone. The muscle afferent drawing illustrates the terminations of a single C-afferent fiber from the gastrocnemius muscle recorded in the L5 DRG. This fiber extended about 10 mm (two or three spinal segments) rostrocaudally along the dorsal surface and gave off terminal collaterals to laminae I, II, and the DF. Visceral afferent fibers from the celiac ganglion area terminated in laminae I, II, V, X ipsilaterally and in laminae V, X contralaterally (not shown), extending over 20 mm rostrocaudally in the spinal cord.

---

fibers characteristically transmit pain and other sensations from muscle organs with more somatotopic sharpness than do visceral afferents, but more vaguely and in a more widespread fashion than do cutaneous afferents.

ACKNOWLEDGMENTS

We thank Mr. Y. Shiraishi for his assistance in creating the illustrations.

REFERENCES

Abrahams VC, Swett JE. The pattern of spinal and medullary projections from a cutaneous nerve and muscle nerve of the forelimb of the cat: a study using the transganglionic transport of HRP. *J Comp Neurol* 1986; 246:70–84.

Alvarez FJ, Kavookjian AM, Light AR. Ultrastructural morphology, synaptic relationships, and CGRP immunoreactivity of physiologically identified C-fiber terminals in the monkey spinal cord. *J Comp Neurol* 1993; 329:472–490.

Brown AG, Fyffe REW. The morphology of group Ib afferent fiber collaterals in the spinal cord of the cat. *J Physiol* 1979; 296:215–228.

Brushart TM, Henry EW, Mesulam M-M. Reorganization of muscle afferent projection accompanies peripheral nerve regeneration. *Neuroscience* 1981; 6:2053–2061.

Craig AD, Mense S. The distribution of afferent fibers from the gastrocnemius-soleus muscle in the dorsal horn of the cat, as revealed by the transport of horseradish peroxidase. *Neurosci Lett* 1983; 41:233–238.

Hirakawa M, McCabe JT, Kawata M. Time-related changes in the labeling pattern of motor and sensory neurons innervating the gastrocnemius muscle, as revealed by the retrograde transport of the cholera toxin B subunit. *Cell Tissue Res* 1992; 267:419–427.

Hoheisel U, Lehmann-Willenbrock E, Mense S. Termination 1 patterns of identified group II and III afferent fibres from deep tissues in thc spinal cord of the cat. *Neuroscience* 1989; 28:495–507.

Hoheisel U, Mense S. Response behaviour of cat dorsal horn neurons receiving input from skeletal muscle and other deep somatic tissues. *J Physiol* 1990; 426:265–280.

Ishizuka N, Mannen H, Hongo T, Sasaki S. Trajectory of group Ia afferent fibers stained with horseradish peroxidase in the lumbosacral spinal cord of the cat: three dimensional reconstructions from serial sections. *J Comp Neurol* 1979; 186:189–212.

Kalia M, Mei SS, Kao FF. Central projections from ergoreceptors (C fibers) in muscle involved in cardiopulmonary responses to static exercise. *Circ Res* 1981; 48:48–62.

McMahon SB, Wall PD. The distribution and central termination of single cutaneous and muscle unmyelinated fibers in rat spinal cord. *Brain Res* 1985; 359:39–48.

Mense S. Nociception from skeletal muscle in relation to clinical muscle pain. *Pain* 1993; 54:241–289.

Mense S, Craig AD. Spinal and supraspinal terminations of primary afferent fibers from the gastrocnemius-soleus muscle in the cat. *Neuroscience* 1988; 26:1023–1035.

Nyberg G, Blomqvist A. The central projection of muscle afferent fibers to the lower medulla and upper spinal cord: an anatomical study in the cat with the transganglionic transport method. *J Comp Neurol* 1984; 230:99–109.

Sugiura Y, Lee CL, Perl ER. Central projections of identified, unmyelinated (C) afferent fibers innervating mammalian skin. *Science* 1986; 234:358–361.

Sugiura Y, Terui N, Hosoya Y. Difference in distribution of central terminals between visceral and somatic unmyelinated (C) primary afferent fibers. *J Neurophysiol* 1989; 62:834–840.

Sugiura Y, Terui N, Hosoya Y, et al. Quantitative analysis of central terminal projections of visceral and somatic unmyelinated (C) primary afferent fibers in the guinea pig. *J Comp Neurol* 1993; 332:315–325.

Torre GD, Lucchi ML, Burnetti O, et al. Central projection and entries of capsaicin-sensitive muscle afferents. *Brain Res* 1995; 713:223–231.

Zimmermann M. Ethical guideline for investigation of experimental pain in conscious animals. *Pain* 1983; 16:109–110.

Correspondence to: Yasuo Sugiura, MD, PhD, Department of Functional Anatomy and Neuroscience, Nagoya University Graduate School of Medicine, 65 Tsurumaicho, Showaku, Nagoya 466-8550, Japan. Tel: 81-52-744-2014; Fax: 81-52-744-2027; email: ysugiura@med.nagoya-u.ac.jp.

Proceedings of the 10th World Congress on Pain,
Progress in Pain Research and Management, Vol. 24,
edited by Jonathan O. Dostrovsky, Daniel B. Carr, and
Martin Koltzenburg, IASP Press, Seattle, © 2003.

20

Absence of Substance P and CGRP in the Dorsal Root Ganglia of Naked Mole Rats Correlates with an Absence of Hyperalgesia to Heat

Ying Lu,[a] Thomas Park,[b] Frank L. Rice,[c] and Charles E. Laurito[a]

Departments of [a]Anesthesiology and [b]Biological Science, University of Illinois at Chicago, Chicago, Illinois, USA; [c]Department of Pharmacology and Neuroscience, Albany Medical College, Albany, New York, USA

Activation of nociceptive primary afferents induces the release of neurotransmitters, such as amino acids, substance P (SP), and calcitonin gene-related peptide (CGRP) (Yaksh 1988; Lawand et al. 2000; Yeomans et al. 2000). The neuropeptides SP and CGRP coexist in the same neurons in the dorsal root ganglia (DRG; Gulbenkian et al. 1986). They are expressed by primary afferent fibers and released from the central terminals in the spinal cord by the application of noxious stimuli, including capsaicin injection (Mantyh et al. 1995). SP appears to be released by activation of unmyelinated (C-fiber), but not of myelinated (Aδ-fiber), thermonociceptors (Zachariou et al. 1997). Intraspinal release of immunoreactive SP is evoked by electrical stimulation of unmyelinated C-afferent fibers in peripheral nerves and by thermal or mechanical noxious stimuli applied to the skin (Go and Yaksh 1987; Duggan et al. 1988, 1992; Collin et al. 1991). CGRP also increases the nociceptive flexion reflex mediated via C-afferent fibers in the spinal cord (Woolf and Wiesenfeld-Hallin 1986). Most of the CGRP-binding sites were expressed in unmyelinated DRG neurons (Schaible et al. 2002). Thus, different nociceptor types make and release different ensembles of neurotransmitters (Lawson 1995). SP and CGRP are predominantly made and released by unmyelinated C-afferent nociceptors.

African naked mole rats are subterranean rodents with cutaneous C fibers and small DRG cells that congenitally lack both SP and CGRP, substances that are present in rats and other mammals (Davis et al. 1997; Park et al. 2003). In contrast, the skin of naked mole rats has an abundance of presumptive Aδ fibers. Selective absence of these peptidergic neurotransmitters raises questions about the capacity of response to nociceptive stimuli and the differential effect of Aδ- and C-fiber activation. Our experiments investigate the effects of the natural absence of both SP and CGRP on the nociceptive response and attempt to determine whether the absence of these two peptides differentially affects C-fiber or Aδ-nociceptor activity.

METHODS

Experimental animals. The study used 18 naked mole rats (35–45 g) and 15 Swiss-Webster mice (20–30 g). The mole rats were housed under semi-natural conditions in an artificial burrow system within a colony room that was maintained under dim rad light at 30°C and 45–65% relative humidity (Artwohl et al. 2002). The University of Illinois at Chicago Institutional Animal Care and Use Committee approved animal protocols.

Aδ- versus C-fiber nociception test. Naked mole rats were lightly anesthetized with pentobarbital (50 mg/kg, i.p.). Foot-withdrawal responses evoked by thermal activation of Aδ (with 6.5°C/second high heating rate) and C nociceptors (with 0.9°C/second low heating rate) were separately assessed. Baseline response latencies were measured in response to high- or low-rate skin heating. Approximately 10 minutes after topical application of 2 mM capsaicin on the unilateral hindpaw skin and at 15-minute intervals thereafter, foot withdrawal latencies were remeasured over approximately 1 hour to determine the nociceptive effects of tonic activation of C fibers.

Long-term inflammatory pain model. Naked mole rats received an injection of complete Freund's adjuvant (CFA, 50%, pH 7.0, in saline, 50 μL) in the unilateral hindpaw. We measured foot-withdrawal latencies before injection and 3 days after injection.

RESULTS

In the behavioral foot-withdrawal test, the baseline latencies of naked mole rats were the same as in mice. After topical application of low-dose capsaicin, the low heating rate associated with C-fiber activation decreased the latencies for mice but not for naked mole rats. No changes occurred for Aδ-fiber-mediated responses evoked by a high heating rate (Fig. 1).

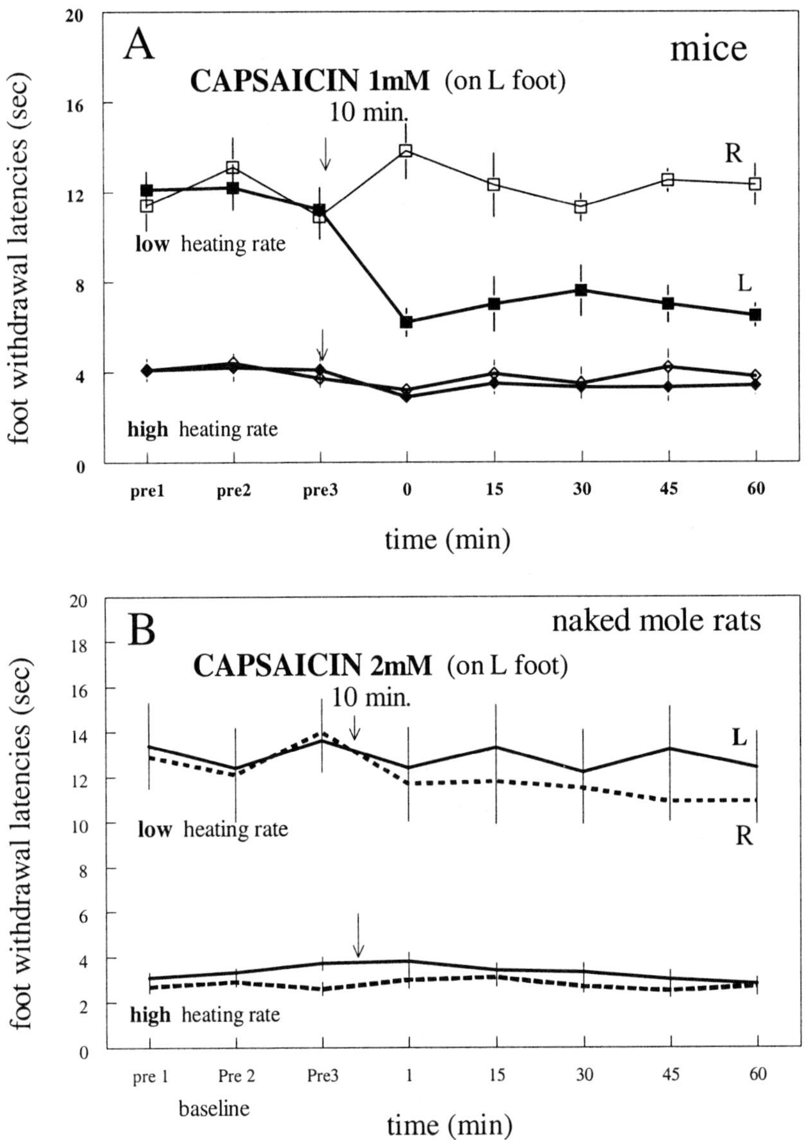

Fig. 1. (A) Ten minutes after topical application of 1 mM capsaicin, withdrawal latencies of the treated left feet of mice ($n = 8$) were significantly decreased by the low heating rate of 0.9°C/second ($P < 0.05$, one-way ANOVA) but not by the high heating rate of 6.5°C/second ($P > 0.05$). (B) In naked mole rats ($n = 6$), withdrawal latencies of the treated left foot showed no changes with both the low ($P > 0.05$) and high ($P > 0.05$) heating rate after topical application of 2 mM capsaicin. Vehicle phosphate-buffered saline had no effect on foot-withdrawal latencies of naked mole rats (data not shown; $P > 0.05$, ANOVA).

In the CFA-induced long-term inflammatory model, naked mole rats showed no changes in foot-withdrawal responses to either a low or high heating rate before or after CFA injection. Mice, however, showed a significant decrease of foot-withdrawal latencies evoked by C-fiber activation (Fig. 2).

DISCUSSION

Previous studies have provided evidence that behavioral nociceptive responses produced by different rates of skin heating are mediated by different classes of nociceptive afferents. More specifically, low (0.9°C/second) skin heating rates may evoke responses mediated by the activation of C-nociceptive afferents, whereas high (6.5°C/second) skin heating rates may produce responses mediated by Aδ nociceptive afferents (Yeomans and Proudfit 1994a, 1996a,b). The treatment of the foot skin with a low concentration of capsaicin (2 mM), which should selectively sensitize C-fiber nociceptors (LaMotte et al. 1992; Lynn et al. 1992; Yeomans and Proudfit 1996b), decreased the latency of responses to the low heating rate, but did not alter the latencies of responses to the high heating rate.

Our results demonstrate that after topical application of low-dose capsaicin on foot skin, ongoing pain behavior and hyperalgesia appeared for C-fiber response activated by low heating rates in mice but not in naked mole rats. These results are consistent with the finding that hyperalgesia to heating (and punctate mechanical stimuli) at a capsaicin-treated skin site are mediated by unmyelinated nociceptors, as revealed by experiments in which conduction in myelinated fibers was blocked differentially (Culp et al. 1989; Koltzenburg et al. 1992). Evidence indicates that cultured DRG release immunoreactive SP and immunoreactive CGRP (iCGRP) in response to stimulation with capsaicin (Dymshitz and Vasko 1994a,b; Huang and Neher 1996). Capsaicin evoked concentration-dependent increases in iCGRP release. A competitive capsaicin receptor antagonist, capsazepine, significantly inhibited capsaicin-evoked release of iCGRP (Flores et al. 2001). Intrathecal injection of the SP antagonist CP96,345 increased the latencies of foot-withdrawal responses to the low heating rate but did not affect responses evoked by the high heating rate (Yeomans and Proudfit 1994b). Consistent with these observations, naked mole rats naturally lack SP and CGRP immunoreactivity in their cutaneous C-fiber peripheral and central terminals (Park et al. 2003). These animals experienced significantly decreased nociceptive behavioral responses to capsaicin-evoked C-fiber activation. This finding indicates that SP and CGRP are important peptidergic neurotransmitters

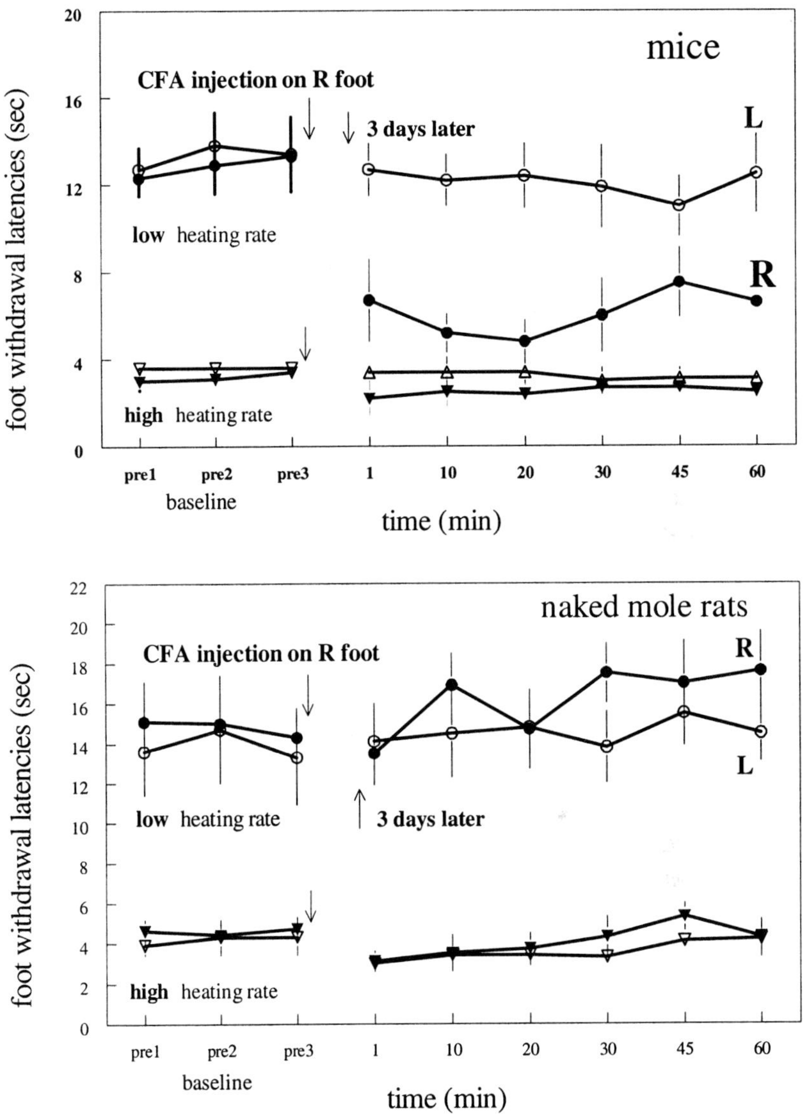

Fig. 2. (A) 72 hours after injection of complete Freund's adjuvant (CFA), mice (n = 7) showed significant decreases of foot-withdrawal latencies evoked by the low heating rate on the treated right foot ($P < 0.05$, one-way ANOVA). The contralateral untreated foot showed no changes in foot-withdrawal responses ($P > 0.05$). (B) Naked mole rats (n = 6) showed no changes in foot-withdrawal latencies evoked by either the high or low heating rate ($P > 0.05$).

released from DRG neurons and play a robust role in nociceptive responses mediated by C fibers. Absence of these peptides selectively affects C-fiber activation but not Aδ-fiber-transmitted nociception.

In the CFA-induced long-term inflammatory pain model, naked mole rats showed no changes in foot-withdrawal responses to either the low or high heating rate before and 3 days after CFA injection. Mice, however, appear to have hyperalgesia to low heating stimuli. Under normal conditions, stimulus-evoked intraspinal release of SP and CGRP occurs after induction of inflammation (Schaible et al. 1990, 1994; Collin et al. 1993). The synthesis of SP and CGRP is upregulated during chronic inflammation (Hanesch et al. 1993, 1995a,b), as is evidenced by the increase in SP mRNA (McCarson and Krause 1994, 1996) and in CGRP mRNA (Seybold et al. 1995) in the spinal cord. This functional plasticity of upregulation and enhanced release of the excitatory neuropeptides SP and CGRP may contribute significantly to the neuronal basis of hyperalgesia and allodynia in animals with chronic inflammation (Dubner and Ruda 1992; Schaible and Grubb 1993). The absence of SP and CGRP in naked mole rats exerts both short- and long-term effects on behavioral nociceptive responses, and selectively alters the animal's nociceptive responses to noxious stimuli, specifically the effects of C-fiber activation evoked by a low heating rate.

In summary, our studies have shown that the hyperalgesia to low rate heating produced by capsaicin and by CFA is markedly reduced in naked mole rats. These findings are consistent with the results of previous studies implicating release of SP and CGRP under these conditions and thus provide further support for their involvement in mediating these changes.

ACKNOWLEDGMENTS

The experimental work of the author and her colleagues was supported by the Department of Anesthesiology, University of Illinois at Chicago.

REFERENCES

Allen BJ, Rogers SD, Ghilardi JR, et al. Noxious cutaneous thermal stimuli induce a graded release of endogenous substance P in the spinal cord: imaging peptide action in vivo. *J Neurosci* 1997; 17(15):5921–5927.

Allen BJ, Li J, Menning PM, et al. Primary afferent fibers that contribute to increased substance P receptor internalization in the spinal cord after injury. *J Neurophysiol* 1999; 81(3):1379–1390.

Artwohl J, Hill T, Comer C, Park T. Naked mole-rats. Unique opportunities and husbandry challenges. *Lab Anim (NY)* 2002; 31(5):32–36.

Collin E, Mauborgne A, Bourgoin S, et al. In vivo tonic inhibition of spinal substance P (-like material) release by endogenous opioid(s) acting at delta receptors. *Neuroscience* 1991; 44(3):725–731.

Collin E, Mantelet S, Frechilla D, et al. Increased in vivo release of calcitonin gene-related peptide-like material from the spinal cord in arthritic rats. *Pain* 1993; 54(2):203–211.

Culp WJ, Ochoa J, Cline M, Dotson R. Heat and mechanical hyperalgesia induced by capsaicin. Cross modality threshold modulation in human C nociceptors. *Brain* 1989; 112(Pt 5):1317–1331.

Davis BM, Fundin BT, Albers KM, et al. Overexpression of nerve growth factor in skin causes preferential increases among innervation to specific sensory targets. *J Comp Neurol* 1997; 387(4):489–506.

Dubner R, Ruda MA. Activity-dependent neuronal plasticity following tissue injury and inflammation. *Trends Neurosci* 1992; 15(3):96–103.

Duggan AW, Hendry IA, Morton CR, Hutchison WD, Zhao ZQ. Cutaneous stimuli releasing immunoreactive substance P in the dorsal horn of the cat. *Brain Res* 1988; 451(1–2):261–273.

Dymshitz J, Vasko MR. Nitric oxide and cyclic guanosine 3', 5'-monophosphate do not alter neuropeptide release from rat sensory neurons grown in culture. *Neuroscience* 1994a; 62(4):1279–1286.

Dymshitz J, Vasko MR. Endothelin-1 enhances capsaicin-induced peptide release and cGMP accumulation in cultures of rat sensory neurons. *Neurosci Lett* 1994b; 167 (1–2):128–132.

Flores CM, Leong AS, Dussor GO, et al. Capsaicin-evoked CGRP release from rat buccal mucosa: development of a model system for studying trigeminal mechanisms of neurogenic inflammation. *Eur J Neurosci* 2001; 14(7):1113–1120.

Go VL, Yaksh T. Release of substance P from the cat spinal cord. *J Physiol* 1987; 391:141–167.

Gulbenkian S, Merighi A, Wharton J, Varndell IM, Polak JM. Ultrastructural evidence for the coexistence of calcitonin gene-related peptide and substance P in secretory vesicles of peripheral nerves in the guinea pig. *J Neurocytol* 1986; 15(4):535–542.

Hanesch U, Pfrommer U, Grubb BD, Heppelmann B, Schaible HG. The proportion of CGRP-immunoreactive and SP-mRNA containing dorsal root ganglion cells is increased by a unilateral inflammation of the ankle joint of the rat. *Regul Pept* 1993; 46(1-2):202–203.

Hanesch U, Blecher F, Stiller RU, et al. The effect of a unilateral inflammation at the rat's ankle joint on the expression of preprotachykinin-A mRNA and preprosomatostatin mRNA in dorsal root ganglion cells—a study using non-radioactive in situ hybridization. *Brain Res* 1995a; 700(1-2):279–284.

Hanesch U, Schaible HG. Effects of ankle joint inflammation on the proportion of calcitonin gene-related peptide (CGRP)-immunopositive perikarya in dorsal root ganglia. *Prog Brain Res* 1995b; 104:339–347.

Huang LY, Neher E. Ca(2+)-dependent exocytosis in the somata of dorsal root ganglion neurons. *Neuron* 1996; 17(1):135–145.

Koltzenburg M, Lundberg LE, Torebjork HE. Dynamic and static components of mechanical hyperalgesia in human hairy skin. *Pain* 1992; 51(2):207–219.

LaMotte RH, Lundberg LE, Torebjork HE. Pain, hyperalgesia and activity in nociceptive C units in humans after intradermal injection of capsaicin. *J Physiol* 1992; 448:749–764.

Lawand NB, McNearney T, Westlund KN. Amino acid release into the knee joint: key role in nociception and inflammation. *Pain* 2000; 86(1–2):69–74.

Lawson SN. Neuropeptides in morphologically and functionally identified primary afferent neurons in dorsal root ganglia: substance P, CGRP and somatostatin. *Prog Brain Res* 1995; 104:161–173.

Lynn B, Ye W, Cotsell B. The actions of capsaicin applied topically to the skin of the rat on C-fibre afferents, antidromic vasodilatation and substance P levels. *Br J Pharmacol* 1992; 107(2):400–406.

Mantyh PW, DeMaster E, Malhotra A, et al. Receptor endocytosis and dendrite reshaping in spinal neurons after somatosensory stimulation. *Science* 1995; 268(5217):1629–1632.

McCarson KE, Krause JE. NK-1 and NK-3 type tachykinin receptor mRNA expression in the rat spinal cord dorsal horn is increased during adjuvant or formalin-induced nociception. *J Neurosci* 1994; 14(2):712–720.

McCarson KE, Krause JE. The neurokinin-1 receptor antagonist LY306,740 blocks nociception-induced increases in dorsal horn neurokinin-1 receptor gene expression. *Mol Pharmacol* 1996; 50(5):1189–1199.

Park T, Comer C, Carol A, Hong H-S, Rice FL. Somatosensory organization and behavior in naked mole-rats. II: Peripheral structures, innervation, and selective lack of neuropeptides associated with thermoregulation and pain. *J Comp Neurol* 2003; in press.

Schaible HG, Grubb BD. Afferent and spinal mechanisms of joint pain. *Pain* 1993; 55(1):5–54.

Schaible HG, Jarrott B, Hope PJ, Duggan AW. Release of immunoreactive substance P in the spinal cord during development of acute arthritis in the knee joint of the cat: a study with antibody microprobes. *Brain Res* 1990; 529(1–2):214–223.

Schaible HG, Hope PJ, Lang CW, Duggan AW. Calcitonin gene-related peptide causes intraspinal spreading of substance P released by peripheral stimulation. *Eur J Neurosci* 1992: 4(8):750–757.

Schaible HG, Freudenberger U, Neugebauer V, Stiller RU. Intraspinal release of immunoreactive calcitonin gene-related peptide during development of inflammation in the joint in vivo—a study with antibody microprobes in cat and rat. *Neuroscience* 1994; 62(4):1293–1305.

Schaible HG, Ebersberger A, Von Banchet GS. Mechanisms of pain in arthritis. *Ann NY Acad Sci* 2002; 66:343–354.

Seybold VS, Galeazza MT, Garry MG, Hargreaves KM. Plasticity of calcitonin gene related peptide neurotransmission in the spinal cord during peripheral inflammation. *Can J Physiol Pharmacol* 1995; 73(7):1007–1014.

Woolf C, Wiesenfeld-Hallin Z. Substance P and calcitonin gene-related peptide synergistically modulate the gain of the nociceptive flexor withdrawal reflex in the rat. *Neurosci Lett* 1986; 66(2):226–230.

Yaksh T. Substance P release from knee joint afferent terminals: modulation by opioids. *Brain Res* 1988; 458(2):319–324.

Yaksh T, Go VL. Survey of distribution of substance P, vasoactive intestinal polypeptide, cholecystokinin, neurotensin, Met-enkephalin, bombesin and PHI in the spinal cord of cat, dog, sloth and monkey. *Peptides* 1988; 9(2):357–372.

Yeomans DC, Proudfit H. Characterization of the foot withdrawal response to noxious radiant heat in the rat. *Pain* 1994a; 59(1):85–94.

Yeomans DC, Proudfit HK. Selective effects of the SP antagonist CP96,345 on nociceptive responses to low skin heating rates: evidence for mediation by C fiber activity. *Soc Neurosci Abstracts* 1994b; 20.

Yeomans DC, Proudfit H. Nociceptive responses to high and low rates of noxious cutaneous heating are mediated by different nociceptors in the rat: electrophysiological evidence. *Pain* 1996; 68(1):141–150.

Yeomans DC, Pirec V, Proudfit HK. Nociceptive responses to high and low rates of noxious cutaneous heating are mediated by different nociceptors in the rat: behavioral evidence. *Pain* 1996; 68(1):133–140.

Yeomans DC, Lu Y, Peters M, Whitely M, Laurito CE. Differential spinal release of amino acid neurotransmitters following selective activation of C or Ad thermonociceptors. In: Devor M, Rowbotham MC, Wiesenfeld-Hallin Z (Eds). *Proceedings of the 9th World Congress on Pain,* Progress in Pain Research and Management, Vol. 16. Seattle: IASP Press, 2000, pp 335–341.

Zachariou V, Goldstein BD, Yeomans DC. Low but not high rate noxious radiant skin heating evokes a capsaicin-sensitive increase in spinal cord dorsal horn release of substance P. *Brain Res* 1997; 752(1-2):143–150.

Correspondence to: Ying Lu, MD, Department of Anesthesiology, University of Illinois at Chicago, 1740 West Taylor Street, Suite 3200 West, Chicago, IL 60612-7239, USA. Tel: 312-413-9669; Fax: 312-355-3616; email: yinglu@ uic.edu.

Proceedings of the 10th World Congress on Pain, Progress in Pain Research and Management, Vol. 24, edited by Jonathan O. Dostrovsky, Daniel B. Carr, and Martin Koltzenburg, IASP Press, Seattle, © 2003.

21

In Vivo Patch-Clamp Analysis of Norepinephrine Effects on Nociceptive Transmission in Substantia Gelatinosa Neurons of the Rat Spinal Cord

Hidemasa Furue,[a] Motoki Sonohata,[a] Akitoshi Ito,[a] Yasuhiko Kawasaki,[b] Hiroshi Baba,[c] and Megumu Yoshimura[a]

[a]Department of Integrative Physiology, Graduate School of Medical Sciences, Kyushu University, Fukuoka, Japan; [b]Department of Physiology, Saga Medical School, Saga, Japan; and [c]Department of Anesthesiology, Niigata University School of Medicine, Niigata, Japan

Although many studies have demonstrated that the descending noradrenergic pathway originating in the nucleus locus ceruleus of the brainstem modulates nociceptive transmission at the spinal cord level, only a few studies have attempted to resolve this mechanism at the single-cell level. Our previous studies using a slice preparation of the rat spinal cord with an attached dorsal root demonstrate that norepinephrine decreases excitatory transmission to substantia gelatinosa (SG) neurons through Aδ and C-afferent fibers by activating the α_2-adrenoceptor on the presynaptic terminals (Kawasaki et al. 2001). Norepinephrine also enhances inhibitory transmitter release from the terminals of GABAergic and glycinergic interneurons by activating the α_1-adrenoceptor (Baba et al. 2000a,b). In addition, norepinephrine directly hyperpolarizes SG neurons by activating the α_2-adrenoceptor expressed at the postsynaptic membranes (North and Yoshimura 1984). It remains, however, to be settled what kind of sensory modality is subserved by norepinephrine.

To investigate the modulatory effect of norepinephrine, we developed an in vivo patch-clamp technique to record from dorsal horn neurons (Furue et al. 1999) and investigated the effect of norepinephrine on excitatory transmission evoked by cutaneous mechanical noxious stimuli.

METHODS

PREPARATION

Experiments were carried out in 7–10-week-old male Sprague-Dawley rats. Each rat was anesthetized with urethane (i.p.; 1.5 g/kg). After placing the rat under artificial ventilation, we performed laminectomy at the level of L4 and L5 and then placed the animal in a stereotactic apparatus. We cut the pia-arachnoid membrane to make a window that allowed us to position the patch electrode in the spinal cord. We irrigated the surface of the spinal cord with Krebs solution (117 mM NaCl, 3.6 mM KCl, 2.5 mM $CaCl_2$, 1.2 mM $MgCl_2$, 1.2 mM NaH_2PO_4, 11 mM glucose, and 25 mM $NaHCO_3$) equilibrated with a combination of 95% O_2 and 5% CO_2 at 38°C. We added norepinephrine to the perfusing Krebs solution for 1–2 minutes without changing the perfusion rate or temperature.

WHOLE-CELL PATCH-CLAMP RECORDING

Whole-cell voltage-clamp recordings were made from SG neurons with patch-pipettes filled with a solution with the following composition: 110 mM Cs_2SO_4, 5 mM tetraethylammonium (TEA), 0.5 mM $CaCl_2$, 2 mM $MgCl_2$, 5 mM EGTA, 5 mM HEPES, 5 mM Mg-ATP, and 1 mM guanosine-5´-0-(2-thiodiphosphate) (GDP-β-S). This pipette solution blocked the postsynaptic action of norepinephrine. To analyze synaptic potentials and action potentials under a current-clamp condition, the patch pipette was filled with a solution at pH 7.2 with the following composition: 135 mM K-gluconate, 5 mM KCl, 0.5 mM $CaCl_2$, 2 mM $MgCl_2$, 5 mM EGTA, 5 mM ATP-Mg, and 5 mM HEPES-KOH. The electrode was advanced at an angle of 30° into the spinal dorsal horn through the window in the pia-arachnoid membrane and then a giga-ohm sealing (~10 GΩ) was performed from SG neurons. All the experiments were conducted in accordance with the Kyushu University Guideline for Animal Experimentation and the Guiding Principles for the Care and Use of Animals in the Field of Physiological Science of the Physiological Society of Japan.

RESULTS

SYNAPTIC RESPONSE OF SUBSTANTIA GELATINOSA NEURONS EVOKED BY CUTANEOUS PINCH STIMULATION

Whole-cell patch-clamp recordings could be obtained from in vivo preparations for more than 12 hours, and stable recordings were made from SG neurons for up to 3 hours. All SG neurons examined exhibited spontaneous excitatory postsynaptic currents (EPSCs) at a holding potential of –70 mV. Pinch stimuli applied to the skin of the hindlimb elicited a barrage of EPSCs (Fig. 1B). As reported previously (Furue et al. 1999), the spontaneous and pinch-evoked EPSCs were suppressed by CNQX (a non-NMDA receptor antagonist), and no slow response was elicited (data not shown). Under current-clamp conditions, pinch stimuli evoked excitatory postsynaptic potentials (EPSPs). Some stimuli initiated a train of action potentials (Fig. 1A).

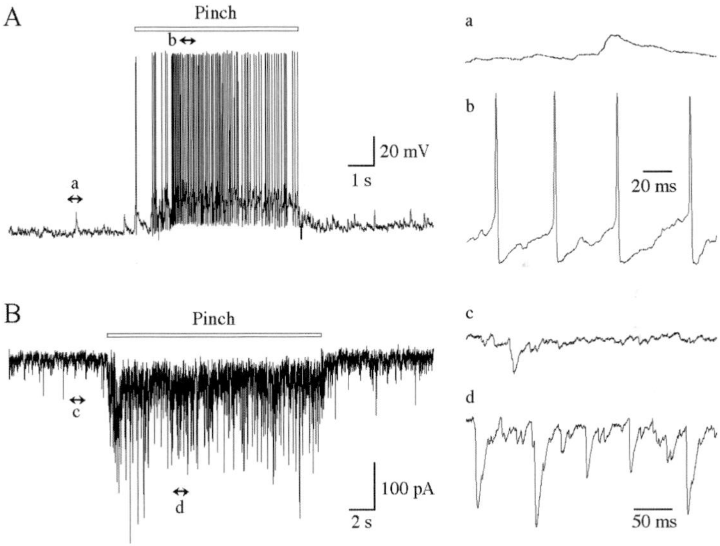

Fig. 1. Action potentials and excitatory postsynaptic currents (EPSCs) of substantia gelatinosa (SG) neurons in response to pinch stimuli. (A) Pinch stimuli applied to the skin of the hindlimb produced excitatory postsynaptic potentials (EPSPs), some of which initiated action potentials under a current-clamp condition. (B) Under a voltage-clamp condition at a holding potential of –70 mV, pinch stimuli elicited a barrage of EPSCs. Insets in panels A and B show EPSPs and action potentials in an expanded time scale, indicated by a, b, c, and d. The records shown were obtained from the same neuron.

EFFECT OF NOREPINEPHRINE ON PINCH-EVOKED EPSCS

To analyze the presynaptic action of norepinephrine, we used the pipette solution containing GDP-β-S together with Cs and TEA. Under voltage-clamp conditions at a holding potential of –70 mV, norepinephrine applied by superfusion to the surface of the spinal cord at a concentration of 50 μM induced an outward current in ~80% of SG neurons examined shortly after establishment of whole-cell configuration (data not shown). No outward current was observed when norepinephrine was administered 10 minutes later, indicating blockade of the postsynaptic action of norepinephrine by intrasomatic injection of GDP-β-S, Cs, and TEA (North and Yoshimura 1984; Baba et al. 2000a). The presynaptic effect of norepinephrine on pinch responses was analyzed more than 10 minutes after the establishment of the whole-cell configuration. Fig. 2 demonstrates the effect of 50 μM norepinephrine on pinch-evoked EPSCs. The pinch-evoked EPSCs were reversibly reduced in amplitude by norepinephrine. The effect of norepinephrine was rapid (<20 s), as was recovery after washout (<60 s), indicating that the effect was due to a direct action to the spinal cord and was not mediated by blood circulation.

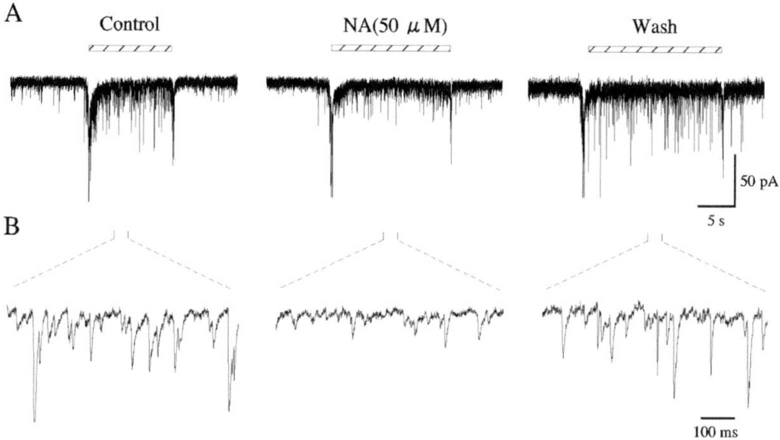

Fig. 2. Effect of norepinephrine on EPSCs evoked by cutaneous pinch stimuli. (A) EPSCs evoked by pinch stimuli were inhibited by norepinephrine (NA) in a reversible manner. (B) EPSCs, shown in an expanded time scale, for a period indicated by marks shown below each of the chart recordings in panel A. Holding potential = – 70 mV. Note that norepinephrine suppresses the amplitude of pinch-evoked EPSCs without affecting the frequency.

DISCUSSION

The present study, conducted in SG neurons of the spinal cord in vivo, reveals that norepinephrine reduces the amplitude of EPSCs evoked by cutaneous pinch stimuli. This is the first study showing the effect of norepinephrine on EPSCs evoked by mechanical noxious stimuli in spinal dorsal horn neurons in vivo. Our previous studies using spinal cord slices suggest that the activation of primary afferent Aδ and C fibers results in production of EPSCs in SG neurons monosynaptically (Yoshimura and Jessell 1990). Our previous findings also indicate that the superfusion of norepinephrine to spinal cord slices inhibits the amplitude of both Aδ- and C-fiber-evoked EPSCs by activating α_2-adrenoceptors on the presynaptic terminals of the afferents (Kawasaki et al. 2001). Based on these observations, we propose a possible mechanism for the modulation of sensory transmission in the SG by norepinephrine. As shown in Fig. 3, mechanical noxious information is conveyed to the SG through Aδ and C fibers. Norepinephrine acts on the presynaptic terminals of the afferents and decreases glutamate release to SG neurons. This presynaptic action could contribute to the analgesic effects of norepinephrine. In addition to its action on excitatory synaptic transmission, norepinephrine facilitates inhibitory transmission in the SG of the spinal cord

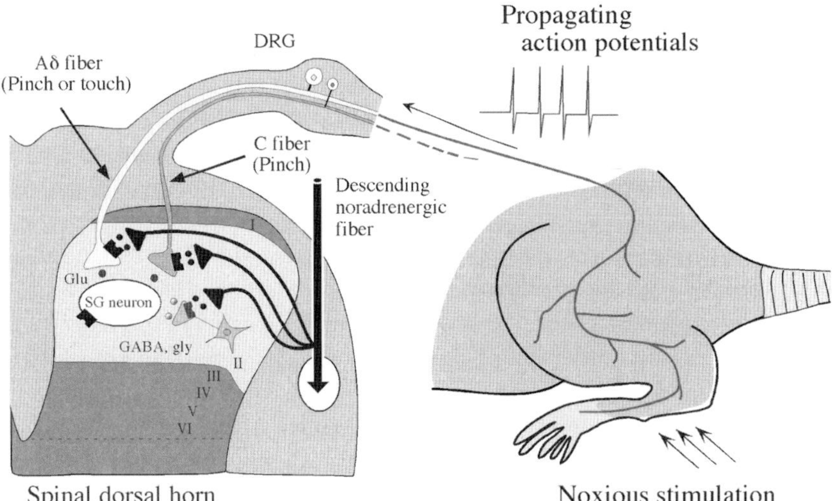

Fig. 3. Possible mechanisms for the modulation by norepinephrine on excitatory transmission in the SG. Noxious mechanical information is conveyed by glutamatergic Aδ- or C-afferents to SG neurons from the periphery. Norepinephrine released from descending noradrenergic fibers acts on α_2-adrenoceptors located at Aδ- and C-afferent terminals and then decreases the release of L-glutamate.

(Baba et al. 2000a,b). While we know that non-noxious mechanical stimulation evokes inhibitory postsynaptic currents mediated by GABA or glycine in the majority of SG neurons (Narikawa et al. 2000), the effect of norepinephrine on the inhibitory responses in the SG in vivo remains to be investigated.

ACKNOWLEDGMENTS

The present study was supported by Grant-in-Aid for Scientific Research to H. Furue and M. Yoshimura from the Ministry of Education, Science, Sports, Culture, and Technology of Japan.

REFERENCES

Baba H, Goldstein PA, Okamoto M, et al. Norepinephrine facilitates inhibitory transmission in substantia gelatinosa of adult rat spinal cord (Part 2): effects on somatodendritic sites of GABAergic neurons. *Anesthesiology* 2000a; 92(2):485–492.

Baba H, Shimoji K, Yoshimura M. Norepinephrine facilitates inhibitory transmission in substantia gelatinosa of adult rat spinal cord (part 1): effects on axon terminals of GABAergic and glycinergic neurons. *Anesthesiology* 2000b; 92(2):473–484.

Furue H, Narikawa K, Kumamoto E, et al. Responsiveness of rat substantia gelatinosa neurones to mechanical but not thermal stimuli revealed by in vivo patch-clamp recording. *J Physiol* 1999; 521 Pt 2:529–535.

Kawasaki Y, Kumamoto E, Furue H, et al. Cellular mechanisms for inhibition by noradrenaline of pain transmission in the spinal dorsal horn. *Pain Res* 2001; 16:69–75.

Narikawa K, Furue H, Kumamoto E, et al. In vivo patch-clamp analysis of IPSCs evoked in rat substantia gelatinosa neurons by cutaneous mechanical stimulation. *J Neurophysiol* 2000; 84(4):2171–2174.

North RA, Yoshimura M. The actions of noradrenaline on neurones of the rat substantia gelatinosa in vitro. *J Physiol* 1984; 349:43–55.

Yoshimura M, Jessell T. Amino acid-mediated EPSPs at primary afferent synapses with substantia gelatinosa neurones in the rat spinal cord. *J Physiol* 1990; 430:315–335.

Correspondence to: Hidemasa Furue, PhD, Department of Integrative Physiology, Graduate School of Medical Sciences, Kyushu University, 3-1-1 Maidashi, Higashi-ku, Fukuoka 812-8582, Japan. Tel: 81-92-642-6089; Fax: 81-92-642-6093; email: furueh@physiol.med.kyushu-u.ac.jp.

Proceedings of the 10th World Congress on Pain,
Progress in Pain Research and Management, Vol. 24,
edited by Jonathan O. Dostrovsky, Daniel B. Carr, and
Martin Koltzenburg, IASP Press, Seattle, © 2003.

22

Descending Modulation after Injury[1]

Mary M. Heinricher,[a] Antti Pertovaara,[b] and Michael H. Ossipov[c]

[a]*Department of Neurological Surgery, Oregon Health Sciences University, Portland, Oregon, USA;* [b]*Department of Physiology, University of Turku, Turku, Finland;* [c]*Department of Pharmacology, University of Arizona, Arizona Health Sciences Center, Tucson, Arizona, USA*

It has been over three decades since the initial demonstration that electrical stimulation within the ventral periaqueductal gray (PAG) in the midbrain produces potent antinociception in rats (Mayer et al. 1971; Mayer and Liebeskind 1974). This antinociception is blocked by naloxone given systemically, and sites supporting analgesia produced by electrical stimulation are also responsive to focal application of morphine (Akil et al. 1976; Lewis and Gebhart 1977). These observations, in concert with the discovery of the endogenous opioid peptides, stimulated intense interest in the idea of an "analgesia system" within the brainstem that is the substrate for opioid analgesic drugs. Work from many groups subsequently provided strong behavioral, pharmacological, anatomical, and electrophysiological evidence supporting the now generally accepted view that the PAG is part of a descending pain inhibition system, with an essential relay in the rostral ventromedial medulla (RVM) (Fields et al. 1988; Fields and Basbaum 1999).

The idea that this system might have a more general modulatory role, which would include descending facilitation as well as inhibition, was not widely discussed. Although observations pointing to descending facilitation could be found scattered through the literature, these received relatively little attention, or were interpreted within the pain inhibition framework. Moreover, although the physiological advantage of an inhibitory system was readily appreciated from an evolutionary standpoint, the value to the organism

---

[1]Based on a Congress workshop.

of a facilitatory influence was not obvious. However, as the focus of pain research in general has shifted in recent years toward understanding mechanisms of hyperalgesia and persistent pain states, increasing interest has focused on the idea that supraspinal modulatory systems could facilitate nociception. With this new emphasis has come an increasing body of work showing that the RVM contributes actively to enhanced nociceptive responding in animal models of hyperalgesia and chronic pain.

ACTIVATION OF THE RVM CAN FACILITATE NOCICEPTION

One of the earliest clear demonstrations of bidirectional control arising from the RVM was the observation that low-intensity electrical stimulation applied at some sites in the RVM facilitated the tail-flick reflex or dorsal horn responses to noxious heat, whilst higher-intensity stimulation at the same site inhibited the reflex (Zhuo and Gebhart 1990, 1992). Comparable bidirectional effects were elicited by chemical stimulation of the RVM with different concentrations of glutamate, *N*-methyl D-aspartate (NMDA), or neurotensin (Urban and Smith 1993; Smith et al. 1997; Zhuo and Gebhart 1997; Urban et al. 1999). Interestingly, descending facilitation from the RVM, like descending inhibition, is prevented by intrathecal administration of methysergide (Zhuo and Gebhart 1991), indicating that spinal serotonergic transmission is important for both facilitatory and inhibitory effects of RVM activation.

DESCENDING FACILITATION DRIVES INFLAMMATORY AND NEUROPATHIC PAIN

The demonstration that direct manipulation of the RVM can facilitate nociceptive responses suggests that this region might contribute to enhanced pain behaviors under physiological and pathological conditions. Accumulating evidence now supports this idea. The RVM is required for the facilitation of nociceptive reflexes during naloxone-precipitated withdrawal, during prolonged exposure of the tail to noxious heat, or during illness (Kaplan and Fields 1991; Morgan et al. 1994; Wiertelak et al. 1997). In each case, facilitation of nociception is attenuated or blocked by lidocaine microinjected into the RVM. Inactivation of the RVM by focal application of lidocaine or α-amino-3-hydroxy-5-methyl-4-isoxazole propionate (AMPA)/kainate receptor blockade also prevents facilitation of nociceptive reflexes by electrical stimulation within the anterior cingulate cortex (Calejesan et al. 2000).

The possibility that supraspinal sites contribute to the exaggerated responsiveness characteristic of neuropathic and inflammatory pain models has received support from experiments in which transection of the spinal cord attenuates or prevents increased responding. For example, spinal transection abolished the heightened responses to mechanical or cold stimuli in rats with peripheral nerve injury, although hyperalgesia to heat was not blocked and in one experiment was even enhanced (Bian et al. 1998; Kauppila et al. 1998; Sung et al. 1998). A similar reduction in exaggerated nociceptive responses was seen following disruption of the ipsilateral dorsolateral funiculus, which includes the descending projection from the RVM. Unlike spinal transection, this lesion does not alter normal locomotor or grooming behaviors (Ossipov et al. 2000). Allodynia and hyperalgesia in mustard oil and carrageenan inflammation models were also reduced in spinalized animals, as was the increased excitability of dorsal horn neurons (Mansikka and Pertovaara 1997; Kauppila et al. 1998; Pertovaara 1998).

Studies focusing on the brainstem point to a specific contribution of the RVM to the descending facilitation revealed by spinal lesions. General inactivation of the RVM itself by microinjection of lidocaine interferes with tactile allodynia in animals with a spinal nerve ligation (Pertovaara et al. 1996; Kovelowski et al. 2000). The RVM is also required for the secondary hyperalgesia and enhanced sensitivity of dorsal horn neurons in several inflammatory models (Urban and Gebhart 1999; Pertovaara 2000). Both NMDA and cholecystokinin (CCK) transmission within the RVM play a role. Thus, block of NMDA receptors within the RVM attenuates the expression of tactile and thermal hypersensitivities (Urban and Gebhart 1999). Microinjection of the CCK_B antagonist L365,260 into the RVM similarly prevents tactile and thermal hypersensitivity in the spinal nerve ligation (SNL) model, and administration of CCK into the RVM mimicked these behavioral signs of neuropathic pain (Kovelowski et al. 2000).

Although the activation of descending facilitation from the RVM is a critical element driving the maintenance of neuropathic pain behavior, a recent study suggests that this phenomenon is not essential for the initiation and early manifestation of neuropathic pain (Burgess et al. 2002). Animals with lesions of the dorsolateral funiculus performed prior to L5/L6 SNL showed signs of tactile and thermal hypersensitivity only for the first 4 days after the nerve injury, whereas these behaviors were maintained for at least 14 days in control animals. Thus, animals with a physical disruption of descending pathways developed, but failed to maintain, neuropathic pain behaviors. Studies focusing more specifically on the RVM showed a similar time course: an acute lidocaine block of this region was without effect if performed 3 days after the SNL treatment, but reversed tactile and thermal hypersensitivity at 6, 9, or 12 days after the nerve injury. A comparable time-dependent contribution of the RVM was observed with selective downregulation of μ-opioid-expressing neurons in this region.

The RVM-dependent maintenance phase of neuropathic pain demonstrates a time course consistent with the upregulation of spinal dynorphin, which promotes enhanced pain states (Bian et al. 1999; Claude et al. 1999). Spinal dynorphin levels are increased significantly by day 5 post-injury, with a peak at day 10 (Malan et al. 2000). Lesions of the dorsolateral funiculus and microinjection of dermorphin-saporin conjugate into the RVM to downregulate μ-opioid-expressing neurons block this upregulation of spinal dynorphin (Burgess et al. 2002). These observations raise the possibility that the facilitating output of the RVM works at least in part by stimulating dynorphin upregulation at the level of the spinal cord. Consistent with this idea, prodynorphin knockout mice showed tactile and thermal hypersensitivity on the second day after SNL was performed, but these behavioral signs were not maintained beyond the sixth day. In contrast, the wild-type mice maintained behavioral signs of neuropathic pain throughout the entire 14-day observation period, with upregulation of spinal dynorphin at 10, but not 2, days after the SNL treatment (Wang et al. 2001).

Thus, the RVM is not involved in early behavioral changes, but is necessary at later times after the nerve injury. This finding may mean that continuing injury discharge from the nerve itself (Han et al. 2000; Liu et al. 2000), or within the dorsal horn, is sufficient to mediate behaviorally measurable hyperresponsiveness at early time points. If so, a facilitating input from the RVM, even if present, might have no additional effect. An alternative possibility is that the circuitry within the RVM develops a novel bias toward expressing a facilitatory output over a period of days after the nerve injury. This second alternative would resemble the plasticity recently demonstrated within the RVM during development of hindpaw inflammation produced by complete Freund's adjuvant (Miki et al. 2002). Reorganization within the RVM would presumably be triggered by the intense ascending barrage associated with the nerve ligation procedure (Wei and Pertovaara 1999). Enhanced descending facilitation from the RVM could then potentiate the spinal sensitization that had been triggered by the initial injury inputs, at least in part by causing upregulation of spinal dynorphin. This would in turn lead to increased input to the RVM, which would most likely maintain, if not further enhance, the descending facilitation. In this manner the effects of the initial insult could be maintained for a prolonged period by a positive feedback process that includes the RVM.

NEURAL BASIS FOR DESCENDING FACILITATION FROM THE RVM

Functional studies show very clearly that descending modulation from the RVM contributes to facilitated responding in both inflammatory and neuropathic models. Yet the net effect of electrical stimulation or opioid microinjection in the RVM is antinociception, and the RVM is known to be recruited as part of the circuitry mediating "stress-induced" analgesia. A possible explanation for this apparent contradiction lies in the diverse cell population within the RVM. Single-unit recording within this region in lightly anesthetized animals without inflammation or nerve injury reveals some neurons whose activity is positively correlated with nociceptive responding ("on-cells"), and others that exhibit a negative correlation ("off-cells"). Cells of a third class, "neutral cells," show no change in activity correlated with nocifensive responses. Based on these firing patterns, one could propose that the pronociceptive influence of the RVM reflects activation of on-cells (Fields and Heinricher 1985). Although correlative data are supportive (Fields 1992), the suggestion has been criticized. Thurston and Randich (1995) contend that excitation of on-cells inhibits pain, and the Cardiff group also concludes, on the basis of correlative data, that neurons in the lateral aspect of the RVM that are activated by noxious stimuli (and may therefore be "on-cells") inhibit pain (Li et al. 1998; Azami et al. 2001). In contrast, Mason (2001) argues that on- and off-cells are unlikely to have any role in descending nociceptive modulation, in part because they may respond to inputs in addition to noxious stimulation.

Resolution of this controversy requires an experimental approach in which the firing of RVM neurons is manipulated, and the effects of this manipulation on nociceptive responding are determined. This technique is performed routinely in awake behaving animals with drug microinjection into the RVM. However, interpretation of such experiments is limited because it is impossible to know with certainty which cell class or classes are affected by the manipulation to produce the behavioral effect. To solve this problem, we have adopted a microinjection approach that allowed us to monitor simultaneously the activity of an identified RVM neuron and nociceptive responses (as indicated by withdrawal reflexes) in the same lightly anesthetized animal. We are therefore able to verify the effects of a behaviorally significant drug application on the different RVM cell classes. Using this approach, we previously demonstrated that off-cells are the inhibitory output neuron of the RVM (Heinricher et al. 1994; Heinricher et al. 2001b).

We have now used this technique to address the question of whether on-cells are in fact the facilitating output neuron of the RVM. Pertovaara and colleagues have shown that the RVM is required for sensitization of dorsal horn neurons and for the accompanying secondary tactile allodynia following mustard oil application to the limb (Mansikka and Pertovaara 1997; Pertovaara 1998). Using this inflammatory model, we recently demonstrated a reliable thermal hyperalgesia on the ipsilateral hindpaw that is correlated with a robust and prolonged activation of on-cells, and a small but significant decrease in the firing of off-cells. Selective block of the enhanced on-cell firing by local application of the NMDA-receptor antagonist AP5 demonstrated that increased on-cell activity is required for hyperalgesia in this model. The decrease in off-cell firing was unchanged after AP5 application, indicating that diminished off-cell firing is not sufficient to produce measurable hyperalgesia in the lightly anesthetized animal (Kincaid et al. 2001).

Further evidence that the on-cells are the facilitatory output neuron of the RVM comes from experiments using microinjection of a dermorphin-saporin conjugate into the RVM to selectively downregulate those neurons that express the μ-opioid receptor (Porreca et al. 2001). It is likely that the neurons primarily affected by this treatment are the on-cells, because these are the only RVM neurons that respond directly to μ-opioid agonists (Heinricher et al. 1992). Application of the toxin blocked expression of tactile and thermal hypersensitivity in animals with SNL, whether given before or after the ligation procedure. These experiments show that the selective lesion of RVM neurons expressing the μ-opioid receptor blocks enhanced nociceptive responding, demonstrating that this population contributes to descending facilitation. This study thus provides additional support for the idea that on-cells are the facilitatory output from the region. Importantly baseline responses to acute noxious or innocuous stimuli are not altered in the toxin-treated animals (Porreca et al. 2001), or following acute suppression of the firing of on-cells (Heinricher and McGaraughty 1998). Thus, descending facilitation from the RVM is not critical to normal nociceptive responses, but is recruited as part of the mechanism of abnormal, facilitated pain states.

Surprisingly, the spontaneous firing patterns and evoked responses of on-cells are not altered in animals subjected to SNL (Pertovaara and Wei 2000; Pertovaara et al. 2001). Nevertheless, hyperalgesia in these ligated animals apparently requires on-cell activity, as already noted. It may be that the contribution of these neurons is not evident in firing parameters measured over a short time period in anesthetized animals.

The previous observations thus demonstrate that activation of on-cells is essential for secondary hyperalgesia in the mustard oil inflammation model, and quite likely following nerve injury as well. In these situations, on-cell activation functions as part of a positive feedback process, and presumably both reflects and contributes to enhanced processing at the lumbar dorsal horn. However, this leaves open the question of whether direct activation of on-cells, or activation via pathways that do not involve nociceptive input as a triggering mechanism, is sufficient to produce a measurable hyperalgesia. Based on behavioral observations from Urban, Smith, and colleagues (Urban and Smith 1993; Smith et al. 1997), we hypothesized that focal application of low doses of neurotensin within the RVM would activate on-cells selectively, and that this activation in turn would produce hyperalgesia (again as measured by the latency of paw withdrawal to noxious heat). This hypothesis has been confirmed (Heinricher et al. 2001a). Microinjection of a low dose of neurotensin activated on-cells selectively, and significantly decreased paw-withdrawal latency. Higher doses of neurotensin activated off-cells as well as on-cells, and in agreement with earlier work (Smith et al. 1997), resulted in inhibition of the withdrawal reflex. Thus, direct activation of the on-cells is sufficient to produce hyperalgesia, whereas the net effect of activating both on- and off-cells results in antinociception.

SUMMARY AND CONCLUSIONS

Since its first description as a critical relay in the descending modulatory pathway, the RVM has been primarily considered to mediate descending inhibition. Until fairly recently, this uneven focus has obscured recognition of the ability of the RVM to facilitate nociception. The data summarized above demonstrate clearly that descending facilitation from the RVM is critical for enhanced nociceptive responses in various models of hyperalgesia and persistent pain. Moreover, direct evidence now shows that the RVM neurons responsible for this effect are the on-cells. These new data support a role for the RVM as part of a positive feedback system in which injury or inflammation sensitizes spinal nociception. Injury-induced afferent discharges and the resultant spinal sensitization shift the balance of activity within the RVM so that facilitation predominates.

This suprasegmental positive feedback loop parallels and reinforces the sensitization process that has been clearly documented in the dorsal horn. Furthermore, many of the processes that have been implicated in sensitization within the dorsal horn (e.g., NMDA-receptor-mediated activation) are likely to be brought into play in the RVM as well. Thus, it will be important to understand not only the properties of the RVM and dorsal horn, but also how they interact with each other. The physiologically and functionally diverse cell population within the RVM provides a neural basis for bidirectional control: recruitment of on-cells will have a net facilitating effect, whereas activation of off-cells will have a net suppressive effect. The challenge presented is to identify the conditions under which the two cell classes are activated, and the inputs that are responsible.

ACKNOWLEDGMENTS

This work was supported in part by grants from NIDA.

REFERENCES

Akil H, Mayer DJ, Liebeskind JC. Antagonism of stimulation-produced analgesia by naloxone, a narcotic antagonist. *Science* 1976; 191:961–962.

Azami J, Green DL, Roberts MH, Monhemius R. The behavioural importance of dynamically activated descending inhibition from the nucleus reticularis gigantocellularis pars alpha. *Pain* 2001; 92:53–62.

Bian D, Ossipov MH, Zhong C, Malan TP Jr, Porreca F. Tactile allodynia, but not thermal hyperalgesia, of the hindlimbs is blocked by spinal transection in rats with nerve injury. *Neurosci Lett* 1998; 241:79–82.

Bian D, Ossipov MH, Ibrahim M, et al. Loss of antiallodynic and antinociceptive spinal/supraspinal morphine synergy in nerve-injured rats: restoration by MK-801 or dynorphin antiserum. *Brain Res* 1999; 831:55–63.

Burgess SE, Gardell LR, Ossipov MH, et al. Time-dependent descending facilitation from the rostral ventromedial medulla maintains, but does not initiate, neuropathic pain. *J Neurosci* 2002; 22:5129–5136.

Calejesan AA, Kim SJ, Zhuo M. Descending facilitatory modulation of a behavioral nociceptive response by stimulation in the adult rat anterior cingulate cortex. *Eur J Pain* 2000; 4:83–96.

Claude P, Gracia N, Wagner L, Hargreaves KM. Effect of dynorphin on iCGRP release from capsaicin-sensitive fibers. *Abstracts: 9th World Congress on Pain.* Seattle: IASP Press, 1999, p 262.

Fields HL. Is there a facilitating component to central pain modulation? *APS J* 1992; 1:71–78.

Fields HL, Basbaum AI. Central nervous mechanisms of pain modulation. In: Wall PD, Melzack R (Eds). *Textbook of Pain.* Edinburgh: Churchill Livingston, 1999, pp 309–329.

Fields HL, Heinricher MM. Anatomy and physiology of a nociceptive modulatory system. *Philos Trans R Soc Lond B Biol Sci* 1985; 308:361–374.

Fields HL, Barbaro NM, Heinricher MM. Brain stem neuronal circuitry underlying the antinociceptive action of opiates. *Prog Brain Res* 1988; 77:245–257.

Han HC, Lee DH, Chung JM. Characteristics of ectopic discharges in a rat neuropathic pain model. *Pain* 2000; 84:253–261.

Heinricher MM, McGaraughty S. Analysis of excitatory amino acid transmission within the rostral ventromedial medulla: implications for circuitry. *Pain* 1998; 75:247–255.

Heinricher MM, Morgan MM, Fields HL. Direct and indirect actions of morphine on medullary neurons that modulate nociception. *Neuroscience* 1992; 48:533–543.

Heinricher MM, Morgan MM, Tortorici V, Fields HL. Disinhibition of off-cells and antinociception produced by an opioid action within the rostral ventromedial medulla. *Neuroscience* 1994; 63:279–288.

Heinricher MM, Kincaid W, Neubert MJ. Neural substrate for analgesic and hyperalgesic actions of neurotensin within the rostral ventromedial medulla. *Soc Neurosci Abstr* 2001a; 27:161.7.

Heinricher MM, Schouten JC, Jobst EE. Activation of brainstem n-methyl-d-aspartate receptors is required for the analgesic actions of morphine given systemically. *Pain* 2001b; 92:129–138.

Kaplan H, Fields HL. Hyperalgesia during acute opioid abstinence: evidence for a nociceptive facilitating function of the rostral ventromedial medulla. *J Neurosci* 1991; 11:1433–1439.

Kauppila T, Kontinen VK, Pertovaara A. Influence of spinalization on spinal withdrawal reflex responses varies depending on the submodality of the test stimulus and the experimental pathophysiological condition in the rat. *Brain Res* 1998; 797:234–242.

Kincaid W, Xu M, Kim CJ, et al. Medullary substrate of secondary hyperalgesia produced by mustard oil in lightly anesthetized rats. *Soc Neurosci Abstr* 2001; 27:161.5.

Kovelowski CJ, Ossipov MH, Sun H, et al. Supraspinal cholecystokinin may drive tonic descending facilitation mechanisms to maintain neuropathic pain in the rat. *Pain* 2000; 87:265–273.

Lewis VA, Gebhart GF. Evaluation of the periaqueductal central gray (PAG) as a morphine-specific locus of action and examination of morphine-induced and stimulation-produced analgesia at coincident PAG loci. *Brain Res* 1977; 124:283–303.

Li HS, Monhemius R, Simpson BA, Roberts MH. Supraspinal inhibition of nociceptive dorsal horn neurones in the anaesthetized rat: tonic or dynamic? *J Physiol* 1998; 506:459–469.

Liu CN, Wall PD, Ben-Dor E, et al. Tactile allodynia in the absence of c-fiber activation: altered firing properties of DRG neurons following spinal nerve injury. *Pain* 2000; 85:503–521.

Malan TP, Ossipov MH, Gardell LR, et al. Extraterritorial neuropathic pain correlates with multisegmental elevation of spinal dynorphin in nerve-injured rats. *Pain* 2000; 86:185–194.

Mansikka H, Pertovaara A. Supraspinal influence on hindlimb withdrawal thresholds and mustard oil-induced secondary allodynia in rats. *Brain Res Bull* 1997; 42:359–365.

Mason P. Contributions of the medullary raphe and ventromedial reticular region to pain modulation and other homeostatic functions. *Annu Rev Neurosci* 2001; 24:737–777.

Mayer DJ, Liebeskind JC. Pain reduction by focal electrical stimulation of the brain: an anatomical and behavioral analysis. *Brain Res* 1974; 68:73–93.

Mayer DJ, Wolfle TL, Akil H, Carder B, Liebeskind JC. Analgesia from electrical stimulation in the brainstem of the rat. *Science* 1971; 174:1351–1354.

Miki K, Zhou QQ, Guo W, et al. Changes in gene expression and neuronal phenotype in brain stem pain modulatory circuitry after inflammation. *J Neurophysiol* 2002, 87:750–760.

Morgan MM, Heinricher MM, Fields HL. Inhibition and facilitation of different nocifensor reflexes by spatially remote noxious stimuli. *J Neurophysiol* 1994; 72:1152–1160.

Ossipov MH, Hong Sun T, Malan P Jr, Lai J, Porreca F. Mediation of spinal nerve injury induced tactile allodynia by descending facilitatory pathways in the dorsolateral funiculus in rats. *Neurosci Lett* 2000; 290:129–132.

Pertovaara A. A neuronal correlate of secondary hyperalgesia in the rat spinal dorsal horn is submodality selective and facilitated by supraspinal influence. *Exp Neurol* 1998; 149:193–202.

Pertovaara A. Plasticity in descending pain modulatory systems. *Prog Brain Res* 2000; 129:231–242.

Pertovaara A, Wei H. Attenuation of ascending nociceptive signals to the rostroventromedial medulla induced by a novel α_2-adrenoceptor agonist, MPV-2426, following intrathecal application in neuropathic rats. *Anesthesiology* 2000; 92:1082–1092.

Pertovaara A, Wei H, Hamalainen MM. Lidocaine in the rostroventromedial medulla and the periaqueductal gray attenuates allodynia in neuropathic rats. *Neurosci Lett* 1996; 218:127–130.

Pertovaara A, Keski-vakkuri U, Kalmari J, Wei H, Panula P. Response properties of neurons in the rostroventromedial medulla of neuropathic rats: attempted modulation of responses by [1DMe]NPYF, a neuropeptide FF analogue. *Neuroscience* 2001; 105:457–468.

Porreca F, Burgess SE, Gardell LR, et al. Inhibition of neuropathic pain by selective ablation of brainstem medullary cells expressing the micro-opioid receptor. *J Neurosci* 2001; 21:5281–5288.

Smith DJ, Hawranko AA, Monroe PJ, et al. Dose-dependent pain-facilitatory and -inhibitory actions of neurotensin are revealed by SR 48692, a nonpeptide neurotensin antagonist: influence on the antinociceptive effect of morphine. *J Pharmacol Exp Ther* 1997; 282:899–908.

Sung B, Na HS, Kim YI, et al. Supraspinal involvement in the production of mechanical allodynia by spinal nerve injury in rats. *Neurosci Lett* 1998; 246:117–119.

Thurston CL, Randich A. Responses of on and off cells in the rostral ventral medulla to stimulation of vagal afferents and changes in mean arterial blood pressure in intact and cardiopulmonary deafferented rats. *Pain* 1995; 62:19–38.

Urban MO, Gebhart GF. Supraspinal contributions to hyperalgesia. *Proc Natl Acad Sci USA* 1999; 96:7687–7692.

Urban MO, Smith DJ. Role of neurotensin in the nucleus raphe magnus in opioid-induced antinociception from the periaqueductal gray. *J Pharmacol Exp Ther* 1993; 265:580–586.

Urban MO, Coutinho SV, Gebhart GF. Involvement of excitatory amino acid receptors and nitric oxide in the rostral ventromedial medulla in modulating secondary hyperalgesia produced by mustard oil. *Pain* 1999; 81:45–55.

Wang Z, Gardell LR, Ossipov MH. Pronociceptive actions of dynorphin maintain chronic neuropathic pain. *J Neurosci* 2001; 21:1779–1786.

Wei H, Pertovaara A. MK-801, an NMDA receptor antagonist, in the rostroventromedial medulla attenuates development of neuropathic symptoms in the rat. *Neuroreport* 1999; 10:2933–2937.

Wiertelak EP, Roemer B, Maier SF, Watkins LR. Comparison of the effects of nucleus tractus solitarius and ventral medial medulla lesions on illness-induced and subcutaneous formalin-induced hyperalgesias. *Brain Res* 1997; 748:143–150.

Zhuo M, Gebhart GF. Characterization of descending inhibition and facilitation from the nuclei reticularis gigantocellularis and gigantocellularis pars alpha in the rat. *Pain* 1990; 42:337–350.

Zhuo M, Gebhart GF. Spinal serotonin receptors mediate descending facilitation of a nociceptive reflex from the nuclei reticularis gigantocellularis and gigantocellularis pars alpha in the rat. *Brain Res* 1991; 550:35–48.

Zhuo M, Gebhart GF. Characterization of descending facilitation and inhibition of spinal nociceptive transmission from the nuclei reticularis gigantocellularis and gigantocellularis pars alpha in the rat. *J Neurophysiol* 1992; 76:1599–1614.

Zhuo M, Gebhart GF. Biphasic modulation of spinal nociceptive transmission from the medullary raphe nuclei in the rat. *J Neurophysiol* 1997; 78:746–758.

Correspondence to: Michael H. Ossipov, PhD, Department of Pharmacology, University of Arizona, Arizona Health Sciences Center, P.O. Box 245050, Tucson, AZ 85724-5050, USA. Email: michaelo@u.arizona.edu.

Proceedings of the 10th World Congress on Pain,
Progress in Pain Research and Management, Vol. 24,
edited by Jonathan O. Dostrovsky, Daniel B. Carr, and
Martin Koltzenburg, IASP Press, Seattle, © 2003.

23

Imaging Visceral Sensations[1]

Karen D. Davis,[a,b,d] M. Catherine Bushnell,[e] Irina A. Strigo,[e] Gary H. Duncan,[f] Chun L. Kwan,[a,d] Nicholas E. Diamant,[a,c,d] Sanchoy Sarkar,[g] Lloyd Gregory,[g,h] and Qasim Aziz[g,i]

[a]Institute of Medical Science, and Departments of [b]Surgery and [c]Medicine, University of Toronto, Toronto, Ontario, Canada; [d]Toronto Western Research Institute, Toronto Western Hospital, University Health Network, Toronto, Ontario, Canada; [e]Department of Anesthesiology, McGill University, Montreal, Quebec, Canada; [f]Faculty of Dentistry, University of Montreal, Montreal, Quebec, Canada; [g]Hope Hospital, University of Manchester, Salford, United Kingdom; [h]Neuroimaging Group, Institute of Psychiatry, London, United Kingdom; [i]GI Sciences, Department of Medicine, University of Manchester, Manchester, United Kingdom

Visceral sensations arising from the digestive tract are an everyday occurrence and range from nonpainful sensations such as pressure or a sense of urgency to defecate to pain. Painful visceral sensations and hyperalgesia are a hallmark of disorders such as inflammatory bowel disease, irritable bowel disorder, and esophageal disease. However, little is known of the brain mechanisms underlying visceral sensations under normal and injured states, and how they differ from cutaneous sensations. Over the last decade, functional brain imaging has been adopted for the study of acute and chronic pain, typically arising from the skin. Imaging of visceral sensations poses several challenges due to the internal location of the site to be stimulated. The three studies presented in this chapter demonstrate that visceral imaging studies not only are feasible but also represent a valuable approach to understanding basic mechanisms of visceral sensations compared to cutaneous sensations under normal and pathological conditions. First, Bushnell and colleagues present psychophysical and brain imaging data that highlight

[1] Based on a Congress workshop.

differences between cutaneous and visceral (esophageal) pain. Next, Qasim and colleagues review models of functional gastrointestinal (GI) disorders and presents data from imaging studies of the impact of emotion on esophageal stimulation. Finally, Davis and colleagues discuss a method to identify cortical responses related to specific types of rectal-evoked sensations.

HOW DO VISCERAL AND CUTANEOUS PAINS DIFFER?

The widespread convergence of information from visceral and cutaneous tissues leads to an important dilemma: how can we distinguish visceral pain from that originating in other tissues of the body? There is extensive viscerosomatic convergence in the spinothalamic, spinoreticular, and spinomesencephalic tracts (McMahon et al. 1995) and in the dorsal column postsynaptic pathway (Bradshaw and Berkley 2000), which is thought be particularly important for visceral pain (Al Chaer et al. 1996; Berkley 1997; Nauta et al. 1997). Similar convergence is found in the medial, lateral, and posterior thalamus (Chandler et al. 1992; Berkley et al. 1993; Kawakita et al. 1993; Bruggemann et al. 1994; Berkley et al. 1995), as well as in the primary somatosensory and ventrolateral orbital cortices (Snow et al. 1992; Follett and Dirks 1994, 1995). Although purely somatic cells exist in the central nervous system (CNS), neurons with exclusive visceral inputs appear to be virtually absent (Bruggemann et al. 1994; Bradshaw and Berkley 2000).

Despite this ubiquitous convergence in the CNS, clinical evidence suggests that the experience of visceral pain differs substantially from that of cutaneous pain. Whereas cutaneous pain is localizable and has distinct sensory qualities consistent with the type of tissue damage (e.g., burning, pricking, or pinching), visceral pain is difficult to localize, is often referred to a distant region (e.g., cardiac ischemia often is felt as pain in the arm), and is frequently described as variable, difficult to define, but with a strong affective component (Schott 1994; McMahon et al. 1995). Most strikingly, visceral and cutaneous pains often elicit highly divergent behavioral and autonomic responses. Whereas cutaneous pain usually evokes quick protective reflexes, tachycardia, hypertension, and increased alertness, some visceral pains produce quiescence, bradycardia, hypotension, and loss of interest in the environment (described by Lewis 1942).

To investigate why visceral and cutaneous pain experiences differ, despite CNS convergence, we first performed quantitative within-subject psychophysical studies examining similarities and differences in pain evoked by esophageal distension and cutaneous heat. Then we used functional magnetic resonance imaging (fMRI) to determine the neural correlates of the observed perceptual similarities and differences.

In our studies, healthy male and female volunteers were subjected to esophageal balloon distension and cutaneous heat pain in the zone of referral for esophageal stimulation (Strigo et al. 2002). Esophageal stimulation was performed by distending a custom-designed polyethylene balloon that was 8 cm in length, 6 cm in diameter, with a maximum volume of 70–80 mL, which was attached to a multilumen polyvinyl esophageal catheter 10 cm above the tip. The upper chest was thermally stimulated with a 9-cm^2 Peltier-type contact thermode, using a 5°/second rate of temperature increase. For each subject, we identified a temperature and a pressure that produced a standard level of moderate nonpainful sensation, rated at approximately 5 on a 10-point scale of nonpainful sensation. We also identified for each subject a temperature and a pressure that produced similar intensities of pain, rated at 4–5 on a 10-point scale of pain sensation. The resulting nonpainful and painful temperatures were approximately 40°C and 46°C, whereas the pressures were approximately 18 and 36 mm Hg, respectively (Fig. 1). Stimuli were presented in quasi-random and counterbalanced orders. In the psychophysical studies, subjects rated pain intensity and unpleasantness on a visual analogue scale (VAS), quality of sensation with words chosen from the McGill Pain Questionnaire, temporal properties of the pain sensation on an electronic online VAS, and spatial extent of the pain (on dermatome sketches) (Strigo et al. 2002).

As shown in Fig. 2, our psychophysical studies revealed that for painful stimuli perceived as equally intense, subjects rated esophageal pain as being significantly more unpleasant than heat pain (Strigo et al. 2002). Further,

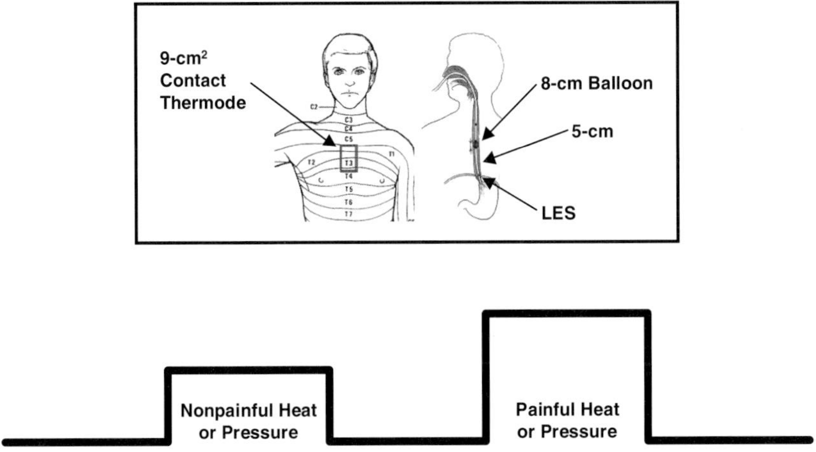

Fig. 1. Experimental design for esophageal and cutaneous stimulation (adapted from Strigo et al. 2002).

subjects chose more affective words to describe the esophageal pain, with the most commonly chosen affective words being "suffocating" and "tiring." Despite the similar duration and surface area of stimulation, the pain of visceral origin was perceived as more diffuse, both temporally and spatially, compared to that arising from the cutaneous thermal stimulation. Perception of cutaneous heat pain followed closely the temporal profile of the noxious thermal stimulus, but pain evoked by the esophageal distension remained near its maximum well after termination of the stimulus, with significant levels of visceral pain persisting for approximately 20 seconds (Fig. 3). Similarly, perception of the cutaneous heat pain was restricted to the site of stimulation, whereas perception of visceral pain, associated with the esophageal distension, extended to the chest and back, in addition to the esophagus (Fig. 3).

To examine the neural basis of the similarities and differences in visceral and cutaneous pain perception, we performed fMRI studies using the same stimulation paradigm as used for the psychophysical studies (Strigo et al. 2001). A similar neural network, including the secondary somatosensory (S2) and parietal cortices, thalamus, basal ganglia, and cerebellum, was activated by visceral and cutaneous painful stimuli. Such similarities could underlie the common construct of "pain" that is used to describe the experience associated with both the cutaneous heat and esophageal distension stimuli. However, despite these similarities, cutaneous and visceral pain showed differential activation patterns in both sensory and limbic cortical regions. For example, in the insular cortex, cutaneous pain evoked significantly higher activation bilaterally in the anterior aspect of the insula, whereas the peak activation for the esophageal stimulation was in a mid-insular region. This

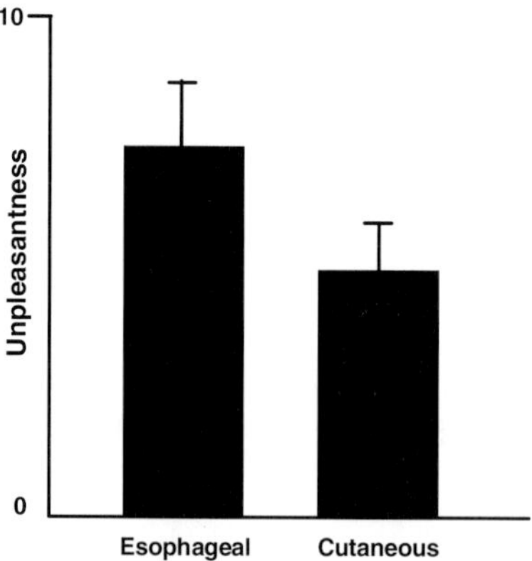

Fig. 2. Stimulation-evoked unpleasantness during painful esophageal distension and cutaneous heat of equal perceived intensities. Subjects rated the visceral stimuli as significantly more unpleasant than the cutaneous stimuli (adapted from Strigo et al. 2002).

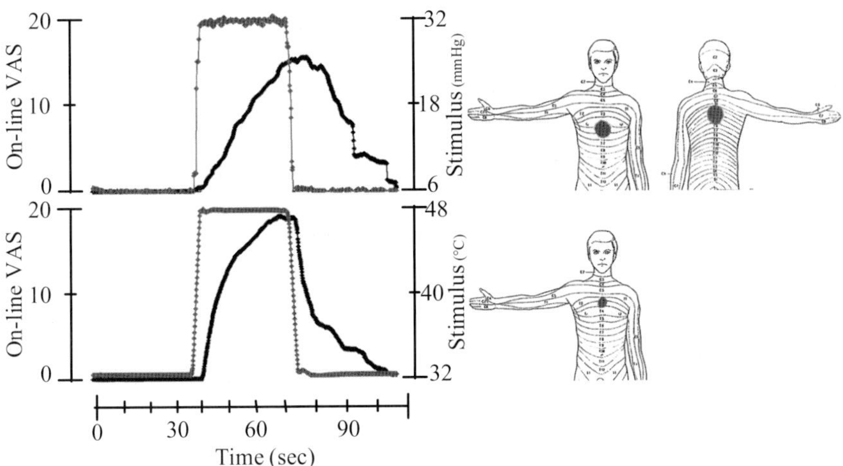

Fig. 3. Temporal profile of stimulus-evoked sensations (left) and regions of perceived pain (right) during painful esophageal and cutaneous stimulation. Subjects gave continuous ratings of pain intensity by moving a sliding bar along a pain scale from "no pain sensation" to "extremely intense pain sensation" (adapted from Strigo et al. 2002).

differentiation of peak activation foci could be related to different autonomic or emotional responses evoked by cutaneous and visceral pain. In the anterior cingulate cortex, visceral pain activated a more anterior region than did cutaneous stimulation. Again, the different locations could subserve different emotional aspects of the cutaneous and visceral pain experiences, or they could be related to different expected behavioral reactions. Topographic differences in activation were also observed in the primary somatosensory cortex (S1), and these differences are consistent with tactile somatotopy. Fig. 4 shows that the peak activation evoked by the cutaneous heat pain was located in the chest region of S1, and that the peak activation evoked by the esophageal distension pain was located near the intra-abdominal region. Interestingly, painful esophageal stimulation produced a secondary activation in the chest region of S1, which could form the neural underpinnings of the referred pain sensation. On the other hand, cutaneous heat pain on the chest did not activate the esophageal region of S1, consistent with the observation that the cutaneous pain was well localized and did not spread to other regions.

Results of these studies demonstrate that visceral and cutaneous pains of similar intensity have different perceptual profiles related to affective qualities of the sensation and to temporal and spatial indices that help define sensory aspects of pain sensation. Brain imaging, conducted under identical stimulus conditions, reveals a differential representation of visceral and cutaneous

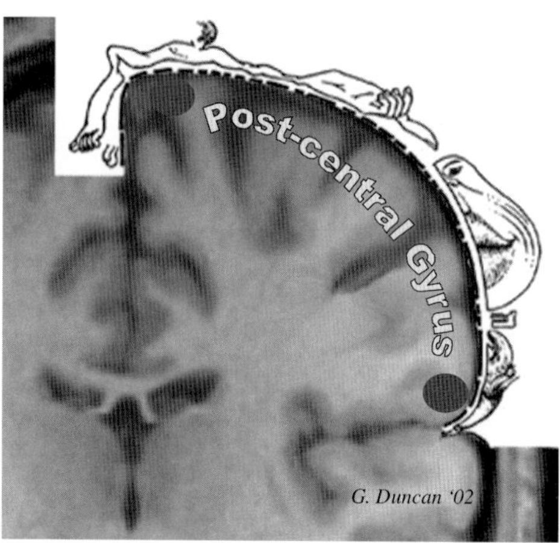

Fig. 4. Sensory homunculus. Regions that we found to be activated during painful heat on the chest and painful esophageal distension are shown by the upper left and lower right filled circles, respectively.

heat pain in somatosensory, motor, and limbic areas of the brain, which could underlie the differential perceptions and reactions associated with stimulation of skin and viscera. However, similarities in activation sites evoked by the visceral and cutaneous stimuli, within the S2 and posterior-parietal cortices, as well as the thalamus, basal ganglia, and cerebellum, suggest the existence of a common cortical and subcortical network that identifies a stimulus as painful, independent of the nature of that pain.

M. Catherine Bushnell, Irina A. Strigo, and Gary H. Duncan

UNDERSTANDING FUNCTIONAL GASTROINTESTINAL DISORDERS

THE IMPACT OF FUNCTIONAL GASTROINTESTINAL DISORDERS ON PATIENTS AND HEALTH RESOURCES

Functional gastrointestinal disorder (FGID) is the clinical term given to a number of conditions that are primarily characterized by abdominal pain without any underlying organic cause. In clinical practice, common examples of a functional disorder of the GI tract are irritable bowel syndrome (IBS), noncardiac chest pain, and functional dyspepsia. FGIDs can cause distress and feelings of helplessness and frustration for both patient and physician. Even for individuals who do not seek health care, FGIDs are associated with significant work absenteeism and impaired health quality of life (Drossman et al. 1999). FGIDs also produce a huge financial burden on the health service, with approximately 41 billion U.S. dollars being spent annually in eight leading industrialized Western nations (Fullerton 1998) in order to manage these disorders. Yet despite the high incidence of FGIDs (8–23%), little is known about their pathophysiology.

DIAGNOSTIC CRITERIA

FGIDs are characterized by chronic intermittent symptoms. These include recurrent abdominal or chest pain, altered frequency of defecation, and abdominal distension and bloating. Heightened perception of visceral sensation (hypersensitivity) and altered GI motility are two pathophysiological abnormalities that appear to underlie these symptoms. Furthermore, psychiatric illness occurs in approximately 50–80% of FGID patients (Creed and Guthrie 1987). Depression, hysteria, and obsessive-compulsive traits occur commonly in IBS patients and that psychological stress frequently exacerbates symptoms (Ringel et al. 2001).

Several hypotheses have been proposed to explain the etiology of hypersensitivity in FGIDs. These include (1) sensitization of GI afferent nerves, (2) sensitization of spinal cord dorsal horn neurons, and (3) aberrant brain processing of a visceral sensation such that a non-noxious sensation is misinterpreted as noxious due to cognitive and emotional biasing within the CNS. The following sections are devoted to the theory and techniques currently employed to ascertain the role of peripheral and central sensitization and cerebral processing in visceral hypersensitivity in FGID.

GASTROINTESTINAL AFFERENT PATHWAY SENSITIZATION

Unlike most internal organs, the gut is constantly exposed to a combination of potentially pathogenic organisms and a cocktail of digestive chemicals. It is therefore not surprising that damage commonly occurs to the gut in the form of infection (food poisoning) or inflammation (esophagitis, Crohn's disease). However, while treatment of these conditions can appear successful, patients often complain of symptoms, such as pain, long after the original insult has passed. Recent research suggests that this persistence of pain is due to sensitization of nerves, both within the gut (peripheral sensitization) and within the spinal cord (central sensitization). The effect of peripheral and central sensitization is that a stimulus that may have been previously nonpainful is now perceived as painful. It is likely that a similar mechanism is responsible for the hypersensitivity observed in some patients with FGID.

We have now developed a consistent model for human visceral hypersensitivity in the esophagus (Sarkar et al. 2000). Our studies show that infusion of hydrochloric acid into the healthy esophagus reduces the pain threshold not only in the acid-exposed region (primary hyperalgesia) but also in the adjacent unexposed region (secondary hyperalgesia). This esophageal hyperalgesia lasts for up to 5 hours after 30 minutes of acid exposure. Primary hyperalgesia is likely to occur due to sensitization of GI afferents, while secondary hyperalgesia is likely to result from central sensitization of spinal dorsal horn neurons. Furthermore, we have demonstrated a reduction in latency of cortical evoked potentials from the area of secondary hyperalgesia, which suggests that facilitation of esophageal afferent pathways occurs in our model (Sarkar et al. 2001). These experiments suggest that in susceptible patients, even brief periods of esophageal injury can lead to both peripheral and central sensitization and could be the pathophysiological basis for visceral hypersensitivity in FGIDs. Indeed, in a preliminary study (Sarkar et al. 2000), we found that acid-induced injury caused significantly greater esophageal hyperalgesia in noncardiac chest pain patients as compared to healthy subjects.

CEREBRAL PROCESSING OF VISCERAL SENSATIONS

William Beaumont first described a clear relationship between brain and GI function in 1833 when he observed that a change in emotion or mood produced a concomitant change in mucosal color, gastric secretion, and motility (Beaumont 1959). The pioneering experiments of the Russian physiologists Ivan Pavlov (1910) and Konstantine Bykov (1957) have demonstrated in a systematic and scientific manner the role that cognition plays in GI tract motility. More recently, the work of Thomas Almy and colleagues (1950) has demonstrated the importance of the environment and of psychological state in modulating visceral responses.

Craig (1999) suggests that a broad range of emotions accompany pain to provide a context for the experience itself. The way in which an individual appraises the context in which autonomic arousal occurs has been considered to be important in some theories of emotion (Schachter and Singer 1962). When patients experience specific GI symptoms, the way in which they appraise the emotional context may determine their emotional symptoms, which may, in turn, affect the perceived severity of their GI symptoms.

Cognitive influences on the perception of visceral sensation have recently been viewed as potential contributors to the pathogenesis of FGIDs (Ness and Gebhart 1990; Mayer and Gebhart 1994; Gwee et al. 1999; Hollerbach et al. 1999). In IBS, for example, several findings favor a psychological rather than a purely biological basis for increased pain sensitivity. First, IBS patients rate even sham distensions as painful (Silverman et al. 1997), and second, manipulation of their attention and changes in their arousal level produced by stress and relaxation alter the perceived intensity of distension-related sensations (Prior et al. 1990; Ford et al. 1995; Accarino et al. 1997). Finally, somatization, defined as the tendency to notice many bodily sensations and to interpret them as symptoms of disease without any apparent physical cause, occurs in IBS patients (Heaton et al. 1992; Gwee et al. 1999) and correlates significantly and substantially with pain thresholds (Whitehead and Palsson 1997). This finding suggests that selective attention (an attentional bias) to gut sensations (Latimer 1981; Mayer and Raybould 1990) may be the psychological mechanism responsible for the lowered pain thresholds observed in FGIDs.

FUNCTIONAL BRAIN IMAGING

The advent of techniques such as positron emission tomography (PET) and functional magnetic resonance imaging (fMRI) allows neuroscientists and clinicians to observe the human brain as it reacts to various stimuli including visceral sensations.

Recently, studies using functional brain imaging techniques have provided insight into the role that cognitive and emotional factors play in modulating the brain processing of somatic sensation (Derbyshire et al. 1998; Peyron et al. 1999; Ploghaus et al. 2000). These studies highlight the importance of the neural network integrating cognitive and sensory information. Functional brain imaging techniques have also been used to identify brain areas that process human esophageal sensation (Aziz et al. 1997, 2000; Aziz and Thompson 1998; Furlong et al. 1998; Hobson et al. 2000). These studies show that cortical processing of esophageal sensation involves initial processing in the primary and secondary somatosensory cortices for sensory discrimination, with subsequent involvement of the anterior cingulate and prefrontal cortices for affect and cognition, respectively. This finding indicates that not only are we able to localize the site of our gut sensation, but we are also able to give it emotional valence.

Our research examining the influence of emotional context on the cerebral processing of nonpainful esophageal sensation has demonstrated that visceral sensation is modulated by the emotional context in which it is perceived. We have shown that the dorsal anterior cingulate gyrus and anterior insula integrate emotionally salient information and gut sensory information. As context becomes more negative as subjects view a series of faces depicting progressively more fearful expressions, sensory input is amplified such that a nonpainful visceral stimulus is interpreted as more noxious (Phillips et al. 2003). This work has significant clinical relevance to our understanding of unexplained functional gut pain where negative emotional states may contribute to visceral hyperalgesia in FGID patients so that non-noxious sensation is perceived as noxious. Treatment of emotional disturbances may be useful in managing visceral hyperalgesia in these patients. Our ongoing work suggests that cognitive factors such as attention and anticipation also modulate brain processing of esophageal sensation.

CONCLUSIONS

By understanding the contribution that central and peripheral sensitization and cognitive and emotional factors play in the etiology of visceral hypersensitivity in FGID, a clearer picture will emerge as to how to manage functional GI disorders. For example, if cognitive and emotional biasing is responsible for the symptoms reported, then suitable psychological treatment strategies could be targeted at alleviating symptom severity. Conversely, if central or peripheral sensitization is found to be the root cause of visceral hypersensitivity in FGID, then pharmacological agents could be used. However, it is extremely likely that visceral hypersensitivity results from a combination of the two causes, in which case a multidimensional treatment strategy will be required.

QASIM AZIZ, SANCHOY SARKAR, AND LLOYD GREGORY

LINKING THE PERCEPTION OF VISCERAL SENSATIONS WITH CORTICAL ACTIVITY

The last decade has seen an explosion of fMRI studies of pain. Some of the earliest studies reported pain-related brain responses in individual subjects. These studies revealed intersubject variability, particularly when using thermal stimuli (see Davis 2000). Intersubject variability is a critically important consideration for the application of fMRI to assessing clinical conditions. One contributing factor to variability in brain response is that the quality and intensity of the pain experience evoked by such stimuli differ from subject to subject. Furthermore, stimulus-evoked sensations may not share an identical temporal signature with the stimulus itself. Therefore, fMRI analysis techniques that only identify activations that occur during the duration of the stimulus are not well suited to situations in which many covarying sensations are evoked by a stimulus, or when the time course of the stimulus and that of the evoked sensation(s) do not completely coincide. Both of these potential confounds are relevant to the study of sensations that arise from the rectum. Therefore, we have used a unique approach that we refer to as "percept-related fMRI" (Davis et al. 2002) to identify cortical responses that are associated with the intensity and temporal signature of particular sensations evoked by rectal distension.

METHODS

Psychophysical and fMRI studies of rectal-evoked sensations were performed in both healthy volunteers and IBS patients. All subjects provided informed consent, and all procedures received ethics approval from the University Health Network. Isobaric rectal stimuli were delivered via a computer-controlled barostat and a 10-cm polystyrene balloon catheter (for details, see Kwan et al. 2002). Each subject underwent several series of stimuli consisting of either 30-second distensions (interleaved with a 30-second baseline pressure level), or prolonged (140—300-second) stimuli. Each series consisted of either low-intensity stimuli (to evoke urge) or moderate-intensity stimuli (to evoke pain or unpleasantness). Throughout all series, subjects made continuous ratings of urge to defecate, pain intensity, or unpleasantness. For the fMRI experiments, we acquired whole-brain anatomical and functional images with a 1.5-Tesla MRI "echospeed" system. Details of preprocessing and statistical analysis were performed using BrainVoyager software (see Davis et al. 2002; Downar et al. 2002). Percept-related fMRI was used to extract brain activations associated with particular sensations (Davis et al. 2002). The following steps were used to create a functional brain map that reflects a perceptual experience across a group of subjects. First, subjects were instructed in the use of a trackball that controlled a computerized 100-point VAS (visible via a head-stage mounted mirror) to continuously rate a particular component of the feelings evoked by the rectal stimuli (urge, pain intensity, or unpleasantness). These ratings were then convolved with a standard hemodynamic response function. The convolved ratings signature for each subject was then used as a predictor in a general linear model analysis of the data across the subject group. For comparative purposes, the intensity and time course of the stimulus pressure (convolved with the hemodynamic response function) were also used as predictors.

DISCUSSION

The psychophysical experiments in healthy subjects revealed a similar onset and duration of evoked sensations compared to the short rectal stimuli.

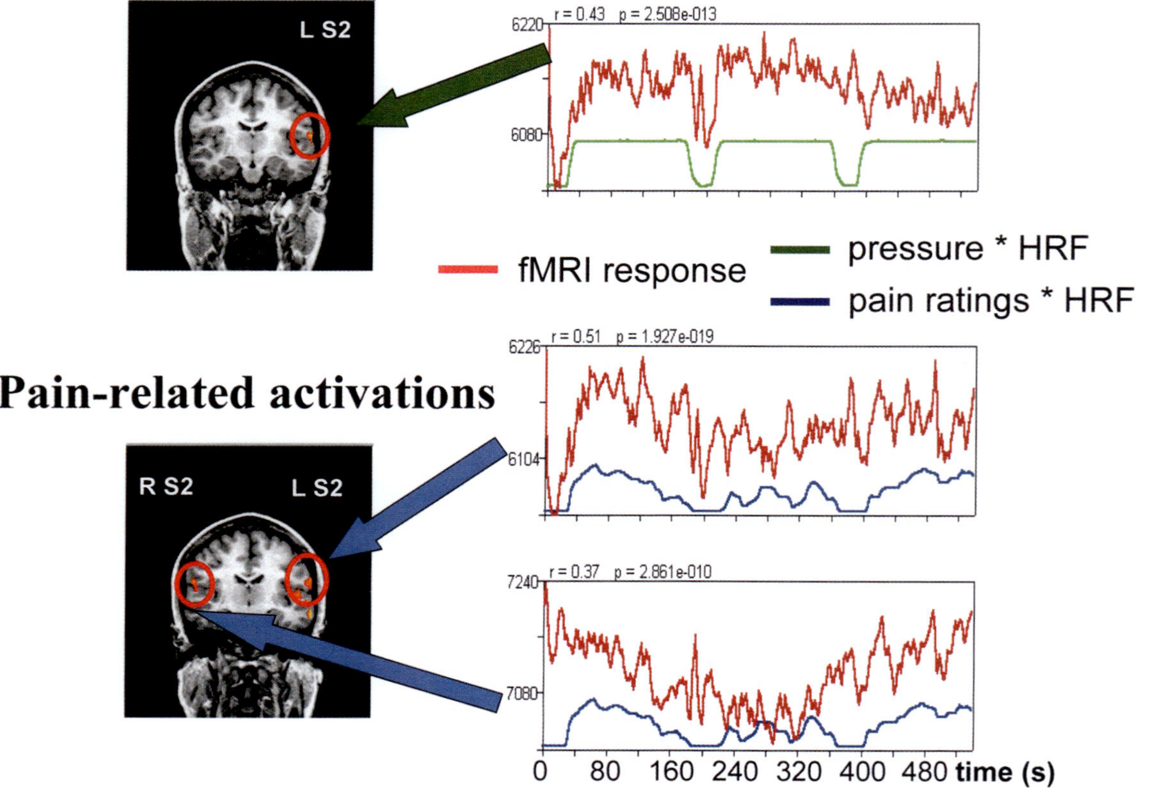
Pressure-related activation
L S2
r = 0.43 p = 2.508e-013
6220
6080
fMRI response
pressure * HRF
pain ratings * HRF
Pain-related activations
R S2
L S2
r = 0.51 p = 1.927e-019
6226
6104
r = 0.37 p = 2.861e-010
7240
7080
0 80 160 240 320 400 480 time (s)

← **Fig. 5.** fMRI responses to rectal distension. Regions of activations are shown (left panels) that are correlated to the rectal stimulus profile (top) or the pain reported by the subject (bottom). The right panel shows the response within the regions of interest (red curves, ordinate scale is in arbitrary MRI units). Correlation functions used in the analysis were derived from either the barostat pressure (green) or pain rating (blue) convolved with standard hemodynamic response function.

However, when the stimuli were prolonged, the reported sensations tended to wax and wane during each stimulus (see Kwan et al. 2002). The uncoupling between stimulus and perception was even more striking in the IBS patients. The patients tended to report intense urge, pain, and unpleasantness, which started at the onset of the first rectal distension but continued throughout the stimulus and interstimulus intervals. These findings highlight the importance of using online ratings of evoked sensations, rather than the period of stimulation, to identify cortical responses associated with rectal sensations.

Using the percept-related fMRI approach, we extracted cortical activations associated with the profile of online ratings (an example is shown in Fig. 5). Activations associated with urge were identified in the frontal cortex, S1, insula, anterior cingulate cortex (ACC), and supplemental motor area (SMA); activations associated with pain intensity were identified in the frontal cortex, S2, ACC, and SMA; and activations associated with unpleasantness were identified in the frontal cortex, S1, S2, ACC, and SMA. These findings suggest that particular sets of brain regions are associated with the conscious perception of rectal distension-evoked urge, pain intensity, and unpleasantness. The percept-related activations were distinct from those associated with the pressure stimulus profile. Stimulus-related activations included sites in the frontal cortex, ACC, SMA, S2, and also the insula. In those cases in which the subject's perception roughly synchronized with the stimulus, a distinction between stimulus- and percept-related cortical response could not be clearly made. The function of the stimulus-related activations is not known, but it may relate to unconscious homeostatic or reflective mechanisms (Craig 2002). Therefore, in situations where there is an uncoupling between the time course of rectal distension and rectal-evoked sensations, a method such as percept-related fMRI can be useful to identify cortical responses related to specific types of evoked perceptions.

Karen D. Davis, Chun L. Kwan, and Nicholas E. Diamant

REFERENCES

Accarino AM, Azpiroz F, Malagelada JR. Attention and distraction: effects on gut perception. *Gastroenterology* 1997; 113:415–422.

Al Chaer ED, Lawand NB, Westlund KN, Willis WD. Visceral nociceptive input into the ventral posterolateral nucleus of the thalamus: a new function for the dorsal column pathway. *J Neurophysiol* 1996; 76:2661–2674.

Almy TP, Abbot FK, Hinkle LE. Alterations in colonic function in man under stress. IV: Hypomotility of the sigmoid colon and its relationship to the mechanism of functional diarrhea. *Gastroenterology* 1950; 15:95–105.

Aziz Q, Thompson DG. Brain-Gut axis in health and disease. *Gastroenterology* 1998; 114:559–578.

Aziz Q, Andersson JL, Valind S, et al. Identification of human brain loci processing oesophageal distension using positron emission tomography. *Gastroenterology* 1997; 113:50–60.

Aziz Q, Thompson DG, Ng VW, et al. Cortical processing of human somatic and visceral sensation. *J Neurosci* 2000; 20:2657–2663.

Berkley KJ. On the dorsal columns: translating basic research hypotheses to the clinic. *Pain* 1997; 70:103–107.

Berkley KJ, Hubscher CH, Wall PD. Neuronal responses to stimulation of the cervix, uterus, colon, and skin in the rat spinal cord. *J Neurophysiol* 1993; 69:545–556.

Berkley KJ, Benoist JM, Gautron M, Guilbaud G. Responses of neurons in the caudal intralaminar thalamic complex of the rat to stimulation of the uterus, vagina, cervix, colon and skin. *Brain Res* 1995; 695:92–95.

Beaumont W. Experiments and observations on the gastric juice and physiology of digestion. New York: Dover, 1959.

Bradshaw HB, Berkley KJ. Estrous changes in responses of rat gracile nucleus neurons to stimulation of skin and pelvic viscera. *J Neurosci* 2000; 20:7722–7727.

Bruggemann J, Shi T, Apkarian AV. Squirrel monkey lateral thalamus. II. Viscerosomatic convergent representation of urinary bladder, colon, and esophagus. *J Neurosci* 1994; 14:6796–6814.

Bykov KM. The cerebral cortex and the internal organs. Gantt WH (Translator). New York: Chemical Publishing Co., 1957.

Chandler MJ, Hobbs SF, Fu QG, et al. Responses of neurons in ventroposterolateral nucleus of primate thalamus to urinary bladder distension. *Brain Res* 1992; 571:26–34.

Craig AD. How do you feel? Interoception: the sense of the physiological condition of the body. *Nat Rev Neurosci* 2002; 3:655–666.

Craig KD. Emotions and psychology. In: Wall PD, Melzack R (Eds). *Textbook of Pain,* 4th ed. Edinburgh: Churchill Livingstone, 1999, pp 331–344.

Creed F, Guthrie E. Psychological factors in the irritable bowel syndrome. *Gut* 1987; 28:1307–1318.

Davis KD. The neural circuitry of pain as explored with functional MRI. *Neurological Res* 2000; 22:313–317.

Davis KD, Pope GE, Crawley AP, Mikulis DJ. Neural correlates of prickle sensation: a percept-related fMRI study. *Nat Neurosci* 2002; in press.

Derbyshire SW, Vogt BA, Jones AK. Pain and Stroop interference tasks activate separate processing modules in anterior cingulate cortex. *Exp Brain Res* 1998; 118:52–56.

Downar J, Crawley AP, Mikulis DJ, Davis KD. A cortical network sensitive to stimulus salience in a neutral behavioral context across multiple sensory modalities. *J Neurophysiology* 2002; 87:615–620.

Drossman DA. The functional gastrointestinal disorders and the Rome II process. *Gut* 1999; 45(Suppl II):II1–II5.

Follett KA, Dirks B. Characterization of responses of primary somatosensory cerebral cortex neurons to noxious visceral stimulation in the rat. *Brain Res* 1994; 656:27–32.

Follett KA, Dirks B. Responses of neurons in ventrolateral orbital cortex to noxious visceral stimulation in the rat. *Brain Res* 1995; 669:157–162.

Ford MJ, Camilleri M, Zinsmeister AR, Hanson RB. Psychosensory modulation of colonic sensation in the human transverse and sigmoid colon. *Gastroenterology* 1995; 109:1772–1780.

Fullerton S. Functional digestive disorders (FDD) in the year 2000-economic impact. *Eur J Surg* 1998; (Suppl 5)82:62–64.

Furlong PL, Aziz Q, Singh KD, et al. Cortical localization of magnetic fields evoked by oesophageal distension. *Electroencephalogr Clin Neurophysiol* 1998; 108:234–243.

Gwee K-A, Leong YL, Graham C, et al. The role of psychological and biological factors in postinfective gut dysfunction. *Gut* 1999; 44:400–406.

Heaton KW, O'Donnell LJ, Braddon FE, et al. Symptoms of irritable bowel syndrome in a British urban community: consulters and nonconsulters. *Gastroenterology* 1992; 102:1962–1967.

Hobson AR, Sarkar S, Furlong PL, Thompson DG, Aziz Q. A cortical evoked potential study of afferents mediating human oesophageal sensation. *Am J Physiol Gastrointest Liver Physiol* 2000; 279:G139–G147.

Hollerbach S, Fitzpatrick D, Shine G, et al. Cognitive evoked potentials to anticipated oesophageal stimulus in humans: quantitative assessment of the cognitive aspects of visceral perception. *Neurogastroenterol Motil* 1999; 11:37–46.

Kawakita K, Dostrovsky JO, Tang JS, Chiang CY. Responses of neurons in the rat thalamic nucleus submedius to cutaneous, muscle and visceral nociceptive stimuli. *Pain* 1993; 55:327–338.

Kwan CL, Mikula K, Diamant NE, Davis KD. The relationship between rectal pain, unpleasantness, and urge to defecate in normal subjects. *Pain* 2002; 97:53–63.

Latimer PR. Irritable bowel syndrome: a behavioral model. *Behav Res Ther* 1981; 19:475–483.

Lewis T. *Pain*. New York: MacMillan, 1942.

Mayer E, Gebhart G. Basic and clinical aspects of visceral hyperalgesia. *Gastroenterology* 1994; 107:271–293.

Mayer E, Raybould H. Role of visceral afferent mechanisms in functional bowel disorders. *Gastroenterology* 1990; 99:1688–1704.

McMahon SB, Dmitrieva N, Koltzenburg M. Visceral pain. *Br J Anaesth* 1995; 75:132–144.

Ness T, Gebhart G. Visceral pain: a review of experimental studies. *Pain* 1990; 41:167–234.

Nauta HJ, Hewitt E, Westlund KN, Willis WD Jr. Surgical interruption of a midline dorsal column visceral pain pathway. Case report and review of the literature. *J Neurosurg* 1997; 86:538–542.

Pavlov I. *The Work of Digestive Glands*. Thompson WH (Translator). London: Griffin, 1910.

Peyron R, Garcia-Larrea L, Gregoire MC, et al. Haemodynamic brain responses to acute pain in humans sensory and attentional networks. *Brain* 1999; 122:1765–1779.

Phillips ML, Gregory LJ, Cullen S, et al. The effect of negative emotional context on neural and behavioural responses to oesophageal stimulation. *Brain* 2003; in press.

Ploghaus A, Tracey I, Clare S, et al. Learning about pain: the neural substrate of the prediction error for aversive events. *Proc Natl Acad Sci USA* 2000; 97:9281–9286.

Prior A, Colgan SM, Whorwell PJ. Changes in rectal sensitivity after hypnotherapy in patients with irritable bowel syndrome. *Gut* 1990; 31:896–898.

Ringel Y, Sperber AD, Drossman DA. Irritable bowel syndrome. *Annu Rev Med* 2001; 52:319–338.

Sarkar S, Aziz Q, Woolf CJ, Hobson AR, Thompson DG. Contribution of central sensitisation to the development of non-cardiac chest pain. *Lancet* 2000; 356:1154–1159.

Sarkar S, Hobson AR, Furlong PL. Mediating human visceral hypersensitivity. *Am J Physiol Gastrointest Liver Physiol* 2001; 281(5):G1196–1202.

Schachter S, Singer JE. Cognitive, social, and physiological determinants of emotional states. *Psych Rev* 1962; 69:379–399.

Schott GD. Visceral afferents: their contribution to 'sympathetic dependent' pain. *Brain* 1994; 117:397–413.

Silverman D, Munakata JA, Ennes H, et al. Regional cerebral activity in normal and pathological perception of visceral pain. *Gastroenterology* 1997; 112:64–72.

Snow PJ, Lumb BM, Cervero F. The representation of prolonged and intense, noxious somatic and visceral stimuli in the ventrolateral orbital cortex of the cat. *Pain* 1992; 48:89–99.

Strigo IA, Bushnell MC, Boivin M, Duncan GH. Cerebral activity during painful stimulation of skin and viscera. *Soc Neurosci Abstr* 27; 2001.

Strigo IA, Bushnell MC, Boivin M, Duncan GH. Psychophysical analysis of visceral and cutaneous pain in human subjects. *Pain* 2002; 97:235–246.

Whitehead W, Palsson O. Is rectal pain sensitivity a biological marker for irritable bowel syndrome: psychological influences on perception. *Gastroenterology* 1997; 115:1263–1271.

Correspondence to: Karen D. Davis, PhD, Division of Neurosurgery, Toronto Western Hospital, University Health Network MP14-306, 399 Bathurst Street, Toronto, Ontario, Canada M5T 2S8. Tel: 416-603-5662; Fax: 416-603-5745; email: kdavis@uhnres.utoronto.ca.

Proceedings of the 10th World Congress on Pain,
Progress in Pain Research and Management, Vol. 24,
edited by Jonathan O. Dostrovsky, Daniel B. Carr, and
Martin Koltzenburg, IASP Press, Seattle, © 2003.

24

Cognitive Modulation of Cortical Responses to Pain[1]

Roland Peyron,[a] Pierre Rainville,[b]
Predrag Petrovic,[c] and Luis Garcia-Larrea[d]

[a]Department of Neurology, Bellevue Hospital, St-Etienne, France; [b]Department of Stomatology, Faculty of Dental Medicine, University of Montreal, Montreal, Quebec, Canada; [c]Department of Clinical Neuroscience, Karolinska Institute, Karolinska Hospital, Stockholm, Sweden; [d]CERMEP, Lyon, France

Brain responses to pain have been widely investigated over the past 10 years through positron emission tomography (PET) and functional magnetic resonance imaging (fMRI) studies. Experiments in which normal volunteers undergo brain scans during a painful experience have allowed investigators to perform precise spatial mapping of brain responses. Two meta-analyses that reviewed brain activations to nociceptive stimuli have clearly identified discrete brain regions where activation is consistently found during the application of noxious stimuli and/or the experience of pain (Derbyshire 2000; Peyron et al. 2000b). Thus, the question of which brain regions show pain-related changes in activity can now be answered within the framework of a relatively stable functional map and a limited number of activated brain regions. The questions of "when" brain areas are activated during pain and "what" is the functional contribution of those areas to pain cannot be so easily answered by PET and fMRI techniques.

Despite recent improvements in temporal resolution with functional imaging, the timing of pain-related activations in humans is largely extrapolated from electrophysiological data. Nevertheless, several lines of evidence suggest that different processes or components of the brain's response to nociceptive stimuli can occur both in parallel and in series in a normal brain

[1] Based on a Congress workshop.

during the temporal window of functional imaging techniques (Frot et al. 1999; Frot and Mauguiere 1999; Timmermann et al. 2001). Thus, the question of "when" applied to the observation of brain responses to pain by functional imaging is still largely open. A first step in answering this question is to pool data collected by different techniques including PET, fMRI, and electrophysiology (Peyron et al. 2002). However, a definitive answer to this question is most likely to come from the integration of electrophysiological and magnetophysiological methods such as magnetoencephalography (with high temporal resolution) and functional brain imaging methods such as PET and fMRI (with high spatial resolution).

PET and fMRI methods, used alone with dedicated experimental paradigms, have nevertheless provided some partial answers to the problem of the functional contribution of the multiple brain areas activated during pain. Investigations have focused on brain responses to the following processes: sensory discrimination, attention to pain, affective modulation of pain, anticipation or expectation of pain, and motor control. This chapter discusses these aspects of the nociceptive matrix (Fig. 1) in light of results obtained by our different teams in an attempt to understand the individual contributions of the various brain regions activated by a painful stimulus to the multidimensional experience of pain.

SENSORY-DISCRIMINATIVE ASPECTS OF PAIN PROCESSING AND ITS MODULATION

A major component of the pain-related response relates to the encoding of the sensory-discriminative aspects of the stimulus, including the quality of the stimulus, the evoked sensation, and its intensity. In their factorial design, Peyron et al. (1999) identified a network related to the encoding of noxious heat intensity (regardless of attention) and involving the anterior insular cortices bilaterally. These findings are in accordance with results from other groups showing that anterior insular activity correlates with thermal intensity for both cold stimuli (Craig et al. 2000) and heat pain (Coghill et al. 1999). These data also are compatible with findings from other PET and fMRI studies showing that, compared to other brain regions, the insular and secondary somatosensory (S2) cortex regions demonstrate the most reliable pain-related activations across subjects and different experimental paradigms (for a review, see Peyron et al. 2000b). Indirectly, if the insular and S2 cortices are the most reliably activated area across experimental paradigms, and because pain is the common denominator in all pain experiments, it seems reasonable to assume that this cortical area is involved in encoding

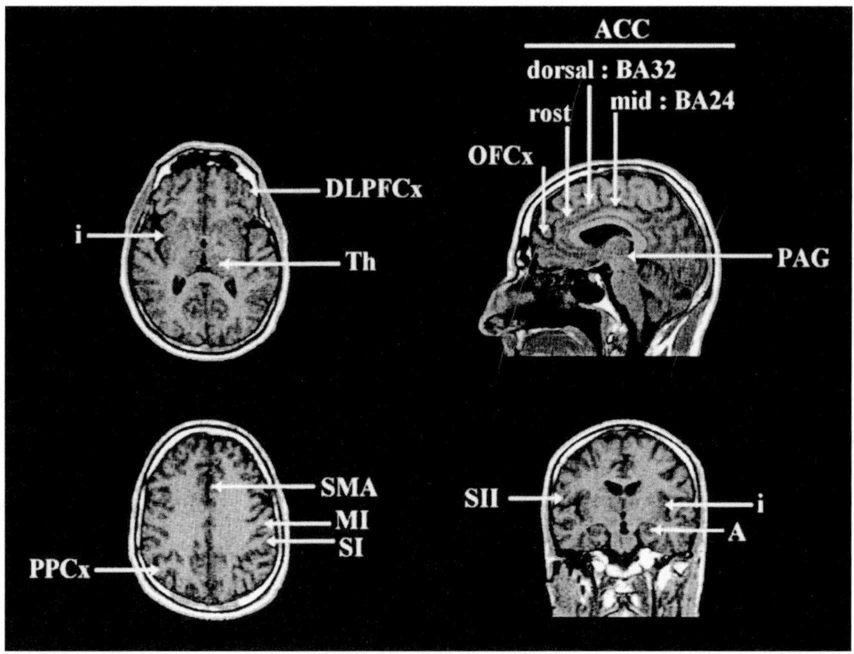

Fig. 1. A three-dimensional anatomical MRI showing the main brain regions that have been described as pertaining to the "nociceptive matrix." For each of these regions, in agreement with what is known of their functions, a summary of their involvement in pain or in pain-associated processes has been labeled. This is not an exhaustive list of functions associated with pain integration, and the functions listed here are not exclusive in a given brain region. Moreover, a given brain region may participate equally in several functions, and these functions may occur at different times. In addition, some functions have been deliberately omitted in order to simplify the presentation of the figure. Functions and explanations of abbreviations are as follows: insula (i): somatovisceral integration, intensity coding, autonomic function, cold perception (including noxious), emotion. Dorsolateral prefrontal cortex (DLPFCx): cognition, working memory, attention. Orbitofrontal cortex (OFCx): modulation of affective-emotional response, pain anticipation, motivation. Thalamus (Th): gating sensory information (arousal, attention, sensory), motivation, consciousness. Anterior cingulate cortex (ACC): rost (rostral): somatovisceral responses; mid (BA24): motor behavior, unpleasantness, attentional shift, orientation, intrusion; dorsal (BA32): cognitive modulation, sustained attention. Periaqueductal gray (PAG): descending regulation, emotion. Secondary somatosensory cortex and operculum (SII): sensory. Primary somatosensory cortex (SI): sensory, attention, anticipation. Primary motor area (MI) and supplementary motor area (SMA): regulation of motor response. Posterior parietal cortex (PPCx) (BAs 40, 5, 7): oriented/spatial attention. Amygdala (A): fear-associated behavior, fear-induced analgesia, aversive conditioning, emotion.

thermal and/or pain intensity. In addition, this region is known from invasive neurophysiological techniques in humans to be involved in the encoding of pain intensity to a noxious heat laser stimulus (Frot and Mauguiere 2003).

PET has been used to study three situations in which the sensory-discriminative system of pain either is abnormal or is experimentally manipulated. The first was the "thermal grill" experiment, whereby non-noxious cold and warm stimuli were alternated spatially to generate an illusion of pain (Craig et al. 1996). In Craig's experiment, physical stimuli were misinterpreted by a normal discriminative system (the sensation was perceived as painful while all individual stimuli were non-noxious); both the discrimination and the intensity of the real stimulus were distorted. This illusion was associated with significantly increased regional cerebral blood flow (rCBF) in the anterior cingulate, S2, and insular cortices, suggesting that these three regions might have contributed to the distorted sensation. The second situation was clinical, and involved patients with neuropathic pain in whom the discriminative system was damaged and unable to analyze correctly the physical characteristics of the stimulus. Such patients often cannot detect whether the stimulus is cold, warm, or neutral, or even say whether or not they have been touched by the examiner; however, they immediately feel pain when an innocuous tactile stimulus grazes their skin. In this particular model of sensory distortion, called allodynia, reliable abnormal activity was reported in the insular and S2 cortices (Peyron et al. 1998, 2000a; Petrovic et al. 1999), suggesting postlesion reorganization in a system devoted to the discriminative aspect of pain. In a third situation, the intensity of perceived pain was decreased as attention was diverted from pain with the consequence of decreased activity in the anterior insular and S2 cortices (Petrovic et al. 2000; Frankenstein et al. 2001). This region did not pertain to the attentional network (Peyron et al. 1999; Frankenstein et al. 2001), and thus modulation of insular/S2 activity could be considered to be contributing to the pain intensity coding system. However, three important considerations are that (1) the illusion of pain produced by the thermal grill is associated with unpleasant feelings characteristic of pain, (2) allodynic pain is typically very unpleasant, and (3) distraction usually modulates both pain intensity and unpleasantness (see Miron et al. 1989). Therefore, these paradigms do not exclude a contribution of the S2 and insular cortices to both sensory and affective aspects of pain (for a review, see Phan et al. 2002).

Evidence for the participation of other cortical areas to sensory-discriminative aspects of pain has been less consistent. In particular, activation of the primary somatosensory (S1) cortex during pain has been observed in about half of the studies reviewed by Peyron et al. (2000b). Physical characteristics of the stimulus (e.g., skin contact, cold, heat, movement, and surface area of stimulation) have been argued to influence S1 responses (Jones and Derbyshire 1995; Peyron et al. 2000b). However, other processes associated with pain also modify rCBF in the S1 cortex, namely anticipation (which could be considered as an attentional process) and attention. Attention to pain and the suggestion of increased pain perception increase S1 activity (Bushnell et al. 1999), as shown at the neuronal level in single-unit recording studies (Steinmetz et al. 2000; Niebur et al. 2002). Anticipation of a painful as well as an innocuous stimulus was shown to decrease rCBF in the ipsilateral S1 cortex and also in the contralateral S1 cortex in the somatotopic subdivision that is not affected by the site of stimulation (Drevets et al. 1995). Similar results were observed in the ipsilateral S1 in an attentional experiment that concurrently included some amount of anticipation of a phasic painful stimulus (Peyron et al. 1999). Taken together, these functional imaging data sets suggest that the S1 cortex participates in several functions including discrimination of painful stimuli, spatial attention to pain, and anticipation of pain, and in their mutual interactions.

THE ATTENTIONAL COMPONENT OF THE NOCICEPTIVE MATRIX AND ITS MODULATION

The modulation of pain perception by attention is a well-known effect (Miron et al. 1989). The brain responses that may support such an effect were first identified by PET (Peyron et al. 1999), subsequently confirmed by fMRI (Peyron et al. 2000c), and also observed using laser-evoked potentials (Garcia-Larrea et al. 1997). Several other imaging studies have confirmed the role of the posterior parietal cortex (Brodmann's area [BA] 40) and prefrontal cortex (BAs 44–47) in pain-related attentional processes (Petrovic et al. 2000; Bornhovd et al. 2002). These studies found that the modulation was independent of pain intensity. The interactions between pain and the attentional matrices have been described (Petrovic et al. 2000; Frankenstein et al. 2001). While activity levels in other components of the pain matrix were reduced as the pain intensity decreased, the anterior portion of the cingulate gyrus was activated as the subjects' attention was diverted from pain (Bantick et al. 2002). In this situation, the anterior cingulate cortex (ACC) could be involved in intermittent attention shifts from the target task to the intrusive pain (Peyron et al. 1999). These findings are consistent with a role of the ACC in experiments specifically testing attention shifting (Posner 1994) and divided attention processes (Pardo et al. 1990; Corbetta et al. 1991; Bench et al. 1993; Petrovic et al. 2000). They are also in accordance with the hypothesis that increased activity in the ACC could reflect a modulation of other brain regions involved in nociceptive processing.

Subcortical regions such as the thalamus (Peyron et al. 1999) and periaqueductal gray (PAG; Tracey et al. 2002) also may participate in the attentional network, possibly via increased arousal as reported in other sensory modalities (Fredrikson et al. 1995; Nobre et al. 1997; Portas et al. 1998; Paus 2000).

DISSOCIATION OF THE SENSORY AND AFFECTIVE DIMENSIONS OF PAIN

The role of pain-related structures in the sensory and affective dimensions of pain has been examined in several studies using self-reports of pain intensity and unpleasantness. In accordance with the results of the meta-analyses discussed above, blood flow measures of brain activity in the S1, S2, insular, and anterior cingulate cortices have consistently shown a monotonic relation with self-reports of pain intensity (Derbyshire et al. 1997; Coghill et al. 1999, 2001). A series of studies using various hypnotic suggestions (Rainville et al. 1999a) has further demonstrated that the specific manipulation of pain unpleasantness modulates pain-related activity in the ACC (Rainville et al. 1997), while the manipulation of pain intensity modulates pain-related activity mainly in the S1 cortex (Hofbauer et al. 2001). This finding is consistent with impairments in pain sensation (but preservation of pain affect) following lesions in the S1 cortex in humans (Ploner et al. 1999). It is also compatible with the results of electrophysiological studies showing task-relevant precise coding of noxious stimulus intensity in S1 neurons in monkeys (Kenshalo et al. 1988). The finding that ACC modulation is associated with changes in pain intensity suggests that the modulation of pain-related ACC activity (Rainville et al. 1997) did not merely reflect a nonspecific aspect of the hypnotic procedure (e.g., attention) and emphasizes the specific encoding of pain unpleasantness in the ACC. Although there may not be a simple correspondence between a function or an experiential dimension and a brain area activated during pain, the evidence reviewed here is consistent with a contribution of the S1, S2, and insular cortices to the sensory-discriminative aspect of pain, while the ACC appears to be mainly concerned with affective and cognitive dimensions of the experience.

ROLE OF THE ANTERIOR CINGULATE CORTEX IN PAIN AFFECT AND ATTENTION

The association of the ACC with pain unpleasantness may seem to contradict a specific role for the ACC in attention, independent of pain. Yet it is clear that higher levels of pain unpleasantness are likely to be accompanied by increased attention to pain or to the source of noxious stimulation so that most studies are unable to discriminate between attention and pain unpleasantness. However, in the study mentioned above on the hypnotic modulation of pain unpleasantness (Rainville et al. 1999a) , attention was directed toward the sensation, and the subjects received suggestions to attend to the sensation and reinterpret it as being more or less unpleasant. In this condition, pain intensity ratings remained unchanged, a finding that is inconsistent with previous studies of attention showing comparable modulation of pain intensity and unpleasantness by a difficult task designed to distract the subjects from the pain (Miron et al. 1989). One possible interpretation involves a distinction between subsectors of the ACC associated with pain and attention.

A functional segregation of subsectors of the ACC likely depends on the type of input processed and the specific processing and output mechanisms engaged, as previously suggested (Bush et al. 2000; Paus 2000, 2001; Picard and Strick 2001). Spinothalamocortical input to the ACC is found in the ventral aspect of the supracallosal ACC, within BA 24 (Vogt et al. 1993). Consistent with this anatomical projection, pain-related activation frequently is reported in the ventral part of the supracallosal ACC (Peyron et al. 2000b). The significance of increased activity in the ventral portion of BA24 is still a matter of debate. This area may be more specifically involved in conditions where the afferent input is of somatic origin and has an *intrinsic* affective value, as suggested previously (Rainville 2002). It may also be involved in orienting attention from one task to another, particularly for intrusive events such as pain (Peyron et al. 2000b). In this condition, pain may be conceived as a highly distracting concurrent stimulus that constitutes a potential hindrance to the optimal performance of the task and to the instruction given to the subjects to "perform the cognitive task as well as you can." In the case of a distractive task, ventral BA24 activation could not be attributed to pain affect because distraction is known to decrease both pain intensity and pain unpleasantness. Therefore, ventral BA24 may be involved in processes resulting in increased pain affect and increased intrusion in cognitive processes.

In contrast, the role of the dorsal sector of the ACC (BA32) seems to be more consistently activated in difficult, attention-demanding cognitive tasks (Davis et al. 1997; Paus et al. 1998), which involve sustained, rather than phasic, attention (for review, see Peyron et al. 2000b), including cognitive processes related to the implementation of the hypnotic suggestions (Rainville 2002). BA32 may be involved in conditions where *extrinsic*, or secondary, positive or negative affective value is attributed to the distracting stimuli relevant to the task performed. Such distraction may call upon additional attentional resources and may increase activity within the cognitive division of the ACC. Understanding the relation between pain and ACC activity may require that we take into account the functional specificity of different areas of the ACC, as well as the goal set by the experimental context and the potentially detrimental effect of pain on performance.

HYPNOTIC STATES AND THE HYPNOTIC MODULATION OF PAIN

Turning now to mechanisms underling hypnotic analgesia, we first consider the general effects of hypnotic induction. Before analgesic suggestions are given, hypnosis typically involves suggestions for the establishment of a relaxed and focused mental state that produces the characteristic subjective experience of mental ease and absorption (Price 1996). Hypnotic relaxation and mental absorption result in changes in rCBF in the brainstem, the thalamus, and the ACC, as well as in the right inferior frontal cortex, the right posterior parietal cortex, and the occipital cortices (Rainville et al. 2002). These changes in brain activity produced by the hypnotic state appear to share some common characteristics with states of decreased vigilance (correlated with the increases in subjective levels of relaxation and mental ease), concurrent with increases in focal attention (correlated with increases in subjective levels of mental absorption). Although hypnotic induction procedures without specific suggestions of altered pain may not be sufficient to induce changes in pain perception (see Rainville et al. 1997, 1999a,b; Hofbauer et al. 2001), the induction of hypnotic states may facilitate the effects of analgesic suggestions (Price 1996).

Additional results of hypnosis studies reveal nonspecific effects of hypnotic suggestions for increases or decreases in pain intensity (P. Rainville, unpublished observations) or unpleasantness (Rainville et al. 1999b). The nonspecific, suggestion-related, activation within parts of the prefrontal cortices and the dorsal sector of the anterior ACC (BA32) could reflect cognitive processes responsible for the implementation of hypnotic suggestions for pain modulation and the recruitment of self-regulatory mechanisms underlying the modulation of pain-related activity (Rainville 2002). Specific mechanisms could involve (1) cortico-cortical interactions between the dorsal and ventral parts of the ACC and with the prefrontal cortices, (2) cortical influences on thalamocortical projections to the ACC and S1, and (3) descending projections to subcortical structures such as the PAG. Consistent with this last possibility, suggestions for hypnotic analgesia have been shown to modulate pain-related autonomic responses (Rainville et al. 1999b) as well as the RIII reflex, a spinally mediated nociceptive reflex (Kiernan et al.

1995; Danziger et al. 1998). These additional effects attest to the participation of descending mechanisms possibly involving the PAG, autonomic nuclei of the brainstem and spinal cord, the rostroventral medulla, and spinal nociceptive processes. Although the specific effects of hypnotic states on the self-implementation of analgesic suggestions remain to be clarified, these studies clearly point to robust physiological effects underlying the production of hypnotic states and the hypnotic modulation of pain. These mechanisms may be *partly* shared with other forms of cognitive interventions such as distraction or placebo, but the specificity of the effects of each type of cognitive intervention remains to be examined in a within-study design.

THE ANTICIPATION COMPONENT OF THE NOCICEPTIVE MATRIX

As discussed above in the sensory-discriminative and the attentional sections, anticipation of predictable pain is likely to add one component to the pain matrix. Compared to other components of the pain matrix, the most striking findings of these studies are the frequently reported decreases in activity in brain areas that are parts of the pain matrix, or at least a coexistence of increased and decreased activity in adjacent subdivisions of a brain structure.

Drevets et al. (1995) first demonstrated that the expectation of either an innocuous or a painful stimulus could lead to a bilateral decrease in rCBF in S2 and in the sensory-motor cortices to stimulation in subdivisions that were not congruent with the localization of the stimulus itself. Localized rCBF decreases adjacent to the activated area in the contralateral S1 were hypothesized to enhance the detection of stimuli. Decreased activity in the ipsilateral S1 has been described in two experiments that examined the changes induced by anticipation of tickling (Carlsson et al. 2000) or pain (Porro et al. 2002).

Conversely, other brain areas are likely to mediate other aspects of anticipation to pain. Anticipation to a simple cognitive task (in nonpainful situations) is known to activate the ACC (Murtha et al. 1999), and thus it is not surprising that this area and the adjacent medial prefrontal cortex were found to be regularly associated with anticipation of pain (Porro et al. 1998, 2002; Chua et al. 1999; Hsieh et al. 1999; Ploghaus et al. 1999, 2001). In medial prefrontal cortices, including the rostral part of the ACC (rACC; i.e., the perigenuate area), changes in activity were found in experiments that included some amount of anticipatory anxiety (Chua et al. 1999), coping strategy (Hsieh et al. 1999), differences in predictability, or uncertainty of events (Sawamoto et al. 2000). These activations thus are likely to mediate other aspects of anticipation such as cognitive or affective aspects, including stress and anxiety.

A common finding in anticipation studies is the presence of regions of decreased activity. This phenomenon was first reported during pain anticipation in the S2 cortex in the same region that is reliably activated during painful stimulation. In the S1 cortex, the situation is probably more complex, because areas of both decreased and increased activity may coexist simultaneously within this region. Processes that might either increase or decrease activity in the sensory-motor cortices cannot be easily differentiated in most experiments, and the resulting changes in activity therefore reflect a summation of these processes. This could explain why S1 activation is not a consistent finding across studies. Coexistence of increased and decreased activities has also been repeatedly reported in anterior cingulate and medial prefrontal cortices (Porro et al. 1998, 2002; Hsieh et al. 1999; Simpson et al. 2001b), possibly related to stress or anxiety (Simpson et al. 2001a). Interestingly, these imaging findings match data from single-unit recordings in macaques (Koyama et al. 1998) and humans (Hutchison et al. 1999) that show that nociceptive neurons in the ACC also respond to pain anticipation.

BEHAVIORAL ASPECTS OF PAIN: MOTOR-RELATED ACTIVATIONS

Recent neuro-imaging studies have devoted little attention to the cerebral correlates of the motor component of the pain response. Withdrawal is a motor response to pain frequently observed in daily life situations, and, to a lesser degree, in the experimental pain conditions of neuro-imaging studies, particularly for severe pain intensities. It is well known that such painful stimuli elicit spinally mediated nociceptive withdrawal reflexes to escape from the painful stimulus (Willer 1977). This behavioral aspect of the pain response recruits a motor network that includes the vermis, right S2 and premotor cortices, and the posterior cingulate, posterior parietal, S1, and primary motor (M1) cortices, bilaterally (Peyron et al. 2001). This (motor) component, similar to the other components listed above, is likely to participate in the nociceptive matrix for pain intensities severe enough to induce a withdrawal. This motor component of the network could participate not only in motor control during severe pain and in escape behavior, but probably also in top-down control of pain processes as discussed elsewhere in this chapter.

THE PLACEBO EFFECT

The study of placebo analgesia contributes to our understanding of the interaction between higher-order cognitive systems and mechanisms involved in pain modulation. Placebo analgesia has been studied for several decades and is therefore behaviorally well described (Price 1999; Wall 1999). The 1978 finding that naloxone can partially block placebo analgesia suggests the involvement of an endogenous opioid system (Levine et al. 1978; Benedetti and Amanzio 1997). The pharmacology and mechanisms of the endogenous opioid system are beginning to be well characterized (Fields and Basbaum 1999), making it possible to unravel some of the underlying processes in placebo analgesia.

The opioid system in the brain comprises a network involving the brainstem and other subcortical structures and a cortical network (Fields and Basbaum 1999). Briefly, some divisions of the PAG have a pivotal role in the regulation of pain-related activity. The PAG receives ascending noxious input from the spinal cord and descending afferents from higher-order brain areas (e.g., the amygdala and cingulate cortex). The PAG modulates the activity of neurons in the rostral ventromedial medulla, which sends descending projections to the spinal cord involving the opioid system. Other nuclei in the pons, such as the parabrachial area, may also interact with these regions during opioid analgesia.

Opioid receptor imaging studies in humans have shown extensive concentrations of the receptors in several regions in the cortex (see, for example, Jones et al. 1991; Willoch et al. 1999), with especially high concentrations in the rACC and the anterior insula. Several functional imaging studies have shown that these same regions show increased activity when the subjects are given opioids (Firestone et al. 1996; Adler et al. 1997; Casey et al. 2000; Petrovic et al. 2002).

It may be asked why cortical regions involved in higher-order cognitive processes also are involved in opioid mechanisms. One basic hypothesis would be that cognitive processes have access to the opioid network and use it to achieve higher-order cognitive goals. The lower brainstem opioid network may then be viewed as a more primitive network. Logically, these networks should interact, especially when higher-order opioid-dependent processes use the lower-order opioid mechanisms. Such a functional interaction has been hypothesized between the ACC and the brainstem in general (Vogt et al. 1993). Such interactions should be even more important in higher-order cognitive processes that also use the endogenous opioid system, such as placebo analgesia.

These suggestions were recently tested in a PET study (Petrovic et al. 2002). Subjects were given either remifentanil (a short-acting opioid activating μ-opioid receptors), a placebo (saline), or no treatment during a pain state or a control state. They were told that both treatments were potent analgesic drugs and that one was an opioid. The subjects showed extensive activations in the anterior insula and the ACC (especially the rostral ACC) when given opioids. During placebo analgesia the subjects also activated the rostral ACC. Moreover, there was a covariation between the rACC and the lower pons/medulla (and a similar finding for the PAG) in both the opioid analgesia and placebo analgesia conditions, but no such findings were observed during untreated pain. Although no causal relationship was shown, these data suggest that the rACC may modulate the lower-order opioid network during placebo analgesia in a similar way as when opioids are given. Thus, the evidence indicates that higher-order cognitive processes can indeed interact with lower-order opioid networks.

The ACC is a region involved in many different cognitive processes (Bush et al. 2000; Miller 2000; Paus 2000). Together with the prefrontal cortex, it may allocate resources toward long-term goals when different processes are competing in the brain (Carter et al. 1999). It may therefore be suggested that the ACC is involved in the cognitively mediated regulation of opioid-mediated processes. In this light, placebo analgesia may be viewed as the result of cognitive processing in higher-order areas including the ACC.

Another region that shows increased activity during placebo analgesia is the orbitofrontal cortex (Petrovic et al. 2002). The orbitofrontal cortex is involved in relational associations between primary and secondary reinforcers, thus creating a motivational bias signal for the organism (Tremblay and Schultz 1999; Rolls 2000; O'Doherty et al. 2001; Schoenbaum and Setlow 2001). It may modulate distant activity in order to achieve this goal (Fuster 1997; Schoenbaum and Setlow 2001). Both the rACC and the orbitofrontal cortex have increased activity when pain is modulated during cognitive tasks (Rainville et al. 1999b; Petrovic et al. 2000, 2002; Bantick et al. 2002). It may therefore be hypothesized that these regions belong to a network involved in higher-order cognitive interactions with pain.

Finally, a substantial interindividual variability in the response to opioids may partly explain the differences in placebo responses (Amanzio et al. 2001). This finding is in line with the variability seen in opioid receptor availability and endogenous opioid system activity in response to pain (Zubieta et al. 2001), and with different cortical activations seen during opioid treatment in placebo responders compared to nonresponders (Petrovic et al. 2002). Thus, a possible explanation to why some subjects respond well to a placebo while others do not may depend on the underlying biology of the endogenous opioid system.

ACKNOWLEDGMENTS

The authors' studies reported in this chapter were supported by the Swedish Research Council and the Petrus and Augusta Hedlunds Foundation, the Projet Hospitaliers de Recherche Clinique 1999–2002, and the Institut UPSA de la Douleur.

REFERENCES

Adler LJ, Gyulai FE, Diehl DJ, et al. Regional brain activity changes associated with fentanyl analgesia elucidated by positron emission tomography. *Anesth Analg* 1997; 84:120–126.

Amanzio M, Pollo A, Maggi G, Benedetti F. Response variability to analgesics: a role for non-specific activation of endogenous opioids. *Pain* 2001; 90:205–215.

Bantick SJ, Wise RG, Ploghaus A, et al. Imaging how attention modulates pain in humans using functional MRI. *Brain* 2002; 125:310–319.

Bench CJ, Frith CD, Grasby, et al. Investigations of the functional anatomy of attention using the Stroop test. *Neuropsychologia* 1993; 31:907–922.

Benedetti F, Amanzio M. The neurobiology of placebo analgesia: from endogenous opioids to cholecystokinin. *Prog Neurobiol* 1997; 52:109–125.

Bornhovd K, Quante M, Glauche V, et al. Painful stimuli evoke different stimulus-response functions in the amygdala, prefrontal, insula and somatosensory cortex: a single-trial fMRI study. *Brain* 2002; 125:1326–1336.

Bush G, Luu P, Posner MI. Cognitive and emotional influences in anterior cingulate cortex. *Trends Cogn Sci* 2000; 4:215–222.

Bushnell MC, Duncan GH, Hofbauer, et al. Pain perception: is there a role for primary somatosensory cortex? *Proc Natl Acad Sci USA* 1999; 96:7705–7709.

Carlsson K, Petrovic P, Skare S, Petersson KM, Ingvar M. Tickling expectations: neural processing in anticipation of a sensory stimulus. *J Cogn Neurosci* 2000; 12:691–703.

Carter CS, Botvinick MM, Cohen JD. The contribution of the anterior cingulate cortex to executive processes in cognition. *Rev Neurosci* 1999; 10:49–57.

Casey KL, Svensson P, Morrow TJ, et al. Selective opiate modulation of nociceptive processing in the human brain. *J Neurophysiol* 2000; 84:525–533.

Chua P, Krams M, Toni I, Passingham R, Dolan R. A functional anatomy of anticipatory anxiety. *Neuroimage* 1999; 9:563–571.

Coghill RC, Sang CN, Maisog JM, Iadarola MJ. Pain intensity processing within the human brain: a bilateral, distributed mechanism. *J Neurophysiol* 1999; 82:1934–1943.

Coghill RC, Gilron I, Iadarola MJ. Hemispheric lateralization of somatosensory processing. *J Neurophysiol* 2001; 85:2602–2612.

Corbetta M, Miezin FM, Dobmeyer S, Shulman GL, Petersen SE. Selective and divided attention during visual discriminations of shape, color, and speed: functional anatomy by positron emission tomography. *J Neurosci* 1991; 11:2383–23402.

Craig AD, Reiman EM, Evans A, Bushnell MC. Functional imaging of an illusion of pain. *Nature* 1996; 384:258–260.

Craig AD, Chen K, Bandy D, Reiman EM. Thermosensory activation of insular cortex. *Nat Neurosci* 2000; 3:184–190.

Danziger N, Fournier E, Bouhassira D, et al. Different strategies of modulation can be operative during hypnotic analgesia: a neurophysiological study. *Pain* 1998; 75:85–92.

Davis KD, Taylor SJ, Crawley AP, Wood ML, Mikulis DJ. Functional MRI of pain and attention-related activations in the human cingulate cortex. *J Neurophysiol* 1997; 77:3370–3380.

Derbyshire SW. Exploring the pain "neuromatrix." *Curr Rev Pain* 2000; 4:467–477.

Derbyshire SW, Jones AK, Gyulai F, et al. Pain processing during three levels of noxious stimulation produces differential patterns of central activity. *Pain* 1997; 73:431–445.

Drevets WC, Burton H, Videen TO, et al. Blood flow changes in human somatosensory cortex during anticipated stimulation. *Nature* 1995; 373:249–252.

Fields H, Basbaum A. Central nervous system mechanisms of pain modulation. In: Wall PD, Melzack R (Eds). *Textbook of Pain*. Churchill Livingstone, 1999, pp 309–329.

Firestone LL, Gyulai F, Mintun M, et al. Human brain activity response to fentanyl imaged by positron emission tomography. *Anesth Analg* 1996; 82:1247–1251.

Frankenstein UN, Richter W, McIntyre MC, Remy F. Distraction modulates anterior cingulate gyrus activations during the cold pressor test. *Neuroimage* 2001; 14:827–836.

Fredrikson M, Wik G, Fischer H, Andersson J. Affective and attentive neural networks in humans: a PET study of Pavlovian conditioning. *Neuroreport* 1995; 7:97–101.

Frot M, Mauguiere F. Operculo-insular responses to nociceptive skin stimulation in humans. A review of the literature. *Neurophysiol Clin* 1999; 29:401–410.

Frot M, Mauguiere F. Dual representation of pain in the operculo-insular cortex in humans. *Brain* 2003; 126:438–450.

Frot M, Rambaud L, Guenot M, Mauguiere F. Intracortical recordings of early pain-related CO_2-laser evoked potentials in the human second somatosensory (SII) area. *Clin Neurophysiol* 1999; 110:133–145.

Fuster JM. *The Prefrontal Cortex: Anatomy, Physiology, and Neuropsychology of the Frontal Lobe*. New York: Lippincott-Raven, 1997, pp 333.

Garcia-Larrea L, Peyron R, Laurent B, Mauguiere F. Association and dissociation between laser-evoked potentials and pain perception. *Neuroreport* 1997; 8:3785–3789.

Hofbauer RK, Rainville P, Duncan GH, Bushnell MC. Cortical representation of the sensory dimension of pain. *J Neurophysiol* 2001; 86:402–411.

Hsieh JC, Stone-Elander S. Ingvar M. Anticipatory coping of pain expressed in the human anterior cingulate cortex: a positron emission tomography study. *Neurosci Lett* 1999; 262:61–64.

Hutchison WD, Davis KD, Lozano AM. Tasker RR, Dostrovsky JO. Pain-related neurons in the human cingulate cortex. *Nat Neurosci* 1999; 2:403–405.

Jones AK, Qi LY, Fujirawa T, et al. In vivo distribution of opioid receptors in man in relation to the cortical projections of the medial and lateral pain systems measured with positron emission tomography. *Neurosci Lett* 1991; 126:25–28.

Jones AKP, Derbyshire SWG. Cortical and thalamic imaging in normal volunteers and patients with chronic pain. In: Besson JM, Guilbaud G, Ollat H (Eds). *Forebrain Areas Involved in Pain Processing*. Paris: John Libbey Eurotext, 1995, pp 229–238.

Kenshalo DR Jr, Chudler EH, Anton F, Dubner R. SI nociceptive neurons participate in the encoding process by which monkeys perceive the intensity of noxious thermal stimulation. *Brain Res* 1988; 454:378–382.

Kiernan BD, Dane JR, Phillips LH, Price DD. Hypnotic analgesia reduces R-III nociceptive reflex: further evidence concerning the multifactorial nature of hypnotic analgesia. *Pain* 1995; 60:39–47.

Koyama T, Tanaka YZ, Mikami A. Nociceptive neurons in the macaque anterior cingulate activate during anticipation of pain. *Neuroreport* 1998; 9:2663–2667.

Levine JD, Gordon NC, Fields HL. The mechanism of placebo analgesia. *Lancet* 1978; 2:654–657.

Miller EK. The prefrontal cortex and cognitive control. *Nat Rev Neurosci* 2000; 1:59–65.

Miron D, Duncan GH, Bushnell MC. Effects of attention on the intensity and unpleasantness of thermal pain. *Pain* 1989; 39:345–352.

Murtha S, Chertkow H, Beauregard M, Evans A. The neural substrate of picture naming. *J Cogn Neurosci* 1999; 11:399–423.

Niebur E, Hsiao SS, Johnson KO. Synchrony: a neuronal mechanism for attentional selection? *Curr Opin Neurobiol* 2002; 12:190–194.

Nobre AC, Sebestyen GN, Gitelman DR, et al. Functional localization of the system for visuospatial attention using positron emission tomography. *Brain* 1997; 120(Pt 3):515–533.

O'Doherty J, Kringelbach ML, Rolls ET, Hornak J, Andrews C. Abstract reward and punishment representations in the human orbitofrontal cortex. *Nat Neurosci* 2001; 4:95–102.

Pardo JV, Pardo PJ, Janer KW, Raichle ME. The anterior cingulate cortex mediates processing selection in the Stroop attentional conflict paradigm. *Proc Natl Acad Sci USA* 1990; 87:256–259.

Paus T. Functional anatomy of arousal and attention systems in the human brain. *Prog Brain Res* 2000; 126:65–77.

Paus T. Primate anterior cingulate cortex: where motor control, drive and cognition interface. *Nat Rev Neurosci* 2001; 2:417–424.

Paus T, Koski L, Caramanos Z, Westbury C. Regional differences in the effects of task difficulty and motor output on blood flow response in the human anterior cingulate cortex: a review of 107 PET activation studies. *Neuroreport* 1998; 9:R37–47.

Petrovic P, Ingvar M, Stone-Elander S, et al. A PET activation study of dynamic mechanical allodynia in patients with mononeuropathy. *Pain* 1999; 83:459–470.

Petrovic P, Petersson KM, Ghatan PH, Stone-Elander S, Ingvar M. Pain-related cerebral activation is altered by a distracting cognitive task. *Pain* 2000; 85:19–30.

Petrovic P, Kalso E, Petersson KM, Ingvar M. Placebo and opioid analgesia—imaging a shared neuronal network. *Science* 2002; 295:1737–1740.

Peyron R, Garcia-Larrea L, Gregoire MC, et al. Allodynia after lateral-medullary (Wallenberg) infarct: a PET study. *Brain* 1998; 121:345–356.

Peyron R, Garcia-Larrea L, Gregoire MC, et al. Haemodynamic brain responses to acute pain in humans: sensory and attentional networks. *Brain* 1999; 122:1765–1780.

Peyron R, Garcia-Larrea L, Gregoire MC, et al. Parietal and cingulate processes in central pain: a combined positron emission tomography (PET) and functional magnetic resonance imaging (fMRI) study of an unusual case. *Pain* 2000a; 84:77–87.

Peyron R, Laurent B, Garcia-Larrea L. Functional imaging of brain responses to pain: a review and meta-analysis. *Neurophysiol Clin* 2000b; 30:263–288.

Peyron R, Schneider F, Giraux P, et al. Brain responses to thermal pain in normals: a comparison of PET and 1-Tesla fMRI results. *Proceedings of the Society for Neuroscience Meeting, New Orleans.* Society for Neuroscience, 2000c.

Peyron R, Jehl JL, Schneider F, et al. Pain-related cerebral responses evoked by the nociceptive flexion reflex (RIII) in man: fMRI study. *Neuroimage* 2001; 13:S1237.

Peyron R, Frot M, Schneider F, et al. Role of operculoinsular cortices in human pain processing: converging evidence from PET, fMRI, dipole modeling, and intracerebral recordings of evoked potentials. *Neuroimage* 2002; 17:1336–1346.

Phan KL, Wager T, Taylor SF, Liberzon I. Functional neuroanatomy of emotion: a meta-analysis of emotion activation studies in PET and fMRI. *Neuroimage* 2002; 16:331–348.

Picard N, Strick PL. Imaging the premotor areas. *Curr Opin Neurobiol* 2001; 11:663–672.

Ploghaus A, Tracey I, Gati JS, et al. Dissociating pain from its anticipation in the human brain. *Science* 1999; 284:1979–1981.

Ploghaus A, Narain C, Beckmann, et al. Exacerbation of pain by anxiety is associated with activity in a hippocampal network. *J Neurosci* 2001; 21:9896–9903.

Ploner M, Freund HJ, Schnitzler A. Pain affect without pain sensation in a patient with a postcentral lesion. *Pain* 1999; 81:211–214.

Porro CA, Cettolo V, Francescato MP, Baraldi P. Temporal and intensity coding of pain in human cortex. *J Neurophysiol* 1998; 80:3312–3320.

Porro CA, Baraldi P, Pagnoni G, et al. Does anticipation of pain affect cortical nociceptive systems? *J Neurosci* 2002; 22:3206–3214.

Portas CM, Rees G, Howseman AM, et al. A specific role for the thalamus in mediating the interaction of attention and arousal in humans. *J Neurosci* 1998; 18:8979–8989.

Posner MI. Attention: the mechanisms of consciousness. *Proc Natl Acad Sci USA* 1994; 91:7398–73403.

Price DD. Hypnotic analgesia: psychological and neural mechanisms. In: Barber J (Ed). *Hypnosis and Suggestions in the Treatment of Pain.* New York: Norton, 1996, pp 67–84.

Price DD. Placebo analgesia. In: Price DD (Ed). *Psychological Mechanisms of Pain and Analgesia,* Progress in Pain Research and Management, Vol. 15. Seattle: IASP Press, 1999, pp 155–181.

Rainville P. Brain mechanisms of pain affect and pain modulation. *Curr Opin Neurobiol* 2002; 12:195–204.

Rainville P, Duncan GH, Price DD, Carrier B, Bushnell MC. Pain affect encoded in human anterior cingulate but not somatosensory cortex. *Science* 1997; 277:968–971.

Rainville P, Carrier B, Hofbauer RK, Bushnell MC, Duncan GH. Dissociation of sensory and affective dimensions of pain using hypnotic modulation. *Pain* 1999a; 82:159–171.

Rainville P, Hofbauer RK, Paus T, et al. Cerebral mechanisms of hypnotic induction and suggestion. *J Cogn Neurosci* 1999b; 11:110–125.

Rainville P, Hofbauer RK, Bushnell MC, Duncan GH, Price DD. Hypnosis modulates activity in brain structures involved in the regulation of consciousness. *J Cogn Neurosci* 2002; 14:887–901.

Rolls ET. The orbitofrontal cortex and reward. *Cereb Cortex* 2000; 10:284–294.

Sawamoto N, Honda M, Okada T, et al. Expectation of pain enhances responses to nonpainful somatosensory stimulation in the anterior cingulate cortex and parietal operculum/posterior insula: an event-related functional magnetic resonance imaging study. *J Neurosci* 2000; 20:7438–7445.

Schoenbaum G, Setlow B. Integrating orbitofrontal cortex into prefrontal theory: common processing themes across species and subdivisions. *Learn Mem* 2001; 8:134–147.

Simpson JR Jr, Drevets WC, Snyder AZ, Gusnard DA, Raichle ME. Emotion-induced changes in human medial prefrontal cortex: II. During anticipatory anxiety. *Proc Natl Acad Sci USA* 2001a; 98:688–693.

Simpson JR Jr, Snyder A, Gusnard DA, Raichle ME. Emotion-induced changes in human medial prefrontal cortex: I. During cognitive task performance. *Proc Natl Acad Sci USA* 2001b; 98:683–687.

Steinmetz PN, Roy A, Fitzgerald PJ. et al. Attention modulates synchronized neuronal firing in primate somatosensory cortex. *Nature* 2000; 404:187–190.

Timmermann L, Ploner M, Haucke K, et al. Differential coding of pain intensity in the human primary and secondary somatosensory cortex. *J Neurophysiol* 2001; 86:1499–1503.

Tracey I, Ploghaus A, Gati JS, et al. Imaging attentional modulation of pain in the periaqueductal gray in humans. *J Neurosci* 2002; 22:2748–2752.

Tremblay L, Schultz W. Relative reward preference in primate orbitofrontal cortex. *Nature* 1999; 398:704–708.

Vogt BA, Sikes RW, Vogt LJ. Anterior cingulate cortex and the medial pain system. In: Vogt BA, Gabriel M (Eds). *Neurobiology of Cingulate Cortex and Limbic Thalamus: A Comprehensive Handbook.* Boston: Birkhäuser, 1993, pp 313–344.

Wall PD. The placebo and the placebo response. In: Wall PD, Melzack R (Eds.). *Textbook of Pain*. Churchill Livingstone, 1999, pp 1419–1430.

Willer JC. Comparative study of perceived pain and nociceptive flexion reflex in man. *Pain* 1977; 3:69–80.

Willoch F, Tolle TR, Wester, HJ, et al. Central pain after pontine infarction is associated with changes in opioid receptor binding: a PET study with ^{11}C-diprenorphine. *AJNR Am J Neuroradiol* 1999; 20:686–690.

Zubieta JK, Smith YR, Bueller JA, et al. Regional mu opioid receptor regulation of sensory and affective dimensions of pain. *Science* 2001; 293:311–315.

Correspondence to: Roland Peyron, MD, PhD, Department of Neurology, Bellevue Hospital, Boulevard Pasteur, 42055 St Etienne, France. Email: Roland.Peyron@univ-st-etienne.fr.

Proceedings of the 10th World Congress on Pain,
Progress in Pain Research and Management, Vol. 24,
edited by Jonathan O. Dostrovsky, Daniel B. Carr,
and Martin Koltzenburg, IASP Press, Seattle, © 2003.

25

Functional Magnetic Resonance Imaging of Capsaicin-Induced Thermal Hyperalgesia

Jonathan C.W. Brooks,[a,b] William E. Bimson,[b] Neil Roberts,[b] and Turo J. Nurmikko[a]

[a]Pain Research Institute, Clinical Sciences Centre, and [b]Magnetic Resonance and Image Analysis Research Centre, University of Liverpool, Liverpool, United Kingdom

Most clinical pain is associated with increased sensitivity to external stimuli. In both inflammatory and neuropathic conditions, pain may be evoked by touch, pressure, movement, heat, or cold. Essentially, these phenomena represent reduced thresholds for eliciting pain and are termed allodynia, when pain is caused by innocuous stimuli, and hyperalgesia, when an exaggerated response follows application of a normally painful stimulus. Several animal models of neuropathic pain have been developed to investigate these pain syndromes (Devor and Seltzer 1999). Recent studies have described human pain models (Liu et al. 1998; Petersen and Rowbotham 1999) that share some characteristics of neuropathic pain and thus provide an opportunity to study clinical pain under controlled conditions. Our previous functional magnetic resonance imaging (fMRI) studies used intrinsically painful stimuli (thermal pain applied via a contact thermode) and healthy subjects, and thus primarily address physiological pain (Brooks et al. 2002). Results from these studies do not necessarily tell us much about clinical pain, in which multiple functional alterations occur in central and peripheral pain-signaling pathways.

Simone and colleagues (1989) addressed the need for a human pain model by injecting capsaicin solution intradermally to produce regions of primary and secondary hyperalgesia. This approach allows observation of areas of mechanical allodynia and hyperalgesia to punctate stimuli (Liu et al. 1998). Three previous neuroimaging studies (Iadarola et al. 1998; Baron et al. 1999; Witting et al. 2001) have used this technique to elicit mechanical allodynia, but with inconsistent results. These discrepancies may be related to differences in the pain levels evoked by stimulation, prior exposure to the capsaicin stimulus, type of pain investigated (e.g., dynamic versus punctate allodynia), or variability in the delay between capsaicin injection and recording functional data. We used the capsaicin model of Petersen and Rowbotham (1999) to investigate whether heat hyperalgesia modifies patterns of pain-related brain activity and to address some of the technical difficulties of previous studies. We sensitized skin with capsaicin cream and used a thermode to produce heat hyperalgesia and evoke physiological pain. We measured brain activity by blood oxygenation-level-dependent (BOLD) fMRI. This chapter discusses the relation between the data we obtained and possible mechanisms for central sensitization.

METHODS

Sixteen healthy subjects (six female) were recruited, screened for the presence of neurological disease, and given a general health check. All subjects were right-handed and between 20 and 37 years of age. The local ethics committee approved the study, and subjects consented to thermal stimulation and capsaicin application to the thenar eminence of the right hand.

EXPERIMENT 1: PHYSIOLOGICAL HEAT PAIN

We evaluated heat pain thresholds prior to fMRI investigation. Thermal stimuli were applied using a 3 × 3 cm^2 Peltier thermode adapted for use in the MRI scanner. Before scanning, we recorded for each subject the temperature giving rise to a visual analogue scale (VAS) rating of between 5 and 7 (of 10), corresponding to moderate to severe pain. Subjects were blind to the applied temperature of the thermode. This temperature (T_{PAIN}) was then used in the first part of the fMRI study.

We used a 1.5-Tesla scanner. Subjects were placed in the standard quadrature head coil, with the head restrained by suitable placement of foam padding. After acquiring localizer images, we placed 24 axial oblique slices, each 6 mm thick, parallel to the anterior-posterior commissure line for functional imaging. To obtain fMRI data, we used a gradient echo echo-planar imaging sequence with 64 by 64 matrix, 19-cm field of view, echo time/repetition time (TE/TR) = 40/3000 ms, and flip angle of 90°.

The thermode was attached to the subject's right palm, and an MRI-compatible potentiometer was placed in the left hand to provide on-line VAS rating of pain experience. VAS data were recorded with an analogue-to-digital converter connected to a laptop computer and in-house software, and the relative position of the potentiometer was used to generate a value between 0 and 100 on a linear VAS. The minimum position of the VAS was labeled with "no pain" and the maximum value labeled with "worst pain imaginable." We used a projector to back-project the VAS onto a screen visible to subjects in the scanner room.

We applied stimuli in a block design (Brooks et al. 2002) with an interstimulus interval of 30 seconds. Experiments commenced with a baseline epoch (stimulus temperature 35°C), followed by 9 seconds of painful stimulation (at the predetermined value, T_{PAIN}, the pain epoch). Immediately after stimulation the VAS was displayed on the screen for 9 seconds, followed by a 12-second baseline epoch. Experiments consisted of 10 cycles of alternating rest, stimulation, and VAS rating, for a total scan time of 300 seconds and acquisition of 100 brain volumes.

EXPERIMENT 2: EXPERIMENTAL THERMAL HYPERALGESIA

Following the first experiment, we removed the subject from the scanner and administered capsaicin (Petersen and Rowbotham 1999). Briefly, the thenar eminence of the right hand was first stimulated with the thermode, which was maintained at a constant 45°C for 5 minutes. Following thermal stimulation, 0.075% capsaicin was applied topically to the same area and covered with a Tegaderm dressing. The dressing remained in place for approximately 45 minutes, after which the capsaicin was removed and the skin cleaned. Subsequently, we reassessed thermal pain thresholds with the subject blind to the applied temperature. We noted the new temperature giving rise to a VAS rating of between 5 and 7 (T_{CAPS}), and then returned the subject to the scanner.

We then repeated fMRI as in the first part of the experiment, with one modification, an applied temperature during the pain epochs of T_{CAPS}.

DATA ANALYSIS

Statistical parametric mapping software allowed us to correct functional imaging data for motion. This step involved a six-parameter rigid body transformation. Subsequently data were normalized using a 12-parameter affine transformation, and smoothed using a 9-mm full-width half-maximum gaussian kernel. We used the general linear model approach to model changes in BOLD signal intensity (Worsley et al. 1992; Friston et al. 1994; Worsley et al. 1996), and included motion parameters as covariates of no interest. We determined representative group activation maps for pre- and postcapsaicin scans by using a random effects model (one-sample t test) and reported data at an uncorrected $P < 0.001$. A region of interest (ROI) analysis determined the specificity of observed difference in group activation maps (Smith et al. 2000). Using bilateral ROIs previously defined in the anterior/middle/posterior insula (Brooks et al. 2002) and in the prefrontal cortex (Iadarola et al. 1998; Witting et al. 2001) and parietal cortex (Witting et al. 2001), we recorded regional activity in response to stimulus lateralization and experimental condition (precapsaicin versus postcapsaicin). We analyzed mean signal amplitudes from each of the ROIs by using a repeated-measures general linear model approach in SPSS software, and defined within-subject factors for "experiment" (pre- versus postcapsaicin), "side" (left versus right hemisphere), and "location" (corresponding to the five different ROIs). A significance level of $P < 0.05$ was adopted.

RESULTS

The average temperature T_{PAIN} used for precapsaicin fMRI was 47.2°C (SD = 2.4), whereas the average postcapsaicin temperature T_{CAPS} was 44.9°C (3.1). Despite a significant difference between T_{PAIN} and T_{CAPS} (paired t test, $P = 0.01$), psychophysics data acquired outside the scanner demonstrated remarkable similarity between VAS scores (pre = 63, SD = 8; and post = 63 [7], paired t test, $P = 0.92$). Online recording of VAS data confirmed this finding (pre = 60 [16] and post = 62 [15], $P = 0.77$). No subject reported any significant spontaneous pain following application of capsaicin cream. The main change caused by capsaicin sensitization was the generation of thermal hyperalgesia, as evidenced by the significant differences in T_{PAIN} and T_{CAPS}, while pain ratings remained constant.

Fig. 1 presents the different patterns of brain activity following thermal stimulation pre- and postcapsaicin. Postcapsaicin, we observed increased activity bilaterally in the prefrontal cortex and ipsilateral (right) parietal regions compared to noxious thermal stimulation prior to capsaicin treatment. The specific locations, Brodmann areas (BAs), and Talairach coordinates of activated brain regions are given in Table I. A repeated-measures general linear model and ROI data revealed significant interactions between "experiment" (pre- versus postcapsaicin) and "location" (of the ROIs), and between "side" (hemisphere) and "location," but not between "side" and

Table I
Description and Talairach coordinates for the main regions of activity observed following physiological pain (precapsaicin) and after capsaicin sensitization (postcapsaicin)

Region	Talairach Coordinates X (R-L)	Y (A-P)	Z (I-S)	Brodmann Area
Precapsaicin				
Anterior insula	36	18	7	
Anterior insula	–33	6	–1	
Cingulate gyrus	3	–28	29	23
Medial frontal gyrus	3	17	52	6
Inferior frontal gyrus	–45	–1	30	44
Middle frontal gyrus	51	8	47	6/8
Inferior parietal lobule	36	–45	46	40
Cerebellum	–27	–60	–25	
Cerebellum	36	–68	–19	
Thalamus	0	–3	8	
Superior frontal gyrus	33	48	28	9
Postcapsaicin				
Anterior insula	39	20	–9	
Anterior insula	–39	20	–6	
Middle frontal gyrus	42	47	12	10
Middle frontal gyrus	–45	45	17	46
Inferior parietal lobule	42	–44	55	40
Cingulate gyrus	3	17	41	32
Cerebellum	–12	–80	–24	

Note: Identification of activated regions was based on the stereotactic atlas of Talairach and Tournoux (1988). Only activated regions with a cluster size greater than 10 voxels are reported. Brodmann areas are given where appropriate.

"experiment." Paired *t* tests allowed further comparisons (Table II). The insular ROIs showed no significant difference between activation pre- and postcapsaicin, whereas the prefrontal and parietal ROIs were significantly more active postcapsaicin. In addition, we observed significant rightward asymmetry of the BOLD response in the anterior insula and prefrontal cortex (postcapsaicin). The only region exhibiting leftward asymmetry was the posterior insula, as we have previously reported (Brooks et al. 2002). Fig. 2 shows the average BOLD signal amplitude recorded from each subject for those regions exhibiting a dependence on capsaicin sensitization, namely, the prefrontal and parietal ROIs.

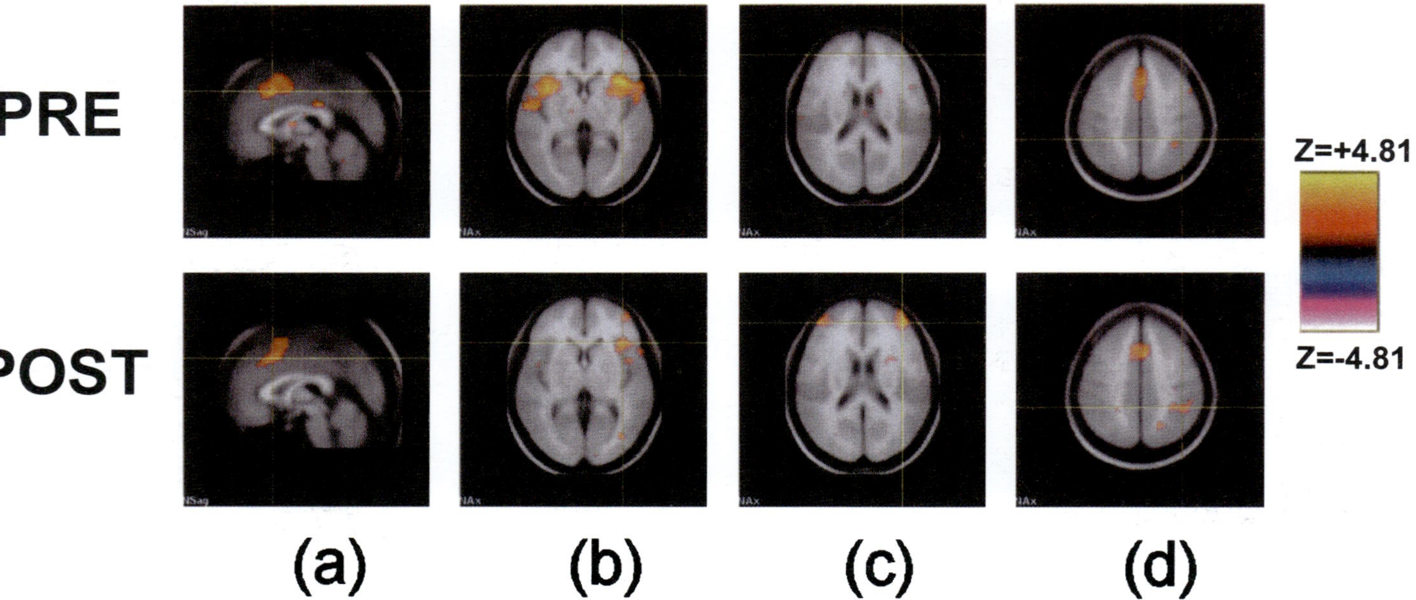

Fig. 1. Sagittal and axial sections through the Montreal Neurological Institute average brain, with pre- and postcapsaicin activation maps superimposed. Activations in four main areas are shown: (a) anterior cingulate gyrus, (b) anterior insula, (c) prefrontal cortex, and (d) parietal lobe. Activations in (c) and (d) are only associated with postcapsaicin activation maps. The activation maps correspond to the output from a second-level analysis, thresholded at an uncorrected $P < 0.001$. Please note that the stimulus was delivered to the right hand and that the right side of the figures is the right side of the brain.

Table II
Results of paired *t* tests for each region of interest, examining the main effects of "experiment" (pre- versus postcapsaicin) and "side" (left versus right hemisphere)

Region of Interest	"Experiment"		"Side"	
	Right	Left	Pre	Post
Anterior insula	0.579	0.986	**0.025** (R>L)	**0.034** (R>L)
Middle insula	0.620	0.780	0.932	0.874
Posterior insula	0.732	0.900	**0.043** (L>R)	0.107
Prefrontal	**0.017**	0.353	0.150	**0.003** (R>L)
Parietal	**0.049**	**0.016**	0.188	0.492

Note: In the column labeled "Experiment," "right" (ipsilateral to stimulus) and "left" refer to laterality of the ROI, while in the column labeled "Side" comparisons were made between left and right ROIs, and are distinguished by the experimental condition during data collection, i.e., pre- or postcapsaicin. Where a significant asymmetry of BOLD response was found, the nature of the asymmetry is indicated. Capsaicin sensitization has the greatest effect in the prefrontal and parietal ROIs of the right hemisphere. Asymmetrical BOLD response was found primarily in the anterior insula, which is in keeping with neuroanatomical data (Craig 1998) and our previous study (Brooks et al. 2002). Activity within posterior insula is contralateral to the stimulation site for precapsaicin stimulation only, while for the prefrontal cortex, rightward asymmetry was observed following capsaicin sensitization. Significant findings ($P < 0.05$) are shown in boldface type.

DISCUSSION

Previous experiments using intradermal capsaicin injection have demonstrated similar patterns of activity to those observed in the current study. Using positron emission tomography (PET), Iadarola et al. (1998) imaged spontaneous pain caused by capsaicin injection and compared it to activation maps obtained by light brushing of the treated area after the injection pain had subsided. Their subjects reported experiencing allodynic pain to light brushing, which was associated with activation across the pain matrix. However, the main difference between brush-evoked touch and allodynia conditions was bilateral activation of the superior frontal gyrus. Baron et al. (1999) reported similar findings after using fMRI to study mechanical allodynia, and in a study using PET, Witting et al. (2001) found that the main difference between allodynic and capsaicin pain was increased activity in the contralateral posterior parietal cortex (BA 7). A PET study of mechanical allodynia in patients with mononeuropathy (Petrovic et al. 1999) found the greatest blood flow differences in the primary somatosensory cortex, but also found increased blood flow in the contralateral posterior parietal cortex (BA 7). Additional evidence supporting this observation comes from a PET study of patients with lateral-medullary (Wallenberg) infarct

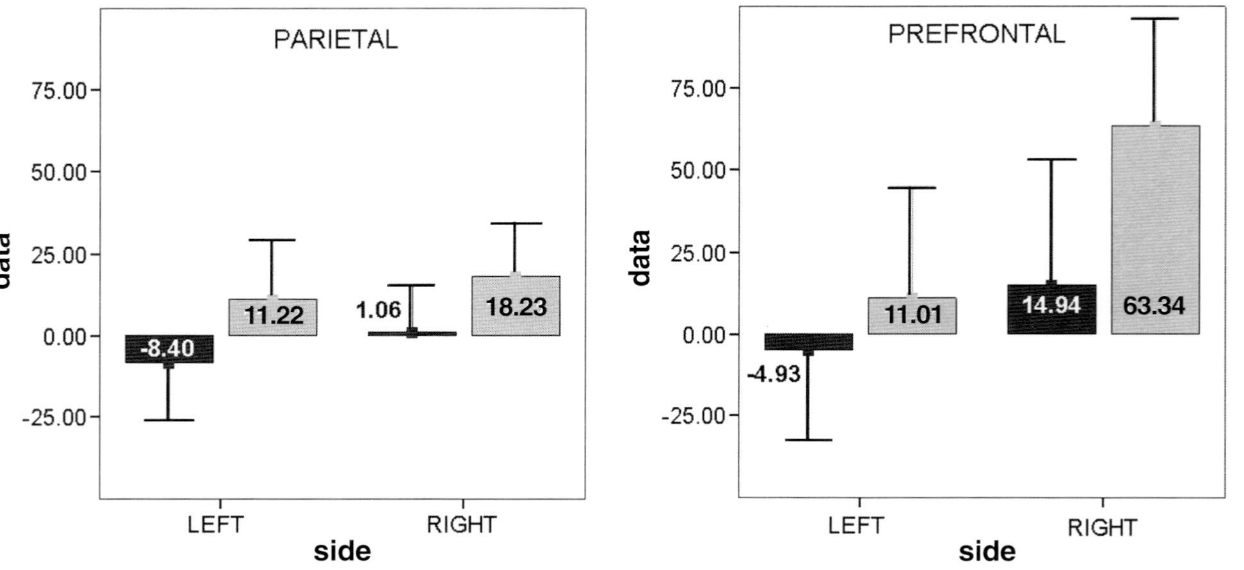

Fig. 2. Regions of interest (ROI) analysis for parietal (A) and frontal (B) activation. By defining ROIs in prefrontal and parietal cortices we were able to extract the amplitude of the BOLD fMRI response for each region. Bar graphs show plots of mean activation for each ROI (in either the right [ipsilateral] or left hemisphere) and for each condition (pre- or postcapsaicin). Error bars represent 2 SEM. For each pair of bars the left (dark gray) and right (light gray) bar corresponds to pre- and postcapsaicin experiments, respectively. Postcapsaicin, a significant increase in activation was found for left and right parietal ROIs and for the right prefrontal ROI, which was the largest activation increase. *P* values were calculated using a two-tailed paired *t* test.

(Peyron et al. 1998). They showed increased activation in the inferior parietal cortex during a comparison of mechanical/cold allodynia to identical stimulation of the unaffected side.

CONCLUSIONS

We used a model of neuropathic pain, which synergistically combines mild warming of the skin and topical application of 0.075% capsaicin ointment to produce cutaneous heat hyperalgesia, and fMRI to demonstrate significant modulation of the cortical pain network. When compared to activation maps produced by an intrinsically painful hot stimulus, the brain response to heat hyperalgesia showed significantly increased activity in ipsilateral prefrontal (BA 10) and bilateral parietal (BA 40) regions. By recording VAS pain levels inside and outside the scanner, we were able to discount the possibility that the observed change in brain activation was due to altered subjective pain experienced postcapsaicin. The similarity between the pattern of activity recorded in this study and those previously reported in experimental studies on hyperalgesia and clinical case studies suggests that these areas may be specifically involved in processing of altered sensory input, such as that seen after tissue damage.

REFERENCES

Baron R, Baron Y, Disbrow E, Roberts T. Brain processing of capsaicin-induced secondary hyperalgesia. *Neurology* 1999; 53:548–557.

Brooks J, Nurmikko T, Bimson W, et al. fMRI of thermal pain: effects of stimulus laterality and attention. *Neuroimage* 2002; 15:293–301.

Craig AD. A new version of thalamic disinhibition hypothesis of central pain. *Pain Forum* 1998; 7:1–14.

Devor M, Seltzer Z. Pathophysiology of damaged nerves in relation to chronic pain. In: Wall P, Melzack R (Eds). *Textbook of Pain*, 4th ed. Edinburgh: Churchill Livingstone, 1999, pp 129–164.

Friston K, Worsley K, Frakowiak R, et al. Assessing the significance of focal activations using their spatial extent. *Hum Brain Map* 1994; 1:214–220.

Iadarola M, Berman K, Zeffiro T, et al. Neural activation during acute capsaicin-evoked pain and allodynia assessed with PET. *Brain* 1998; 121:931–947.

Liu M, Max M, Robinovitz E, et al. The human capsaicin model of allodynia and hyperalgesia: sources of variability and methods for reduction. *J Pain Symptom Manage* 1998; 16:10–20.

Petersen K, Rowbotham M. A new human experimental pain model: the heat/capsaicin sensitization model. *Neuroreport* 1999; 10:1511–1516.

Petrovic P, Ingvar M, Stone-Elander S, et al. A PET activation study of dynamic mechanical allodynia in patients with mononeuropathy. *Pain* 1999; 83:459–470.

Peyron R, Garcia-Larrea L, Gregoire M, et al. Allodynia after lateral-medullary (Wallenberg) infarct. A PET study. *Brain* 1998; 121:345–356.

Simone D, Baumann T, LaMotte R. Dose-dependent pain and mechanical hyperalgesia in humans after intradermal injection of capsaicin. *Pain* 1989; 38:99–107.

Smith A, Scott-Samuel N, Singh K. Global motion adaptation. *Vision Res* 2000; 40:1069–1075.

Talairach J, Tournoux P. *Co-planar Stereotaxic Atlas of the Human Brain*. New York: Thieme Medical Publishers, 1988.

Witting N, Kupers R, Svensson P, et al. Experimental brush-evoked allodynia activates posterior parietal cortex. *Neurology* 2001; 57:1817–1824.

Worsley K, Evans A, Marrett S, Neelin P. A three-dimensional statistical analysis for CBF activation studies in human brain. *J Cereb Blood Flow Metab* 1992; 12:900–918.

Worsley K, Marrett S, Neelin P, et al. A unified statistical approach for determining significant signals in images of cerebral activation. *Hum Brain Map* 1996; 4:58–73.

Correspondence to: Jonathan Brooks, PhD, Department of Human Anatomy and Genetics, University of Oxford, South Parks Road, Oxford OX1 3QX, United Kingdom. Tel: 44-(0)1865-282675; Fax: 44-(0)1865-272183; email: jonathan.brooks@anat.ox.ac.uk.

Proceedings of the 10th World Congress on Pain,
Progress in Pain Research and Management, Vol. 24,
edited by Jonathan O. Dostrovsky, Daniel B. Carr, and
Martin Koltzenburg, IASP Press, Seattle, © 2003.

26

Anesthetic Effect of Barbiturates Microinjected into the Brainstem: Neuroanatomy

Inna Sukhotinsky, Vladimir Zalkind, and Marshall Devor

Department of Cell and Animal Biology, Institute of Life Sciences, Hebrew University of Jerusalem, Israel

Bilaterally symmetrical microinjection of minute quantities of the barbiturate general anesthetic pentobarbital into a restricted region of the rat brainstem tegmentum induces a state of general anesthesia (Devor and Zalkind 2001). Characteristics include loss of postural support and the righting reflex, failure to respond to both noxious stimuli (antinociception) and strong acoustic and visual stimuli, and synchronization of the cortical electroencephalogram (EEG). Barbiturate microinjections outside this locus failed to produce anesthesia. We refer to this region as the mesopontine tegmental anesthesia area (MPTA). The anesthetic effect of pentobarbital was reproduced by other molecules that enhance GABAergic neurotransmission, including the barbiturate phenobarbital and the neurosteroids alphaxalone/alphadolone (Alphathesin, Glaxo), and also by the direct $GABA_A$-receptor ($GABA_A$-R) selective agonist muscimol. To better understand the mechanisms by which barbiturates affect posture, nociception, and arousal, we have begun to investigate the neuroanatomical connections of the MPTA and its immunohistochemical fingerprint, with a focus on GABAergic circuitry.

METHODS

To trace neuroanatomical connections of the MPTA, we microinjected anterograde and retrograde tracers into the MPTA region in adult male Sabra strain rats (275–500 g). Biotinylated dextran amine (BDA, 10%, injection volume 10–30 nL) was used to trace anterograde connections. The retrograde tracer was horseradish peroxidase conjugated to either wheat germ agglutinin (WGA-HRP, 5%, injection volume 10–20 nL) or cholera toxin β subunit (CTB-HRP, 1% or 3%, 15–30 nL). After appropriate survival times the rats were deeply anesthetized and perfused transcardially with aldehyde fixatives. Following dissection and cryoprotection, we made frozen serial transverse brain and spinal cord sections (40 or 50 μm) and processed them for peroxidase localization with tetramethylbenzidine (TMB) as chromogen. Series of sections containing labeled neurites and neuronal somata were traced using Neurolucida software (Microbrightfield). In addition, frozen sections through the MPTA were immunolabeled with antibodies to GABA (provided by P. Somogyi, Oxford), or to the α_1 subunit of the $GABA_A$-R (provided by J.-M. Fritschy, Zurich) using the avidin-biotin-peroxidase reaction (ABC Elite kit, Vector Laboratories) and diaminobenzidine (DAB) as chromogen. Specificity and selectivity of the antibodies are known from negative controls including omission of primary antibody and preabsorption (quenching) of antiserum with the target antigen (Hodgson et al. 1985; Somogyi et al. 1985; Benke et al. 1991a,b). The $GABA_A$-R is composed of a variable combination of α, β, γ, and other subunits. However, $GABA_A$-R species containing the α_1 subunit are the most abundant type in the brainstem (Fritschy and Mohler 1995; for review see Hevers and Luddens 1998, Pirker et al. 2000).

RESULTS

Anterograde projections. In rats in which BDA was placed in the MPTA, we found ascending anterogradely labeled axons in the caudoputamen, globus pallidus, septal nuclei, lateral preoptic area, perifornical lateral hypothalamus and medial forebrain bundle, posterior hypothalamus, zona incerta, cerebral peduncle, intralaminar and midline thalamic nuclei, posterior thalamic nuclear group, lateral posterior nucleus, deep superior colliculus, and the pretectal area. Projections were densest ipsilaterally, but we found examples of bilateral input in each target site. We found no direct projections to any part of the cerebral cortex or the amygdaloid complex (Fig. 1).

Upper brainstem and descending bulbospinal projection areas included the mesencephalic reticular formation, pars reticulata and compacta of the substantia nigra, the lateral part of the periaqueductal gray, the central tegmental tract, the contralateral MPTA, more caudal parts of the pontine reticular formation including PnO and PnC, the pedunculopontine tegmental nucleus, parts of the parabrachial complex, widespread areas of the ventromedial

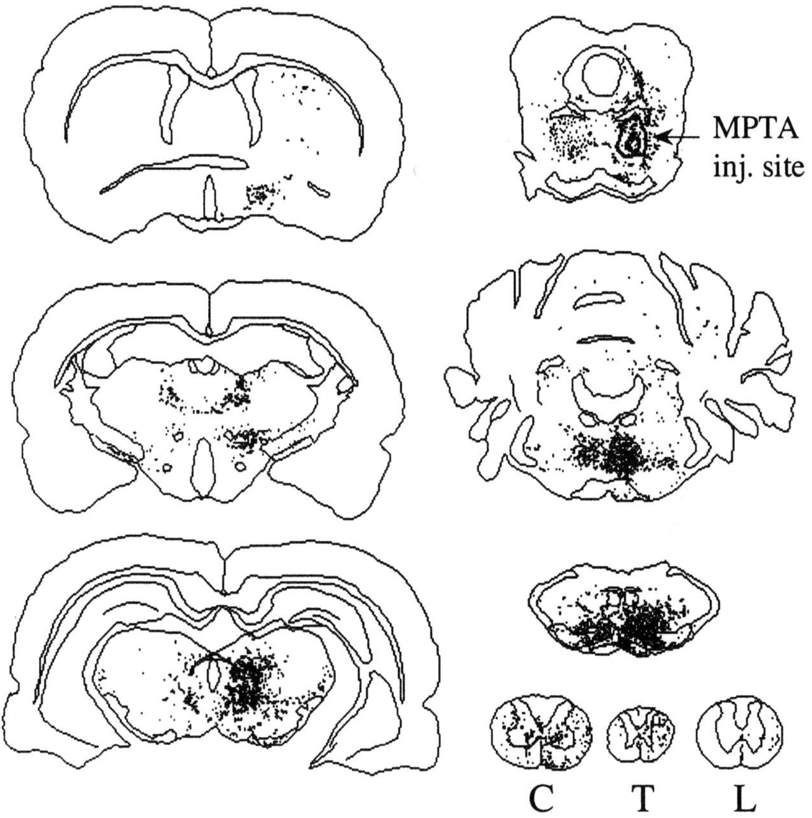

Fig. 1. Representative brain and spinal cord sections showing anterograde axonal projections following biotinylated dextran amine (BDA) microinjection into the mesopontine tegmental anesthesia area (MPTA).

medullary reticular formation, the superior cerebellar peduncle, deep cerebellar nuclei, and cerebellar cortex. Like most of the ascending projections, descending projections were densest ipsilaterally, although a significant crossed projection also occurred. In the spinal cord we found labeling at all segmental levels, including sacral segments, with the density of labeling declining toward the sacral spinal cord. Labeled axons were concentrated in the lateral and the anterior quadrants of the spinal white matter, and ended mostly in deep laminae of spinal gray matter (laminae V–IX).

Retrograde projections. In rats microinjected with retrograde tracers, we found labeled neuronal somata and axons in the cingulate and medial frontal cortex, in restricted areas of the diencephalon (central amygdaloid nucleus, substantia innominata, lateral hypothalamic area, and zona incerta), and in the brainstem (substantia nigra pars reticulata and compacta), periaqueductal gray, deep layers of the superior colliculus, parabrachial nuclei, locus ceruleus, deep cerebellar nuclei, and the mesencephalic, pontine, and medullary reticular formation). Labeling was predominantly ipsilateral, but most of these areas contained labeled cells bilaterally.

GABA and GABA$_A$-R immunolabeling. GABA-immunolabeled cell bodies in the MPTA were of small diameter, were mostly fusiform, and were scattered throughout the MPTA region (Fig. 2). Based on observations of Nissl stained sections, we estimate that up to about 10% of MPTA neurons were GABA immunoreactive. Numerous immunopositive axons, variously

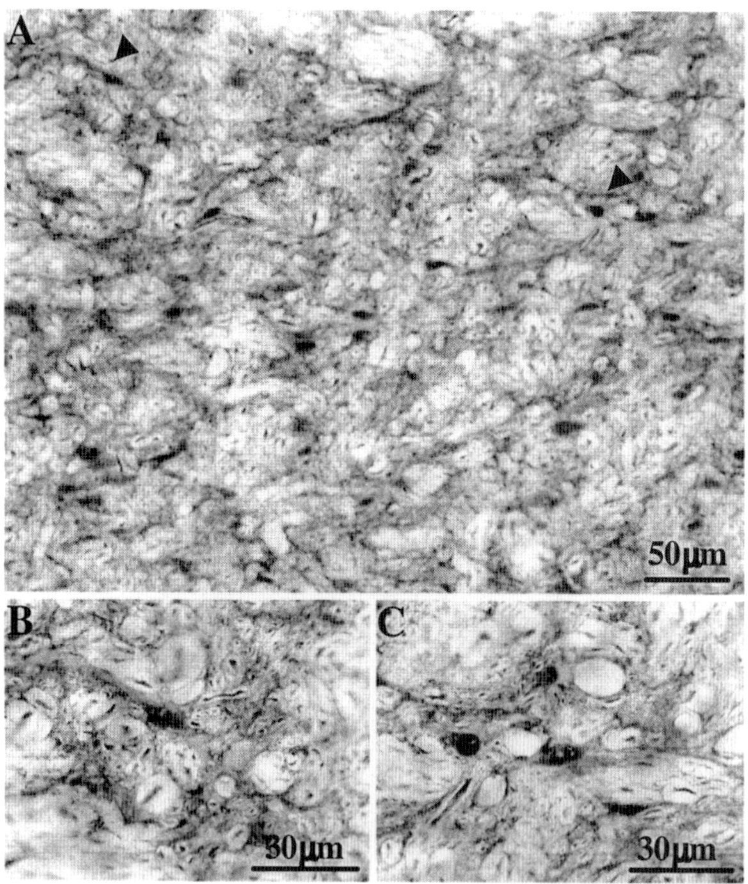

Fig. 2. GABA-immunolabeled neurons in the MPTA. Arrowheads in part (A) indicate cells that are shown at higher magnification in parts (B) and (C).

orientated, were also visible, as was significant punctate staining in the neuropil, which may represent axon terminals.

GABA$_A$-R α_1 subunit immunolabeled neurons were also abundant, and homogeneously scattered throughout the MPTA. Neuronal somata tended to be multipolar, and much larger that the GABA-immunopositive cells. They constituted roughly 20–30% of MPTA neurons (Fig. 3). In many cells variously oriented proximal dendrites were labeled. Numerous immunopositive puncta were richly scattered throughout the neuropil, which suggests postsynaptic receptor aggregates on smaller dendritic processes.

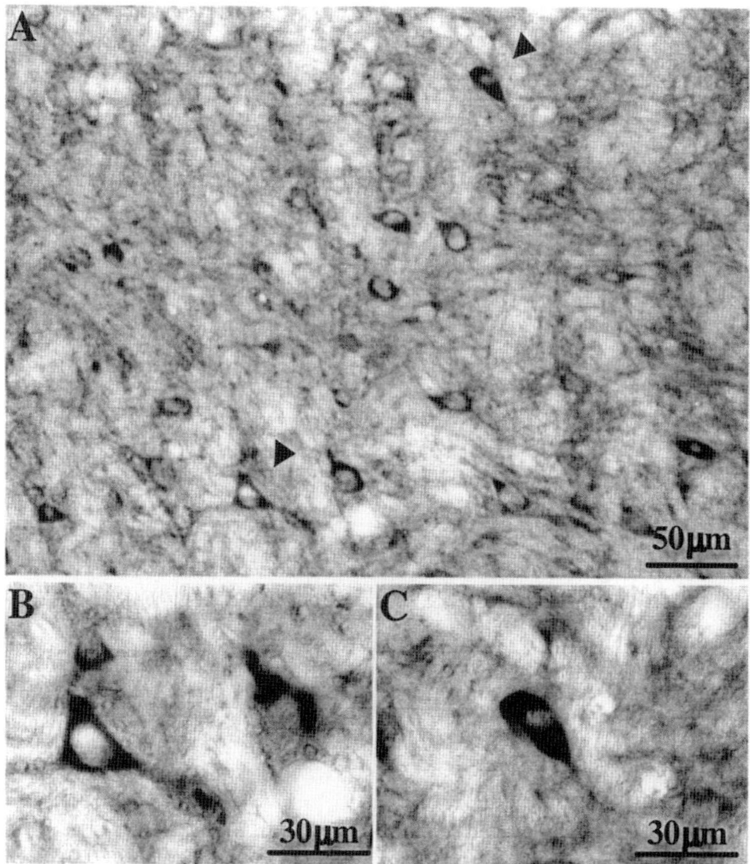

Fig. 3. GABA$_A$-R-immunolabeled neurons in the MPTA based on an antibody that recognizes the receptor α_1 subunit. Arrowheads in part (A) indicate cells that are shown at higher magnification in parts (B) and (C).

DISCUSSION

Several neuroanatomical tracer studies have addressed connectivity of the upper brainstem in rats, but these have focused either on the general architecture of the region or on connections of specific brainstem nuclei or brainstem projection areas (e.g., Jones and Yang 1985; Rye et al.1987; Shammah-Lagnado et al. 1987; Semba and Fibiger 1992; Krout et al. 2002). No prior studies have specifically focused on the MPTA, as only recently has research revealed the functional importance of this area as a possible integrator of motor, sensory, and arousal functions (Devor and Zalkind 2001).

Diversity of projections. Although both outputs from and inputs to the MPTA are diverse, and include components of a variety of functional subsystems, the connections of the MPTA are not ubiquitous. A variety of areas that we might have predicted to be intimately connected with the MPTA are not, most notably the thalamic "relay" nuclei and the cerebral convexity. Behavioral responsiveness to multisensory inputs are suppressed following pentobarbital microinjection into the MPTA, and the cerebral EEG is transformed from the low-voltage, high-frequency "wake" pattern to the high-voltage, low-frequency "slow-wave sleep" pattern. We therefore suspect the presence of powerful MPTA connectivity with thalamocortical or basal forebrain cortical circuitry. These connections, however, are likely to be multisynaptic. A second general feature of MPTA connectivity is that it is largely bilateral, albeit with ipsilateral predominance. This feature suggests that the MPTA on either side may control motor, sensory, and arousal functions on both sides. Finally, although we did not find direct projections from the MPTA to the cerebral cortex, prominent MPTA projections go directly to the spinal cord. Sensorimotor suppression during anesthesia induced by MPTA microinjection may thus be due to descending spinal pathways.

Descending projections. Projections descending to the spinal cord in the lateral and anterior columns terminate in laminae V–IX. Thus, they may directly, or indirectly via segmental interneurons, affect ascending nociceptive signaling by inhibitory actions on wide-dynamic-range spinobulbothalamic neurons of the deep dorsal horn and intermediate gray. The absence of a prominent MPTA projection to the nociceptive-selective neurons of laminae I and II (substantia gelatinosa) is noteworthy. Likewise, direct descending projections to motor neurons or premotor interneurons of the ventral horn could contribute to the behavioral suppression of self-initiated rhythmic motor patterns, of postural reflexes, and of nocifensive responses to noxious stimuli. However, the presence of these direct MPTA bulbospinal projections in no way precludes the possibility that the MPTA region in fact modulates sensory and motor responsiveness indirectly via one or more of the numerous other descending bulbospinal pathways known to be involved in antinociception, rhythmogenesis, and postural atonia (e.g., during REM sleep). For example, stimulation of several pontine and medullary sites elicits atonia (Hajnik et al. 2000). The MPTA may produce atonia indirectly by activating one or more of these. Finally, sensorimotor suppression could be due to actions at supraspinal levels.

Ascending projections. The MPTA has ascending projections to multiple mesencephalic, diencephalic, and (subcortical) telencephalic structures that may mediate its effects on behavioral and electrographic arousal. These projection areas include several of the key cell groups known to have widespread direct and indirect projections to the cortical mantle and prominent effects on cerebral arousal. We note three families of such projections.

The first includes the direct, cortically projecting neurons of the upper brainstem and limbic forebrain. Among these are the histaminergic neurons of the tuberomamillary nucleus, the orexin-containing neurons of the perifornical hypothalamus, the dopaminergic neurons of the basal mesencephalon, the serotonergic neurons of the midline raphe, and the noradrenergic neurons of the locus ceruleus and associated clusters. Part of the regions that contain these cell groups receive input from the MPTA, although double-labeling experiments will be required to confirm that MPTA neurons form synaptic endings directly on them. Interestingly, the MPTA also projects prominently to the lateral preoptic area, a region with executive control over a variety of the direct nonthalamic afferents to the cortex (Saper et al. 2001).

The second family of ascending arousal systems operates via thalamocortical projections, with particular recent attention focused on the thalamic reticular nucleus (Steriade and McCarley 1990). Ascending MPTA projections might access thalamocortical circuitry directly, or indirectly via relays such as the (cholinergic) pedunculopontine and lateral dorsal nuclei. The direct nonthalamic pathways to the cortex, as well as the thalamocortical systems, may play an important role in arousal functions in the context of sleep-wakefulness cycles (Saper et al. 2001).

Finally, an ascending system with brainstem derivatives in the pedunculopontine area, and in the region of the MPTA itself, may control arousal functions of the hippocampal formation and associated areas of limbic cortex. This pathway, which may have intermediate relays in mamillary and supramamillary cell groups, and in the medial septum/vertical limb of the diagonal band of Broca, controls the hippocampal theta rhythm (Vertes and Kocsis 1997; Bland and Oddie 1998).

GABAergic neurons and neurons with GABA$_A$-receptors. In addition to our own work on the effects of pentobarbital microinjection into the MPTA, several recent studies have focused attention on the potential role for GABAergic inhibition in arousal circuitry (Maloney et al. 1999; Xi et al. 1999; Nelson et al. 2002). At liminal concentration, barbiturates act at a modulatory site on the $GABA_A$-R to potentiate the action of endogenous GABA. Indeed, we have demonstrated the presence of GABAergic neurons in the MPTA. GABA-immunopositive cells are small and may constitute inhibitory interneurons with synaptic endings on the larger $GABA_A$-R-bearing neurons in the MPTA.

Most functional $GABA_A$ receptors are formed from a pentameric combination of α, β, and γ subunits, each of which exists in several variants. The preferred pentameric combinations are [2α, 2β, γ] and [2α, β, 2γ] (for review see Hevers and Luddens 1998). We have documented the presence of cells positively labeled for the α_1 subunit, the most common $GABA_A$-R α subunit in the brain. Neurons bearing $GABA_A$-Rs are abundant in the MPTA. Moreover, they are relatively large neurons, which suggests that they might be among those that project to distant loci. Confirmation of this conclusion will require immunolabeling of cells simultaneously marked as projection neurons by retrograde labeling. Pending such data, we propose a working model whereby barbiturates microinjected into the MPTA induce the various changes characteristic of general anesthesia by an inhibitory action on MPTA projection neurons bearing $GABA_A$-Rs. These, in turn, modulate the activity of a variety of spinal, brainstem, and diencephalic centers that regulate movement, posture, nociception, and arousal.

ACKNOWLEDGMENTS

This work was supported by the Whitehall Foundation and the Israel Science Foundation.

REFERENCES

Benke D, Cicin-Sain A, Mertens S, Mohler H. Immunohistochemical identification of the alpha1- and alpha 3-subunits of the GABAA-receptor in rat brain. *J Recept Res* 1991a; 11:407–424.

Benke D, Mertens S, Trzeciak A, Gillessen D, Mohler H. GABAA-receptors display association of gamma 2-subunit with alpha 1- and beta 2/3-subunits. *J Biol Chem* 1991b; 266:4478–4483.

Bland BH, Oddie SD. Anatomical, electrophysiological and pharmacological studies of ascending brainstem hippocampal synchronizing pathways. *Neurosci Biobehav Rev* 1998; 22:259–273.

Devor M, Zalkind V. Reversible atonia, analgesia and loss of consciousness on bilateral intracerebral injection of pentobarbital. *Pain* 2001; 94:101–112.

Fritschy JM, Mohler H. GABAA-receptor heterogeneity in the adult rat brain: differential regional and cellular distribution of seven major subunits. *J Comp Neurol* 1995; 359:154–194.

Hajnik T, Lay YY, Siegel JM. Atonia related regions in the rodent pons and medulla. *J Neurophysiol* 2000; 84:1942–1948.

Hevers W, Luddens H. The diversity of GABA-A receptors. *Mol Neurobiol* 1998; 18:35–86.

Hodgson AJ, Penke B, Erdei A, Chubb IW, Somogyi P. Antisera to γ-aminobutyric acid. I. Production and characterization using a new model system. *J Histochem Cytochem* 1985; 33:229–239.

Jones BE, Yang TZ. The efferent projections from the reticular formation and the locus coeruleus studied by anterograde and retrograde axonal transport in the rat. *J Comp Neurol* 1985; 242:56–92.

Krout KE, Belzer RE, Loewy AD. Brainstem projections to midline and intralaminar thalamic nuclei of the rat. *J Comp Neurol* 2002; 448:53–101.

Nelson LE, Guo TZ, Lu J, et al. The sedative component of anesthesia is mediated by $GABA_A$ receptors in an endogenous sleep pathway. *Nat Neurosci* 2002; 5:979–984.

Maloney KJ, Mainville L, Jones BE. Differential c-Fos expression in cholinergic, monoaminergic, and GABAergic cell groups of the pontomesencephalic tegmentum after paradoxical sleep deprivation and recovery. *J Neurosci* 1999; 19:3057–3072.

Pirker S, Schwarzer C, Wieseltahler A, Sieghart W, Sperk G. GABAA-receptors: immunocytochemical distribution of 13 subunits in the adult rat brain. *Neuroscience* 2000; 101:815–850.

Rye DB, Saper CB, Lee HJ, Wainer BH. Pedunculopontine tegmental nucleus of the rat: cytoarchitecture, cytochemistry, and some extrapyramidal connections of the mesopontine tegmentum. *J Comp Neurol* 1987; 259:483–528.

Saper CB, Chou TC, Scammel TE. The sleep switch: hypothalamic control of sleep and wakefulness. *Trends Neurosci* 2001; 24:726–731.

Semba K, Fibiger HC. Afferent connections of the laterodorsal and the pedunculopontine tegmental nuclei in the rat: a retro- and anterograde transport and immunohistochemical study. *J Comp Neurol* 1992; 323:387–410.

Shammah-Lagnado SJ, Negrao N, Silva BA, Ricardo JA. Afferent connections of the nuclei reticularis pontis oralis and caudalis: a horseradish peroxidase study in the rat. *Neuroscience* 1987; 20:961–989.

Somogyi P, Hodgson AJ, Chubb IW, Penke B, Erdei A. Antisera to γ-aminobutyric acid. II. Immunocytochemical application to the central nervous system. *J Histochem Cytochem* 1985; 33:240–248.

Steriade M, McCarley RW. *Brainstem Control of Wakefulness and Sleep*. New York: Plenum Press, 1990.

Vertes RP, Kocsis B. Brainstem-diencephalo-septohippocampal systems controlling the theta rhythm of the hippocampus. *Neuroscience* 1997; 81:893–926.

Xi MC, Morales FR, Chase MH. A GABAergic pontine reticular system is involved in the control of wakefulness and sleep. *Sleep Res Online* 1999; 2(2):43–48.

Correspondence to: Inna Sukhotinsky, Department of Cell and Animal Biology, Institute of Life Sciences, Hebrew University of Jerusalem, Jerusalem 91904, Israel. Tel: 972 (2) 6586436; Fax: 972 (2) 6520261; email: sinna@vms.huji.ac.il.

Proceedings of the 10th World Congress on Pain,
Progress in Pain Research and Management, Vol. 24,
edited by Jonathan O. Dostrovsky, Daniel B. Carr,
and Martin Koltzenburg, IASP Press, Seattle, © 2003.

27

Placebo Analgesia: From Physiological Mechanisms to Clinical Implications

Fabrizio Benedetti,[a,b] Antonella Pollo,[a,b] Giuliano Maggi,[c] Sergio Vighetti,[a] and Innocenzo Rainero[a,d]

[a]*Department of Neuroscience,* [b]*Clinical and Applied Physiology Program,* [c]*Division of Thoracic Surgery, and* [d]*Neurology III, Headache Center, University of Turin Medical School, Turin, Italy*

The placebo effect helps us to understand how the context around a therapy influences the treatment outcome. A placebo is a dummy medical treatment that simulates a real treatment, so that the patient believes that a therapy is being administered. Several lines of evidence indicate that placebo analgesia is mediated by the endogenous opioid systems. In this chapter we review these findings to make it clear that the placebo effect is worthy of scientific inquiry.

DEFINITION AND ASSESSMENT OF THE PLACEBO EFFECT

The placebo effect is a change in the body, or the body-mind unit, that occurs as a result of the symbolic significance attributed to an event or object in the healing environment (Brody 2000). To be more specific, a placebo is a dummy medical treatment and the placebo effect is the response to it. It is important to point out that the effect is not due to the inertness of the treatment per se. In fact, an inert medical treatment is administered within a context and it is the context that plays the crucial role. When we talk about context, basically we are talking about everything to do with a medical treatment, such as the words uttered by doctors and nurses, the smell of a drug, the sight of hospitals and room layouts, or the touch of a needle or a complex apparatus. In other words, the context surrounding a therapy is represented by any clue that leads to the knowledge that the therapy is being performed (Benedetti and Amanzio 1997; Benedetti and Pollo 2001; Benedetti 2002). The terms "context effects," "nonspecific effects," and "placebo effects" can be used, at least in part, interchangeably, but the term "context effect" is advisable to make it clear that it is the context that influences the specific treatment (Di Blasi et al. 2001). A positive context can reduce a symptom (placebo effect), while a negative context can increase it (nocebo effect), as reviewed in detail recently (White et al. 1985; Harrington 1997; Guess et al. 2002).

In order to assess a placebo effect, spontaneous remission of the symptom must be ruled out, and this can be achieved by including a "natural history" or no-treatment group (Fields and Levine 1984). The difference between a group that receives no treatment and a group that receives the placebo represents the real placebo effect. Of course, this is true not only for drugs, but also for procedural treatments (e.g., surgery and physical therapy) and behavioral interventions (e.g., psychotherapy). If these methodological rules are not followed, many wrong interpretations and conclusions may occur, and spontaneous remission may be erroneously interpreted as a placebo effect.

ENDOGENOUS OPIOIDS MEDIATE PLACEBO ANALGESIA

Several lines of evidence indicate that the context around an analgesic treatment activates the endogenous opioid systems. In other words, the administration of a dummy painkilling therapy (placebo) together with the appropriate verbal instructions ("your pain is going to decrease") is capable of inducing a pain reduction via the opioid receptors. An important step in understanding the neurobiological mechanisms of the placebo effect was made when Levine et al. (1978) found that placebo analgesia is mediated by endogenous opioids. These pioneering findings have been confirmed by other studies (Grevert et al. 1983; Levine and Gordon 1984; Benedetti 1996). Today we know that placebo analgesia has both opioid and non-opioid components, depending on the procedure used to induce the placebo response (Amanzio and Benedetti 1999). In fact, by using the experimental ischemic arm pain model, we found that if the placebo response is induced after repeated administrations of morphine, it can be blocked by the opioid antagonist naloxone. In contrast, if the placebo response is induced after repeated administrations of the non-opioid analgesic ketorolac, naloxone is ineffective.

Whereas nothing is known about the non-opioid component, we are beginning to understand some of the mechanisms of opioid-mediated placebo analgesia. For example, we now know that highly specific placebo responses can be obtained in different parts of the body (Montgomery and Kirsch 1996; Price et al. 1999) and that these analgesic responses are naloxone reversible (Benedetti et al. 1999b). If four noxious stimuli are applied to the hands and feet and a placebo cream is applied to one hand only, pain is reduced only on the hand where the placebo cream was applied. This highly specific effect is blocked by naloxone, suggesting that the placebo-activated endogenous opioid systems have a precise and somatotopic organization (Benedetti et al. 1999b). Another line of research suggests that the placebo-activated endogenous opioids interact with endogenous cholecystokinin (CCK). In fact, on the basis of the anti-opioid action of CCK (Benedetti 1997), we found that CCK antagonists are capable of potentiating the placebo analgesic effect (Benedetti et al. 1995; Benedetti 1996). An additional study supporting the involvement of endogenous opioids in placebo analgesia was performed by Lipman et al. (1990) in chronic pain patients. These authors found that patients who responded to a placebo administration showed higher concentrations of peak β-endorphin in the cerebrospinal fluid compared with patients who did not respond to the placebo.

A likely candidate for the mediation of opioid-dependent placebo analgesia is an opioid neuronal network in the cerebral cortex and brainstem (Fields and Basbaum 1999; Price 1999). This opioid network belongs to a descending pain-modulating pathway that directly or indirectly connects the cerebral cortex to the brainstem. In particular, the anterior cingulate cortex (ACC) and the orbitofrontal cortex (OrbC) project to the periaqueductal grey (PAG), which, in turn, modulates the activity of the rostral ventromedial medulla (RVM). The ACC and the PAG, together with other nuclei in the brainstem (e.g., the parabrachial nuclei), are rich in opioid receptors and could play an important role in placebo analgesia. In fact, context-related cognitive cues could activate this opioid network in the cerebral cortex and the brainstem. This hypothesis is supported by a recent brain imaging study with positron emission tomography (Petrovic et al. 2002). These authors found that the very same brain regions in the cerebral cortex and in the brainstem are affected by both placebo analgesia and the rapidly acting opioid agonist remifentanil, thus indicating a related mechanism in placebo and opioid analgesia. In particular, the administration of a placebo induced the activation of the rostral ACC (rACC) and the OrbC. Moreover, there was a significant covariation in activity between the rACC and the lower pons/medulla, and a subsignificant covariation between the rACC and the PAG, thus suggesting that the descending rACC/PAG/RVM pain-modulating circuit is involved in placebo analgesia, as previously hypothesized by Fields and Price (1997).

The placebo-activated endogenous opioids also yield a typical side effect of opioids, that is, respiratory depression (Benedetti et al. 1999a). After repeated administrations of analgesic doses of buprenorphine in the postoperative phase, which induces a mild decrease in respiration, a placebo is capable of mimicking the same respiratory depressant response. Most interesting, this respiratory placebo response can be blocked totally by naloxone, indicating that it is mediated by endogenous opioids. Thus placebo-activated opioid systems act not only on pain mechanisms, but also on the respiratory centers.

Finally, in a recent study we analyzed the sympathetic and parasympathetic systems of the heart during placebo analgesia (Pollo et al. 2003). In the clinical setting, we found that the placebo analgesic response to a phasic noxious stimulus was accompanied by a reduced heart rate response. In order to investigate this effect from a pharmacological viewpoint, we reproduced the same effect in the laboratory setting by using tonic noxious stimulation. We found that the opioid antagonist naloxone completely antagonized both placebo analgesia and the concomitant reduced heart rate response, whereas the β-adrenergic blocker propranolol antagonized the placebo heart rate reduction but not placebo analgesia. By contrast, both placebo responses were present during muscarinic blockade with atropine, indicating no involvement of the parasympathetic system. In order to better understand the effects of naloxone and propranolol, we performed a spectral analysis of the heart rate variability to identify the sympathetic and parasympathetic components, and found that the β-adrenergic low-frequency (0.15 Hz) spectral component was reduced during placebo analgesia, an effect that was reversed by naloxone. These findings indicate that opioid-mediated placebo analgesia is accompanied by a complex cascade of events that affect the cardiovascular system.

MECHANISMS OF ENDOGENOUS OPIOID ACTIVATION

It appears clear from the above findings that there is an intimate relationship between the context and the endogenous opioid network. Although researchers are now in general agreement that, at least for pain, placebos trigger the release of endogenous opioids, the mechanisms through which this activation occurs are not clear. There are at least two possibilities. First, according to the cognitive theory or response expectancy theory, the placebo response is due to the expectation of pain relief. In other words, the expectation of a positive outcome would be represented by a cognitive neural network that involves the opioid systems in the cortex and brainstem (Kirsch

1985, 1999; Price 1999). Second, the conditioning theory proposes that the placebo response is a conditioned response due to repeated associations between a conditioned stimulus (e.g., the context itself) and an unconditioned stimulus (e.g., morphine). After repeated associations, the context around morphine can produce an analgesic effect through the same receptors to which morphine binds (Herrnstein 1962; Voudouris et al. 1989; Ader 1997; Siegel 2002). One theory does not necessarily rule out the other. In fact, the repeated associations of conditioned and unconditioned stimuli could increase the expectation of an analgesic effect.

OPEN AND HIDDEN ANALGESIC TREATMENTS

The importance of context in any analgesic treatment is shown by the fact that its elimination influences the therapeutic outcome. In order to eliminate the context around a medical treatment the patient must be completely unaware that a therapy is being applied. To do this, drugs are administered through hidden infusions by machines (Levine et al. 1981; Gracely et al. 1983; Levine and Gordon 1984; Amanzio et al. 2001). It is possible to perform a hidden infusion of a drug by means of a computer-controlled infusion pump that is preprogrammed to deliver the drug at the desired time. The crucial point is that the patient is not aware that any drug is being injected. The computer-controlled infusion pump can deliver analgesics automatically, without any doctor or nurse in the room, and with the patient being completely unaware that an analgesic treatment has been started.

In postoperative pain following the extraction of the third molar, Levine et al. (1981) and Levine and Gordon (1984) found that a hidden injection of a 6–8-mg dose of morphine corresponds to an open injection of saline solution in full view of the patient. In other words, injecting a saline solution while telling the patient that a painkiller is being injected is as potent as 6–8 mg of morphine. Only by increasing the hidden morphine dose to 12 mg was its analgesic effect stronger than the placebo effect observed. These authors concluded that an open injection of morphine in full view of the patient, which represents usual medical practice, is more effective than a hidden one because in the latter the placebo component is absent.

Our group recently made a careful analysis of the differences between open and hidden injections in the postoperative setting (Amanzio et al. 2001). We analyzed the effects of four widely used analgesics (buprenorphine, tramadol, ketorolac, and metamizol), which were administered with either open or hidden injections. The open injection was carried out by a doctor at the bedside who told the patient that the injection was a powerful analgesic and that the pain was going to subside in a few minutes. By contrast, the hidden injection of the same analgesic dose was performed by an automatic infusion machine that started the painkilling infusion without any doctor or nurse in the room. Thus these patients were completely unaware that an analgesic therapy had been started. We found that the time course of post-surgical pain was significantly different between open and hidden injections. In fact, during the first hour after the injection, pain ratings were much higher with a hidden injection than with an open one.

In the same study (Amanzio et al. 2001), we also investigated the difference between open and hidden injections in the laboratory setting by using the experimental model of ischemic arm pain in healthy volunteers. As occurred in the clinical setting, we found that a hidden injection of the non-opioid painkiller, ketorolac, was less effective than an open one. We added a 10-mg dose of the opioid antagonist naloxone to an open injection of ketorolac and found that the effect was reduced as much as with a hidden injection of ketorolac. This interesting finding suggests that an open injection in full view of the patient, during the routine doctor-patient interaction, activates the endogenous opioid systems, which enhance the effects of the injected painkiller.

The importance of these findings is twofold. First, by eliminating the context (at least its component that produces the patient's perception of the administration of the agent) by means of a hidden administration of a medical treatment, we reduce the effectiveness of the treatment itself. Second, the effects of the context can be blocked psychologically, by means of hidden administration, or pharmacologically through the opioid antagonist naloxone, thus indicating that the context affects the endogenous opioid systems.

USING PLACEBOS TO REDUCE OPIOID INTAKE

Experimental evidence suggests that the placebo effect may be harnessed to the patient's advantage. For example, we conducted a study to investigate the effects of different types of placebo administration on the intake of opioids (Pollo et al. 2001). In this study, we treated several postoperative patients with buprenorphine, on request, for three consecutive days, and with a basal infusion of saline solution. However, the symbolic meaning of this saline basal infusion varied in three different groups of patients. The first group was told that the infusion was a rehydrating solution (natural history or no-treatment group), the second was told that it could be either a potent analgesic or a placebo (classic double-blind administration), and the third group was told that the infusion was a potent painkiller (deceptive administration). The placebo effect of the saline basal infusion was measured by recording the doses of buprenorphine requested over the 3-day treatment period. It is important to point out that the double-blind group received uncertain verbal instructions ("It can be either an inert substance or a painkiller"), whereas the deceptive administration group received certain instructions ("It is a painkiller"). We found a decrease in buprenorphine intake with the double-blind administration and even more with the deceptive administration of the saline basal infusion. In fact, the reduction of buprenorphine requests in the double-blind group was as large as 20.8% compared with the natural history group, and the reduction in the deceptive administration group was even larger (33.8%). It is important to point out that the time course of pain was the same in the three groups over the 3-day period of treatment. Thus, the same analgesic effect was obtained with different doses of buprenorphine. Although further experimental and clinical work is needed, this study clearly shows that those patients who are under the effect of strong expectations of analgesia request lower doses of drugs than those who are not.

CONCLUSIONS

The placebo effect is an interesting model by which to study the therapeutic effects of complex social interactions, in particular the doctor-patient relationship. Although the investigation of placebo analgesia represents a good model in which the endogenous opioid systems can be analyzed, it is important to remember that the activation of endogenous substances by placebos is a phenomenon that is not confined to the field of pain. In fact, the administration of a placebo to Parkinsonian patients triggers the release of dopamine in the striatum (de la Fuente-Fernandez et al. 2001), and some experimental evidence suggests that serotonin is involved in the placebo response of depressed patients (Mayberg et al. 2002). Our group has also started exploring the mechanisms of the placebo effect in Parkinson's disease (Pollo et al. 2002). We believe that the integration of the findings in the field of pain with those in other pathological conditions will help us better understand the intricate mechanisms that link mind, brain, and body.

ACKNOWLEDGMENTS

This work was supported by grants from the Italian Ministry of University and Research, and by the National Research Council (CNR) projects "Trigeminal pain" and "Neuroscience."

REFERENCES

Ader R. The role of conditioning in pharmacotherapy. In: Harrington A (Ed). *The Placebo Effect: An Interdisciplinary Exploration*. Cambridge, MA: Cambridge University Press, 1997, pp 138–165.

Amanzio M, Benedetti F. Neuropharmacological dissection of placebo analgesia: expectation-activated opioid systems versus conditioning-activated specific sub-systems. *J Neurosci* 1999; 19:484–494.

Amanzio M, Pollo A, Maggi G, Benedetti F. Response variability to analgesics: a role for non-specific activation of endogenous opioids. *Pain* 2001; 90:205–215.

Benedetti F. The opposite effects of the opiate antagonist naloxone and the cholecystokinin antagonist proglumide on placebo analgesia. *Pain* 1996; 64:535–543.

Benedetti F. Cholecystokinin type-A and type-B receptors and their modulation of opioid analgesia. *News Physiol Sci* 1997; 12:263–268.

Benedetti F. How the doctor's words affect the patient's brain. *Eval Health Prof* 2002; 25:369–386.

Benedetti F, Amanzio M. The neurobiology of placebo: from endogenous opioids to cholecystokinin. *Prog Neurobiol* 1997; 52:109–125.

Benedetti F, Pollo A. The pharmacology of placebos. *Int J Pain Med Palliative Care* 2001; 1:42–48.

Benedetti F, Amanzio M, Maggi G. Potentiation of placebo analgesia by proglumide. *Lancet* 1995; 346:1231.

Benedetti F, Amanzio M, Baldi S, Casadio C, Maggi G. Inducing placebo respiratory depressant responses in humans via opioid receptors. *Eur J Neurosci* 1999a; 11:625–631.

Benedetti F, Arduino C, Amanzio M. Somatotopic activation of opioid systems by target-directed expectations of analgesia. *J Neurosci* 1999b; 19:3639–3648.

Brody H. *The Placebo Response*. New York: Harper Collins, 2000.

de la Fuente-Fernandez R, Ruth TJ, Sossi V, et al. Expectation and dopamine release: mechanism of the placebo effect in Parkinson's disease. *Science* 2001; 293:1164–1166.

Di Blasi Z, Harkness E, Ernst E, Georgiou A, Kleijnen J. Influence of context effects on health outcomes: a systematic review. *Lancet* 2001; 357:757–762.

Fields HL, Basbaum AI. Central nervous system mechanisms of pain modulation. In: Wall PD, Melzack R (Eds). *Textbook of Pain*. Edinburgh: Churchill Livingstone, 1999, pp 309–329.

Fields HL, Levine JD. Placebo analgesia—a role for endorphins? *Trends Neurosci* 1984; 7:271–273.

Fields HL, Price DD. Toward a neurobiology of placebo analgesia. In: Harrington A (Ed). *The Placebo Effect: An Interdisciplinary Exploration*. Cambridge, MA: Harvard University Press, 1997, pp 93–116.

Gracely RH, Dubner R, Wolskee PJ, Deeter WR. Placebo and naloxone can alter postsurgical pain by separate mechanisms. *Nature* 1983; 306:264–265.

Grevert P, Albert LH, Goldstein A. Partial antagonism of placebo analgesia by naloxone. *Pain* 1983; 16:129–143.

Guess HA, Kleinman A, Kusek JW, Engel LW (Eds). *The Science of the Placebo: Toward an Interdisciplinary Research Agenda*. London: Medical Journal Books, 2002.

Harrington A (Ed). *The Placebo Effect: An Interdisciplinary Exploration*. Cambridge, MA: Harvard University Press, 1997.

Herrnstein RJ. Placebo effect in the rat. *Science* 1962; 38:677–678.

Kirsch I. Response expectancy as a determinant of experience and behavior. *Am Psychol* 1985; 40:1189–1202.

Kirsch I (Ed). *How Expectancies Shape Experience*. Washington, DC: American Psychological Association, 1999.

Levine JD, Gordon NC. Influence of the method of drug administration on analgesic response. *Nature* 1984; 312: 755–756.

Levine JD, Gordon NC, Fields HL. The mechanisms of placebo analgesia. *Lancet* 1978; 2:654–657.

Levine JD, Gordon NC, Smith R, Fields HL. Analgesic responses to morphine and placebo in individuals with postoperative pain. *Pain* 1981; 10:379–389.

Lipman JJ, Miller BE, Mays KS, et al. Endorphin concentration in cerebrospinal fluid: reduced in chronic pain patients and increased during the placebo response. *Psychopharmacology* 1990; 102:112–116.

Mayberg HS, Silva AJ, Brannan SK, et al. The functional neuroanatomy of the placebo effect. *Am J Psychiatry* 2002; 159:728–737.

Montgomery GH, Kirsch I. Mechanisms of placebo pain reduction: an empirical investigation. *Psychol Sci* 1996; 7:174–176.

Petrovic P, Kalso E, Petersson KM, Ingvar M. Placebo and opioid analgesia—imaging a shared neuronal network. *Science* 2002; 295:1737–1740.

Pollo A, Amanzio M, Arslanian A, et al. Response expectancies in placebo analgesia and their clinical relevance. *Pain* 2001; 93:77–84.

Pollo A, Torre E, Lopiano L, et al. Expectation modulates the response to subthalamic nucleus stimulation in Parkinsonian patients. *Neuroreport* 2002; 13:1383–1386.

Pollo A, Vighetti S, Rainero I, Benedetti F. Placebo analgesia and the heart. *Pain* 2003; in press.

Price DD. *Psychological Mechanisms of Pain and Analgesia,* Progress in Pain Research and Management, Vol. 15. Seattle: IASP Press, 1999.

Price DD, Milling LS, Kirsch I, et al. An analysis of factors that contribute to the magnitude of placebo analgesia in an experimental paradigm. *Pain* 1999; 83:147–156.

Siegel S. Explanatory mechanisms for placebo effects: Pavlovian conditioning. In: Guess HA, Kleinman A, Kusek JW, Engel LW (Eds). *The Science of the Placebo: Toward an Interdisciplinary Research Agenda.* London: British Medical Journal Books, 2002, pp 133–157.

Voudouris NJ, Peck CL Coleman G. Conditioned response models of placebo phenomena: further support. *Pain* 1989; 38:109–116.

White L, Tursky B, Schwartz GE (Eds). *Placebo: Theory, Research, and Mechanisms.* New York: Guilford Press, 1985.

Correspondence to: Fabrizio Benedetti, MD, Dipartimento di Neuroscienze, Università di Torino, Corso Raffaello 30, 10125 Torino, Italy. Tel: 39-011-670-7709; Fax: 39-011-670-7708; email: fabrizio.benedetti@unito.it.

Part IV

Mechanisms of Central Sensitization

Proceedings of the 10th World Congress on Pain,
Progress in Pain Research and Management, Vol. 24,
edited by Jonathan O. Dostrovsky, Daniel B. Carr, and
Martin Koltzenburg, IASP Press, Seattle, © 2003.

28

Sensitization of Nociceptor-Specific Neurons by Capsaicin or Mustard Oil: Effect of $GABA_A$-Receptor Blockade

Esther Garcia-Nicas, Jennifer M.A. Laird,
and Fernando Cervero

*Department of Physiology, University of Alcalá,
Alcalá de Henares, Madrid, Spain*

The sensory alterations that characterize postinjury hypersensitivity include a change in the modality of sensation evoked by low-threshold mechanoreceptors (allodynia or "touch-evoked pain") and an increase in magnitude of the pain sensations evoked by mechanically sensitive nociceptors (hyperalgesia) (LaMotte et al. 1991). In areas of hyperalgesia remote from the injury site (secondary hyperalgesia), both of these changes are due to alterations in the central processing of sensory input and are induced and maintained by the arrival in the central nervous system of the afferent barrage evoked by the originating injury in peripheral nociceptors (LaMotte et al. 1991; Torebjörk et al. 1992).

Most models of secondary hyperalgesia revolve around the notion of "central sensitization," whereby injury discharges in nociceptive afferents cause spinal cord neurons to enhance their excitability and/or to increase their responsiveness to other peripheral drives (Woolf and Thompson 1991; Dubner and Ruda 1992). Increases in neuronal excitability after an injury have also been suggested to change the afferent properties of nociceptor-specific neurons (Simone et al. 1989; Woolf et al. 1994). In this case the process would include the expression of previously inhibited low-threshold inputs as part of a general mechanism of central sensitization.

Some years ago, we proposed a new model of allodynia based on a central presynaptic interaction between low-threshold mechanoreceptors and nociceptors. In this model, light touch of the skin evokes action potentials in Aβ fibers, which in turn activate the central terminals of nociceptive afferents (see Cervero and Laird 1996b). The central presynaptic link between these two kinds of afferent fiber contains at least one GABAergic interneuron and evokes primary afferent depolarization (PAD) of the nociceptive afferents when low-threshold mechanoreceptors are stimulated. In hyperalgesic states, the PAD produced in the nociceptive afferents can be intense enough to generate spike activity. This activation would be conducted antidromically in the form of dorsal root reflexes (DRRs), evoking localized flares in the area of secondary hyperalgesia via antidromic activation of nociceptors, but would also be conducted forward, activating second-order neurons normally driven by nociceptors (see Fig. 1).

In previous investigations we obtained supporting evidence for this model by showing that selective activation of low-threshold mechanoreceptors or of primary afferent Aβ fibers, both in human volunteers and in rats, evokes vasodilatations in areas of secondary hyperalgesia. We ascertained that this touch-evoked flare is dependent on a central connection via dorsal roots

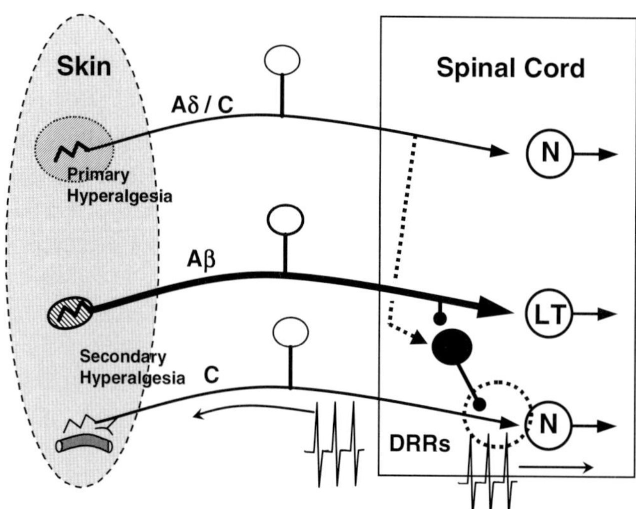

Fig. 1. Model of allodynia based on presynaptic interactions between low-threshold mechanoreceptors (Aβ fibers) and nociceptors (Aδ/C fibers). An injury to the periphery activates and sensitizes nociceptors, resulting in primary hyperalgesia. Discharges from this area arrive at the spinal cord and sensitize the interneurons that mediate presynaptic inhibition (solid black neuron in the diagram). This sensitization results in enhanced primary afferent depolarization of the terminals of nociceptors (N) when low-threshold (LT) mechanoreceptors are activated. The depolarization can be intense enough to produce spike activity that will be conducted antidromically as dorsal root reflexes (DRRs)—causing localized peripheral vasodilatations—and centrally, activating nociceptive neurons, thus triggering touch-evoked pain. Based on the model of Cervero and Laird (1996b).

(Cervero and Laird 1996a; Garcia-Nicas et al. 2001). This chapter describes a study in which we tested the hypothesis in anesthetized rats by examining the effects of mechanical and electrical stimulation of Aβ fibers on nociceptor-specific (NS) neurons before and after producing cutaneous secondary hyperalgesia by applying an irritant (capsaicin or mustard oil). We also examined the effects of antagonists of the $GABA_A$ receptor, bicuculline and picrotoxin.

MATERIALS AND METHODS

Wistar adult rats of either sex were anesthetized with pentobarbital sodium. One catheter was placed in the left carotid artery for continuous arterial blood pressure recording and another in the left jugular vein for injection of anesthetic and other compounds. The trachea was cannulated to allow artificial ventilation and continuous end-tidal CO_2 recordings. Rectal temperature was kept constant at 38°C with a feedback-controlled electric blanket. The left sciatic nerve was dissected and prepared for stimulation through bipolar silver electrodes. A laminectomy was performed to expose the T13–L2 segments of the spinal cord. Before nerve stimulation, the animal was paralyzed with pancuronium bromide and artificially ventilated.

Cord dorsum potential measurements were used to locate the terminal field of the sciatic nerve in the spinal cord. Single-unit electrical activity was recorded from spinal neurons through glass micropipettes filled with 4 M NaCl (10–15 MΩ). Each neuron was characterized by its responses to natural mechanical stimulation of the skin receptive field on the paw and to electrical stimulation of the sciatic nerve. Mechanical stimulation of the receptive field included innocuous stimuli such as brushing and touching with a cotton bud, as well as noxious stimuli such as pinching. Mechanical thresholds were determined using calibrated von Frey monofilaments applied to the receptive field of the neuron. The extent of the high-threshold excitatory receptive field was mapped with small forceps or pinprick. The threshold and latency of the response to electrical stimulation of the sciatic nerve were also noted. Nociceptor-specific (NS) neurons with excitatory responses to electrical stimulation of C fibers were selected for further analysis. Most of these neurons were located in lamina I of the superficial dorsal horn. For comparison, some NS neurons were also recorded in the deep dorsal horn.

The recording protocol was as follows: (1) recording of the background activity of the neuron; (2) 20-second periods of stimulation of the receptive field with a brush, cotton bud, or pinch (~3.3 N applied to a surface of 8.9 mm^2), separated by not less than 20 seconds of interstimulus rest;

and (3) electrical stimulation of the sciatic nerve at twice the threshold (2 T) and at 40 T. An experimental inflammation was then induced by topical application of mustard oil in one or two doses of 5 μL each, diluted at 50% in ethanol or by intradermal injection of capsaicin in one or two doses of 20 μL each, diluted at 0.3%. Forty-five minutes after the induction of inflammation, each neuron was completely characterized again, and the series of mechanical and electrical tests was repeated in order to assess inflammation-induced changes in responsiveness of the neuron. Finally, to examine whether any change observed was mediated by $GABA_A$ receptors, the actions of $GABA_A$-receptor antagonists were tested. Cumulative doses of picrotoxin (0.5, 1 mg/kg) were administrated systemically. In another series of animals, cumulative doses of bicuculline were given intrathecally (i.t.; 0.03–0.3 μg).

RESULTS

Of the 29 NS neurons tested with capsaicin or mustard oil, none showed responses to innocuous mechanical stimulation or were excited by afferent Aβ fibers before the application of these agents to their receptive fields. We considered that a neuron had been mechanically sensitized after the application of an irritant when it responded with a minimum of 10 spikes during the 20 seconds of the innocuous mechanical stimulation (see Fig. 2) or when it showed a previously absent response to electrical stimulation at an intensity sufficient to excite Aβ afferent fibers.

Of the 29 NS neurons tested, 21 were sensitized mechanically and/or electrically after the application of capsaicin or mustard oil. The mechanical threshold measured showed a significant decrease ($P < 0.05$) after application of the irritant. The median mechanical threshold for sensitized NS neurons was 181 mN before application of the irritant and 45.3 mN after application. Seventeen of the 21 sensitized neurons were located in the superficial layers of the dorsal horn (laminae I–II), and 4 neurons were located in deep layers (laminae V–VI). Both sensitized and nonsensitized neurons had a C-fiber input and responded to stimulation of Aδ fibers. After the injection of capsaicin or application of mustard oil, all neurons were excited at 2 T intensity, consistent with activation by Aβ fibers (see Fig. 3C). The threshold for C-fiber activation did not change after application of the irritants.

Administration of picrotoxin (i.v.) produced a dose-dependent reversal of the mechanical sensitization in five neurons (Figs. 2 and 3A). Administration of bicuculline (i.t.) was also tested in six neurons and produced a reversal of mechanical sensitization (Fig. 3B). We also observed a reduction in the strength of the novel Aβ-fiber drive after i.t. administration of bicuculline (Fig. 3C).

DISCUSSION

Our results show that after application of an irritant to their cutaneous receptive field, NS neurons acquire a novel Aβ-fiber input and respond to low-intensity mechanical stimulation of their receptive fields. We have shown here that this sensitization of NS neurons to innocuous stimuli involves $GABA_A$ receptors.

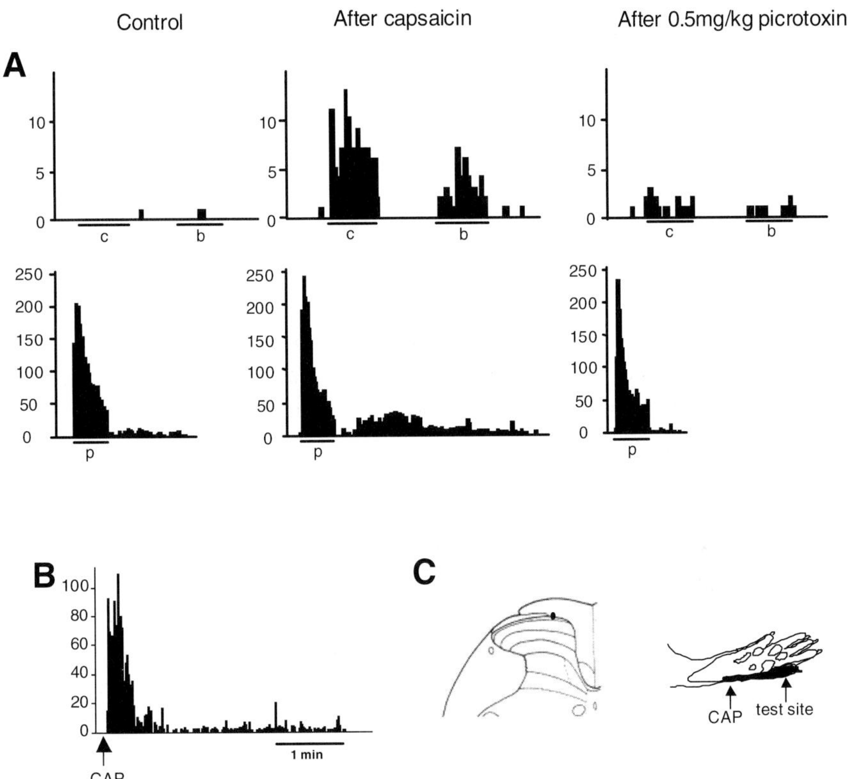

Fig. 2. Panel A shows responses of a nociceptor-specific (NS) neuron to innocuous (top) and noxious (bottom) stimulation of its receptive field (shown in C). Also shown in panel C is the location of the NS neuron in the superficial dorsal horn of the spinal cord. This neuron did not respond to innocuous cotton bud (c) or brushing (b) stimulation of the receptive field in the control situation, but did respond after intradermal injection of capsaicin in its receptive field (injection site shown as CAP in C). Each stimulation period is 20 seconds long. These novel responses were reduced after i.v. administration of picrotoxin. The response of the neuron to pinch (p in bottom diagrams of panel A, also 20 seconds long) was enhanced after capsaicin, the effect being also reversed by picrotoxin. Panel B shows the response of the neuron to the capsaicin injection.

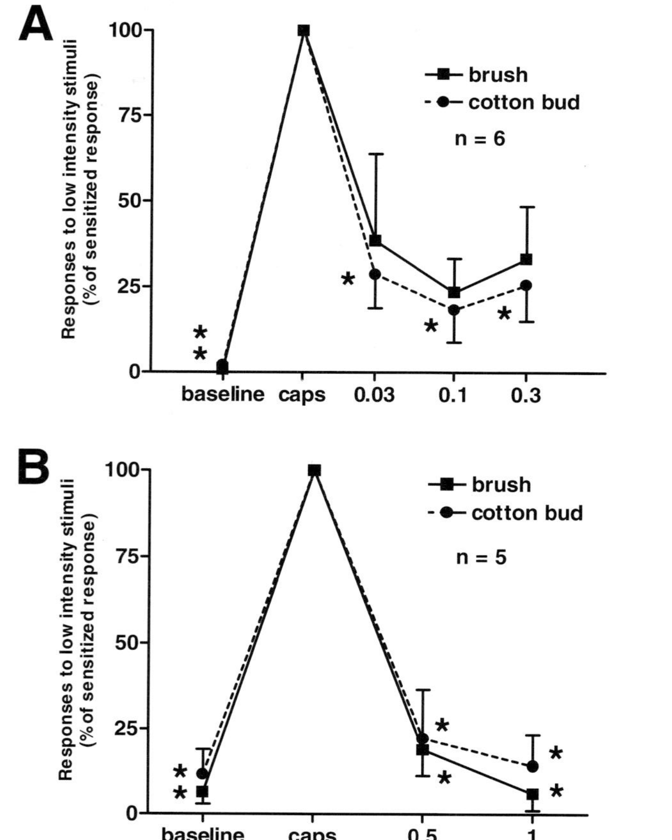
A
Responses to low intensity stimuli (% of sensitized response)
100
75
50
25
0
brush
cotton bud
n = 6
baseline
caps
0.03
0.1
0.3
B
Responses to low intensity stimuli (% of sensitized response)
100
75
50
25
0
brush
cotton bud
n = 5
baseline
caps
0.5
1

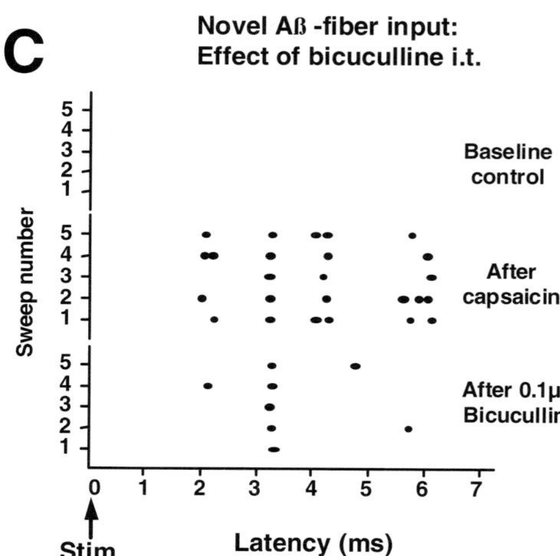
C
Novel Aß -fiber input:
Effect of bicuculline i.t.
Sweep number
Baseline control
After capsaicin
After 0.1µg Bicuculline
0 1 2 3 4 5 6 7
Stim.
Latency (ms)

Previous reports have described sensitization of NS neurons following the application of capsaicin to their receptive fields or after an experimental injury or inflammation of the skin. For instance, Simone et al. (1989) described, in the cat, an enhancement of excitability in both NS and wide-dynamic-range (WDR) dorsal horn neurons after intradermal injection of capsaicin. Equally, Woolf et al. (1994) showed that NS neurons in the superficial dorsal horn of the rat could acquire novel low-threshold inputs following the application of mustard oil outside their receptive fields. More recently, Khasabov et al. (2001) described enhanced excitability of NS neurons to heat and cold stimuli following a freeze injury to the skin.

All previous reports concluded that the expression of a new low-threshold input by NS neurons could be a mechanism for touch-evoked allodynia. In our experiments we have confirmed that NS neurons can become sensitized after capsaicin or mustard oil and that this sensitization correlates with the expression of a new Aβ-fiber afferent input. In line with other authors, we also believe that the expression of a novel low-threshold input by neurons that are normally activated only by nociceptors can contribute to the touch-evoked pain sensitivity that characterizes secondary hyperalgesia. However, the details of the mechanism remain to be clarified.

We do not believe that touch-evoked pain can be attributed to a generalized increase in the excitability of all dorsal horn neurons, including NS and WDR neurons. Such a general increase would be difficult to reconcile with the precise sensory alterations of secondary hyperalgesia, which include static and dynamic components of allodynia and selective hyperalgesia to mechanical, but not thermal, stimuli (see Treede et al. 1992 for review). It is likely that a more precise mechanism is involved, with selective activation of NS neurons by low-threshold afferents.

Our model of presynaptic interaction between low-threshold and high-threshold afferents (Cervero and Laird 1996b) offers such selectivity and is supported by the data presented here. In our experiments, NS neurons showed no Aβ-fiber afferent input or low-threshold mechanical activation prior to the application of the sensitizing stimuli to their receptive fields. The appearance of

---

← **Fig. 3.** Effects of $GABA_A$ antagonists on the responses of NS neurons to innocuous stimulation of their receptive fields. Panels A and B show the responses of the neurons to brushing and cotton bud stimulation before and after intradermal injections of capsaicin (caps) and the effects on these responses of increasing doses of bicuculline (µg, i.t.) (panel A) and picrotoxin (mg/kg, i.v.) (panel B). Panel C shows the responses (dot raster) of a single neuron to repetitive electrical stimulation (five stimulations at the time indicated by the arrow) of the sciatic nerve at Aβ-fiber intensity. Note (from top to bottom) the complete lack of an Aβ-fiber input in control conditions (baseline), the appearance of a new Aβ-fiber input after capsaicin, and the partial reversal of the Aβ-fiber input by bicuculline.

such low-threshold input was very rapid after the application of capsaicin or mustard oil and could be reversed by low doses of $GABA_A$ antagonists, indicating a synaptic GABAergic effect. As the postsynaptic actions of GABA on dorsal horn neurons are normally inhibitory, the effects of GABA antagonists shown here can only be explained by reference to a presynaptic rather than a postsynaptic effect. Moreover, the effects observed with i.t. application of GABA antagonists would rule out a generalized effect of the antagonists or a supraspinal site of action.

We therefore conclude that our results are consistent with a spinal presynaptic mechanism for touch-evoked pain. This could be a simple, and in some respects more efficient, way for low-threshold Aβ fibers to access nociceptive neurons in the spinal cord. The mechanism is fast and can also be quickly reversed, both of these features being characteristic components of secondary hyperalgesia.

ACKNOWLEDGMENTS

This study was supported by the Madrid Regional Government (Contrato Programa) and the Ministry of Science and Technology, Spain (SAF-2000-0199). E. Garcia-Nicas holds a Postgraduate Fellowship from the Madrid Regional Government. J.M.A. Laird was a Ramón y Cajal Investigator (Ministry of Science and Technology, Spain). The authors are grateful to María-José García for expert technical assistance.

REFERENCES

Cervero F, Laird JMA. Mechanisms of allodynia: interactions between sensitive mechanoreceptors and nociceptors. *NeuroReport* 1996a; 7:526–528.

Cervero F, Laird JMA. Mechanisms of touch-evoked pain (allodynia): a new model. *Pain* 1996b; 68:13–23.

Dubner R, Ruda MA. Activity-dependent neuronal plasticity following tissue injury and inflammation. *Trends Neurosci* 1992; 15:96–103.

Garcia-Nicas E, Laird JMA, Cervero F. Vasodilatation in hyperalgesic rat skin evoked by stimulation of afferent Aβ-fibers: further evidence for a role of dorsal root reflexes in allodynia. *Pain* 2001; 94:283–291.

Khasabov SG, Cain DM, Thong D, Mantyh PW, Simone DA. Enhanced responses of spinal dorsal horn neurons to heat and cold stimuli following mild freeze injury to the skin. *J Neurophysiol* 2001; 86:986–996.

LaMotte RH, Shain CN, Simone DA, Tsai E-FP. Neurogenic hyperalgesia: psychophysical studies of underlying mechanisms. *J Neurophysiol* 1991; 66:190–211.

Simone DA, Baumann TK, Collins JG, LaMotte RH. Sensitization of cat dorsal horn neurons to innocuous mechanical stimulation after intradermal injection of capsaicin. *Brain Res* 1989; 486:185–189.

Torebjörk HE, Lundberg LER, LaMotte RH. Central changes in processing of mechanoreceptive input in capsaicin-induced secondary hyperalgesia in humans. *J Physiol (Lond)* 1992; 448:765–780.

Treede R-D, Meyer RA, Raja SN, Campbell JN. Peripheral and central mechanisms of cutaneous hyperalgesia. *Prog Neurobiol* 1992; 38:397–421.

Woolf CJ, Thompson SWN. The induction and maintenance of central sensitization is dependent on N-methyl-D-aspartic acid receptor activation; Implications for the treatment of post-injury pain hypersensitivity states. *Pain* 1991; 44:293–299.

Woolf CJ, Shortland P, Sivilotti LG. Sensitization of high mechanothreshold superficial dorsal horn and flexor motor neurones following chemosensitive primary afferent activation. *Pain* 1994; 58:141–155.

Correspondence to: Prof. Fernando Cervero, MD, PhD, DSc, Anesthesia Research Unit, McGill University, McIntyre Medical Building, Room 1207, 3655 Promenade Sir William Osler, Montreal, Quebec, Canada H3G 1Y6. Tel: 514-398-5764; Fax: 514-398-8241; email: fernando.cervero@mcgill.ca.

Proceedings of the 10th World Congress on Pain,
Progress in Pain Research and Management, Vol. 24,
edited by Jonathan O. Dostrovsky, Daniel B. Carr, and
Martin Koltzenburg, IASP Press, Seattle, © 2003.

29

What the Brain Tells the Spinal Cord: Lamina I/III NK1-Expressing Neurons Control Spinal Activity via Descending Pathways

Rie Suzuki,[a] Sara Morcuende,[b] Mark Webber,[b]
Stephen P. Hunt,[b] and Anthony H. Dickenson[a]

[a]Department of Pharmacology and [b]Department of Anatomy and Developmental Biology, University College London, London, United Kingdom

The long-term increase in pain sensitivity that frequently follows tissue or nerve injury is thought to be due to alterations in synaptic transmission and morphology within the spinal cord and to changes in descending controls from the brainstem (Hunt and Mantyh 2001). Neurokinin-1 (NK1) receptors, which are highly expressed in the superficial dorsal horn, form part of several important ascending pathways. Although NK1-expressing lamina I neurons make collateral projections to the deeper dorsal horn (Light et al. 1993; Cheunsuang and Morris 2000), they are also predominantly nociceptive-specific projection neurons terminating extensively within the parabrachial area (PB), with other terminations in the periaqueductal gray area, thalamus, and reticular formation (Todd et al. 2000; Gauriau and Bernard 2002; Lima and Almeida 2002). The PB accesses areas of the brain such as the amygdala and hypothalamus that modulate descending monoaminergic pathways from the brainstem and regulate nociceptive processing at spinal levels (Hunt 2000). Input from the periphery is therefore under continuous modulation by descending influences from the brainstem and intrinsic spinal mechanisms. We have used the molecular microneurosurgical technique of substance P/saporin (SP-SAP) to ablate lamina I and/or III (I/III) NK1 projection neurons (Mantyh et al. 1997) and show their significant effect on both descending controls and local spinal circuits.

ABLATION OF NEURONS EXPRESSING NK1-R RESULTS IN ALTERED PAIN BEHAVIORS FOLLOWING TISSUE AND NERVE INJURY

Elegant studies by Mantyh and colleagues (1997) showed that spinal SP-SAP selectively and markedly depletes NK1-expressing neurons in the superficial dorsal horn. Animals treated with SP-SAP display long-lasting changes in pain sensitivity, characterized by an attenuation of pain behaviors following local inflammation or nerve injury produced by L5/L6 spinal nerve ligation (Nichols et al. 1999).

SP-SAP LESION REDUCES THE EXCITABILITY OF DEEP DORSAL HORN NEURONS

To extend these behavioral observations, we conducted in vivo electrophysiological studies 1 month after infusion of the conjugate. Loss of the NK1 receptor was verified in a separate group of animals to confirm a selective and marked depletion of lamina I/II NK1 immunoreactivity, with no abnormal glial hypertrophy. Recordings were made from wide-dynamic-range (WDR) neurons in the deep dorsal horn of halothane-anesthetized rats.

Electrophysiological analysis revealed that ablation of lamina I/III NK1 neurons abolishes wind-up of deep dorsal horn neurons and reduces receptive field (RF) size for low- and high-intensity von Frey filaments (Suzuki et al. 2002). Consistent with behavioral reports (Nichols et al. 1999), SP-SAP dramatically reduced the second phase of the formalin response in spinal neurons, a correlate of the *N*-methyl-D-aspartate (NMDA)-receptor-mediated, frequency-dependent increase in neuronal activity (known as *wind-up*).

Characterization of neuronal responses to natural stimuli similarly revealed deficits in the coding of mechanical (von Frey 30–75 g) and thermal (42°–48°C) stimuli, selectively for the mildly noxious to noxious range (Suzuki et al. 2002). For heat, the graded response seen normally in deep dorsal horn neurons following application of increasing temperatures was lost, resulting in an abrupt stimulus-response curve. Thus, ablation of superficial NK1 neurons impaired the ability of deep dorsal horn neurons to accurately code for the intensity of mechanical and thermal stimuli. These electrophysiological changes were somewhat surprising because the behavior of these animals indicates that acute nociception remains unaltered (Nichols et al. 1999). However, behavioral studies measure threshold responses, while electrophysiological studies measure responses to suprathreshold stimuli; hence the reduced neuronal stimulus-response may still generate sufficient activity in spinal neurons to elicit withdrawal reflexes to threshold stimuli in SP-SAP-treated rats.

PHARMACOLOGICAL BLOCK OF THE 5-HT3 RECEPTOR USING ONDANSETRON REPRODUCES THE EFFECT OF SP-SAP LESION

What could underlie the plasticity seen in deep WDR neurons following ablation of lamina I/III NK1 neurons? Lamina I neurons form part of an important ascending pathway projecting to the brainstem that indirectly drives descending serotoninergic (5-HT) inputs to the cord (Bowker et al. 1983; Polgar et al. 2002). We hypothesized that alterations in descending controls may account for the pronounced changes seen in deep dorsal horn neurons following treatment with SP-SAP. To test this hypothesis, we blocked the spinal action of 5-HT at the excitatory ionotropic 5-HT3 receptor by using ondansetron, a selective 5-HT3-receptor antagonist. The 5-HT3 receptors have a pronociceptive function in the spinal cord (Green et al. 2000; Zeitz et al. 2002) and are localized in the superficial dorsal horn, where they are preferentially expressed by a subgroup of small-diameter primary afferents (Kidd et al. 1993; Zeitz et al. 2002).

We observed striking results in SAP-injected rats after intrathecal ondansetron administration. Both the second-phase formalin response and natural (mechanical/thermal) responses were reduced by the antagonist to exactly mimic the stimulus-response relation seen in the SP-SAP group (Fig. 1). The only exception was wind-up, which remained unaffected by the antagonist. In rats with ablation of lamina I/III NK1 neurons, spinally administered ondansetron produced little or no effect on any neuronal measure. These results thus provide novel evidence for a 5-HT3-receptor-mediated descending excitatory influence on the mechanical and thermal responses of deep dorsal horn neurons. Most electrophysiological alterations that accompany SP-SAP treatment can be reproduced by a pharmacological block of the 5-HT3 receptor; thus, these lamina I/III neurons must activate descending excitatory circuits that act through spinal excitatory 5-HT3 receptors to allow deep WDR cells to code peripheral inputs (Fig. 2). Importantly, wind-up does not depend on a descending facilitatory influence, in keeping with many studies showing that it is an intrinsic spinal event.

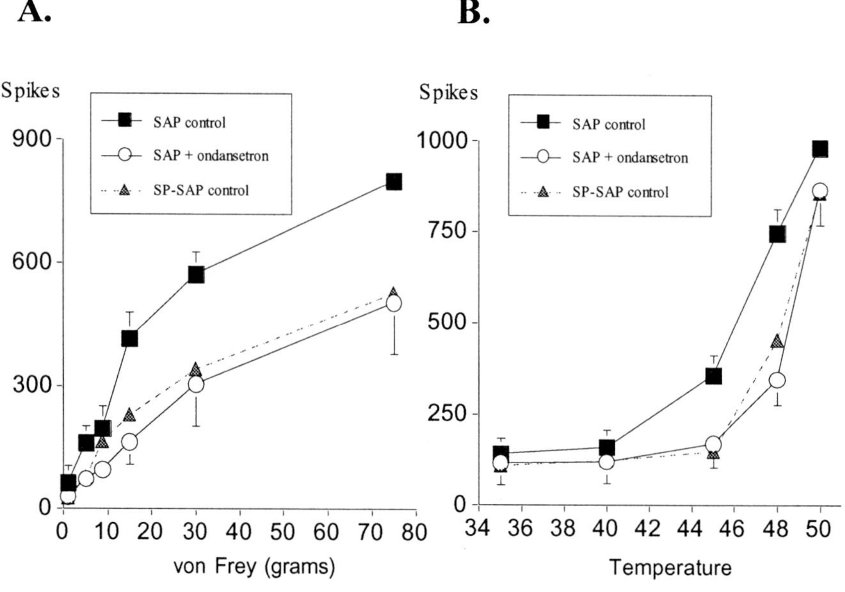
A.
B.
Spikes
SAP control
SAP + ondansetron
SP-SAP control
900
600
300
0
0 10 20 30 40 50 60 70 80
von Frey (grams)
Spikes
1000
750
500
250
0
34 36 38 40 42 44 46 48 50
Temperature

C.
D.

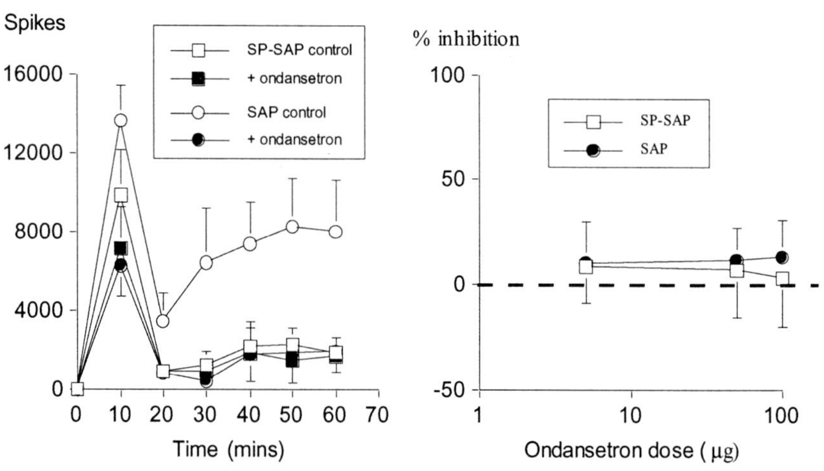
Spikes
SP-SAP control
+ ondansetron
SAP control
+ ondansetron
16000
12000
8000
4000
0
0 10 20 30 40 50 60 70
Time (mins)
% inhibition
SP-SAP
SAP
100
50
0
-50
1 10 100
Ondansetron dose (μg)

DESCENDING CONTROLS ARE LOST FOLLOWING SP-SAP TREATMENT

If SP-SAP attenuates descending excitatory pathways, it can be envisaged that descending inhibitory controls, which also require intact descending pathways, are similarly disrupted. This surmise led us to investigate whether the phenomenon of diffuse noxious inhibitory control (DNIC, a widespread inhibition of WDR neurons triggered by heterotopic noxious stimulation) is attenuated in rats treated with SP-SAP. Examination of *c-fos* expression in the cervical cord following noxious thermal stimulation of the forepaw alone or of both the fore- and hindpaw revealed a loss of DNIC in rats treated with SP-SAP. Furthermore, Fos immunoreactivity (Fos-IR) following noxious fore- and hindpaw stimulation was reduced in the nucleus raphe magnus of SP-SAP-treated rats, compared to SAP-treated controls. Finally, we showed that *c-fos* expression in 5-HT-containing neurons in the nucleus raphe magnus was reduced after ablation of NK1 lamina I/III neurons. Taken together, these results support the idea of a loss of descending 5-HT-mediated control following ablation of lamina I/III NK1 neurons.

CONCLUSIONS

Lamina I/III NK1 projection cells represent important links between peripheral afferent traffic and the full sensory repertoire of WDR neurons, and their destruction has a significant effect on the responses of deep dorsal horn neurons to polymodal stimuli. The gate control theory of pain originally described by Melzack and Wall (1965) proposed that the spinal cord acts like a gate that can facilitate or inhibit sensory transmission through a

---

← **Fig. 1.** Spinal ondansetron administration mimics the effect of substance P/saporin (SP-SAP) treatment in SAP-injected rats. (A) Mechanical coding and (B) thermal coding are disrupted following SP-SAP treatment (dashed line) and are reproduced by pharmacological block of the excitatory 5-HT3 receptor using ondansetron in SAP-injected rats (open circles). (C) Similarly, the second phase of the formalin response was markedly reduced in rats treated with SP-SAP (open squares), compared to SAP-treated controls (open circles), following ablation of superficial NK1 neurons. Following ondansetron administration, the already-reduced formalin response remained unaltered in SP-SAP-treated rats. Remarkably, the formalin second phase of SAP-injected rats was dramatically reduced following ondansetron, to exactly overlay the SP-SAP control-response curve. (D) Following ablation of lamina I/III NK1 neurons, wind-up was dramatically reduced in deep dorsal horn neurons of SP-SAP-treated rats. Administration of spinal ondansetron produced little or no effect on this measure in SP-SAP-treated rats. In SAP-treated control rats, wind-up was similarly unaffected by ondansetron, a finding that was in marked contrast to the inhibitions seen with the mechanical, thermal, and formalin responses following pharmacological block of 5-HT3 receptors.

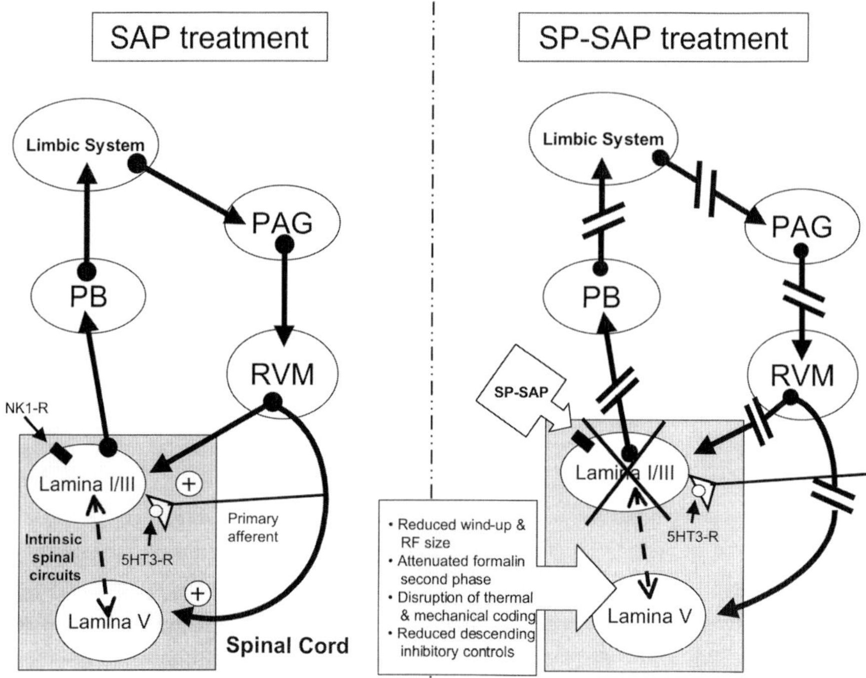

Fig. 2. Proposed circuit for the effect of SP-SAP lesion of NK1 lamina I/III neurons on descending controls from the brainstem. Lamina I/III NK1-expressing neurons are at the origin of the spinal-bulbo-spinal loop. Possible anatomical substrates for this pathway are shown. SP-SAP treatment disrupts descending projections to the spinal cord, in particular, a 5-HT3-receptor-mediated excitatory pathway. The 5-HT3 receptors appear to be localized on the nerve terminals of thinly myelinated fibers and a subset of C fibers (non-VR1, nonpeptidergic) (Zeitz et al. 2002). SP-SAP treatment results in an alteration in the response characteristic of lamina V neurons, through alterations in descending pathways and changes in intrinsic spinal circuits (dashed arrows). NK1-R = NK1 receptor; PAG = periaqueductal gray; PB = parabrachial area; RF = receptive field; RVM = rostroventral medulla.

dynamic influence both from primary afferent input and by descending projections from the brainstem (Melzack and Wall 1965). Our results lend further support to this theory, providing an electrophysiological, pharmacological, and immunohistochemical explanation of the behavioral (Nichols et al. 1999) and neuronal deficits seen after treatment with SP-SAP. Neuronal plasticity observed after SP-SAP treatment is largely explicable in terms of a disruption of descending pathways (Urban and Gebhart 1999) and changes in local spinal circuits. These findings support the hypothesis that lamina I/III neurons are at the origin of the spinal-bulbo-spinal loop. Descending projections are in part serotoninergic, and most of the effects of SP-SAP treatment, with the notable exception of wind-up, were replicated by application of the 5-HT3-receptor antagonist, ondansetron. It thus appears that 5-HT3-receptor-mediated excitatory projections from the brainstem are needed for sensory coding by deep spinal neurons. The attenuated formalin response seen after SP-SAP treatment or ondansetron administration in SAP-injected rats parallels studies in the 5-HT3-receptor knockout mice, where comparable reductions have been reported (Zeitz et al. 2002). The 5-HT3 receptors are preferentially located on nerve terminals (Kia et al. 1995; Miquel et al. 2002; Zeitz et al. 2002), whereas 5-HT inhibitory synapses are mainly on lamina I cell bodies (Polgar et al. 2002), perhaps indicating differential location of inhibitory and excitatory bulbospinal systems. The balance between these converging actions on deep dorsal horn neurons favors facilitatory drives because ablation of NK1 lamina I/III neurons reduced neuronal responses, despite the concomitant loss of descending inhibitions.

Reduction in wind-up of deep dorsal horn neurons by SP-SAP lesion, but not by ondansetron, suggests that wind-up is predominantly mediated through intrinsic spinal circuits. Wind-up results from summation of slow, long depolarizations indicative of peptide actions that allow NMDA-receptor activation through removal of the voltage-dependent Mg^{2+} block (Dickenson 1995). The reduction in formalin response, wind-up, and receptive field sizes may arise from diminished excitability within spinal circuits in concert with the loss of descending excitation. These results reveal a novel network of spinal and supraspinal circuits that interact to allow a changing spinal sensitivity in the behavioral and environmental context. We conclude that NK1-positive spinal projection neurons in the superficial dorsal horn project upon higher brain areas and control central excitability through intrinsic spinal mechanisms and descending pathways from the brainstem.

ACKNOWLEDGMENTS

This work was supported by the Wellcome Trust, by the London Pain Consortium, and by the European Community Marie Curie Fellowship.

REFERENCES

Bowker R, Westlund K, Sullivan M, Wilber J, Coulter J. Descending serotonergic, peptidergic and cholinergic pathways from the raphe nuclei: a multiple transmitter complex. *Brain Res* 1983; 288:33–48.

Cheunsuang O, Morris R. Spinal lamina I neurons that express neurokinin 1 receptors: morphological analysis. *Neuroscience* 2000; 97:335–345.

Dickenson AH. Spinal cord pharmacology of pain. *Br J Anaesth* 1995; 75:193–200.

Gauriau C, Bernard J. Pain pathways and parabrachial circuits in the rat. *Exp Physiol* 2002; 87:251–2518.

Green G, Scarth J, Dickenson A. An excitatory role for 5-HT in spinal inflammatory nociceptive transmission; state-dependent actions via dorsal horn 5-HT3 receptors in the anaesthetized rat. *Pain* 2000; 89:81–88.

Hunt S. Pain control: breaking the circuit. *Trends Pharmacol Sci* 2000; 21:284–286.

Hunt S, Mantyh P. The molecular dynamics of pain control. *Nature Reviews* 2001; 2:83–91.

Kia H, Miquel M-C, McKernan R, et al. Localization of 5HT3 receptors in the rat spinal cord: immunohistochemistry and in situ hybridization. *Neuroreport* 1995; 6:257–261.

Kidd E, Laporte A, Langlois X, et al. 5HT3 receptors in the rat central nervous system are mainly located on nerve fibres and terminals. *Brain Res* 1993; 612:289–298.

Light A, Sedivec M, Casale E, Jones S. Physiological and morphological characteristics of spinal neurones projecting to the parabrachial region of the cat. *Somatosens Mot Res* 1993; 10:309–325.

Lima D, Almeida A. The medullary dorsal reticular nucleus as a pronociceptive centre of the pain control system. *Prog Neurobiol* 2002; 66:81–108.

Mantyh P, Rogers S, Honore P, et al. Inhibition of hyperalgesia by ablation of lamina I spinal neurons expressing the substance P receptor. *Science* 1997; 278:275–279.

Melzack R, Wall P. Pain mechanisms: a new theory. *Science* 1965; 150:971–979.

Miquel M, Emerit M, Nosjean A, et al. Differential subcellular localization of the 5HT3-As receptor subunit in the rat central nervous system. *Eur J Neurosci* 2002; 15:449–457.

Nichols M, Allen B, Rogers S, et al. Transmission of chronic nociception by spinal neurons expressing the substance P receptor. *Science* 1999; 286:1558–1561.

Polgar E, Puskar Z, Watt C, Matesz C, Todd A. Selective innervation of lamina I projection neurones that possess the neurokinin 1 receptor by serotonin-containing axons in the rat spinal cord. *Neuroscience* 2002; 109:799–809.

Suzuki R, Morcuende S, Webber M, Hunt S, Dickenson A. Superficial NK1 expressing neurones control spinal excitability by activation of descending pathways. *Nat Neurosci* 2002; 12:1319–1326.

Todd A, McGill M and Shehab S. Neurokinin 1 receptor expression by neurons in laminae I, III and IV of the rat spinal dorsal horn that project to the brainstem. *Eur J Neurosci* 2000; 12:689–700.

Urban M, Gebhart G. Supraspinal contributions to hyperalgesia. *Proc Natl Acad Sci USA* 1999; 95:2630–2635.

Zeitz K, Guy N, Malmberg A, et al. The 5-HT3 subtype of serotonin receptor contributes to nociceptive processing via a novel subset of myelinated and unmyelinated nociceptors. *J Neurosci* 2002; 22:1010–1019.

Correspondence to: Rie Suzuki, PhD, Neuropharmacology of Pain Group, Department of Pharmacology, University College London, Gower Street, London WC1E 6BT, United Kingdom. Tel: 0207-679-3737; Fax: 0207-679-3742; email: ucklrsu@ucl.ac.uk.

Proceedings of the 10th World Congress on Pain,
Progress in Pain Research and Management, Vol. 24,
edited by Jonathan O. Dostrovsky, Daniel B. Carr, and
Martin Koltzenburg, IASP Press, Seattle, © 2003.

30

Purinergic and NMDA-Receptor Mechanisms Underlying Tooth Pulp Stimulation-Induced Central Sensitization in Trigeminal Nociceptive Neurons

Chen Yu Chiang,[a] Bo Hu,[a] Soo Joung Park,[a]
Sun Zhang,[a] Chun L. Kwan,[a] James W. Hu,[a]
Jonathan O. Dostrovsky,[b] and Barry J. Sessle[a,b]

Faculties of [a]Dentistry and [b]Medicine, University of Toronto, Toronto, Canada

Nociceptive neurons in spinal nociceptive pathways (e.g., the dorsal horn and ventrobasal thalamus) may undergo a prolonged period of increased excitability following injury or inflammation of spinally innervated tissues. These changes reflect a neuroplasticity or "central sensitization" of nociceptive neuronal circuits and represent important processes in the development of chronic pain (Ren and Dubner 1999; Vos et al. 2000; Ji and Woolf 2001). While NMDA-receptor mechanisms are critical to this central sensitization process, recent studies raise the possibility that purinergic receptor mechanisms involving adenosine triphosphate (ATP) and P2X receptor (P2XR) modulation of glutamate release from presynaptic nociceptive afferents in the central nervous system also may play a role (MacDermott et al. 1999; McCleskey and Gold 1999; Burnstock 2000; Nakatsuka and Gu 2001).

Seven P2XR subtypes have been cloned, and some occur as heteromultimers (e.g., $P2X_2/P2X_3R$, $P2X_1/P2X_5R$, and $P2X_4/P2X_6R$). $P2X_1R$ through $P2X_6R$ are all expressed in neurons of sensory ganglia, and with the exception of $P2X_3R$, they are also found in dorsal and ventral regions of the spinal cord. $P2X_2R$, $P2X_4R$, and $P2X_6R$ in particular are expressed within lamina II of the dorsal horn. $P2X_1R$ and $P2X_3R$ are both highly sensitive (eliciting fast currents) and have rapidly desensitizing responses to ATP and its agonist

α,β-methylene ATP (meATP). The heteromeric form $P2X_{2/3}R$ is also sensitive but with a slow current, and is characterized by slow desensitization kinetics and potentiation by low pH. $P2X_2R$, $P2X_4R$, and $P2X_6R$ are much less sensitive and mediate a nondesensitizing response (Lewis et al. 1995; Ueno et al. 1998, 1999; McCleskey and Gold 1999; North and Surprenant 2000; Khakh et al. 2001). The trinitrophenyl analogue of ATP, 2',3'-O-(2,4,6-trinitrophenyl)adenosine 5'-triphosphate (TNP-ATP), is a highly selective antagonist for $P2X_1R$, $P2X_3R$, and $P2X_{2/3}R$, but not for other P2XRs; TNP-ATP is 1,000-fold more effective when blocking ATP-induced currents at $P2X_1R$ or $P2X_3R$ than at $P2X_2R$, $P2X_4R$, or $P2X_7R$ (see North and Suprenant 2000).

One of the most common pains in the body is toothache resulting from injury or inflammation of the tooth pulp, yet information is limited regarding the central neural consequences of pulpal injury and inflammation. Nonetheless, it is established that pulp afferent inputs project onto nociceptive brainstem neurons in the trigeminal subnucleus caudalis (Vc, also termed the medullary dorsal horn, MDH), and the subnucleus oralis (Vo). As in the spinal dorsal horn, central sensitization can be induced in Vc and Vo nociceptive neurons by the application of small-fiber excitants and inflammatory irritants such as mustard oil (MO) to cutaneous or deep tissues (Hu et al. 1992; Ren and Dubner 1999; Sessle 2000). In an effort to understand the central mechanisms involved in inflammatory toothache, we initiated a series of studies to determine (1) if central sensitization can be induced in nociceptive neurons in Vc and Vo by application of MO to the tooth pulp, and (2) whether NMDA and purinergic receptor mechanisms are involved in the MO-induced effects.

METHODS

The methods used have been detailed previously (Chiang et al. 1998, 2002a; Park et al. 2001; Hu et al. 2002) and were approved by the University of Toronto Animal Care Committee. Briefly, neuronal activity was recorded from histologically confirmed sites in Vc or Vo of urethane/α-chloralose-anesthetized male adult rats. A wide range of graded mechanical stimuli (brush, pressure, and pinch) and noxious radiant heat (51°–53°C) was used to classify single neurons into wide-dynamic-range (WDR), nociceptive-specific (NS), or low-threshold mechanoreceptive (LTM) neurons. Baseline values were first determined for the neuronal mechanoreceptive field (RF), spontaneous activity, mechanical activation threshold, and suprathreshold responses to graded pinch or heavy pressure (20–200 g) stimuli. A segment (0.5 mm) of dental paper point soaked with either 0.2 μL MO (allyl isothiocyanate, 95%) or mineral oil (which served as control) was applied to the exposed ipsilateral maxillary molar pulp. Three minutes after the MO or mineral oil application, spontaneous activity, RF, and response properties were repeatedly determined at intervals of 8–10 minutes over a 40–60-minute period. Data were expressed as mean ± SE or median with 25th and 75th percentiles. In some rats, in which neuronal recordings were made in Vc or Vo, 10–35 minutes prior to MO application we administered either the NMDA-receptor antagonist MK-801 or a P2XR agonist by intrathecal microinjection into the rostral Vc or by intranuclear microinjection into the Vo. In other rats, in which neuronal recordings were made in Vo, we instead administered the synaptic blocker $CoCl_2$ or a P2XR antagonist by microinjection to the Vc 20 minutes after MO application. Differences in chemical-induced effects were treated statistically by analysis of variance (ANOVA), and individual pair data were treated by the *t* test or Mann-Whitney test; a *P* value < 0.05 was considered statistically significant.

RESULTS

NMDA-receptor-dependent central sensitization in the Vc. Possible MO-induced central sensitization in the Vc was first tested by application of saline vehicle (10 μL) to the surface of the rostral Vc, followed by MO application to the molar pulp. This treatment produced central sensitization in all four WDR and eight NS neurons tested (but not in LTM neurons), as reflected by a prolonged significant decrease in mechanical activation threshold as well as significant increases in neuronal spontaneous activity, pinch and/or tactile RF size, and suprathreshold responses to graded pinch stimuli; many of the NS neurons developed a MO-induced novel tactile RF (Fig. 1; Table I). Mineral oil application to the pulp did not produce any significant neuronal changes over the 40–60 minute observation period. Pretreatment with MK-801 (10 μg/10 μL) applied to the rostral Vc significantly reduced or abolished the MO-induced neuroplastic changes (Fig. 1) (Chiang et al. 1998).

NMDA-receptor-dependent central sensitization in the Vo. As in the case of the Vc neurons, mineral oil application to the pulp was ineffective, but pretreatment with saline vehicle microinjection (0.3 μL) into the Vo, followed by MO pulp application, was associated with significant increases in spontaneous activity, pinch and/or tactile RF size, and responses to graded pinch stimuli, as well as a significant decrease in mechanical threshold of all Vo nociceptive neurons tested (three WDR, five NS neurons). Furthermore,

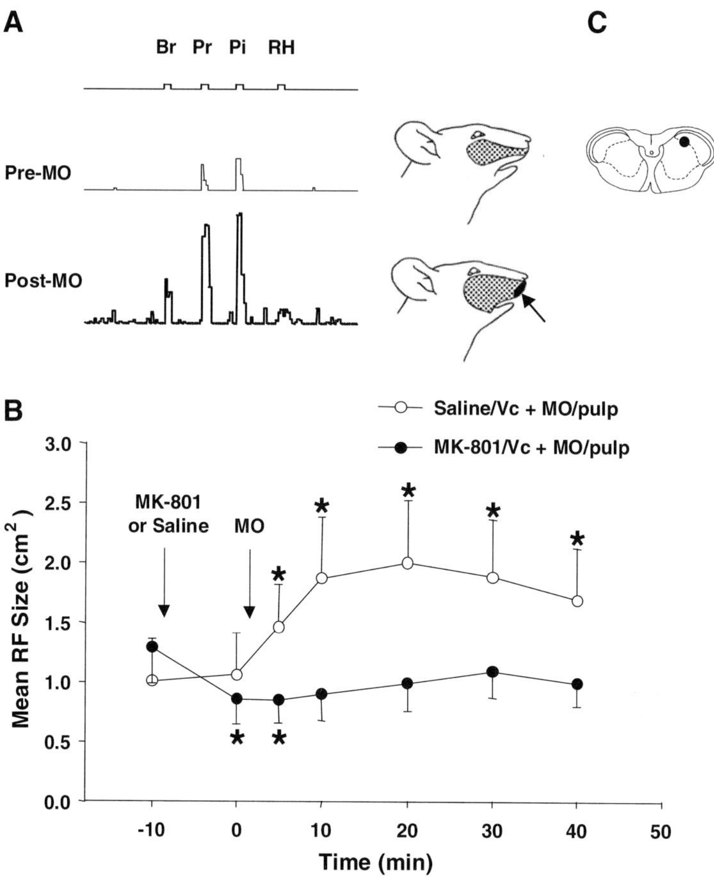

Fig. 1. Neuroplastic changes in trigeminal subnucleus caudalis (Vc) neuronal mechanoreceptive field (RF) and response properties following mustard oil (MO) application to the right maxillary molar pulp, and their attenuation by pretreatment of MK-801 to the Vc (saline as control). (A) Responses of a nociceptive-specific (NS) neuron to mechanical and thermal stimuli applied to the cutaneous RF. Upper trace is a marker of Br (brush), Pr (pressure), Pi (pinch), and RH (radiant heat). Middle trace shows neuronal responses in control conditions (i.e., pre-MO, before MO application). Lower trace shows neuronal responses to similar stimuli 20 minutes after MO application (i.e., post-MO, after MO application). (B) Time course of MO-induced neuroplastic changes in mean pinch RF size of Vc nociceptive neurons. Note that the pinch RF sizes of the Saline/Vc group (n = 12) significantly increased throughout the 40-minute observation period following MO application ($^*P < 0.05$; repeated-measures ANOVA), while those of the MK-801/Vc group (n = 9) were unchanged. In addition, in the MK-801/Vc group, the value at 10 minutes (i.e., 0 minutes in the graph) after MK-801 application is significantly lower than the baseline value, indicating that pretreatment with MK-801 (10 µg, i.t.) reduces the pinch RF size. (C) MO-induced expansion of cutaneous pinch RF as well as transient appearance of tactile RF. Dotted area represents pinch RF size before MO application; black area shows appearance of tactile RF 10 minutes after MO application. The drawing of a transverse section at the rostral Vc illustrates the histologically retrieved neuronal recording site.

Table I
Effects of NMDA and purinergic receptor agonists and antagonists on mustard oil-induced central sensitization

Neuron Type	Experimental Procedure	Spontaneous Activity	RF Size	Response to Noxious Stimulus	Mechanical Activation Threshold	Reference
Vc	MO	↑	↑	↑	↓	
	MK801/Vc + MO	X	X	X	X	Chiang et al. 1998
Vo	MO	↑	↑	↑	↓	
	MK801/Vo + MO	X	X	X	X	Park et al. 2001
	$CoCl_2$/Vc + MO	X	X	X	X	
	$CoCl_2$/Vi + MO	↑	↑	↑	↓	Chiang et al. 2002
	TNP-ATP/Vc + MO	X	X	X	X	
	α,β-meATP/Vc	↑	↑	↑	↓	
	α,β-meATP/Vc + MO	X	X	X	X	
	β,γ-meATP/Vc	O	O	O	O	
	β,γ-meATP/Vc + MO	↑	↑	↑	↓	Hu et al. 2002
Thal. VPM	MO	↑	↑	↑	↓	
	$CoCl_2$/Vc + MO	X	X	X	X	Unpublished data

Symbols and abbreviations: ↑ prolonged increase; ↓ prolonged decrease; X blocking effect; O no effect; Vc = trigeminal subnucleus caudalis; Vo = subnucleus oralis; thal. VPM = thalamic nucleus ventralis posteromedialis; MO = mustard oil.

pretreatment with MK-801 microinjection (3 μg/0.3 μL) into the Vo close to the recording site significantly reduced the MO-induced neuroplastic changes reflecting Vo central sensitization (Park et al. 2001).

The pulp-induced central sensitization in the Vo must depend on the functional integrity of the Vc because microinjection of $CoCl_2$ (5 mM, 0.3 μL) into the ipsilateral Vc produced a reversible blockade of the MO-induced Vo neuroplastic changes. In control experiments, microinjection of vehicle into the ipsilateral Vc or microinjection of $CoCl_2$ outside the Vc (e.g., into the subnucleus interpolaris, Vi) did not affect the MO-induced neuroplastic changes in the Vo (Chiang et al. 2002a).

P2X-receptor-dependent central sensitization. Administration to the rostral Vc of the selective $P2X_1R$, $P2X_3R$, and $P2X_{2/3}R$ antagonist TNP-ATP (2 μg/10 μL) significantly and reversibly attenuated the MO-induced neuroplastic changes in all Vo nociceptive neurons tested (eight WDR neurons), whereas

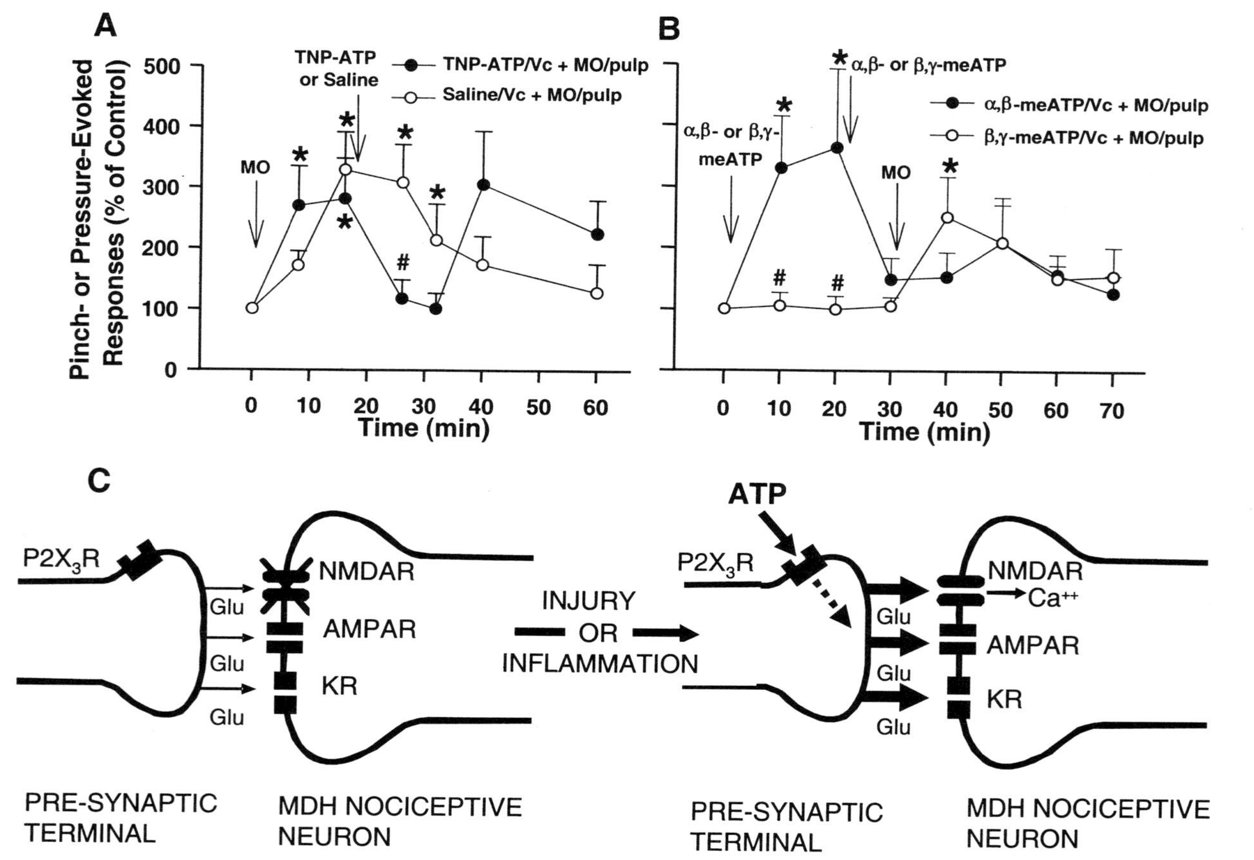

A
B
Pinch- or Pressure-Evoked Responses (% of Control)
500
400
300
200
100
0
MO
TNP-ATP or Saline
TNP-ATP/Vc + MO/pulp
Saline/Vc + MO/pulp
0 10 20 30 40 50 60
Time (min)
α,β- or β,γ-meATP
α,β- or β,γ-meATP
α,β-meATP/Vc + MO/pulp
β,γ-meATP/Vc + MO/pulp
MO
0 10 20 30 40 50 60 70
Time (min)
C
P2X3R
Glu
NMDAR
AMPAR
KR
PRE-SYNAPTIC TERMINAL
MDH NOCICEPTIVE NEURON
INJURY OR INFLAMMATION
ATP
P2X3R
Glu
NMDAR
Ca++
AMPAR
KR
PRE-SYNAPTIC TERMINAL
MDH NOCICEPTIVE NEURON

saline administration had no effect (Fig. 2A). Administration to the rostral Vc of the selective $P2X_1R$, $P2X_3R$, and $P2X_{2/3}R$ agonist α,β-meATP (1 μg/10 μL) produced significant neuroplastic changes in the Vo nociceptive neurons tested (eight WDR neurons), followed by neuronal desensitization as evidenced by the ineffectiveness of a second application of α,β-meATP and subsequent application of MO to the pulp (e.g., Fig. 2B). Administration of the selective $P2X_1R$ agonist β,γ-meATP (1 μg/10 μL) was ineffective (e.g., Fig. 2B) (Hu et al. 2002). Table I summarizes the various findings in the Vc and Vo.

DISCUSSION

MO application to the tooth pulp produced significant increases in spontaneous activity, RF size, and suprathreshold responses, and a decrease in mechanical activation threshold in over 90% of WDR and NS neurons in both the Vc and Vo (Chiang et al. 1998, 2002a; Park et al. 2001; Hu et al. 2002). These results indicate that the MO-induced activation of molar pulpal afferents can produce profound neuroplastic changes that reflect central sensitization in both Vc and Vo nociceptive neurons. These changes may contribute to the hyperalgesia, allodynia, and spread of pain that can be associated

← **Fig. 2.** (A) Time course of MO-induced neuroplastic changes in responses to a pinch or pressure stimulus in Vo nociceptive neurons, and their attenuation by the P2X antagonist TNP-ATP applied to the Vc (the medullary dorsal horn, MDH) 20 minutes after MO (saline as control). Significant differences (*$P < 0.05$) were found between baseline values (0 minutes) and values at different time points after MO application (repeated measures ANOVA) and significant differences (# $P < 0.05$) in values 26-minutes after MO application between the effects of TNP-ATP/Vc and Saline/Vc groups (*t* test). The RF size increase and activation threshold decrease induced by MO were similarly antagonized by TNP-ATP (not illustrated). (B) Time course of neuroplastic changes in responses to a pinch or pressure stimulus induced by application to the Vc of α,β-meATP, but not of β,γ-meATP, and attenuation of the MO/pulp-induced neuroplastic changes following previous α,β-meATP application. Significant differences (*$P < 0.05$) were found between baseline values (0 minutes) and values at different time points after α,β-meATP application (repeated measures ANOVA), but not with β,γ-meATP application. Additional significant differences (# $P < 0.05$) in values 10 and 20 minutes after agonist application (time 0) were found between these two P2XR agonists (*t* test). MO produced a significant increase in pinch- or pressure-evoked responses in the β,γ-meATP/Vc group, but no effect was found in the α,β-meATP/Vc group. The RF size increase and activation threshold decrease were similarly affected by α,β-meATP, which also attenuated the subsequent MO-induced changes (not illustrated). (C) Working schema based on the literature and our current data showing that, after peripheral tissue injury or inflammation, ATP acts on presynaptic P2XRs, which increases the release of the excitatory neurotransmitter glutamate, which in turn acts on NMDA receptors (NMDAR) on nociceptive neurons to produce the neuroplastic changes associated with central sensitization. AMPAR = AMPA receptors; KR = kainate receptors.

with pulpal injury and inflammation. Furthermore, we have recently found evidence that MO application to the pulp induces central sensitization in 35 nociceptive neurons tested in the thalamic nucleus ventralis posteromedialis (VPM), and as in the Vo, we noted that central sensitization in the VPM is secondary to and dependent on the functional integrity of the Vc (Chiang et al. 2002b; Table I). These findings are consistent with the major role of the Vc in trigeminal nociceptive processing by virtue of its neuronal circuitry, its neurochemical receptor processes (e.g., NMDA, neurokinin), and its ascending projections to both the VPM and Vo (see Sessle 2000).

We found that central sensitization in both the Vc and Vo can be antagonized by application of MK-801. This finding is consistent with previous studies demonstrating that NMDA-dependent central sensitization can be selectively induced in trigeminal brainstem nociceptive neurons by MO or other algesic chemicals applied to the craniofacial skin or deep tissues, and that it is accompanied by enhanced jaw electromyographic activity that is dependent on the functional integrity of the Vc and on NMDA-receptor mechanisms in the Vc (see Hu et al. 1992; Yu et al. 1996; Ren and Dubner 1999; Sessle 2000; Cairns et al. 2001).

In addition to the importance of NMDA-receptor mechanisms in central sensitization and in the initiation and maintenance of chronic pain, recent evidence indicates that ATP also plays an important role (see MacDermott et al. 1999, McCleskey and Gold 1999; Burnstock 2000). ATP may activate P2Y metabotropic receptors and P2X ionotropic receptors. Also, spinal studies indicate that ATP activates spinal dorsal neurons at the central terminals of primary afferents and may modulate glutamate release and alter neuronal responses to peripheral afferent inputs through presynaptic actions on specific P2XR subtypes, in particular $P2X_3R$ and $P2X_{2/3}R$ (MacDermott et al. 1999; McCleskey and Gold 1999; Burnstock 2000; Nakatsuka and Gu 2001). Other than observations of $P2X_3Rs$ in tooth pulp sensory neurons and presumably their central endings (Cook et al. 1997; Alavi et al. 2001), there have been no published reports of purinergic receptor mechanisms in central trigeminal nociceptive processes. Our initial studies on this topic with the use of selective $P2X_1R$, $P2X_3R$, and $P2X_{2/3}R$ agonists and antagonists have revealed that application to the Vc of the selective $P2X_1R$, $P2X_3R$, and $P2X_{2/3}R$ agonist α,β-meATP, but not the selective $P2X_1R$ agonist β,γ-meATP, can evoke neuroplastic changes indicative of central sensitization in Vo nociceptive neurons. These findings suggest that the initiation of central sensitization depends on the release of endogenous ATP in the Vc. Our findings that TNP-ATP can reversibly block the ongoing neuroplastic changes induced by MO application suggest that the maintenance of central sensitization also depends on the existence of endogenous ATP.

Heteromeric $P2X_{2/3}Rs$ are expressed mostly on capsaicin-insensitive, medium-sized cells in the dorsal root ganglion (DRG; Ueno et al. 1999; Petruska et al. 2000; Tsuda et al. 2000). These receptors have slow desensitization kinetics, are less sensitive to α,β-meATP, are potentiated by low pH, and are readily distinguished from the $P2X_3R$ in vitro. In particular, ATP- and α,β-meATP-evoked inward currents are dramatically decreased for more than 10 minutes by a second application of the agonist in the case of $P2X_1R$ or $P2X_3R$, but little or no such decrease occurs in the case of $P2X_{2/3}R$ (Lewis et al. 1995; Ueno et al. 1998, 1999). In our studies the initial effect produced by α,β-meATP could not be reproduced by a second application, consistent with behavioral findings (Tsuda et al. 1999) suggesting that $P2X_3Rs$, rather than $P2X_{2/3}Rs$, are involved in eliciting the central sensitization observed. This finding also suggests that the effects observed are due to a presynaptic action on capsaicin-sensitive nociceptive primary afferents because only the capsaicin-sensitive DRG neurons display marked desensitization to repeated applications of α,β-meATP, as shown by in vitro studies (Ueno et al. 1999).

Taken together with the current literature on purinergic receptor mechanisms, our findings strongly indicate that endogenous ATP and $P2X_3Rs$ play a key role in the initiation and maintenance of central sensitization, possibly through a presynaptic regulation of excitatory neurotransmitters (e.g., glutamate) that act on NMDA receptors to produce central sensitization (diagrammed in Fig. 2C). Future studies in our laboratory will directly assess P2XR mechanisms in Vc nociceptive neurons and determine their possible regulation of glutamate release and postsynaptic NMDA-receptor activation.

ACKNOWLEDGMENTS

This study was supported by NIH grant DE-04786. B.J. Sessle holds a Canada Research Chair.

REFERENCES

Alavi AM, Dubyak GR, Burnstock G. Immunohistochemical evidence for ATP receptors in human dental pulp. *J Dent Res* 2001; 80:476–483.

Burnstock G. P2X receptors in sensory neurones. *Br J Anaesth* 2000; 204:476–488.

Cairns BE, Sessle BJ, Hu JW. Temporomandibular-evoked jaw muscle reflex: role of brain stem NMDA and non-NMDA receptors. *Neuroreport* 2001; 12:1875–1878.

Chiang CY, Park SJ, Kwan CL, Hu JW, Sessle BJ. NMDA receptor mechanisms contribute to neuroplasticity induced in caudalis nociceptive neurons by tooth pulp stimulation. *J Neurophysiol* 1998; 80:2621–2631.

Chiang CY, Hu B, Hu JW, Dostrovsky JO, Sessle BJ. Central sensitization of nociceptive neurons in trigeminal subnucleus oralis depends on integrity of subnucleus caudalis. *J Neurophysiol* 2002a; 88:256–264.

Chiang CY, Park SJ, Zhang S, et al. Central sensitization in VPM thalamic nociceptive neurons depends on trigeminal (V) subnucleus caudalis. *Soc Neurosci Abstr* 2002b; 28:656.16.

Cook SP, Vulchanova L, Hargreaves KM, Elde R, McCleskey EW. Distinct ATP receptors on pain-sensing and stretch-sensing neurons. *Nature* 1997; 387:505–508.

Hu JW, Sessle BJ, Raboisson P, Dallel R, Woda A. Stimulation of craniofacial muscle afferents induces prolonged facilitatory effects in trigeminal nociceptive brain-stem neurones. *Pain* 1992; 48:53–60.

Hu B, Chiang CY, Hu JW, Dostrovsky JO, Sessle BJ. P2X receptors in trigeminal subnucleus caudalis modulate central sensitization in trigeminal subnucleus oralis. *J Neurophysiol* 2002; 88:1614–1624.

Ji RR, Woolf CJ. Neuronal plasticity and signal transduction in nociceptive neurons: implications for the initiation and maintenance of pathological pain. *Neurobiol Dis* 2001; 8:1–10.

Khakh BS, Burnstock G, Kennedy C, et al. International union of pharmacology. XXIV. Current status of the nomenclature and properties of P2X receptors and their subunits. *Pharmacol Rev* 2001; 53:107–118.

Lewis CJ, Neidhart S, Holy C, et al. Coexpression of P2X2 and P2X3 receptor subunits can account for ATP-gated currents in sensory neurons. *Nature* 1995; 377:432–435.

MacDermott AB, Role LW, Siegelbaum SA. Presynaptic ionotropic receptors and the control of transmitter release. *Annu Rev Neurosci* 1999; 22:443–485.

McCleskey EW, Gold MS. Ion channels of nociception. *Annu Rev Physiol* 1999; 61:835–856.

Nakatsuka T, Gu JG. ATP P2X receptor-mediated enhancement of glutamate release and evoked EPSCs in dorsal horn neurons of the rat spinal cord. *J Neurosci* 2001; 21:6522–6531.

North RA, Surprenant A. Pharmacology of cloned P2X receptors. *Annu Rev Pharmacol Toxicol* 2000; 40:563–580.

Park SJ, Chiang CY, Hu JW, Sessle BJ. Neuroplasticity induced by tooth pulp stimulation of nociceptive neurons in trigeminal subnucleus oralis involves NMDA receptor mechanisms. *J Neurophysiol* 2001; 85:1836–1846.

Petruska JC, Napaporn J, Johnson RD, Gu JG, Cooper BY. Subclassified acutely dissociated cells of rat DRG: histochemistry and patterns of capsaicin-, proton-, and ATP-activated currents. *J Neurophysiol* 2000; 84:2365–2379.

Ren K, Dubner R. Central nervous system plasticity and persistent pain. *J Orofac Pain* 1999; 13:155–163.

Sessle BJ. Acute and chronic craniofacial pain: brainstem mechanisms of nociceptive transmission and neuroplasticity, and their clinical correlates. *Crit Rev Oral Biol Med* 2000; 11:57–91.

Tsuda M, Ueno S, Inoue K. In vivo pathway of thermal hyperalgesia by intrathecal administration of a,b-methylene ATP in mouse spinal cord: involvement of the glutamate-NMDA receptor system. *Br J Pharmacol* 1999; 127:449–456.

Tsuda M, Koizumi S, Kita A, et al. Mechanical allodynia caused by intraplantar injection of P2X receptor agonist in rats: involvement of heteromeric $P2X_{2/3}$ receptor signaling in capsaicin-insensitive primary afferent neurons. *J Neurosci* 2000; 20:RC90 (1–5).

Ueno S, Koizumi, S, Inoue K. Characterization of Ca2+ influx through recombinant P2X receptor in C6BU-1 cells. *Br J Pharmacol* 1998; 124:1484–1490.

Ueno S, Tsuda M, Iwanaga T, Inoue K. Cell type-specific ATP-activated responses in rat dorsal root ganglion neurons. *Br J Pharmacol* 1999; 126:429–436.

Vos BP, Benoist JM, Gautron M, Guilbaud G. Changes in neuronal activities in the two ventral posterior medial thalamic nuclei in an experimental model of trigeminal pain in the rat by constriction of one infraorbital nerve. *Somatosens Mot Res* 2000; 17:109–122.

Yu XM, Sessle BJ, Haas DA, et al. Involvement of NMDA receptor mechanisms in jaw electromyographic activity and plasma extravasation induced by inflammatory irritant application to temporomandibular joint region of rats. *Pain* 1996; 68:169–178.

Correspondence to: Barry J. Sessle, BDS, MDS, PhD, FRSC, Faculty of Dentistry, University of Toronto, 124 Edward Street, Toronto, Ontario M5G 1G6, Canada. Tel: 416-979-4910; Fax: 416-979-4936; email: barry.sessle@ utoronto.ca.

Proceedings of the 10th World Congress on Pain,
Progress in Pain Research and Management, Vol. 24,
edited by Jonathan O. Dostrovsky, Daniel B. Carr, and
Martin Koltzenburg, IASP Press, Seattle, © 2003.

31

Enhanced AMPA Receptor GluR1 Subunit Expression and Neuronal Activation within Brainstem Pain Modulatory Circuitry after Inflammation

Cynthia L. Renn, Yun Guan, Ronald Dubner, and Ke Ren

Department of Oral and Craniofacial Biological Sciences and Program in Neuroscience, Dental School, University of Maryland, Baltimore, Maryland, USA

Supraspinally organized descending pathways within the central nervous system (CNS) modulate the ascending transmission of nociceptive information at the level of the spinal dorsal horn (for reviews see Willis 1988; Fields and Basbaum 1999). Although progress has been made in understanding the function of the descending pathways in response to transient noxious stimuli (Willis 1988; Fields and Basbaum 1999), less is known about their function during persistent noxious stimulation after inflammation. Descending pain modulation is not a fixed process but displays dynamic, temporal changes in response to persistent noxious input, yielding an enhanced net inhibition of hyperalgesia and nocifensive behavior (for reviews see Dubner and Ren 1999; Ren and Dubner 2002). However, research has not yet clarified the changes in the neurochemical mechanisms and neuronal activation within the brainstem pain modulatory circuitry that underlie the enhanced pain modulation during inflammation.

The rostral ventromedial medulla (RVM), which includes the nucleus raphe magnus (NRM), nucleus reticularis gigantocellularis pars alpha (GiA), and nucleus paragigantocellularis lateralis (LPGi), is a major component of the descending pain modulatory circuitry (for reviews see Dubner and Bennett 1983; Duggan and Morton 1988; Fields and Basbaum 1999). Neuronal activity within the RVM increases along with enhanced descending modulation of pain as persistent inflammatory hyperalgesia develops (Schaible et al. 1991; Ren and Dubner 1996, 2002; Dubner and Ren 1999; Urban et al. 1999; Hurley and Hammond 2000; Terayama et al. 2000). Neurons within the RVM express the α-amino-3-hydroxy-5-methylisoxazole-4-propionic acid (AMPA) subtype of glutamate receptors. Glutamate receptors mediate excitatory neurotransmission in the mammalian CNS (Nakanishi 1992; Hollmann and Heinemann 1994). During persistent inflammation, AMPA receptors become activated and the strength of AMPA-mediated synaptic transmission in the RVM increases, accompanied by enhanced inhibition of hyperalgesia and nocifensive behavior (Urban et al. 1999; Guan et al. 2002). Of the four receptor subunits (GluR1–GluR4) that assemble to form heteromeric AMPA receptors, the GluR1 and GluR2 subunits are key components that play a role in postsynaptic AMPA-receptor function (Suarez et al. 1997; Banke et al. 2000).

Inflammation-induced synaptic plasticity within the RVM pain modulatory circuitry may result from an increased expression of AMPA receptors in neurons and/or from increased activation of neurons in the RVM. To test this hypothesis, we examined nocifensive behavior in response to AMPA microinjection, changes in expression of the AMPA-receptor GluR1 subunit, and changes in Fos protein expression in the RVM of rats after inflammation.

METHODS

Animals. Adult male Sprague-Dawley rats (250–350 g) were used. The research protocol followed the International Association for the Study of Pain guidelines for investigations of pain in animals (Zimmerman 1983). The Institutional Animal Care and Use Committee of the University of Maryland Dental School approved the experiments.

Inflammation. Inflammation was induced by a subcutaneous injection of complete Freund's adjuvant (CFA; 0.5 μg/μL *Mycobacterium tuberculosis* in a 1:1 oil : saline emulsion) into the plantar surface of one hindpaw for behavioral testing (0.2 mL) and immunohistochemistry (0.3 mL) or both hindpaws (0.2 mL/paw) for Western blot analysis. After CFA injection, an intense inflammation developed, characterized by erythema, edema, and hyperalgesia. The signs of inflammation were evident 1 hour after injection, remained localized to the injected hindpaw, and persisted for 2 weeks (Iadarola et al. 1988).

Behavioral nociceptive testing. For behavioral testing, the rats were initially anesthetized by intraperitoneal (i.p.) injection of pentobarbital sodium (Nembutal; 45 mg/kg) for insertion of an intravenous (i.v.) catheter into the jugular vein. Throughout the experiment, a light level of anesthesia was maintained by a continuous i.v. infusion of pentobarbital sodium, 3–10 mg/kg/hour (Fields et al. 1983; Sandkühler and Gebhart 1984; Terayama et al. 2002).

We tested the nocifensive behavioral response of the rats to a noxious thermal stimulus by a method modified from Hargreaves et al. (1988). The anesthetized rat was placed in a stereotactic apparatus (David Kopf model 900) situated on a glass platform with the glass temperature maintained at 25°C. The heat source for the thermal stimulus was a high-intensity projector lamp bulb (Osram 58-8007; 8 V, 50 W) located beneath the glass with the light beam directed at either the plantar surface of a hindpaw or the underside of the tail. The stimulus intensity was set to produce paw-withdrawal latencies within 9–11 seconds in naive animals, with a preset 20-second cut-off to minimize the potential for tissue damage. Paw-withdrawal latencies were examined at 0, 3, 5, and 24 hours after inflammation.

Immunohistochemistry. At 0, 3, and 24 hours after inflammation, the rats were deeply anesthetized with pentobarbital (100 mg/kg i.p.) and perfused transcardially with 200 mL of cold 0.9% saline followed by 600 mL of 4% paraformaldehyde (PFA) in 0.1 M phosphate-buffered saline (PBS) at pH 7.4. The brainstem tissue was removed, and frozen coronal tissue sections (30 μm) were cut from a segment of the medulla (Bregma –10.80 to Bregma –11.60; Paxinos and Watson 1998). We used the avidin-biotin method of Hsu et al. (1981) to process the free-floating tissue sections for Fos protein (1:20,000; Oncogene) and GluR1 (1:800; Chemicon) immunohistochemistry. We used the chromogen diaminobenzidine (DAB) with nickel to visualize Fos protein, which appeared black, and DAB alone to visualize GluR1, which appeared brown.

We examined the tissue under bright-field microscopy at 200× magnification. Fos-labeled neurons in the NRM were counted in three randomly selected sections from each rat. To determine the staining intensity of GluR1-like immunoreactivity (GluR1-LI), we used Scion Image to analyze computer-acquired images of the tissue. The pixel densities of all positively stained neurons and 10 unstained background neurons in the NRM of each tissue section were combined to generate one histogram for each group of animals to verify that neurons identified by the investigator as being positively stained for GluR1 were different from background staining. A clear demarcation between background and GluR1-LI neurons was evident in each histogram (for example, see Fig. 3). Only the pixel density measurements of neurons demonstrating an increase in GluR1-LI when compared to background staining were used for analysis. The measured neuronal pixel density minus the background pixel density was calculated as the staining intensity. We used the mean pixel densities of each animal for statistical analysis.

Intracerebral drug microinjection. Following the method of Terayama et al. (2000), we stereotactically placed a 26-gauge stainless steel guide cannula in the RVM (midline, interaural –2 mm, cerebellum surface –9 mm; Paxinos and Watson 1998). A 33-gauge internal cannula was inserted through the lumen, extended 1 mm beyond the tip of the guide cannula, and was connected to a 10-μL Hamilton syringe. All microinjections of drug or vehicle (0.5 μL) were delivered slowly over 1–2 minutes. At the end of the experiment, coronal sections through the RVM (40 μm) were Nissl stained for verification of the cannula location. The (s)-AMPA zwitterion (Sigma-RBI) was the active drug and 0.9% saline was the vehicle control, delivered by microinjection. Cumulative doses of AMPA (0.1, 1, 10, 50, 100 pmol) were given at 30-minute intervals, which allowed response latencies to return to baseline between doses.

Western blot analysis. GluR1 protein levels in RVM tissue were analyzed from naive animals and 2 hours, 5 hours, 24 hours, 3 days, 7 days, and 14 days after inflammation. The rats were overdosed with pentobarbital (100 mg/kg i.p.). Fresh brainstem tissue from a segment of the medulla (interaural –1.33 to interaural –2.5 mm; Paxinos and Watson 1998) was removed and immediately flash-frozen. A punch of RVM tissue (including the NRM, GiA, and LPGi, and excluding the facial nucleus and inferior olive) was obtained from the medullary segment.

The tissue was homogenized and centrifuged. The decanted supernatant was used for all Western blot analyses. Protein concentration was determined by a detergent-compatible protein assay with a bovine serum albumin standard. The proteins were fractionated on a 7.5% (weight/volume) SDS-PAGE gel and transferred to a nitrocellulose membrane (Amersham) by a Trans-Blot Transfer Cell system (Bio-Rad). The membranes were incubated with a rabbit polyclonal antibody to GluR1 (1:1000, Chemicon), followed by incubation with a goat anti-rabbit horseradish peroxidase-conjugated IgG (1:2000, Santa Cruz Biotechnology). Immunoreactivity was detected by enhanced chemiluminescence (Amersham). Computer-assisted densitometry quantified the intensity of immunoreactivity of the autoradiograms. Equal protein loading into the gel lanes was verified by Coumassie blue staining.

Data analysis. Data from all experiments are presented as the mean ± SEM. One-way ANOVA was used to compare the pixel density of GluR1 staining, the intensity of Western blot immunoreactivity, the number of Fos-labeled cells, and withdrawal latency changes in different groups of animals. Fisher's protected least significant difference test was used to identify significance. A priori, statistical significance was set at $P < 0.05$.

RESULTS

Injection of CFA produced an intense inflammation that was restricted to the injected hindpaw. The presence of inflammation was determined by the development of erythema and an increase in the dorsal/plantar paw diameter from 5.1 ± 0.1 mm preinjection to 10.7 ± 0.2 mm at 2 hours postinjection. There was no erythema or change in paw diameter in the noninjected hindpaw.

Cumulative dosing studies in naive and inflamed animals examined the effect of AMPA on the behavioral response to a noxious thermal stimulus. Intra-RVM microinjection of AMPA dose-dependently increased paw-withdrawal latencies at all time points (Fig. 1; Guan et al. 2003), while saline

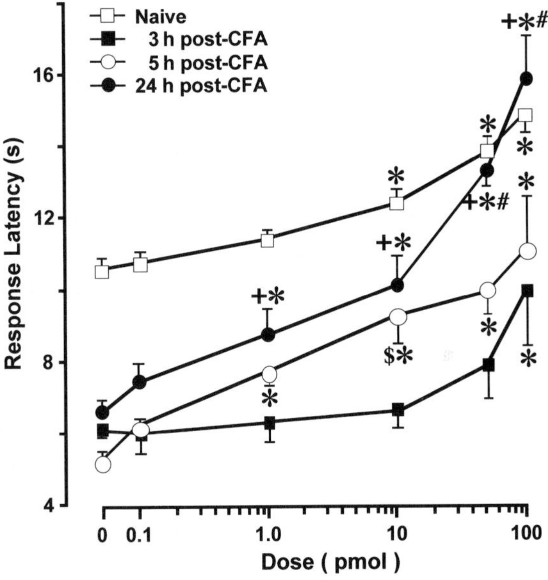

Fig. 1. Microinjection of AMPA into the rostral ventromedial medulla (RVM) increased paw-withdrawal latency in naive rats and inflamed rats 3, 5, and 24 hours after complete Freund's adjuvant (CFA, (n = 6–8 rats per group) (Guan et al. 2002a). Cumulative dosing of AMPA (0.1–100 pmol) was used in these experiments. Intra-RVM microinjection of AMPA produced dose-dependent increases in response latencies at all time points. Low-dose AMPA (1.0, 10 pmol) produced significant increases in paw-withdrawal latencies at 5 and 24 hours post-CFA (*), but was without effect 3 hours post-CFA. High-dose AMPA (50, 100 pmol) produced significant increases in response latencies in naive and inflamed rats 5 and 24 hours post-CFA (*), while 3 hours post-CFA, AMPA produced a significant increase only at the 100 pmol dose (*). At the 50 and 100 pmol doses, a significant leftward shift occurred in the dose-response curve from 3 hours to 5 hour (+), with a further significant shift from 5 hours to 24 hours (#) post-CFA. Symbols indicate significance ($P < 0.05$). Adapted from Guan et al. (2003), with permission.

microinjection had no modulatory effect (Guan et al. 2002). Compared to the predrug baseline, the increase in paw-withdrawal latency became significant for the naive group following the 10-pmol dose ($P < 0.05$) and for the 5-hour and 24-hour groups at 1.0 pmol ($P < 0.05$). The increased paw-withdrawal latency for the 3-hour group did not reach significance until after the 100-pmol dose was given ($P < 0.05$). Further, Fig. 1 demonstrates a significant leftward shift of the dose-response curve occurring from 3 hours to 5 hours ($P < 0.05$), with a further significant shift from 5 hours to 24 hours ($P < 0.05$) after inflammation. We did not compare the dose-response curve of the naive group to the curves of the inflamed groups due to its significant difference in baseline latency.

The findings from the behavioral experiments suggest an increase in AMPA-mediated synaptic transmission within the RVM after inflammation. We next examined whether changes occurred in the amount of GluR1 protein that was expressed in the RVM after inflammation. Western blot analysis showed a time-dependent upregulation of GluR1 protein levels in the RVM (Fig. 2A; Guan et al. 2003). The results of the Western blot analyses ($n = 5$ per time point) were quantified (Fig. 2B). Each bar represents the GluR1 protein levels of inflamed groups as a percentage of the GluR1 protein level of the naive group. While earlier increases in GluR1 protein levels were not statistically significant, a significant increase in GluR1 protein occurred at 24 hours (332.1 ± 119.9%, $P < 0.05$) and 3 days (266.6 ± 53.6%, $P < 0.01$) post-CFA, as compared to that of naive animals (Fig. 2B). The GluR1 protein levels returned to baseline between 7 and 14 days post-CFA.

Immunohistochemistry further confirmed the inflammation-induced upregulation of the GluR1 subunit and localized it to NRM neurons (Fig. 3; Renn et al. 2002). To quantify GluR1, we compared the staining intensities of NRM neurons. Fig. 3D shows a histogram derived from the measurements acquired from the naive group. The arrow indicates a clear demarcation between the pixel densities of background neurons and the pixel densities of neurons identified by the investigator as being positively stained. A baseline level of GluR1 expression in NRM neurons was evident in the absence of inflammation (Fig. 3A). Quantification of GluR1-LI demonstrated a significant increase in staining intensity at 24 hours postinflammation as compared to naive animals (Fig. 3B), as previously reported (Guan et al. 2002). The number of neurons expressing GluR1 following inflammation did not change.

We then examined neuronal activation in the NRM following inflammation by using Fos protein expression as a marker for neuronal activation (Hunt et al. 1987; Menetrey et al. 1989; Wei et al. 1999). The persistent inflammation induced a significant increase in the number of Fos-LI neurons

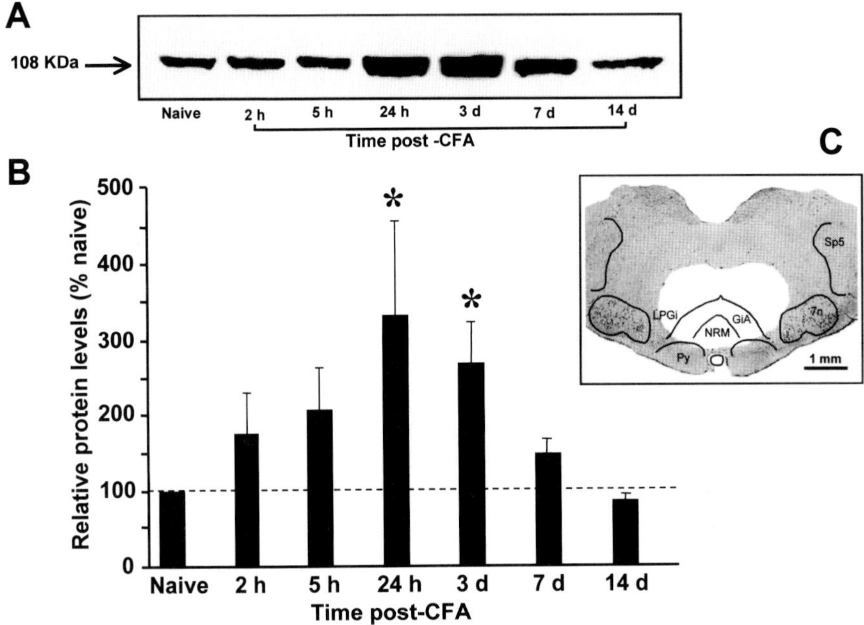

Fig. 2. Inflammation increased GluR1 protein expression in the RVM. (A) An example of Western blot using polyclonal antibodies directed against the AMPA receptor GluR1 subunit. The blot shows GluR1 protein levels at different time points (naive, 2 hours to14 days) after CFA injection. (B) Bar graph summarizing the relative GluR1 protein levels in rat RVM tissue after inflammation, compared to naive animals. Asterisks denote significant differences between experimental and naive groups (ANOVA, $P < 0.05$; $n = 5$ per time point). (C) The RVM tissue, including the NRM, GiA, LPGi and excluding the facial nucleus (7n), pyramidal tract (Py), and inferior olive, was removed by the punch method from a segment of the medulla (interaural –1.3 to interaural –2.5 mm; Paxinos and Watson 1998). Adapted from Guan et al. (2003), with permission.

in the NRM at 3 hours and 24 hours after CFA injection as compared to naive animals (Fig. 4A; Renn et al. 2002). A further significant increase occurred from 3 hours to 24 hours after inflammation.

Finally, we examined whether the upregulation of the GluR1 subunit occurred in activated neurons by testing the staining intensity of GluR1-LI in Fos-expressing neurons. Fig. 3C shows a tissue section that has been double-labeled for Fos protein and GluR1. Both double-labeled neurons (vertical arrows) and single-labeled neurons (horizontal arrows) are clearly evident. We measured the pixel densities of neuronal cell bodies, omitting the nucleus of Fos-labeled neurons. The presence of persistent inflammation induced an increase in GluR1-LI in double-labeled neurons, demonstrated by a significant rightward shift of the distribution curve of pixel densities of

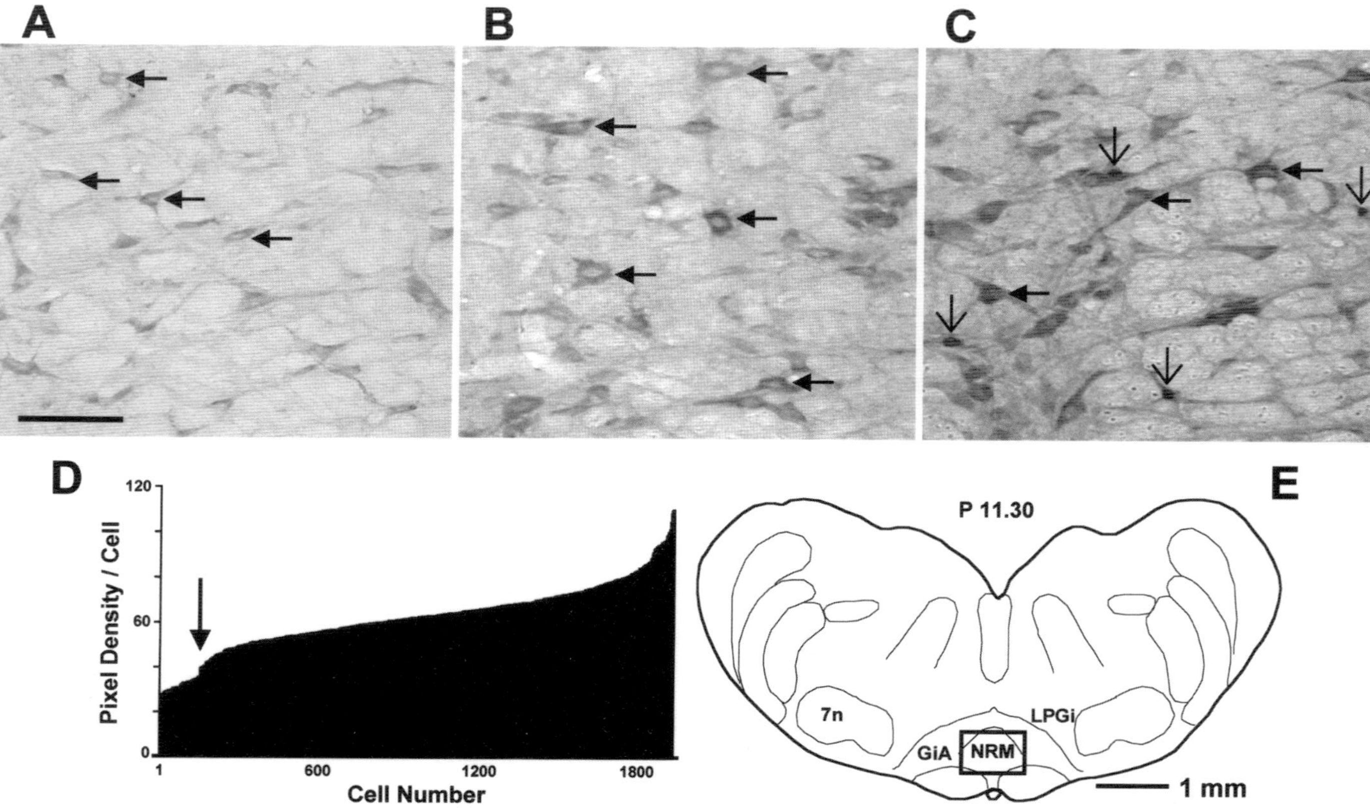

A
B
C
D
Pixel Density / Cell
120
60
0
1
600
1200
1800
Cell Number
E
P 11.30
7n
LPGi
GiA
NRM
1 mm

← **Fig. 3.** Inflammation-induced an increase in GluR1 immunoreactivity in the nucleus raphe magnus (NRM) (Renn et al. 2002). (A) Single-labeled tissue from a naive rat demonstrating GluR1-like immunoreactivity (GluR1-LI) in the NRM. Staining for GluR1-LI is evident in the cytoplasm (arrows) while the nuclei are unstained. Scale bar 200 μm. (B) Single-labeled tissue from an inflamed rat at 24 hours after CFA. Staining for GluR1-LI in the cytoplasm (arrows) appears darker than the staining in naive animals. (C) Tissue from an inflamed rat 24 hours after CFA double-labeled for GluR1 and Fos protein. Single-labeled (horizontal arrows) neurons demonstrate GluR1-LI only and double-labeled (vertical arrows) neurons demonstrate GluR1-LI (cytoplasm) and Fos-LI (nucleus). (D) Histogram of the pixel densities of all stained neurons and a sample of unstained neurons in 18 tissue sections from naive rats. The arrow indicates the demarcation between background unstained neurons and positively stained neurons. The cell number was arbitrarily assigned according to staining intensity. (E) Drawing of the RVM 11.30 mm posterior to Bregma (Paxinos and Watson 1998). The box indicates the site of the analysis in the NRM region. Scale bar 1 mm. GiA = nucleus reticularis gigantocellularis pars alpha; LPGi = nucleus paragigantocellularis lateralis. Adapted from Renn et al. (2003), with permission.

GluR1-LI from naive to 3 hours with a further significant shift from 3 hours to 24 hours (Fig. 4B; Renn et al. 2002). The increase in GluR1-LI staining intensity was also shown by a significant increase in the overall mean pixel density from naive to 3 hours and from 3 hours to 24 hours after inflammation (Fig. 4 inset).

DISCUSSION

We have shown that persistent inflammation induced a time-dependent increase in sensitivity to AMPA microinjected into the RVM, the amount of GluR1 protein expressed in the RVM, the number of activated neurons in the NRM, and the level of GluR1 expression within the activated neurons. These findings suggest that neuronal activation and GluR1 expression may play a role in the development of activity-induced plasticity within the brainstem pain modulatory circuitry and contribute to an enhanced descending pain modulation.

Our results demonstrate that persistent inflammation induces changes in neuronal plasticity in the RVM pain modulatory circuitry, indicated by a time-dependent increase in the level of inhibition produced by microinjection of AMPA into the NRM. Further, our results provide evidence of increased neuronal activation in the NRM after hindpaw inflammation, as measured by Fos protein expression. Descending pain modulation shows dynamic changes during persistent noxious input (Dubner and Ren 1999; Hurley and Hammond 2000; Terayama et al. 2000). Early in the inflammatory process, the net modulatory effect is inhibitory, with a facilitatory component (Terayama et al. 2000; Urban and Gebhart 1999; for reviews see also

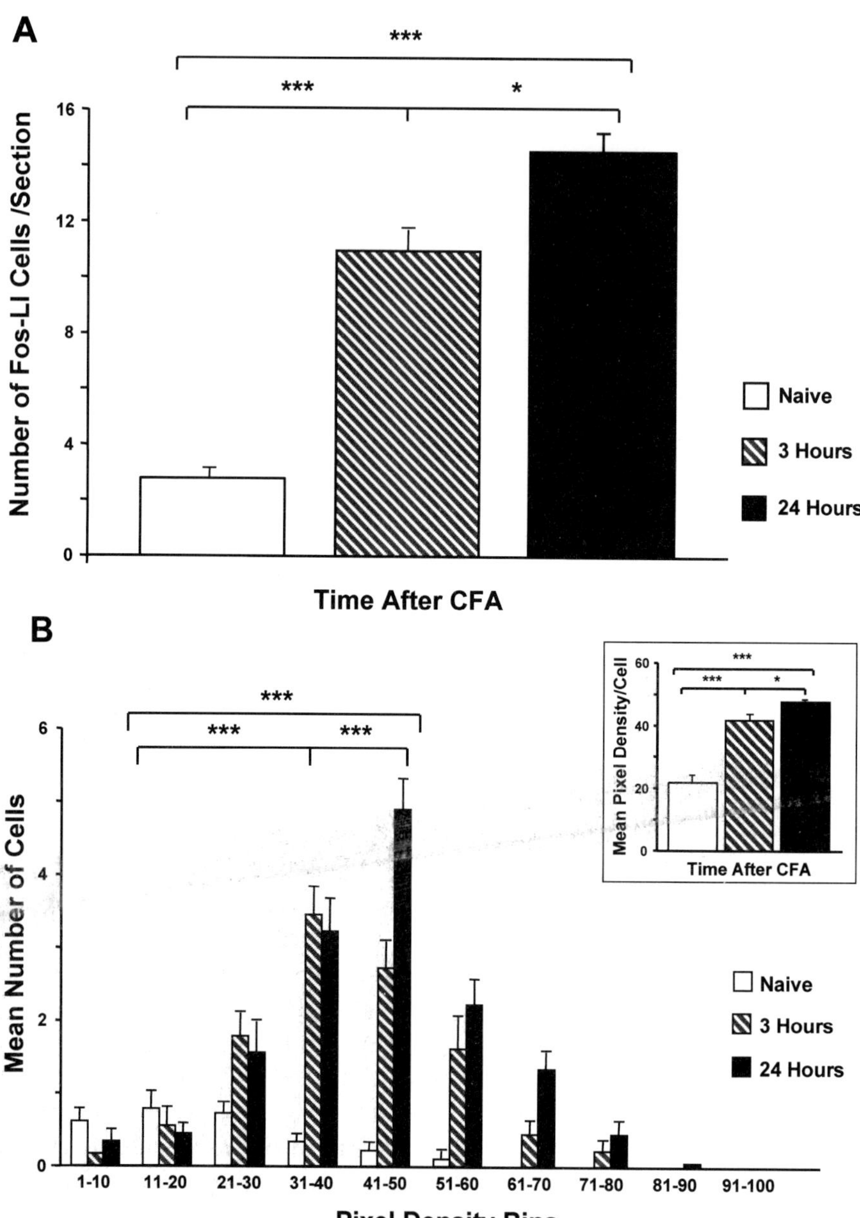
A
***
***
*
16
12
8
4
0
Number of Fos-LI Cells /Section
Naive
3 Hours
24 Hours
Time After CFA
B
***
***
***
6
4
2
0
Mean Number of Cells
60
40
20
0
Mean Pixel Density/Cell
Time After CFA
Naive
3 Hours
24 Hours
1-10
11-20
21-30
31-40
41-50
51-60
61-70
71-80
81-90
91-100
Pixel Density Bins

← **Fig. 4.** Inflammation increased Fos-LI and GluR1-LI in the NRM (Renn et al. 2002). (A) Effect of hindpaw inflammation on the number of Fos-LI neurons in the NRM 0, 3, and 24 hours after CFA injection ($n = 6$ per group). The number of NRM neurons exhibiting Fos-LI increased significantly at 3 hours and 24 hours after CFA compared to naive animals (ANOVA, $P < 0.001$). There was a further significant increase from 3 hours to 24 hours (ANOVA, $P < 0.05$). (B) Effect of hindpaw inflammation on the distribution of GluR1-LI pixel densities in activated (Fos-LI) neurons in the NRM at 0, 3, and 24 hours after CFA injection ($n = 6$ per group). The pixel density curve of GluR1-LI staining in activated neurons shifted significantly (ANOVA, $P < 0.001$) to the right at 3 hours and 24 hours compared to naive. A further significant shift (ANOVA, $P < 0.001$) occurred from 3 hours to 24 hours. The mean pixel density (inset) of GluR1-LI staining in all neurons increased significantly (ANOVA, $P < 0.001$) at 3 hours and 24 hours compared to naive. A further significant increase (ANOVA, $P < 0.05$) occurred from 3 hours to 24 hours. Adapted from Renn et al. (2003), with permission.

Porreca et al. 2002; Ren and Dubner 2002). As the inflammatory process continues, the modulatory effects shift to a greater increase in net inhibition (Hurley and Hammond 2000; Terayama et al. 2000). The findings of these experiments are consistent with our previous study that demonstrated increased activity and a phenotypic change in pain modulatory neurons within the RVM (Miki et al. 2002).

Excitatory amino acids (EAAs) play a key role in the mechanisms underlying descending pain modulation (Aimone and Gebhart 1986; Heinricher et al. 1999; Urban and Gebhart 1999; Terayama et al. 2000; Guan et al. 2002; Miki et al. 2002). The GluR1 subunit is a major component of heteromeric AMPA receptors and is important in postsynaptic AMPA receptor function (Suarez et al. 1997; Banke et al. 2000). Our studies demonstrate an increase in GluR1 staining intensity in activated neurons and an increase in GluR1 protein levels in the RVM after inflammation. The total number of GluR1-LI neurons did not significantly increase after inflammation (Guan et al. 2003), and thus it is likely that the increase in GluR1 expression is occurring in the same group of GluR1-expressing neurons, rather than recruiting non-GluR1-expressing neurons found in the absence of inflammation.

The upregulation of GluR1 protein could be a mechanism underlying the increased inhibitory effect of AMPA in the NRM. Together with an increase in NMDA-receptor activation (Terayama et al. 2000; Miki et al. 2002), the increased AMPA neurotransmission in the RVM leads to an increase in excitability in pain modulatory circuitry. This activity-dependent plasticity mirrors similar changes in excitability found at the spinal level, often referred to as central sensitization (Woolf and Thompson 1991; Dubner and Ruda 1992). Our findings support the hypothesis that plasticity occurs at the RVM level in response to inflammation and may be a common property of structures involved in nociceptive processing at different levels of the CNS following tissue injury.

ACKNOWLEDGMENTS

Sources of support for the study come from the National Institute on Drug Abuse (DA10275) and the National Institute of Nursing Research (NR07837).

REFERENCES

Aimone LD, Gebhart GF. Stimulation-produced spinal inhibition from the midbrain in the rat is mediated by an excitatory amino acid neurotransmitter in the medial medulla. *J Neurosci* 1986; 6:1803–1813.

Banke TG, Bowie D, Lee H, et al. Control of GluR1 AMPA receptor function by cAMP-dependent protein kinase. *J Neurosci* 2000; 20:89–102.

Dubner R, Bennett GJ. Spinal and trigeminal mechanisms of nociception. *Ann Rev Neurosci* 1983; 6:381–418.

Dubner R, Ren K. Endogenous mechanisms of sensory modulation. *Pain (Suppl)* 1999; 6:S45–S53.

Dubner R, Ruda MA. Activity-dependent neuronal plasticity following tissue injury and inflammation. *Trends Neurosci* 1992; 15:96–103.

Duggan AW, Morton CR. Tonic descending inhibition and spinal nociceptive transmission. *Prog Brain Res* 1988; 77:193–211.

Fields HL, Basbaum AI. Central nervous system mechanisms of pain modulation. In: Wall PD, Melzack R (Eds). *Textbook of Pain*. London: Churchill Livingstone, 1999, pp 309–329.

Fields HL, Bry J, Hentall I, Zorman G. The activity of neurons on the rostral medulla of the rat during withdrawal from noxious heat. *J Neurosci* 1983; 3:2545–2552.

Guan Y, Terayama R, Dubner R, Ren K. Plasticity in excitatory amino acid receptor-mediated descending pain modulation after inflammation. *J Pharm Exp Ther* 2002; 300:513–520.

Guan Y, Guo W, Zou S-P, Dubner R, Ren K. Inflammation-induced upregulation of AMPA receptor subunit expression in brainstem pain modulatory circuitry. *Pain* 2003; in press.

Hargreaves K, Dubner R, Brown F, Flores C, Joris J. A new and sensitive method for measuring thermal nociception in cutaneous hyperalgesia. *Pain* 1988; 32:77–88.

Heinricher MM, McGaraughty S, Farr DA. The role of excitatory amino acid transmission within the rostral ventromedial medulla in the antinociceptive actions of systemically administered morphine. *Pain* 1999; 81:57–65.

Hollmann M, Heinemann S. Cloned glutamate receptors. *Ann Rev Neurosci* 1994; 17:31–108.

Hsu SM, Raind L, Fanger H. Use of avidin-biotin-peroxidase complex (ABC) in immunoperoxidase technique: a comparison between ABC and unlabeled antibody (PAP) procedures. *J Histochem Cytochem* 1981; 29:577–580.

Hunt SP, Pini A, Evan G. Induction of c-fos like protein in spinal cord neurons following sensory stimulation. *Nature* 1987; 328:632–634.

Hurley RW, Hammond DL. The analgesic effects of supraspinal μ and δ opioid receptor agonists are potentiated during persistent inflammation. *J Neurosci* 2000; 20:1249–1259.

Iadarola MJ, Brady LS, Draisci G, Dubner R. Enhancement of dynorphin gene expression in spinal cord following experimental inflammation: stimulus specificity, behavioral parameters and opioid receptor binding. *Pain* 1988; 35:313–326.

Menetery D, Gannon A, Levine JD, Basbaum AI. Expression of c-fos protein in interneurons and projection neurons of the rat spinal cord in response to noxious somatic and visceral stimulation. *J Comp Neurol* 1989; 285:177–195.

Miki K, Zhou QQ, Guo W, et al. Changes in gene expression and neuronal phenotype in brainstem pain modulatory circuitry after inflammation. *J Neurophysiol* 2002; 87:750–760.

Nakanishi S. Molecular diversity of glutamate receptors and implications for brain function. *Science* 1992; 258:597–603.

Paxinos G, Watson C. *The Rat Brain in Stereotaxic Coordinates,* 4th ed. New York: Academic Press, 1998.

Porreca F, Ossipov MH, Gebhart GF. Chronic pain and medullary descending facilitation. *Trends Neurosci* 2002; 25:319–325.

Ren K, Dubner R. Enhanced descending modulation of nociception in rats with persistent hindpaw inflammation. *J Neurophysiol* 1996; 76:3025–3057.

Ren K, Dubner R. Descending modulation in persistent pain: an update. *Pain* 2002; 100:1–6.

Renn C, Dubner R, Ren K. Enhanced AMPA receptor GluR1 subunit expression and neuronal activation within brainstem pain modulatory circuitry after inflammation. *Abstracts: 10th World Congress on Pain.* Seattle: IASP Press, 2002, p 265.

Renn CL, Dubner R, Ren K. Neuronal activation and GluR1 expression in the nucleus raphe magnus after inflammation. *Neuroreport* 2003; in press.

Sandkühler J, Gebhart GF. Characterization of inhibition of a spinal nociceptive reflex by stimulation medially and laterally in midbrain and medulla in the pentobarbital-anesthetized rat. *Brain Res* 1984; 305:67–76.

Schaible HG, Neugebauer V, Cervero F, Schmidt RF. Changes in tonic descending inhibition of spinal neurons with articular input during the development of acute arthritis in the cat. *J Neurophysiol* 1991; 66:1021–1032.

Suarez I, Bodega G, Fernandez B. Modulation of AMPA receptor subunits GluR1 and GluR2/3 in the rat cerebellum in an experimental hepatic encephalopathy model. *Brain Res* 1997; 778:346–353.

Terayama R, Guan Y, Dubner R, Ren K. Activity-induced plasticity in brainstem pain modulatory circuitry after inflammation. *Neuroreport* 2000; 11:1915–1919.

Terayama R, Dubner R, Ren K. The roles of NMDA receptor activation and nucleus reticularis gigantocellularis in the time-dependent changes in descending inhibition after inflammation. *Pain* 2002; 97:171–181.

Urban MO, Gebhart GF. Supraspinal contributions to hyperalgesia. *Proc Natl Acad Sci USA* 1999; 96:7687–7692.

Urban MO, Coutinho SV, Gebhart GF. Involvement of excitatory amino acid receptors and nitric oxide in the rostral ventromedial medulla in modulating secondary hyperalgesia produced by mustard oil. *Pain* 1999; 81:45–55.

Willis WD. Anatomy and physiology of descending control of nociceptive responses of dorsal horn neurons: a comprehensive review. *Prog Brain Res* 1988; 77:1–29.

Woolf CJ, Thompson SWN. The induction and maintenance of central sensitization is dependent on *N*-methyl-D-aspartate acid receptor activation: implications for the treatment of post-injury pain hypersensitivity states. *Pain* 1991; 44:293–299.

Zimmerman M. Ethical guidelines for investigations of experimental pain in conscious animals. *Pain* 1983; 16:109–110.

Correspondence to: Ke Ren, PhD, Department of Oral and Craniofacial Biological Sciences, Room 5-A-12, Dental School, University of Maryland, 666 West Baltimore Street, Baltimore, MD 21201-1586, USA. Tel: 410-706-3250; Fax: 410-706-4172; email: kren@umaryland.edu.

Proceedings of the 10th World Congress on Pain,
Progress in Pain Research and Management, Vol. 24,
edited by Jonathan O. Dostrovsky, Daniel B. Carr, and
Martin Koltzenburg, IASP Press, Seattle, © 2003.

32

Immune and Glial Involvement in Physiological and Pathological Exaggerated Pain States

Linda R. Watkins, Erin D. Milligan, and Steven F. Maier

Department of Psychology and Center for Neuroscience, University of Colorado at Boulder, Boulder, Colorado, USA

Until recently, glia (microglia and astrocytes) were assumed to have little or no role in neural signaling. However, over the past decade, it has become apparent that glial regulation of neuronal function in general (Vernadakis 1996; Hatton 1999), and pain modulation in particular (Watkins et al. 2001), has been underestimated. Under normal conditions, spinal cord glia are quiescent. Disruption of glial function or blockade of the actions of glially derived substances, such as proinflammatory cytokines (PICs), has no effect on pain thresholds for thermal or mechanical stimuli (Meller et al. 1994; Milligan et al. 2000, 2001b). Thus, glia do not appear to play a role in normal pain processing.

However, the role of glia changes under conditions that show evidence of pain enhancement. Under such conditions, microglia and astrocytes become activated and begin to affect pain. Microglia and astrocytes activate in response to widely diverse pain-enhancing manipulations, including inflammation of or trauma to body tissues (Meller et al. 1994; Fu et al. 1999; Schwei et al. 1999), peripheral nerves (Colburn et al. 1999), spinal roots (Hashizume et al. 2000), and the spinal cord (Milligan et al. 2001b). Such activation appears to be more than merely correlated with the presence of exaggerated pain states. Indeed, glial activation appears to be important for both the creation and maintenance of pathological pain. Disruption of glial activation (Meller et al. 1994; Watkins et al. 1997; Milligan et al. 2000) or pharmacological blockade of glial products (DeLeo et al. 1996; Watkins et al. 1997; Arruda et al. 2000; Milligan et al. 2001b; Sweitzer et al. 2001b) prevents or reverses exaggerated pain induced by inflammation of bodily tissues, inflammation of and trauma to peripheral and spinal nerves, and bacterial and viral activation of glia in the spinal cord.

Activated glia are well positioned to regulate neural activity because they encapsulate synapses and contact neuronal dendrites and somas (Vernadakis 1996). This juxtaposition allows substances released by activated glia to alter neuronal function. Activated glia release a wide array of pain-enhancing substances, including PICs (Koka et al. 1995), reactive oxygen species (Torreilles et al. 1999), nitric oxide (NO) (Koka et al. 1995), arachidonic acid and its metabolites (Levi et al. 1998), and enkephalinases (Lucius et al. 1995). Activated glia can also rapidly increase extracellular levels of pain-enhancing excitatory amino acids (EAAs) both by reducing uptake and by active release (Vesce et al. 1997). Furthermore, glially derived substances can release "pain" transmitters from primary afferents (Inoue et al. 1999). Together, this profile of effects is impressive in that many of these released substances either transmit pain signals or create exaggerated pain states.

How does this occur? What activates glia? They express a wide array of receptors, not only for viruses and bacteria, but also for pain-enhancing substances. Glia can express receptors for or become activated by substance P (Luber-Narod et al. 1994), calcitonin gene-related peptide (CGRP; Reddington et al. 1995), EAAs (Kommers et al. 1998), NO (Holguin et al. 2002), prostaglandins (Repovic and Benveniste 1992), cholecystokinin (Muller et al. 1997), and other substances. The implications of such a list are striking. When exaggerated pain states are inhibited by antagonists of substance P, EAAs, and other substances, such pain control may reflect blockade of glial as well as neuronal activation.

To illustrate how, and potentially why, glia are involved in pain regulation, we will sequentially describe the involvement of glia in three diverse exaggerated pain states resulting (1) as a natural component of the sickness response, (2) in response to viral activation of spinal cord glia, and (3) in response to inflammation of otherwise healthy peripheral nerves. We then will discuss the implications of glial activation for clinical pain syndromes and drug development.

HISTORICAL OVERVIEW

Our focus on glial regulation of pathological pain was a natural outgrowth of our interest in central nervous system (CNS)/immune system interactions and in the effect of stress on immune function (Maier et al. 1994). This interest in CNS regulation of immunity began to shift in the mid-1990s as it became clear that communication between the CNS and immune system was, in fact, bidirectional, and that each system can dramatically alter the function of the other (Maier and Watkins 1998). Immune activation in response to viral and bacterial infections, tissue damage, and the like exert profound effects on brain and behavior, including enhancement of pain responses (Maier and Watkins 1998; Watkins and Maier 2000).

An entire constellation of changes occurs rapidly in response to immune activation. Together, these changes are referred to as the sickness response. This evolutionarily old, phylogenetically ubiquitous defense response enhances host survival (Maier and Watkins 1998). It involves a series of physiological changes (e.g., fever, increased white blood cell count, alterations in blood carrier proteins and ions, increased sleep), endocrine changes (e.g., activation of the hypothalamo-pituitary axis and the sympathetic nervous system), and behavioral changes (e.g., decreased social interaction and sexual activity, enhanced pain) (Maier and Watkins 1998).

It is striking that these sickness responses are, by and large, created by the CNS in response to signals received from the immune system. We have been attempting to define the immunological and neural mechanisms involved in the creation of sickness responses. Given the topic of this chapter, discussion of immune-to-brain communication will be restricted to enhanced pain, that is, sickness-induced hyperalgesia (Watkins and Maier 2000). Understanding the mechanisms underlying this phenomenon will lay the groundwork for understanding how pathological pain may arise in response to bodily infection and damage, CNS infection and damage, and so forth. Such pathological pain responses may potentially occur because conditions that create pathological pain drive the ancient immune system-to-CNS pathways that evolved to enhance host survival.

SICKNESS-INDUCED HYPERALGESIA AS A NATURAL COMPONENT OF THE SICKNESS RESPONSE

As noted above, microbial products and tissue damage activate the sickness response. In bacterial infection, for example, one of the earliest events is detection of the foreign invaders by specialized immune cells called macrophages. Detection of bacteria causes macrophage activation, leading to engulfment and destruction of the bacteria by these immune cells. In addition, the activated macrophages release PICs: tumor necrosis factor alpha (TNF-α), interleukin-1 beta (IL1-β), and IL6. These molecules are "pro-inflammatory" as they stimulate and orchestrate the early immune response (Maier and Watkins 1998).

In addition, PICs signal the CNS to trigger the sickness response. The importance of PICs is reflected by the failure of immunological challenges to trigger sickness responses if the actions of PICs are pharmacologically blocked (Maier and Watkins 1998). Furthermore, administration of PICs is sufficient to create all of the sickness responses (Maier and Watkins 1998), including sickness-induced hyperalgesia (Watkins and Maier 2000).

The pathways by which the PICs signal the CNS have been a matter of great debate. Both blood-borne and neural signaling pathways have been identified (Watkins et al. 1995b). Both may be expected to elicit sickness-induced hyperalgesia, but only neural pathways have been examined to date. The most extensively studied neural pathway is activated by intraperitoneal injection of bacterial cell walls or PICs. In either case, the result is PIC binding to sensory organs called paraganglia (Goehler et al. 2000). These paraganglia are scattered throughout the thorax and abdomen, positioned to receive signals from immune cells. Paraganglia form sensory (afferent) synapses with vagal nerve fibers and activate them upon binding of immune-derived substances (Goehler et al. 2000). This process creates an immune-driven signal to the nucleus tractus solitarius, the site of termination of afferent vagal fibers (Goehler et al. 2000). This medullary structure has been referred to as the "hub of sickness" as its axons project to diverse brain and spinal cord sites, leading to the creation of sickness responses (Maier and Watkins 1998).

The CNS pathway mediating sickness-induced hyperalgesia has been defined through a combination of lesion and immediate early gene activation studies. These studies have revealed that sickness-induced hyperalgesia is created by a pathway from the nucleus tractus solitarius through the ventral medial medulla to the dorsal lateral funiculus (Watkins and Maier 2000). In spinal cord, sickness-induced hyperalgesia is created via the release of NO, EAAs, and substance P (Watkins and Maier 2000). The ventral medial medulla is the most likely source of substance P and EAAs for creation of sickness-induced hyperalgesia (Watkins et al. 1994).

Interestingly, the brain creates sickness responses by de novo synthesis and release of PICs (Maier and Watkins 1998). Glia (and possibly some neurons) are activated in response to immune-to-brain signals, leading to release of PICs. These brain-derived PICs, in turn, participate in the creation of sickness responses (Maier and Watkins 1998). Thus, we tested whether peripheral immune challenge activates glia in the spinal cord dorsal horn and, if so, whether sickness-induced hyperalgesia is dependent upon spinal glial activation and PIC release. Indeed, that was the case, because blocking glial activation with the glial metabolic inhibitor fluorocitrate and blocking

PIC action with an interleukin-1 receptor antagonist each prevented sickness-induced hyperalgesia (Watkins et al. 1995a, 1997).

PATHOLOGICAL PAIN IN RESPONSE TO SPINAL IMMUNE CHALLENGE

These developments encouraged us to determine whether spinal cord glial activation might be sufficient to create pathological pain in the absence of bodily infection, inflammation, or tissue damage. To test this possibility, we took advantage of the fact that glia are immunocompetent cells that express receptors for, and become activated by, viruses and bacteria.

We chose to examine glial activation in response to the human immunodeficiency virus 1 (HIV-1) glycoprotein, gp120, the portion of HIV-1 that activates astrocytes and microglia. HIV-1 gp120 was also chosen based on its potential clinical relevance. HIV-1 is frequently neurotropic as it "homes" to and becomes resident in the CNS, including the spinal cord (Atwood et al. 1993). HIV-1 invasion is insidious because drugs used to treat acquired immunodeficiency syndrome (AIDS) do not cross the blood-brain barrier (Hartman et al. 1990; VanLeeuwen et al. 1996). Thus, the AIDS virus continues to stimulate glia unhindered by such drugs. Furthermore, nearly all AIDS patients suffer from pain (Breitbart et al. 1996). In a surprisingly large number of cases, a source for the pain cannot be identified in the periphery (Thuluvath et al. 1991). This situation raises the possibility that the pain may not arise from peripheral abnormalities, but rather as a direct result of spinal cord glial activation driven by HIV-1. It also suggests that even with identifiable causes of pain associated with HIV-1 (e.g., neuropathies, opportunistic infections, and cancers), the ongoing spinal glial activation may amplify those pain signals.

Indeed, intrathecal (i.t.) HIV-1 gp120 produces thermal hyperalgesia, low-threshold mechanical allodynia, and dynamic allodynia in rats (Milligan et al. 2000, 2001b). In addition, gp 120 activates dorsal horn astrocytes and microglia, as evidenced by upregulation of cell-type-specific activation markers (Milligan et al. 2001b). Indeed, activation of glia is required for gp120-induced pain changes to occur (Milligan et al. 2000).

Could HIV-1 gp120 create pathological pain by "tapping into" the pain enhancement circuit already defined for sickness-induced hyperalgesia? If so, then PICs should again be involved. Indeed, the dose of gp120 that produces exaggerated pain states elevates (1) mRNA for TNF-α, IL1-β, and IL6 protein; (2) dorsal spinal cord TNF-α, IL1-β, and IL6; and (3) release of

TNF-α, IL1-β, and IL6, as evidenced by their accumulation in lumbosacral cerebrospinal fluid (Milligan et al. 2001b; Holguin et al. 2002). Demonstrating release of PICs is important because these proteins are often produced but not released (Watkins et al. 1995b). Release of PICs means that they may be physiologically relevant to the pain changes that ensue. Blocking TNF-α or IL1-β by i.t. administration of selective antagonists blocks gp120-induced exaggerated pain (Milligan et al. 2001b). In further support of PIC involvement, i.t. and systemic CNI-1493 each block gp120-induced pain (Milligan et al. 2000, 2001a). CNI-1493 is a member of the class of compounds called CSAIDs (cytokine-suppressive anti-inflammatory drugs). CSAIDs all inhibit p38 mitogen-activated protein (MAP) kinase, which is involved in PIC signaling and production (Bhat et al. 1998).

We are extending these studies to define the cascade of events that ultimately creates exaggerated pain responses. What we know to date is that very early generation of NO is critical for gp120-induced effects (Holguin et al. 2002). Indeed, this gp120-induced NO is being created by NO synthase (NOS) type I, also commonly but inaccurately referred to as neuronal NOS (nNOS). NOS-I (nNOS) is constitutively expressed by spinal cord astrocytes and by neurons (Holguin et al. 2002). The relative importance of astrocyte-derived and neuron-derived NOS-I is not yet known. What is clear is that NOS-I generated NO is essential for all gp120-induced effects such as elevated PIC mRNAs, tissue content, and release, and for exaggerated pain (Holguin et al. 2002).

As noted above, activation of glia or PICs also increases extracellular levels of EAAs (Vesce et al. 1997) and enhances release of substance P from synaptic terminals (Inoue et al. 1999). Hence, we are examining the potential role of substance P and EAAs in gp120-induced exaggerated pain states. While EAAs are involved in gp120-induced effects, the relative role of *N*-methyl D-aspartate (NMDA) and calcium-permeable α-amino-3-hydroxy-5-methyl-4-isoxazole propionate (AMPA) receptors in thermal hyperalgesia and mechanical allodynia is complex. The effectiveness of selective antagonists varies both with the pain measure and with time after a dose of gp120 (Milligan et al. 2001c). In contrast, the role of substance P is straightforward. Intrathecal CP-96345, an NK-1 receptor antagonist, prevents gp120-induced thermal hyperalgesia and mechanical allodynia (E.D. Milligan, S.F. Maier, and L.R. Watkins, unpublished observations). Tissues have been collected to assess whether this compound alters gp120-induced PIC production. Failure of CP-96345 to alter PIC production would argue that substance P effects are distal to the actions of the cytokines.

PATHOLOGICAL PAIN IN RESPONSE TO SCIATIC INFLAMMATORY NEUROPATHY

As reviewed above, enhanced pain is a natural physiological consequence of immune-to-brain communication, wherein immune signals activate a vagus-to-brain-to-spinal cord circuit. Such pain is also created pathologically as a consequence of spinal immune challenges that activate spinal cord glia in their role as immunocompetent cells. In either case, glial activation leads to the release of PICs that create exaggerated pain. In addition, NO, substance P, and EAAs are involved in the creation of these physiological and pathological pain states. These similarities between sickness-induced hyperalgesia and gp120-induced pathological pain support the speculative concept that pathological pain can occur as a consequence of pathogens tapping into the ancient circuit that evolved to enhance host survival through the creation of sickness responses.

Are pathogens, such as bacteria and viruses, the only way to tap into this circuitry? No, clearly not. Neural activity induced by peripheral neuropathies can also activate a glially and PIC-mediated enhanced pain state. We will review what is known to date about pathological pain induced by sciatic inflammatory neuropathy (SIN).

We developed the SIN model because approximately half of all neuropathies are inflammatory rather than traumatic in etiology (Said and Hontebeyrie-Joskowicz 1992). In contrast, virtually all animal models developed to study neuropathic pain involve physical trauma to peripheral nerves (Seltzer et al. 1990; Kim and Chung 1992; DeLeo et al. 1994; Tal and Bennett 1994). Our rat model is distinct in several aspects. First, we wrapped a single healthy sciatic nerve at mid-thigh level with a soft gelatin sponge and attached it to an external catheter system. We used isoflurane anesthesia during the surgery as it has minimal effects on immune function compared to other commonly used laboratory animal anesthetics. The catheter system allows the animals to recover fully from the acute trauma of surgery and anesthesia. To activate the localized immune response around the enwrapped nerve in awake unrestrained animals, we injected zymosan (yeast cell walls) into the gelfoam to attract immune cells to the site. The immune cells bind zymosan and become activated. The gelfoam can be harvested at the termination of the experiment to allow examination of the perisciatic immune cells and their products.

The behavioral responses to perisciatic immune activation are stimulus and dose dependent. Mechanical allodynia occurs, but not thermal hyperalgesia (Chacur et al. 2001). Low levels of immune activation create a unilateral mechanical allodynia ipsilateral to the site of zymosan injection. Higher levels of immune activation create a bilateral allodynia, both ipsilateral and "mirror image" (Chacur et al. 2001). The expansion of allodynia to the contralateral paw is not due to spread of zymosan to the systemic circulation, but rather reflects a local change within the sciatic nerve that then drives the CNS to create a bilateral change in pain responsivity (Chacur et al. 2001; Gazda et al. 2001). Extraterritorial allodynia also occurs in the skin innervated by the neighboring, unaffected saphenous nerve (Chacur et al. 2001). The occurrence of robust extraterritorial and mirror image pain in the SIN model is exciting because such "anatomically impossible" pain changes are reported in many human pathological pain conditions, yet virtually nothing is known about the underlying mechanisms (Watkins and Maier 2002).

To date, the SIN model has revealed several intriguing facts about what is happening at the level of the peripheral immune cells, peripheral nerve, and spinal cord. We will consider each in turn.

At the level of the peripheral nerve, the immune system responds to the injected zymosan as if it were a natural infection. Neutrophils are the first immune cells recruited, and neutrophils and macrophages predominate at the site (Gazda et al. 2001). These immune cells respond to zymosan by releasing a variety of factors. A low dose of zymosan releases mostly TNF-α. In contrast, a higher dose releases high levels of TNF-α, IL1-β, and reactive oxygen species (Gazda et al. 2001). While this study did not measure complement activation, zymosan is a classic activator of the alternative complement pathway, leading to the generation of membrane attack complexes (Austen and Fearon 1979). Preliminary studies of complement and PIC blockers reveal that these immune products have a significant role in the generation of inflammatory neuropathy-induced pain (Schoeniger et al. 2002).

How these, and potentially other, immune products interact with the sciatic nerve to create pain is not yet known. Complement activation can result in the formation of membrane attack complexes that literally punch holes in cell membranes including myelin sheaths, thereby increasing axonal excitability (Koski 1992). PICs are thought to increase the permeability of sodium and calcium ion channels and to create cation channels via insertion of these immune-derived proteins into the cell membrane (Kagan et al. 1992; Wilkinson et al. 1996; Qiu et al. 1998). Primary afferent neurons also express mRNA for PIC receptors (Pollock et al. 2002), but whether these receptors are expressed along their axons is unknown. Whatever the mechanism, SIN creates marked dose-dependent differences in the anatomy of the sciatic nerve 24 hours after zymosan injection (Gazda et al. 2001). When unilateral (ipsilateral) allodynia occurs, the zymosan-exposed sciatic nerve appears identical to control nerves. In contrast, with bilateral (ipsilateral and mirror image) allodynia, edema (swelling) occurs along the outer edge of the nerve that contacts immune cells and immune-derived substances (Gazda et al. 2001). Edema is an early pathological change in nerves (Stoll et al. 2002). Thus, it is clear that immune activation near otherwise healthy peripheral nerves can alter both nerve form and function.

Immune-induced alteration in peripheral nerve activity, in turn, creates mechanical allodynia via activation of spinal cord glia. As reviewed above, the glial metabolic inhibitor fluorocitrate prevented sickness-induced hyperalgesia and i.t. HIV-1 gp120-induced pain changes (Watkins et al. 1997; Milligan et al. 2001b). Fluorocitrate likewise prevents SIN-induced pain changes (Milligan et al. 2003). Importantly, this glial inhibitor blocked not only ipsilateral allodynia, but also extraterritorial allodynia and even mirror-image allodynia. This finding implicates spinal cord glia in the creation of "anatomically impossible" forms of pain in which pain expands beyond the site of inflammation or trauma.

Glia create these pain phenomena via the release of PICs. Blocking the action of TNF-α, IL1-β, or IL6 blocks or reverses ipsilateral, extraterritorial, and mirror image SIN-induced allodynias (Milligan et al. 2003). Importantly, the acute SIN model can be modified to a chronic condition by repeatedly delivering the zymosan over the sciatic nerve via the indwelling catheter. This process maintains sciatic inflammation and the resultant allodynia for weeks (Milligan et al. 2003). Even under these conditions, a single dose of an IL1-β receptor antagonist over the spinal cord reverses the chronic allodynia for a period of time (Milligan et al. 2003) and supports the conclusion that PICs are key to the maintenance of pathological pain, not just its creation. With regard to other potential mediators, present knowledge suggests that substance P again has an important role (Johnston et al. 2002).

The involvement of glial PICs in extraterritorial and mirror-image pain is consistent with their paracrine-like action. They diffuse far from their sites of release, potentially enabling them to interact with spinal terminations of neighboring nerves. The involvement of glial PICs in these "anatomically impossible" pains may also reflect involvement of gap junctions. Glia are electrically linked into widespread networks via gap junctions. Activation of glia at one site rapidly leads to a wave of activation spreading across the network (Araque et al. 1999). The result is that glia, quite distant from the site of initial stimulation, are activated and begin releasing PICs and other pain-enhancing substances (Araque et al. 1999).

FRACTALKINE: A NEURON-TO-GLIA SIGNAL FOR PATHOLOGICAL PAIN

A mystery remains, however. Recall that in the SIN model, immune activation occurs around a single healthy peripheral nerve at mid-thigh level. How does an inflamed sciatic nerve trunk lead to spinal cord glial activation? Clearly, some signal to glia must arise from neurons, either from the incoming afferent neuron or from the pain transmission neuron. The candidate signals can belong to, at minimum, three classes of substances: neurotransmitters released at afferent synapses, neuromodulators such as NO or prostaglandins that diffuse from either afferent terminals or pain transmission neurons, or glial modulators such as fractalkine that are released by neurons (Chapman et al. 2000). Neurotransmitters are a possibility as glia in general, and glia in the spinal cord in particular, express receptors for neurotransmitters released by afferent pain fibers, including EAAs, substance P, and adenosine triphosphate (Marriott et al. 1991; Ziak et al. 1998; Fam et al. 2000). Neuromodulators are possible, given their recent implication in other glially mediated pain states (Holguin et al. 2002).

An additional intriguing possibility is that neurons release a substance that serves as a specific activation signal for glia. Fractalkine is an excellent candidate for such a signal. Fractalkine is a protein that is tethered to the outer surface of neurons (Asensio and Campbell 1999). When neurons are strongly activated, fractalkine breaks free and diffuses away in the extracellular fluid (Chapman et al. 2000; Hughes et al. 2002). Microglia express receptors for fractalkine and become activated in response to it, which suggests that fractalkine could serve as a neuron-to-glia signal (Milligan et al. 2002b). We have found that i.t. delivery of fractalkine causes dramatic thermal hyperalgesia and mechanical allodynia (Milligan et al. 2002b). Importantly, endogenous fractalkine also creates pathological pain. For example, i.t. delivery of a fractalkine antagonist (a neutralizing antibody to the fractalkine receptor) prevents SIN-induced pain changes (Milligan et al. 2002b). Anatomically, fractalkine is expressed both by sensory afferents and by neurons intrinsic to the spinal cord (Milligan et al. 200b). Fractalkine receptors are expressed on dorsal horn microglia (Milligan et al. 2002b), in keeping with prior observations in the brain (Asensio and Campbell 1999). Intriguingly, microglial activation and fractalkine receptor expression increase in parallel in the superficial dorsal horn in response to SIN (Milligan et al. 2002b). Furthermore, fractalkine creates both thermal hyperalgesia and mechanical allodynia via the i.t. release of IL1-β, a receptor antagonist that blocks both pain changes (Milligan et al. 2002b). This effect is duplicated in vitro. We have recently developed cell cultures of microglia isolated from adult rat dorsal spinal cord. These cells do indeed respond to fractalkine by releasing IL1-β (Wiesler-Frank et al. 2002). It thus appears that this neuron-to-glia signal may well be one way to "tap into" the circuitries described above for sickness-induced hyperalgesia and gp120-induced exaggerated pain responses.

IMPLICATIONS FOR CLINICAL PAIN AND DRUG DEVELOPMENT

Any discussion of the clinical relevance of this work is speculative. However, an effort to address the implications for human pathological pain appears warranted given that (1) glial activation occurs in diverse animal models of pathological pain, (2) blockade of glial activation disrupts diverse enhanced pain states, and (3) spinal cord PICs are implicated in the creation and maintenance of diverse enhanced pain states.

The implications of the animal data are clear. First, glia may be an as-yet-unrecognized source of pain in various infectious diseases during which viruses or bacteria take up residence in the spinal cord. Such infections would be expected to activate glia and release spinal PICs, which, in turn, could either cause or contribute to pathological pain. Second, glia and PICs may drive pathological pain states created by peripheral inflammation and trauma. This effect would be especially noteworthy for neuropathic pain, which is poorly controlled by drug therapies that target neurons. Third, glial activation and spinal PICs may be responsible, at least in part, for expanding the body region involved in pain perception, for example, extraterritorial and mirror image pain phenomena. Such "anatomically impossible" pains are reported in a wide array of chronic pain syndromes including complex regional pain syndrome type I (Maleki et al. 2000) and type II (Shir and Seltzer 1991), atypical facial pain (Woda and Pionchon 2000), idiopathic facial arthromyalgia (Woda and Pionchon 2000), and stomatodynia (Woda and Pionchon 2000). Such anatomically impossible pain reports have prompted many referrals for psychiatric evaluation due to lack of a logical neurological explanation for such pain patterns.

How can the information be used to go from bench to bedside? Some of the drugs used in animal studies are inappropriate for human use. Glial metabolic inhibitors such as fluorocitrate, for example, are inappropriate for humans, or even for animal studies if administered at high doses or over prolonged periods. Other drugs used in the above experiments are not easily applied to humans as they do not cross the blood-brain barrier (e.g., IL1-β receptor antagonist, TNF-α-soluble receptors, IL6 antiserum, and anti-inflammatory cytokines such as IL10) or are not adequately selective (e.g., matrix metalloproteinase inhibitors).

Two classes of drugs, however, can cross the blood-brain barrier and are either in, or have passed, clinical trials for other uses. The first are the cytokine-suppressive anti-inflammatory drugs (CSAIDs), a family of compounds that was first identified by their ability to disrupt PIC production and signaling (Bhat et al. 1998). Subsequently it became clear that these drugs exerted such effects because they were all p38 MAP kinase inhibitors (Lee et al. 2000). Given that p38 MAP kinase is important both for PIC production and signaling (Lee et al. 2000), we can anticipate that p38 MAP kinase would disrupt PIC-driven pain. Indeed they do. CNI-1493 is a member of this family of drugs that disrupts enhanced pain induced by inflammation of peripheral tissues (Watkins et al. 1997), peripheral nerves (Milligan et al. 2003), or spinal cord (Milligan et al. 2000). It is effective after either i.t. or systemic administration (Milligan et al. 2001a), which demonstrates that at least this member of the CSAID family can cross the blood-brain barrier.

The second class of drugs is composed of xanthine derivatives, including propentofylline and pentoxifylline. Compounds in this family have passed clinical trials for other purposes and are known to cross the blood-brain barrier (Mielke et al. 1998; Bath et al. 2000). They have multiple effects, including but not limited to inhibiting the production of PICs, NO, reactive oxygen species, and prostaglandins (Banati et al. 1994; Schubert and Rudolphi 1998; Suzumura et al. 1998). Although these drugs have a complex profile of effects, they work in the appropriate direction for pain control. Indeed, these drugs are effective in animal models of pathological pain (Sweitzer et al. 2001a).

One problem with these drugs is that systemic administration will, by necessity, disrupt immune system functioning in the periphery along with disrupting spinal cord glia. Chronic disruption of immune function is not desirable, for obvious reasons. The alternative would be an indwelling spinal catheter to allow selective spinal delivery, but this approach also has drawbacks.

An ideal solution would be to (1) selectively deliver the drug to the spinal cord, leaving the peripheral immune system unaltered; (2) selectively disrupt PIC production by activated glia, leaving basal functioning of glia unaltered; and (3) maintain normal functioning of neurons. In an attempt to realize this ideal, we are exploring i.t. gene therapy by using a viral vector to deliver the interleukin-10 (IL10) gene sequence to drive the chronic spinal production and release IL10, which is the most powerful member of the anti-inflammatory cytokine family in that it suppresses the transcription, translation, post-translational processing, and release of all the PICs (Moore et al. 2001). IL10 also downregulates expression of membrane-bound signaling receptors for PICs, upregulates soluble ("decoy") receptors for PICs, and upregulates the expression of other anti-inflammatory cytokines (Moore et al. 2001). Thus, IL10 simultaneously disrupts PIC production and signaling at multiple levels of gene activation and expression. Importantly, neurons do not express receptors for IL10 in either normal or inflamed spinal cord (Ledeboer 2002; Ledeboer et al., in press), so IL10 will have no direct effect on neuron function. Disadvantages of IL10 are its short half-life, inability to cross the blood-brain barrier, and high production costs. Perhaps gene therapy will provide a way to induce the spinal cord to constantly create its own IL10 over prolonged periods, an approach that appears quite promising. Intrathecal gene therapy to create IL10 release prevents or reverses pathological pain induced by i.t. HIV-1 gp120, sciatic inflammatory neuropathy, and sciatic traumatic neuropathy induced by chronic constrictive injury (Milligan et al. 2002a).

In conclusion, the growing recognition of the power and importance of glial activation to pain modulation provides hope. It does so because pathological pain is, overall, poorly managed by the therapies now available. All centrally acting therapies for pathological pain were developed explicitly to target neurons. Shifting the focus of drug therapies to include disruption of glial activation and spinal PIC production provides a novel approach to pain control worthy of clinical consideration.

ACKNOWLEDGMENTS

This work was supported by grants MH01558, NS38020, MH55283, NS40696, and DA015656.

REFERENCES

Araque A, Parpura V, Sanzgiri RP, Haydon PG. Tripartite synapses: glia, the unacknowledged partner. *Trends Neurosci* 1999; 22:208–215.

Arruda JL, Rutkowski MD, Sweitzer SM, DeLeo JA. Antibody and IgG attenuates mechanical allodynia in a mononeuropathy model in the rat: potential role of immune modulation in neuropathic pain. *Brain Res* 2000; 879:216–225.

Asensio VC, Campbell IL. Chemokines in the CNS: plurifunctional mediators in diverse states. *Trends Neurosci* 1999; 22:504–512.

Atwood WJ, Berger JR, Kaderman R, Tornatore CS, Major EO. Human immunodeficiency virus type 1 infection of the brain. *Clin Microbiol Rev* 1993; 6:339–366.

Austen KF, Fearon DT. A molecular basis of activation of the alternative pathway of human complement. *Adv Exp Med Biol* 1979; 120B.

Banati RB, Schubert P, Rothe G, et al. Modulation of intracellular formation of reactive oxygen intermediates in peritoneal macrophages and microglia/brain macrophages by propentofylline. *J Cereb Blood Flow Metab* 1994; 14:145–149.

Bath PM, Bath FJ, Asplund K. Pentoxifylline, propentofylline and pentifylline for acute ischaemic stroke. *Cochrane Database Syst Rev* 2000; CD000162.

Bhat NR, Zhang P, Lee JC, Hogan EL. Extracellular signal-regulated kinase and p38 subgroups of mitogen-activated protein kinases regulate inducible nitric oxide synthase and tumor necrosis factor-alpha gene expression in endotoxin-stimulated primary glial cultures. *J Neurosci* 1998; 18:1633–1641.

Breitbart W, McDonald MV, Rosenfeld B, et al. Pain in ambulatory AIDS patients. I: Pain characteristics and medical correlates. *Pain* 1996; 68:315–321.

Chacur M, Milligan ED, Gazda LS, et al. A new model of sciatic inflammatory neuritis (SIN): induction of unilateral and bilateral mechanical allodynia following acute unilateral peri-sciatic immune activation in rats. *Pain* 2001; 94:231–244.

Chapman GA, Moores K, Harrison D, et al. Fractalkine cleavage from neuronal membranes represents an acute event in the inflammatory response to excitotoxic brain damage. *J Neurosci* 2000; 20:RC87 (81–85).

Colburn RW, Rickman AJ, DeLeo JA. The effect of site and type of nerve injury on spinal glial activation and neuropathic pain behavior. *Exp Neurol* 1999; 157:289–304.

DeLeo JA, Coombs DW, Willenbring S, et al. Characterization of a neuropathic pain model: sciatic cryoneurolysis in the rat. *Pain* 1994; 56:9–16.

DeLeo JA, Colburn RW, Nichols M, Malhotra A. Interleukin (IL)-6 mediated hyperalgesia/allodynia and increased spinal IL-6 in a rat mononeuropathy model. *J Interferon Cytokine Res* 1996; 16:695–700.

Fam SR, Gallagherm CJ, Salter MW. P2Y(1) purinoceptor-mediated Ca(2+) signaling and Ca(2+) wave propagation in dorsal spinal cord astrocytes. *J Neurosci* 2000; 20:2800–2808.

Fu K-Y, Light AR, Matsushima GK, Maixner W. Microglial reactions after subcutaneous formalin injection into the rat hind paw. *Brain Res* 1999; 825:59–67.

Gazda LS, Milligan ED, Hansen MK, et al. Sciatic inflammatory neuritis (SIN): behavioral allodynia is paralleled by peri-sciatic proinflammatory cytokine and superoxide production. *J Periph Nerv Sys* 2001; 6:1–19.

Goehler LE, Gaykema RPA, Hansen MK, et al. Vagal immune-to-brain communication: a visceral chemosensory pathway. *Autonom Neurosci* 2000; 85:49–59.

Hartman NR, Yarchoan R, Pluda JM, Thomas RV, Marczyk KS. Pharmacokinetics of 2',3'-dideoxyadenosine and 2',3'-dideoxyinosine in patients with severe human immunodeficiency virus infection. *Clin Pharmacol Ther* 1990; 47:647–654.

Hashizume H, DeLeo JA, Colburn RW, Weinstein JN. Spinal glial activation and cytokine expression after lumbar root injury in the rat. *Spine* 2000; 25:1206–1217.

Hatton GI. Astroglial modulation of neurotransmitter/peptide release from the neurohypophysis: present status. *J Chem Neuroanat* 1999; 16:203–221.

Holguin A, O'Connor KA, Hansen MK, et al. Nitric oxide mediates HIV-1 gp120-induced spinal proinflammatory cytokine production and low threshold mechanical allodynia. *J Pain* 2002; 3(Suppl 1):29.

Hughes PM, Batham MS, Frentzel S, Mir A, Perry VH. Expression of fractalkine (CX3CL1) and its receptor (CX3CR1), during acute and chronic inflammation in the rodent CNS. *Glia* 2002; 37:314–327.

Inoue A, Ikoma K, Morioka N, et al. Interleukin-1beta induces substance P release from primary afferent neurons through the cyclooxygenase-2 system. *J Neurochem* 1999; 73:2206–2213.

Johnston IN, Milligan ED, Sloane E, Maier SF, Watkins LR. Spinal neurochemistry of sciatic inflammatory neuritis (SIN). *Proc Soc Neurosci* 2002; 28:455.1.

Kagan BL, Baldwin RL, Munoz D, Wisnieski BJ. Formation of ion-permeable channels by tumor necrosis factor-alpha. *Science* 1992; 255:1427–1430.

Kim SH, Chung JM. An experimental model for peripheral neuropathy produced by segmental spinal nerve ligation in the rat. *Pain* 1992; 50:355–363.

Koka P, He K, Zack JA, et al. Human immunodeficiency virus 1 envelope proteins induce interleukin 1, tumor necrosis factor alpha, and nitric oxide in glial cultures derived from fetal, neonatal and adult human brain. *J Exp Med* 1995; 182:941–951.

Kommers T, Vinade L, Pereira C, et al. Regulation of the phosphorylation of glial fibrillary acidic protein (GFAP) by glutamate and calcium ions in slices of immature rat spinal cord: comparison with immature hippocampus. *Neurosci Lett* 1998; 248:141–143.

Koski CL. Peripheral neuropathy: new concepts and treatments. Humoral mechanisms in immune neuropathies. *Neurol Clin* 1992; 10:629–649.

Ledeboer A. Interleukin-10 and interleukin-10 receptor in neuroinflammation. Dissertation. Amsterdam: Department of Medical Pharmacology, Research Institute Neurosciences, VU University Medical Center, 2002.

Ledeboer A, Wierinckx A, Bol JGJM, et al. Regional and temporal expression patterns of interleukin-10, interleukin-10 receptor and adhesion molecules in the rat spinal cord during chronic relapsing EAE. *J Neuroimmunol;* in press.

Lee JC, Kumar S, Griswold DE, et al. Inhibition of p38 MAP kinase as a therapeutic strategy. *Immunopharmacology* 2000; 47:185–201.

Levi G, Minghetti L, Aloisi F. Regulation of prostanoid synthesis in microglial cells and effects of prostaglandin E2 on microglial functions. *Biochimie* 1998; 80:899–904.

Luber-Narod J, Kage R, Leeman SE. Substance P enhances the secretion of tumor necrosis factor-alpha from neuroglial cells stimulated with lipopolysaccharide. *J Immunol* 1994; 152:819–824.

Lucius R, Sievers J, Mentlein R. Enkephaline metabolism by microglial aminopeptidase N (CD13). *J Neurochem* 1995; 64:1841–1847.

Maier SF, Watkins LR, Fleshner M. Psychoneuroimmunology: the interface between behavior, brain and immunity. *Am Psychol* 1994; 49:1004–1018.

Maier SF, Watkins LR. Cytokines for psychologists: implications of bi-directional immune-to-brain communication for understanding behavior, mood, and cognition. *Psych Rev* 1998; 105:83–107.

Maleki J, LeBel AA, Bennett GJ, Schwartzman RJ. Patterns of spread in complex regional pain syndrome, type I (reflex sympathetic dystrophy). *Pain* 2000; 88:259–266.

Marriott DR, Wilkin GP, Wood JN. Substance P-induced release of prostaglandins from astrocytes: regional specialisation and correlation with phosphoinositol metabolism. *J Neurochem* 1991; 56:259–265.

Meller ST, Dyskstra C, Grzybycki D, Murphy S, Gebhart GF. The possible role of glia in nociceptive processing and hyperalgesia in the spinal cord of the rat. *Neuropharmacology* 1994; 33:1471–1478.

Mielke R, Moller HJ, Erkinjuntti T, et al. Propentofylline in the treatment of vascular dementia and Alzheimer-type dementia: overview of phase I and phase II clinical trials. *Alzheimer Dis Assoc Disord* 1998; 12:S29–S35.

Milligan ED, Mehmert KK, Hinde JL, et al. Thermal hyperalgesia and mechanical allodynia produced by intrathecal administration of the Human Immunodeficiency Virus-1 (HIV-1) envelope glycoprotein, gp120. *Brain Res* 2000; 861:105–116.

Milligan ED, O'Connor KA, Armstrong CB, et al. Systemic administration of CNI-1493, a p38 mitogen-activated protein kinase inhibitor, blocks intrathecal human immunodeficiency virus-1 gp120-induced enhanced pain states in rats. *J Pain* 2001a; 2:326–333.

Milligan ED, O'Connor KA, Nguyen KT, et al. Intrathecal HIV-1 envelope glycoprotein gp120 enhanced pain states mediated by spinal cord proinflammatory cytokines. *J Neurosci* 2001b; 21:2808–2819.

Milligan ED, O'Connor KA, Twining CM, et al. Spinal NMDA and Ca^{2+} permeable channels are partially involved with HIV-1 gp120-induced exaggerated pain states. *Proc Soc Neurosci* 2001c; 27.

Milligan ED, O'Connor KA, Hammack SE, et al. A novel gene therapy approach for controlling pathological pain states: intrathecal (i.t.) delivery in rats of viral vectors encoding the anti-inflammatory cytokine, interleukin-10 (IL10). *Abstracts: 10th World Congress on Pain.* Seattle: IASP Press, 2002a, p 134.

Milligan ED, Twining C, Chapman GA, et al. Spinal cord fractalkine, a chemokine, is involved in exaggerated pain states. *Brain Behav Immun* 2002b; 16:201.

Milligan ED, Twining C, Chacur M, et al. Spinal glia and proinflammatory cytokines mediate "anatomically impossible" (mirror-image) neuropathic pain. *J Neurosci* 2003; in press.

Moore KW, de Waal Malefyt R, Coffman RL, O'Garra A. Interleukin-10 and the interleukin-10 receptor. *Annu Rev Immunol* 2001; 19:683–765.

Muller W, Heinemann U, Berlin K. Cholecystokinin activates CCKB-receptor-mediated Ca-signaling in hippocampal astrocytes. *J Neurophysiol* 1997; 78:1997–2001.

Pollock J, McFarlane SM, Connell MC, et al. TNF-alpha receptors simultaneously activate Ca^{2+} mobilisation and stress kinases in cultured sensory neurones. *Neuropharmacology* 2002; 42:93–106.

Qiu Z, Sweeney DD, Netzeband JG, Gruol DL. Chronic interleukin-6 alters NMDA receptor-mediated membrane responses and enhances neurotoxicity in developing CNS neurons. *J Neurosci* 1998; 18:10445–10456.

Reddington M, Priller J, Treichel J, Haas C, Kreutzberg GW. Astrocytes and microglia as potential targets for calcitonin gene related peptide in the central nervous system. *Can J Physiol Pharmacol* 1995; 73:1047–1049.

Repovic P, Benveniste EN. Prostaglandin e2 is a novel inducer of oncostatin-m expression in macrophages and microglia. *J Neurosci* 1992; 22:5334–5343.

Said G, Hontebeyrie-Joskowicz M. Nerve lesions induced by macrophage activation. *Res Immunol* 1992; 143:589–599.

Schoeniger D, Twining C, Milligan E, et al. Peri-sciatic proinflammatory cytokines mediate allodynia produced by sciatic inflammatory neuropathy (SIN). *Proc Soc Neurosci* 2002; 28:455.2.

Schubert P, Rudolphi K. Interfering with the pathologic activation of microglial cells and astrocytes in dementia. *Alzheimer Dis Assoc Disord* 1998; 12:S21–S28.

Schwei MJ, Honore P, Rogers SD, et al. Neuro chemical and cellular reorganization of the spinal cord in a murine model of bone cancer pain. *J Neurosci* 1999; 19:10886–10897.

Seltzer Z, Dubner G, Shir Y. A novel behavioral model of neuropathic pain disorders produced in rats by partial sciatic nerve injury. *Pain* 1990; 43:205–218.

Shir Y, Seltzer Z. Effects of sympathectomy in a model of causalgiform pain produced by partial sciatic nerve injury in rats. *Pain* 1991; 45:309–320.

Stoll G, Jander S, Myers RR. Degeneration and regeneration of the peripheral nervous system: from Augustus Waller's observations to neuroinflammation. *J Peripher Nerv Syst* 2002; 7:13–27.

Suzumura A, Sawada M, Makino M, Takayanagi T. Propentofylline inhibits production of TNF alpha and infection of LP-BM5 murine leukemia virus in glial cells. *J Neurovirol* 1998; 4:553–559.

Sweitzer SM, Schubert P, DeLeo JA. Propentofylline, a glial modulating agent, exhibits anti-allodynic properties in a rat model of neuropathic pain. *J Pharmacol Exp Ther* 2001a; 297:1210–1217.

Sweitzer SM, Martin D, DeLeo JA. Intrathecal interleukin-1 receptor agonist in combination with soluble tumor necrosis factor receptor exhibits an anti-allodynic action in a rat model of neuropathic pain. *Neuroscience* 2001b; 103:529–539.

Tal M, Bennett GJ. Extra-territorial pain in rats with a peripheral mononeuropathy: mechano-hyperalgesia and mechano-allodynia in the territory of an uninjured nerve. *Pain* 1994; 57:375–382.

Thuluvath PJ, Connolly GM, Forbes A, Gazzard BG. Abdominal pain in HIV infection. *Q J Med* 1991; 78:275–285.

Torreilles F, Salman-Tabcheh S, Guerin M, Torreilles J. Neurodegenerative disorders: the role of peroxynitrite. *Brain Res Brain Res Rev* 1999; 30:153–163.

VanLeeuwen R, Katlama C, Kitchen V, Boucher CA, Tubiana R. Evaluation of safety and efficacy of 3TC (lamivudine) in patients with asymptomatic or mildly symptomatic human immunodeficiency virus infection: a phase I/II study. *J Infect Dis* 1996; 171:1166–1171.

Vernadakis A. Glia-neuron intercommunications and synaptic plasticity. *Prog Neurobiol* 1996; 49:185–214.

Vesce S, Bezzi P, Rossi D, Meldoleis J, Volterra A. HIV-1 gp120 glycoprotein affects the astrocyte control of extracellular glutamate by both inhibiting the uptake and stimulating the release of the amino acid. *FASEB Lett* 1997; 411:107–109.

Watkins LR, Maier SF. The pain of being sick: implications of immune-to-brain communication for understanding pain. *Annu Rev Psych* 2000; 51:29–57.

Watkins LR, Maier SF. Beyond neurons: evidence that immune and glial cells contribute to pathological pain states. *Physiol Rev* 2002; 82:981–1011.

Watkins LR, Wiertelak EP, Goehler L, et al. Neurocircuitry of illness-induced hyperalgesia. *Brain Res* 1994; 639:283–299.

Watkins LR, Deak T, Silbert L, et al. Evidence for involvement of spinal cord glia in diverse models of hyperalgesia. *Proc Soc Neurosci* 1995a; 21:897.

Watkins LR, Maier SF, Goehler LE. Cytokine-to-brain communication: a review and analysis of alternative mechanisms. *Life Sci* 1995b; 57:1011–1026.

Watkins LR, Martin D, Ulrich P, Tracey KJ, Maier SF. Evidence for the involvement of spinal cord glia in subcutaneous formalin induced hyperalgesia in the rat. *Pain* 1997; 71:225–235.

Watkins LR, Milligan ED, Maier SF. Glial activation: a driving force for pathological pain. *Trends Neurosci* 2001; 24:450–455.

Wiesler-Frank JL, Cheepsunthorn P, Milligan ED, et al. Characterization of adult rat microglia and astrocyte response properties: toward an understanding of how glia produce pathological pain. *Abstracts: 10th World Congress on Pain*. Seattle: IASP Press, 2002, p 134.

Wilkinson MF, Earle ML, Triggle CR, Barnes S. Interleukin-1 beta, tumor necrosis factor-alpha, and LPS enhance calcium channel current in isolated vascular smooth cells of rat tail artery. *FASEB J* 1996; 10:785–791.

Woda A, Pionchon P. A unified concept of idiopathic orofacial pain: pathophysiologic features. *J Orofac Pain* 2000; 14:196–212.

Ziak D, Chvatal A, Sykova E. Glutamate-, kainate- and NMDA-evoked membrane currents in identified glial cells in rat spinal cord slice. *Physiol Res* 1998; 47:365–375.

Correspondence to: Linda R. Watkins, PhD, Department of Psychology, Campus Box 345, University of Colorado at Boulder, Boulder, CO 80309-0345, USA. Tel: 303-492-7034; Fax: 303-492-2967; email: lwatkins@psych. colorado.edu.

Proceedings of the 10th World Congress on Pain,
Progress in Pain Research and Management, Vol. 24,
edited by Jonathan O. Dostrovsky, Daniel B. Carr, and
Martin Koltzenburg, IASP Press, Seattle, © 2003.

33

Animal Models of Neuropathic Pain Induce Apoptosis and a Loss of GABAergic Inhibition in the Spinal Dorsal Horn

Joachim Scholz,[a] Daniel C. Broom,[a] Tatsuro Kohno,[a] Helena A. Lekan,[b] Richard E. Coggeshall,[b] and Clifford J. Woolf[a]

[a]*Neural Plasticity Research Group, Department of Anesthesia, Massachusetts General Hospital, Charlestown, Massachusetts, USA;* [b]*Department of Anatomy and Neuroscience, University of Texas Medical Branch, Galveston, Texas, USA*

Neuropathic pain is a frequent complication in a variety of clinical conditions including infections, metabolic diseases, and traumatic injuries of peripheral nerves or the central nervous system (Koltzenburg 1998). As analgesic drugs are only partially effective, neuropathic pain represents a therapeutic challenge, particularly because it persists chronically in the majority of patients (Woolf and Mannion 1999). In some cases, the persistence of neuropathic pain may be related to the underlying etiology, for example in conditions like diabetes mellitus, but it is unclear why pain becomes chronic after traumatic nerve damage or persists after the reactivation of *Varicella zoster* virus in postherpetic neuralgia. We have investigated the hypothesis that decreased inhibition of afferent input in the spinal dorsal horn promotes neuropathic pain by allowing unchecked nociceptive transmission, and have attempted to determine whether reduced inhibition is attributable to the death of inhibitory interneurons. A loss of inhibitory interneurons would represent a permanent change and hence provide an explanation for ongoing pain after nerve injury.

SPINAL INHIBITORY CONTROL OF SENSORY INPUT

Sensory input from the periphery is processed in the dorsal horn of the spinal cord before being transmitted to higher centers of the brain. The dorsal horn integrates information from facilitating pathways and inhibitory modulation originating in supraspinal centers (Hunt and Mantyh 2001). At the spinal level, interneurons from the same or neighboring segments exert an important tonic and phasic inhibitory influence on dorsal horn neurons. The amino acids γ-aminobutyric acid (GABA) and glycine are the major inhibitory neurotransmitters in the dorsal horn (Willis and Coggeshall 1991). In superficial laminae I–III, inhibitory interneurons containing GABA, glycine, or both form axoaxonic contacts with the central terminals of primary afferents. GABA and glycine are also involved in postsynaptic inhibition of spinal transmission neurons expressing $GABA_A$ receptors, G-protein-coupled $GABA_B$ receptors, and glycine receptors. Low-threshold and nociceptive sensory afferents can activate these interneurons, evoking longer-lasting GABAergic inhibitory postsynaptic currents (IPSCs) and short currents elicited by glycine (Yoshimura and Nishi 1995, Narikawa et al. 2000).

Animal models of nerve injury and clinical studies have demonstrated the significance of inhibitory control mechanisms in nociception and neuropathic pain (reviewed in Moore et al. 2001). Baclofen, a $GABA_B$ agonist, reduces the release of the excitatory transmitter glutamate from nociceptive afferents. Application of the $GABA_A$-receptor antagonist bicuculline produces hypersensitivity of dorsal horn neurons to glutamate. Intrathecal administration of $GABA_A$ or $GABA_B$-receptor antagonists, or of the glycine-receptor antagonist strychnine, provokes an increased reaction to painful stimuli (hyperalgesia) and a withdrawal response to normally innocuous mechanical stimulation (mechanical allodynia) in the rat (Malan et al. 2002). Following a chronic constriction injury (CCI) of the rat sciatic nerve (Bennett and Xie 1988), GABA levels in the dorsal horn decrease, accompanied by behavioral changes indicating mechanical allodynia. Reduced immunoreactivity of the GABA-synthesizing enzyme, glutamic acid decarboxylase (GAD) after CCI or sciatic nerve transection (SNT) suggests a reduction in the synthesis of this inhibitory transmitter (Eaton et al. 1998). On the other hand, $GABA_A$- and $GABA_B$-receptor agonists attenuate mechanical allodynia and thermal hyperalgesia induced by spinal nerve ligation (SNL) (Malan et al. 2002). Similar results have been reported for glycine and related compounds in the CCI model of neuropathic pain and after partial ligation of the sciatic nerve. In patients with severe neuropathic pain, an analgesic effect of intrathecally administered baclofen has been reported (Zuniga et al. 2000).

However, this method of treatment is limited by its costs and by side effects such as motor weakness when baclofen is given in higher doses.

GABAERGIC INHIBITION IS REDUCED AFTER PARTIAL PERIPHERAL NERVE INJURY

Despite biochemical and pharmacological evidence of reduced GABA levels in the dorsal horn after nerve injury and a role for glycine in nociceptive transmission, it was not clear whether changes in the inhibitory control of afferent input are involved in conditions of neuropathic pain.

We have therefore examined afferent-evoked IPSC in the dorsal horn in various models of nerve injury. Animals were studied 2 weeks after spared nerve injury (SNI), CCI, or SNT and compared with naive controls. The SNI model induces profound, and in contrast to CCI, persistent, behavioral changes indicating mechanical allodynia, pinprick hyperalgesia, and cold allodynia (Decosterd and Woolf 2000). Transverse slices of the lumbar spinal cord with the ipsilateral L4 dorsal root attached were isolated and transferred into preoxygenated Krebs solution. Electrodes for whole-cell recording were placed in lamina II. The dorsal root was stimulated using a constant current, and afferent-evoked IPSCs and excitatory postsynaptic currents (EPSCs) were recorded (see Moore et al. 2002 for details).

EPSCs evoked by stimulation of Aβ fibers or Aδ and C fibers remained largely unchanged after partial (SNI, CCI) or complete (SNT) nerve injury. In contrast, significantly fewer neurons exhibited primary afferent-evoked IPSCs in spinal cord slices from animals after SNI (IPSCs absent in 28% of neurons) or CCI (17%). Following SNI or CCI, the amplitudes of IPSCs were decreased to 47 ± 7 pA or 113 ± 12 pA, respectively, compared to 159 ± 13 pA in naive controls ($P < 0.05$). Moreover, IPSC kinetics shifted toward the glycinergic component. In controls, pharmacological blockade with either strychnine or bicuculline demonstrated that the predominant IPSC component is generated by activation of $GABA_A$ receptors (rise time 6.9 ± 0.8 ms, decay time constant $\tau = 30.8 \pm 3.2$ ms) and that glycinergic currents (rise time 4.8 ± 0.6 ms, $\tau = 9.2 \pm 0.8$ ms) contribute less. The average rise time of IPSCs was reduced to 4.2 ± 0.4 ms following SNI and 4.2 ± 0.2 ms following CCI ($P < 0.05$). The decay time τ was 11.0 ± 0.3 ms following SNI and 17.5 ± 0.2 ms following CCI compared to 30.4 ± 0.3 ms in the control group ($P < 0.05$) (Fig. 1). Analysis of miniature $GABA_A$-evoked IPSCs showed a diminished frequency in the dorsal horn following SNI or CCI whereas amplitudes were unchanged, pointing to a reduction in the

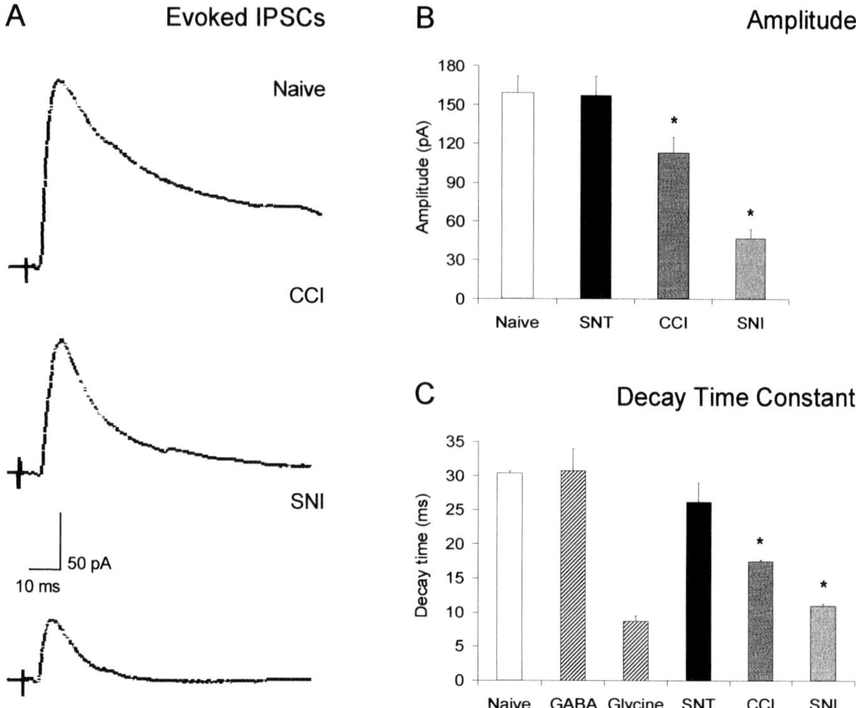

Fig. 1. (A) Representative afferent-evoked inhibitory postsynaptic currents (IPSCs) recorded in spinal cord slices from naive rats and from rats 2 weeks after chronic constriction injury (CCI) or spared nerve injury (SNI). (B) Amplitude and duration of IPSCs are markedly decreased following CCI and SNI, but not after complete sciatic nerve transection (SNT). (C) Analysis of the decay time constant reveals a shift towards the pharmacologically (5–10 μmol/L bicuculline) isolated glycinergic component of IPSCs in naive control animals. By contrast, in uninjured animals, the decay time constant corresponds to the GABAergic component recorded in the presence of 0.5 μmol/L strychnine.

presynaptic release of GABA with preserved postsynaptic receptor status. Importantly, the proportion of neurons with IPSCs did not change after complete transection of the sciatic nerve, nor did the amplitudes or the kinetics of IPSCs after SNT differ from those in naive control animals.

DECREASED EXPRESSION LEVELS OF GAD65

In parallel experiments, the expression levels of the two GAD isoforms, GAD65 and GAD67, were examined over 4 weeks following sciatic nerve lesions. After transcardial perfusion with Zamboni's fixative, the lumbar spinal cord was dissected, and frozen sections (20 μm) of the spinal segment

L4 were cut. Tissue sections were stained for GAD65 and GAD67, and immunofluorescence was quantified using the IPLab Image Analysis software. Western blots were performed on homogenized tissue samples of the ipsilateral L4 dorsal horn with ERK42 (p42 extracellular signal-regulated kinase) serving as loading control (Moore et al. 2002).

Two weeks following surgery, GAD65 immunofluorescence showed a decrease of approximately 30% ($P < 0.05$) in both the SNI and the CCI model. GAD67 immunolabeling was slightly reduced to 90% after CCI compared with naive controls ($P < 0.05$); no significant change was found after SNI. Western blotting revealed a significant decrease of GAD65 in the SNI and CCI models, with a maximum reduction of approximately 40% at 9 days following surgery ($P < 0.05$). GAD65 levels remained lowered over 4 weeks after SNI but returned to baseline levels in the CCI group. In contrast, only minor, transient differences from control tissue concentrations of GAD67 were found.

These results suggest a downregulation of GAD65 and, to a lesser degree, of GAD67. Alternatively, the reduction in GAD65 levels could indicate of a loss of GABAergic inhibitory interneurons, accompanied by a compensatory increase of GAD67 expression in surviving cells. Another interpretation could be that if not all interneurons express both GAD isoforms, the subpopulation carrying GAD65 could be specifically affected.

APOPTOTIC CELL DEATH IN THE DORSAL HORN

A combination of terminal deoxynucleotidyl transferase-mediated biotinylated UTP nick end labeling (TUNEL) and chromatin staining with bisbenzimide was used to detect DNA strand breaks and nuclear pyknosis or chromatin fragmentation, which are characteristic features of apoptotic cell death. To identify those apoptotic profiles that stem from neurons, we used immunostaining for neuronal nuclei protein (NeuN). One 10-μm section of the L4 spinal segment was randomly selected from every second 100-μm interval, and the average number of apoptotic profiles was determined.

On day 7 after SNI, we found 1.48 ± 0.08 TUNEL-positive profiles per section with nuclear signs of apoptosis in the ipsilateral dorsal horn (laminae I–III) (Fig. 2). Only a fraction of these profiles (0.16 ± 0.03) also stained for NeuN, indicating neurons undergoing apoptotic cell death (Fig. 2). It is widely recognized that any cell marker protein will be degraded during apoptosis. Therefore, it is likely that the number of NeuN-immunoreactive profiles represents an underestimate of the actual proportion of apoptotic neurons, although it cannot be ruled out that profiles of non-neuronal cells are included in the total number of apoptotic profiles.

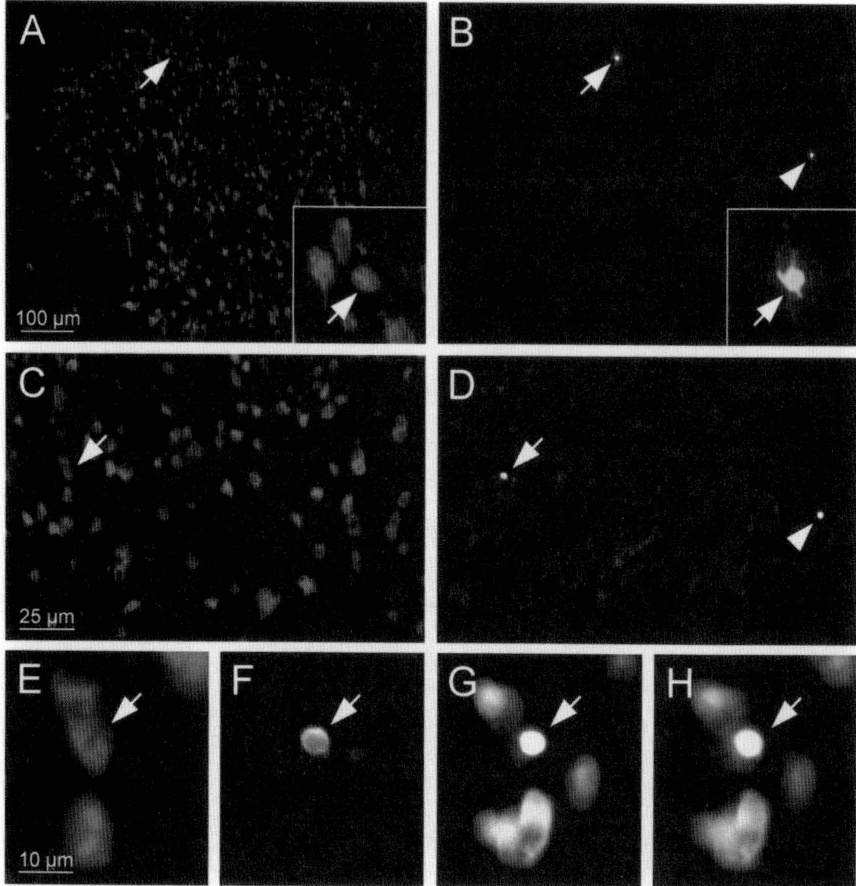

Fig. 2. Partial peripheral nerve injury induces apoptosis in neurons of the superficial dorsal horn. Panels A–B and C–H show examples of TUNEL-positive profiles in lamina I and III, respectively, of the ipsilateral dorsal horn 1 week after SNI. Arrows point to TUNEL-positive neurons (B,D,F), identified by NeuN-immunolabeling (A,C,E). Chromatin staining with bisbenzimide revealed nuclear pyknosis indicative of apoptotic cell death (G). Panel H represents an overlay of the different fluorescent signals shown in panels E–G.

Fig. 3. A schematic representation of mechanisms involved in spinal disinhibition following partial peripheral nerve injury. (A) Under physiological conditions, inhibitory interneurons containing GABA, glycine, or both modulate sensory transmission in the dorsal horn. Presynaptic inhibition through GABA acting on the central terminals of primary afferents has been established, while it remains to be shown whether there is also a glycinergic component. (B) After nerve injury, levels of GAD65 decrease and GABA synthesis is reduced. (C) Spontaneous activity of injured and neighboring afferents, together with enhanced sensitivity to noxious or innocuous stimuli, may lead to an increased release of glutamate in the dorsal horn and excitotoxic cell death. A loss of GABAergic interneurons would produce a fixed state of disinhibition. ⟶

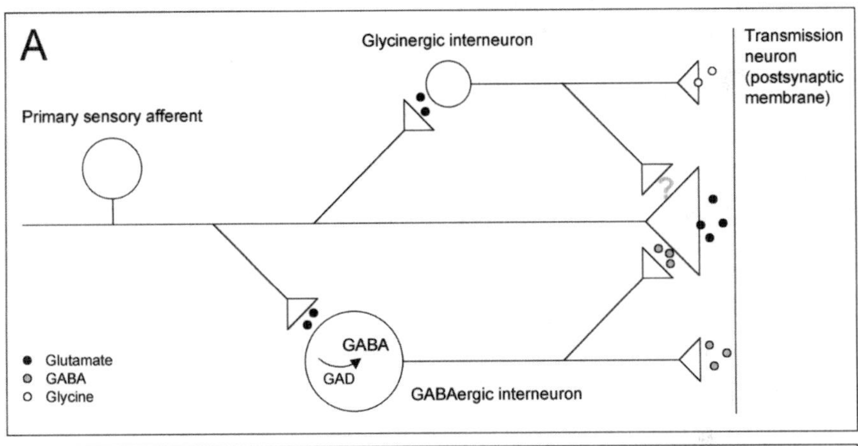
A
Glycinergic interneuron
Transmission neuron (postsynaptic membrane)
Primary sensory afferent
?
GABA
GAD
GABAergic interneuron
Glutamate
GABA
Glycine

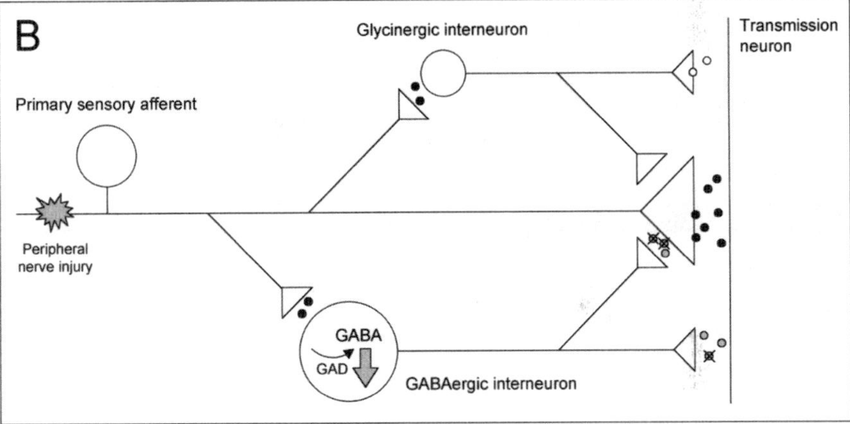
B
Glycinergic interneuron
Transmission neuron
Primary sensory afferent
Peripheral nerve injury
GABA
GAD
GABAergic interneuron

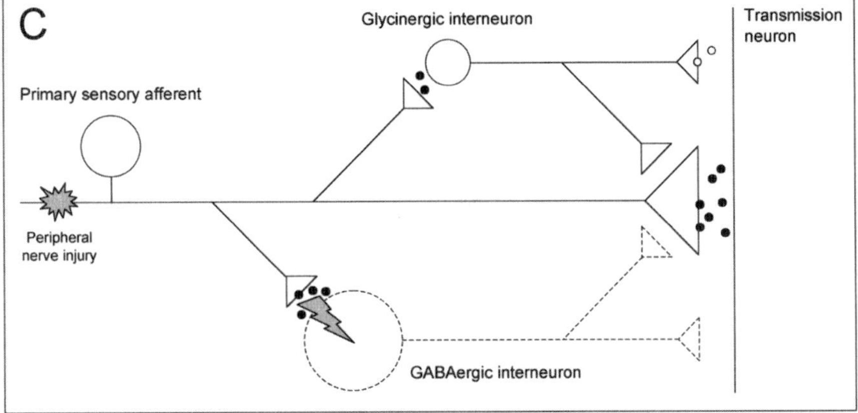
C
Glycinergic interneuron
Transmission neuron
Primary sensory afferent
Peripheral nerve injury
GABAergic interneuron

The occurrence of apoptotic profiles in the ipsilateral dorsal horn following CCI has been described previously. Whiteside and Munglani (2001) found a similar number of TUNEL-positive profiles one week after CCI. Apoptosis in the dorsal horn induced by CCI has also been reported by Kawamura et al. (1997). Technical differences may account for the very high number of TUNEL-positive profiles reported in this study, differing by a factor of about 100 from our results and those of Whiteside and Munglani (2001). In both previous studies, it was not specified whether TUNEL-positive profiles were of neuronal origin. MK-801, a noncompetitive NMDA-type glutamate-receptor antagonist, reduced the average number of apoptotic profiles after CCI, suggesting that the induction of apoptosis depends on the release of glutamate in the dorsal horn, presumably from primary afferents (Whiteside and Munglani 2001). An excessive release of glutamate from afferent terminals may trigger apoptosis through excitotoxic effects (Nicotera and Lipton 1999). Using electron microscopy and stereological counts of neurons, we have recently shown that electrical stimulation of primary afferents in the rat sciatic nerve induces substantial neuron loss in the dorsal horn, whereas no reduction of neurons was observed 4 weeks after complete nerve transection (Coggeshall et al. 2001).

CONCLUSION

Partial, but not complete, lesions of a peripheral nerve result in a loss of inhibition in the ipsilateral dorsal horn. Our electrophysiological data suggest that this finding is attributable to a decrease in the release of GABA while the glycinergic component of afferent-evoked IPSCs is preserved. The present results, demonstrating a reduction in the expression level of GAD65, and previous biochemical studies indicate that the synthesis of GABA is impaired. We have now found apoptosis of dorsal horn neurons in a model of partial sciatic nerve injury, associated with persistent neuropathic pain-like behavior. Preliminary evidence points to an excitotoxic effect of glutamate, which might be excessively released as primary sensory afferents become spontaneously active or exhibit increased responses to painful and nonpainful stimuli following nerve injury (Fig. 3). Further investigations are currently underway to quantify the loss of neurons by stereological counts. We will also determine whether, in agreement with our hypothesis, inhibitory interneurons undergo apoptosis and whether this process affects GABAergic interneurons in particular.

ACKNOWLEDGMENTS

This work is supported by grants from the National Institutes of Health and the Alexander von Humboldt-Foundation (J. Scholz).

REFERENCES

Bennett GJ, Xie YK. A peripheral mononeuropathy in rat that produces disorders of pain sensation like those seen in man. *Pain* 1988; 33:87–107.

Coggeshall RE, Lekan HA, White FA, Woolf CJ. A-fiber sensory input induces neuronal cell death in the dorsal horn of the adult rat spinal cord. *J Comp Neurol* 2001; 435:276–282.

Decosterd I, Woolf CJ. Spared nerve injury: an animal model of persistent peripheral neuropathic pain. *Pain* 2000; 87:149–158.

Eaton MJ, Plunkett JA, Karmally S, et al. Changes in GAD- and GABA-immunoreactivity in the spinal dorsal horn after peripheral nerve injury and promotion of recovery by lumbar transplant of immortalized serotonergic precursors. *J Chem Neuroanat* 1998; 16:57–72.

Hunt SP, Mantyh PW. The molecular dynamics of pain control. *Nat Rev Neurosci* 2001; 2:83–91.

Kawamura T, Akira T, Watanabe M, Kagitani Y. Prostaglandin E1 prevents apoptotic cell death in superficial dorsal horn of rat spinal cord. *Neuropharmacology* 1997; 36:1023–1030.

Koltzenburg M. Painful neuropathies. *Curr Opin Neurol* 1998; 11:515–521.

Malan TP, Mata HP, Porreca F. Spinal $GABA_A$ and $GABA_B$ receptor pharmacology in a rat model of neuropathic pain. *Anesthesiology* 2002; 96:1161–1167.

Moore KA, Kohno T, Scholz J, Karchewski LA, Woolf CJ. Spinal disinhibition: a role in neuropathic pain? *Neurosci News* 2001; 4:5–11.

Moore KA, Kohno T, Karchewski LA, et al. Partial peripheral nerve injury promotes a selective loss of GABAergic inhibition in the superficial dorsal horn of the spinal cord. *J Neurosci* 2002; 22:6724–6731.

Narikawa K, Hidemasa F, Kumamoto E, Yoshimura M. In vivo patch-clamp analysis of IPSCs evoked in rat substantia gelatinosa neurons by cutaneous mechanical stimulation. *J Neurophysiol* 2000; 84:2171–2174.

Nicoteira P, Lipton SA. Excitotoxins in neuronal apoptosis and necrosis. *J Cereb Blood Flow Metab* 1999; 19:583–591.

Whiteside GT, Munglani R. Cell death in the superficial dorsal horn in a model of neuropathic pain. *J Neurosci Res* 2001; 64:168–173.

Willis WD, Coggeshall RE. Functional organization of dorsal horn interneurons. In: Willis WD, Coggeshall RE (Eds). *Sensory Mechanisms of the Spinal Cord*, 2nd ed. New York: Plenum Press, 1991, pp 153–215.

Woolf CJ, Mannion RJ. Neuropathic pain: aetiology, symptoms, mechanisms, and management. *Lancet* 1999; 353:1959–1964.

Yoshimura M, Nishi S. Primary afferent-evoked glycine- and GABA-mediated IPSPs in substantia gelatinosa neurones in the rat spinal cord in vitro. *J Physiol* 1995; 482:29–38.

Zuniga RE, Schlicht CR, Abram SE. Intrathecal baclofen is analgesic in patients with chronic pain. *Anesthesiology* 2000; 92:876–880.

Correspondence to: Joachim Scholz, MD, Neural Plasticity Research Group, Department of Anesthesia and Critical Care, Massachusetts General Hospital and Harvard Medical School, 149 13th Street, Room 4309, Charlestown, MA 02129, USA. Tel: 617-724-3633; Fax: 617-724-3632; email: scholz.joachim@mgh.harvard.edu.

Proceedings of the 10th World Congress on Pain,
Progress in Pain Research and Management, Vol. 24,
edited by Jonathan O. Dostrovsky, Daniel B. Carr, and
Martin Koltzenburg, IASP Press, Seattle, © 2003.

34

Differential Role of Spinal Prostaglandin Receptor Subtypes EP1–EP4 in Rats with Normal and Inflamed Knee Joints

Andrea Ebersberger, Karl-Jürgen Bär, Philipp Teschner, Alejandro Telleria-Diaz, Enrique Vasquez, and Hans-Georg Schaible

Department of Physiology, University of Jena, Jena, Germany

Pain sensitivity during inflammatory joint diseases is enhanced by the generation of hypersensitivity in nociceptive neurons in the peripheral nervous system (peripheral sensitization), and it is also increased by nociceptive neurons in the spinal cord that develop a state of hyperexcitability (central sensitization) (McMahon et al. 1993; Schaible and Grubb 1993). Prostaglandin E_2 (PGE_2) is a major inflammatory mediator that sensitizes nociceptors (Vane 1971; Julius and Basbaum 2001). However, PGE_2 also causes allodynia and hyperalgesia when it is administered intrathecally (Vanegas and Schaible 2001; Svensson and Yaksh 2002). An important role of endogenous spinal PGE_2 in spinal nociceptive processing during peripheral inflammation has recently been established. Cyclooxygenases are expressed in dorsal root ganglia and in the spinal cord (Willingale et al. 1997; Inoue et al. 1999). During joint inflammation, spinal cyclooxygenase-2 is upregulated (Beiche et al. 1998a), and the intraspinal release of PGE_2 is enhanced (Ebersberger et al. 1999; Samad et al. 2001). The spinal application of PGE_2 induces a state of hyperexcitability in spinal cord neurons similar to that resulting from peripheral inflammation, and spinal application of the prostaglandin synthesis inhibitor indomethacin attenuates central sensitization during experimental inflammation (Vasquez et al. 2001).

PGE_2 effects are mediated by G-protein-coupled prostanoid (EP) receptors. Because all four receptor types (EP1–4) are present in the spinal cord, it is of considerable interest to study their role in the generation of spinal hyperexcitability. EP1 (Oida et al. 1995), EP3 (Beiche et al. 1998b), and EP4 (Oida et al. 1995) receptors are expressed in dorsal root ganglion neurons. Prostaglandins may thus influence the release of transmitters from primary afferent fibers. EP2 receptors are expressed in spinal cord neurons (Kawamura et al. 1997), indicating postsynaptic effects of PGE_2 (Baba et al. 2001; Ahmadi et al 2002). Activation of the EP1 receptor leads to calcium influx. The stimulation of EP2 and EP4 receptors enhances intracellular cyclic adenosine monophosphate (cAMP) through adenylate cyclase, but activation of the EP3 receptor, in particular the EP3α and EP3β subtypes, reduces the intracellular cAMP concentration (Negishi et al. 1995; Narumiya et al. 1999).

This chapter describes a study in which we use topical application of recently developed specific agonists to the spinal cord to show that all spinal EP receptors have a role in spinal nociception and, importantly, that the relative importance of these receptors is different under normal and inflammatory conditions.

METHODS

PREPARATION

Male Wistar rats (n = 68, 200–350 g) were anesthetized with 85–115 mg/kg intraperitoneal sodium thiopentone. Vital parameters were kept within physiological range. Spinal cord segments L1–L4 were exposed by laminectomy. A small trough (30 µL) was formed over the region of recordings by tightly sealing a rubber ring onto the cord surface with silicone gel. The trough was surrounded by 3% agar in physiological solution. In 23 rats an inflammation was induced in the left knee joint 7–11 hours before recordings by injection of 70 µL of a 4% kaolin suspension and thereafter 70 µL of a 2% carrageenan solution into the joint cavity (Neugebauer et al. 1993).

RECORDING FROM NEURONS

Action potentials of individual dorsal horn neurons were extracellularly recorded using glass-insulated carbon filaments. Dorsal horn neurons were selected that responded to pressure applied to the ipsilateral knee but not to brushing or squeezing of the skin over the knee (Neugebauer et al. 1993; Schaible and Grubb 1993). The receptive fields and mechanical thresholds of neurons were determined using mechanical stimulation of skin and deep tissue. For the test protocol we used a calibrated mechanical device that compressed the knee joint in the mediolateral axis with innocuous intensity (1.9 N/40 mm^2, corresponding to the pressure produced by holding the joint) or noxious intensity (7.8 N/40 mm^2 or 5.9 N/40 mm^2, felt as painful when applied to the experimenter's fifth finger) for 15 seconds. Additionally, mediolateral compression of the ankle joint and dorsoventral compression of the middle of the paw (1.1 N/20 mm^2 for innocuous stimulation, 5.8 N/20 mm^2 for noxious stimulation) were applied with modified crocodile clips.

EXPERIMENTAL PROTOCOL

Every 5 minutes innocuous and noxious test stimuli were applied sequentially to the knee, ankle, and paw for 15 seconds each. After we had established the neuronal baseline responses, we replaced the vehicle solution (0.07% ethanol in physiological solution) in the spinal trough with 30 μL of a solution containing one specific EP receptor agonist, and the stimulation protocol was continued. After 50 minutes, the next higher concentration of the agonist was administered, followed by the mechanical stimulation protocol. The agonists were ONO-DI-004, an EP1 agonist, at concentrations of 0.1 ng/μL (2.36 μM) to 100 ng/μL (2.36 mM); butaprost, an EP2 agonist, at 0.1 ng/μL (2.44 μM) to 100 ng/μL (2.44 mM); ONO-AE-248, an EP3α agonist, at 1 ng/μL (26.28 μM) to 100 ng/μL (2.628 mM); and ONO-AE1-329, an EP4 receptor agonist, at 1 ng/μL (21.9 μM) to 100 ng/μL (2.199 mM). In each experiment we tested one neuron with a single compound. The recently characterized compounds ONO-DI-004, ONO-AE-248, and ONO-AE1-329 have been used in various studies (Yamamoto et al. 1999; Suzawa et al. 2000; Maruyama et al. 2001; Shinomiya et al. 2001). In some experiments, we tested whether the EP3α receptor agonist would alter the responses to PGE_2 by administering 30 μL PGE_2 at 100 ng/μL (3.525 mM) to the spinal cord prior to administering ONO-AE-248 at 10 ng/μL (0.263 mM) and 100 ng/μL (2.628 mM).

DATA ANALYSIS

Averaged test responses to each type of stimulus in the 25 minutes preceding drug application served as the baseline, and averaged test responses during the last 25 minutes of EP receptor agonist application were compared to baseline using the Wilcoxon matched-pairs signed-rank test. Significance was accepted at $P < 0.05$.

RESULTS

SPINAL HYPERSENSITIVITY DURING ADMINISTRATION OF AGONISTS AT THE EP1, EP2, AND EP4 RECEPTOR

When PGE_2 is applied to the spinal cord, nociceptive spinal cord neurons develop enhanced responses to mechanical stimulation of the tissue, and their receptive fields expand (Vasquez et al. 2001). Topical application of the EP1, EP2, and EP4 receptor agonists to the spinal cord produced a similar dose-dependent effect (Fig. 1A). The responses of the neurons to mechanical stimulation of the knee joint increased. In addition, we noted an expansion of the receptive field toward the ankle and/or the paw in three neurons after administering the EP1 agonist, and in three neurons after administering the EP2 agonist. Long-term recordings without agonist application showed stable responses over 175 minutes. During peripheral inflammation that had been induced 7–11 hours before the recordings, we found a different pattern of effects of EP agonists. Only the EP1 receptor agonist enhanced the responses of the neurons to knee stimulation (Fig. 1B) in a similar way to that which occurs under normal conditions.

THE ROLE OF EP3 RECEPTORS

Of particular interest was the effect of the EP3 agonist, an agonist at the EP3α receptor subtype. When the knee joint was normal, the EP3 agonist did not significantly alter the responses of the neurons. However, when the knee joint was inflamed, the EP3 agonist significantly reduced neuronal responses to knee and ankle stimulation (innocuous knee stimulation at 10 ng/μL, noxious knee stimulation at 1 ng/μL, and noxious ankle stimulation at 100 ng/μL; Fig. 2). The agonist also reduced responses to spinal PGE_2. During application of PGE_2 to the spinal cord of normal rats, the responses to noxious pressure showed a gradual and persistent increase (Fig. 3A), as we have shown previously (Vasquez et al. 2001). When PGE_2 was administered first, the subsequent coadministration of the EP3α agonist caused a significant and dose-dependent attenuation of the effect of PGE_2 (the effect reaches significance 25–50 minutes following administration of 10 ng/μL of agonist; Fig 3B).

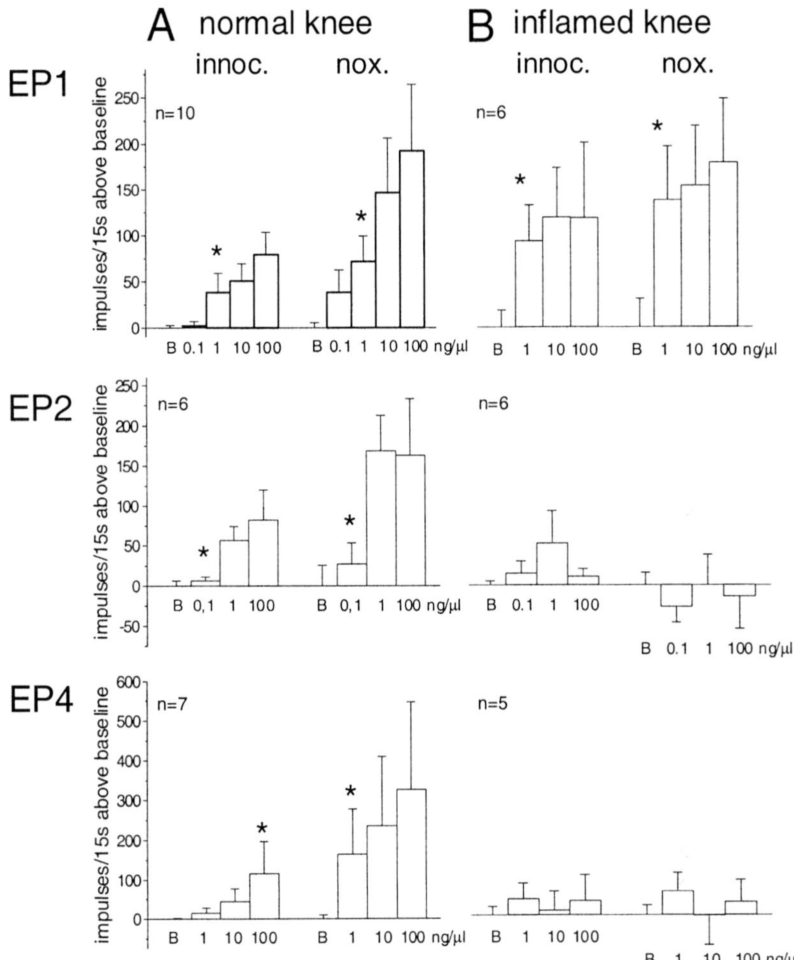

Fig. 1. Effect of spinal application of EP1, EP2, and EP4 agonists in rats with normal and inflamed knee joints. (A) EP1, EP2, and EP4 receptor agonists (ONO-DI-004, butaprost, and ONO-AE1 329, respectively) induce spinal hyperexcitability in normal rats. Columns show the average increase (over a 50-minute interval, mean ± SEM) of the responses of neurons during innocuous (innoc.) and noxious (nox.) pressure onto the knee joint after different concentrations of the agonists. The baseline (B) was set to zero. The predrug baseline values were (impulses/15 seconds, mean ± SEM): innocuous pressure on the knee joint, 46 ± 21 (EP1), 19 ± 11 (EP2), and 16 ± 11 (EP4); noxious pressure on the knee joint 153 ± 36 (EP1), 243 ± 98 (EP2), and 183 ± 76 (EP4). (B) The effect of EP receptor agonists in rats with acute inflammation of the knee joint, displayed as in Fig. 1A. The predrug baseline values were (impulses/15 seconds, mean ± SEM): innocuous pressure on the knee joint, 247 ± 75 (EP1), 79 ± 30 (EP2), and 265 ± 84 (EP4); noxious pressure on the knee joint, 770 ± 162 (EP1), 355 ± 98 (EP2), and 618 ± 135 (EP4); n = number of neurons. Asterisks show the lowest concentration of the agonist that caused a significant increase of the response to the mechanical stimulation compared to baseline (Wilcoxon's matched-pairs signed-rank test, $P < 0.05$).

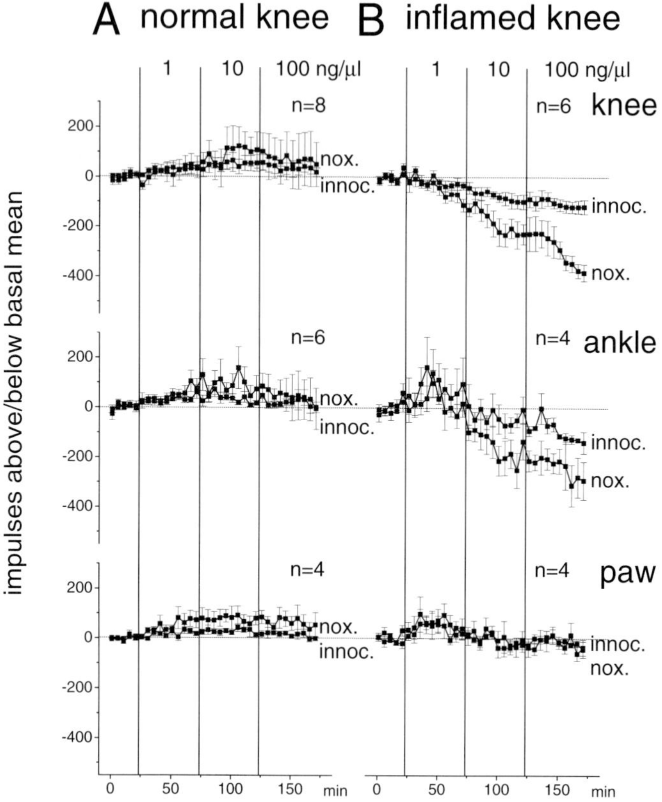

Fig. 2. Time course of the different effects of EP3α receptor agonist under normal and inflammatory conditions. Dose-dependent effects of the EP3α receptor agonist ONO-AE-248 on the responses to innocuous and noxious pressure onto the normal knee joint, ankle, and paw (A); and onto the inflamed knee joint, ankle, and paw (B). The predrug baseline values were (impulses/15 seconds, mean ± SEM): innocuous pressure on the knee joint, 61 ± 30 (normal knee), 147 ± 29 (inflamed knee); noxious pressure on the knee joint, 345 ± 73 (normal knee), 506 ± 35 (inflamed knee); innocuous pressure on the ankle, 35 ± 18 (normal knee), 238 ± 54 (inflamed knee); noxious pressure on the ankle 159 ± 58 (normal knee), 520 ± 114 (inflamed knee); innocuous pressure on the paw, 17.8 ± 10.4 (normal knee), 105.2 ± 61.4 (inflamed knee); noxious pressure on the paw 24.2 ± 13.6 (normal knee), 147.1 ± 55.3 (inflamed knee).

DISCUSSION

FACILITATORY EFFECTS OF AGONISTS AT THE EP1, EP2, AND EP4 RECEPTOR

The spinal application of EP1, EP2, and EP4 receptor agonists mimicked the facilitatory effect of spinal PGE_2 (Vasquez et al. 2001), suggesting

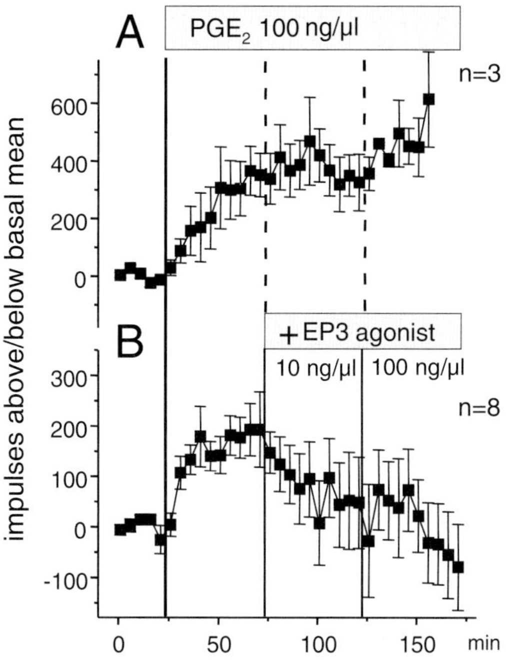

Fig. 3. Effect of EP3α agonist on PGE_2-induced spinal hyperexcitability. (A) Long-term increase of the responses to noxious pressure onto the normal knee during topical application of PGE_2 to the spinal cord surface. (B) Facilitation of the responses by PGE_2 and partial reversal of this effect by coadministration of the EP3α agonist in two doses.

that these receptors may mediate the PGE_2 effect in the generation of central sensitization. The pattern of sensitization was similar whether the process was set in motion by agonists at the EP1, EP2, or EP4 receptor. This similarity suggests that PGE_2 can initiate the process of facilitation by acting at pre- and postsynaptic sites. EP1 and EP4 receptors are located in primary afferent neurons (Oida et al. 1995), and PGE_2 enhances stimulation-evoked substance P and calcitonin gene-related peptide release from cultured or native DRG neurons, while cyclooxygenase inhibitors reduce the release (Nicol et al. 1992; Andreeva and Rang 1993; Southall et al. 1998). EP2 receptors are located on dorsal horn neurons (Kawamura et al. 1997), and PGE_2 excites spinal cord intrinsic neurons directly (Baba et al. 2001) and blocks inhibitory glycinergic neurotransmission in the dorsal horn (Ahmadi et al. 2002). Unfortunately, it is impossible to assess the relative contribution of these EP receptors to the process of inflammation-evoked central sensitization because no specific antagonists are available for the different EP receptors.

DIFFERENT PATTERN OF AGONISTS AT EP RECEPTORS DURING PERIPHERAL INFLAMMATION

When the joint was inflamed, only the EP1 agonist facilitated the responses, as in non-inflamed animals. Moreover, the EP3α agonist reduced the responses to stimulation of the inflamed joint. This different pattern of effects might explain why spinal application of PGE_2 facilitates responses to mechanical stimulation to a lesser extent when the joint is inflamed (Vasquez et al. 2001). Interestingly, the change in the pattern of effect was observed for the agonists at those receptors that are coupled to cAMP signaling, namely the EP2, EP3, and EP4 receptors (Negishi et al. 1995; Narumiya et al. 1999). Elevation of cAMP and actions of protein kinase A are critically involved in spinal nociceptive processes and hyperexcitability (Cerne et al. 1992; Malmberg et al. 1997), suggesting that the regulation of cAMP is an important mechanism involved in nociception. We propose the following sequence of events. When inflammation develops in the joint, PGE_2 is released in the spinal cord (Yang et al. 1996; Ebersberger et al. 1999). This release activates EP1 receptors, leading to increased excitation. It is also likely to enhance cAMP levels through activation of EP2 and EP4 receptors, which will facilitate responses to stimulation (as in Fig. 1A). Initially, activation of EP3α receptors, which downregulates the cAMP level, probably has no effect because cAMP levels are still low. However, after development of inflammation and central sensitization, PGE_2 activation of the EP2 and EP4 receptors no longer facilitates synaptic transmission (as in Fig. 1B). Either the receptors are desensitized, or second-messenger pathways are uncoupled, or cAMP effects have reached a maximum so that further stimulation of the receptors will not produce additional effects. On the other hand, the EP3α receptors that are coupled to G_i-proteins can now reduce cAMP. The combination of the changes of the effects at EP2, EP4, and EP3α receptors will reduce facilitatory PGE_2 effects after hyperexcitability has developed. It is possible that PGE_2 itself and/or the cAMP level determines the effects of EP receptor activation. The rapid reduction of the facilitatory effect of PGE_2 by the agonist at the EP3α receptor (Fig. 3) suggests such an interaction. Further changes such as up- and downregulation of different receptor types may also contribute.

These data emphasize the importance of spinal hyperexcitability in the generation of inflammatory joint pain and show an interesting role of EP receptors in this process. Through the action of EP1, EP2, and EP4 receptors, PGE_2 generates spinal hyperexcitability. However, once inflammation-evoked hyperexcitability is established, PGE_2 may actively attenuate its own effect by acting on EP3α receptors. Thus, spinal PGE_2 has pronociceptive as well as antinociceptive effects, depending on the presence or absence of peripheral inflammation. It will be of interest to find out whether the spinal EP3α receptor may be used as a target for analgesic treatment.

ACKNOWLEDGMENTS

The authors thank Ono Pharmaceutical Co., Ltd., Shimamoto, Mishima, Osaka, Japan, for the donation of the compounds ONO-DI-004, ONO-AE-248, and ONO-AE1-329. We thank Mrs. G. Cuny for skillful assistance, and acknowledge the Deutsche Forschungsgemeinschaft for funding. E. Vasquez held fellowships from the Deutscher Akademischer Austauschdienst and the Venezuelan Consejo Nacional de Investigaciones Cientificas y Tecnologicas.

REFERENCES

Ahmadi S, Lippross S, Neuhuber WL, Zeilhofer HU. PGE(2) selectively blocks inhibitory glycinergic neurotransmission onto rat superficial dorsal horn neurons. *Nature Neurosci* 2002; 5:34–40.

Andreeva L, Rang HP. Effect of bradykinin and prostaglandins on the release of calcitonin gene-related peptide-like immunoreactivity from the spinal cord in vitro. *Br J Pharmacol* 1993; 108:185–190.

Baba H, Kohno T, Moore KA, Woolf CJ. Direct activation of rat spinal dorsal horn neurons by prostaglandin E2. *J Neurosci* 2001; 21:1750–1756.

Beiche F, Brune K, Geisslinger G, Goppelt-Struebe M. Expression of cyclooxygenase isoforms in the rat spinal cord and their regulation during adjuvant-induced arthritis. *Inflamm Res* 1998a; 47:482–487.

Beiche F, Klein T, Nüsing R, Neuhuber W, Goppelt-Struebe M. Localization of cyclooxygenase-2 and prostaglandin E2 receptor EP3 in the rat lumbar spinal cord. *J Neuroimmunol* 1998b; 89:26–34.

Cerne R, Jiang M, Randic M. Cyclic adenosine 3´5´-monophosphate potentiates excitatory amino acid and synaptic responses of rat spinal dorsal horn neurons. *Brain Res* 1992; 596:111–123.

Cerne R, Rusin KI, Randic M. Enhancement of the *N*-methyl-D-aspartate response in spinal dorsal horn neurons by cAMP-dependent protein kinase. *Neurosci Lett* 1993; 161:124–128.

Ebersberger A, Grubb BD, Willingale HL, et al. The intraspinal release of prostaglandin E2 in a model of acute arthritis is accompanied by up-regulation of cyclo-oxygenase-2 in the spinal cord. *Neuroscience* 1999; 93:775–781.

Inoue A, Ikoma K, Morioka N, et al. Interleukin-1β induces substance P release from primary afferent neurons through the cyclooxygenase-2 system. *J Neurochem* 1999; 73:2206–2213.

Julius D, Basbaum AI. Molecular mechanisms of nociception. *Nature* 2001; 413:203–210.

Kawamura T, Yamauchi T, Koyama M, et al. Expression of prostaglandin EP2 receptor mRNA in the rat spinal cord. *Life Sci* 1997; 61:2111–2116.

Malmberg AB, Brandon EP, Idzerda RI, et al. Diminished inflammation and nociceptive pain with preservation of neuropathic pain in mice with a targeted mutation of the type I regulatory subunit of cAMP-dependent protein kinase. *J Neurosci* 1997; 17:7462–7470.

Maruyama T, Asada M, Shiraishi T, et al. Design and synthesis of a highly selective EP4-receptor agonist. Part 1: 3,7-dithiaPG derivates with high selectivity. *Bioorg Med Chem Lett* 2001; 11:2029–2031.

McMahon SB, Lewin GR, Wall PD. Central hyperexcitability triggered by noxious inputs. *Curr Opin Neurobiol* 1993; 3:602–610

Narumiya S, Sugimoto Y, Ushikubi F. Prostanoid receptors: structures, properties, and functions. *Physiol Rev* 1999; 79:1193–1226.

Negishi M, Sugimoto Y, Ichikawa A. Molecular mechanisms of diverse actions of prostanoid receptors. *Biochim Biophys Acta* 1995; 1259:109–120.

Neugebauer V, Lücke T, Schaible H-G. N-methyl-D-aspartate (NMDA) and non-NMDA receptor antagonists block the hyperexcitability of dorsal horn neurons during development of acute arthritis in rat's knee joint. *J Neurophysiol* 1993; 70:1365–1377.

Nicol GD, Klingberg DK, Vasko MR. Prostaglandin E2 increases calcium conductance and stimulates release of substance P in avian sensory neurons. *J Neurosci* 1992; 12:1917–1927.

Oida H, Namba T, Sugimoto Y, et al. In situ hybridization studies of prostacyclin receptor mRNA expression in various mouse organs. *Br J Pharmacol* 1995; 116:2828–2837.

Samad TA, Moore KA, Sapirstein A, et al. Interleukin-β-mediated induction of COX-2 in the CNS contributes to inflammatory pain hypersensitivity. *Nature* 2001; 410:471–475.

Schaible H-G, Grubb BD. Afferent and spinal mechanisms of joint pain. *Pain* 1993; 55:5–54.

Shinomiya S, Naraba H, Ueno A, et al. Regulation of TNFα and interleukin-10 production by prostaglandins I2 and E2: studies with prostaglandin receptor-deficient mice and prostaglandin E-receptor subtype-selective synthetic agonists. *Biochem Pharmacol* 2001; 61:1153–1160.

Southall MD, Michael RL, Vasko MR. Intrathecal NSAIDs attenuate inflammation-induced neuropeptide release from rat spinal cord slices. *Pain* 1998; 78:39–48.

Suzawa T, Miyaura C, Inada M, et al. The role of prostaglandin E receptor subtypes (EP1, EP2, EP3, and EP4) in bone resorption: an analysis using specific agonists for the respective EPs. *Endocrinology* 2000; 141:1554–1559.

Svensson CI, Yaksh TL. The spinal phospholipase-prostanoid cascade in nociceptive processing. *Annu Rev Toxicol* 2002; 42:553–583.

Vane JR. Inhibition of prostaglandin synthesis as a mechanism of action for aspirin-like drugs. *Nature New Biol* 1971; 231:232–235.

Vanegas H, Schaible H-G. Prostaglandins and cyclooxygenases in the spinal cord. *Prog Neurobiol* 2001; 64:327–363.

Vasquez E, Bär K-J, Ebersberger A, et al. Spinal prostaglandins are involved in the development but not the maintenance of inflammation-induced spinal hyperexcitability. *J Neurosci* 2001; 21:9001–9008.

Willingale HL, Gardiner NJ, McLymont N, et al. Prostanoids synthesized by cyclooxygenase isoforms in rat spinal cord and their contribution to the development of neuronal hyperexcitability. *Br J Pharmacol* 1997; 122:1593–1604.

Yamamoto H, Maruyama T, Sakata K, et al. Novel four selective agonists for prostaglandin E receptor subtypes. *Prostaglandins Lipid Mediators* 1999; 59:150.

Yang LC, Marsala M, Yaksh TL. Characterization of time course of spinal amino acids, citrulline and PGE_2 release after carrageenan/kaolin-induced knee joint inflammation: a chronic microdialysis study. *Pain* 1996; 67:345–354.

Correspondence to: Andrea Ebersberger, Dr. rer. nat., Department of Physiology I, University of Jena, Teichgraben 8, D-07743 Jena, Germany. Tel: 49-3641-938814; Fax: 49-3641-938812; email: aebe@mti-n.uni-jena.de.

Proceedings of the 10th World Congress on Pain,
Progress in Pain Research and Management, Vol. 24,
edited by Jonathan O. Dostrovsky, Daniel B. Carr, and
Martin Koltzenburg, IASP Press, Seattle, © 2003.

35

Perceptual Correlates of Long-Term Potentiation in the Spinal Cord

Thomas Klein,[a,b] Walter Magerl,[a] Ursula Mantzke,[c] Hanns-Christian Hopf,[b] Jürgen Sandkühler,[d] and Rolf-Detlef Treede[a]

[a]Institute of Physiology and Pathophysiology, [b]Department of Neurology, and [c]Department of Anesthesiology, Johannes Gutenberg University, Mainz, Germany; [d]Brain Research Institute, Vienna University Medical School, Vienna, Austria

It is well known that the efficacy of nociceptive transmission to dorsal horn neurons is enhanced following a strong painful stimulus (Simone et al. 1991; Brennan et al. 1996; Dougherty et al. 1998). This central sensitization leads to an increase in pain sensitivity in a large area around the conditioned skin site (neurogenic secondary hyperalgesia; LaMotte et al. 1991). Neurogenic hyperalgesia also forms an integral part of some neuropathic pain states caused by dysfunction and/or lesion of the peripheral or central nervous system (Treede et al. 1992; Fields et al. 1998; Baumgärtner et al. 2002). Brief incidents such as tissue or nerve injury may enhance pain perception for many hours or even months and years. It is thus tempting to propose that long-term potentiation (LTP) of synaptic strength in nociceptive pathways, at least in part, may underlie neurogenic hyperalgesia and chronic pain (Randic et al. 1993; Willis 1997; Miletic and Miletic 2000; Sandkühler 2000; Woolf and Salter 2000).

LTP represents an ubiquitous phenomenon of synaptic plasticity that has been extensively studied in the hippocampus and neocortex (Bliss and Collingridge 1993). An *N*-methyl D-aspartate (NMDA)-receptor dependent form of homosynaptic LTP of C-fiber input was recently found in nociceptive pathways of the spinal cord (Randic et al. 1993; Liu and Sandkühler 1997; Svendsen et al. 1998).

Despite evidence in animal experiments, the role of nociceptive LTP in *human* pain perception is unknown. Fortunately, functionally specialized classes of nociceptive primary afferents (Aδ and C fibers) can be excited selectively by noninvasive stimuli in awake humans (Schmidt et al. 1995; Magerl et al. 2001), and pain ratings can serve as reliable output measures (Mayer et al. 1975). Taking advantage of these circumstances, we have studied plasticity of human pain perception using electrical stimulus protocols that reliably elicit LTP in intact animals.

METHODS

SUBJECTS

Eight subjects (mean age 30 years) each participated in two sessions of electrical stimulation. Another five subjects (mean age 24 years) participated in experiments on the effect of the NMDA-receptor antagonist ketamine. All subjects consented in writing to the investigation, which was approved by the local ethics committee.

CONDITIONING STIMULI

Electrical stimuli delivered by a constant current stimulator were applied on the forearm by a circular array of 10 punctate electrodes (200 μm diameter each; Fig. 1A). Stimulus intensity was adjusted to multiples of the detection threshold (*T*). Conditioning pulse trains of 100 Hz (monophasic, cathodal, 2 ms pulse width) for 1 second repeated five times at 10-second intervals (high-frequency stimulation [HFS] at 10× and 20× *T*) were used to elicit LTP. To demonstrate excitation of peptidergic afferents by HFS, which is essential for the induction of LTP (Liu and Sandkühler 1997), increase of blood flow after electrical conditioning stimulation was measured by laser Doppler perfusion imaging (Fig. 1B; Magerl et al. 1987). Although instantaneous discharge frequencies of up to 190 Hz in human peptidergic afferents have been reported under certain circumstances (Weidner et al. 2002), high-discharge frequencies induced by HFS are usually not transmitted unaltered to the spinal cord. Nevertheless, HFS (100 Hz) of peptidergic afferents ensures a maximum of spinal nociceptive input.

TEST STIMULI

Sensitivity of the conditioned nociceptive pathway was tested by single electrical test stimuli through the conditioning electrode (2 ms pulse width

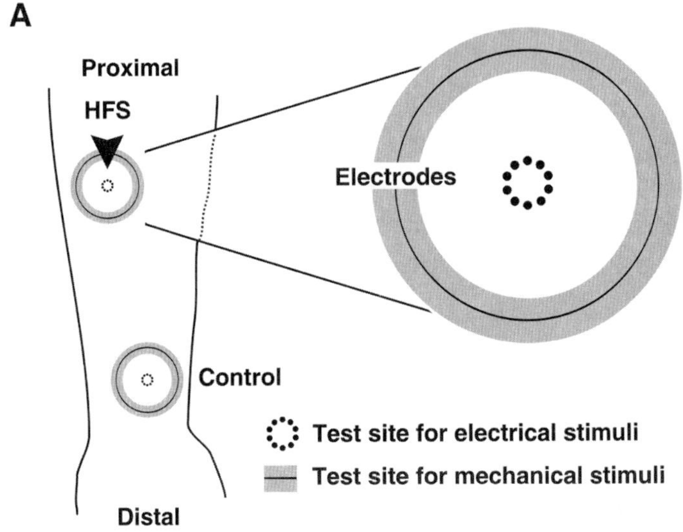

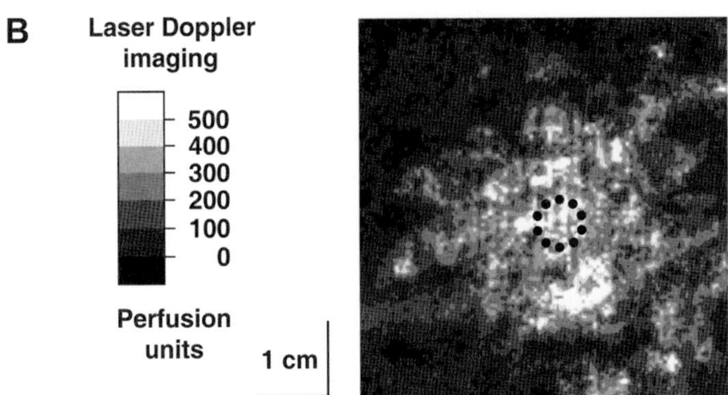

Fig. 1. (A) Experimental set-up. Conditioning high-frequency stimulation (HFS) was applied to the proximal forearm via a circular array of electrodes at 10× and 20× the detection threshold (*T*). Perceptual effects of HFS on nociception mediated by the conditioned pathway were tested with single electrical test pulses at 10× *T* through the conditioning electrode, effects outside the conditioned pathway were tested with mechanical pin prick stimuli (a series of seven forces: 8–512 mN). Subjects rated the magnitude of pain on 0–100 numerical rating scales. Ratings were compared to ratings evoked at an unconditioned control site. (B) HFS at 20× *T* evoked a substantial flare around the electrode array indicating sufficient activation of peptidergic afferents.

at 10× *T*). Stimulus-response functions for pricking pain were obtained adjacent to the conditioned skin site (but essentially outside the area of increased blood flow, i.e., in a nonconditioned pathway; cf. Magerl et al.

2001) with a series of punctate mechanical stimulators (200 μm diameter, 8–512 mN), which preferentially activate Aδ nociceptors (Ziegler et al. 1999). Subjects estimated the magnitude of pain on numerical rating scales (0, nonpainful; 100, most intense pain imaginable).

Mechanical and electrical test stimuli were applied in runs alternating between the conditioned skin site and the unconditioned control site (Fig. 1A) over a period of 40 minutes before (baseline) and 60 minutes after conditioning electrical stimulation (test period).

In the pharmacological study, the NMDA-receptor antagonist ketamine (0.25 mg/kg, i.v., administered over a period of 1 minute) was injected 4 minutes before HFS (at 20× *T*). Mechanical and electrical testing resumed 15 minutes after conditioning stimulation when the psychomimetic effect of ketamine on cognitive performance had subsided, as tested by a mental arithmetic task. Each subject took part in a separate control experiment.

DATA EVALUATION AND STATISTICS

Data were pooled across both intensities (10× *T* and 20× *T*). Pain ratings were transformed into decadic logarithmic values to achieve normally distributed data and homogeneity of variance. To avoid loss of zero values, a small constant (0.1) was added to all ratings (Magerl et al. 1998). Ratings were then normalized to the mean baseline value. Post hoc paired *t* tests were performed to compare values at each time point after conditioning stimulation with the average baseline value.

RESULTS AND DISCUSSION

Conditioning painful HFS of superficial peripheral nerve endings induced a substantial flare around the conditioning electrode (Fig. 1B). This finding indicates activation of peptidergic C fibers, which is a prerequisite for the induction of LTP in animals and of secondary hyperalgesia in humans (Liu and Sandkühler 1997; Ziegler et al. 1999; Magerl et al. 2001). HFS was followed by a significant increase of perceived pain evoked by electrical test stimuli at the site of conditioning stimulation (+46% compared to control; Fig. 2B). The increase persisted until the end of the observation period and was blocked by ketamine (–1% compared to controls vs. +47% in experiments without ketamine; Fig. 3A). Because electrical test stimuli activated the same afferents that were excited by conditioning stimulation, it is likely that the enhanced pain perception to such stimuli depends on *homosynaptic* long-term changes at synapses between nociceptive primary afferents

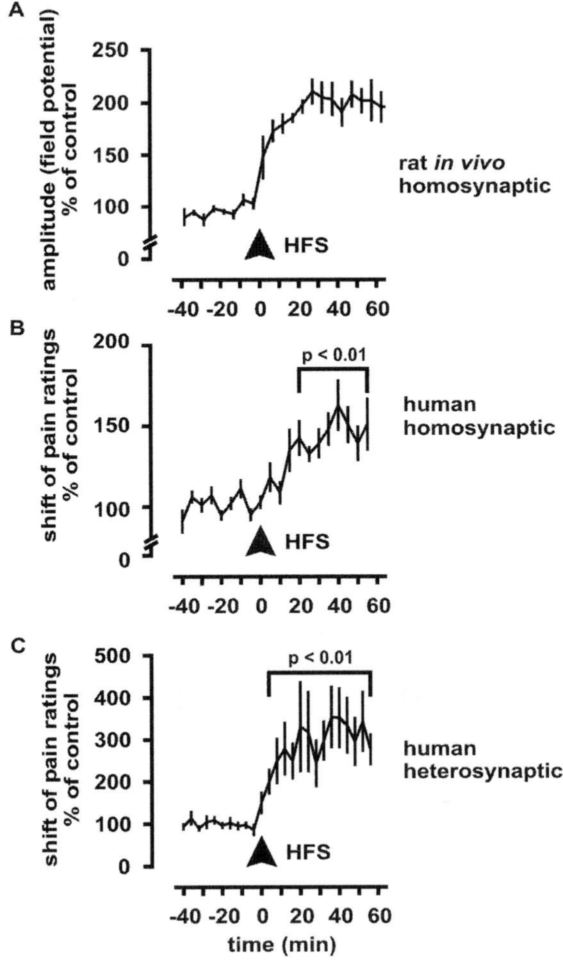

Fig. 2. Long-term changes in spinal cord synaptic strength and perceived pain intensity following HFS. (A) Typical example of long-term potentiation (LTP) of C-fiber field potentials in rat dorsal horn following HFS in vivo. After conditioning HFS of the sural nerve (4 × 1 second at 100 Hz at 10-second intervals), the amplitude of C-fiber-evoked field potentials increased up to 100% above baseline within the first 20 minutes and remained potentiated throughout the observation period (adapted from Sandkühler and Liu 1998). Mean ± SEM (n = 5). (B) In human subjects HFS of superficial peptidergic afferents (5 × 1 second at 100 Hz at 10-s intervals) induced an increase of pain ratings to single electrical test pulses through the conditioning electrode by about 50% compared to a control site. This facilitation also lasted until the end of the observation period. Mean ± SEM (n = 7). (C) HFS also induced a marked increase (about 200%) of pinprick-evoked pain in the area surrounding the conditioned electrode (as compared with an unconditioned control site). Mean ± SEM (n = 8). Each dot in panels B and C represents the shift of normalized pain ratings averaged over 5 minutes compared to the unconditioned control site.

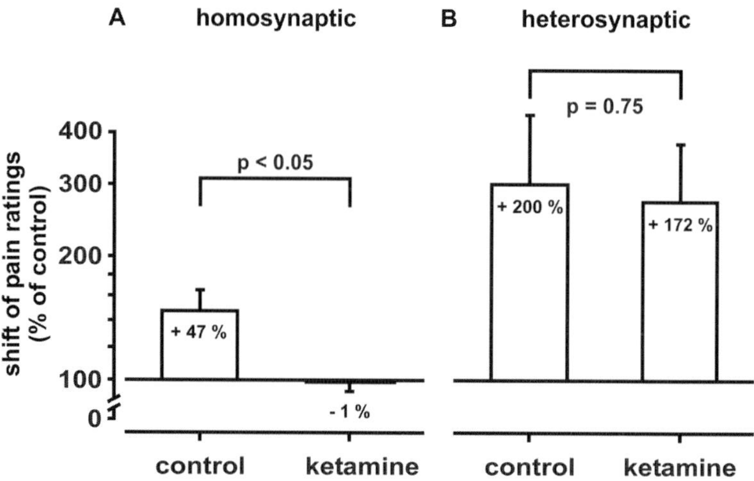

Fig. 3. Effect of the NMDA-receptor antagonist ketamine. (A) Ketamine (0.25 mg/kg i.v.) given immediately prior to conditioning HFS prevented the enhancement of electrical evoked pain at the site of conditioning stimulation (–1% under ketamine vs. +47% without ketamine compared to a control site). (B) In contrast, enhancement of pinprick-evoked pain remained unaffected by ketamine (+172% vs. +200%). The differential effects of ketamine suggest multiple mechanisms of nociceptive perceptual LTP. Mean ± SEM (n = 5). Each bar represents the shift of normalized pain ratings 15 minutes after HFS averaged over 60 minutes compared to the unconditioned control site.

and second-order spinal cord neurons. Taken together, the activation of peptidergic C-fiber afferents, the time course of the enhanced pain perception, and the sensitivity to NMDA-receptor blockade resemble features of LTP of C-fiber-evoked field potentials generated in superficial spinal cord laminae (Fig. 2A). These findings suggest homosynaptic LTP at NMDA-sensitive glutamatergic synapses as the underlying mechanism (*homosynaptic perceptual LTP*).

HFS was also followed by an increase of pain evoked by pinpricks adjacent to the conditioned skin area (neurogenic secondary hyperalgesia, +220% compared to control; Fig. 2C). Its time course was similar to that of homosynaptic LTP at the conditioned skin site. In contrast to homosynaptic changes, however, neurogenic secondary hyperalgesia must involve *heterosynaptic* mechanisms of LTP for several reasons. First, the facilitated input is spatially remote from the conditioning pathway. Second, it involves two electrophysiologically and pharmacologically separate input pathways—the conditioning pathway relies on capsaicin-sensitive peptidergic C fibers, whereas the facilitated input is carried by capsaicin-insensitive Aδ fibers (Ziegler et al. 1999; Magerl et al. 2001). This finding suggests an interaction between subclasses of primary afferents that express the capsaicin receptor

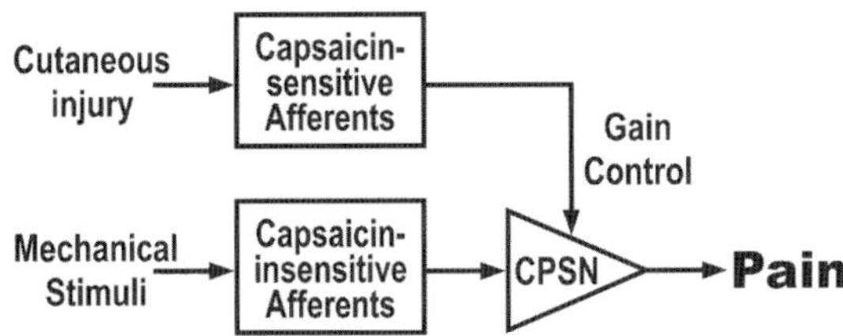

Fig. 4. Gain control model for heterosynaptic LTP (secondary hyperalgesia). Capsaicin-insensitive nociceptive afferents project to central pain-signaling neurons (CPSNs). Mechanical stimulation of the nociceptor terminals of these afferents leads to the perception of pinprick pain in normal skin. Activity in unmyelinated capsaicin-sensitive afferents (e.g., due to an adjacent injury or capsaicin injection) leads to an increase in the gain (or facilitation) of these CPSNs. Mechanical stimulation of the terminals of capsaicin-insensitive afferents now leads to enhanced pain (secondary hyperalgesia). A similar augmentation occurs for capsaicin-insensitive, low-threshold mechanoreceptors, leading to allodynia (from Magerl et al. 2001 by permission of Oxford University Press).

TRPV1 (vanilloid receptor subtype 1, formerly termed VR1) and those that do not (Fig. 4). Thus, the secondary pin-prick hyperalgesia constitutes a correlate of heterosynaptic LTP within the human nociceptive system (*heterosynaptic perceptual LTP*). In addition to pinprick hyperalgesia, HFS also induced long-lasting pain following light tactile stimuli (allodynia, tested at the same site; data not shown) based on heterosynaptic LTP-like facilitation of low-threshold mechanoreceptive Aβ fibers.

Secondary hyperalgesia to pinprick (heterosynaptic perceptual LTP) was not affected by NMDA-receptor blockade by ketamine (+172% vs. +200%; Fig. 3B), suggesting a non-NMDA-dependent mechanism of heterosynaptic LTP. Nociceptive neuropeptides, which are essential for the induction of LTP in spinal cord neurons (Liu and Sandkühler 1997) and for the induction of secondary hyperalgesia (Laird et al. 2001), are likely candidates. Substance P released into extrasynaptic space can survive for a long time, can spread over considerable distances in the spinal cord (Duggan et al. 1995), and eventually can act at extrasynaptic receptors of adjacent neurons or even neurons in adjacent laminae.

CONCLUSIONS

HFS of C-fiber afferents, which induces LTP of C-fiber input in the rat spinal cord, causes two different forms of perceptual LTP in humans. The first is an NMDA-receptor-dependent enhancement of pain perception to electrical test stimuli at the site of conditioning stimulation. This may be the perceptual correlate that parallels homosynaptic glutamatergic LTP as previously described in animal models (*homosynaptic perceptual LTP*). The second form of perceptual LTP evoked by HFS in human subjects is an NMDA-receptor-independent increase of pain evoked by pinpricks in adjacent skin areas (neurogenic secondary hyperalgesia). Because induction and perception of neurogenic secondary hyperalgesia relies on two separate input pathways (nociceptive C- and Aδ-fiber afferents, respectively), the perceptual changes must be based on heterosynaptic synaptic plasticity (*heterosynaptic perceptual LTP*).

Whereas spinal LTP would be sufficient to account for these perceptual changes, plasticity in ascending nociceptive pathways to the thalamus and cortex also may contribute to the observed effects. HFS of primary nociceptive afferents may transiently change their excitability (over a period of less than 1 minute), but peripheral mechanisms cannot explain the observed long-lasting perceptual changes (lasting for at least 1 hour).

The LTP-like mechanism of secondary hyperalgesia, which is a surrogate model of neuropathic pain, points to a role of LTP in the pathophysiology of at least some forms of neuropathic pain. Thus, our findings on perceptual LTP induced by HFS may provide the missing link between a basic neurobiological mechanism (nociceptive LTP) and clinical observations in humans (chronic pain and neurogenic hyperalgesia).

ACKNOWLEDGMENTS

Supported by the Pain Research Program of the Medical Faculty of Heidelberg and the Forschungsfond of the University of Mainz. We thank F.K. Pierau (Max-Planck-Institute for Physiological and Clinical Research, Bad Nauheim, Germany) for providing access to the laser Doppler imager.

REFERENCES

Baumgärtner U, Magerl W, Klein T, Hopf HC, Treede RD. Neurogenic hyperalgesia versus painful hypoalgesia: two distinct mechanisms of neuropathic pain. *Pain* 2002; 96:141–151.

Bliss TVP, Collingridge GL. A synaptic model of memory: long-term potentiation in the hippocampus. *Nature* 1993; 361:31–39.

Brennan TJ, Vandermeulen EP, Gebhart GF. Characterization of a rat model of incisional pain. *Pain* 1996; 64:493–501.

Dougherty PM, Willis WD, Lenz FA. Transient inhibition of responses to thermal stimuli of spinal sensory tract neurons in monkeys during sensitization by intradermal capsaicin. *Pain* 1998; 77:129–136.

Duggan AW, Riley RC, Mark MA, MacMillan SJ, Schaible HG. Afferent volley patterns and the spinal release of immunoreactive substance P in the dorsal horn of the anaesthetized spinal cat. *Neuroscience* 1995; 65:849–858.

Fields HL, Rowbotham M, Baron R. Postherpetic neuralgia: irritable nociceptors and deafferentation. *Neurobiol Dis* 1998; 5:209–227.

Laird JMA, Roza C, DeFelipe C, Hunt SP, Cervero F. Role of central and peripheral tachykinin NK1 receptors in capsaicin-induced pain and hyperalgesia in mice. *Pain* 2001; 90:97–103.

LaMotte RH, Shain CN, Simone DA, Tsai EFP. Neurogenic hyperalgesia: psychophysical studies of underlying mechanisms. *J Neurophysiol* 1991; 66:190–211.

Liu XG, Sandkühler J. Characterization of long-term potentiation of C-fiber evoked potentials in spinal dorsal horn of adult rat: essential role of NK1 and NK2 receptors. *J Neurophysiol* 1997; 78:1973–1982.

Magerl W, Szolcsányi J, Westerman RA, Handwerker HO. Laser Doppler measurements of skin vasodilation elicited by percutaneous electrical stimulation of nociceptors in humans. *Neurosci Lett* 1987; 82:349–354.

Magerl W, Wilk SH, Treede RD. Secondary hyperalgesia and perceptual wind-up following intradermal injection of capsaicin in humans. *Pain* 1998; 74:257–268.

Magerl W, Fuchs PN, Meyer RA, Treede RD. Roles of capsaicin-insensitive nociceptors in pain and secondary hyperalgesia. *Brain* 2001; 124:1754–1764.

Mayer DJ, Price DD, Becker DP. Neurophysiological characterization of the anterolateral spinal cord neurons contributing to pain perception in man. *Pain* 1975; 1:51–58.

Miletic G, Miletic V. Long-term changes in sciatic-evoked A-fiber dorsal horn field potentials accompany loose ligation of the sciatic nerve in rats. *Pain* 2000; 84:353–359.

Randic M, Jiang MC, Cerne R. Long-term potentiation and long-term depression of primary afferent neurotransmission in the rat spinal cord. *J Neurosci* 1993; 13:5228–5241.

Sandkühler J. Learning and memory in pain pathways. *Pain* 2000; 88:113–118.

Sandkühler J, Liu X. Induction of long-term potentiation at spinal synapses by noxious stimulation or nerve injury. *Eur J Neurosci* 1998; 10:2476–2480.

Schmidt R, Schmelz M, Forster C, et al. Novel classes of responsive and unresponsive C nociceptors in human skin. *J Neurosci* 1995; 15:333–341.

Simone DA, Sorkin LS, Oh U, et al. Neurogenic hyperalgesia: central neural correlates in responses of spinothalamic tract neurons. *J Neurophysiol* 1991; 66:228–246.

Svendsen F, Tjolsen A, Hole K. AMPA and NMDA receptor-dependent spinal LTP after nociceptive tetanic stimulation. *Neuroreport* 1998; 9:1185–1190.

Treede RD, Meyer RA, Raja SN, Campbell JN. Peripheral and central mechanisms of cutaneous hyperalgesia. *Prog Neurobiol* 1992; 38:397–421.

Weidner C, Schmelz M, Schmidt R, et al. Neural signal processing: the underestimated contribution of peripheral human C-fibers. *J Neurosci* 2002; 22:6704–6712.

Willis WD. Is central sensitization of nociceptive transmission in the spinal cord a variety of long-term potentiation? *Neuroreport* 1997; 8:R3.

Woolf CJ, Salter MW. Neuronal plasticity: increasing the gain in pain. *Science* 2000; 288:1765–1769.

Ziegler EA, Magerl W, Meyer RA, Treede RD. Secondary hyperalgesia to punctate mechanical stimuli: central sensitization to A-fibre nociceptor input. *Brain* 1999; 122:2245–2257.

Correspondence to: Prof. Dr. Rolf-Detlef Treede, Institute of Physiology and Pathophysiology, Johannes Gutenberg University, Saarstr. 21, D-55099 Mainz, Germany. Tel: 49-6131-392-5715; Fax: 49-6131-392-5902; email: treede@uni-mainz.de.

Part V

Pharmacological Approaches

Proceedings of the 10th World Congress on Pain,
Progress in Pain Research and Management, Vol. 24,
edited by Jonathan O. Dostrovsky, Daniel B. Carr, and
Martin Koltzenburg, IASP Press, Seattle, © 2003.

36

New Targets for Analgesic Drugs

Raymond G. Hill

Neuroscience Research Centre, Merck Sharp and Dohme,
Terlings Park, Harlow, Essex, United Kingdom

The explosion of information on the functions of the nervous system we have recently experienced because of our improved knowledge of integrative physiology and the sequencing of the human and other mammalian genomes would reasonably have been expected to lead to the production of improved analgesic drugs. This promise has not yet been realized, and although we do have an abundance of information on the complexities of the transduction machinery for sensory neurotransmission, it has not been reduced to practice in terms of benefit to the patient in pain. There is real justification for optimism in the long term that tangible benefits will derive from our new biological understanding (see Boyce et al. 2001; Hopkins and Groom 2002; Wise et al. 2002). In the short and medium term, however, the best chance for improved therapies comes from exploiting the technologies for drug discovery that molecular biology has provided in order to improve on existing treatment options. This goal can be achieved in a variety of ways (Fig. 1). We could refine existing therapies to increase pharmacological specificity so as to maximize wanted effects while reducing those that are unwanted. Good examples are the development of the triptans from ergot to improve the treatment of migraine or the derivation of the COX-2-selective inhibitors (coxibs) from the nonsteroidal anti-inflammatory drugs (NSAIDs) to improve the treatment of inflammatory and other pains (see Boyce et al. 2001). In the case of the coxibs, progress was extremely rapid once COX-2 had been isolated and cloned (Hla and Neilson 1992), and selective COX-2-blocking drugs are now available for treating clinical pain (see FitzGerald and Patrono 2001 for review). More effective treatment may also come from an improved kinetic or metabolic profile in a drug without any change in its basic pharmacology, for example by using morphine for terminal pain in a slow-release formulation. Further consideration of these aspects is outside

- Improved formulation
  - controlled release oral morphine
- Improved kinetic or metabolic characteristics
  - remifentanil
- Refinement of a known mechanism of action
  - COX-2 blockers
  - triptans
- Novel pharmacological mechanism
  - NK1 antagonists
- Elucidation of unknown mechanism
  - anticonvulsants and antidepressants

Fig. 1. Strategies to produce new drugs for the treatment of pain.

the scope of the present chapter, however. Completely novel pharmacological approaches are less common but are becoming more feasible as our repertoire of new receptor, channel, and enzyme targets continues to increase (see Oliver et al. 2000; Hopkins and Groom 2002; Wise et al. 2002). Neurokinin-1 (NK1) receptor antagonists, which block the effects of the neuropeptide substance P, illustrate this approach (Boyce and Hill 2000; Boyce et al. 2001). Such novel approaches involve a step into the unknown and cannot rely on the precedent of previous clinical experience. It is also possible to improve on existing treatments that have been introduced empirically, such as the use of anticonvulsants and antidepressants for neuropathic pain, by studying their unique molecular mechanisms in the laboratory and then using the information gained to design analogues that are optimized for the chosen target.

If we look at agents that are now in the development pipeline, the landscape looks all too familiar. A recent review (Mealy et al. 2002) described 94 drugs in development for treatment of pain. Most of these were variations on the theme of opioids or NSAIDs or were reformulations or combinations of existing drugs. There were some newly fashionable but pharmacologically traditional approaches such as cannabinoids and some agents with a limited application such as invertebrate neurotoxins. The novel approaches (exemplified by coxibs and NO-NSAIDs) were very much in the minority. With few exceptions, the mechanisms of the drugs described were the product of pregenomic research and owed their origin to previous therapeutic agents rather than to innovative science.

It is reasonable to ask why we have not yet discovered more and better novel pain-relieving drugs. Compared with other medical needs in clinical neuroscience such as the psychoaffective disorders, pain may be considered an easy target. Animals and humans respond in a similar, aversive way to noxious stimuli, and this response can be measured objectively and quantified. We have a good and improving understanding of the anatomy and physiology underlying nociception (Hill 2001; Hunt and Mantyh 2001). However, the emotional aspects of pain that lead to suffering can only be adequately studied in humans, and the study of the genetics of pain perception is in its infancy. The methodology that will allow both of these aspects to be explored is now readily available but is not fully utilized.

The need for new analgesics is axiomatic, and the very existence of a World Congress on Pain is the best evidence of a continued requirement for better treatment options. We are increasingly aware of the plastic nature of the pain-sensing machinery, and this is a threat and a barrier to effective therapy, as it may render a particular drug less effective over time. It is also an opportunity, because the ability to modulate a system that might only be turned on during a chronic pain state may allow effective pain relief while minimizing the potential for side effects. It has been suggested that some transduction pathways may only be used for nociception and, if true, these would be especially attractive targets.

Recent advances in neurobiology have given us insights that are already helping to improve understanding of the events that lead to a patient experiencing pain and may also produce more successful treatment strategies. Peripheral nerve fibers become activated following tissue damage or inflammation. They carry voltage-gated and ligand-gated ion channels which, together with associated G-protein-coupled receptors (GPCRs), are responsible for the generation of the nerve impulses that travel into the central nervous system (CNS) and carry sensation to the level of consciousness. The unmyelinated sensory C fibers, in addition to containing the transduction elements common to all sensory fibers, are now known to have some specific channels and receptors not found on larger myelinated sensory fibers or on neurons within the CNS. Cytokine and neurotrophin systems are activated by tissue damage, resulting in transducer upregulation or in some cases de novo induction. It is now recognized that glial cells are critically involved in these functions in both peripheral and central nervous systems (Watkins and Maier 2002; Watkins, this volume). The nature of the neurotransmission process changes with maintained tissue damage or inflammation and leads to activation of sensory fibers that are normally silent (silent nociceptors) and, in some cases, recruits large sensory fibers, which normally do not signal pain, into the pain-signaling process. At the level of the spinal cord, excitatory neurotransmitters are released that activate relay neurons that connect via ascending synaptic pathways to higher brain centers. Large and small primary afferent fibers share some of the same signaling systems within the spinal dorsal horn, but small fibers have neurotransmitters, including neuropeptides, that are not found in larger non-nociceptive fibers (at least under normal circumstances). Part of the change in response seen in reaction to persistent nociceptive signaling caused by maintained inflammation or tissue damage and leading to intractable chronic pain (Cervero and Laird 1991; Fig. 2) is due to a reprogramming of the way in which the dorsal horn of the spinal cord and other central circuits respond to sensory inputs. This reprogramming can be due to an upregulation of presynaptic transmitter synthesis and release, to induction or upregulation of postsynaptic receptors or channels (see Yu and Salter 1999), or to a physical rewiring of circuitry caused by the expression of factors leading to sprouting of afferent fiber terminals or the production of additional postsynaptic dendritic spines (Bergman et al. 1999; Hatada et al. 2000). Synapses that are normally silent may become active (Li and Zhuo 1998). Some of the processes involved in chronic pain are similar to those involved in long-term potentiation, believed by many to underlie the laying down of memory. Areas known to be involved in somatosensory perception are activated after noxious stimuli, but so are areas in the limbic system, perhaps related to the distress and suffering aspects of pain and other areas important in autonomic function and defense reactions (see Hutchison et al. 1999). The complexity of the human forebrain limits the value of observations in lower animals at

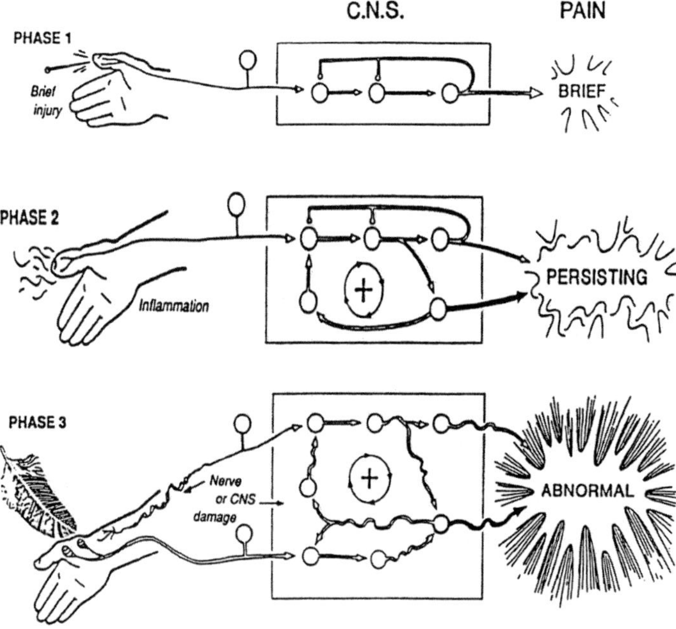

Fig. 2. Mechanistic classification of pain (after Cervero and Laird 1991).

this level, whereas at the spinal level, where more is understood about structure and function, there are fewer differences between higher and lower mammalian species. Knowledge of the function of supraspinal circuits in human pain perception is now improving as a result of data from imaging techniques (PET and fMRI). These methods can visualize evoked activity in areas of the brain, such as the anterior cingulate cortex, which are activated in response to pain but not to peripheral sensory inputs of lower intensity (Hutchison et al. 1999). Sometimes pain can arise centrally (e.g., thalamic pain); such pain may be a result of ischemic damage following a stroke. The mechanism probably involves a loss of inhibitory control because inhibitory interneurons are generally the most sensitive to ischemia. Impulse traffic into and within the CNS is controlled, as well as by local inhibitory circuits, by descending inhibitory pathways coming down to the spinal cord from the brain. The effectiveness of this inhibition may be an important factor in determining the intensity of pain. New targets can arise from all aspects of the neurotransmission process and at all levels from the periphery up to the level of consciousness.

FINDING NEW PAIN TARGETS

Molecular neurobiology has provided tools that allow us to detect changes in gene expression, both peripherally and centrally, in response to activity in sensory neurons, and to locate areas of induced gene expression and translation in the peripheral and central nervous systems. These tools facilitate the study of the localization and function of specific protein products of gene translation (see Wood 2000). The proteins of interest can now readily be expressed transiently or in immortalized cell lines by gene transfection (e.g., Hans et al. 1999; Jordt et al. 2000). Moreover, site-directed mutagenesis (e.g., Jordt et al. 2000) can be used to alter the composition of a protein to establish areas of critical functionality. Also, the assembly of protein subunits into functional heteromers (Hans et al. 1999) can be examined. The study of human genetics can provide evidence for the importance of some molecular systems in pain perception, for example, in the case of those rare individuals with a chronic insensitivity to pain (Indo et al. 1996) or with painful disorders with a strong familial component, such as migraine headache (see Ophoff et al. 1998; Hans et al. 1999). It is tempting to suggest that there must be an important genetic component in many chronic pain states; for example, not every patient who experiences a zoster infection suffers the distress of postherpetic neuralgia, and injury to peripheral nerves does not automatically lead to neuropathic pain. There are sex-related differences in the perception of pain in humans (e.g., see Cairns et al. 2001) and in the response to some opioid analgesic drugs (Gear et al. 1999; Zubieta et al. 2002). If we could understand at the genetic level why some patients are more likely to be victims of intractable pain, treatments might be improved. The evaluation of the effects of peripheral nerve lesions or local inflammation on nociceptive behavior has recently developed into a detailed examination of the effects of these insults on the regulation of gene expression. A large number of papers presented at the 10th World Congress on Pain attested to the popularity of this approach. In some cases it is unquestioned that such investigations help us validate drug targets or elucidate novel mechanisms of action. This is usually the case when specific questions are asked about the regulation of a small number of mechanistically related genes. The increased availability of gene arrays has allowed global studies on the effects on thousands of genes in parallel (see Wang et al. 2002). Such studies generate enormous data sets showing downregulation of some genes and upregulation of others, contributing to the overall message that chronic pain results from a complex, interconnected series of events (Costigan and Woolf 2000; Hill 2001). Proteomics is also adding to the wealth of information on how proteins are arranged in complex interdependent groupings associated, for example, with postsynaptic receptor complexes (Sheng and Lee 2000). It is not possible to adequately describe the status of research in this area in this short chapter or to attempt to list all the putative targets, but I will describe a few key observations that have resulted from the gene identification approach as examples of potential drug discovery targets.

A practical use of genetics for the pain scientist is in the production of mutant animals with gene deletion or gene overexpression to ask direct questions about the importance of particular systems coded by these genes (see Sands 2002). The cloning and sequencing of novel genes expressing proteins with relevance to nociception has also allowed the manufacture of very selective antibodies raised to synthetic peptides that represent a unique nonoverlapping part of the protein sequence. This advance has allowed high-resolution histology of the location of the target proteins in the nervous systems of a number of species, including humans (see Oliver et al. 2000; Wise et al. 2002). In the case of GPCRs it has also allowed the study of function, because activation of many of these receptors is signaled by internalization of the antibody-labeled receptor. This internalization also allows neurotransmitter-coupled toxins to be used to specifically lesion populations of neurons bearing the receptor (see Nichols et al. 1999).

SELECTING THE MOST FEASIBLE TARGET

We now have an impressive array of tools derived from genomics that can be used to help us validate drug targets. In addition, the technology for high throughput screening (HTS) has been refined to the point where once a cell line expressing the protein target has been engineered then hundreds of thousands of compounds can rapidly be screened as activators or blockers (see Hopkins and Groom 2002; Wise et al. 2002). Such agents, once discovered, are often the most useful target validation tools of all, although care must be taken to ensure that they are not only potent but also selective for the chosen target. The most abundant targets remain GPCRs, and new members of this group continue to be discovered, although we are probably close to knowing the identity of all of the genes coding this family of proteins. For example, the Mas-related gene (Mrg) or sensory-neuron-specific (SNSR) receptors (Dong et al. 2001; Lembo et al. 2002) have recently been discovered. These receptors are specifically located on small (presumably nociceptive) sensory neurons and are substrates for a number of naturally occurring neuropeptides with the highest affinity to a family of opioid peptides known as bovine adrenal medulla peptides (BAMs). However, their binding is not opioid-like as it is not sensitive to opioid receptor antagonists (Lembo et al. 2002). Recently it has been shown that an active fragment of BAM, BAM 8-22, is a potent agonist at rat SNSRs. When given intrathecally, BAM 8-22 dose-dependently increases the excitability of the spinal flexor reflex (Cao et al., this volume), suggesting that antagonists at this receptor might have analgesic properties. The relative value of the SNSRs/Mrgs as drug targets is hard to judge because there are marked species differences in the number of these receptors and in the precise populations of dorsal root ganglion (DRG) cells on which they are found. Some of the other recently discovered targets are complex and do not lend themselves to a conventional drug discovery approach. The recent discovery of the involvement of the proteinase-activated receptor-2 (PAR2) in the generation of hyperalgesia, and the observation that its mechanism of action is through sensory neuropeptide regulation (Vergnolle et al. 2001), provide one example. The proteinases involved in the activation of PARs are more commonly associated with protein degradation and include thrombin (which cleaves PAR1, PAR3, and PAR4), trypsin (PAR2 and PAR4), and tryptase (PAR2). Sixty percent of DRG neurons express PAR2 immunoreactivity, and many of these also express calcitonin gene-related peptide (CGRP) and substance P, the two major neuropeptides contained in nociceptive C fibers innervating superficial laminae of the spinal cord. Activation of PARs causes rapid intracellular neuronal Ca^{2+}

mobilization. Trypsin, tryptase, and PAR2-selective agonists cause the release of CGRP and substance P from C fibers in peripheral tissues and in the spinal cord (see Oliver and Hill 2002 for review). Vergnolle et al. (2001) found that PAR2 agonists reduced paw-withdrawal latencies in thermal and mechanical hyperalgesia tests, as did intraplantar administration of trypsin and tryptase. Confirmation that these were PAR2-specific phenomena came from the lack of effect in PAR2-deficient transgenic mice when in wild-type animals, subinflammatory doses of PAR2-activating peptides were hyperalgesic even in the absence of edema. The direct involvement of PAR2-expressing nociceptive neurons in hyperalgesia was suggested by increased Fos-immunoreactivity in spinal cord laminae I and II following intraplantar injection of PAR2 agonists or tryptase. A central mechanism of action for PAR2 hyperalgesia was suggested because inhibition of PGE_2 synthesis in the paw, or local block of substance P activity, using the NK1-receptor antagonists had no effect on PAR2-agonist-induced hyperalgesia. However, systemic suppression of cyclooxygenase or spinal injection of NK1 antagonists profoundly inhibited the thermal hyperalgesia. NK1-receptor-deficient mice and preprotachykinin-A-deficient mice displayed no PAR2-agonist-induced hyperalgesia (Vergnolle et al. 2001).

PAR2 does not fulfill the criteria for an ideal target. This receptor is not exclusively localized to sensory nociceptors: expression of PAR2 mRNA has been demonstrated in gastrointestinal tissues; in the prostate gland, heart, lung, and trachea; and in the CNS (Oliver and Hill 2002). Whether PAR2-inhibitor drugs will be useful therapeutically will depend on their clinical profile, and specifically the ratio of beneficial effects (analgesia) and unwanted effects (actions on nontarget tissues). Clinical relief of pain and headache is readily achieved by agents such as opioids and triptans acting as agonists at presynaptic GPCRs, which (like the PARs) regulate the release of multiple neuropeptides such as CGRP and substance P, so PAR2 inhibitors should in theory produce pain relief.

Another challenging type of target is exemplified by DREAM (downstream regulatory element antagonistic modulator), which is a Ca^{2+}-regulated transcriptional repressor (Carrión et al. 1999). It has four Ca^{2+}-binding domains, which, when occupied, block its ability to bind to the downstream regulatory element and therefore prevent its repressor activity. DREAM suppresses transcription from the human prodynorphin and *c-fos* genes. A gene deletion mutant mouse lacking functional DREAM has now been engineered (Cheng et al. 2002) that shows a striking reduction in its responses both to acute noxious stimuli and to inflammatory hyperalgesia, but otherwise has a wild-type behavioral phenotype. The role of dynorphin in controlling nociceptive threshold is complex; it can be antinociceptive by acting as an agonist at κ-opioid receptors but can also be pronociceptive through a facilitatory action at *N*-methyl-D-aspartate (NMDA) receptors (see Vogt 2002). The decreased sensitivity to noxious stimuli in DREAM knock-out mice seems to be due to increased activity of dynorphin at κ-opioid receptors because it was restored to the level seen in wild-type mice by administration of the selective κ-opioid-receptor antagonist nor-binaltorphimine (Cheng et al. 2002). It is difficult at present to see a practical way in which a DNA-binding protein such as DREAM could be addressed as a drug discovery target. It is not yet clear what controls the expression of DREAM, and it is not known whether or how it is regulated during nociception. No existing drugs using similar mechanisms exist as benchmarks (Vogt 2002).

Another, superficially attractive, downstream target identified recently is ubiquitin C-terminal hydrolase (UCH), which has now been found to be upregulated in the spinal cord of rats with a chronic constriction injury (CCI) to one sciatic nerve (Moss et al. 2002). UCH acts with the proteolytic enzyme complex called the proteosome to facilitate degradative processes within the cell. Known proteosome inhibitors attenuate allodynia and hyperalgesia in CCI rats, and these compounds thus may be potentially useful for treating neuropathic pain (Moss et al. 2002). Proteosome inhibitors are available as experimental tools and are just starting to be evaluated clinically in treatment of cancer. These findings are a further example of plasticity in pain-sensing mechanisms and provide evidence of commonality of changes taking place after neuropathy and in neurodegeneration (Wang et al. 2002).

It is thus clear that there is a plethora of pain targets. The number of traditional targets such as GPCRs and ion channels continues to increase as we work our way through the relevant portions of the genome. More challenging targets are being discovered, for example transcription and repression factors such as DREAM (see Vogt 2002). It necessary for the pain scientist engaged in drug discovery to become skilled at triage so that efforts are expended only on those targets most likely to lead to a new drug (see Boyce et al. 2001 and Fig. 3).

BLOCKADE OF NOVEL RECEPTORS

Substance P has been known since the 1950s to be widespread in the CNS. It is more abundant in dorsal than in ventral roots and has been associated with pain because it can be found in the smaller, unmyelinated sensory fibers. Exogenous substance P, applied to dorsal horn sensory relay neurons, has a slow and prolonged excitatory action resembling excitation seen after peripheral noxious stimuli. Multiple messengers often coexist in

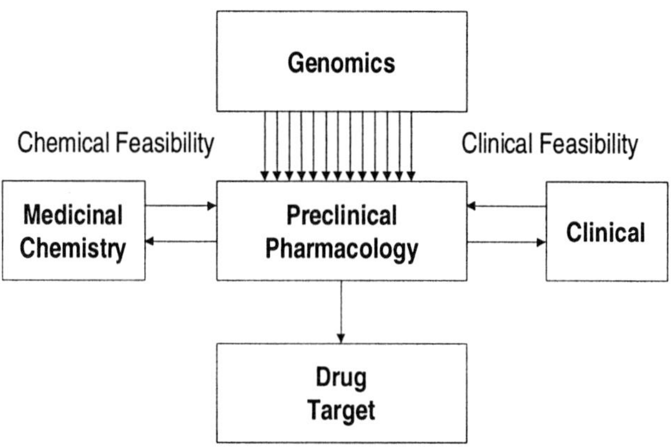

Fig. 3. Selection of the most feasible target (after Boyce et al. 2001).

the same DRG neurons along with substance P, and the activation of nociception within the dorsal horn of the spinal cord may be the result of a parallel release of numerous transmitters and modulators from the terminals of primary afferent fibers. Only if a single, released substance has a dominant role will the specific pharmacological blockade of its effects result in analgesia. It is now well accepted that sensory neurotransmission is plastic, that synthesis of transmitters and their receptors, including that of substance P, can be upregulated by conditions such as inflammation that cause pain, and that synaptic connections often change after nerve injury (Woolf and Mannion 1999). The evidence that substance P has a dominant role in nociception must be carefully examined, and transgenic mice have been helpful in this endeavor.

The preprotachykinin knockout mouse (which lacks both substance P and neurokinin A) has attenuated responses to intense noxious stimuli. NK1-receptor knockout mice show no changes in acute nociception tests but display reduced responses to inflammatory stimuli (Ma and Hill 1999). NK1-receptor antagonists can be shown to have antinociceptive effects in the presence of nerve injury or inflammation but not in acute tests such as the hot-plate test (Rupniak and Hill 1999). The profile of these compounds is similar to that of NSAIDs, which are well known to be analgesic in humans. However, despite this profile, clinical trials have failed to show reproducible analgesic effects with NK1 antagonists so far studied in human subjects (Hill 2000). This finding might be explained by species differences in the physiology of substance P or distribution of NK1 receptors, or by differences between clinical pain and the type of noxious stimulus and response studied experimentally in small animals (Ma and Hill 1999; Hill 2000). However, most of the differences in substance P and NK1-receptor distribution between species are expressed at supraspinal sites, with remarkable similarities in distribution of both the peptide and NK1 receptors in the dorsal horn of the spinal cord. Also, animal tests that have revealed antinociceptive activity with NK1 antagonists have recently been reliably predictive of analgesic activity in humans, for example, in the case of the COX-2 inhibitors (Boyce et al. 2001). It is possible that there are particular human pain states where the role of substance P is dominant and where these agents may be effective analgesics. This may be true, for example, in cases where substance P interacts with other neurotransmitters. It has been accepted for many years that norepinephrine is a key neurotransmitter in the descending inhibitory systems by which the brainstem controls the sensitivity of the dorsal horn of the spinal cord to nociceptive sensory inputs (see Hill 2002 for review). Synaptically released norepinephrine acts through α_2 adrenoceptors to reduce the sensitivity of dorsal horn relay neurons to noxious but not to non-noxious stimuli; it also potentiates the effects of opioid drugs, such as morphine. Jasmin et al (2002) have studied mice in which the gene for dopamine-β-hydroxylase (DBH, the enzyme which converts dopamine to norepinephrine) had been genetically deleted. These mice can have their normal noradrenergic function restored by dosing with L-threo-3,4-dihydroxyphenylserine (DOPS), a synthetic amino acid precursor of norepinephrine that can be converted to norepinephrine by aromatic amino acid decarboxylase. Nociceptive testing of the DBH knockout mice revealed that they were thermally hyperalgesic compared with control animals but had normal responses to mechanical stimuli. When inflammation was produced in a paw, then the DBH knockout animals displayed mechanical hyperalgesia, but to a similar extent to control animals. Restoring norepinephrine in the CNS, by giving DOPS plus carbidopa, abolished the thermal hyperalgesia in DBH knockout mice, but this treatment had no effect on control mice. Drugs that blocked the action of substance P at its target NK1 receptors reversed the thermal hyperalgesia seen in DBH knockout mice, but not in control mice (Jasmin et al. 2002). These findings provide yet more evidence for a pivotal role of substance P in nociception in the mouse and for a critical interaction with descending noradrenergic systems.

We must consider whether our current animal models of nociception are insufficiently predictive. If one regards the noxious stimuli used in the animal behavioral studies as stressful stimuli, then the published work on nociception links well with experimental work supporting the antidepressant actions of NK1 antagonists (Rupniak and Kramer 1999). This combined analysis suggests that NK1 receptor blockade *can* reliably attenuate the behavioral response of small animals to a variety of stressors, but may not be sufficient to result in clinical analgesia in humans. It also adds support to the suggestion by Jasmin et al. (2002) that there are important interactions between substance P and noradrenergic systems. It is relevant to review our inability to accurately predict from animal experiments, including those on gene deletion mutants, the lack of clinical analgesic properties of NK1-receptor antagonists and to consider how this problem may affect our evaluation of other novel pain targets.

TARGETS DERIVED FROM AN UNKNOWN MECHANISM OF ACTION OF AN EXISTING DRUG

We have known for many years that some, but not all, anticonvulsant and antidepressant drugs are useful in the treatment of pain. They are especially useful in treating chronic neuropathic pain where conventional analgesics may be suboptimal (see Boyce et al. 2001). However, we urgently need better agents that are more potent and have fewer side effects than those currently available. As an example of how our improved knowledge of molecular biology can be used together with empirical knowledge of clinical properties to generate a novel drug target, I shall focus on the anticonvulsants. It has been accepted for some time that a cardinal mechanism of anticonvulsant action is blockade of voltage-gated Na^+ channels. It is therefore timely to look at the family of recently cloned Na^+ channels (see Catterall 2000) and to ask whether any of these might be good targets for the analgesic properties of anticonvulsants. It has recently been discovered that the tetrodotoxin-resistant (TTX-r) Na^+ channel Na_v 1.8 is found almost exclusively in small, nociceptive primary afferent fibers (Akopian et al. 1999) and therefore might be an attractive drug discovery target. The TTX-r currents are sensitive to blockade by anticonvulsants, but these agents also block tetrodotoxin-sensitive (TTX-s) Na^+ currents in primary afferent and many other neurons. In the absence of selective blocking drugs, Wood and his colleagues (Akopian et al. 1999) engineered a null mutant mouse in which Na_v 1.8 was nonfunctional. These mice were normal in appearance, fertile, and healthy. They showed no obvious neurological or behavioral deficits, but had elevated thresholds to mechanical and thermal noxious stimuli and less thermal hyperalgesia after peripheral inflammation than did wild-type littermates (Akopian et al. 1999). It was subsequently found that the TTX-s current Na_v 1.7 was upregulated in the Na_v 1.8 null mutants (Akopian et al. 1999) and that a second TTX-r current, Na_v 1.9, was still functional in sensory neurons (see Fang et al. 2002). It was therefore not possible to assess the full contribution of the TTX-r currents to nociception from the phenotype of the null mutants, although antisense experiments (Lai et al. 2002) suggested that Na_v 1.8 was the most important nociceptive channel in rat sensory neurons. It was therefore necessary to also use the ability to construct cell lines expressing individual Na^+ channels with all necessary accessory subunits in a fully functional form (see Okuse et al. 2002) to screen for agents with improved selectivity and potency for use in proof of concept experiments and as chemical leads for drug discovery. WIN 17317-3 (Wanner et al. 1999), although synthesized as a K^+ channel blocker, is one of the most potent Na^+ channel blockers ever described, with little functional effect on other ion channels, yet it is a small molecule producing use-dependent block. It is not selective between Na^+ channels, yet in isolated sensory fibers from nerve-injured rats it reduces the spontaneous action potentials recorded from single C fibers (Ali et al. 2002). WIN 17317-3 also reduced the mechanical hyperalgesia seen in behavioral experiments in nerve-injured rats at doses that had no effect on motor performance (Ali et al. 2002). This finding indicates that it may not be necessary to have complete selectivity between Na^+ channel subtypes in order to achieve a significant improvement over anticonvulsants currently used in treating pain, such as phenytoin, carbamazepine, and lamotrigine. Small molecules that do have greater potency for TTX-r than for TTX-s Na^+ currents are now starting to be found, such as the secretolytic agent, ambroxol (Weiser and Wilson 2002). These molecules may be a good starting point for drug discovery.

Gabapentin is an anticonvulsant that has proved very useful for treating neuropathic pain (Chong et al. 2002) but is without important effects on Na^+ channels. It was originally designed to be an agonist at γ-aminobutyric acid (GABA) receptors, but it is now known to have no agonist properties at GABA-A (Ng et al. 2001) or GABA-B receptors (Lanneau et al. 2001; Jensen et al. 2002). Gabapentin blocks the release of neurotransmitters from brain slices in a similar manner to removing Ca^{2+} from the bathing medium (Dooley et al. 2000). It was therefore of great interest when gabapentin was shown to bind to the $\alpha_2\delta$ subunit of the voltage-gated Ca^{2+} channels, having the highest affinity for the $\alpha_2\delta$-1 subtype (Marais et al. 2001). In an elegant series of electrophysiology experiments, Sutton and colleagues (2002) have shown that gabapentin can inhibit high-threshold Ca^{2+} currents in cultured sensory neurons. This effect depended on culture conditions and on the precise Ca^{2+}-channel subunit expression in the cell being recorded from (Martin et al. 2002). This may not be the whole story for the mechanism of gabapentin as it has also been shown to act via the glycine site of the NMDA-receptor complex (Jun and Yaksh 1998) and to affect amino acid uptake into cells (Uchino et al. 2002). However, it seems likely that we will soon have the information needed to design improved analogues of this useful and unique drug.

THE FUTURE?

Twenty years ago we suffered from a lack of information on the molecular pharmacology and integrative physiology of pain perception, whereas today we literally have too much information. One recent gene array study on rats with neuropathy produced by spinal nerve lesions found a total of 148 genes that were either up- or downregulated more than twofold in DRG (Wang et al. 2002). The genes affected included those coding neuropeptides, cell cycle regulation and cell death, neuroinflammation, ion channels, receptors and signaling molecules, transcription factors, and genes involved in tissue maintenance and plasticity. In order to have a framework in which we can correctly evaluate such a density of information and decide which of the located gene products might be valid drug discovery targets, we must put them in an appropriate context where information derived from clinical observations is considered along with that derived from genomics and from carefully conducted preclinical pharmacology (Loeser 2000; Boyce et al. 2001; Fig. 4). Many of the factors to be considered apply to all modern drug discovery efforts and are not only of concern in the study of pain. The complexities and plastic nature of pain transduction are becoming ever more apparent, and awareness is increasing that there is overlap between those processes concerned with pain and those associated with inflammation, cognitive function,

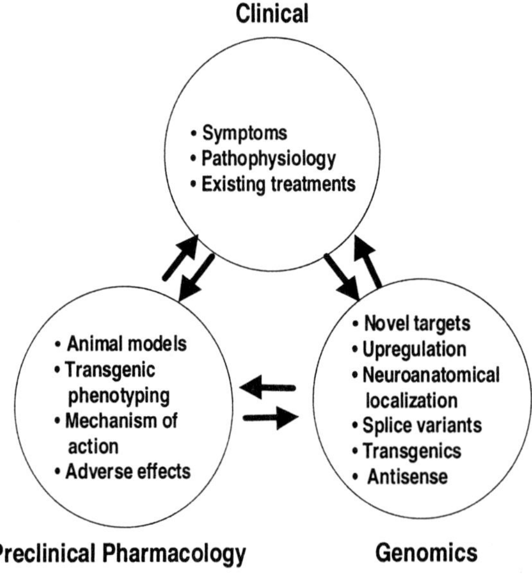

Fig. 4. The modern approach to drug discovery (after Boyce et al. 2001).

and neurodegeneration (see Hill 2001; Wang et al. 2002). The likelihood of any system, whether enzyme, receptor, or ion channel, being completely exclusive to nociception seems slim.

The apparent lack of predictability of preclinical animal studies in the case of the failure to find a clinical analgesic indication for the NK1-receptor antagonists gives pause for thought (Hill 2000). However, this is an isolated example, and in other cases, such as for the coxibs, preclinical experiments have been reliably predictive of analgesic efficacy in humans (see Boyce et al. 2001). The need for better animal models is unquestioned, and much elegant work on disease-relevant models is in progress (see Mantyh et al., this volume). The improvements seen in functional imaging in the recent past also hold the hope of experimental paradigms that can be used both in small animals and in humans, thus closing the gap between preclinical and clinical studies. This possibility would clearly increase the probability that observations made in animals could be duplicated in humans. Borsook and his colleagues (Becerra et al. 2001) have shown that fMRI recordings following noxious stimuli in human volunteers can reveal activity in brain areas coding aversion and reward as well as sensation. They were also able to dissect the multiple effects of morphine and show that it increased the signal in that part of the n. accumbens associated with reward at the same time that it reduced input to those neocortical areas associated with nociception. This approach opens the way to objective assessment of the whole pain experience, including the action of analgesic drugs (Becerra et al. 2001).

ACKNOWLEDGMENTS

I am grateful to all my colleagues in Pain Research over the last 25 years at Bristol University, at Parke-Davis, Cambridge and at Merck. Special thanks are due to Sue Boyce, Zahid Ali, Nadia Rupniak, Kathy Sutton (ex-Pfizer Group Research), and David Borsook (MGH/Descartes Pharmaceuticals) for participating in discussions and sharing data with me during the preparation of this chapter.

REFERENCES

Akopian AN, Souslova V, England S, et al. The tetrodotoxin-resistant sodium channel SNS has a specialized function in pain pathways. *Nat Neurosci* 1999; 2:541–548.

Ali Z, Clark SA, Ash A, et al. Effects of the sodium channel blockers CO102862 and WIN17317-3 in in-vivo and in-vitro models of nerve injury in the rat. *Abstracts: 10th World Congress on Pain.* Seattle: IASP Press, 2002, p 160.

Becerra L, Breiter HC, Wise R, Gonzalez RG, Borsook D. Reward circuitry activation by noxious thermal stimuli. *Neuron* 2001; 32:927–946.

Bergman E, Carlsson K, Liljeborg A, et al. Neuropeptides, nitric oxide synthase and GAP-43 in B4-binding and RT97 immunoreactive primary sensory neurons: normal distribution pattern and changes after peripheral nerve transection and aging. *Brain Res* 1999; 832:63–83.

Boyce S, Hill RG. Discrepant results from preclinical and clinical studies on the potential of substance P-receptor antagonist compounds as analgesics. In: Devor M, Rowbotham MC, Wiesenfeld-Hallin Z (Eds). *Proceedings of the 9th World Congress on Pain,* Progress in Pain Research and Management, Vol. 16. Seattle: IASP Press, 2000, pp 313–324.

Boyce S, Ali Z, Hill RG. New developments in analgesia. *Drug Discovery World* 2001; 2:31–35.

Cairns BE, Hu JW, Arendt-Nielsen L, et al. Sex-related differences in human pain and rat afferent discharge evoked by injection of glutamate into the masseter muscle. *J Neurophysiol* 2001; 86:782–791.

Carrión AM, Link WA, Ledo F, Mellström B, Naranjo JR. DREAM is a Ca^{2+}-regulated transcriptional repressor. *Nature* 1999; 398:80–84.

Catterall WA. From ionic currents to molecular mechanisms: the structure and function of voltage-gated sodium channels. *Neuron* 2000; 26:13–25.

Cervero F, Laird JMA. One pain or many pains? A new look at pain mechanisms. *News Physiol Sci* 1991; 6:268–273.

Cheng H-YM, Pitcher GM, Laviolette SR, et al. DREAM is a critical transcriptional repressor for pain modulation. *Cell* 2002; 108:31–43.

Chong MS, Smith TE, Hanna M. Case reports—reversal of sensory deficit associated with pain relief after treatment with gabapentin. *Pain* 2002; 96:329–333.

Costigan M, Woolf CJ. Pain: molecular mechanisms. *J Pain* 2000; 1:35–44.

Dong X, Han S-K, Zylka MJ, Simon MI, Anderson DJ. A diverse family of GPCRs expressed in specific subsets of nociceptive sensory neurons. *Cell* 2001; 106:619–632.

Dooley DJ, Donovan CM, Pugsley TA. Stimulus-dependent modulation of [^{3}H]norepinephrine release from rat neocortical slices by gabapentin and pregabalin. *J Pharmacol Exp Ther* 2000; 295:1086–1093.

Fang X, Djouhri L, Black JA, et al. The presence and role of the tetrodotoxin-resistant sodium channel $Na_v1.9$ (NaN) in nociceptive primary afferent neurons. *J Neuroscience* 2002; 22:7425–7433.

FitzGerald GA, Patrono C. The coxibs, selective inhibitors of cyclooxygenase-2. *N Engl J Med* 2001; 345:433–442.

Gear RW, Miaskowski C, Gordon NC, et al. The kappa opioid nalbuphine produces gender- and dose-dependent analgesia and antianalgesia in patients with postoperative pain. *Pain* 1999; 83:339–345.

Hans M, Luvisetto S, Williams ME, et al. Functional consequences of mutations in the human α_{1A} calcium channel subunit linked to familial hemiplegic migraine. *J Neurosci* 1999; 19:1610–1619.

Hatada Y, Wu F, Sun Z-Y, Schacher S, Goldberg DJ. Presynaptic morphological changes associated with long-term synaptic facilitation are triggered by actin polymerization at preexisting varicosities. *J Neurosci* 2000; 20(RC82):1–5.

Hill RG. NK1 (substance P) receptor antagonists—why are they not analgesic in humans? *Trends Pharmacol Sci* 2000; 21:244–246.

Hill RG. Molecular basis for the perception of pain. *Neuroscientist* 2001; 7:282–292.

Hill RG. Substance P, opioid, and catecholamine systems in the mouse central nervous system (CNS). *Proc Natl Acad Sci USA* 2002; 99:549–551.

Hla T, Neilson K. Human cyclooxygenase-2 cDNA. *Proc Natl Acad Sci USA* 1992; 89:7384–7388.

Hopkins AL, Groom CR. The druggable genome. *Nat Rev Drug Discovery* 2002; 1:727–730.

Hunt SP, Mantyh PW. The molecular dynamics of pain control. *Nat Rev Neurosci* 2001; 2:83–91.

Hutchison WD, Davis KD, Lozano AM, Tasker RR, Dostrovsky JO. Pain-related neurons in the human cingulate cortex. *Nat Neurosci* 1999; 2:403–405.

Indo Y, Tsuruta M, Hayashida Y, et al. Mutations in the *TRKA*/NGF receptor gene in patients with congenital insensitivity to pain with anhidrosis. *Nat Genet* 1996; 13:485–488.

Jasmin L, Tien D, Weinshenker D, et al. The NK1 receptor mediates both the hyperalgesia and the resistance to morphine in mice lacking noradrenaline. *Proc Natl Acad Sci USA* 2002; 99:1029–1034.

Jensen AA, Mosbacher J, Elg S, et al. The anticonvulsant gabapentin (neurontin) does not act through γ-aminobutyric acid-B receptors. *Mol Pharmacol* 2002; 61:1377–1384.

Jordt S-E, Tominaga M, Julius D. Acid potentiation of the capsaicin receptor determined by a key extracellular site. *Proc Natl Acad Sci USA* 2000; 97:8134–8139.

Jun JH, Yaksh TL. The effect of intrathecal gabapentin and 3-isobutyl γ-aminobutyric acid on the hyperalgesia observed after thermal injury in the rat. *Anesth Analg* 1998; 86:348–354.

Lai J, Gold MS, Kim C-S, et al. Inhibition of neuropathic pain by decreased expression of the tetrodotoxin-resistant sodium channel, $Na_v1.8$. *Pain* 2002; 95:143–152.

Lanneau C, Green A, Hirst WD, et al. Gabapentin is not a $GABA_B$ receptor agonist. *Neuropharmacology* 2001; 41:965–975.

Lembo PMC, Grazzini E, Groblewski T, et al. Proenkephalin A gene products activate a new family of sensory neuron-specific GPCRs. *Nat Neurosci* 2002; 5:201–209.

Li P, Zhuo M. Silent glutamatergic synapses and nociception in mammalian spinal cord. *Nature* 1998; 393:695–698.

Loeser JD. Perils in the pursuit of mechanisms. *Pain* 2000; 86:1–2.

Ma Q-P, Hill RG. Neurokinin antagonists as potential agents for use in pain management. *Curr Opin CPNS Investig Drugs* 1999; 1:65–71.

Mantyh PW, Yaksh TL. Sensory neurons are PARtial to pain. *Nat Med* 2001; 7:772–773.

Marais E, Klugbauer N, Hofmann F. Calcium channel $\alpha_2\delta$ subunits—structure and gabapentin binding. *Mol Pharmacol* 2001; 59:1234–1248.

Martin DJ, McClelland D, Herd MB, et al. Gabapentin-mediated inhibition of voltage-activated Ca^{2+} channel currents in cultured sensory neurones is dependent on culture conditions and channel subunit expression. *Neuropharmacology* 2002; 42:353–366.

Mealy NE, Martin L, Castañer R, et al. Treatment of pain. *Drugs Future* 2002; 27:403–434.

Moss A, Blackburn-Munro G, Garry EM, et al. A role of the ubiquitin-proteasome system in neuropathic pain. *J Neurosci* 2002; 22:1363–1372.

Ng GYK, Bertrand S, Sullivan R, et al. γ-Aminobutyric acid type B receptors with specific heterodimer composition and postsynaptic actions in hippocampal neurons are targets of anticonvulsant gabapentin action. *Mol Pharmacol* 2001; 59:144–152.

Nichols ML, Allen BJ, Rogers SD, et al. Transmission of chronic nociception by spinal neurons expressing the substance P receptor. *Science* 1999; 286:1558–1561.

Okuse K, Malik-Hall M, Baker MD, et al. Annexin II light chain regulates sensory neuron-specific sodium channel expression. *Nature* 2002; 417:653–656.

Oliver KR, Hill RG. Feeling below PAR: proteinase-activated receptors and the perception of neuroinflammatory pain. *Pharmacogenomics J* 2002; 2:10–11.

Oliver KR, Sirinathsinghji DJS, Hill RG. From basic research on neuropeptide receptors to clinical benefit. *Drug News Perspect* 2000; 13:530–542.

Ophoff RA, Terwindt GM, Frants RR, Ferrari MD. P/Q-type Ca^{2+} channel defects in migraine, ataxia and epilepsy. *Trends Pharmacol Sci* 1998; 19:121–126.

Rupniak NMJ, Hill RG. Neurokinin antagonists. In: Sawynok J, Cowan A (Eds). *Novel Aspects of Pain Management: Opioids and Beyond.* New York: Wiley-Liss, 1999, pp 135–155.

Rupniak NMJ, Kramer MS. Discovery of the anti-depressant and anti-emetic efficacy of substance P receptor (NK1) antagonists. *Trends Pharmacol Sci* 1999; 20:485–490.

Sands AT. Industrializing breakthrough discovery. *Current Drug Discovery* 2002; Aug:21-23.

Sheng M, Lee SH. Growth of the NMDA receptor industrial complex. *Nat Neurosci* 2000; 3:633–635.

Sutton KG, Martin DJ, Pinnock RD, Lee K, Scott RH. Gabapentin inhibits high-threshold calcium channel currents in cultured rat dorsal root ganglion neurones. *Br J Pharmacol* 2002; 135:257–265.

Uchino H, Kanai Y, Kim DY, et al. Transport of amino acid-related compounds mediated by L-type amino acid transporter 1 (LAT1): insights into the mechanisms of substrate recognition. *Mol Pharmacol* 2002; 61:729–737.

Vergnolle N, Bunnett, NW, Sharkey KA, et al. Proteinase-activated receptor-2 and hyperalgesia: a novel pain pathway. *Nat Med* 2001; 7:821–826.

Vogt BA. Knocking out the DREAM to Study Pain. *N Engl J Med* 2002; 347:362–364.

Wang H, Sun H, Della Penna K, et al. Chronic neuropathic pain is accompanied by global changes in gene expression and shares pathobiology with neurodegenerative diseases. *Neuroscience* 2002; 114:529–546.

Wanner SG, Glossmann H, Knaus H-G, et al. WIN 17317-3, a new high-affinity probe for voltage-gated sodium channels. *Biochemistry* 1999; 38:11137–11146.

Watkins LR, Maier SF. Beyond neurons: evidence that immune and glial cells contribute to pathological pain states. *Physiol Rev* 2002; 82:1–31.

Weiser T, Wilson N. Inhibition of tetrodotoxin (TTX)-resistant and TTX-sensitive neuronal Na^+ channels by the secretolytic ambroxol. *Mol Pharmacol* 2002; 62:433–438.

Wise A, Gearing K, Rees S. Target validation of G-protein coupled receptors. *Drug Discovery Today* 2002; 7:235–246.

Wood JN (Ed). *Molecular Basis of Pain Induction*. New York; Wiley-Liss, 2000.

Woolf CJ, Mannion RJ. Neuropathic pain: aetiology, symptoms, mechanisms, and management. *Lancet* 1999; 353:1959–1964.

Yu X-M, Salter MW. Src, a molecular switch governing gain control of synaptic transmission mediated by *N*-methyl-D-aspartate receptors. *Proc Natl Acad Sci USA* 1999; 96:7697–7704.

Zubieta J-K, Smith YR, Bueller JA, et al. μ-Opioid receptor-mediated antinociceptive responses differ in men and women. *J Neurosci* 2002; 22:5100–5107.

Correspondence to: Raymond G. Hill, PhD, Neuroscience Research Centre, Merck Sharp and Dohme Research Laboratories, Eastwick Road, Terlings Park, Harlow, Essex CM20 2QR, United Kingdom. Email: hillr@merck.com.

Proceedings of the 10th World Congress on Pain,
Progress in Pain Research and Management, Vol. 24,
edited by Jonathan O. Dostrovsky, Daniel B. Carr,
and Martin Koltzenburg, IASP Press, Seattle, © 2003.

37

Cannabinoids and Pain

Andrew S.C. Rice, W. Paul Farquhar-Smith,
Daniel Bridges, and Jason W. Brooks

Pain Research Group, Department of Anaesthetics, Faculty of Medicine, Imperial College of Science, Technology and Medicine, Chelsea and Westminster Hospital Campus, London, United Kingdom

This chapter reviews the laboratory evidence supporting the putative analgesic effects of cannabinoids. It focuses on strategies for divorcing analgesia from psychotropic actions of cannabinoids, for instance by targeting spinal cord and peripheral cannabinoid receptors.

The last three decades have seen considerable advances in the pharmacology of cannabinoids, including identification of the psychoactive constituents of *Cannabis sativa,* the synthesis of synthetic cannabinoids, the characterization of receptors through which cannabinoids act, the discovery of the endogenous ligands at these receptors (endocannabinoids), and elucidation of the biochemical mechanisms for synthesis and degradation of endocannabinoids (see Pertwee 2001; Rice 2001a; Di Marzo 2002). The potential physiological roles of this novel system are only just beginning to be elucidated, but the fact that cannabinoid receptor knockout mice (Ledent et al. 1999; Zimmer et al. 1999; Buckley et al. 2000) display only subtle physiological deviations from the norm suggests that endocannabinoids play a modulatory, albeit important, rather than a primary physiological function. Endocannabinoids do appear to regulate processes such as cognition and memory, motor coordination, temperature homeostasis, sleep, the inflammatory response, and appetite (Di Marzo 2002). These nonanalgesic effects, particularly on brain functions (which we generically refer to as "psychotropic"), are important and present a considerable impediment to the development of therapeutically useful cannabinoid-based analgesics. Furthermore, the strength of laboratory data contrasts with the weaker clinical evidence in this area, partly because a paucity of cannabinoids with sufficient and consistent bioavailability and an acceptable therapeutic index mitigates against the initiation of clinical trials.

HISTORICAL ASPECTS

Cannabis sativa has been a valuable source of strong hemp fiber for many thousands of years, and use of its psychoactive constituents has also long been evident in many cultures (Iversen 2000). One of the first references to the therapeutic use of cannabis occurs in the Chinese pharmacopoeia *Pen Ts'ao,* elements of which date as far back as 2800 B.C., with analgesia among the effects described. Indian writings in the *Athera Veda,* which were based on an oral tradition dating to about 2000 B.C., also refer to the therapeutic effects of cannabis. Archaeological evidence from the Middle East suggests that cannabis was used therapeutically during obstructed childbirth, possibly as an analgesic (Zias et al. 1993). In the Greek and Roman eras, both the herbal of Dioscorides and the writings of Galen refer to the therapeutic effects of cannabis. Cannabis came to Western medicine far later, although Culpepper's medieval herbal does mention cannabis. The physician William O'Shaughnessy is credited with introducing cannabis for medicinal use to the West after his observations of its therapeutic use in India (Bridge 1988; D. Wujastyk, unpublished manuscript). In his 1939 account, he describes how he first investigated the adverse effects of cannabis in animals, then reports the therapeutic effects of this plant in a range of human diseases, with frequent mentions of analgesia (O'Shaugnessy 1839). The Victorians subsequently used tincture of cannabis for a wide range of indications, including analgesia, and it may have been prescribed to Queen Victoria for relief of pelvic pain. The medicinal use of cannabis faded with the advent of superior alternative medications and legitimate concerns regarding side effects and abuse potential. It was removed from the U.S. Pharmacopoeia in 1942, but continued to be included in the British Pharmacopoeia until 1976 when it was reclassified as a schedule 1 drug (of no therapeutic benefit). In the last decade a patient lobby has forced a reevaluation of cannabinoids as potential therapeutics. Several influential bodies have considered this issue and have reached similar broad conclusions that the strong scientific data and anecdotal clinical reports of the therapeutic use of herbal cannabis and cannabinoids justify further investigation and refinement (Select Committee on Science and Technology and House of Lords 1998).

ENDOCANNABINOID SYSTEM

Two cannabinoid (CB) receptors have been described, both members of the G-protein-coupled superfamily (Fig. 1). The CB_1 receptor, which is mainly expressed by neurons, was the first to be characterized and cloned (Matsuda et al. 1990), quickly followed by the description of receptor CB_2, expressed by immune cells (Munro et al. 1993). Research has identified the genes encoding these proteins (Onaivi et al. 1996, 2002) and created knockout mice lacking the genes encoding the CB_1 (Ledent et al. 1999; Zimmer et al. 1999) and CB_2 receptor (Buckley et al. 2000). Evidence pointing to hitherto uncharacterized CB receptors is based largely on residual pharmacological activity in CB_1 knockout mice or following the administration of receptor

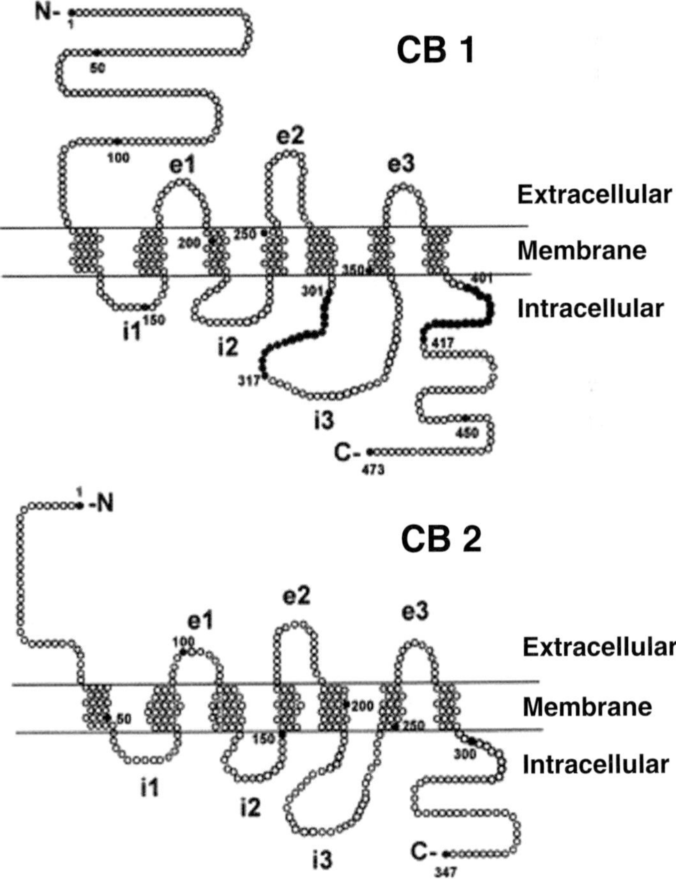

Fig. 1. Sequence of CB_1 and CB_2 receptors.

antagonists in naive rodents (Di Marzo et al. 2000; Breivogel et al. 2001; Brooks et al. 2002b). For instance, a CB_2-like receptor sensitive to SR144528 (a CB_2-receptor antagonist) may mediate the analgesic actions of palmitoylethanolamide (Calignano et al. 2001; Farquhar-Smith and Rice 2001a; Farquhar-Smith et al. 2002). Evidence also suggests a novel murine G-protein-coupled receptor in the brain at which both anandamide and the synthetic cannabinoid WIN 55,212-2 are agonists and SR141716A (a CB_1-receptor antagonist) is an antagonist (Di Marzo et al. 2000; Breivogel et al. 2001). The major psychoactive ingredient of herbal cannabis, Δ^9 tetrahydrocannabinol (Δ^9 THC), is inactive at this receptor. A splice variant of CB_1 has also been isolated from a human lung cDNA library (Shire et al. 1995). Although an obvious strategy to identify these novel receptors is to search databases for a receptor with structural homology to CB_1 or CB_2, this approach has not yet yielded a result, which may not be too surprising considering that CB_1 and CB_2 only share 44% sequence homology.

CB_1 is one of the most abundant receptors in the central nervous system (CNS) and is primarily expressed by neurons (Herkenham et al. 1991; Matsuda et al. 1993; Tsou et al. 1998; Egertova and Elphick 2000). Of particular relevance to sensory systems is the expression of CB_1 in the spinal cord (Hohmann et al. 1999a; Ong and Mackie 1999; Sanudo-Pena et al. 1999; Farquhar-Smith et al. 2000) and dorsal root ganglia (Sanudo-Pena et al. 1999; Hohmann and Herkenham 1999b; Ahluwalia et al. 2000, 2002; Bridges et al. 2003; Ross et al. 2001), which is discussed in detail below. However, CB_1 mRNA and protein also have been identified in the spleen of mice, but not rats, although the precise significance of this finding is unknown (Schatz et al. 1997). In the brain, the results of in vitro ligand-binding studies first suggested the existence of CB_1 (Devane et al. 1988) and led to its subsequent identification and cloning (Matsuda et al. 1990). The receptor distribution was then mapped by autoradiography (Herkenham et al. 1991; Mailleux and Vanderhaeghen 1992), in situ hybridization (Mailleux and Vanderhaeghen 1992; Matsuda et al. 1993), and immunocytochemistry (Pettit et al. 1998; Tsou et al. 1998; Egertova and Elphick 2000). These studies have revealed an exceptionally widespread distribution of CB_1 in the brain. The presence of CB_1 in the periaqueductal grey, rostroventromedial medulla, and thalamus has notable implications for antinociception (for further discussion see Pertwee 2001).

At a molecular level, CB_1 receptors influence, via $G_{i/o}$ proteins, several signal transduction pathways, including negative coupling to adenylate cyclase (for a general review of this area see McAllister and Glass 2002). Nie and Lewis (2002) have elucidated the conformational properties required for G-protein coupling. Among other consequences of CB_1-receptor agonism are inhibition of presynaptic voltage-dependent Ca^{2+} channels (particularly N and P/Q types) (Mackie et al. 1993), augmentation of inwardly rectifying K^+ channels (Mackie et al. 1995; McAllister and Glass 2002), ceramide production (Guzman et al. 2001), and positive coupling to mitogen-activated protein kinase and subsequent induction of the expression of transcription factor Krox-24 (see Childers and Breivogel 1998; Howlett 1998; McAllister and Glass 2002). Thus, the net effect of CB_1-receptor activation is to augment membrane hyperpolarization and inhibit neurotransmitter release. Phosphorylation of the serine 317 site of the CB_1 receptor, via a protein kinase C-mediated mechanism, disrupts the transduction of CB_1 effects (Garcia et al. 1998). Furthermore, activity at CB_1 receptors sequesters $G_{i/o}$ proteins from a common pool, preventing signal transduction at other $G_{i/o}$-protein-coupled receptors (e.g., adrenergic and somatostatin receptors) (Vasquez and Lewis 1999). The CB_1 receptor exists in a variety of conformation states, dictated by binding to different ligands, which in turn determines which transduction mechanism operates (Howlett 1998). The receptor-ligand complex for CB_1 is rapidly internalized and eventually recycled, a process that may underlie the observed development of tolerance to cannabinoids (Hsieh et al. 2000; Coutts et al. 2001; Kouznetsova et al. 2002).

At a synaptic level, at least in the cerebellum and hippocampus, strong evidence suggests that endocannabinoids are synthesized "on demand" in postsynaptic neurons in response to depolarization and then are rapidly released into the extracellular domain where they act as short-range retrograde modulators of neurotransmitter release from presynaptic neurons, via a CB_1-dependent inhibition of Ca^{2+} influx (Kreitzer and Regehr 2001; Ohno-Shosaku et al. 2001; Wilson and Nicoll 2001; Wilson et al. 2001; for reviews, see Christie and Vaughan 2001; Montgomery and Madison 2001; Wilson and Nicoll 2002) (Fig. 2). This phenomenon also occurs in response to metabotropic glutamate type 1 receptor activation in the hippocampus (Varma et al. 2001) and cerebellum (Maejima et al. 2001). This mechanism operates at both hippocampal GABAergic (essentially inhibitory) (Ohno-Shosaku et al. 2001; Wilson and Nicoll 2001) and cerebellar glutaminergic (essentially excitatory) synapses (Kreitzer and Regehr 2001; Ohno-Shosaku et al. 2001). Endocannabinoids thus may be strong candidates for the molecular substrates of depolarization-induced suppression of inhibition (DSI) (Ohno-Shosaku et al. 2001; Wilson and Nicoll 2001; Yoshida et al. 2002) and depolarization-induced suppression of excitation (DSE) (Kreitzer and Regehr 2001; Maejima et al. 2001). A logical extension to this line of investigation was the subsequent revelation that endocannabinoids facilitate the physiological process of long-term potentiation in the hippocampus (Carlson et al. 2002) and long-term depression in the striatum (Gerdeman et al. 2002). A

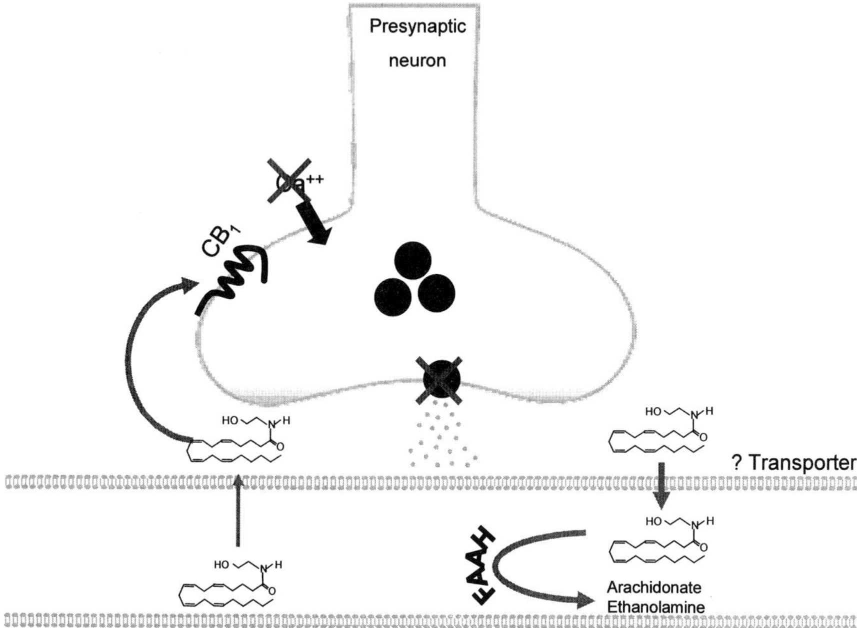

Fig. 2. Schematic depicting endocannabinoids acting as short-range retrograde modulators of neurotransmitter release. Upon depolarization of the postsynaptic neuron, anandamide (AEA) is rapidly synthesized in a calcium-dependent process. As befits its high lipophilicity, AEA rapidly crosses the neuronal membrane to gain access to the synaptic cleft. AEA then interacts with presynaptic CB_1 receptors to induce a block of calcium channels and consequent inhibition of neurotransmitter release. This effect occurs at both glutaminergic and GABAergic synapses. AEA is inactivated by facilitated diffusion into the postsynaptic neuron (and also possibly microglia), probably involving a membrane transporter, where it is hydrolyzed by fatty acid amide hydrolase (FAAH).

similar role has recently been revealed for the extinction of aversive memories at GABAergic synapses in the amygdala (Kouznetsova et al. 2002). It remains to be seen whether these revelations are relevant to the regulation of nociceptive signaling, particularly at the level of the spinal cord, although it is known that exogenous cannabinoids suppress release of neurotransmitters in systems that are fundamentally linked to the suppression of nociceptive activity in the brainstem. They do so by suppressing GABAergic activity in the rostroventromedial medulla (Vaughan et al. 1999) and both GABAergic and glutaminergic transmission in the periaqueductal grey (Vaughan et al. 2000).

CB_2 receptors are generally expressed by immune cells. CB_2 shares only 44% overall sequence homology with CB_1, although this increases to 68% in the transmembrane regions. As for CB_1, the CB_2 receptor is negatively coupled to adenylate cyclase via $G_{i/o}$ proteins (Munro et al. 1993; Schatz et al. 1997). CB_2 was originally identified in macrophages in the marginal zone of the spleen (Munro et al. 1993), but later was found to be highly expressed in the tonsils (Galiegue et al. 1995). Of the circulating human immune cells, the B-lymphocytes and natural killer cells are particularly rich in CB_2 mRNA, with moderate expression in monocytes and minimal expression in polymorphs (Galiegue et al. 1995). Evidence also suggests CB_2 expression on T-cell lines (Schatz et al. 1997). The gene encoding CB_2 and its protein have also been identified in rat peritoneal mast cells, and activation of CB_2 downregulates mast cell function (Facci et al. 1995). CB_2 is also expressed on microglia (Walter et al. 2001, 2002).

ENDOCANNABINOIDS

Anandamide (AEA) was the first endocannabinoid to be identified (Devane et al. 1992), followed by 2-arachidonoylglycerol (2-AG). Since then, an increasing list of endocannabinoid molecules has evolved, for example noladin ether (Hanus et al. 2001) and virodhamine (Porter et al. 2002). Palmitoylethanolamide (PEA) is another long-chain fatty acid with cannabimimetic properties, but it does not bind strongly to known CB receptors. (See Table I for a list of cannabinoids.)

AEA, first isolated from porcine brain (Devane et al. 1992), is widely distributed (Felder et al. 1996). It binds to cannabinoid receptors and evokes the classical "tetrad" (antinociception, catalepsy, hypothermia, and hypolocomotion; Martin et al. 1991) of cannabinoid effects (Crawley et al. 1993; Calignano et al. 1998; Jaggar et al. 1998). AEA induces stimulation of GTPγS binding to G proteins, indicating that it exerts its effects via a G-protein-coupled apparatus (Breivogel et al. 1998; Kearn et al. 1999). AEA evokes the cellular and molecular consequences of cannabinoid receptor activation, including inhibition of adenylyl cyclase (Felder et al. 1993; Bayewitch et al. 1995), inhibition of N-type, P/Q-type, and L-type voltage-gated Ca^{2+} channels (Felder 1993; Mackie et al. 1993, 1995; Gebremedhin et al. 1999), activation of inwardly rectifying K^+ channels (Mackie et al. 1995; McAllister et al. 1999), and inhibition of neurotransmitter release (Shen et al. 1996; Vaughan et al. 2000). However, at low doses AEA appears to act in a manner counter classical cannabinoids and to antagonize the actions of Δ^9 THC, perhaps by acting as a partial agonist or via its effects at the TRPV1 (VR1) vanilloid receptor (see below) (Fride et al. 1995; Di Marzo and Deutsch 1998; Hillard 2000). AEA binds to the CB_1 receptor (K_i ~ 89 nM) but has less affinity for CB_2 (~371 nM); it does not appear to evoke CB_2-mediated effects to a biologically significant degree (Felder et al. 1993; Di Marzo and

Table I
Cannabinoids mentioned in the text

2-AG = 2-arachidonylglycerol. Endogenous cannabinoid agonist.
AEA = Anandamide (arachidonylethanolamide). Prototypical endogenous cannabinoid agonist.
AM1241 = Synthetic CB_2-selective agonist.
AM374 = Palmitylsulfonyl fluoride. Selective FAAH inhibitor.
AM404 = Anandamide transport inhibitor.
CP55,940 = Synthetic cannabinoid agonist.
CT3 = 1',1' dimethylheptyl-Δ^8-THC-11-oic acid. Synthetic cannabinoid agonist.
Δ^9 THC = Δ^9 tetrahydrocannabinol. Naturally occurring cannabinoid agonist.
HU210 = Synthetic cannabinoid agonist.
HU211 = Synthetic cannabinoid agonist.
HU308 = Synthetic selective CB_2 agonist.
Methanandamide = Stable synthetic anandamide analogue. Cannabinoid agonist.
Noladin ether = 2-Arachidonyl glycerol ether (HU310). Endogenous cannabinoid agonist.
O-1057 = Synthetic water-soluble cannabinoid agonist.
PEA = Palmitoylethanolamide (N-(2-hydroxyethyl)hexadecanamide). Endogenous analogue of AEA.
SR141716A = Synthetic CB_1-receptor antagonist (inverse agonist).
SR144528 = Synthetic CB_2-receptor antagonist.
WIN 55,212-2 = Synthetic cannabinoid agonist.
Virodhamine = O-Arachidonylethanolamine. Endogenous cannabinoid agonist.

Deutsch 1998). AEA also has a weak affinity (K_i ~ 10 μM) and agonist activity at the TRPV1 noxious heat-gated ion channel (Zygmunt et al. 1999; Smart et al. 2000), and it might be the case that CB_1 represents the metabotropic receptor for AEA, or a closely related molecule, while TRPV1 is the ionotropic AEA receptor.

The monoacylglycerol 2-AG was first isolated from canine gut and later brain (where it is found in concentrations 170-fold greater than AEA). It binds to cannabinoid receptors and exhibits cannabimimetic effects (Mechoulam et al. 1995; Stella et al. 1997). Appreciable concentrations of 2-AG have also been measured in dorsal root ganglia and spinal cord (Huang et al. 1999). 2-AG is a full agonist at the CB_1 receptor (K_i 14 nM) and appears to be the best candidate as the natural ligand at the CB_2 receptor (K_i 58 nM) (Hillard 2000; Sugiura et al. 2000; McAllister and Glass 2002).

Palmitoylethanolamide (PEA) accumulates in inflamed tissue and in areas of demyelination of spinal cord and brain, downregulates mast cell degranulation (at least in vivo, but not in vitro) (Granberg et al. 2001), prevents edema formation, protects cerebellar granule cells against glutamate-induced excitotoxity, and has analgesic properties (Facci et al. 1995; Mazzari et al. 1996; Calignano et al. 1998, 2001; Jaggar et al. 1998; Baker et al. 2001). While PEA did not bind to CB_1 receptors (Lambert et al. 1999), it displaced cannabinoids from binding sites in a mast cell line in which the CB_2 transcript was identified (Facci et al. 1995). However, later studies indicate that PEA and analogues do not bind with high affinity to CB_2 (K_i 14 μM) (Lambert et al. 1999). Nevertheless, the CB_2-receptor antagonist SR144528 prevents the antihyperalgesic actions of PEA (Calignano et al. 2001; Farquhar-Smith and Rice 2001a; Conti et al. 2002; Farquhar-Smith et al. 2002). Several possible explanations under active investigation could account for this paradox, including a PEA metabolite active at CB_2, the existence of a putative non-CB_1, non-CB_2 receptor at which PEA is an agonist and SR144528 acts as an antagonist (Calignano et al. 1998; Farquhar-Smith and Rice 2001a; Farquhar-Smith et al. 2002), or a permissive role for PEA in enhancing the activity of other endocannabinoids, perhaps by inhibiting their degradation by acting as a competitive substrate for fatty acid amide hydrolase (FAAH; see below) (Ben Shabat et al. 1998; Lambert and Di Marzo 1999; Petrocellis et al. 2000; Jonsson et al. 2001; Lambert et al. 2002).

BIOSYNTHESIS OF ENDOCANNABINOIDS

It was initially thought that the major biosynthetic pathway for AEA was the condensation of arachidonic acid and ethanolamine (Deutsch and Chin 1993), possibly catalyzed by FAAH catalyzing the AEA degradation reaction in reverse (Kurahashi et al. 1997). However, researchers doubted whether this pathway was capable of synthesizing AEA in biologically relevant concentrations (Bisogno et al. 1997; Di Marzo and Deutsch 1998; De Petrocellis et al. 2000). More recently the balance of evidence has favored the model that membrane depolarization and consequent Ca^{2+} influx activate the intracellular cleavage of *N*-arachidonylphosphatidylethanolamine (NAPE) by phospholipase D, with AEA rapidly synthesized "on demand" rather than stored in synaptic vesicles (Childers and Breivogel 1998; Piomelli et al. 1998). It is possible that PEA is synthesized by a similar mechanism for cleavage of *N*-palmitylphosphatidylethanolamine (Bisogno et al. 1997; Di Marzo and Deutsch 1998; Piomelli et al. 1998). Uncertainty surrounds the synthesis of 2-AG, but the most plausible model suggests the hydrolysis of certain diacylglycerols by diacylglycerol lipase. However, alternative explanations exist, and the nature of 2-AG biosynthesis remains to be fully elucidated (Di Marzo and Deutsch 1998; Piomelli et al. 1998). While many of the data for endocannabinoid synthesis relate to neurons, evidence also points to synthesis of endocannabinoids by immune cells, especially basophils, microglia, and macrophages (Bisgono et al. 1997; De Petrocellis et al. 2000; Walter et al. 2001).

INACTIVATION OF ENDOCANNABINOIDS

The major degradation pathway for AEA described to date involves facilitated diffusion into postsynaptic cells (possibly by a putative uptake transporter) and subsequent hydrolysis by an intracellular enzyme (FAAH, also known previously as AEA amidase and AEA amidohydrolase) to arachidonic acid and ethanolamine (Fowler et al. 2001). PEA is probably inactivated by a similar, but not identical, mechanism to AEA, although simple diffusion probably plays a greater role than for AEA. It is therefore less likely that the uptake mechanism for PEA is substantially regulated by FAAH activity (see below) (Fowler et al. 2001; Jacobsson and Fowler 2001).

Deutsch and Chinn (1993) first noted that FAAH could hydrolyze AEA, and Cravatt and colleagues (Cravatt et al. 1996; Giang and Cravatt 1997) characterized and cloned this enzyme. Membrane-bound FAAH activity has been observed in intracellular locations (e.g., microsomes and mitochondria) in a range of tissues, especially in the liver, but also in brain, kidney, gut, testis, and immune cells (Di Marzo et al. 1994; Beltramo et al. 1997; Katayama et al. 1997; Thomas et al. 1997). FAAH expression has been best characterized in the brain (Di Marzo and Deutsch 1998); FAAH activity, and both protein and mRNA expression, are widespread in the brain, particularly in the cerebellum, choroid plexus, hippocampus, and globus pallidus. In general its pattern of expression is complementary to that of the CB_1 receptor (Thomas et al. 1997; Egertova et al. 1998; Egertova et al. 2000; Romero et al. 2002). FAAH knockout mice have almost negligible levels of AEA hydrolytic activity and 15-fold higher brain concentrations of AEA than do wild types (Cravatt et al. 2001). These mice also display evidence of tonic analgesia, presumably a phenomenon related to the increased concentration of AEA, and a significant augmentation in the CB_1-mediated analgesic response to exogenous AEA.

The uptake of AEA by neurons is rapid ($t_{1/2}$ 2.5 minutes), temperature dependent, saturable, and selective, suggesting the presence of a specific transporter, although it has yet to be formally identified and cloned (Di Marzo et al. 1994; Beltramo et al. 1997; for review see Fowler and Jacobsson 2002). However, this hypothesis is controversial, and an alternative explanation suggests that the facilitated diffusion of AEA is driven by FAAH activity maintaining a concentration gradient (Day et al. 2001).

Inhibitors of endocannabinoid degradation are an alternative approach to receptor agonists in the drive to develop therapeutically useful cannabinoid-based drugs (Fowler et al. 2001; Deutsch et al. 2002; Fowler and Jacobsson 2002). This approach recently received added impetus when a mouse model of multiple sclerosis showed selectively elevated concentrations of PEA, 2-AG, and AEA in areas of neuronal injury (Baker et al. 2001). Various inhibitors of FAAH include phenylmethylsulfonyl fluoride, but most have been hampered by a lack of selectivity for FAAH or an unfavorable toxicity profile (Di Marzo and Deutsch 1998; Fowler et al. 2001; Deutsch et al. 2002). AM374 (palmitylsulfonyl fluoride) is a selective FAAH inhibitor (Deutsch et al. 1997) and has alleviated spasticity in a mouse model of multiple sclerosis (Baker et al. 2001). Intriguingly, certain nonsteroidal analgesics, such as ibuprofen and ketorolac, in addition to their cyclooxygenase inhibiting properties, behave as FAAH inhibitors at concentrations achievable after oral administration (Fowler et al. 1997, 1999, 2001). Another approach is to explore inhibitors of the putative AEA transporter, for instance AM404, which enhanced the antinociceptive and hypotensive effects of AEA in vivo (Beltramo et al. 1997; Calignano et al. 1997) and alleviated signs of spasticity in a model of multiple sclerosis (Baker et al. 2001).

ANALGESIC EFFECTS OF CANNABINOIDS

Analgesic sites of action for cannabinoids have been identified in brain areas such as the rostroventromedial medulla and periaqueductal gray (Lichtman et al. 1996; Martin et al. 1996; Meng et al. 1998; Tsou et al. 1998; Vaughan et al. 1999, 2000; Egertova and Elphick 2000), in the spinal cord, and in the periphery. For the purposes of developing clinically useful analgesics with an acceptable therapeutic index, the spinal cord and periphery are possibly more attractive targets and are thus the focus of this review. However, these sites probably do not act independently of each other; for example, brain sites may influence spinally mediated effects by means of descending control (Meng et al. 1998).

SPINAL ANALGESIA

Following the initial reports of localization of CB_1 in the spinal cord in rodents and primates (Tsou et al. 1998; Hohmann et al. 1999a; Ong and Mackie 1999; Sanudo-Pena et al. 1999), we made a detailed immunohistochemical analysis of spinal CB_1-receptor expression (Farquhar-Smith et al.

2000). This analysis demonstrated expression of CB_1 in areas important for nociceptive processing, particularly the dorsolateral funiculus, the superficial dorsal horn, and lamina X. In the dorsal horn, CB_1 expression was evident as a bilayer in laminae I and II_I that overlapped with the central terminals of the nerve growth factor (NGF)-dependent peptidergic class of primary afferent nociceptor. The exact cellular location of spinal CB_1 receptors requires further elucidation, but the available evidence from both lesioning and electrophysiological studies suggests the existence of populations of CB_1 receptors in the spinal and medullary dorsal horn on both the central terminals of primary afferent neurons (Hohmann et al. 1999a; Morisset and Urban 2001; Morisset et al. 2001) and on intrinsic spinal neurons (Farquhar-Smith et al. 2000; Salio et al. 2001, 2002b), including GABAergic and NOS-containing interneurons. Some data suggest that CB_1 is expressed by spinal astrocytes (Salio et al. 2002b). Further supporting the existence of CB_1-expressing intrinsic spinal cord neurons is the finding of minimal change in CB radioligand binding following destruction of primary afferent nociceptors by neonatal capsaicin therapy (Hohmann and Herkenham 1998) or dorsal rhizotomy (Farquhar-Smith et al. 2000). However, radioligand binding in cervical spinal cord harvested from animals subjected to a more extensive rhizotomy suggests that about 50% of spinal CB_1 expression occurs on primary afferent neurons, but postsynaptic changes in response to such an extensive rhizotomy may have complicated this picture (Hohmann et al. 1999a). Electrophysiological studies arrived at similar conclusions with evidence of CB_1 expression on both interneurons inhibiting the release of GABA and glycine (Jennings et al. 2000) and primary afferent neurons inhibiting glutamate release (Morisset and Urban 2001).

Other electrophysiological data support the concept of spinal antinociceptive effects of CBs: noxious thermal and mechanical-evoked activity in spinal wide-dynamic-range (WDR) neurons is attenuated by systemically and intrathecally administered WIN 55,212-2 (Hohmann et al. 1995, 1998, 1999b). Systemic administration of this compound also reduced the augmented activity ("wind-up") in dorsal horn neurons evoked by a sustained noxious input (Strangman and Walker 1999).

Further evidence supporting the hypothesis of spinally mediated effects of cannabinoids is the finding that systemically administered Δ^9 THC retains its antinociceptive properties following spinal transection (Smith and Martin 1992). Hargreaves and colleagues have demonstrated that intrathecal administration of AEA blocked the thermal hyperalgesia associated with carrageenan injection into the skin of the hindpaw, at doses that did not alter sensory thresholds to noxious heat in the absence of inflammation (Richardson et al. 1998a). Intrathecal administration of the potent synthetic cannabinoid

HU210 was more effective in attenuating the characteristic pain behavior associated with subcutaneous formalin injection than was morphine, again at doses that were not associated with adverse motor effects (Guhring et al. 2001). WIN 55,212-2 delivered intrathecally also attenuated pain behavior following formalin injection via a CB_1- but not a CB_2-receptor mechanism (Rice et al. 2002). Finally, spinal intrathecal administration of WIN 55,212-2 reversed the mechanical hyperalgesia that is associated with the partial sciatic nerve ligation model of neuropathic pain (Fox et al. 2001). Biodisposition studies reveal that intrathecally administered cannabinoids tend to remain at the site of action and are not rapidly redistributed to the brain (Martin and Lichtman 1998). Spinal intrathecal administration of the water-soluble CB 0-1057 has been associated with antinociception (Pertwee et al. 2000) and systemic administration of Δ^9 THC accompanied by intrathecal administration of an α_2 noradrenergic antagonists. These findings suggest that the anti-nociceptive effects of cannabinoids are mediated, at least partly, by a descending noradrenergic mechanism (Lichtman and Martin 1991). Other evidence suggests that endocannabinoids regulate the effects of glutamate (NMDA)-mediated central sensitization (Richardson et al. 1998b). Intrathecal administration of WIN 55,212-2 reversed the mechanical allodynia and prevented the appearance of Fos-like immunoreactivity in spinal neurons, which follows subcutaneous injection of complete Freund's adjuvant into the hindpaw (Martin et al. 1999). Systemic administration of WIN 55,212-2, AEA, or PEA has prevented the appearance of Fos immunoreactivity in the dorsal horn following intravesical turpentine (W.P. Farquhar-Smith, S.I. Jaggar, and A.S.C. Rice, unpublished observations) or NGF therapy (Farquhar-Smith et al. 2002) and subcutaneous formalin injection (Tsou et al. 1996).

It has recently become clear that not only neurons, but also microglia, play a role in the CNS responses to the inflammation and peripheral nerve injury that underlie persistent pain (DeLeo and Yezierski 2001; Watkins et al. 2001). Microglia express functional CB_2 receptors and synthesize endocannabinoids and modulate microglial cell migration (Stella et al. 2001; Walter et al. 2001, 2002). Furthermore, cannabinoids block cytokine mRNA expression in cultured microglial cells, although this effect is not mediated by known cannabinoid receptors (Puffenbarger et al. 2000).

It has been suggested that the endogenous opioid and cannabinoid systems interact to produce analgesia (Manzanares et al. 1999). At a spinal level naloxone antagonizes the effects of Δ^9 THC (Welch 1994) and the release of dynorphin A by Δ^9 THC (Manzanares et al. 1999; Mason et al. 1999) and dynorphin B by both CP55,940 and Δ^9 THC (Pugh et al. 1997). A κ-receptor antagonist and dynorphin antisera block Δ^9 THC-induced i.t.

antinociception (Smith et al. 1994; Pugh et al. 1995; Welch et al. 1995b) and further implicate the release of dynorphins in the mechanism of spinal antinociception of some cannabinoids (Welch et al. 1995a). Additionally, the coadministration of i.t. morphine and Δ^9 THC results in a synergistic antinociceptive effect in the tail-flick test (Welch and Stevens 1992), potentially via Δ^9 THC activation of endogenous opiates acting at κ and δ receptors (Pugh et al. 1996).

PERIPHERAL ANALGESIC EFFECTS

An increasing body of evidence supports the hypothesis of a peripheral analgesic action of cannabinoids, particularly during inflammation, and presents an obvious target for the development of cannabinoid-based analgesics. The primary line of evidence comes from studies that have demonstrated analgesic effects of locally delivered cannabinoids at doses that were not systemically effective. For instance, locally administered AEA attenuated carrageenan-induced thermal hyperalgesia, an effect that was sensitive to the CB_1-receptor antagonist SR141716A, although CB_2-mediated effects were not excluded (Richardson et al. 1998c). In the formalin model of cutaneous inflammatory hyperalgesia, Piomelli and colleagues have shown that local administration of WIN 55,212-2, HU210, and methanandamide attenuated both phases of the behavioral response to subcutaneous formalin injection, via a CB_1, but not CB_2 or opioid-receptor-mediated mechanism (Calignano et al. 1998). AEA was similarly active, although only for the first phase of the behavioral response, probably reflecting its rapid degradation. PEA also reduced both phases of the response, but by an SR144528-sensitive, mechanism. In the partial sciatic nerve ligation model of neuropathic pain, WIN 55,212-2 reversed mechanical hyperalgesia associated with painful neuropathy. The suggestion of a peripheral component to this effect derives from the observation that, at the 30-μg dose, WIN 55,212-2 was much more effective when administered into the paw ipsilateral to the site of nerve injury than when given into the contralateral paw. Again, while the local effect of WIN 55,212-2 was antagonized by SR141716A, a CB_2-receptor-mediated effect was not excluded.

Evidence suggests that both CB_2 and CB_1 receptors may participate in the local analgesic effects of cannabinoids. Strong evidence indicates that rat primary afferent neurons express cannabinoid receptors; for instance, cannabinoid binding sites are transported along axons in peripheral nerves (Hohmann and Herkenham 1999a), and immunocytochemistry and flow cytometry have revealed the presence of CB_1 in cultured DRG cells and in the F-11 cell line (Ross et al. 2001). However, confirmation of the exact phenotype of CB_1 expressing dorsal root ganglion cells has been more elusive. In situ hybridization (Hohmann and Herkenham 1999b; Bridges et al. 2003) and immunohistochemistry of intact lumbar dorsal root ganglia, using a polyclonal antibody directed against the C-terminal 13 amino acids of CB_1 (Bridges et al. 2003), suggest that most CB_1-expressing cells are of medium to large diameter and co-stain for neurofilament 200. A smaller population of small-diameter CB_1-expressing DRG cells co-stain for markers of nociceptive neurons, such as CGRP, IB4, trkA, and TRPV1. Conversely, immunocytochemistry of cultured DRG cells using an antibody directed against the N-terminal of CB_1 suggests a very high degree of co-localization and exclusive with markers of primary afferent nociceptors, particularly with TRPV1 (Ahluwalia et al. 2000, 2002). Immunocytochemistry has also shown that both CB_1 and CB_2 receptors (using antibodies raised against the 77 N-terminal amino acids of cloned rat CB_1 or cloned human CB_2 receptors) are expressed in cell cultures of neonatal rat DRGs and in an F-11 cell line with characteristics of DRG cells. Functional data implied that at least some of these cells have a nociceptor phenotype (Ross et al. 2001). Evidence of functionally active CB_1 receptors was seen in the inhibitory effect of WIN 55,212-2 on the voltage-activated Ca^{2+} currents and antagonism of this effect by the CB_1-selective inverse agonist SR141716A. No evidence of functional CB_2-mediated effects were found in these neurons, which suggests that the expression of CB_2 in neonatal DRG cultures is on cells other than primary afferent neurons. Chapman has also provided evidence that DRG cells express functional CB receptors by demonstrating that cannabinoids inhibit the capsaicin-evoked influx of Ca^{2+} into cultured DRG cells (Millns et al. 2001).

Cannabinoids also modulate release of neuropeptides from primary afferent nociceptors. AEA prevents both capsaicin- and K^+-evoked release of the CGRP from primary afferent nociceptors (Richardson et al. 1998a). Use of an in vitro hemisected spinal cord preparation has also demonstrated that WIN 55,212-2 inhibits electrically evoked release of CGRP via CB_1 receptors (Brooks et al. 2002a). Furthermore, this abstract also reported experiments that examined AMPA-induced inhibition of electrically evoked CGRP release and showed that a CB_1-receptor antagonist prevents this phenomenon, which suggests that endocannabinoids act presynaptically to inhibit CGRP release from primary sensory neurons (Brooks et al. 2002a). Studies using the same preparation have provided evidence of tonic modulation of spinal nociceptive systems by cannabinoids (Lever and Malcangio 2002).

Agonist activity at CB_2 receptors generally down modulates activity of immune cells and thus could contribute to the local antihyperalgesic effects of cannabinoids in inflammation and following peripheral nerve injury. While several immune cell mechanisms could contribute to this CB_2-mediated effect, most of the evidence supports such a phenomenon in mast cells, neutrophils, and macrophages. Mast cells are critical to the key NGF-mediated component of inflammatory hyperalgesia, probably via NGF-induced degranulation that effectively "amplifies" the NGF signal (Woolf et al. 1996; Nilsson et al. 1997; Tal and Liberman 1997). Data suggest that CB_2 (or CB_2-like) mechanisms may modulate this mast-cell-mediated amplification of the NGF signal in a process dubbed "autacoid local inflammation antagonism" (ALIA) (Levi-Montalcini et al. 1996). The gene encoding CB_2-receptor mRNA and the protein itself have also been identified in rat peritoneal mast cells, and activation of CB_2 receptors downregulates mast cell function (Facci et al. 1995). However, while some evidence indicates that the actions of PEA may be attributable to an influence on mast cell degranulation, little direct evidence suggests that the same is true for other cannabinoids.

Neutrophil migration is also a key component of the NGF-mediated component of inflammatory hyperalgesia (Bennett et al. 1998). PEA, by an SR144528-sensitive mechanism, decreases NGF-evoked cutaneous thermal hyperalgesia and neutrophil accumulation, as measured by the myeloperoxidase assay (Farquhar-Smith and Rice 2001b). Other investigators have shown that a synthetic cannabinoid attenuates spontaneous and induced migration of rat peritoneal macrophages, mainly via a CB_2-mediated mechanism, although CB_1-mediated effects could not be discounted, at least in vitro (Sacerdote et al. 2000). In the RAW 264.7 macrophage cell line (which expresses transcripts for CB_2, but not CB_1), Δ^9 THC inhibits the inducible nitric oxide synthase (iNOS) transcription and nitric oxide formation associated with lipopolysaccharide stimulation (Jeon et al. 1996). In the same cell line, Ross and colleagues showed that both WIN 55,212-2 and PEA reduced lipopolysaccharide-induced nitric oxide production (Ross et al. 2000).

STRESS-INDUCED ANALGESIA

While the physiological importance of an endocannabinoid-mediated "analgesic tone" is controversial (for discussion see Rice 2001a), Hohmann and colleagues (2002) have provided preliminary evidence for a physiological role of endocannabinoids in analgesia. They have demonstrated that the nonopioid-mediated component of stress-induced analgesia is mediated by endocannabinoids. By using an electrical foot shock paradigm to induce analgesia and the tail-flick test to measure nociception, they were able to show that the CB_1-receptor antagonist SR141716A blocked stress-induced analgesia. An opioid receptor antagonist or CB_2-receptor antagonist had no such effect, indicating a CB_1-mediated mechanism. Conversely, Δ^9 THC and the AEA uptake inhibitor AM404 enhanced stress-induced analgesia.

STUDIES IN ANIMAL MODELS OF HUMAN DISEASE

Ample evidence points to cannabinoid-induced antinociceptive activity in animal models in which a physiological response to an ephemeral noxious stimulus, for example the tail-flick test, was examined (Pertwee 2001). However, these models are rather poor reflections of the clinical state because the excitability of a dynamic nervous system is considerably altered by the consequences of tissue inflammation or peripheral nerve injury. To obtain a closer prediction of clinical usefulness, it is necessary to examine the analgesic effect of cannabinoids in animal models that encompass a significant persistent inflammatory or peripheral nerve injury component.

SOMATIC INFLAMMATION

The behavioral response to an injection of dilute formalin into the skin of the rodent hindpaw is a widely used model of acute pain. Following injection of formalin, a characteristic biphasic behavioral response occurs. The first phase lasts about 15 minutes and may represent the acute response to injection of the noxious chemical. After a short quiescent phase, a second response lasting about 50 minutes represents sensitization of primary afferent and spinal components of the nociceptive "pathway." AEA and PEA dose dependently attenuate the second phase of this response in the rat (Jaggar et al. 1998). Such findings of analgesic activity in the formalin test have also been confirmed for WIN 55,212-2, methanandamide, and HU210, for which a CB_1-mediated effect was identified (Calignano et al. 1998). In this latter study, the effects of AEA were restricted to the first phase of the behavioral response, probably reflecting its limited duration of action. PEA attenuated both phases of the response, and SR144528 antagonized its effects. Other studies have shown that the CB_2 agonist HU308 reduces the second phase of the formalin test by an SR144528-sensitive mechanism (Hanus et al. 1999) and that formalin behavior and the associated increase in the number of dorsal horn cells staining immunopositive for Fos protein are attenuated by WIN 55,212-2 (Tsou et al. 1996). CT3 (1',1'dimethylheptyl-Δ^8-THC-11-oic acid) also has analgesic effects in the mouse formalin test (Burstein et al. 1998). Finally, formalin injection activates the endocannabinoid system, as suggested by the observation that it is associated with release of AEA in the periaqueductal gray matter of the brain (Walker et al. 1999).

Carrageenan injection to the skin of the hindpaw evokes a thermal hyperalgesia that is attenuated by locally or intrathecally administered AEA, via a CB_1-mediated mechanism, although CB_2-mediated effects were not excluded (Richardson et al. 1998a,c). Cannabinoids similarly attenuate the hyperalgesia that is associated with capsaicin injection (Ko and Woods 1999; Li et al. 1999).

The mechanical hyperalgesia and spinal Fos expression related to cutaneous or intra-articular injection of complete Freund's adjuvant is attenuated by intrathecal administration of exogenous cannabinoids (Smith et al. 1998; Martin et al. 1999). Evidence also indicates that AEA attenuates NGF-induced cutaneous thermal hyperalgesia (Farquhar-Smith and Rice 2000). In a collagen-induced murine model of rheumatoid arthritis, cannabidiol has a potent antiarthritic effect via both an anti-inflammatory and immunosuppressive action (Malfait et al. 2000).

PERSISTENT VISCERAL INFLAMMATION

Visceral pain and somatic pain differ significantly in their clinical and pathophysiological aspects, which predicates that each requires study using appropriate models (McMahon 1997). The effects of cannabinoids in persistent visceral pain have been studied in a model of acute cystitis that shares features of a more persistent condition, interstitial cystitis (Jaggar et al. 1998; Farquhar-Smith and Rice 2001a; Farquhar-Smith et al. 2002). In this model inflammation is accompanied by: (1) an increase in excitability of the spinal reflexes that control micturition (viscero-visceral hyper-reflexia) (McMahon and Abel 1987); (2) sensitization of primary afferent neurons (McMahon 1988; McMahon and Koltzenburg 1993); (3) dorsal horn neuronal sensitization (McMahon 1988); (4) referred hyperalgesia (Scott et al. 1998; Jaggar et al. 1999); and (5) an increase in the number of dorsal horn neurons displaying Fos-like immunoreactivity (Birder and De Groat 1992; Cruz et al. 1994; Dmitrieva et al. 1996).

Cannabinoids (AEA, PEA, and WIN 55,212-2) attenuate the viscero-visceral hyper-reflexia, spinal Fos expression, and referred hyperalgesia associated with cystitis at doses that do not interfere with normal micturition (Jaggar et al. 1998; Farquhar-Smith and Rice 2001a; Farquhar-Smith et al. 2002). NGF is crucial to the development of inflammatory hyperalgesia in this model (Dmitrieva and McMahon 1996; Dmitrieva et al. 1997; Jaggar et al. 1999). Both AEA and PEA dose dependently prevent the viscero-visceral hyper-reflexia associated with NGF treatment of the urinary bladder (Farquhar-Smith et al. 2002). The effects of AEA are reversed by SR141716A and partially by SR144528, which implies that its effects may be mediated by both CB_1 and CB_2 receptors. The antihyperalgesic effect of PEA is only antagonized by SR144528, further supporting a CB_2-like effect of PEA. As confirmation, we have also obtained evidence that cannabinoids prevent the appearance of Fos protein in the spinal dorsal horn following NGF treatment of the bladder (Farquhar-Smith et al. 2002). Evidence also suggests cannabinoid efficacy in various models of peritoneal irritation (see Table III in Pertwee 2001).

NEUROPATHIC PAIN

The chronic pain that occasionally follows peripheral nerve injury differs fundamentally from inflammatory pain and is an area of considerable unmet therapeutic need (Bridges et al. 2001b). Although controversial, it is generally accepted that opioid analgesics are less effective for treating neuropathic pain than for treating inflammatory pain. One explanation is a depletion of opioid receptor expression in the spinal dorsal horn following peripheral nerve injury (Besse et al. 1992a,b; Hohmann and Herkenham1998). Destruction of afferent input to the dorsal horn by dorsal rhizotomy (Farquhar-Smith et al. 2000), neonatal capsaicin therapy (Hohmann and Herkenham 1998), or sciatic axotomy (Bridges et al. 2002) is not associated with such a depletion of CB_1-receptor-like immunoreactivity or binding, thus giving cannabinoids a potential therapeutic advantage over cannabinoids in neuropathic pain. Upregulation of CB_1 expression in the thalamus following tibial nerve axotomy has also been reported (Siegling et al. 2001). In the DRG, sciatic axotomy results in a 70% reduction in the number of cells that immunostain for CB_1, not only ipsilaterally, but also to a lesser extent contralaterally (Bridges et al. 2002). Such contralateral effects have previously been reported (Oaklander and Belzberg 1997; Oaklander et al. 1998). Experiments are examining whether similar changes occur in the L5 and adjacent ganglia following section of the L5 spinal nerve.

The effectiveness of cannabinoids has been examined in several animal models of neuropathic pain (Table II): WIN 55,212-2 attenuated the thermal hyperalgesia and the mechanical and cold allodynia that developed 8 days after chronic constriction injury of the rat sciatic nerve (Herzberg et al. 1997). Antagonism of the effects of WIN 55,212-2 by SR141716A confirmed a CB_1-mediated effect, but CB_2 effects were not excluded. We have investigated WIN 55,212-2 in the spinal nerve ligation model (Bridges et al. 2001a). Systemic administration of WIN 55,212-2 dose-dependently reversed the thermal hyperalgesia and the mechanical and cold allodynia by a CB_1-mediated, but not CB_2-mediated, effect. Similar results have been described for the partial sciatic nerve ligation model for WIN 55,212-2, CP55,940, and HU210 (Fox et al. 2001). The effect of WIN 55,212-2 was antagonized by a CB_1-receptor antagonist, but the possibility of CB_2-mediated effects was not examined. This paper also reported the effectiveness of WIN 55,212-2 after intrathecal and peripheral administration and suggested that a spinal or

Table II
Published evidence supporting of cannabinoids in rat models of neuropathic pain

Model	Measurement	Cannabinoid (Route, Dose)	CB_1 Effect	CB_2 Effect
Sciatic axotomy (Zeltser et al. 1991)	Autotomy	HU211+ cupric chloride (i.p. and s.c., 2.5 mg/kg); also tested HU203	NR	NR
CCI (Herzberg et al. 1997)	Thermal hyperalgesia (radiant heat); mechanical hyperalgesia (pinprick); mechanical allodynia (mechanical von Frey); cold allodynia (acetone)	WIN 55,212-2 (i.p., 0.43–4.3 mg/kg)	Yes (SR141716A)	NR
CCI (Mao et al. 2000)	Thermal hyperalgesia (radiant heat)	Δ^9THC (spinal i.t., 5–160 μg)	Yes (SR141716A)	NR
PSL (Fox et al. 2001)	Mechanical hyperalgesia (Randall-Selitto); tactile allodynia (mechanical von Frey); thermal hyperalgesia (radiant heat)	WIN 55,212-2 (s.c., 0.3–3 mg/kg); WIN 55,212-2 (spinal i.t., 100 μg); WIN 55,212-2 (i.pl., 30–100 μg; CP55,940 (s.c., 0.03–0.3 mg/kg); HU210 (s.c., 0.001–0.03 mg/kg)	Yes (SR141716A), WIN 55,212-2 only	NR
SNL (Bridges et al. 2001)	Cold allodynia (acetone); mechanical allodynia (electronic von Frey); thermal hyperalgesia (radiant heat)	WIN 55,212-2 (i.p., 0.1–5 mg/kg)	Yes (SR141716A)	No (SR144528)

Abbreviations: CCI = chronic constriction injury of sciatic nerve; i.p. = intraperitoneal; i.pl. = intraplantar; i.t. = intrathecal; NR = not reported; PSL = partial sciatic nerve ligation; s.c. = subcutaneous; SNL = spinal nerve ligation.
Note: There are also two abstracts that present evidence of cannabinoid efficacy of the synthetic cannabinoid AM1241 in the SNL model (Ibrahim et al. 2001) and palmitoylethanolamide (PEA) in the CCI model (Mazzari et al. 1995).

peripheral site of action may be exploited to divorce the psychotropic effects of cannabinoids from their analgesic effects. A preliminary report has suggested that a selective CB_2-receptor agonist may have useful analgesic properties in neuropathic pain while avoiding the psychotropic side effects of CB_1-receptor agonists (Ibrahim et al. 2001). A preliminary report has shown that PEA reduces mechanical hyperalgesia in the chronic sciatic nerve constriction model. Although the role of cannabinoid receptors in this effect was not investigated, this finding does lend some weight to the arguments supporting a possible peripheral CB_2-like analgesic effect of PEA in neuropathic pain (Mazzari et al. 1995).

CLINICAL EVIDENCE OF ANALGESIA

In contrast to the strong preclinical data, the published clinical trial evidence supporting cannabinoid-induced analgesia is of insufficient quality to allow informed opinions to be voiced (Campbell et al. 2001; Rice 2001a), and we were unable to identify any published studies of cannabinoids in human volunteer models of pain. Interesting reports describe a large (636 subjects), 31-day clinical trial in sciatica patients that compared the effectiveness of oral PEA 300 mg/day or 600 mg/day with placebo, but because these data are yet to be published in a peer-reviewed format, assessment of the trial quality is not possible (see Jack 1996; Rice 2001a). However, PEA was more effective at reducing pain intensity scores than was placebo, and the study presented evidence of a dose-response relationship. This finding lends further support to the hypothesis that PEA or its analogues may provide analgesia without the psychotropic side effects associated with CB_1-receptor antagonists.

Before cannabinoid-based drugs can be used therapeutically in humans, they must be proven both effective and safe in long-term regular use. Well-designed clinical trials are required, but are perhaps premature until suitable cannabinoids, with a satisfactory therapeutic index for analgesia and proven bioavailability when administered by a practical route of administration, are available for human study. For cannabinoids possessing CNS activity, studies also will need to carefully consider the significance of an association of cannabis use with psychiatric disease (Arseneault et al. 2002; Patton et al. 2002; Zammit et al. 2002). Such clinical trials should be performed in an area of therapeutic need, such as neuropathic pain or in situations such as postoperative or cancer pain management where the side effects of cannabinoids might confer additional benefit over existing therapies, for example by exploiting their anti-inflammatory or anti-emetic properties. For chronic pain patients in whom fear contributes to abnormal pain behavior, another intriguing possibility has begun to emerge in the ability of endocannabinoids to extinguish aversive fear-related memories (Marsicano et al. 2002).

Possible drug development strategies for achieving cannabinoids with an acceptable therapeutic index with regard to brain-mediated side effects include: (1) targeting spinal and peripheral sites, for example CB_2 (Malan et al. 2003); (2) FAAH or transporter inhibitors to augment the effects of endocannabinoids (Fowler et al. 2001; Deutsch et al. 2002; Fowler and Jacobsson 2002; Kathuria et al. 2003); (3) targeting novel cannabinoid receptors, for which strong circumstantial evidence exists, if and when they are formally identified; and (4) further investigation of the potential of PEA (Lambert et al. 2002). The problem of bioavailability may perhaps be overcome by the further development of inhaled, sublingually, or intranasally delivered aerosols (Wilson et al. 2002), or of water-soluble cannabinoids with antinociceptive properties (Pertwee et al. 2000).

ACKNOWLEDGMENTS

We gratefully acknowledge funding for our laboratory from the Medical Research Council, The Wellcome Trust, The *British Journal of Anaesthesia*, The Royal College of Anaesthetists, The Association of Anaesthetists of Great Britain and Northern Ireland, and Novartis.

REFERENCES

Ahluwalia J, Urban L, Capogna M, et al. Cannabinoid 1 receptors are expressed in nociceptive primary sensory neurones. *Neuroscience* 2000; 100:685–688.

Ahluwalia J, Urban L, Bevan S, et al. Cannabinoid 1 receptors are expressed by nerve growth factor- and glial cell-derived neurotrophic factor-responsive primary sensory neurones. *Neuroscience* 2002; 110:747–753.

Arseneault L, Cannon M, Poulton R, et al. Cannabis use in adolescence and risk for adult psychosis: longitudinal prospective study. *BMJ* 2002; 325:1212–1213.

Baker D, Pryce G, Croxford JL, et al. Endocannabinoids control spasticity in a multiple sclerosis model. *FASEB J* 2001; 2001:300–302.

Bayewitch M, Avidor Reiss T, Levy R, et al. The peripheral cannabinoid receptor: adenylate cyclase inhibition and G protein coupling. *FEBS Lett* 1995; 375:143–147.

Beltramo M, Stella N, Calignano A, et al. Functional role of high-affinity anandamide transport, as revealed by selective inhibition. *Science* 1997; 277:1094–1097.

Bennett G, al Rashed S, Hoult JR, Brain SD. Nerve growth factor induced hyperalgesia in the rat hind paw is dependent on circulating neutrophils. *Pain* 1998; 77:315–322.

Besse D, Lombard MC, Besson JM. Time-related decreases in mu and delta opioid receptors in the superficial dorsal horn of the rat spinal cord following a large unilateral dorsal rhizotomy. *Brain Res* 1992a; 578:115–127.

Besse D, Lombard MC, Perrot S, Besson JM. Regulation of opioid binding sites in the superficial dorsal horn of the rat spinal cord following loose ligation of the sciatic nerve: comparison with sciatic nerve section and lumbar dorsal rhizotomy. *Neuroscience* 1992b; 50:921–933.

Birder LA, de Groat WC. Increased c-fos expression in spinal neurones after irritation of the lower urinary tract in the rat. *J Neurosci* 1992; 12:4878–4883.

Bisogno T, Maurelli S, Melck D, et al. Biosynthesis, uptake, and degradation of anandamide and palmitoylethanolamide in leukocytes. *J Biol Chem* 1997; 272:3315–3323.

Breivogel CS, Selley DE, Childers SR. Cannabinoid receptor agonist efficacy for stimulating [35S]GTPgammaS binding to rat cerebellar membranes correlates with agonist-induced decreases in GDP affinity. *J Biol Chem* 1998; 273:16865–16873.

Breivogel CS, Griffin G, Di Marzo V, Martin BR. Evidence for a new G-protein coupled cannabinoid receptor in mouse brain. *Mol Pharmacol* 2001; 60:155–163.

Bridge JA. Sir William Brooke O'Shaugnessy: a biographical appreciation by an electrical engineer. *Notes Rec R Soc Lond* 1988; 52:103–120.

Bridges D, Ahmad KS, Rice ASC. The synthetic cannabinoid WIN 55,212-2 attenuates hyperalgesia and allodynia in a rat model of neuropathic pain. *Br J Pharmacol* 2001a; 133:586–594.

Bridges D, Thompson SWN, Rice ASC. Mechanisms of neuropathic pain. *Br J Anaesth* 2001b; 87:12–26.

Bridges D, Rice ASC, Egertova M, et al. The distribution of cannabinoid CB1 receptor within the dorsal root ganglion following peripheral nerve injury. *Abstracts: 10th World Congress of Pain.* Seattle: IASP Press, 2002, p 128.

Bridges D, Rice ASC, Egertová M, et al. Localisation of CB_1 cannabinoid receptor in rat dorsal root ganglion using in situ bybridisation and immunohistochemistry. *Neuroscience* 2003; in press.

Brooks JW, Rice ASC, Thompson SWN, Malcangio M. Inhibition of electrically evoked calcitonin gene-related peptide (CGRP) release from the rat dorsal horn by (S)-AMPA: a role for the endocannabinoid system? *Abstracts: 10th World Congress of Pain.* Seattle: IASP Press, 2002a, p 490.

Brooks JW, Pryce G, Bisogno T, et al. Arvanil-induced inhibition of spasticity and persistent pain: evidence for therapeutic sites of action different from the vanilloid VR1 receptor and cannabinoid CB1/CB2 receptors. *Eur J Pharmacol* 2002b; 439:83–92.

Buckley NE, McCoy KL, Mezey E, et al. Immunomodulation by cannabinoids is absent in mice deficient for the cannabinoid CB(2) receptor. *Eur J Pharmacol* 2000; 396:141–149.

Burstein SH, Friderichs E, Kogel B, et al. Analgesic effects of 1',1' dimethylheptyl-delta8-THC-11-oic acid (CT3) in mice. *Life Sci* 1998; 63:161–168.

Calignano A, La Rana G, Beltramo M, et al. Potentiation of anandamide hypotension by the transport inhibitor, AM404. *Eur J Pharmacol* 1997; 337:R1–2.

Calignano A, La Rana G, Giuffrida A, Piomelli D. Control of pain initiation by endogenous cannabinoids. *Nature* 1998; 394:277–281.

Calignano A, La Rana G, Piomelli D. Antinociceptive activity of the endogenous fatty acid amide, palmitoylethanolamide. *Eur J Pharmacol* 2001; 419:191–198.

Campbell F, Tramer M, Carroll D, et al. Are cannabinoids an effective and safe option in the management of pain? A qualitative systematic review. *BMJ* 2001; 323:13–16.

Carlson G, Wang Y, Ali Z. Endocannabinoids facilitate the induction of LTP in the hippocampus. *Nat Neurosci* 2002; 5(8):723–724.

Childers SR, Breivogel CS. Cannabis and endogenous cannabinoid systems. *Drug Alcohol Depend* 1998; 51:173–187.

Christie MJ, Vaughan CW. Cannabinoids act backwards. *Nature* 2001; 410:527–530.

Conti S, Costa B, Colleoni M, et al. Antiinflammatory action of endocannabinoid palmitoylethanolamide and the synthetic cannabinoid nabilone in a model of acute inflammation in the rat. *Br J Pharmacol* 2002; 135:181–187.

Coutts AA, Anavi-Goffer S, Ross RA, et al. Agonist-induced internalisation and trafficking of cannabinoid CB1 receptors in hippocampal neurons. *J Neurosci* 2001; 21:2425–2433.

Cravatt BF, Giang DK, Mayfield SP, et al. Molecular characterization of an enzyme that degrades neuromodulatory fatty-acid amides. *Nature* 1996; 384:83–87.

Cravatt BF, Demarest K, Patricelli MP, et al. Supersensitivity to anandamide and enhanced endogenous cannabinoid signaling in mice lacking fatty acid amide hydrolase. *Proc Natl Acad Sci USA* 2001; 98:9371–9376.

Crawley JN, Corwin RL, Robinson JK, et al. Anandamide, an endogenous ligand of the cannabinoid receptor, induces hypomotility and hypothermia in vivo in rodents. *Pharmacol Biochem Behav* 1993; 46:967–972.

Cruz F, Avelino A, Lima D, Coimbra A. Activation of the c-fos proto-oncogene in the spinal cord following noxious stimulation of the urinary bladder. *Somatosens Mot Res* 1994; 11:319–325.

Day TA, Rakhshan F, Deutsch DG, Barker EL. Role of fatty acid amide hydrolase in the transport of the endogenous cannabinoid anandamide. *Mol Pharmacol* 2001; 59:1369–1375.

De Petrocellis L, Melck D, Bisogno T, Di Marzo V. Endocannabinoids and fatty acid amides in cancer, inflammation and related disorders. *Chem Phys Lipids* 2000; 108:191–209.

DeLeo JA, Yezierski RP. The role of neuroinflammation and neuroimmune activation in persistent pain. *Pain* 2001; 90:1–6.

Deutsch DG, Chin SA. Enzymatic synthesis and degradation of anandamide, a cannabinoid receptor agonist. *Biochem Pharmacol* 1993; 46:791–796.

Deutsch DG, Lin S, Hill WA, et al. Fatty acid sulfonyl fluorides inhibit anandamide metabolism and bind to the cannabinoid receptor. *Biochem Biophys Res Commun* 1997; 231:217–221.

Deutsch DG, Ueda N, Yamamoto S. The fatty acid amide hydrolase (FAAH). *Prostaglandins Leukot Essent Fatty Acids* 2002; 66:201–210.

Devane WA, Dysarz FA3, Johnson MR, et al. Determination and characterization of a cannabinoid receptor in rat brain. *Mol Pharmacol.* 1988; 34:605–613.

Devane WA, Hanus L, Breuer A, et al. Isolation and structure of a brain constituent that binds to the cannabinoid receptor. *Science* 1992; 258:1946–1949.

Di Marzo V (Ed). Endocannabinoids in the new millennium. *Prostaglandins Leukot Essent Fatty Acids* 2002; 66:91–391.

Di Marzo V, Deutsch DG. Biochemistry of the endogenous ligands of cannabinoid receptors. *Neurobiol Dis* 1998; 5:386–404.

Di Marzo V, Fontana A, Cadas H, et al. Formation and inactivation of endogenous cannabinoid anandamide in central neurons. *Nature* 1994; 372:686–691.

Di Marzo V, Breivogel CS, Tao Q, et al. Levels, metabolism, and pharmacological activity in CB_1 cannabinoid receptor knock out mice. *J Neurochem* 2000; 75:2343–2444.

Dmitrieva N, McMahon SB. Sensitisation of visceral afferents by nerve growth factor in the adult rat. *Pain* 1996; 66:87–97.

Dmitrieva N, Iqbal R, Shelton D, McMahon SB. C-fos induction in a rat model of cystitis: role of NGF. *Soc Neurosci Abstr* 1996; 22:301.6.

Dmitrieva N, Shelton D, Rice ASC, McMahon SB. The role of nerve growth factor in a model of visceral inflammation. *Neuroscience* 1997; 78:449–459.

Egertova M, Elphick MR. Localisation of cannabinoid receptors in the rat brain using antibodies to the intracellular C-terminal of CB_1. *J Comp Neurol* 2000; 422:159–171.

Egertova M, Cravatt BF, Elphick MR. Fatty acid amide hydrolase expression in rat choroid plexus: possible role in regulation of the sleep-inducing action of oleamide. *Neurosci Lett* 2000; 282:13–16.

Egertova M, Giang DK, Cravatt BF, Elphick MR. A new perspective on cannabinoid signalling: complementary localization of fatty acid amide hydrolase and CB1 receptor in brain. *Proc R Soc Lond* 1998; 265:2081–2085.

Facci L, Dal Toso R, Romanello S, et al. Mast cells express a peripheral cannabinoid receptor with differential sensitivity to anandamide and palmitoylethanolamide. *Proc Natl Acad Sci USA* 1995; 92:3376–3380.

Farquhar-Smith WP, Rice ASC. Anandamide attenuates a nerve growth factor-induced hyperalgesia via cannabinoid CB_1 receptors. *J Physiol Lond* 2000; 528:66.

Farquhar-Smith WP, Rice ASC. Administration of endocannabinoids prevents a referred hyperalgesia associated with inflammation of the urinary bladder. *Anesthesiology* 2001a; 94:507–513.

Farquhar-Smith WP, Rice ASC. The effects of endocannabinoids on peripheral NGF-induced neutrophil accumulation in rat skin. In: *2001 Symposium on the Cannabinoids.* International Cannabinoid Research Society, 2001b, p 76.

Farquhar-Smith WP, Egertova M, Bradbury EJ, et al. Cannabinoid CB_1 receptor expression in rat spinal cord. *Mol Cell Neurosci* 2000; 15:510–521.

Farquhar-Smith WP, Jaggar SI, Rice ASC. Attenuation of nerve growth factor-induced visceral hyperalgesia via cannabinoid CB1 and CB2-like receptors. *Pain* 2002; 97:11–21.

Felder CC, Briley EM, Axelrod J, et al. Anandamide, an endogenous cannabimimetic eicosanoid, binds to the cloned human cannabinoid receptor and stimulates receptor- mediated signal transduction. *Proc Natl Acad Sci USA* 1993; 90:7656–7660.

Felder CC, Nielsen A, Briley EM, et al. Isolation and measurement of the endogenous cannabinoid receptor agonist, anandamide, in brain and peripheral tissues of human and rat. *FEBS Lett* 1996; 393:231–235.

Fowler CJ, Jacobsson SOP. Cellular transport of anandamide, 2-arachidonoylglycerol and palmitoylethanolamide—target for drug development? *Prostaglandins Leukot Essent Fatty Acids* 2002; 66:193–200.

Fowler CJ, Stenstrom A, Tiger G. Ibuprofen inhibits the metabolism of the endogenous cannabimimetic agent anandamide. *Pharmacol Toxicol* 1997; 80:103–107.

Fowler CJ, Janson U, Johnson RM, et al. Inhibition of anandamide hydrolysis by the enantiomers of ibuprofen, ketorolac and flurbiprofen. *Arch Biochem Biophys* 1999; 362:191–196.

Fowler CJ, Jonsson K-O, Tiger G. Fatty acid amid hydrolase: biochemistry, pharmacology and therapeutic possibilities for an enzyme hydrolysing anandamide, 2-arachidonylglycerol, palmitoylethanolamide and oleamide. *Biochem Pharmacol* 2001; 62:517–526.

Fox A, Kesingland A, Gentry C, et al. The role of central and peripheral cannabinoid_1 receptors in the antihyperalgesic activity of cannabinoids in a model of neuropathic pain. *Pain* 2001; 92:91–100.

Fride E, Barg J, Levy R, et al. Low doses of anandamide inhibit pharmacological effects of delta 9-tetrahydrocannabinol. *J Pharmacol Exp Ther* 1995; 272:699–707.

Galiegue S, Mary S, Marchand J, et al. Expression of central and peripheral cannabinoid receptors in human immune tissues and leukocyte subpopulations. *Eur J Biochem* 1995; 232:54–61.

Garcia DE, Brown S, Hille B, Mackie K. Protein kinase C disrupts cannabinoid activity by phosphorylation of the CB1 cannabinoid receptor. *J Neurosci* 1998; 18:2834–2848.

Gebremedhin D, Lange AR, Campbell WB, et al. Cannabinoid CB1 receptor of cat cerebral arterial muscle functions to inhibit L-type Ca^{2+} channel current. *Am J Physiol* 1999; 276:H2085–H2093.

Gerdeman GL, Ronesi J, Lovinger DM, Aanonsen L. Postsynaptic endocannabinoid release is critical to long-term depression in the striatum. *Nat Neurosci* 2002; 5:446–450.

Giang DK, Cravatt BF. Molecular characterization of human and mouse fatty acid amide hydrolases. *Proc Natl Acad Sci USA* 1997; 94:2238–2242.

Granberg M, Fowler CJ, Jacobsson SOP. Effects of the cannabimimetic fatty acid derivatives 2-arachidonylglycerol, anandamide, palmitoylethanolamide and methanandamide upon IgE-dependent antigen-induceδ β-hexosaminidase, serotonin and TNF α release from rat RBL-2H3 basophilic leukaemia cells. *Naunyn Schmiedebergs Arch Pharmacol* 2001; 364:66–73.

Guhring H, Schuster J, Hamza M, et al. HU210 shows higher efficacy and potency than morphine after intrathecal administration in the mouse formalin test. *Eur J Pharmacol* 2001; 429:127–134.

Guzman M, Galve-Roperh I, Sanchez C. Ceramide: a new second messenger of cannabinoid action. *Trends Pharmacol Sci* 2001; 22:19–22.

Hanus L, Breuer A, Tchilibon S, et al. HU 308: A specific agonist for CB(2), a peripheral cannabinoid receptor. *Proc Natl Acad Sci USA* 1999; 96:14228–14233.

Hanus L, Abu-lafi S, Fride E, et al. 2-Arachidonyl glycerol ether, an endogenous agonist of the cannabinoid CB1 receptor. *PNAS* 2001; 98:3662–3665.

Herkenham M, Lynn AB, Johnson MR, et al. Characterization and localization of cannabinoid receptors in rat brain: a quantitative in vitro autoradiographic study. *J Neurosci* 1991; 11:563–583.

Herzberg U, Eliav E, Bennett GJ, Kopin IJ. The analgesic effects of R(+)-WIN55,212-2 mesylate, a high affinity cannabinoid agonist, in a rat model of neuropathic pain. *Neurosci Lett* 1997; 221:157–160.

Hillard CJ. Biochemistry and pharmacology of the endocannabinoids arachidonylethanolamide and 2-arachidonylglycerol. *Prostaglandins Other Lipid Mediat* 2000; 61:3–18.

Hohmann AG, Herkenham M. Regulation of cannabinoid and mu opioid receptors in rat lumbar spinal cord following neonatal capsaicin treatment. *Neurosci Lett* 1998; 252:13–16.

Hohmann AG, Herkenham M. Cannabinoid receptors undergo axonal flow in sensory nerves. *Neuroscience* 1999a; 92:1171–1175.

Hohmann AG, Herkenham M. Localization of central cannabinoid CB1 receptor messenger RNA in neuronal subpopulations of rat dorsal root ganglia: a double-label in situ hybridization study. *Neuroscience* 1999b; 90:923–931.

Hohmann AG, Martin WJ, Tsou K, Walker JM. Inhibition of noxious stimulus-evoked activity of spinal cord dorsal horn neurons by the cannabinoid WIN 55,212-2. *Life Sci* 1995; 56:2111–2118.

Hohmann AG, Tsou K, Walker JM. Cannabinoid modulation of wide dynamic range neurons in the lumbar dorsal horn of the rat by spinally administered WIN55, 212. *Neurosci Lett* 1998; 257:119–122.

Hohmann AG, Briley EM, Herkenham M. Pre- and postsynaptic distribution of cannabinoid and mu opioid receptors in rat spinal cord. *Brain Res* 1999a; 822:17–25.

Hohmann AG, Tsou K, Walker JM. Cannabinoid suppression of noxious heat-evoked activity in wide dynamic range neurons in the lumbar dorsal horn of the rat. *J Neurophysiol* 1999b; 81:575–583.

Hohmann AG, Neely MH, Suplita RL, et al. Endocannabinoid mechanisms of stress-induced analgesia. In: *2002 Symposium on the Cannabinoids.* International Cannabinoid Research Society, 2002, p 30.

Howlett AC. The CB1 cannabinoid receptor in the brain. *Neurobiol Dis* 1998; 5:405–416.

Hsieh C, Brown S, Derleth C, Mackie K. Internalisation and recycling of the CB1 cannabinoid receptor *J Neurochem* 2000; 732:501–

Huang SM, Strangman NM, Walker JM. Liquid chromatographic-mass spectrometric measurement of the endogenous cannabinoid 2-arachidonylglycerol in the spinal cord and peripheral nervous system. *Acta Pharmacol Sin* 1999; 20:1098–1102.

Ibrahim MM, Mata HP, Deng H, et al. AM1241, a selective cannabinoid CB2 receptor antagonist, relieves neuropathic pain. *Soc Neurosci Abstr* 2001; 27:716.16.

Iversen L. *The Science of Marijuana.* Oxford: Oxford University Press, 2000.

Jack DB. Alaimides: a new approach to the treatment of inflammation *Drugs News Perspect* 1996; 9:93–98.

Jacobsson SOP, Fowler CJ. Characterisation of palmitoylethanolamide transport in mouse neuro-2a neuroblastoma cells and rat RBL-2H3 basophilic leukaemia cells: comparison with anandamide. *Br J Pharmacol* 2001; 132:1743–1754.

Jaggar SI, Hasnie FS, Sellaturay S, Rice ASC. The anti-hyperalgesic actions of the cannabinoid anandamide and the putative CB2 agonist palmitoylethanolamide investigated in models of visceral and somatic inflammatory pain. *Pain* 1998; 76:189–199.

Jaggar SI, Scott HCF, Rice ASC. Inflammation of the rat urinary bladder is associated with a referred thermal hyperalgesia which is nerve growth factor dependent. *Br J Anaesth* 1999; 83:442–448.

Jennings EA, Vaughan CW, Christie MJ. Effects of cannabinoids on neurons in the superficial medullary dorsal horn of the rat. *Soc Neurosci Abstr* 2000; 26:812.13.

Jennings EA, Vaughan CW, Christie MJ. Cannabinoid actions on rat superficial medullary dorsal horn neurons in vitro. *J Physiol (Lond)* 2001; 534:805–812.

Jeon YJ, Yang KH, Pulaski JT, Kaminski NE. Attenuation of inducible nitric oxide synthase gene expression by delta 9-tetrahydrocannabinol is mediated through the inhibition of nuclear factor- kappa B/Rel activation. *Mol Pharmacol* 1996; 50:334–341.

Katayama K, Ueda N, Kurahashi Y, et al. Distribution of anandamide amidohydrolase in rat tissues with special reference to small intestine. *Biochim Biophys Acta* 1997; 1347:212–218.

Kathuria S, Gaetani S, Fegley D, et al. Modulation of anxiety through blockade of anandamide hydrolysis. *Nat Med* 2003; 9(1):76–81.

Kearn CS, Greenberg MJ, DiCamelli R, et al. Relationships between ligand affinities for the cerebellar cannabinoid receptor CB1 and the induction of GDP/GTP exchange. *J Neurochem* 1999; 72:2379–2387.

Ko MC, Woods JH. Local administration of delta9-tetrahydrocannabinol attenuates capsaicin-induced thermal nociception in rhesus monkeys: a peripheral cannabinoid action. *Psychopharmacology (Berl)* 1999; 143:322–326.

Kouznetsova M, Kelley B, Shen M, Thayer SA. Desensitization of cannabinoid-mediated presynaptic inhibition of neurotransmission between rat hippocampal neurons in culture. *Mol Pharmacol* 2002; 61:477–485.

Kreitzer AC, Regehr WG. Retrograde inhibition of presynaptic calcium influx by endogenous cannabinoids at excitatory synapses onto Purkinje cells. *Neuron* 2001; 29:717–727.

Kurahashi Y, Ueda N, Suzuki H, et al. Reversible hydrolysis and synthesis of anandamide demonstrated by recombinant rat fatty-acid amide hydrolase. *Biochem Biophys Res Commun* 1997; 237:512–515.

Lambert DM, Di Marzo V. The palmitoylethanolamide and oleamide enigmas: are these two fatty acid amides cannabimimetic? *Curr Med Chem* 1999; 6:757–773.

Lambert DM, DiPaolo FG, Sonveaux P, et al. Analogues and homologues of N-palmitoylethanolamide, a putative endogenous CB(2) cannabinoid, as potential ligands for the cannabinoid receptors. *Biochim Biophys Acta* 1999; 1440:266–274.

Lambert DM, Vandevoorde S, Jonsson K-O, Fowler CJ. The palmitoylethanolamide family: a new class of anti-inflammatory agent. *Curr Med Chem* 2002; 9:663–674.

Ledent C, Valverde O, Cossu G, et al. Unresponsiveness to cannabinoids and reduced addictive effects of opiates in CB1 receptor knockout mice. *Science* 1999; 283:401–404.

Lever IJ, Malcangio M. CB1 receptor antagonist SR141716A increases capsaicin-evoked release of substance P from the adult mouse spinal cord. *Br J Pharmacol* 2002; 135:21–24.

Levi-Montalcini R, Skaper SD, Dal Toso R, Petrelli L, Leon A. Nerve growth factor: from neutrophin to neurokine. *Trends Neurosci* 1996; 19:514–520.

Li J, Daughters RS, Bullis C, et al. The cannabinoid receptor agonist WIN 55,212-2 blocks the development of hyperalgesia produced by capsaicin in rats. *Pain* 1999; 81:25–34.

Lichtman AH, Martin BR. Cannabinoid-induced antinociception is mediated by a spinal alpha 2-noradrenergic mechanism. *Brain Res* 1991; 559:309–314.

Lichtman AH, Cook SA, Martin BR. Investigation of brain sites mediating cannabinoid-induced antinociception in rats: evidence supporting periaqueductal gray involvement. *J Pharmacol Exp Ther* 1996; 276:585–593.

Mackie K, Devane WA, Hille B. Anandamide, an endogenous cannabinoid, inhibits calcium currents as a partial agonist in N18 neuroblastoma cells. *Mol Pharmacol* 1993; 44:498–503.

Mackie K, Lai Y, Westenbroek R, Mitchell R. Cannabinoids activate an inwardly rectifying potassium conductance and inhibit Q-type calcium currents in AtT20 cells transfected with rat brain cannabinoid receptor. *J Neurosci* 1995; 15:6552–6561.

Maejima T, Hashimoto K, Yoshida T, et al. Presynaptic inhibition caused by retrograde signal from metabotropic glutamate to cannabinoid receptors. *Neuron* 2001; 31:463–475.

Mailleux P, Vanderhaeghen JJ. Distribution of neuronal cannabinoid receptor in the adult rat brain: a comparative receptor binding radioautography and in situ hybridization histochemistry. *Neuroscience* 1992; 48:655–668.

Malan TP, Ibrahim MM, Lai J, et al. CB2 cannabinoid receptor agonists: pain relief without the psychoactive effects? *Curr Opin Pharmacol* 2003; 3:62–67.

Malfait AM, Gallily R, Sumariwalla PF, et al. The nonpsychoactive cannabis constituent cannabidiol is an oral anti-arthritic therapeutic in murine collagen-induced arthritis. *Proc Natl Acad Sci USA* 2000; 97:9561–9566.

Manzanares J, Corchero J, Romero J, et al. Pharmacological and biochemical interactions between opioids and cannabinoids. *Trends Pharmacol Sci* 1999; 20:287–294.

Mao J, Price DD, Lu J, et al. Two distinctive antinociceptive systems in rats with pathological pain. *Neurosci Lett* 2000; 280:13–16.

Marsicano G, Wotjak CT, Azad SC, et al. The endogenous cannabinoid system controls extinction of aversive memories. *Nature* 2002; 418:530–534.

Martin BR, Lichtman AH. Cannabinoid transmission and pain perception. *Neurobiol Dis* 1998; 5:447–461.

Martin BR, Compton DR, Thomas BF, et al. Behavioral, biochemical, and molecular modeling evaluations of cannabinoid analogs. *Pharmacol Biochem Behav* 1991; 40:471–478.

Martin WJ, Hohmann AG, Walker JM. Suppression of noxious stimulus-evoked activity in the ventral posterolateral nucleus of the thalamus by a cannabinoid agonist: correlation between electrophysiological and antinociceptive effects. *J Neurosci* 1996; 16:6601–6611.

Martin WJ, Loo CM, Basbaum AI. Spinal cannabinoids are anti-allodynic in rats with persistent inflammation. *Pain* 1999; 82:199–205.

Mason D-JJ, Lowe J, Welch SP. Cannabinoid modulation of dynorphin A: correlation to cannabinoid-induced antinociception. *Eur J Pharmacol* 1999; 378:237–248.

Matsuda LA, Lolait SJ, Brownstein MJ, et al. Structure of a cannabinoid receptor and functional expression of the cloned cDNA. *Nature* 1990; 346:561–564.

Matsuda LA, Bonner TI, Lolait SJ. Localization of cannabinoid receptor mRNA in rat brain. *J Comp Neurol* 1993; 327:535–550.

Mazzari S, Canella R, Leon A. N-(2-hydroxyethyl)hexadecamide reduces mechanical hyperalgesia following sciatic nerve constriction injury *Soc Neurosci Abstr* 1995; 21:263.15.

Mazzari S, Canella R, Petrelli L, et al. N-(2-Hydroxyethyl)hexadecanamide is orally active in reducing edema formation and inflammatory hyperalgesia by down-regulating mast cell activation. *Eur J Pharmacol* 1996; 300:227–236.

McAllister SD, Glass M. CB(1) and CB(2) receptor-mediated signalling: a focus on endocannabinoids. *Prostaglandins Leukot Essent Fatty Acids* 2002; 66:161–171.

McAllister SD, Griffin G, Satin LS, Abood ME. Cannabinoid receptors can activate and inhibit G protein-coupled inwardly rectifying potassium channels in a xenopus oocyte expression system. *J Pharmacol Exp Ther* 1999; 291:618–626.

McMahon SB. Neuronal and behavioural consequences of chemical inflammation of rat urinary bladder. *Agents Actions* 1988; 25:231–233.

McMahon SB. Are there fundamental differences in the peripheral mechanisms of visceral and somatic pain? *Behav Brain Sci* 1997; 20:381–391.

McMahon SB, Abel C. A model for the study of visceral pain states: chronic inflammation of the chronic decerebrate rat urinary bladder by irritant chemicals. *Pain* 1987; 28:109–127.

McMahon SB, Koltzenburg M. Changes in the afferent innervation of the inflamed urinary bladder. In: Mayer EA, Raybould EA (Eds). *Basic and Clinical Aspects of Abdominal Pain.* Amsterdam, Elsevier, pp 155–172.

Mechoulam R, Ben Shabat S, Hanus L, et al. Identification of an endogenous 2-monoglyceride, present in canine gut, that binds to cannabinoid receptors. *Biochem Pharmacol* 1995; 50:83–90.

Meng ID, Manning BH, Martin WJ, Fields HL. An analgesic circuit activated by cannabinoids. *Nature* 1998; 395:381–383.

Millns PJ, Chapman V, Kendall DA. Cannabinoid inhibition of the capsaicin-induced calcium response in rat dorsal root ganglion neurones. *Br J Pharmacol* 2001; 132:969–971.

Montgomery JM, Madison DW. The grass roots of synapse suppression. *Neuron* 2001; 29:567–570.

Morisset V, Urban L. Cannabinoid-induced presynaptic inhibition of glutamatinergic EPSCs in substantial gelatinosa neurons of the rat spinal cord. *J Neurophysiol* 2001; 86:40–48.

Morisset V, Ahluwalia J, Nagy I, Urban L. Possible mechanisms of cannabinoid-induced antinociception in the spinal cord. *Eur J Pharmacol* 2001; 429:93–100.

Munro S, Thomas KL, Abu Shaar M. Molecular characterization of a peripheral receptor for cannabinoids. *Nature* 1993; 365:61–65.

Nie J, Lewis DL. The proximal and distal-terminal tail domains of the CB1 cannabinoid receptor mediate G protein coupling. *Neuroscience* 2002; 107:161–176.

Nilsson G, Forsberg Nilsson K, Xiang Z, et al. Human mast cells express functional trkA and are a source of nerve growth factor. *Eur J Immunol* 1997; 27:2295–2301.

O'Shaugnessy WB. On the preparations of the Indian hemp or gunjah (*Cannabis indica):* their effects on the animal system in health, and their utility in the treatment of tetanus and other convulsive diseases. *Trans Med Phys Soc Bengal, 1838–1840* 1839:421–461.

Oaklander AL, Belzberg AJ. Unilateral nerve injury down-regulates mRNA for Na+ channel SCN10A bilaterally in rat dorsal root ganglia. *Brain Res Mol Brain Res* 1997; 52:162–165.

Oaklander AL, Romans K, Horasek S, et al. Unilateral postherpetic neuralgia is associated with bilateral sensory neuron damage. *Ann Neurol* 1998; 44:789–795.

Ohno-Shosaku T, Maejima T, Kano M. Endogenous cannabinoids mediate retrograde signals from depolarized postsynaptic neurons to presynaptic terminals. *Neuron* 2001; 29:729–738.

Onaivi ES, Chakrabarti A, Chaudhuri G. Cannabinoid receptor genes. *Progress Neurobiol* 1996; 48:275–305.

Onaivi ES, Leonard CM, Ishiguro H, et al. Endocannabinoids and cannabinoid receptor genetics. *Progress Neurobiol* 2002; 66:307–344.

Ong WY, Mackie K. A light and electron microscopic study of the CB1 cannabinoid receptor in the primate spinal cord. *J Neurocytol* 1999; 28:39–45.

Patton GC, Coffey C, Carlin JB, et al. Cannabis use and mental health in young people: cohort study. *BMJ* 2002; 325:1195–1198.

Pertwee RG. Cannabinoids and pain. *Progress Neurobiol* 2001; 63:569–611.

Pertwee RG, Gibson TM, Stevenson LA, et al. 0-1057, a potent water-soluble cannabinoid receptor agonist with antinociceptive properties. *Br J Pharmacol* 2000; 129:1577–1584.

Pettit DA, Harrison MP, Olson JM, et al. Immunohistochemical localization of the neural cannabinoid receptor in rat brain. *J Neurosci Res* 1998; 51:391–402.

Piomelli D, Beltramo M, Giuffrida A, Stella N. Endogenous cannabinoid signaling. *Neurobiol Dis* 1998; 5:462–473.

Porter AC, Sauer JM, Knierman MD, et al. Characterization of a novel endocannabinoid, virodhamine, with antagonist activity at the CB1 receptor. *J Pharmacol Exp Ther* 2002; 301:1020–1024.

Puffenbarger R, Boothe AC, Cabral GA. Cannabinoids inhibit LPS-inducible cytokine mRNA expression in rat microglial cells. *Glia* 2000; 29:58–69.

Pugh GJ, Abood ME, Welch SP. Antisense oligodeoxynucleotides to the kappa-1 receptor block the antinociceptive effects of delta 9-THC in the spinal cord. *Brain Res* 1995; 689:157–158.

Pugh GJ, Smith PB, Dombrowski DS, Welch SP. The role of endogenous opioids in enhancing the antinociception produced by the combination of delta 9-tetrahydrocannabinol and morphine in the spinal cord. *J Pharmacol Exp Ther* 1996; 279:608–616.

Pugh GJ, Mason D-JJ, Combs V, Welch SP. Involvement of dynorphin B in the antinociceptive effects of the cannabinoid CP55,940 in the spinal cord. *J Pharmacol Exp Ther* 1997; 281:730–737.

Rice ASC. Cannabinoids and pain. *Current Opinion in Investigational Drugs* 2001a; 2:399–414.

Rice ASC, Brooks JW, Thompson SWN. Spinal intrathecal administration of the cannabinoid WIN55,212-2 attenuates pain behaviour in the formalin model. *Abstracts: 10th World Congress on Pain.* Seattle: IASP Press, 2002, p 282.

Richardson JD, Aanonsen L, Hargreaves KM. Antihyperalgesic effects of spinal cannabinoids. *Eur J Pharmacol* 1998a; 345:145–153.

Richardson JD, Aanonsen L, Hargreaves KM. Hypoactivity of the spinal cannabinoid system results in NMDA-dependent hyperalgesia. *J Neurosci* 1998b; 18:451–457.

Richardson JD, Kilo S, Hargreaves KM. Cannabinoids reduce hyperalgesia and inflammation via interaction with peripheral CB1 receptors. *Pain* 1998c; 75:111–119.

Romero J, Hillard CJ, Calero M, Rabano A. Fatty acid amide hydrolase localization in the human central nervous system: an immunohistochemical study. *Mol Brain Res* 2002; 100:85–93.

Ross RA, Brockie HC, Pertwee RG. Inhibition of nitric oxide production in RAW264.7 macrophages by cannabinoids and palmitoylethanolamide. *Eur J Pharmacol* 2000; 401:121–130.

Ross RA, Coutts AA, McFarlane SM, et al. Actions of cannabinoid receptor ligands on rat cultured sensory neurones: implications for antinociception. *Neuropharmacology* 2001; 40:221–232.

Sacerdote P, Massi P, Panerai AE, Parolaro D. In vivo and in vitro treatment with the synthetic cannabinoid CP55, 940 decreases the in vitro migration of macrophages in the rat: involvement of both CB1 and CB2 receptors. *J Neuroimmunol* 2000; 109:155–163.

Salio C, Fischer J, Franzoni MF, et al. CB1-cannabinoid and μ-opioid receptor co-localization on postsynaptic target in the rat dorsal horn. *Neuroreport* 2001; 12:3689–3692.

Salio C, Doly S, Fischer J, et al. Neuronal and astrocytic localization of the cannabinoid receptor-1 in the dorsal horn of the rat spinal cord. *Neurosci Lett* 2002a; 329:13–16.

Salio C, Fischer J, Franzoni MF, Conrath M. Pre- and postsynaptic localizations of the CB1 cannabinoid receptor in the dorsal horn of the rat spinal cord. *Neuroscience* 2002b; 110:755–764.

Sanudo-Pena MC, Strangman NM, Mackie K, et al. CB1 receptor localization in rat spinal cord and roots, dorsal root ganglion and peripheral nerve. *Acta Pharmacol Sin* 1999; 20:1115–1120.

Schatz AR, Lee M, Condie RB, et al. Cannabinoid receptors CB1 and CB2: a characterization of expression and adenylate cyclase modulation within the immune system. *Toxicol Appl Pharmacol* 1997; 142:278–287.

Scott HCF, Jaggar SI, Rice ASC. Mechanical hyperalgesia is referred to the hind limb following inflammation of the urinary bladder in the rat. *J Physiol Lond* 1998; 507:18.

Select Committee on Science and Technology and House of Lords. *Cannabis: The Scientific and Medical Evidence.* London: HMSO, 1998, p 9.

Shen M, Piser TM, Seybold VS, Thayer SA. Cannabinoid receptor agonists inhibit glutamatergic synaptic transmission in rat hippocampal cultures. *J Neurosci* 1996; 16:4322–4334.

Shire D, Carillon C, Kaghad M, et al. An amino-terminal variant of the central cannabinoid receptor resulting from alternative splicing [published erratum appears in *J Biol Chem* 1996; 271(52):33706]. *J Biol Chem* 1995; 270:3726–3731.

Siegling A, Hofmann HA, Denzer D, et al. Cannabinoid CB1 receptor upregulation in a rat model of chronic neuropathic pain. *Eur J Pharmacol* 2001; 415:R5–R7.

Smart D, Gunthorpe MJ, Jerman JC, et al. The endogenous lipid anandamide is a full agonist at the human vanilloid receptor (hVR1). *Br J Pharmacol* 2000; 129:227–230.

Smith PB, Martin BR. Spinal mechanisms of delta 9-tetrahydrocannabinol-induced analgesia. *Brain Res* 1992; 578:8–12.

Smith PB, Welch SP, Martin BR. Interactions between delta 9-tetrahydrocannabinol and kappa opioids in mice. *J Pharmacol Exp Ther* 1994; 268:1381–1387.

Smith FL, Fujimore K, Lowe J, Welch SP. Characterisation of delta 9 tetrahydrocannabinol and anandamide antinociception in nonarthritic and arthritic rats. *Pharmacol Biochem Behav* 1998; 60:183–191.

Stella N, Schweitzer P, Piomelli D. A second endogenous cannabinoid that modulates long-term potentiation. *Nature* 1997; 388:773–778.

Stella N, Franklin A, Mhyre A, et al. Microglial cells produce docosatetraenyethanolamide: evidence for a third endocannabinoid. *2001 Symposium on the Cannabinoids.* Burlington, VT: International Cannabinoid Research Society, 2001, p 23.

Strangman NM, Walker JM. Cannabinoid WIN 55,212-2 inhibits the activity-dependent facilitation of spinal nociceptive responses. *J Neurophysiol* 1999; 82:472–477.

Sugiura T, Kondo S, Kishimoto S, et al. Evidence that 2-arachidonoylglycerol but not N-palmitoylethanolamine or anandamide is the physiological ligand for the cannabinoid CB2 receptor. Comparison of the agonistic activities of various cannabinoid receptor ligands in HL-60 cells. *J Biol Chem* 2000; 275:605–612.

Sugiura T, Kobayashi S, Oka S, Waku K. Biosynthesis and degradation of anandamide and 2-arachidonylglycerol and their possible physiological significance. *Prostaglandins Leukot Essent Fatty Acids* 2002; 66:173–192.

Tal M, Liberman R. Local injection of nerve growth factor (NGF) triggers degranulation of mast cells in rat paw. *Neurosci Lett* 1997; 221:129–132.

Thomas EA, Cravatt BF, Danielson PE, et al. Fatty acid amide hydrolase, the degradative enzyme for anandamide and oleamide, has selective distribution in neurons within the rat central nervous system. *J Neurosci Res* 1997; 50:1047–1052.

Tsou K, Lowitz KA, Hohmann AG, et al. Suppression of noxious stimulus-evoked expression of Fos protein-like immunoreactivity in rat spinal cord by a selective cannabinoid agonist. *Neuroscience* 1996; 70:791–798.

Tsou K, Brown S, Mackie K, et al. Immunohistochemical distribution of cannabinoid CB1 receptors in the rat central nervous system. *Neuroscience* 1998; 83:393–411.

Varma N, Carlson GC, Ledent C, Alger BE. Metabotropic glutamate receptors drive the endocannabinoid system in hippocampus. *J Neurosci* 2001; 21 (188RC):1–5.

Vasquez C, Lewis DL. The CB_1 cannabinoid receptor can sequester G-proteins, making them unavailable to couple to other receptors. *J Neurosci* 1999; 19:9271–9280.

Vaughan CW, McGregor IS, Christie MJ. Cannabinoid receptor activation inhibits GABAergic neurotransmission in rostral ventromedial medulla neurons in vitro. *Br J Pharmacol* 1999; 127:935–940.

Vaughan CW, Connor M, Bagley EE, Christie MJ. Actions of cannabinoids on membrane properties and synaptic transmission in rat periaqueductal gray neurons in vitro. *Mol Pharmacol* 2000; 57:288–295.

Walker JM, Huang SM, Strangman NM, et al. Pain modulation by release of the endogenous cannabinoid anandamide. *Proc Natl Acad Sci USA* 1999; 96:12198–12203.

Walter LA, Franklin A, Myhre A, et al. Microglial cells produce endocannabinoids and express functional cannabinoid receptors. *Soc Neurosci Abstr* 2001; 634.16.

Walter L, Franklin A, Witting A, et al. At the leading edge: non-psychotrophic cannabinoid receptors regulate microglial migration. In: *2002 Symposium on the Cannabinoids.* International Cannabinoid Research Society, 2002, p 45.

Watkins LR, Milligan ED, Maier SF. Spinal cord glia: new players in pain. *Pain* 2001; 93:201–205.

Welch SP. Blockade of cannabinoid-induced antinociception by naloxone benzoylhydrazone (NalBZH). *Pharmacol Biochem Behav* 1994; 49:929–934.

Welch SP, Stevens DL. Antinociceptive activity of intrathecally administered cannabinoids alone, and in combination with morphine, in mice. *J Pharmacol Exp Ther* 1992; 262:10–18.

Welch SP, Dunlow LD, Patrick GS, Razdan RK. Characterization of anandamide- and fluoroanandamide-induced antinociception and cross-tolerance to delta 9-THC after intrathecal administration to mice: blockade of delta 9-THC-induced antinociception. *J Pharmacol Exp Ther* 1995a; 273:1235–1244.

Welch SP, Dunlow LD, Patrick GS, Razdan RK. Characterization of anandamide- and fluoroanandamide-induced antinociception and cross-tolerance to delta 9-THC after intrathecal administration to mice: blockade of delta 9-THC-induced antinociception. *J Pharmacol Exp Ther* 1995b; 273:1235–1244.

Wilson DM, Peart J, Martin BR, et al. Physiochemical and pharmacological characterization of a [Delta]9-THC aerosol generated by a metered dose inhaler. *Drug Alcohol Depend* 2002; 67(3):259–267.

Wilson RI, Nicoll RA. Endogenous cannabinoids mediate retrograde signalling at hippocampal synapses. *Nature* 2001; 410:588–592.

Wilson RI, Nicoll RA. Endocannabinoid signaling in the brain. *Science* 2002; 296:678–682.

Wilson RI, Kunos G, Nicoll RA. Presynaptic specificity of endocannabinoid signaling in the hippocampus. *Neuron* 2001; 31:453–462.

Woolf CJ, Ma QP, Allchorne A, Poole S. Peripheral cell types contributing to the hyperalgesic action of nerve growth factor in inflammation. *J Neurosci* 1996; 16:2716–2723.

Yoshida T, Hashimoto K, Zimmer A, et al. The cannabinoid CB1 receptor mediates retrograde signals for depolarisation-induced suppression of inhibition in cerebellar Purkinje cells. *J Neurosci* 2002; 22:1690–1697.

Zammit S, Allebeck P, Andreasson S, et al. Self reported cannabis use as a risk factor for schizophrenia in Swedish conscripts of 1969: historical cohort study. *BMJ* 2002; 325:1199.

Zeltser R, Seltzer Z, Eisen A, et al. Suppression of neuropathic pain behavior in rats by a non-psychotropic synthetic cannabinoid with NMDA receptor-blocking properties. *Pain* 1991; 47:95-103.

Zias J, Stark H, Sellgman J, et al. Early medical use of cannabis. *Nature* 1993; 363:215.

Zimmer A, Zimmer AM, Hohmann AG, et al. Increased mortality, hypoactivity, and hypoalgesia in cannabinoid CB1 receptor knockout mice. *Proc Natl Acad Sci* 1999; 96:5780–5785.

Zygmunt PM, Petersson J, Andersson DA, et al. Vanilloid receptors on sensory nerves mediate the vasodilator action of anandamide. *Nature* 1999; 400:452–457.

Correspondence to: Andrew S.C. Rice, MBBS, MD, FRCA, Pain Research Group, Department of Anaesthetics, Faculty of Medicine, Imperial College of Science, Technology and Medicine, Chelsea and Westminster Hospital Campus, 369 Fulham Road, London SW10 9NH, United Kingdom. Tel: (0)208-746-8156; Fax: (0)208-237-5109; email: a.rice@imperial.ac.uk.

Proceedings of the 10th World Congress on Pain,
Progress in Pain Research and Management, Vol. 24,
edited by Jonathan O. Dostrovsky, Daniel B. Carr, and
Martin Koltzenburg, IASP Press, Seattle, © 2003.

38

Nociceptin, Nocistatin, and Pain[1]

Hanns Ulrich Zeilhofer,[a] Rainer K. Reinscheid,[b] and Emiko Okuda-Ashitaka[c,d]

[a]*Institute of Experimental and Clinical Pharmacology and Toxicology, University of Erlangen-Nürnberg, Erlangen, Germany;* [b]*Department of Pharmacology, University of California Irvine, Irvine, California, USA;* [c]*Department of Medical Chemistry, Kansai Medical University, Moriguchi, Osaka, Japan;* [d]*Information and Cell Function, PRESTO Japan Science and Technology Corporation, Moriguchi, Osaka, Japan*

The discovery of the first opioid receptor, the δ-opioid receptor, by expression cloning (Kieffer et al. 1992) has led not only to the identification of the expected μ and κ receptors, but also to that of a fourth, unperceived receptor, which does not bind classical opioids (Bunzow et al. 1994; Fukuda et al. 1994; Mollereau et al. 1994; Wang et al. 1994). This "orphan" receptor has therefore been termed opioid-receptor-like 1 (ORL-1) receptor (Mollereau et al. 1994). Only a year later a 17-amino-acid neuropeptide binding to the ORL-1 receptor was identified by two independent groups, which called it nociceptin (Meunier et al. 1995) or orphanin FQ (Reinscheid et al. 1995). The corresponding ORL-1 receptor is now designated N/OFQ peptide (NOP) receptor (Cox et al. 2000). Both the N/OFQ peptide and the NOP receptor share a high degree of homology with classical opioid peptides (namely dynorphin A) and with classical opioid receptors (namely the κ-opioid receptor), respectively. N/OFQ is released after proteolytic cleavage from a larger precursor polypeptide called pre-pro-N/OFQ (ppN/OFQ; Meunier et al. 1995; Saito et al. 1995; Houtani et al. 1996; Nothacker et al. 1996; Pan et al. 1996). In addition to the cleavage sites necessary for the release of N/OFQ, ppN/OFQ contains additional sites, which may give rise to other neuropeptides with potential biological activity. Three of these peptides, N/OFQ2 (Florin et al. 1997), a carboxyl terminal peptide (Mathis et al. 2001; Rossi et

[1] Based on a Congress workshop.

al. 2002), and nocistatin (NST; Okuda-Ashitaka et al. 1998) have been reported to have biological activity, but no receptors have been identified yet.

Both the NOP receptor and the N/OFQ precursor peptide ppN/OFQ are widely expressed throughout the mammalian nervous system. Particularly intense staining is seen in areas involved in nociception such as the spinal cord dorsal horn and around the central canal, as well as in areas involved in fear and stress control such as the amygdala (Neal et al. 1997a,b).

PHARMACOLOGICAL EFFECTS OF N/OFQ AND NST ON NOCICEPTION IN VIVO

Since the discovery of N/OFQ and its receptor, great progress has been made in understanding its role in numerous physiological and pathophysiological processes (for a recent review see Caló et al. 2000). The close structural relationship of N/OFQ and its receptor to classical opioid peptides and their receptors has drawn researchers' attention to their roles in nociception. Meanwhile, numerous studies have reported either pro- or antinociceptive effects of N/OFQ in a variety of animal models of pain, probably depending on the dose and site of administration (Caló et al. 2000; Ito et al. 2000). At the level of the spinal cord, N/OFQ possesses both pro- and antinociceptive actions depending on the dose. Low doses of N/OFQ (0.05 amol–0.5 pmol) injected intrathecally (i.t.) induce allodynia and hyperalgesia (Okuda-Ashitaka et al. 1996; Hara et al. 1997) and aggravate the second phase of 1% formalin-induced pain (Nakano et al. 2000). Higher doses of N/OFQ (0.15–1.5 nmol) inhibit nociceptive behavior in both phases of the formalin test (Erb et al. 1997; Nakano et al. 2000) and in a variety of other pain tests (e.g., Xu et al. 1996; Inoue et al. 1999). The aggravating effect of N/OFQ in the formalin test is blocked by JTC-801 (Muratani et al. 2002), a non-peptidyl N/OFQ-receptor antagonist (Shinkai et al. 2000). The antinociceptive effect of N/OFQ on formalin-evoked pain is absent in NOP-receptor-deficient mice (Ahmadi et al. 2001a).

NST was first characterized as a functional antagonist that reverses the pronociceptive effect of N/OFQ and also that of prostaglandin E_2 (Okuda-Ashitaka et al. 1998). The simultaneous i.t. injection of femto- to picomolar doses of NST attenuates pronociceptive effects induced by 25 fmol N/OFQ, and an anti-NST antibody decreases the threshold for N/OFQ-induced allodynia (Okuda-Ashitaka et al. 1998). NST also blocks the aggravation of formalin-induced pain by N/OFQ at low doses, but does not affect the inhibitory effect of high doses of N/OFQ in the formalin test (Yamamoto and Sakashita 1999; Nakano et al. 2000). Fig. 1 summarizes the relationship between NST and N/OFQ with respect to effective doses and pain in mice. At nanomolar doses, NST can also facilitate nociceptive behavior in the rat formalin test when applied via chronically implanted catheters (Zeilhofer et al. 2000). Meanwhile, several studies have shown that NST can antagonize many biological effects induced by N/OFQ, such as morphine analgesia (Zhao et al. 1999), impairment of learning and memory (Hiramatsu and Inoue 1999), anxiety-like behavior (Gavioli et al. 2002), food intake (Olszewski et al. 2000), and glutamate release (Nicol et al. 1998).

It is a somewhat surprising finding that two peptides derived from the same precursor polypeptide show antagonistic effects in vivo. To better understand the interplay of these two messengers, it is important to learn more about where and under what conditions N/OFQ and NST are produced and released. While both NST and N/OFQ are colocalized in the superficial laminae of the mouse spinal dorsal horn (Okuda-Ashitaka et al. 1998), NST does not bind to NOP receptors and does not affect N/OFQ-evoked inhibition of forskolin-induced cyclic adenosine monophosphate (cAMP) production or N/OFQ-induced increases in cytosolic Ca^{2+}. To identify the putative NST receptor, we used a photoaffinity labeling approach (E. Okuda-Ashitaka et al., unpublished data). Mouse spinal cord membranes were incubated with a ^{125}I-labeled NST analogue, [^{125}I-Tyr^{6}, 4-N_3-Phe^{14}]-bPNP-3. This analogue binds a protein of approximately 33 kDa by photolysis. The 33-kDa protein labeling is decreased by NST but not by N/OFQ. The photoaffinity-labeled protein disappeared after GTPγS treatment, suggesting that the NST-specific photolabeled protein may be associated with a guanosine triphosphate (GTP)-binding protein. The 33-kDa photolabeled protein is abundantly expressed

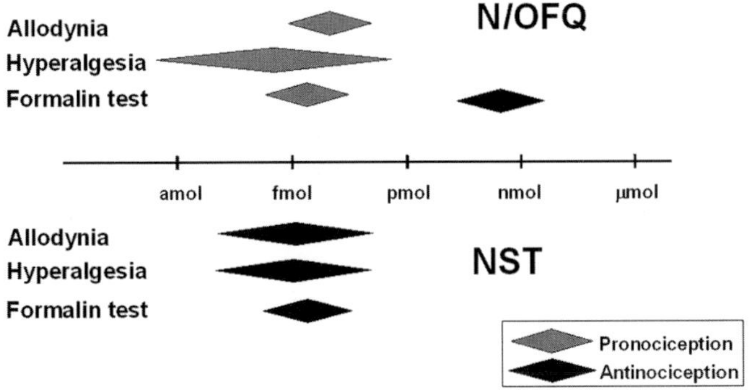

Fig. 1. Relationship between nocistatin (NST) and nociceptin/orphanin FQ (N/OFQ) with respect to effective doses and pain in mice. The dotted column represents pronociception and the closed column represents antinociception. Modified from Ito et al. (2000).

in the spinal cord, brain, and heart. When applied to the left ventricular wall of the heart using dialysis probes, NST reverses N/OFQ block of ouabain-induced cardiac acetylcholine and norepinephrine release (Yamazaki et al. 2001). In summary, NST exhibits biological effects through a specific receptor, not only in the central nervous system but also in the heart.

PROCESSING MECHANISM OF ppN/OFQ

To investigate the production of NST and N/OFQ from ppN/OFQ, we studied the processing of a genetically modified ppN/OFQ polypeptide labeled with the green fluorescent protein (GFP) mutant proteins enhanced cyan fluorescent protein (ECFP) and enhanced yellow fluorescent protein (EYFP) in living cells (E. Okuda-Ashitaka et al., unpublished data). Changes in fluorescence resonance energy transfer (FRET) between ECFP and EYFP were applied to monitor the enzymatic processing of ppN/OFQ. When the tandem fusion construct of (EYFP)-(NST-KR-N/OFQ)-(ECFP) was transfected into Cos7 cells devoid of cleavage activity of NST-KR-N/OFQ, a clear FRET signal was detected, indicating that FRET occurred in the fusion protein with the proximate distance designed for induction of FRET between the two end fluorescent proteins. However, in NG108-15 cells, which are capable of ppN/OFQ processing, the FRET signal decreased, indicating the rapid cleavage of NST and N/OFQ.

Proprotein convertase 1 (PC1) and PC2 are involved in the processing of several neuropeptide precursors such as proinsulin, proenkephalin, and pro-opiomelanocortin. To determine whether PC1 and/or PC2 are implicated in the production of NST and N/OFQ, we constructed fusion precursor proteins tagged with ECFP by directly linking to the COOH terminal of each peptide. NST-, N/OFQ-, and NST-KR-N/OFQ-tagged ECFP proteins were detected in the culture medium of NG108-15 cells expressing these constructs. PC12 cells that lack endogenous PC1 and PC2 were cotransfected with these fusion constructs and with PC1 or PC2. These experiments showed that the cleavage site downstream of N/OFQ was digested by PC1 and PC2 equally, while that located between NST and N/OFQ was dramatically digested by PC1 and (less effectively) by PC2. Although the cleavage site upstream of NST was digested in the absence of PC1 and PC2, cleavage was slightly enhanced by PC1 and PC2. These results suggest that a peptide harboring both NST and N/OFQ is first produced from ppN/OFQ, and then further processed by PC1 and PC2 to yield NST and N/OFQ. Evidence for the involvement of PC2 in the formation of N/OFQ also comes from a study using PC2-deficient mice (Allen et al. 2001). PC1 and PC2 show different tissue and subcellular localization (Seidah and Chrétien 1999), suggesting that region-specific post-translational processing may contribute to regulating the biological functions of NST and N/OFQ.

EMIKO OKUDA-ASHITAKA

SYNAPTIC ACTIONS OF N/OFQ AND NST IN THE SPINAL CORD DORSAL HORN

The superficial layers of the spinal cord dorsal horn, where thinly myelinated and unmyelinated primary afferent nerve fibers terminate, represent a particularly important structure for pain processing. This structure constitutes the first site of synaptic integration in the pain pathway. Protein and mRNA of both the N/OFQ precursor ppN/OFQ and the NOP receptor are highly expressed in this structure, suggesting that at least some of the pain-modulating effects of N/OFQ originate from this area of the central nervous system (CNS). We have therefore concentrated our efforts on identifying the mechanism of action of N/OFQ and NST in pain processing. To understand how N/OFQ and NST modulate spinal nociceptive processing, we have characterized how these neuropeptides affect neuronal excitability or synaptic transmission. In the spinal cord dorsal horn, fast excitatory neurotransmission is primarily mediated by L-glutamate and inhibitory neurotransmission by glycine (together with GABA). In several reports, we have demonstrated that N/OFQ inhibits excitatory glutamatergic neurotransmission (Liebel et al. 1997) without affecting GABA- or glycine receptor-mediated synaptic responses (Zeilhofer et al. 2000). This inhibition is naloxone-insensitive (Liebel et al. 2000), is dose-dependently blocked and partially mimicked by the partial NOP receptor agonist [F/G]N/OFQ$_{(1-13)}$NH$_2$ (Ahmadi et al. 2001b), and is absent in NOP-receptor-deficient mutant mice (Ahmadi et al. 2001a), indicating that it is specifically mediated by NOP receptors. N/OFQ does not affect the responsiveness of postsynaptic α-amino-3-hydroxy-5-methyl-4-isoxazole propionate (AMPA) receptors or that of *N*-methyl-D-aspartate (NMDA) receptors, but it decreases the synaptic release of L-glutamate, which means that it acts via a presynaptic site (Liebel et al. 1997). Inhibition of glutamatergic transmission by N/OFQ is thus remarkably reminiscent of the spinal analgesic mechanism of classical opioids. Inhibition of glutamate release, primarily from C and Aδ fibers (Luo et al. 2002), therefore most likely underlies the now well-accepted antinociceptive action of spinally applied N/OFQ. Nevertheless, synaptic connections targeted by N/OFQ and by classical opioids, such as methionine-enkephalin, are not identical (Schulz et al. 1996; Liebel et al. 1997; Monteillet-Agius et al. 1998). In light of these findings, it is interesting that lower doses of N/

OFQ can also elicit a pronociceptive action in the spinal cord (see above). A possible explanation of its proallodynic action might be a reduction in synaptic release of glycine in the spinal cord dorsal horn, as suggested by Ito et al. (2001). Indeed, other pronociceptive agents such as prostaglandin E_2 do indeed reduce glycinergic neurotransmission (Ahmadi et al. 2002). However, a large set of data unambiguously indicates that N/OFQ does not interfere with GABAergic or glycinergic neurotransmission at the level of the spinal cord (Zeilhofer et al. 2000; Ahmadi et al. 2001a; Luo et al. 2002). Although unproven, an intriguing hypothesis is that a reduction in synaptic glutamate release not only reduces fast excitatory neurotransmission via AMPA and NMDA receptors but also inhibits activation of—perhaps inhibitory—metabotropic glutamate receptors (Neugebauer 2002).

In higher areas of the CNS, the inhibitory action of N/OFQ is not restricted to glutamatergic neurons, but also affects inhibitory GABAergic neurons. The hypothesis has been put forward that in naive animals, inhibition of excitatory glutamatergic and inhibitory GABAergic neurotransmission may compensate for one another (Pan et al. 2000). Interestingly, classical opioids exert part of their supraspinal analgesic action by decreasing GABA release and thereby causing a disinhibition of descending antinociceptive tracts. In animals either treated with opioids or exposed to a stressful environment, N/OFQ might antagonize the action of classical opioids by compensating for the inhibitory action of opioids on GABAergic transmission via an inhibition of glutamate release.

As outlined above, NST antagonizes many in vivo effects of N/OFQ. In order to identify a cellular correlate for the functional antagonism of N/OFQ by NST, we also investigated the effects of NST on fast synaptic transmission in the superficial layers of the spinal cord dorsal horn. NST turned out to be completely ineffective when tested on AMPA-receptor-mediated glutamatergic transmission. However, NST inhibited glycinergic and GABAergic neurotransmission in a reversible and concentration-dependent manner. Inhibition occurs with a half maximum effective concentration of about 450 nM and a maximum inhibition of about 45% (Zeilhofer et al. 2000). This inhibition was again presynaptic in origin, i.e., caused by a reduction in synaptic release of GABA and glycine, as demonstrated with the use of variation analysis (Malinow and Tsien 1990). In contrast to what we have shown for N/OFQ, this inhibition was unaffected by the partial NOP receptor antagonist [F/G]N/OFQ$_{(1-13)}$ and was completely retained in mice lacking the NOP receptor (Ahmadi et al. 2001a,b), indicating that NST's action does not require NOP receptors or N/OFQ. Instead, these results suggest that the action of NST is mediated via a still unidentified receptor. Indeed, the inhibition was completely prevented by preincubation of spinal cord

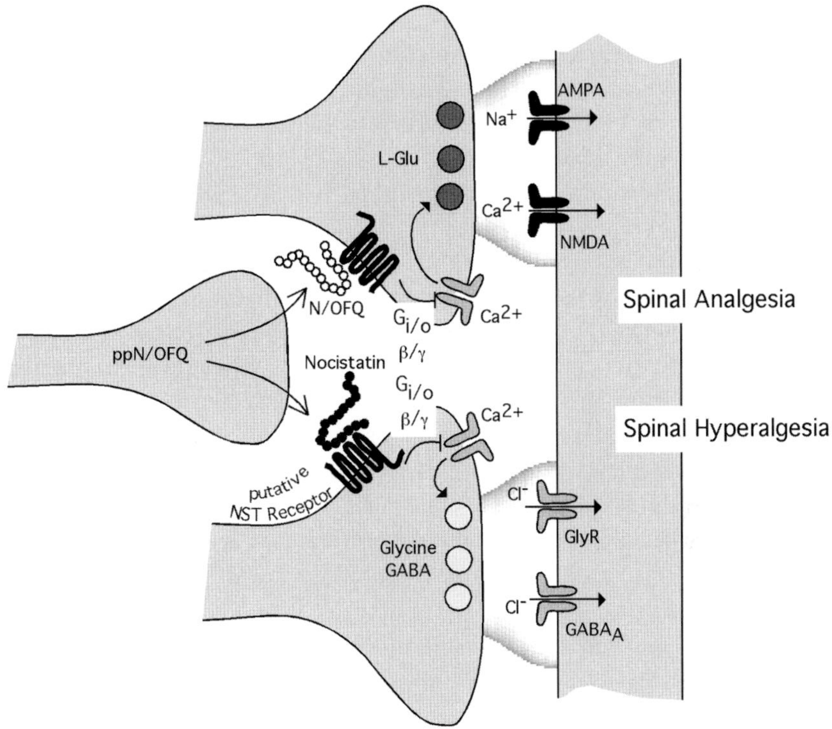

Fig. 2. Schematic showing synaptic actions of N/OFQ and NST in the spinal cord dorsal horn. N/OFQ and NST reduce the synaptic release of the excitatory transmitter L-glutamate and of the inhibitory transmitters glycine and GABA, respectively. Inhibition of postsynaptic responses mediated by AMPA and NMDA receptors and by strychnine-sensitive glycine receptors probably accounts for the anti-and pronociceptive effects of N/OFQ and NST in the spinal cord.

slices with pertussis toxin, an irreversible inhibitor of G proteins of the Gi/Go type.

In summary, in the spinal cord dorsal horn, inhibition by N/OFQ and NST of excitatory and inhibitory synaptic transmission, respectively, might explain at least part of the functional antagonism of N/OFQ and NST seen in vivo (Fig. 2).

HANNS U. ZEILHOFER

MICE LACKING THE N/OFQ PRECURSOR POLYPEPTIDE

Increasing evidence from behavioral and cellular studies indicates that exogenous application of N/OFQ to the CNS of mice and rats modulates nociception and pain-related behavior in a complex manner. Much less is known about the role of endogenous N/OFQ and NST and about the potential contribution of these peptides to pain control. Recent progress has been made through the generation of mice lacking the ppN/OFQ precursor peptide (Köster et al. 1999), which primarily point to an important role of N/OFQ in controlling stress responses.

Central administration of the peptide as well as a synthetic small-molecule agonist can alleviate stress responses, in particular anxiety and stress-induced analgesia (Jenck et al. 1997; Griebel et al. 1999; Jenck et al. 2000). Stress is a healthy response that prepares an organism for "fight or flight" behavior. The most dominant behavioral changes involve an increase of anxiety-like behavior and stress-induced analgesia, the latter being partially produced by release of endogenous opioids. N/OFQ can reverse stress-induced analgesia when administered centrally (Mogil et al. 1996a). N/OFQ can also block opioid-induced analgesia by functionally antagonizing μ-, δ-, and κ-opioid-mediated effects at supraspinal sites (Grisel et al. 1996; Mogil et al. 1996b). Thus, N/OFQ has been classified as a functional anti-opioid, although its effects are not mediated by direct interaction with opioid receptors (Reinscheid et al. 1998).

Phenotypic analysis of knockout mice lacking the N/OFQ precursor protein has provided further insight into the role of N/OFQ in stress-induced analgesia. N/OFQ knockout mice displayed normal pain sensitivity under stress-free conditions when compared to their wild-type littermates (Köster et al. 1999). However, the knockout animals failed to adapt to even mild chronic stress, such as social stress produced by group housing of male mice. In addition, the knockout mice were unable to habituate to repeated acute stress such as forced swimming on consecutive days. While wild-type mice quickly adapted to the stressor, knockout animals displayed the same magnitude of stress response (measured as stress-induced analgesia) after

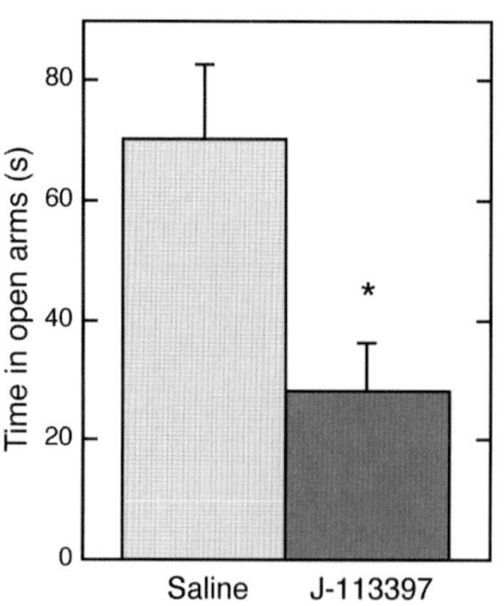

Fig. 3. Anxiety-like behavior in male mice of the C57Bl/6 strain (n = 9 for each group) injected with either saline or J-113397, a synthetic small-molecule N/OFQ antagonist (20 mg/kg, i.p.). Five minutes after injection the animals were placed in a plus maze apparatus. Time spent in the open arms of the maze and the number of transitions were recorded. Mice injected with the N/OFQ antagonist spent significantly less time exploring the open arms, which is indicative of increased anxiety. General locomotor activity did not differ between the two groups. Data are shown as means ± SEM, * $P < 0.02$.

three swim sessions, showing no signs of habituation. Furthermore, N/OFQ knockout mice showed increased anxiety-like behavior in a battery of test paradigms, including the open field, light-dark box, and plus maze tests. In summary, these results support an important role for N/OFQ in modulating neuronal responses to stress.

However, it remains unclear whether endogenous N/OFQ is released during stress responses. Neither the exogenous administration of N/OFQ nor the knockout mouse model can adequately address this question. Recently, a synthetic small-molecule N/OFQ antagonist (J-113397) has become available that is able to cross the blood-brain barrier after peripheral administration (Ozaki et al. 2000). We have started to investigate the effects of J-113397 on stress-related behavior in normal mice. When injected intraperitoneally, J-113397 (20 mg/kg) is able to increase anxiety-like behavior in the plus maze paradigm (Fig. 3). These results demonstrate for the first time that endogenous N/OFQ is released during stress responses and that endogenous N/OFQ might act as an anxiolytic transmitter in vivo.

RAINER K. REINSCHEID

SUMMARY

In summary, more than 5 years after its discovery, our understanding of the role of the N/OFQ-NOP neuropeptide system is far from being complete, not only in pain processing but also in many other physiological and pathophysiological processes. It is very likely that this system will offer many more surprises during forthcoming years.

ACKNOWLEDGMENTS

This work has been supported by a grant from the Deutsche Forschungsgemeinschaft (SFB 353/A8) to H.U. Zeilhofer and by Grants-in-Aid for scientific research from the Ministry of Education, Culture, Sports, Science, and Technology of Japan to E. Okuda-Ashitaka.

REFERENCES

Ahmadi S, Kotalla C, Gühring H, et al. Modulation of synaptic transmission by nociceptin/orphanin FQ and nocistatin in the spinal cord dorsal horn of mutant mice lacking the nociceptin/orphanin FQ receptor. *Mol Pharmacol* 2001a; 59:612–618.

Ahmadi S, Liebel JT, Zeilhofer HU. The role of the ORL1 receptor in the modulation of spinal neurotransmission by nociceptin/orphanin FQ and nocistatin. *Eur J Pharmacol* 2001b; 412:39–44.

Ahmadi S, Lippross S, Neuhuber WL, Zeilhofer HU. PGE_2 selectively blocks inhibitory glycinergic neurotransmission onto rat superficial dorsal horn neurons. *Nat Neurosci* 2002; 5:34–40.

Allen RG, Peng B, Pellegrion MJ, et al. Altered processing of pro-orphanin FQ/nociceptin and pro-opiomelanocortin-derived peptides in the brains of mice expressing defective prohormone convertase 2. *J Neurosci* 2001; 21:5864–5870.

Bunzow JR, Saez C, Mortrud M, et al. Molecular cloning and tissue distribution of a putative member of the rat opioid receptor gene family that is not a mu, delta or kappa opioid receptor type. *FEBS Lett* 1994; 347:284–288.

Caló G, Guerrini R, Rizzi A, et al. Pharmacology of nociceptin and its receptor: a novel therapeutic target. *Br J Pharmacol* 2000; 129:1261–1283.

Cox BM, Chavkin C, Christie MJ, et al. Opioid receptors. In: Girdlestone D (Ed). *The IUPHAR Compendium of Receptor Characterization and Classification.* London: IUPHAR Media, 2000, pp 321–333.

Erb K, Liebel JT, Tegeder I, et al. Spinally delivered nociceptin/orphanin FQ reduces flinching behaviour in the rat formalin test. *NeuroReport* 1997; 8:1967–1970.

Florin S, Suaudeau C, Meunier JC, et al. Orphan neuropeptide NocII, a putative pronociceptin maturation product, stimulates locomotion in mice. *NeuroReport* 1997; 8:705–707.

Fukuda K, Kato S, Mori K, et al. cDNA cloning and regional distribution of a novel member of the opioid receptor family. *FEBS Lett* 1994; 343:42–46.

Gavioli EC, Ras GA, Calo G, et al. Central injections of nocistatin or its C-terminal hexapeptide exert anxiogenic-like effect on behaviour of mice in the plus-maze test. *Br J Pharmacol* 2002; 136:764–772.

Griebel G, Perrault G, Sanger DJ. Orphanin FQ, a novel neuropeptide with anti-stress-like activity. *Brain Res* 1999; 836:221–224.

Grisel JE, Mogil, JS, Belknap JK, Grant KA. Orphanin FQ acts as a supraspinal, but not spinal, anti-opioid peptide. *Neuroreport* 1996; 7:2125–2129.

Hara N, Minami T, Okuda-Ashitaka E, et al. Characterization of nociceptin hyperalgesia and allodynia in conscious mice. *Br J Pharmacol* 1997; 121:401–408.

Hiramatsu M, Inoue K. Effects of nocistatin on nociceptin-induced impairment of learning and memory in mice. *Eur J Pharmacol* 1999; 367:151–155.

Houtani T, Nishi M, Takeshima H, Nukada T, Sugimoto T. Structure and regional distribution of nociceptin/orphanin FQ precursor. *Biochem Biophys Res Commun* 1996; 219:714–719.

Inoue M, Shimohira I, Yoshida A, et al. Dose-related opposite modulation by nociceptin/orphanin FQ of substance P nociception in the nociceptors and spinal cord. *J Pharmacol Exp Ther* 1999; 291:308–313.

Ito S, Okuda-Ashitaka E, Imanishi T, et al. Central roles of nociceptin/orphanin FQ and nocistatin: allodynia as a model of neural plasticity. *Prog Brain Res* 2000; 129:205–218.

Ito S, Okuda-Ashitaka E, Minami T. Central and peripheral roles of prostaglandins in pain and their interactions with novel neuropeptides nociceptin and nocistatin. *Neurosci Res* 2001; 41:299–332.

Jenck F, Moreau JL, Martin JR, et al. Orphanin FQ acts as an anxiolytic to attenuate behavioral responses to stress. *Proc Natl Acad Sci USA* 1997; 94:14854–14858.

Jenck F, Wichmann J, Dautzenberg FM, et al. A synthetic agonist at the orphanin FQ/nociceptin receptor ORL1: anxiolytic profile in the rat. *Proc Natl Acad Sci USA* 2000; 97:4938–4943.

Kieffer BL, Befort K, Gaveriaux-Ruff C, Hirth CG. The delta-opioid receptor: isolation of a cDNA by expression cloning and pharmacological characterization. *Proc Natl Acad Sci USA* 1992; 89:12048–12052.

Köster A, Montkowski A, Schulz S, et al. Targeted disruption of the orphanin FQ/nociceptin gene increases stress susceptibility and impairs stress adaptation in mice. *Proc Natl Acad Sci USA* 1999; 96:10444–10449.

Liebel JT, Swandulla D, Zeilhofer HU. Modulation of excitatory synaptic transmission by nociceptin in superficial dorsal horn neurones of the neonatal rat spinal cord. *Br J Pharmacol* 1997; 121:425–432.

Luo C, Kumamoto E, Furue H, Chen J, Yoshimura M. Nociceptin inhibits excitatory but not inhibitory transmission to substantia gelatinosa neurones of adult rat spinal cord. *Neuroscience* 2002; 109:349–358.

Malinow R, Tsien RW. Presynaptic enhancement shown by whole-cell recordings of long-term potentiation in hippocampal slices. *Nature* 1990; 346:177–3180.

Mathis JP, Rossi GC, Pellegrino MJ, et al. Carboxyl terminal peptides derived from prepro-orphanin FQ/nociceptin (ppOFQ/N) are produced in the hypothalamus and possess analgesic bioactivities. *Brain Res* 2001; 895:89–94.

Meunier JC, Mollereau C, Toll L, et al. Isolation and structure of the endogenous agonist of opioid receptor-like ORL1 receptor. *Nature* 1995; 377:532–535.

Mogil JS, Grisel JE, Reinscheid RK, et al. Orphanin FQ is a functional anti-opioid peptide. *Neuroscience* 1996a; 75:333–337.

Mogil JS, Grisel JE, Zhang G, Belknap JK, Grandy DK. Functional antagonism of μ-, δ- and κ-opioid antinociception by orphanin FQ. *Neurosci Lett* 1996b; 214:131–134.

Mollereau C, Simons MJ, Soularue P, et al. ORL1, a novel member of the opioid receptor family. Cloning, functional expression and localization. *FEBS Lett* 1994; 341:33–38.

Monteillet-Agius G, Fein J, Anton B, Evans CJ. ORL-1 and mu opioid receptor antisera label different fibers in areas involved in pain processing. *J Comp Neurol* 1998; 399:373–383.

Muratani T, Minami T, Enomoto U, et al. Characterization of nociceptin/orphanin FQ-induced pain responses by the novel receptor antagonist *N*-(4-amino-2-methylquinolin-6-yl)-2-(4-ethylphenoxymethyl) benzamide monohydrochloride. *J Pharmacol Exp Ther* 2002; 303:424–430.

Nakano H, Minami T, Abe K, et al. Effect of intrathecal nocistatin on the formalin-induced pain in mice versus that of nociceptin/orphanin FQ. *J. Pharmacol Exp Ther* 2000; 292:331–336.

Neal CR Jr, Mansour A, Reinscheid R, et al. Localization of orphanin FQ (nociceptin) peptide and messenger RNA in the central nervous system of the rat. *J Comp Neurol* 1999a; 406:503–547.

Neal CR Jr, Mansour A, Reinscheid R, et al. Opioid receptor-like (ORL1) receptor distribution in the rat central nervous system: comparison of ORL1 receptor mRNA expression with ^{125}I-[^{14}Tyr]-orphanin FQ binding. *J Comp Neurol* 1999b; 412:563–605.

Neugebauer V. Metabotropic glutamate receptors—important modulators of nociception and pain behavior. *Pain* 2002; 98:1–8.

Nicol B, Lambert DG, Rowbotham DJ, et al. Nocistatin reverses nociceptin inhibition of glutamate release from rat brain slices. *Eur J Pharmacol* 1998; 356:R1–R3.

Nishi M, Houtani T, Noda Y, et al. Unrestrained nociceptive response and disregulation of hearing ability in mice lacking the nociceptin/orphanin FQ receptor. *EMBO J* 1997; 16:1858–1864.

Nothacker HP, Reinscheid RK, Mansour A, et al. Primary structure and tissue distribution of the orphanin FQ precursor. *Proc Natl Acad Sci USA* 1996; 93:8677–8682.

Okuda-Ashitaka E, Tachibana S, Houtani T, et al. Identification and characterization of an endogenous ligand for opioid receptor homologue ROR-C: its involvement in allodynic response to innocuous stimulus. *Mol Brain Res* 1996; 43:96–104.

Okuda-Ashitaka E, Minami T, Tachibana S, et al. Nocistatin, a peptide that blocks nociceptin action in pain transmission. *Nature* 1998; 392:286–289.

Olszewski PK, Shaw TJ, Grace MK, et al. Nocistatin inhibits food intake in rats. *Brain Res* 2000; 872:181–187.

Ozaki S, Kawamoto H, Itoh Y, et al. In vitro and in vivo pharmacological characterization of J-113397, a potent and selective non-peptidyl ORL1 receptor antagonist. *Eur J Pharmacol* 2000; 402:45–53.

Pan YX, Xu J, Pasternak GW. Cloning and expression of a cDNA encoding a mouse brain orphanin FQ/nociceptin precursor. *Biochem J* 1996; 315:11–13.

Pan Z, Hirakawa N, Fields HL. A cellular mechanism for the bidirectional pain-modulating actions of orphanin FQ/nociceptin. *Neuron* 2000; 26:515–522.

Reinscheid RK, Nothacker HP, Bourson A, et al. Orphanin FQ, a neuropeptide that activates an opioid-like G protein-coupled receptor. *Science* 1995; 270:792–794.

Reinscheid RK, Higelin J, Henningsen RA, Monsma FJ Jr, Civelli O. Structures that delineate orphanin FQ and dynorphin A pharmacological selectivities. *J Biol Chem* 1998; 273:1490–1495.

Rossi GC, Pellegrino M, Shane R, et al. Characterization of rat prepro-orphanin FQ/nociceptin$_{(154-181)}$: nociceptive processing in supraspinal sites. *J Pharmacol Exp Ther* 2002; 300:257–264.

Saito Y, Maruyama K, Saido TC, Kawashima S. N23K, a gene transiently up-regulated during neural differentiation, encodes a precursor protein for a newly identified neuropeptide nociceptin. *Biochem Biophys Res Commun* 1995; 217:539–545.

Schulz S, Schreff M, Nuss D, Gramsch C, Hollt V. Nociceptin/orphanin FQ and opioid peptides show overlapping distribution but not co-localization in pain-modulatory brain regions. *Neuroreport* 1996; 7:3021–3025.

Seidah NG, Chrétien M. Proprotein and prohormone convertases: a family of subtilases generating diverse bioactive polypeptides. *Brain Res* 1999; 848:45–62.

Shinkai H, Ito T, Iida T, et al. 4-Aminoquinolines: novel nociceptin antagonists with analgesic activity. *J Med Chem* 2000; 43:4667–4677.

Wang JB, Johnson PS, Imai Y, et al. cDNA cloning of an orphan opiate receptor gene family member and its splice variant. *FEBS Lett* 1994; 348:75–79.

Xu XJ, Hao JX, Wiesenfeld-Hallin Z. Nociceptin or antinociceptin: potent spinal antinociceptive effect of orphanin FQ/nociceptin in the rat. *NeuroReport* 1996; 7:2092–2094.

Yamamoto T, Sakashita Y. Effect of nocistatin and its interaction with nociceptin/orphanin FQ on the rat formalin test. *Neurosci Lett* 1999; 262:179–182.

Yamazaki T, Akiyama T, Mori H. Effects of nociceptin on cardiac norepinephrine and acetylcholine release evoked by ouabain. *Brain Res* 2001; 904:153–156.

Zeilhofer HU, Muth-Selbach U, Gühring H, Erb K, Ahmadi S. Selective suppression of inhibitory synaptic transmission by nocistatin in the rat spinal cord dorsal horn. *J Neurosci* 2000; 20:4922–4929.

Zhao CS, Li BS, Zhao GY, et al. Nocistatin reverses the effect of orphanin FQ/nociceptin in antagonizing morphine analgesia. *NeuroReport* 1999; 10:297–299.

Correspondence to: Prof. Hanns U. Zeilhofer, Dr med, Institut für Experimentelle und Klinische Pharmakologie und Toxikologie, Universität Erlangen-Nürnberg, Fahrstrasse 17, D-91054 Erlangen, Germany. Tel: 49-9131-85-26935; Fax: 49-9131-85-22774; email: zeilhofer@pharmakologie.uni-erlangen.de.

Proceedings of the 10th World Congress on Pain,
Progress in Pain Research and Management, Vol. 24,
edited by Jonathan O. Dostrovsky, Daniel B. Carr, and
Martin Koltzenburg, IASP Press, Seattle, © 2003.

39

Effects of Sumatriptan on Rat Medullary Dorsal Horn Neurons

Ernest A. Jennings,[a] Renae M. Ryan,[a] and MacDonald J. Christie[a,b]

[a]*Department of Pharmacology and* [b]*The Medical Foundation, University of Sydney, Sydney, Australia*

The clinically effective antimigraine drug sumatriptan has both peripheral and central sites of action. Migraine is thought to result from neurogenic inflammation (dilation of the cerebral vessels following release of peptides from the peripheral terminals), and much work to date has therefore focused on sumatriptan's peripheral actions (Goadsby et al. 2002). Migraine pain originates from primary afferent terminals in the dura mater, especially near major blood vessels. These fibers have central terminals in the superficial medullary dorsal horn (nucleus caudalis) (Goadsby et al. 2002). Sumatriptan binds to a subset of serotonin (5-HT) receptor subtypes (5HT-1B, 5HT-1D, and 5HT-1F). In the human nucleus caudalis, sumatriptan binds preferentially to 5HT-1B and 5HT-1F (Castro et al. 1997).

This chapter presents the preliminary results of a study designed to examine the cellular effects of sumatriptan and other specific agonists of the 5HT-1B and 5HT-1D receptor subtypes on neurons in the substantia gelatinosa of the trigeminal nucleus caudalis, and to look for mRNA of these receptor subtypes in trigeminal ganglion neurons.

METHODS

All procedures reported conformed to the University of Sydney Ethics Committee guidelines. The methods used in this study have been published in full elsewhere (Jennings et al. 2001). Briefly, Sprague-Dawley rats (12–19 days old) were anesthetized with halothane and decapitated. Horizontal brain

Table I
Sequences of the forward (F) and reverse (R) primers used to amplify fragments from the 5HT-1B, 5HT-1D, and hypoxanthine phosphoribosyl-transferase (HPRT) DNA, and size (in base pairs) of the expected PCR products

Receptor			Size (bp)
HPRT	F	GCTACTGTAATGATCAGTCAACGGG	394
	R	CAACATCAACAGGACTCCTCGTA	
5HT-1B	F	CCAACAGATCCCTGAATGCTACAG	166
	R	CCAAGATAGAAACCAGGAGGTCGG	
5HT-1D	F	CGACTACATTTACCAGGACTCCATC	215
	R	CCAGCGAGGCGATCAGGTAGTTAG	

slices (250 μm) containing the trigeminal nucleus caudalis were cut (Grudt and Williams 1994). Slices were stored in artificial cerebrospinal fluid (34°C), and recordings were made in a superfusing chamber (32°C; Jennings et al. 2001).

Neurons in the substantia gelatinosa of the trigeminal nucleus caudalis were clearly visible as a translucent band just medial to the spinal trigeminal tract, which enters the slice 5–6 mm rostral to the nucleus caudalis and travels along the lateral edge of the slice (Grudt and Williams 1994). Neurons were visualized using infrared Nomarski optics, and whole-cell patch-clamp recordings (patch electrodes 3–7 MΩ), under voltage clamp (holding potential –74 mV, using a cesium chloride-based internal solution), were made using an Axopatch 200B amplifier. Patch-clamp recordings of postsynaptic currents were performed using a K^+ gluconate internal solution (holding potential –60 mV).

Miniature excitatory postsynaptic currents (mEPSCs) were recorded in the presence of picrotoxin (100 μM), strychnine (3 μM), and tetrodotoxin (TTX; 300 nM). The mEPSC rate and amplitude recorded during a 3-minute period in the presence of sumatriptan were compared with control recordings without sumatriptan.

Electrically evoked EPSCs (eEPSCs) were elicited via bipolar stimulating electrodes placed in the spinal trigeminal tract about 1 mm rostral to the site of recording. Stimuli were delivered once every 15 seconds (0.07 Hz) at intensities in the range of 3–10 V for 0.06–0.2 ms, and were recorded in the presence of picrotoxin (100 μM) and strychnine (3 μM). For paired-pulse experiments, two stimuli of identical strength were applied with an interstimulus interval of 70 ms.

We used 6-cyano-7-nitroquinoxaline-2,3-dione (CNQX) as a control at the end of some of the experiments to check that we were recording mEPSCs/

eEPSCs. CNQX (10 μM) abolishes the mEPSC rate or eEPSC amplitude, depending on what is being recorded.

Stock solutions of all drugs were diluted to working concentrations using artificial cerebrospinal fluid (ACSF) immediately before use and were applied by superfusion. Stock solutions of all drugs were made in distilled water, or added directly to the ACSF. All pooled data are expressed as means ± SEM, and statistical comparisons were made using the paired Student's *t* test, unless otherwise stated.

Reverse transcription polymerase chain reaction (RT-PCR) experiments were performed as previously published (Borgland et al. 2002). Briefly, fresh rat trigeminal ganglia were removed, and total RNA was extracted. For the RT-PCR reaction, 1 μg of RNA was incubated with 1 μg of random primers (oligoDT). The mRNA was reverse transcribed, PCR amplification was performed, and the products were separated on a 2% agarose gel and visualized with ethidium bromide.

RESULTS

The effects of sumatriptan on postsynaptic currents in superficial trigeminal nucleus caudalis neurons were examined using a K^+ gluconate internal solution. Superfusion of sumatriptan (3 μM) produced no significant membrane current (0.2 ± 2 pA; $n = 5$; Fig. 1B) in neurons that were voltage clamped at –60 mV. Superfusion of the opioid agonist met-enkephalin (10 μM) produced a reversible outward current of 19 ± 4 pA in three of the five neurons, producing no current in the remaining two neurons. 5-HT (10 μM) was superfused onto two of the five neurons, resulting in an outward current of 26 and 55 pA. 5HT-1B and 5HT-1D were detected in rat trigeminal ganglion tissue (Fig. 1A).

mEPSCs were recorded in the presence of TTX (0.3 μM), picrotoxin (100 μM), and strychnine (3 μM). mEPSCs had a mean rate of 1.5 ± 0.3 Hz and were abolished by CNQX (10 μM). Superfusion of sumatriptan (3 μM) decreased the mEPSC rate by 36 ± 5% (range, 8–55%; $n = 12$; $P < 0.05$; Fig. 2) in all neurons tested, without affecting the amplitude. The amplitude of mEPSCs was similar in the absence (36 ± 2 pA) and presence of sumatriptan (3 μM; 33 ± 3 pA; $P > 0.05$; $n = 12$). The inhibitory effect of sumatriptan on mEPSC rate was dose dependent, with an EC_{50} of 139 nM.

Glutamatergic EPSCs were recorded in the medullary dorsal horn in the presence of strychnine (5 μM) and picrotoxin (100 μM). Evoked EPSCs had a mean amplitude of 64 pA and 52 pA, respectively, and were abolished by CNQX (10 μM). Superfusion of sumatriptan (3 μM) reduced the eEPSC

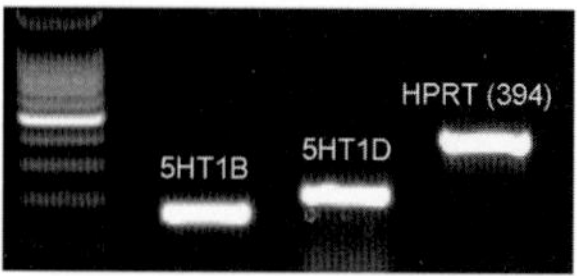

B:

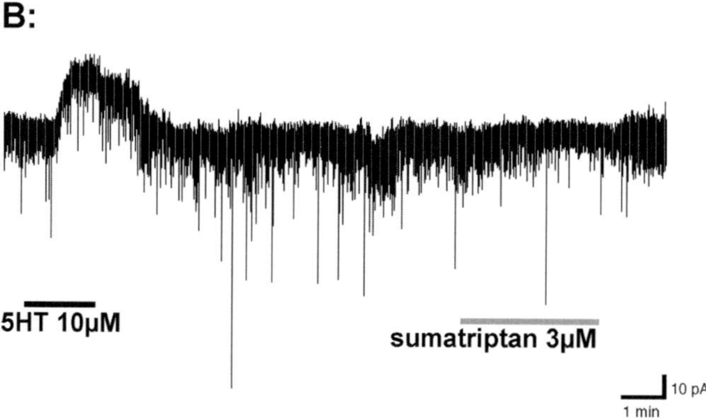

Fig. 1. (A) Representative detection, by RT-PCR, of mRNA from 5HT-1B and 5HT-1D serotonin receptor subtypes in the trigeminal nucleus of rats (the housekeeping enzyme hypoxanthine phosphoribosyltransferase [HPRT] is included as a control). (B) K^+ current recording showing a 26-pA outward current following application of 5-HT (10 μM), but no response in the presence of sumatriptan (3 μM).

amplitude by 18% and 36%, respectively. Under control conditions the ratio of the paired eEPSC (interstimulus interval 70 ms) was 126% and 94%, respectively. Superfusion of sumatriptan (3 μM) produced an increase in the mean ratio of eEPSC2/eEPSC1 of 180% and 115%, respectively.

DISCUSSION

The results presented here demonstrate that sumatriptan acts at central terminals of primary afferents to diminish the release of the excitatory neurotransmitter glutamate by reducing the mEPSC rate (without altering the amplitude). Sumatriptan also reduced the amplitude of evoked EPSCs, and when two identical stimuli were delivered (with an interval of 70 ms), the second eEPSC was relatively larger than the first (paired pulse facilitation), again indicating a presynaptic site of action. Although serotonin induces an outward K^+ current in second-order neurons, sumatriptan does not, suggesting

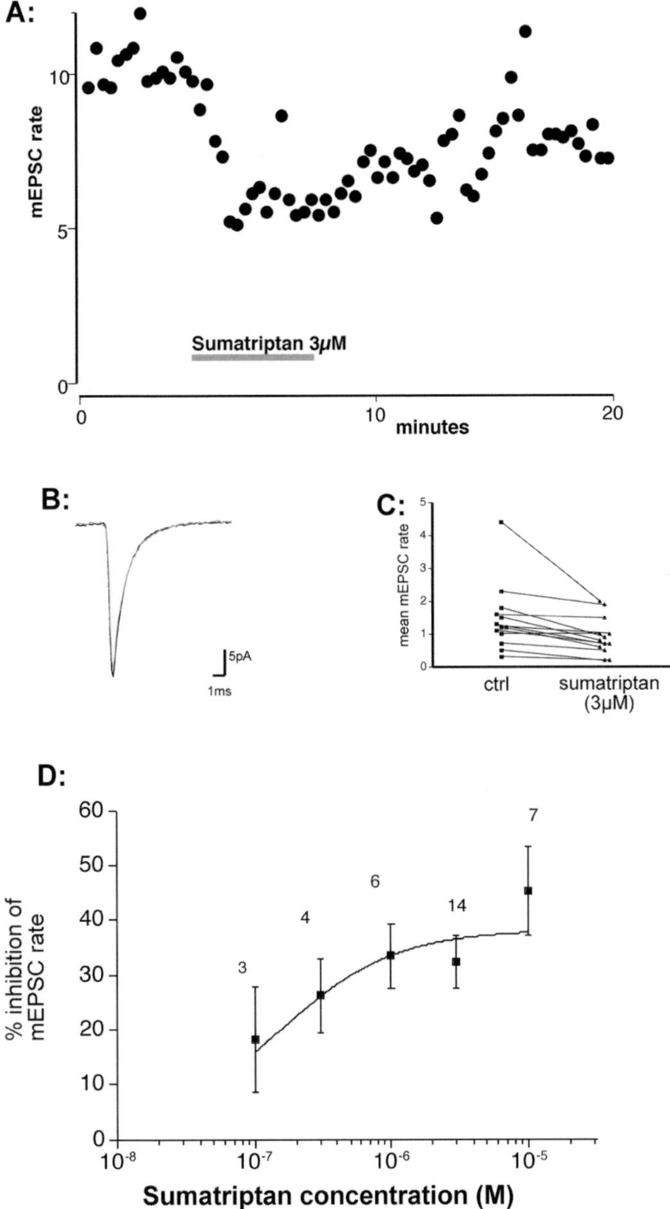

Fig. 2. (A) Time plot showing the miniature excitatory postsynaptic current (mEPSC) rate before and during application of sumatriptan (3 μM). (B) Average amplitudes of mEPSC in the same neuron: black (control), gray (sumatriptan). (C) Plot showing mEPSC rate before and during application of sumatriptan (3 μM) in all neurons from which recordings were taken. (D) Concentration response curve for sumatriptan; EC_{50} (effective concentration to reach 50% of the maximum response) = 139 nM.

that this hyperpolarizing current is acting through different receptor subtypes; indeed, activation of the 5HT-1A receptor subtype has been shown to activate an outward K^+ current in hippocampus neurons (Luscher et al. 1997). Messenger RNA for both 5HT-1B and 5HT-1D receptor subtypes is present in the rat trigeminal ganglion, and presumably the receptor is expressed on the primary afferent fiber.

5HT-1B receptor mRNA has been reported in cerebral blood vessels (Bouchelet et al. 1996) and in peptidergic neurons in the guinea pig trigeminal ganglion (Bonaventure et al. 1998). The peripheral actions of sumatriptan are exerted either by vasoconstriction of cerebral arteries or by a direct effect on inhibition of neurogenic extravasation; both actions are mediated through 5HT-1B receptors (Goadsby et al. 2002). The lack of effect of neurokinin-1 (NK1) antagonists and of specific inhibitors of protein plasma extravasation (Goldstein et al. 1997; Roon et al. 2000) has led some investigators to question the role of antimigraine drugs at the peripheral terminal of the primary afferent fiber.

The data presented here demonstrate that sumatriptan effects reported in the nucleus caudalis are due to presynaptic inhibition of glutamate release from the primary afferent terminals. There is also the possibility that sumatriptan might exert central effects on other nuclei in the brain. Binding studies in the human brainstem have shown that [^{3}H]sumatriptan also binds to both 5HT-1B and 5HT-1D receptors in the dorsal raphe nucleus, periaqueductal gray, and locus ceruleus (Castro et al. 1997).

ACKNOWLEDGMENTS

E.A. Jennings and M.J. Christie are supported by the National Health and Medical Research Council, and M.J. Christie is further supported by The Medical Foundation, Sydney University; R.M. Ryan receives an Australian Postgraduate Award. Sumatriptan was generously donated by GlaxoSmithKline.

REFERENCES

Bonaventure P, Voorn P, Luyten WH, et al. Detailed mapping of serotonin 5-HT1B and 5-HT1D receptor messenger RNA and ligand binding sites in guinea-pig brain and trigeminal ganglion: clues for function. *Neuroscience* 1998; 82:469–484.

Borgland SL, Connor M, Ryan RM, et al. Prostaglandin E(2) inhibits calcium current in two sub-populations of acutely isolated mouse trigeminal sensory neurons. *J Physiol* 2002; 539:433–444.

Bouchelet I, Cohen Z, Case B, et al. Differential expression of sumatriptan-sensitive 5-hydroxytryptamine receptors in human trigeminal ganglia and cerebral blood vessels. *Mol Pharmacol* 1996; 50:219–223.

Castro ME, Pascual J, Romon T, et al. Differential distribution of [H-3]sumatriptan binding sites (5-HT_{1B}, 5-HT_{1D} and 5-HT_{1F} receptors) in human brain—focus on brainstem and spinal cord. *Neuropharmacology* 1997; 36:535–542.

Goadsby PJ, Lipton RB, Ferrari MD. Migraine—current understanding and treatment. *N Engl J Med* 2002; 346:257–270.

Goldstein DJ, Wang O, Saper JR, et al. Ineffectiveness of neurokinin-1 antagonist in acute migraine: a crossover study. *Cephalalgia* 1997; 17:785–790.

Grudt TJ, Williams JT. mu-Opioid agonists inhibit spinal trigeminal substantia gelatinosa neurons in guinea pig and rat. *J Neurosci* 1994; 14:1646–1654.

Jennings EA, Vaughan CW, Christie MJ. Cannabinoid actions on rat superficial medullary dorsal horn neurons in vitro. *J Physiol (Lond)* 2001; 534:805–812.

Luscher C, Jan LY, Stoffel M, et al. G protein-coupled inwardly rectifying K+ channels (GIRKs) mediate postsynaptic but not presynaptic transmitter actions in hippocampal neurons. *Neuron* 1997; 19:687–695.

Roon KI, Olesen J, Diener HC, et al. No acute antimigraine efficacy of CP-122,288, a highly potent inhibitor of neurogenic inflammation: results of two randomized, double-blind, placebo-controlled clinical trials. *Ann Neurol* 2000; 47:238–241.

Correspondence to: Ernest Jennings, PhD, Department of Pharmacology (D06), University of Sydney, Sydney, NSW 2006, Australia. Email: erniej@med.usyd.edu.au.

Proceedings of the 10th World Congress on Pain,
Progress in Pain Research and Management, Vol. 24,
edited by Jonathan O. Dostrovsky, Daniel B. Carr, and
Martin Koltzenburg, IASP Press, Seattle, © 2003.

40

Predictive Validity of Neuropathic Pain Models in Pharmacological Studies with a Behavioral Outcome in the Rat: A Systematic Review

Vesa K. Kontinen[a,b,c] and Theo F. Meert[a]

[a]CNS Pain and Alzheimer, Johnson & Johnson Pharmaceutical Research and Development, Beerse, Belgium; [b]Department of Pharmacology, Institute of Biomedicine, University of Helsinki, Helsinki, Finland; [c]Department of Anesthesia, Jorvi Hospital, Helsinki University Hospital, Helsinki, Finland

Animal models of neuropathic pain are increasingly used for basic research (for review, see Zeltser and Seltzer 1994; Schmalbruch and Krarup 1996) and for screening and preclinical characterization of compounds intended for the treatment or prevention of neuropathic pain. However, few studies have assessed the predictive validity of the animal models.

The validity of an animal model of a human disease comprises face validity, construct validity, and predictive validity (Willner 1984). Face validity means that the model and the condition being modeled have phenomenological similarities. For neuropathic pain models, this is usually described when the models are initially introduced (Bennett and Xie 1988; Seltzer et al. 1990; Kim and Chung 1992; Courteix et al. 1993). Construct validity implies that the model has a sound theoretical rationale, based on current knowledge of the clinical condition. Animal models of neuropathic pain seem to represent the known human pathology relatively well, within the inherent limitation that it is impossible to know what the animals perceive (for references, see Bridges et al. 2001). Predictive validity means that performance of a compound in the preclinical test is prognostic to its performance in the clinical setting. A few experimental studies (Yamamoto and Yaksh 1991, 1992; Courteix et al. 1994; Koch et al. 1996; Malcangio and Tomlinson 1998; Fox et al. 1999; Idänpään-Heikkilä and Guilbaud 1999) and topical reviews (Yaksh et al. 1992; Bennett 1999; Wallace 2001) have explored this aspect, but to our knowledge no systematic reviews exist on this topic. This chapter assesses the predictive validity of the most widely used experimental animal models of neuropathic pain models in light of the available clinical evidence.

METHODS

This review included the chronic constriction injury (CCI) model (Bennett and Xie 1988), the partial sciatic ligation (PSL) model (Seltzer et al. 1990), and the spinal nerve ligation (SNL) model (Kim and Chung 1992) of mononeuropathy (Fig. 1) and the streptozocin-induced diabetes (STZ) model of polyneuropathy (Courteix et al. 1993) in rats (Table Ia). Studies were obtained from the Ovid Technologies, Inc. combined edition of Medline (1966 to September 2001) and PreMedline (up to October 2, 2001), with the key words presented in Table Ia. We only included studies that reported pharmacological data on at least one behavioral outcome, such as heat, cold, or tactile allodynia or mechanohyperalgesia, in awake animals. Thus, electrophysiological or biochemical studies were excluded from the review (Table Ib). In

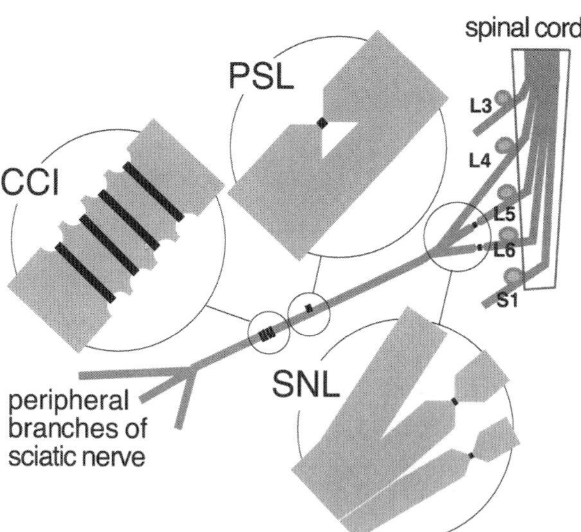

Fig. 1. Schematic illustration of the surgical neuropathic pain models included in the review. The localization of axonal damage in the chronic constriction injury (CCI), the spinal nerve ligation (SNL), and the partial sciatic ligation (PSL) models of neuropathic pain on the rat sciatic nerve is illustrated. In the CCI model predominantly myelinated fibers are affected, whereas the other two models (SNL and PSL) affect all fiber types.

Table I
Paper flow in the review

a) Search Strategy and Results

Terms	Yield
#1: [[[neuropathy OR neuropathic] AND [pain*] OR [mononeuropathy OR mononeuropathic]] AND [rat or rats]	881
#2: [[[chronic constriction injury] OR [CCI] OR [[ligation OR ligature*] AND [sciatic nerve OR loose]] OR [Bennett AND model]] AND [year ≥ 1988]	944
#3: [[[spinal nerve OR L5] AND [ligation OR ligature*]] OR [SNL] OR [Chung AND model]] AND [year ≥ 1991]	258
#4: [[partial sciatic ligation] OR [PSL]] OR [[[ligation OR ligature*] OR [injury]] AND [sciatic OR nerve] AND [partial OR incomplete]] OR [Seltzer AND model]] AND [year ≥ 1990]	832
#5: [[streptozocin OR streptozotocin OR Zanosar OR NCS-85998] OR [diabetic OR diabetes]] AND [[neuropathy OR neuropathic] OR [pain* OR allodynia OR hyperalgesia]] AND [rat OR rats]	760
#1 OR #2 OR #3 OR #4 OR #5	2929

b) Studies Included

Criteria	Applicable Studies
Does the paper contain data on CCI, SNL, PSL or STZ model?	1158
Are there any pharmacological data on treatment of established neuropathy?	357
Are there any data on systemic or intrathecal administration?	288
Is there any clinical evidence in neuropathic pain available on the drug used in the experimental study?	119

Note: All terms were searched as free text words in the title or the abstract. The Ovid Technologies, Inc. combined edition of Medline (1966–September 2001) and PreMedline (to October 2, 2001) was used.

mononeuropathy models, only studies in which the test stimulus was applied on the innervation territory of the injured (sciatic) nerve were included.

Clinical studies in neuropathic pain have been mainly performed in patients who have established neuropathic pain, and therefore experimental studies in which the drug treatment started prior to nerve injury were excluded from this review. For the same reason, only studies in which the compounds were administered either systemically (by the oral, subcutaneous, intraperitoneal, or intravenous route) or intrathecally were included. Thus, studies in which drugs were administered locally (for example directly on the nerve, on the skin, as microinjections to a certain brain region, or intracerebroventricularly) were excluded. Also, studies in which local anesthetics were administered intrathecally were excluded. Only papers published in English were included in this analysis.

Finally, only experimental studies of drug classes for which some published clinical data were identified were included in this analysis. We searched for clinical evidence in Medline using the name of the compound, and if necessary, when we found a large number of studies, we added additional search terms such as "neuropathic pain," "neuralgia," and "nerve injury AND pain." When systematic reviews on the efficacy of certain drug classes in neuropathic pain were available, those were considered to contain the best clinical evidence and were used as the basis for clinical assessment (for methodology of systematic reviews in clinical pain research, see McQuay and Moore 1998).

RESULTS

Three thousand publications were found and screened to identify the applicable studies, representing nine drug classes with different mechanisms of action (Table II). A full listing of the studies included in this review can be obtained from the corresponding author of this chapter. There was substantial heterogeneity in experimental methodology and presentation of results. Therefore, a qualitative "vote counting" procedure was used to estimate predictive validity (Table II).

The sensitivity of the models is generally good, but there are few data for the evaluation of the PSL model. In the CCI model, 94 experimental endpoints were positive out of the 107 that were expected to be positive based on the clinical opinion used for this study. This finding gives a general sensitivity of 88% for the CCI model. There were no experimental endpoints with a negative outcome for the CCI model, but four endpoints were expected to be negative based on the clinical opinion. Specificity of the model, as calculated from these figures, is 0%, which does not seem to be a valid estimate, but reflects the low number of negative studies and lack of clinical evidence on ineffective drugs. The specificity figures for the SNL model were 63 experimental endpoints positive out of 93 predicted positive, with a sensitivity of 68%. The specificity numbers were again poor, with 6 negative studies out of 10 predicted negative (60%). For the PSL model 8 experimental endpoints were positive out of 13 predicted positive, with a sensitivity of 61%. There were no applicable studies for a specificity estimate for the PSL model. For the STZ model, the figures were 26 experimental endpoints positive out of 37 predicted positive, with a sensitivity of 70%. The specificity numbers were again poor, with 2 negative studies out of 3 predicted negative (66%).

DISCUSSION

It is possible to apply methods of evidence-based medicine to experimental pain research data. The neuropathic pain models studied have a relatively good predictive validity in pharmacological studies. The largest body of evidence exists for the CCI model, whereas little information is available on the PSL model. For calculation of validity estimates, it is necessary to form an opinion on the clinical efficacy of treatments. In the case of neuropathic pain, this is often difficult. No drug is effective in all neuropathic pain patients, there are often responders and nonresponders in a group of patients with seemingly similar neuropathic pain, and often only partial pain relief is achieved. In this review, fairly liberal criteria were used for the clinical opinion: if the drug had been shown to be effective in some type of neuropathic pain, it was considered effective for the purpose of the sensitivity calculations. A slightly higher proportion of compounds showed efficacy in the CCI model than in the SNL model; perhaps selecting more rigid criteria for clinical efficacy would have decreased the sensitivity estimate for the CCI model and improved the estimated sensitivity of the SNL model.

Few data were available for the evaluation of the specificity of the models (Table II), due to the small number of published studies with negative controls (drugs expected to be ineffective). This deficiency considerably reduces the power of the specificity estimates. More rigid criteria for clinical efficacy would have increased the number of "ineffective" drugs, which in turn would have improved the quality of the specificity estimates. Excluding studies with methodological problems, such as inadequate dose range or very small study groups (e.g., $n = 3$), would improve the predictive validity of the models. Studies will be scored for quality in the full version of this review.

Development of neurokinin-1 (NK1) receptor antagonists for pain has been a disappointment so far in the clinic, although many of the NK1 antagonist compounds were reported to show efficacy in animal models of various types of pain, including some for neuropathic pain. The lessons learned from this controversy have been reviewed previously (Boyce and Hill 2000; Hill 2000; Urban and Fox 2000). The two clinical studies involving NK1 antagonists for neuropathic pain have been published only in conference abstract format. Humans and rats differ in NK1–receptor-binding characteristics, and the compounds used in the published experimental studies in neuropathic pain models in the rat were not identical to those used in the clinical neuropathic pain studies. Due to these aspects, NK1 antagonists were not included in this systematic review. Generally, it can be argued that the risk of publication bias toward neglecting negative studies is greater in the field of experimental animal studies than in clinical drug research.

Table II
The results of the "vote counting" procedure for each drug group, pain model, and outcome (sensory modality)

Drug Class	Clinical Opinion (Reference)	CCI				SNL				PSL				STZ			
		TA	MH	HH	CA	TA	MH	HH	CA	TA	MH	HH	CA	TA	MH	HH	CA
Opioids																	
Morphine, systemic	Effective (C) (e, o)	1/2	7/8	5/6	1/3	9/10	2/2	1/1	2/2	–	1/1	–	–	3/4	3/5	2/2	1/1
Morphine, spinal	Effective (D) (o)	1/1	2/2	7/8	2/2	1/9	–	–	–	–	–	0/1	–	1/1	–	–	–
Fentanyl	Effective (B) (d)	–	–	–	–	–	–	–	–	–	–	–	–	–	–	–	–
Tramadol	Effective (B) (g)	–	–	–	–	–	–	–	–	–	–	–	–	–	–	–	–
Antidepressants, Tricyclic																	
Amitriptyline	Effective (A) (c, g)	3/3	–	1/1	–	1/4	4/4	–	–	–	–	–	–	2/3	–	–	–
Clomipramine	Effective (B) (c, g)	2/2	–	–	–	–	1/2	–	–	–	–	–	–	–	1/4	–	–
Desipramine	Effective (C) (c, g)	1/1	3/3	–	–	1/1	1/4	–	–	–	–	–	–	–	–	–	–
Antidepressants, Nontricyclic																	
Fenfluramine	Ineffective (D)	–	–	–	–	1/2	–	–	0/1	–	–	–	–	–	–	–	–
Fluoxetine	Ineffective (C) (c, g)	–	–	–	–	1/1	1/1	–	–	–	–	–	–	–	–	–	–
Venlafaxine	Effective (C) (n)	–	–	2/2	–	–	–	–	–	–	–	–	–	–	–	–	–
Anticonvulsants																	
Gabapentin	Effective (A) (g, k)	2/2	3/5	2/2	2/2	5/5	–	–	–	3/4	–	–	–	2/2	1/1	–	–
Pregabalin	Effective (D)	–	–	–	–	–	–	–	–	–	–	–	–	2/2	–	–	–
Lamotrigine	Effective (C) (g, j)	1/1	1/1	–	1/1	0/1	–	–	–	–	1/1	–	–	–	3/3	–	–
Carbamazepine	Effective (B) (b, g)	–	1/1	–	–	0/1	–	–	–	–	–	–	–	–	1/1	–	–
Felbamate	Effective (D)	1/1	1/1	1/1	1/1	0/1	–	–	–	–	–	–	–	–	–	–	–
Topiramate	Ineffective (C) (m)	–	–	–	–	0/2	–	–	–	–	–	–	–	–	–	–	–
Vigabatrin	Effective (D)	–	–	1/1	–	–	–	–	–	–	–	–	–	–	–	–	–
Phenytoin	Effective (C) (b, g)	–	–	–	0/1	0/1	–	–	–	–	–	–	–	–	0/1	–	–
Systemic Local Anesthetics																	
Lidocaine	Effective (A) (f)	–	–	1/1	2/2	4/4	–	–	–	–	–	–	–	–	1/1	–	–
Mexiletine	Effective (C) (f, g)	–	1/1	–	–	1/1	1/1	–	–	–	–	–	–	–	–	–	–
Flecainide	Effective (C) (l)	1/1	–	1/1	–	–	–	–	–	–	–	–	–	–	–	–	–

NMDA-Receptor Antagonists																	
Ketamine	Effective (B) (e, i)	–	–	2/2	–	2/2	1/1	–	1/1	–	–	–	–	0/1	–	–	–
Dextromethorphan	Effective (C) (g, i)	–	–	–	–	–	–	–	–	–	–	–	–	–	–	–	–
Magnesium	Effective (C) (h)	–	–	–	–	1/1	–	–	–	–	–	–	–	–	–	–	–
Memantine	Ineffective (C) (g)	–	0/2	0/1	–	–	–	–	–	–	–	–	–	–	0/1	–	–
MK-801, systemic	Effective (X)	1/1	4/4	3/3	–	–	–	–	–	–	0/1	–	–	1/1	1/1	–	–
MK-801, i.t.	Effective (X)	–	1/1	7/8	–	2/5	–	1/1	–	–	0/1	0/1	–	–	0/1	–	–
Alpha-Adrenergic Agonists																	
Clonidine, systemic	Effective (C) (e)	0/1	1/1	2/3	2/2	–	–	–	–	–	–	–	–	–	–	–	–
Clonidine, spinal	Effective (C) (e)	1/1	–	–	–	10/10	–	–	–	–	–	–	–	–	–	–	–
Tizanidine	Effective (C)	1/1	2/2	1/1	–	–	–	–	–	–	–	–	–	–	–	–	–
Phentolamine	Effective (D)	–	–	1/1	–	3/6	–	–	–	–	–	–	–	–	–	–	–
Drugs Acting on GABA Receptors																	
Baclofen	Effective (C) (a)	1/1	–	1/1	–	2/2	–	–	–	–	3/3	–	–	1/1	0/1	–	–
Clonazepam	Effective (D)	–	–	1/1	–	–	–	–	–	–	–	–	–	–	–	–	–
NSAIDs																	
Acetylsalicylic acid	Ineffective (D)	–	–	–	–	–	–	–	–	–	–	–	–	–	1/1	–	–
Ketoprofen	Ineffective (D)	–	–	–	–	1/1	–	–	–	–	–	–	–	–	–	–	–
Ketorolac	Ineffective (D)	–	–	0/1	0/1	1/1	–	1/1	–	–	–	–	–	–	–	1/1	–
Indomethacin	Ineffective (D)	–	–	–	–	–	–	–	–	–	–	–	–	–	–	–	–
Overall		17/19	27/32	39/45	11/15	46/71	11/15	3/3	3/4	3/4	5/7	0/2	0/0	12/15	12/21	3/3	1/1

Note: The first number is for experimental studies that were in agreement with the clinical opinion, and the second number is the total number of applicable study outcomes in the category. Each outcome (e.g., different pain modality such as tactile or thermal allodynia or hyperalgesia, or results on different administration routes) has been calculated separately, and thus the numbers are not the same as the number of studies.

Abbreviations: CA = cold allodynia; CCI = chronic constriction injury; HH = heat hyperalgesia; MH = mechanohyperalgesia; PSL = partial sciatic ligation; SNL = spinal nerve ligation; STZ = streptozotocin; TA = tactile allodynia.

Coding of the level of the clinical evidence: (A) Strong evidence. Systematic review(s) of multiple methodologically good studies. (B) Moderate evidence. At least one methodologically good study of reasonable size, or several moderate studies. (C) Weak evidence. At least one small or methodologically moderate study. (D) Clinical impression. No published scientific evidence. (X) No direct evidence. There is no clinical experience on MK-801, but as an important experimental research tool it has been included based on clinical evidence on another NMDA–receptor antagonist, ketamine.

References: a, Fromm (1994); b, McQuay et al. (1995); c, McQuay et al. (1996); d, Dellemijn and Vanneste (1997); e, Kingery (1997); f, Kalso et al. (1998); g, Sindrup and Jensen (1999); h, Crosby et al. (2000); i, Hewitt (2000); j, McCleane (2000); k, Tremont-Lukats et al. (2000); l, Ichimata et al. (2001); m, Jensen (2002); n, Tasmuth et al. (2002); o, Kalso (this volume).

The STZ model might provide a good mechanistic model for painful diabetic neuropathy, but some of the symptoms could be related to the poor general health of the animals rather than to peripheral neuropathy (Fox et al. 1999). Maintenance treatment with low doses of insulin improves the general condition of the animals, but does not prevent the development of tactile allodynia in STZ rats (Calcutt et al. 1996). It can be misleading to compare results from experiments where the STZ model has been used without insulin treatment to those obtained from STZ animals treated with insulin.

Clinical studies in neuropathic pain are most often conducted with patients who have a condition like painful diabetic neuropathy or postherpetic neuropathy that may have a different mechanism from that of the allodynia or hyperalgesia seen in the surgical injury models. Furthermore, it is recognized that a dichotomous (effective/ineffective) clinical opinion for the efficacy of the different drugs is at best a gross overall estimate, and that efficacy varies in different clinical situations. Ongoing or spontaneous pain is seldom reported in the experimental studies, whereas it is often an important component of clinical neuropathic pain problems. Despite these inherent problems, the neuropathic pain models reviewed here had surprisingly good predictive validity when used with rigorous scientific methodology, such as adequate controls, sufficiently large study groups, and well-controlled environments. Most importantly, the correct scientific questions should be asked. A good experimental model of neuropathic pain can teach us about the mechanisms of neuropathic pain and provide an idea of the efficacy of a new compound, but nothing more. The models should not be held accountable for unrelated failures in the drug development process.

ACKNOWLEDGMENTS

T.F. Meert is, and V.K. Kontinen has been, an employee of Johnson & Johnson Pharmaceutical Research and Development. We thank Dr. Eija Kalso for her pertinent comments on this manuscript, and many helpful discussions on this topic.

REFERENCES

Bennett GJ. Opioids and painful peripheral neuropathy. In: Kalso E, McQuay HJ, Wiesenfeld-Hallin Z (Eds). *Opioid Sensitivity of Chronic Noncancer Pain,* Progress in Pain Research and Management, Vol. 14. Seattle: IASP Press, 1999, pp 319–326.

Bennett GJ, Xie YK. A peripheral mononeuropathy in rat that produces disorders of pain sensation like those seen in man. *Pain* 1988; 33:87–107.

Boyce S, Hill RG. Discrepant results from preclinical and clinical studies on the potential of substance P-receptor antagonist compounds as analgesics. In: Devor M, Rowbotham MC, Wiesenfeld-Hallin Z (Eds). *Proceedings of the 9th World Congress on Pain,* Progress in Pain Research and Management, Vol. 16. Seattle: IASP Press, 2000, pp 313–324.

Bridges D, Thompson SW, Rice AS. Mechanisms of neuropathic pain. *Br J Anaesth* 2001; 8712–8726.

Calcutt NA, Jorge MC, Yaksh TL, Chaplan SR. Tactile allodynia and formalin hyperalgesia in streptozotocin-diabetic rats: effects of insulin, aldose reductase inhibition and lidocaine. *Pain* 1996; 68:293–299.

Courteix C, Eschalier A, Lavarenne J. Streptozocin-induced diabetic rats: behavioural evidence for a model of chronic pain. *Pain* 1993; 53:81–88.

Courteix C, Bardin M, Chantelauze C, Lavarenne J, Eschalier A. Study of the sensitivity of the diabetes-induced pain model in rats to a range of analgesics. *Pain* 1994; 57:153–160.

Crosby V, Wilcock A, Corcoran R. The safety and efficacy of a single dose (500 mg or 1 g) of intravenous magnesium sulfate in neuropathic pain poorly responsive to strong opioid analgesics in patients with cancer. *J Pain Symptom Manage* 2000; 19:35–39.

Dellemijn PL, Vanneste JA. Randomised double-blind active-placebo-controlled crossover trial of intravenous fentanyl in neuropathic pain. *Lancet* 1997; 349:753–758.

Fox A, Eastwood C, Gentry C, Manning D, Urban L. Critical evaluation of the streptozotocin model of painful diabetic neuropathy in the rat. *Pain* 1999; 81:307–316.

Fromm GH. Baclofen as an adjuvant analgesic. *J Pain Symptom Manage* 1994; 9:500–549.

Hewitt DJ. The use of NMDA-receptor antagonists in the treatment of chronic pain. *Clin J Pain* 2000; 16:S73–S79.

Hill R. NK1 (substance P) receptor antagonists—why are they not analgesic in humans? *Trends Pharmacol Sci* 2000; 21:244–246.

Ichimata M, Ikebe H, Yoshitake S, et al. Analgesic effects of flecainide on postherpetic neuralgia. *Int J Clin Pharmacol Res* 2000; 21:15–9.

Idänpään-Heikkilä JJ, Guilbaud G. Pharmacological studies on a rat model of trigeminal neuropathic pain: baclofen, but not carbamazepine, morphine or tricyclic antidepressants, attenuates the allodynia-like behaviour. *Pain* 1999; 79:281–290.

Jensen TS. Anticonvulsants in neuropathic pain: rationale and clinical evidence. *Eur J Pain* 2002; 6(Suppl A):61–68.

Kalso E, Tramer MR, McQuay HJ, Moore RA. Systemic local-anaesthetic-type drugs in chronic pain: a systematic review. *Eur J Pain* 1998; 2:3–14.

Kim SH, Chung JM. An experimental model for peripheral neuropathy produced by segmental spinal nerve ligation in the rat. *Pain* 1992; 50:355–363.

Kingery WS. A critical review of controlled clinical trials for peripheral neuropathic pain and complex regional pain syndromes. *Pain* 1997; 73:123–139.

Koch BD, Faurot GF, McQuirk JR, Clarke DE, Hunter JC. Modulation of mechano-hyperalgesia by clinically effective analgesics in rats with peripheral mononeuropathy. *Analgesia* 1996; 2:157–164.

Malcangio M, Tomlinson DR. A pharmacologic analysis of mechanical hyperalgesia in streptozotocin/diabetic rats. *Pain* 1998; 76:151–157.

McCleane GJ. Lamotrigine in the management of neuropathic pain: a review of the literature. *Clin J Pain* 2000; 16:321–326.

McQuay HJ, Moore RA. *An Evidence-Based Resource for Pain Relief.* Oxford: Oxford University Press, 1998.

McQuay H, Carroll D, Jadad AR, Wiffen P, Moore A. Anticonvulsant drugs for management of pain: a systematic review. *Br Med J* 1995; 311:1047–1052.

McQuay HJ, Tramer M. Nye BA, et al. A systematic review of antidepressants in neuropathic pain. *Pain* 1996; 68:217–227.

Schmalbruch H, Krarup C. Animal models of neuropathies. *Baillieres Clin Neurol* 1996; 5:77–105.

Seltzer Z, Dubner R, Shir Y. A novel behavioral model of neuropathic pain disorders produced in rats by partial sciatic nerve injury. *Pain* 1990; 43:205–218.

Sindrup SH, Jensen TS. Efficacy of pharmacological treatments of neuropathic pain: an update and effect related to mechanism of drug action. *Pain* 1999; 83:389–400.

Tasmuth T, Hartel B, Kalso E. Venlafaxine in neuropathic pain following treatment of breast cancer. *Eur J Pain* 2002; 6:17–24.

Tremont-Lukats IW, Megeff C, Backonja MM. Anticonvulsants for neuropathic pain syndromes: mechanisms of action and place in therapy. *Drugs* 2000; 60:1029–1052.

Urban LA, Fox AJ. NK1 receptor antagonists—are they really without effect in the pain clinic? *Trends Pharmacol Sci* 2000; 21:462–464, discussion p 465.

Wallace MS. Pharmacologic treatment of neuropathic pain. *Curr Pain Headache Reports* 2001; 5:138–150.

Willner P. The validity of animal models of depression. *Psychopharmacology* 1984; 83:1–16.

Yaksh TL, Yamamoto T, Myers R. Pharmacology of nerve compression evoked hyperalgesia. In: Willis WD (Ed). *Hyperalgesia and Allodynia.* New York: Raven Press, 1992, pp 245–258.

Yamamoto T, Yaksh TL. Spinal pharmacology of thermal hyperesthesia induced by incomplete ligation of sciatic nerve. I. Opioid and nonopioid receptors. *Anesthesiology* 1991; 75:817–826.

Yamamoto T, Yaksh TL. Spinal pharmacology of thermal hyperesthesia induced by constriction injury of sciatic nerve: excitatory amino acid antagonists. *Pain* 1992; 49:121–128.

Zeltser R, Seltzer Z. A practical guide for the use of animal models in the study of neuropathic pain. In: Boivie J, Hansson P, Lindblom U (Eds). *Touch, Temperature, and Pain in Health and Disease: Mechanisms and Assessments,* Progress in Pain Research and Management, Vol. 3. Seattle: IASP Press, 1994, pp 295–338.

Correspondence to: Vesa Kontinen, MD, PhD, Department of Pharmacology, Institute of Biomedicine, University of Helsinki, P.O. Box 63, FIN-00014 Helsinki, Finland. Email: vesa.kontinen@helsinki.fi.

Proceedings of the 10th World Congress on Pain,
Progress in Pain Research and Management, Vol. 24,
edited by Jonathan O. Dostrovsky, Daniel B. Carr, and
Martin Koltzenburg, IASP Press, Seattle, © 2003.

41

Side Effects of COX-2 Inhibitors and Other NSAIDs

Henry J. McQuay and R. Andrew Moore

Pain Research, Nuffield Department of Anaesthetics, University of Oxford, and Pain Relief Unit, Oxford Radcliffe Hospital, The Churchill, Oxford, United Kingdom

Medical knowledge gained and then forgotten is more common than we care to believe. At one time we were involved with the rediscovery of the adverse effects of morphine in kidney failure. The problem had been known for well over 100 years, but was forgotten sometime after the first world war. Perhaps then we should be less surprised than we are by the focus on the gastrointestinal (GI) adverse effects of nonsteroidal anti-inflammatory drugs (NSAIDs), to the exclusion of attention to their effects on the heart and kidneys. There are two reasons why this exclusion deserves attention. The first is that cardiac problems lead to as many hospital admissions as GI problems, and the second is that COX-2 inhibitors (also termed "coxibs") do not protect against cardiac problems.

The advent of the coxibs has led to much more thought about NSAID adverse effects, not least because we now have much more high-quality trial information. Coxibs do what they were designed to do: they provide the same efficacy as nonselective COX inhibitors with better GI safety. While we may argue about the extent of the improvement in GI safety, there seems little biological reason why the coxibs should be any safer than nonselective COX inhibitors for the heart and kidney. If heart problems are as common as GI problems, which although true is not the common medical perception, then coxibs are not a panacea.

This chapter will discuss the GI, cardiac, and renal adverse effects of acute and chronic NSAID use, while avoiding the trap of forgetting the importance of dose.

NSAID SAFETY IN ACUTE USE

MAJOR PROBLEMS

In acute pain the main concerns with NSAIDs are renal and coagulation problems. Acute renal failure can be precipitated when NSAIDs are given to patients with preexisting heart or kidney disease, those on loop diuretics, or those who have lost more than 10% of blood volume.

NSAIDs cause significant lengthening (by about 30%) of the bleeding time, usually still within the normal range. This prolonged bleeding can last for days with aspirin, and while it only lasts for several hours with non-aspirin NSAIDs, it still raises the possibility that these drugs may significantly increase blood loss.

A comparison of ketorolac, diclofenac, and ketoprofen in over 11,000 patients having major surgery, and given injected and then oral doses of one of these three NSAIDs, gave a 1% incidence of increased surgical site bleeding, 0.1% incidence of allergy, 0.1% incidence of acute renal failure, and 0.04% incidence of GI bleeding (Forrest et al. 2002). There was no difference between the three NSAIDs. The problem with the paper is that we do not know what would happen in the absence of NSAIDs. These estimates are in a sense the worst case; they tell us what happens when taking NSAIDs, and confirm that the postoperative risk of acute renal failure (0.1%) with NSAIDs is greater than the risk of GI bleeding (0.04%). Until a study similar in scope to that of Forrest et al. is conducted with coxibs, we will not know whether the 1% risk of surgical site bleeding would be the same with them.

Many orthopedic surgeons worry that NSAIDs may impair bone healing. Some basic science studies suggest such impairment, but such clinical studies as we have are at best inconclusive (Bandolier 2001). As always, it will be difficult to prove a negative.

MINOR PROBLEMS

Oral route. Adverse effects from single-dose oral acute pain studies have been examined systematically for ibuprofen and aspirin (Edwards et al. 1999). Common adverse effects such as nausea, dizziness, or drowsiness were reported more often when diaries were used, and drowsiness was reported more often in dental rather than other pain models. The incidence of any adverse effect with any single dose of analgesic was low, but gastric irritation was two to three times more common with aspirin than with placebo, and the number needed to harm was 22 (95% confidence interval [CI] = 22–174) (Edwards et al. 2000).

Other routes. For injected and rectal administration, commonly reported adverse effects independent of the route of administration were nausea, vomiting, dizziness, drowsiness, sedation, anxiety, dyspepsia, indigestion, and dry mouth (Tramèr et al. 1998). Two studies reported prolongation of bleeding time. In 12 patients with rheumatoid arthritis treated with indomethacin at a dose of 100 mg and 150 mg orally and rectally, respectively, in a crossover design for 2 weeks, endoscopically diagnosed gastric mucosal damage was independent of the route of administration.

Adverse effects related to the route of administration were most often reported for intramuscular and rectal regimens. Discomfort at the site of injection was the most common complaint in relation to intramuscular injections. After rectal administration, diarrhea, rectal irritation, and nonretention of suppositories were reported.

For topical NSAIDs in acute and chronic pain, both local and systemic adverse events, as well as drug-related study dropouts, had a low incidence no different from placebo (Moore et al. 1998).

NSAID SAFETY IN CHRONIC USE

At recommended doses, NSAIDs can cause a number of minor adverse effects, but also can cause major adverse effects—GI, cardiac, and renal. This profile is different for acetaminophen (paracetamol), which at recommended doses can cause minor adverse effects, but no major adverse effects. In overdose, acetaminophen can cause hepatic failure.

With the NSAIDs it is worth recalling that the slope of the dose-response curve for analgesia may not be as steep as, for instance, that of morphine. The important point is that the slope of the dose-response curves for adverse effects need not be the same as the slope for analgesia. If the slope for adverse effects is steeper than that for analgesia, then dose increases to produce greater analgesia may produce a proportionately greater increase in adverse effects.

GASTROINTESTINAL SIDE EFFECTS

Nonselective COX inhibitors. Oral NSAIDs cause ulcers in some people. Some of those who have ulcers, which include bleeding ulcers, also have symptoms. In some of those who have bleeding ulcers, the bleeding is sufficiently severe to result in hospital admission and may cause death. The variables are drug and dose, duration of exposure, and patient characteristics. The total burden is large, with some 106,000 NSAID-related hospital admissions and 16,500 deaths in the United States every year (Singh 1998). Age and sex are the major risk factors for serious GI complications with NSAIDs, though a history of previous ulcers and heart disease is also important. Of the different NSAIDs, some are implicated more than others, though case-control and cohort studies give somewhat different estimates. Both types of study indicate that ibuprofen is among the safest of the NSAIDs.

GI emergencies associated with oral NSAID use constitute a major problem. Two recent studies, each on about 1% of the population of the United Kingdom, indicate, first, that 1.9% of NSAID users might be admitted to hospital each year with upper GI emergencies (Moore and Phillips 1999), and second, that one episode of ulcer bleeding in the elderly will be expected for each 2,823 prescriptions (Hawkey et al. 1997). Another way of putting this is that if oral NSAIDs are taken for at least 2 months, the risk of an endoscopic ulcer is 1 in 5, of a symptomatic ulcer is about 1 in 70, of a bleeding ulcer is about 1 in 150, and of a death from a bleeding ulcer about 1 in 1,300 (Tramèr et al. 2000). None of these risks is associated with topical NSAIDs, which produce much lower plasma concentrations.

Hernandez-Diaz and Rodriguez (2000) reviewed the epidemiological studies associating NSAID use and upper GI problems, published in the 1990s, and pooled the data to give a much clearer picture of risks. To be included, studies had to be case-control or cohort studies on non-aspirin NSAIDs, with data on bleeding, perforation, or another serious upper GI tract event resulting in hospital admission or referral to a specialist, and had to have data to calculate relative risk. Eighteen studies were found, all of which had specific definitions of exposure and outcome and similar ascertainment for comparison groups. All but two attempted to control for potential confounding factors such as age, sex, history of ulcer, or concomitant medicines.

The main results are summarized in Figs. 1 and 2. Compared with nonusers, current NSAID users had a higher risk of upper GI bleeding, and the risk was higher when they were taking a higher dose. The duration of use was unimportant, but different NSAIDs had different risks, with ibuprofen (especially at doses below 2,400 mg a day) being least harmful.

The effect of ulcer history and age is shown in Figs. 3 and 4. Those with a history of ulcer or with a previous bleed who took NSAIDs were at much greater risk than those with no history of ulcer who took NSAIDs. Older patients who took NSAIDs were at greater risk than those under 50 who took NSAIDs.

What can be done to minimize these risks? The risk of GI bleeding with nonselective COX inhibitors may be reduced by coadministration of proton pump inhibitors (such as omeprazole) or misoprostol. GI adverse effects limit the tolerability of misoprostol.

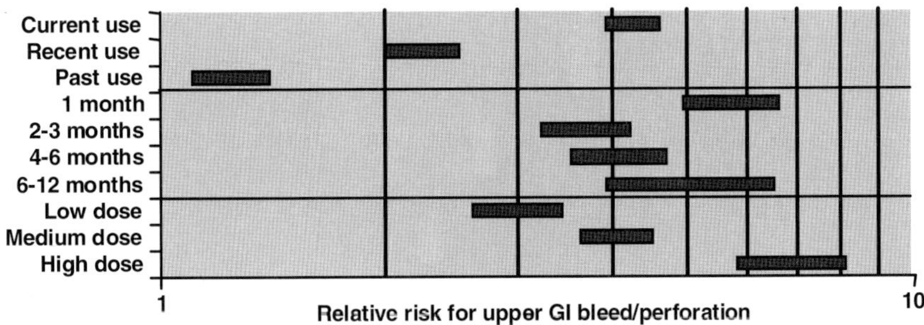

Fig. 1. Risk of upper GI bleeding for NSAID users compared with nonusers. In this and subsequent figures, bars represent 95% confidence intervals (CI) of relative risk.

COX-2 inhibitors. The coxibs reduce, but do not eliminate, the risk of GI bleeding. The evidence that they decrease gastric risk compared with nonselective COX inhibitors came from two large trials, VIGOR (rofecoxib) and the Celecoxib Long-term Arthritis Safety Study (CLASS). These trials have been subject to a great deal of criticism regarding design, analysis, and presentation (Juni et al. 2002), but they have provoked a great deal of thought about NSAID safety.

In the VIGOR trial, rofecoxib at a dose of 50 mg daily resulted in 2.1 confirmed GI events per 100 patient-years compared with 4.5 GI events per 100 patient-years on naproxen at a dose of 500 mg twice daily (relative risk = 0.5; 95% CI = 0.3–0.6), with a median follow-up of 9 months (Bombardier et al. 2000). For these two drugs the respective rates of confirmed complications (perforation, obstruction, and severe upper GI bleeding) were 0.6 per 100 patient-years and 1.4 per 100 patient-years (relative risk = 0.4; 95% CI = 0.2–0.8).

These patients had rheumatoid arthritis, over half were on steroids and over half on methotrexate, and yet the GI event rate on a 50-mg dose of rofecoxib was at the lower end of the range quoted by the U.S. Food and

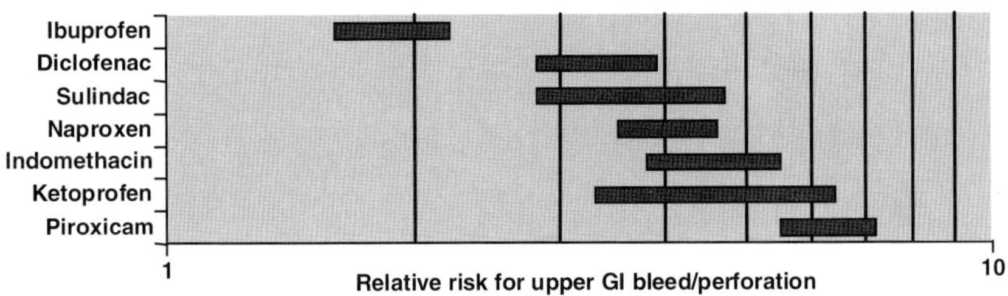

Fig. 2. Risk of upper GI bleeding for particular NSAIDs, compared with risk in nonusers.

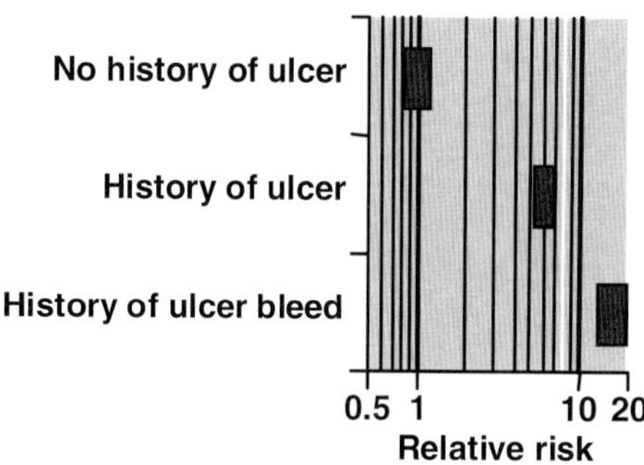

Fig. 3. Effect of history of ulcer in users of NSAIDs.

Drug Administration (FDA) in its NSAID-class label for the general population, 2 to 4% perforations, symptomatic ulcers, and GI bleeds in patients treated for 1 year. This 50-mg dose of rofecoxib is twice the recommended maximal daily dose, which begs the question whether the GI event rate would be reduced at a 25-mg or lower dose in a lower-risk population.

In the CLASS trial, 800 mg of celecoxib per day (n = 3,987 subjects), four times the usual arthritis dose, was compared in one trial with 2,400 mg of ibuprofen per day (n = 1,985 subjects), and in another with 150 mg of diclofenac per day (n = 1,996 subjects) (Silverstein et al. 2000). Results were pooled for the analysis. Patients could take aspirin for cardiovascular prophylaxis at daily doses of 325 mg or less. There was no significant difference in the annualized incidence of upper GI ulcer complications alone or combined with symptomatic ulcers for celecoxib versus ibuprofen and diclofenac. For the subgroup of patients taking aspirin, the annualized incidence rates of upper GI ulcer complications alone or combined with symptomatic ulcers for celecoxib versus NSAIDs were 2.01% versus 2.12% (P = 0.92) and 4.70% versus 6.00% (P = 0.49), respectively. Again, these values fell within the FDA label range. In the subgroup of patients not taking aspirin there were significant reductions in the annualized incidence rates of upper

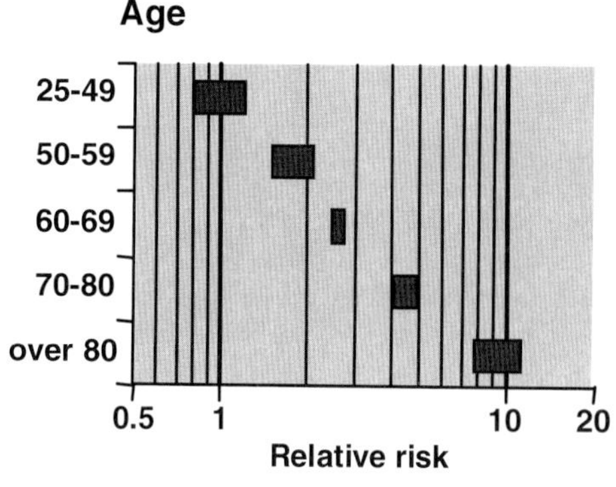

Fig. 4. Effect of age in users of NSAIDs.

GI ulcer complications alone or combined with symptomatic ulcers. These respective incidences for celecoxib versus NSAIDs were 0.44% versus 1.27% ($P = 0.04$) and 1.40% versus 2.91% ($P = 0.02$). One obvious interpretation is that aspirin masked any GI protection afforded by celecoxib. This is a key issue, because arthritis pain predominantly afflicts older people, many of whom take aspirin prophylactically. If the aspirin, even at low dose, negates any GI benefit of coxibs over nonselective COX inhibitors, then the advice must be either not to take the aspirin (heresy), or to use aspirin plus a nonselective COX inhibitor.

The CLASS and VIGOR trials were designed to demonstrate the improved GI safety of coxibs compared with nonselective COX inhibitors. Improved safety was shown for rofecoxib at 50 mg per day versus naproxen at 1,000 mg per day in patients not taking aspirin prophylaxis, and similarly for celecoxib at 800 mg per day versus ibuprofen at 2400 mg and diclofenac at 150 mg, again in the patients not taking aspirin. The rough rule of thumb is that if without an NSAID the incidence of perforations, symptomatic ulcers, and GI bleeds in patients treated for one year is 1% then we can expect a rate of 2% with coxibs and 4% on maximal daily doses of nonselective COX inhibitors. Then of course we must take account of the differences between the different COX-1-inhibiting drugs (Fig. 2), and the data available to compile relative risks as in Fig. 2 often do not include the crucial information about dose.

Summarizing the GI data for coxibs, they reduce the risk of GI adverse events compared with (high-dose) NSAIDs, but they do not eliminate it. At present it appears that this advantage may be lost if COX-2 inhibitors are taken in conjunction with low-dose aspirin. It is important to remember that these data are averages, so that the risks may be higher in the presence of factors such as increased age, previous bleed history, and steroid therapy, and lower in their absence.

The limited evidence available suggests that there are fewer dyspeptic symptoms with coxibs than with NSAIDs (Watson et al. 2000).

CARDIAC SIDE EFFECTS

Congestive heart failure. The second in the triad of major NSAID problems is congestive heart failure (CHF) in older people (Page and Henry 2000). This problem has had a much lower profile than GI bleeding and renal failure. This low profile may be inappropriate, because as many hospital admissions may result from NSAID-induced CHF as from NSAID-induced GI bleeding.

A study at two hospitals in New South Wales (population about 450,000) enrolled consecutive patients between 1993 and 1995 where the medical officer admitting the case and the attending physician agreed that the primary reason for admission was CHF (Page and Henry 2000). Patients admitted for other reasons with incidental CHF were not included. Study nurses ensured that all included cases met Framingham criteria for CHF. Controls (target of two controls per case) were patients of the same sex and within 5 years of the subject's age admitted to the same hospital, but with no clinical or radiological signs of CHF.

There were 365 cases and 658 controls, with a mean age of 76 years. Most cases had moderate or severe CHF. Use of non-aspirin NSAIDs was 17% in the cases in the week before admission, compared with 12% in controls. The adjusted odds ratio was 2.1 (95% CI = 1.2–3.3) for all cases, and 2.8 (95% CI = 1.5–5.1) for the 272 cases with first admission for CHF (Table I).

CHF was far more likely in those patients with a prior history of heart disease, in which the odds ratio was 26 (5.8 to 119). Complicated statistical analysis confirmed the effect of preexisting heart disease, and suggested that NSAIDs with longer half-lives (naproxen, piroxicam, and tenoxicam) had much higher risk than those with shorter half-lives (ibuprofen and diclofenac, for instance), although these conclusions were inferred from small numbers in a subgroup analysis.

The importance of NSAID precipitation of CHF was substantiated by a large study from Sweden (Merlo et al. 2001). Ecological line regression established an increased relative risk of 1.26 (1.23 to 1.28) between outpatient NSAID use and hospitalized heart failure.

Overall, the available data suggest no advantage of coxibs over NSAIDs for CHF.

Hypertensive effects of analgesics. NSAIDs raise blood pressure in some individuals, but to a variable degree (Hillis 2002). Hypertensive patients on NSAIDs were more susceptible to blood pressure increases than were normotensives on NSAIDs, and the mean increase in blood pressure was slightly higher in untreated hypertensive patients than in normotensive patients

Table I
NSAID use and history of heart disease: effect on risk of congestive heart failure

Heart Disease	NSAID Use	Odds Ratio (95% CI)
No history	Nonuser	1
No history	User	1.6 (0.7 to 3.7)
History	Nonuser	2.5 (1.4 to 4.3)
History	User	26 (6 to 119)

(Johnson et al. 1994). Hypertensive patients receiving antihypertensive therapy experienced a greater mean increase in supine blood pressure as a result of NSAID therapy than did uncontrolled hypertensive patients (4.7 mm Hg versus 1.8 mm Hg). Blood pressure increases were greater in patients receiving β-blockers than in those receiving vasodilators and diuretics (Johnson et al. 1994). In normotensive patients, hypertensive effects of conventional NSAIDs appear to be minimal (Pope et al. 1993; Johnson et al. 1994). Coxibs probably have similar effects, but the information is still limited (Hillis 2002).

Summary. Summarizing the cardiovascular data, both NSAIDs and coxibs can cause CHF, hypertension, and pedal edema (see FDA Advisory Committee 2001 for data on rofecoxib and naproxen). Low-dose aspirin reduces the GI benefits of coxibs, and NSAIDs (specifically, ibuprofen) may reduce the cardiac benefits of aspirin (Catella-Lawson et al. 2001). We are left with the controversial question as to whether coxibs cause myocardial infarction. In the VIGOR trial there were statistically significantly more thrombotic cardiovascular serious adverse events with rofecoxib than with naproxen (45/4,047 and 19/4,029, respectively) (FDA Advisory Committee 2001). The defense that this difference was due to a protective effect of naproxen that was not afforded by rofecoxib, a previously unrealized and untested effect, persuades some epidemiologists but not others. If the difference was due to a protective effect of naproxen, then this effect was some five times greater than the protective effect of aspirin seen in the randomized trials. Once again we have a potentially serious effect unmasked in a clinical trial, and we must wait for the evidence from further trials to determine whether it is reproducible and whether it is a class phenomenon.

RENAL SIDE EFFECTS

NSAIDs can cause acute renal failure with acute or chronic use. If renal function depends on prostaglandin "overdrive," then taking NSAIDs that reduce prostaglandin overdrive will impair function. Renal risk factors during acute or chronic NSAID use include preexisting heart or kidney disease, treatment with loop diuretics, or loss of more than 10% of blood volume. A recent estimate of renal risk came from a study conducted among all members of the Tennessee Medicaid program aged 65 years or older, enrolled for at least 1 year during 1987–1991 (Griffin et al. 2000). Those with first admission to hospital for acute renal failure (with a creatinine level of 180 μmol/L or more at admission) were deemed cases of community-acquired acute renal failure. Controls were randomly selected for all persons in the study population. Exclusions were people with end-stage renal disease and those with hospital-acquired acute renal failure. NSAID exposure was ascertained from prescriptions filled in the year before the index date.

There were 1,799 cases, with an annual incidence of community-acquired acute renal failure of 4.5 admissions per 1000. The median hospital stay was 8 days. Thirty-six percent died within 30 days. Forty-two percent were classified as having new renal disease. The remainder were classified as having chronic renal failure with acute exacerbation based on a prior creatinine level above 122 μmol/L, a documented history of chronic renal failure, or imaging studies compatible with chronic renal disease. There were 9,899 controls. Controls were less likely to be nursing home residents or to be 85 years or older.

NSAID use was higher (18%) in cases than in controls (11%). For current NSAID use the odds ratio was 1.6 (95% CI = 1.3–1.9). Those who had stopped using NSAIDs within the past 30 days had no increased risk of renal failure. For certain NSAIDs where there was sufficient information, ibuprofen and indomethacin, there was a dose response for risk. Among individual NSAIDs, ibuprofen, piroxicam, fenoprofen, and indomethacin had the greatest increased risk, with odds ratios of about 2.

A previous detailed study, although with fewer subjects, indicated that preexisting renal disease or gout, but particularly a joint history of gout plus preexisting renal disease were major risks for renal failure with NSAIDs (Henry et al. 1997). Patients using NSAIDs with half-lives of 12 hours or more in the previous week had a particularly high risk of renal failure.

There seems no biological reason why the risk of renal problems should be lower with coxibs than with the COX-1-inhibiting NSAIDs.

PUTTING IT TOGETHER

These three major NSAID risks—GI bleeding, renal failure, and congestive heart failure—are important because increased age is such an important factor in each. The population is aging, arthritis is a disease of older people, and NSAIDs are used to manage the pain of arthritis.

Putting all this into the perspective of an average primary care grouping of 100,000 (Blower et al. 1997), then in this population (3,500 over 65 years old taking NSAIDs), there would be 18 hospital admissions every year for upper GI bleeding, 10 for acute renal failure, and 22 for congestive heart failure. The majority of the renal and heart failure cases would be among those aged 75 and over. For both renal failure and congestive heart failure, NSAIDs "uncover" existing disease problems, and for both there are plausible mechanisms, dose-response relationships, and particular association with NSAIDs with longer half-lives.

Coxibs, however, do not reduce the risk of renal failure or of congestive heart failure, and for these risks there must be a clinical balance between the analgesia provided by a COX-1 or COX-2 inhibitor and the risk of complication. Over half the patients in the CLASS study (FDA 2002) of celecoxib versus COX-1-inhibiting drugs in arthritis were receiving hypertensive drugs, a reminder of the awkward fact that patients with pain will often be hypertensive and hence at risk. There is no evidence that the risk of congestive heart failure is higher with COX-2 than with COX-1 inhibitors, but neither is there evidence that it is lower, and for rofecoxib at least there is debate about thrombotic safety. Equally, there is no evidence that the risk of renal failure is lower with COX-2 than with COX-1 inhibitors. The three risks can only be minimized by sensible matching of drug with patient, followed regularly thereafter by assessment.

REFERENCES

Bandolier. NSAIDs and bone. Available at http:www.jr2.ox.ac.uk/Bandolier/booth/painpag/wisdom/NSAIbone.html. Accessed 2001.

Blower AL, Brooks A, Penn GC, et al. Emergency admissions for upper gastrointestinal disease and their relation to NSAID use. *Aliment Pharmacol Ther* 1997; 11:283–291.

Bombardier C, Laine L, Reicin A, et al. Comparison of upper gastrointestinal toxicity of rofecoxib and naproxen in patients with rheumatoid arthritis. *N Engl J Med* 2000; 343:1520–1528.

Catella-Lawson F, Reilly MP, Kapoor SC, et al. Cyclooxygenase inhibitors and the antiplatelet effects of aspirin. *N Engl J Med* 2001; 345:1809–1817.

Edwards JE, McQuay HJ, Moore RA, Collins SL. Reporting of adverse effects in clinical trials should be improved. Lessons from acute postoperative pain. *J Pain Symptom Manage* 1999; 81:289–297.

Edwards JE, Oldman A, Smith L, et al. Single dose oral aspirin for acute pain. *Cochrane Database Syst Rev* 2000; CD002067.

FDA. Celebrex labeling. Available at www.fda.gov/cder/foi/label/2002/20998s009lbl.pdf. Accessed 2002.

FDA Advisory Committee. VIOXX gastrointestinal safety. Briefing Document NDA 21-042, s007, 2001.

Forrest JB, Camu F, Greer IA, et al. Ketorolac, diclofenac, and ketoprofen are equally safe for pain relief after major surgery. *Br J Anaesth* 2002; 88:227–233.

Griffin MR, Yared A, Ray WA. Nonsteroidal antiinflammatory drugs and acute renal failure in elderly persons. *Am J Epidemiol* 2000; 151:488–496.

Hawkey CJ, Cullen DJ, Greenwood DC, Wilson JV, Logan RF. Prescribing of nonsteroidal anti-inflammatory drugs in general practice: determinants and consequences. *Aliment Pharmacol Ther* 1997; 11:293–298.

Henry D, Page J, Whyte I, et al. Consumption of non-steroidal anti-inflammatory drugs and the development of functional renal impairment in elderly subjects. Results of a case-control study. *Br J Clin Pharmacol* 1997; 44:85–90.

Hernandez-Diaz S, Rodriguez LAG. Association between nonsteroidal anti-inflammatory drugs and upper gastrointestinal tract bleeding/perforation. *Arch Intern Med* 2000; 160:2093–2099.

Hillis WS. Areas of emerging interest in analgesia: cardiovascular complications. *Am J Ther* 2002; 9:259–269.

Johnson AG, Nguyen TV, Day RO. Do nonsteroidal anti-inflammatory drugs affect blood pressure? *Ann Intern Med* 1994; 121:289–300.

Juni P, Rutjes AW, Dieppe PA. Are selective COX 2 inhibitors superior to traditional non steroidal anti-inflammatory drugs? *BMJ* 2002; 324:1287–1288.

Merlo J, Broms K, Lindblad U, et al. Association of outpatient utilisation of non-steroidal anti-inflammatory drugs and hospitalised heart failure in the entire Swedish population. *Eur J Clin Pharmacol* 2001; 57:71–75.

Moore RA, Phillips CJ. Cost of NSAID adverse effects to the UK National Health Service. *J Med Economics* 1999; 2:45–55.

Moore RA, Tramèr MR, Carroll D, Wiffen PJ, McQuay HJ. Quantitive systematic review of topically-applied non-steroidal anti-inflammatory drugs. *BMJ* 1998; 316:333–338.

Page J, Henry D. Consumption of NSAIDs and the development of congestive heart failure in elderly patients. *Arch Intern Med* 2000; 160:777–784.

Pope JE, Anderson JJ, Felson DT. A meta-analysis of the effects of nonsteroidal anti-inflammatory drugs on blood pressure. *Arch Int Med* 1993; 153:477–484.

Silverstein FE, Faich G, Goldstein JL, et al. Gastrointestinal toxicity with celecoxib vs nonsteroidal anti-inflammatory drugs for osteoarthritis and rheumatoid arthritis: the CLASS study: a randomized controlled trial. Celecoxib Long-term Arthritis Safety Study. *JAMA* 2000; 284:1247–1255.

Singh G. Recent considerations in nonsteroidal anti-inflammatory drug gastropathy. *Am J Med* 1998; 105:31S–38S.

Tramèr MR, Williams JE, Carroll D, et al. Comparing analgesic efficacy of non-steroidal anti-inflammatory drugs given by different routes in acute and chronic pain: a qualitative systematic review. *Acta Anaesthesiol Scand* 1998; 42:71–79.

Tramèr MR, Moore RA, Reynolds DJ, McQuay HJ. Quantitative estimation of rare adverse events which follow a biological progression: a new model applied to chronic NSAID use. *Pain* 2000; 85:169–182.

Watson DJ, Harper SE, Zhao P-L, et al. Gastrointestinal tolerability of the selective cyclooxygenase-2 (COX-2) inhibitor rofecoxib compared with nonselective COX-1 and COX-2 inhibitors in osteoarthritis. *Arch Intern Med* 2000; 160:2998–3003.

Correspondence to: Henry J. McQuay, DM, FRCA, FRCP, Pain Relief Unit, Oxford Radcliffe Hospital, The Churchill, Headington, Oxford OX3 7LJ, United Kingdom. Tel: 01865-226161; Fax: 01865-226160; email: henry.mcquay@pru.ox.ac.uk.

Part VI

Genetics and Gene Therapy

Proceedings of the 10th World Congress on Pain,
Progress in Pain Research and Management, Vol. 24,
edited by Jonathan O. Dostrovsky, Daniel B. Carr, and
Martin Koltzenburg, IASP Press, Seattle, © 2003.

42

Genetic Influence on Pain Sensitivity in Humans: Evidence of Heritability Related to Single Nucleotide Polymorphisms in Opioid Receptor Genes

Hyungsuk Kim,[a] John K. Neubert,[a]
Michael J. Iadarola,[a] Anitza San Miguel,[a]
David Goldman,[b] and Raymond A. Dionne[a]

[a]Pain and Neurosensory Mechanisms Branch, National Institute of Dental and Craniofacial Research, National Institutes of Health, Bethesda, Maryland, USA; [b]Laboratory of Neurogenetics, National Institute on Alcohol Abuse and Alcoholism, National Institutes of Health, Rockville, Maryland, USA

The human pain experience is traditionally explained by a variety of factors such as cultural or psychological influences that account for interindividual variation. Recent studies in rodent pain models using hot-plate tests and nerve injury, however, demonstrate phenotypic differences in pain sensitivity that may be due to genetic factors (Mogil 1999; Seltzer et al. 2001). Though species may differ in important ways, converging lines of evidence from animal studies suggest that pain sensitivity is also likely to be heritable in humans (Lariviere et al. 2002) and that polymorphisms at the δ-opioid receptor subtype 1 gene (*OPRD1*) and the μ-opioid receptor subtype 1 gene (*OPRM1*) may affect the variability of pain sensitivity. Despite evidence for genetic factors and even specific genes influencing pain perception in mice (Mogil et al. 1997), the role of genetic factors in the perception, interpretation, and behavioral expression of pain in humans is obscured by genetic and environmental heterogeneity. To investigate a possible role for genetic factors in pain sensitivity, we have measured intraclass correlation coefficients (ICCs) from sibling pairs for experimental pain sensitivity and examined the role of opioid receptor alleles in this domain of human behavior.

METHODS

Normal subjects (294 females and 186 males) were evaluated in the Pain Research Clinic of the National Institute of Dental and Craniofacial Research (NIDCR). The subjects gave informed consent under a human research protocol approved by the NIDCR Institutional Review Board.

We measured pain sensitivity in response to experimental painful thermal stimuli and cold stimuli with separate visual analogue scale (VAS) ratings for pain intensity and unpleasantness. Individuals rated heat pain intensity (HI) and heat pain unpleasantness (HU) following application of thermal stimuli of 43°, 44°, 45°, 46°, 47°, and 49°C for 5 seconds. The thermode probe area was 1 cm in diameter and was mounted in a housing to maintain constant pressure on the skin. Subjects self-applied the probe at six different sites on the volar forearm within an area of ~ 40 × 100 mm. Subjects completed four iterations for each temperature, moving the probe location to eliminate the possibility of sensitization or tissue damage. We predetermined the order of each temperature for each trial, but the order was quasi-random to prevent subjects from anticipating subsequent stimuli. Subjects were blinded with regard to the temperature of the stimulus.

For cold stimuli, cold pain intensity (CI), and cold pain unpleasantness (CU), VAS ratings were measured every 30 seconds following submersion of the subject's hand up to the wrist into an insulated bucket filled with iced water (2–4°C). Subjects kept their hand submerged while clenching and unclenching repeatedly until pain reached an "unbearable level" or submersion time reached 180 seconds, whichever occurred first. Subjects could withdraw their hand at any time. We analyzed CI and CU at 30 seconds. If the subject withdrew his or her hand prior to 30 seconds, CI and CU were recorded at their cold withdrawal time (CWT).

For genotyping, 50 mL of venous blood from each subject was collected. DNA was isolated with the Puregene DNA isolation kit according to the manufacturer's instructions. Polymerase chain reaction (PCR) was performed under the following conditions: two cycles of 50°C, 2 minutes and 95°C, 10 minutes followed by 40 cycles of 95°C, 15 seconds and annealing temperature, 1 minute in a Perkin-Elmer 9600 thermocycler. Annealing temperatures were 61.5°C for *OPRD1* 80, 61°C for *OPRD1* 921, 62°C for *OPRM1* 17, and 65°C for *OPRM1* 118. Each well contained Taqman universal master

Table I
Primer and probe pairs

OPRD1 T80G		
	Primers	F: 5'-GCAGCCCCCCGCTCTT-3'
		R: 5'-GGCCCCGACGCATT-3'
	Probes	G80G: 6FAM-5'-ACCCTAGCGCCTGCCCCAG-3'-TAMRA
		T80T: VIC-5'-ACCCTAGCGCCTTCCCCAGCC-3'-TAMRA
OPRD1 T921C		
	Primers	F: 5'-GCTGCGCTGCACCTGTG-3'
		R: 5'-TGAAGTTCTCGTCGAGGAAAGC-3'
	Probes	T921T: 6FAM-5'-CGCGCTGGGCTACGCCAATA-3'-TAMRA
		C921C: VIC-5'-TCGCGCTGGGTTACGCCAATA-3'-TAMRA
OPRM1 C17T		
	Primers	F: 5'-TCGGTGCTCCTGGCTACCT-3'
		R: 5'-GTTGCCATCTAAGTGGGACAAGTT-3'
	Probes	C17C: 6FAM-5'-CAGCGCTGCCCCCACGA-3'-TAMRA
		T17T: VIC-5'-AGCAGCGCTGTCCCCACGA-3'-TAMRA
OPRM1 A118G		
	Primers	F: 5'-GCCGGTTCCTGGGTCAAC-3'
		R: 5'-GGAGGGCACAGGCTGTCTCT-3'
	Probes	A118A: 6FAM-5'-CCACTTAGATGGCAACCTGTCCGACC-3'-TAMRA
		G118G: VIC-5'-CCACTTAGATGGCGACCTGTCCGAC-3'-TAMRA

mix, 100 nM labeled probe, 900 nM of each primer (Table I), and 50 ng DNA. Following PCR, fluorescence in each well was measured using the ABI Prism 7700 Sequence Detection System. Genotype discrimination was performed using Taqman Sequence Detector version 1.7 software.

We examined pain sensitivity ICCs from 103 sibling pairs by using VAS scores for HI, HU, CI, CU, and CWT. For sets of sibships, wide-sense heritability of a quantitative trait is obtained from the ICC estimated through a one-way analysis of variance (ANOVA). If we assume that common environment plays a minimal role in the sibling-sibling correlations, we can calculate heritability estimate as h^2 (%) = 2 × ICC × 100 (Ott 1999). We used ANOVA with Duncan's post hoc analysis to examine the effect of the three different *OPRD1* T921C genotypes on experimental pain response. The frequencies of the rarer homozygous genotypes were insufficient, so we grouped the common homozygote and the heterozygote for *OPRD1* T80G and *OPRM1* A118G. We used independent t tests to compare differences between common homozygous and heterozygous groups in *OPRD1* T80G and *OPRM1* A118G. Probability of $P < 0.05$ was considered to be significant for statistical comparison.

RESULTS

To assess the genetic factors in human pain sensitivity, we evaluated the ICCs for experimental pain sensitivity. The ICC for CWT (0.23, 95% CI: 0.04–0.40) was the highest; the ICCs for CI (0.17, 95% CI: –0.03 to 0.35), CU (0.16, 95% CI: –0.04 to 0.34), HI (0.11, 95% CI: –0.09 to 0.30), and HU (0.13, 95% CI: –0.06 to 0.32) were somewhat lower.

OPRD1 80G affected pain sensitivity differently depending both on gender and on the modality of the applied stimuli. Male subjects with the homozygous 80T/80T genotype showed higher heat pain sensitivity, including HI and HU ratings, than did 80T/80G heterozygotes (Fig. 1a). Females did not demonstrate this type of association. We observed significant differences in

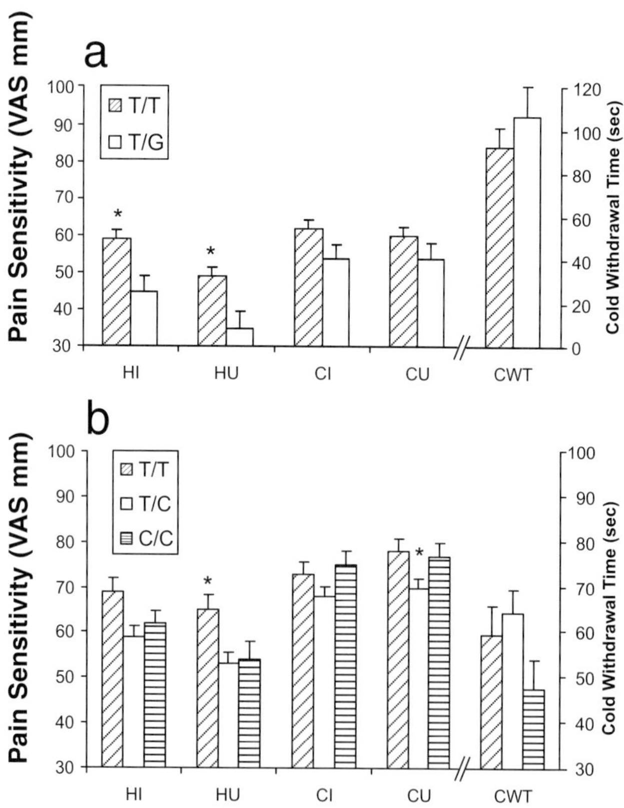

Fig. 1. Genotype association with experimental pain ratings (VAS) and withdrawal time (seconds). (a) *OPRD1* T80G in males. * $P < 0.01$. (b) *OPRD1* T921C in females. * $P < 0.05$. HI = heat pain intensity, HU = heat pain unpleasantness, CI = cold pain intensity, CU = cold pain unpleasantness, CWT = cold withdrawal time, T/T = thymine/thymine allele, T/G = thymine/guanine allele, T/C = thymine/cytosine allele, C/C = cytosine/cytosine allele.

pain unpleasantness for HU and CU for *OPRD1* T921C in female subjects (Fig. 1b), but not in male subjects.

DISCUSSION

Sibling resemblance for complex traits may arise due to genetic transmission or common environment. Studies of different familial constellations, including twins and unrelated individuals raised together, can isolate these effects and also can identify additional nonadditive components of inheritance. However, sibling-sibling correlations can define a portion of trait variance that may present additive heritability, and can therefore identify a potential domain of variance attributable to genetic variation. The ICCs from sibling pairs translate to additive heritability values up to twice as large, depending on the contribution of common family environment to resemblance between siblings in pain sensitivity (Ott 1999).

We found moderate, but significant, ICCs from sibling pairs for pain sensitivity. These moderate correlations are consistent with correlations for inherited traits such as body mass and longevity (Yazdi et al. 2000; Pausova et al. 2001). Human sex differences in experimental pain perception are well documented and were also found in our sample (Table II). Therefore, these moderate correlations for pain sensitivity from siblings suggest an important role for genetic factors in the perception and responses to experimental pain and may help explain diversity of clinical pain presentation.

To uncover sex-specific genetic effects, we analyzed male and female subjects separately for pain sensitivity. *OPRD1* T80G results in a phenylalanine to cysteine substitution at codon 27 in the N-terminal domain of the receptor. *OPRD1* T80G appeared to differ in its association to pain sensitivity

Table II
Sex differences in experimental pain sensitivity using VAS (mean ± standard deviation)

	Female	Male	Significance
HI	62.0 ± 27.2	57.0 ± 25.3	*
HU	55.8 ± 29.6	47.4 ± 28.8	**
CI	70.9 ± 23.5	61.5 ± 23.4	***
CU	73.4 ± 24.3	60.3 ± 26.4	***
CWT	58.4 ± 55.1	93.2 ± 65.0	***

Abbreviations: HI = heat pain intensity; HU = heat pain unpleasantness; CI = cold pain intensity; CU = cold pain unpleasantness; CWT = cold withdrawal time; VAS = visual analogue scale.
* $P < 0.05$, ** $P < 0.01$, *** $P < 0.001$.

depending on gender and on the characteristics of applied stimuli. These findings are consistent with evidence suggesting a sex-specific quantitative trait locus (QTL) on murine chromosome 4 that contains *Oprd1* and mediates acute, thermal nociception as measured with a hot plate (Mogil et al. 1997). A difference in baseline sensitivity in the hot-plate assay between wild-type and *Oprd1* knockout mice has also been reported (Zhu et al. 1999).

OPRD1 T921C is located in transmembrane domain 7 and is a synonymous substitution. Despite the absence of a structural change due to the T921C substitutions, this allelic difference may have influenced the pain unpleasantness found in our samples. It is also conceivable that another closely linked polymorphism, for example within the gene promoter region or a portion of a haplotype, could alter the rate of δ-opioid receptor expression with respect to the mode of expression regulation. These data suggest that gender and genotype of *OPRD1* in our population interact to affect pain sensitivity to thermal and cold stimuli. Dimerization interactions between opioid receptors, including δ-opioid receptors (Gomes et al. 2000; Milligan and White 2001), and some protein-DNA interactions (Smirnov et al. 2001) in *OPRD1,* may provide a mechanism for differential pain sensitivity found in our samples.

We predict that the amino acid changes induced by the *OPRM1* C17T and A118G alleles will alter receptor function. The C17T polymorphism results in an amino acid substitution from alanine to valine in codon 6 of the N-terminal domain, while the A118G results in a substitution from asparagine to aspartate in codon 40 of the same domain of the receptor. The A118G variant receptor binds β-endorphin with approximately three times greater affinity than the most common allelic form of the receptor and results in a threefold increase in potency for agonist-induced activation of G-protein-coupled potassium channels (Bond et al. 1998). This functional alteration in endogenous opioid activity may affect a range of behaviors that involve opioid receptor function, including drug and alcohol dependence, and pain sensitivity. The A118G SNP reduces the potency of morphine's active metabolite, morphine-6-glucuronide, in central opioid effects in humans (Lötsch et al. 2002). However, we did not find significant difference in VAS ratings among the variants of *OPRM1* in either male and female subjects for any experimental pain responses.

Even though we found differences in pain sensitivity to thermal and cold stimuli related to single nucleotide polymorphisms (SNPs) in *OPRD1,* for modest genetic effects and for identification of genotypic subgroups, much larger sample sizes may be required. A sample drawn from only one ethnic group may increase researchers' ability to study phenotype-genotype association (Altmüller et al. 2001). The strength of linkage-based mapping is also its weakness because no mechanism assumptions are possible from these data. However, these functional-level allelic differences may, at some level, be encoded in the genome and segregate.

In conclusion, our observations demonstrate that pain sensitivity is familial and suggest that individual response to pain is heritable. The results also suggest that gender and *OPRD1* genotype act upon one another to affect pain due to thermal and cold stimuli. Larger samples with more subjects for each ethnic group and also functional genomic studies are needed to confirm these associations. Ideally, in vitro functional tests to directly measure the effect of the SNPs are desirable to confirm these findings and to provide a stronger rationale for the relationship to pain sensitivity.

ACKNOWLEDGMENTS

This research was supported by the Division of Intramural Research, NIDCR, NIH.

REFERENCES

Altmüller J, Palmer LJ, Fischer G, Scherb H, Wjst M. Genomewide scans of complex human diseases: true linkage is hard to find. *Am J Hum Genet* 2001; 69:936–950.

Bond C, LaForge K, Tian M, et al. Single-nucleotide polymorphism in the human mu opioid receptor gene alters β-endorphin binding and activity: possible implications for opiate addiction. *Proc Natl Acad Sci USA* 1998; 95:9608–9613.

Gomes I, Jordan BA, Gupta A, et al. Heterodimerization of μ and δ opioid receptors: a role in opiate synergy. *J Neurosci* 2000; 20:1–5.

Lariviere WR, Wilson SG, Laughlin TM, et al. Heritability of nociception. III. Genetic relationships among commonly used assays of nociception and hypersensitivity. *Pain* 2002; 97:75–86.

Lötsch J, Skarke C, Grösch S, et al. The polymorphism A118G of the human mu-opioid receptor gene decreases the pupil constrictory effect of morphine-6-glucuronide but not that of morphine. *Pharmacogenetics* 2002; 12:3–9.

Milligan G, White J. Protein-protein interactions at G-protein-coupled receptors. *Trends Pharmacol Sci* 2001; 22:513–518.

Mogil JS. The genetic mediation of individual differences in sensitivity to pain and its inhibition. *Proc Natl Acad Sci USA* 1999; 96:7744–7751.

Mogil JS, Richards SP, O'Toole LA, et al. Genetic sensitivity to hot-plate nociception in DBA/2J and C57BL/6J inbred mouse strains: possible sex-specific mediation by δ_2-opioid receptors. *Pain* 1997; 70:267–277.

Ott J. *Analysis of Human Genetic Linkage*, 3rd ed. Baltimore: Johns Hopkins University Press, 1999.

Pausova Z, Gossard F, Gaudet D, et al. Heritability estimates of obesity measures in siblings with and without hypertension. *Hypertension* 2001; 38:41–47.

Seltzer Z, Wu T, Max MB, Diehl SR. Mapping a gene for neuropathic pain-related behavior following peripheral neurectomy in the mouse. *Pain* 2001; 93:101–106.

Smirnov D, Im H, Loh HH. δ-Opioid receptor gene: effect of Sp1 factor on transcriptional regulation in vivo. *Mol Pharmacol* 2001; 60:331–340.

Yazdi MH, Rydhmer L, Ringmar-Cederberg E, Lundeheim N, Johansson K. Genetic study of longevity in Swedish Landrace sows. *Livestock Production Science* 2000; 63:255–264.

Zhu Y, King MA, Schuller AG, et al. Retention of supraspinal delta-like analgesia and loss of morphine tolerance in δ opioid receptor knockout mice. *Neuron* 1999; 24:243–252.

Correspondence to: Raymond A. Dionne, DDS, PhD, Pain and Neurosensory Mechanisms Branch, National Institute of Dental and Craniofacial Research, National Institutes of Health, Building 10, Room 1N103, 10 Center Drive, Bethesda, MD 20892, USA. Tel: 301-496-0294; Fax: 301-402-9885; email: rdionne@dir.nidcr.nih.gov.

Proceedings of the 10th World Congress on Pain,
Progress in Pain Research and Management, Vol. 24,
edited by Jonathan O. Dostrovsky, Daniel B. Carr, and
Martin Koltzenburg, IASP Press, Seattle, © 2003.

43

Gene Therapy for Pain: Different Approaches toward a Common Goal[1]

David C. Yeomans,[a] Andrew Mannes,[b] and Youichi Saitoh[c]

[a]*Department of Anesthesia, Stanford University, Stanford, California, USA;* [b]*Department of Anesthesia and Surgical Services, National Institute of Dental and Craniofacial Research, National Institutes of Health, Bethesda, Maryland, USA;* [c]*Department of Neurosurgery, Osaka University, Osaka, Japan*

As lifespan increases and the "baby-boomer" generation approaches senior citizenship, chronic pain is taking an increasing toll on human society. Millions of people suffer from debilitating, persistent pain, at a cost to society in the billions of dollars, indicative of the clear inadequacy of current pharmacotherapies. End of life, whether from cancer or other diseases, can be associated with pain that is refractory to conventional therapies. This pain can be most severe in the final weeks of life (Bonica 1990; Cleeland et al. 1994). It can be associated with the disease itself or may result from the therapies used to treat the disease (chemotherapy, surgery, or radiation therapy). With advanced disease, pain is often widespread and can include visceral, somatic, and neuropathic components. Conventional medical therapies are often effective in symptom management, but a significant number of patients either do not obtain substantial relief or are plagued by side effects preventing adequate pain control. Neurolytic blocks using phenol or ethanol are alternatives for severe pain, but they can be ineffective against widespread pain and can have catastrophic outcomes. Improvements in intrathecal and epidural drug delivery provide profound relief, but these therapies are regionally specific and require additional intervention and risks, increasing the cost and complexity of care at the end of life.

[1] Based on a Congress workshop.

The need for new approaches to this problem is clear. Work described in this chapter investigates the potential clinical utility of an alternate approach to chronic pain, namely gene therapy. The goal of most gene therapy work is to alter the genome of targeted cells, either through replacing nonfunctional genes (as in genetic disease), or through downregulating overexpressed genes that have toxic products (e.g., amyloid plaques). In the pain system, however, gene therapy generally has different goals. The pain system may be functioning correctly, carrying peripheral or central pain information to the brain so that it can be perceived. The goal, instead, is to selectively and permanently manipulate the function of this segment of the nervous system, such that the tone of the chronically active pain system is diminished. Several different approaches have been applied to this problem, all with somewhat different specific goals. This chapter describes three such approaches.

Cell transplantation for the treatment of pain has been under investigation for more than two decades, and has been used successfully to treat cancer pain patients (Pappas et al. 1997). In this procedure, pieces of allogenic adrenal tissue are infused into the spinal subarachnoid space. The chromaffin cells within these tissue pieces secrete a mixture of compounds, some of which have profound analgesic effects. However, as in any transplant from one organism to another, rejection is always a potential problem. In addition, these cells secrete a large number of compounds, some of which may have deleterious effects over which we can have no control. For these reasons, the strategy arose of developing specific, analgesic cell lines for transplantation. Thus, the first section of this chapter describes investigations into the efficacy of transplantation of genetically altered neuronal cells onto the spinal cord as a means of providing a paracrine source of analgesic agents.

The second and third sections of this chapter introduce the use of recombinant viruses to transfect cells that are critical in pain physiology. In this way, genes encoding analgesic peptides or antisense genes to decrease expression of endogenous proalgesic peptides can be introduced into specific sites of the nervous system that are involved in the production and maintenance of pain. Thus, the second section of the chapter deals with administration of adenoviruses encoding the endogenous opioid peptide β-endorphin. Spinal intraparenchymal or intrathecal injections of these viruses can transfect spinal cord neurons or meningeal cells, causing them to express and secrete this peptide. The third section examines the use of recombinant herpes viruses as vectors to selectively alter the genome of primary afferent nociceptors. Each of these strategies has its own peculiar strengths, and each has the potential to provide long-term relief in different chronic pain patients, including those near the end of life.

EX VIVO GENE THERAPY FOR INTRACTABLE PAIN

This section describes the use of transplantation of encapsulated cells. Semipermeable membranes used for the capsules allow the transport of nutrients and neurotransmitters of low molecular mass, but prevent the inward diffusion of both humoral and cellular elements of the immune system. Therefore, cells in the capsules are isolated from the host immune system. This technique has been used in animal models of Parkinson's disease, in treating patients with amyotrophic lateral sclerosis, and in modulating cancer pain.

Pro-opiomelanocortin (POMC) is a precursor of adrenocorticotropic hormone (ACTH) and β-endorphin, a potent endogenous opioid. The mouse neuroblastoma cell line (Neuro2A) possesses converting enzymes so that Neuro2A cells transfected with the POMC gene under simian virus 40 (SV40) promoter secrete equal amounts of ACTH and β-endorphin (Noel et al. 1989). When this cell line was encapsulated in polymer capsules and transplanted into the rat spinal cerebrospinal fluid (CSF) space, the animals demonstrated analgesia in analgesimetric tests. For clinical therapy, it is important that regulated amounts of opioids should be infused into the CSF space. Ideally, transfected genes in the implanted grafts should be regulated intrinsically, leading to delivery of neuropeptides or transmitters on demand. A practical alternative might be to control gene expression of transfected cells exogenously. A transcriptional transactivator, known as rtTA, was developed that fuses the *Herpes simplex* virus transcriptional regulatory protein (VP16) activation domain with a mutant tetracycline (Tet) repressor from *Escherichia coli.* This transactivator requires Tet derivatives such as doxycycline (Dox) to bind a specific target sequence Tet operator. Thus, addition of Tet to cells that constitutively synthesize rtTA increases the expression of genes under the control of rtTA by more than 1,000-fold. This system is called the "Tet-On system" (Gossen and Bujard 1992). Several other systems in which gene expression can be artificially manipulated by exogenous stimuli are available. However, some of these inducers are toxic, and others are endogenous substances not suitable for clinical use. On the other hand, Tet derivatives are minimally toxic at concentrations less than 3 μg/mL, and the Tet regulatory transcriptional system is not present in mammalian cells. Furthermore, with the Tet-On system, gene expression begins shortly after the addition of Tet, and levels of gene expression increase in a dose-dependent manner. Therefore, the Tet-On system appears to be suitable for clinical use in regulating gene expression.

In our study we used plasmids pUHD172-1neo, pUHG16-3, and pUHD10-3 to produce stable Tet-On expression. Stable transfectants of the

Tet-On system were obtained and labeled Neuro2A-Tet-On-LacZ (NLZ) and Neuro2A-Tet-On-POMC (NTP). Plasmid pUHD10-3-neprilysin-1-β-endorphin was constructed to express NL1-β-endorphin fusion protein under the regulation of the Tet-On system. In order to activate the Tet-On system, NLZ cells were cultured in conditioned media. NLZ and NTP cells were seeded on dishes and were treated with Dox at 1,000, 100, 10, 1.0, and 0 ng/mL for 24 hours. To detect *LacZ* gene expression, NLZ cells were fixed with 1% glutaraldehyde and stained in X-gal (5-bromo-4-chloro-3-indoly-β-D-galactopyranoside) buffer. For NTP cells, the amount of ACTH was measured by radioimmunoassay (RIA).

Under an operative microscope, the occipitoatlantal junction of Sprague-Dawley rats was exposed, the dura mater and arachnoid membrane were incised, and a capsule was implanted into the CSF space of the spinal cord in animals treated with either Neuro2A-POMC or NTP. Animals in a control group received the polymer capsules without cells. Polymer capsules (inner diameter, 0.5 mm; length, 10 mm; total volume, 20 μL), permeable to molecules with molecular masses less than 30 kDa, were filled with cells suspended in phosphate buffer solution (PBS) at a density of 5.0×10^6 cells/mL. Analgesia was assessed by the hot-plate test, tail-pinch test, and electrical stimulation.

In vitro, the ratio of ACTH and β-endorphin secretion from Neuro2A-POMC cells was 1:0.82 ± 0.09. ACTH secretion from a capsule was approximately 100 pg/mL in 3 mL conditioned culture media for 24 hours. Rats in the Neuro2A-POMC group revealed significant analgesia in comparison with both the control group and pretransplanted rats in the three analgesimetric tests. Intramuscular injection of naloxone increased pain sensitivity in the Neuro2A-POMC group. Morphological study revealed that the tumor cells in the capsules survived but aggregated, and that the core of the spheroid was necrotic (Saitoh et al. 1995).

Approximately 70% of NLZ cells were stained with X-gal buffer after a 24-hour incubation in 1,000 ng Dox/mL, while very few cells incubated without Dox were stained. The extent of staining varied among cells in the same dish, but overall staining intensity appeared to depend on the dose of Dox. NTP cells secreted ACTH and β-endorphin according to the amount of Dox. However, NTP cells unexpectedly secreted low amounts of β-endorphin, despite the fact that Neuro2A-POMC cells secreted almost equal amounts of ACTH and β-endorphin. It may be that the Tet-On system itself interferes with the processing of POMC specifically or with that of large molecular precursors in general.

To examine whether POMC expression in NTP cells in the rat CSF space can be controlled by administration of Dox, rats in the NTP group were given an intraperitoneal injection of 5.0, 2.0, 0.5, or 0 mg of Dox, four times at 6-hour intervals. The capsules were removed from the animals 6 hours after the last Dox injection and incubated in medium, and the amount of secreted ACTH was measured. The results indicate that POMC expression by NTP cells in the CSF space of rats can be induced by intraperitoneal administration of Dox and also that ACTH levels can be controlled by changing the Dox concentration (Fig. 1). When encapsulated NTP cells stimulated by 5 mg Dox were incubated for a longer period of time in the medium, the level of secreted ACTH gradually declined, returning to almost the basal level after 3 days, which was 16.3% of the level seen on day 1 (Saitoh et al. 1998).

To examine the function of the Tet-On system for a long period, encapsulated NTP cells in vitro were divided into two groups and treated either with continuous or intermittent administration of Dox. With continuous administration, the averaged amount of ACTH secretion from days 4, 7, 14, 21, and 28 at each Dox concentration is shown in Fig. 2. The ACTH secretions appeared to depend on the concentration of administered Dox, but

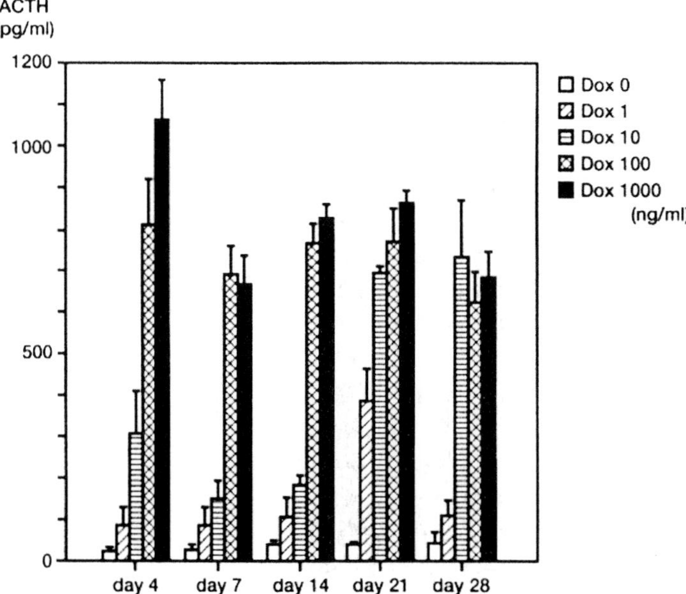

Fig. 1. In vivo pro-opiomelanocortin (POMC) expression by Neuro2A-Tet-On-POMC (NTP) cells implanted in the spinal subarachnoid space of rats. Cerebrospinal fluid levels of adrenocorticotropic hormone (ACTH), a gene product of POMC, were directly dependent on the dose of intraperitoneal administration of doxycycline (Dox). Abbreviations: Dox 5 = 5.0 mg Dox; Dox 2 = 2.0 mg Dox; Dox 0.5 = 0.5 mg Dox.

some fluctuation appeared in the course of the experiment. The reason for this fluctuation was unclear, but there may have been some change of sensitivity to Dox in NTP cells. With intermittent administration of Dox, the high secretions of ACTH obtained with 24-hour Dox administration were seen on days 7, 14, 21, and 28. The Tet-On system appeared to be functionally stable for a month with intermittent administration (Hagihara et al. 1999).

In recent studies we cotransfected pUHD10-3-NL1-β-endorphin and pUHD172-1neo to HEK293, which does not have the POMC-converting enzyme (HEK-Tet-β-endorphin). NL1 is a new cDNA that encodes a peptidase of the same family as neprilysin (Ghaddar et al. 2000). HEK-Tet-β-endorphin secreted β-endorphin depending on the amount of Dox administered. This system can be applicable to any cell line. That cell line can secrete selected neural peptides that can be controlled by the amount of Tet. This technique may be used for clinical ex vivo gene therapy.

YOUICHI SAITOH

ADENOVIRAL GENE THERAPY FOR END OF LIFE PAIN

Our laboratory has examined numerous methods of gene transfer for treating severe pain, utilizing herpes virus, adeno-associated virus (AAV),

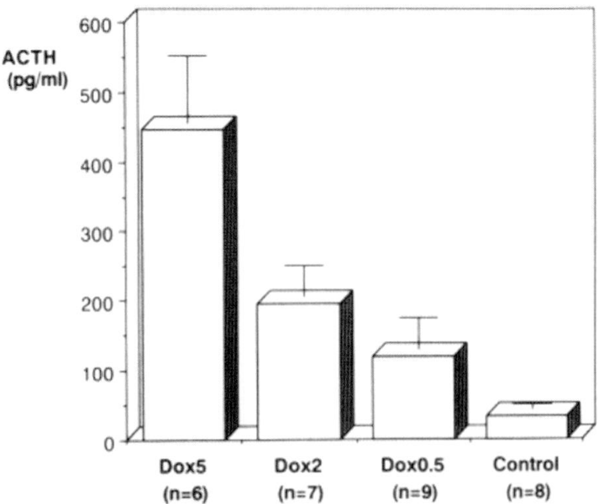

Fig. 2. Examination of the Tet-On expression system in vitro. With continuous administration of Dox, the averaged amount of ACTH secretion from encapsulated NTP cells on days 4, 7, 14, 21, and 28 is shown. The ACTH secretions were dependent on the concentration of administered Dox in most cases.

and retrovirus. We have found that adenovirus is most useful for this approach. As of December 2001, 164 adenovirus-based therapies had been used in clinical trials, including five of eight gene therapy phase III clinical trials (Amalfitano and Parks 2002). Adenovirus is a non-enveloped, 36 kb DNA virus that has been made replication defective by removing varying amounts of native genetic sequences. It has the capacity for one or more moderately sized inserts, can be raised to very high titers, and has robust expression, broad cellular tropism, and, most importantly, rapid expression.

Our initial work with adenovirus utilized two techniques for transferring genes to the rat spinal cord: intrathecal and parenchymal injections (Mannes et al. 1998). Transgene expression using a replication-deficient adenovirus containing a cytomegalovirus (CMV) promoter and *LacZ* reporter gene administered via the two routes was examined with histochemical, immunocytochemical, and biochemical analyses. A highly sensitive fluorometric assay was set up to reliably measure β-galactosidase activity quantitatively using an authentic enzyme as the standard (4-methylum-belliferyl β-D-galactoside [MUG] assay).

Spinal cord injections at the cervical level resulted in high expression of β-galactosidase activity, which was significantly elevated 21-fold over noninjected control tissue 1 day after injection. Activity increased to 57-fold by day 7 and remained elevated at 9.8-fold at 14 days. Significant activity above control was still detectable at day 60, but was greatly diminished in comparison to the first week. Assay of 1-cm spinal cord sections successively further from the injection site showed a time-dependent spread of enzyme activity. At days 1, 3, and 7, activity was largely confined to the 1-cm section containing the injection site. At 14 days, the overall level of expression had diminished from 57-fold (peak) to a 10-fold elevation at the site of injection, but enzyme activity extended caudally into the two adjacent segments, which showed a 5.6- and 0.8-fold elevation, respectively. No significant activity was detected in the remaining spinal cord sections.

In animals that received a single intrathecal injection in which the catheter tip was located at the sacral level, enzyme activity in the spinal cord at 7 days was elevated in the sacral, lumbar, thoracic, and cervical regions as compared to controls. The activity in sacral, lumbar, and thoracic sections was statistically significant, with the highest elevation in the sacral region at the approximate tip of the catheter. The pia mater MUG value represented a significant five-fold increase above the control value ($P < 0.05$).

This study showed that parenchymal injections resulted in robust reporter gene expression in the spinal cord, but that this activity was limited to the injected spinal level. These quantitative data were obtained from a homogenate of spinal cord, and the virally transduced cell types required identification with additional anatomically based methods. Histochemical reactions for *E. coli* β-galactosidase activity showed that motor neurons had the greatest level of expression, with little or no expression in neurons in the sensory laminae of the spinal cord. We made numerous attempts to physically "aim" the viral infusion solution at the dorsal horn in an effort to virally transduce the cells in laminae I or II. None of these experiments yielded any substantial transduction in neurons in the dorsal horn. However, in some of these animals, we did see β-galactosidase histochemical reaction product in the dorsal root ganglion neurons and in afferent fiber terminations in the dorsal horn, suggesting that nociceptive afferents might be potential targets for binding and uptake of adenoviral particles.

Intrathecal injections resulted in expression throughout the spinal cord but at a vastly reduced level in comparison to the parenchymal injections. Histology demonstrated that *LacZ* expression was limited to the pial-glial layer, with minimal tissue penetration. Thus, an intrathecal injection could be used to transfect cells lining this space in order to allow more widespread effects.

Current approaches to treating pain using gene therapy have primarily targeted the primary afferents and the spinal cord (Kawaja et al. 1991; Mannes et al. 1999; Wilson et al. 1999). Modifications to these sites can be used to upregulate or overexpress a native gene to increase sensitivity or modulate the nociceptive signal. We are currently characterizing a cassette containing the μ-opioid receptor driven by the cytomegalovirus (CMV) promoter (Finegold et al. 1999). Antisense gene delivery with an adenoviral therapy has also been used to downregulate a native receptor in the spinal cord (Finegold et al. 2001). While these techniques are effective locally, no efficient method of viral delivery to the spinal cord parenchyma has been demonstrated. Therefore, we have focused on the paracrine model in the spinal cord.

The paracrine model is based on the findings from the previous study (Mannes et al. 1999). The virus can efficiently transfect the pial/glial cells defining the intrathecal space. These cells then produce the potent analgesic β-endorphin. A replication-defective adenovirus containing a fusion of β-endorphin and nerve growth factor (NGF) and the CMV promoter was constructed (AdCMV β-endorphin). Cells transfected with this virus constitutively expressed and secreted β-endorphin extracellularly (into the CSF). This technique is the biological equivalent of an intrathecal infusion pump. Rats were dosed intrathecally with AdCMV β-endorphin. The effect on thermal hyperalgesia of an inflamed hindpaw was assessed on day 7. CSF was sampled and assayed for β-endorphin with a radioimmunoassay. Intrathecal

AdCMV β-endorphin resulted in a normalization of the paw-withdrawal latency in a dose-dependent fashion (Fig. 3). The observed behavioral effects were naloxone reversible, and AdCMV β-endorphin had no effect on the uninflamed paw.

There are continued concerns with implementing an adenoviral-based pain therapy, including questions of safety, concerns about its inflammatory effects, and the problem of transient expression seen in previous studies. Some of these issues are being addressed with a newer generation gutted vector or high-capacity adenovirus (HC-Ad) (Kochanek et al. 2001). Virtually all of the genes responsible for expressing native proteins have been deleted in this virus. The inflammatory response, especially seen with peripheral priming, has been a problem with previous generation vectors. The transient expression seen with early generation vectors has also implicated a T-cell immune response to the non-native (viral) proteins (Mannes et al. 1998). Thomas et al. (2000) have reported reduced inflammation and persistent transgene expression inflammation with the HC-Ad vector (β-galactosidase expression at 6 months) with the gutless vector in the CNS. They similarly showed that adenoviral therapies are effective after a previous or a subsequent adenoviral exposure.

Removing the native DNA of the HC-Ad further increases the capacity of the cassette to 27 kb. This method could allow either multiple genes to be coexpressed or permit multiple copies of the same gene, amplifying the effects.

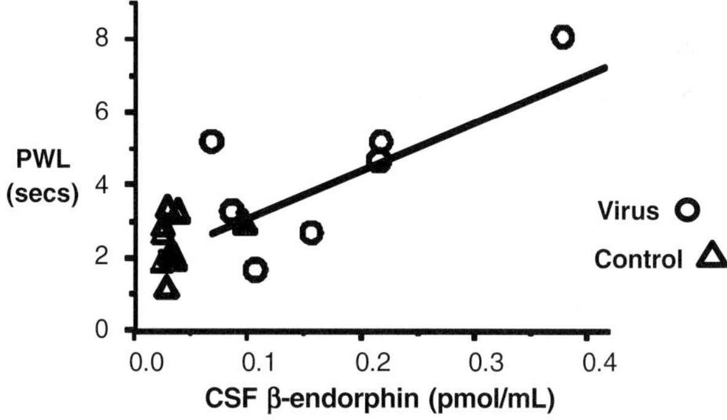

Fig. 3. Correlation of β-endorphin measurements with inflamed paw withdrawal latencies (PWL). Three days prior to the pain test, rats were injected i.t. with 10^{10} particles of AdCMV β-endorphin (circles) or AdCMV β-galactoside (triangles), in a volume of 10 μL. Baseline thermal hyperalgesia tests in unrestrained rats indicated that PWL to a radiant thermal stimulus were 8.7 ± 2.6 seconds for AdCMV β-galactoside, and 8.9 ± 2.5 seconds for AdCMV β-endorphin (mean ± standard error; N = 33 for each virus). Latencies obtained 3 days after injection are plotted against β-endorphin assay of cisternal CSF obtained from the same animal 7 days after injection (to allow cisternal wound healing).

Another improvement in altering tropism is to allow more cell type targeting. More than 50 serotypes have been described, and differential tropism for the various serotypes has been reported. Adenovirus vector design includes modifications to the capsid-cell interaction responsible for binding and internalization of the virus (Wickham 2000). Altering the adenoviral DNA for the protein knob would produce a structure similar to a receptor ligand (Biermann et al. 2001). Another successful technique to modify the targeting is to conjugate a protein or antibody to the capsid that enhances cell-specific internalization (Hoganson et al. 2001).

Despite vast improvements in drugs and delivery systems, we will continue to experience failures in pain symptom management. As an alternative to traditional pharmacotherapy, we propose the use of gene therapy to treat the severe pain seen with end-stage disease. This therapy requires a simple, single procedure that provides long-acting delivery of a potent analgesic. Later generation adenovirus has become more compatible with this approach with its improved safety, more persistent expression, and increased capacity for multiple inserts. Other improvements in the vectors may further improve targeting of specific pain pathways. More work is needed in optimizing this methodology, but continued improvements with adenoviral vectors have made this approach more feasible.

ANDREW MANNES

HERPES VECTOR GENE THERAPY

Herpes simplex virus, type A (HSV) has several native properties that make it particularly well suited as a vector for gene therapy for pain. First, the virus is highly neurotropic, and in fact this tropism appears to be quite selective for primary sensory neurons (Glorioso et al. 1995). Inoculation of the skin or other peripheral tissue of mice with solutions of herpes virus inevitably leads to latent infection in the cell bodies of somatosensory (including pain-transducing) neurons in the trigeminal or dorsal root ganglia. Second, in these latently infected neurons, the DNA of the virus is present in endosomes for the life of the host cell. Typically little or no replication of the virus occurs during latency, and no viral genes or proteins are expressed, with the exception of one genome sequence called the latency-associated transcript (LAT). The LAT segment is transcribed, but no proteins are produced. Finally, HSV is somewhat unique in that large sections of the virus's genome can be deleted without substantially affecting its ability to latently infect neurons (Burton et al. 2001). Thus, transcripts of up to 15 kb of DNA can be readily incorporated, large enough for most genes of interest. In addition, HSV is reasonably straightforward to manipulate in culture (Burton et al. 2001). Thus, HSV can be readily and quite selectively introduced into nociceptive sensory neurons and can take up long-term residence there, bringing with it the potential for long-term manipulation of one or more of the myriad of genes that are important in pain function.

For the experiments reviewed here, we used, as a basis for our vectors, a native variation of the human HSV called the Koss strain, which is substantially less virulent than typical "wild-type" HSV (Glorioso et al. 1995). From this basis, various deletions can be made to limit or eliminate the replication potential and toxicity of HSV infections (Wilson et al. 1999). The recombinant vectors described here have deletions in the thymidine kinase (TK) sequence, which effectively prevents the virus from replicating in cells that do not have appreciable amounts of thymidine, hence nondividing cells such as neurons. Various promoters can also be inserted into the recombination cassette before the transgene of interest. These can be cell specific, of different durations, and of different strengths, depending on the experiment. Vectors used in the studies described here have used the human cytomegalovirus (CMV) immediate early gene promotor/enhancer, a relatively strong, nonspecific promoter. Briefly, a cassette containing the CMV promoter and the transgene of interest is cloned into a plasmid (Wilson et al. 1999). This plasmid is then cloned into the TK locus of the viral DNA. The resultant virus is isolated on a complementing cell line and purified. Various transgenes can be inserted, either in sense or antisense orientation, to form herpes vectors that can be used to alter the genotype of sensory neurons.

For the work described here, we constructed three viruses: KHPE, which encodes the sequence for human preproenkephalin (hPPE); KaCGRP, encoding the gene for rat calcitonin gene-related peptide (CGRP) in antisense orientation; and KHZ, encoding the bacterial reporter gene, *Lac-Z*, which, in these experiments, we used as a control vector (Wilson et al. 1999). The hPPE transgene was chosen because we expected it to induce the transcription, translation, and eventual production of the opioid analgesic peptides leu- and met-enkephalin, and possibly to have an analgesic effect. CGRP, which is located almost exclusively in small-diameter nociceptive neurons, has an important role in the development of central hyperalgesia (Zhang et al. 2001). Therefore, an antisense transgene should inhibit the production of CGRP in infected neurons, and consequently reduce the development of hyperalgesia under conditions that would normally promote it (Wilson and Yeomans 2001). Finally, because the bacterial protein β-galactosidase, which the *Lac-Z* gene codes for, should have no effect on sensory neuronal function, this transgene was chosen so that control administrations could be made.

All viruses were applied to the lightly abraded dorsal surface of the hindpaws of anesthetized Swiss-Webster mice or the feet of Japanese macaque monkeys. After several weeks, the animals were tested to determine whether the surface inoculated would demonstrate a change in nociceptive responsivity. Specifically, we measured the latencies to foot withdrawals in response to either C-fiber or Aδ-fiber thermonociceptive stimulation (Yeomans et al. 1996a,b). In addition, we measured the effects of inoculation of the feet with the viruses on thermal hyperalgesia induced by the topical application of capsaicin to sensitize C-fiber thermonociceptors (Yeomans and Proudfit 1996; Wilson et al. 1999). We retested the animals at various time points (weeks) after viral application to determine the duration of any analgesic effects. At different time points, some animals were euthanized, and the expression of the *Lac*-Z, enkephalin, or CGRP antisense transgenes in primary afferents was examined using X-gal histochemistry for β-galactosidase or immunohistochemistry for enkephalins or CGRP, respectively.

Fig. 4 presents a series of photomicrographs demonstrating transgene expression in primary afferent sensory neurons. As is evident in Fig. 4A–C, introduction of herpes vectors through the skin leads to induction of nonendogenous transgenes in the cell bodies of sensory neurons, including β-galactosidase in mice (Fig. 4A) and leu-enkephalin in macaques (Fig. 4C). Furthermore, inoculation of mouse hindpaw skin with KaCGRP decreases endogenous levels of CGRP in primary afferent terminals in the dorsal horn by 30–40% when compared to afferents that have been infected with a control (KHZ) vector (Fig. 4D,E). Thus, application of HSV encoding either sense or antisense transgenes to the skin can alter the genome and biochemical phenotype of sensory afferents innervating that area of the skin.

Fig. 5 presents graphical demonstrations of the behavioral effects of application of these three vectors to the skin of macaques (Fig. 5A) and mice (Fig. 5B). Topical capsaicin application typically induces a C-fiber hyperalgesia, decreasing the withdrawal latencies in response to heat (Yeomans et al. 1996a). This effect can be seen in both macaques and mice in the decrease in response latencies of skin onto which the control virus, KHZ, was applied 6 weeks previously (Figs. 5A,B). These responses are similar to those of animals to which no virus had been applied (data not shown for simplicity). On the other hand, macaques that had received an application of the KHPE virus 6 weeks before not only did not become hyperalgesic, but instead they became analgesic, as indicated by the increase in response latency up to the maximum (20 seconds). In addition, the reversal of this analgesia by intrathecal injection of the opioid antagonist naloxone in

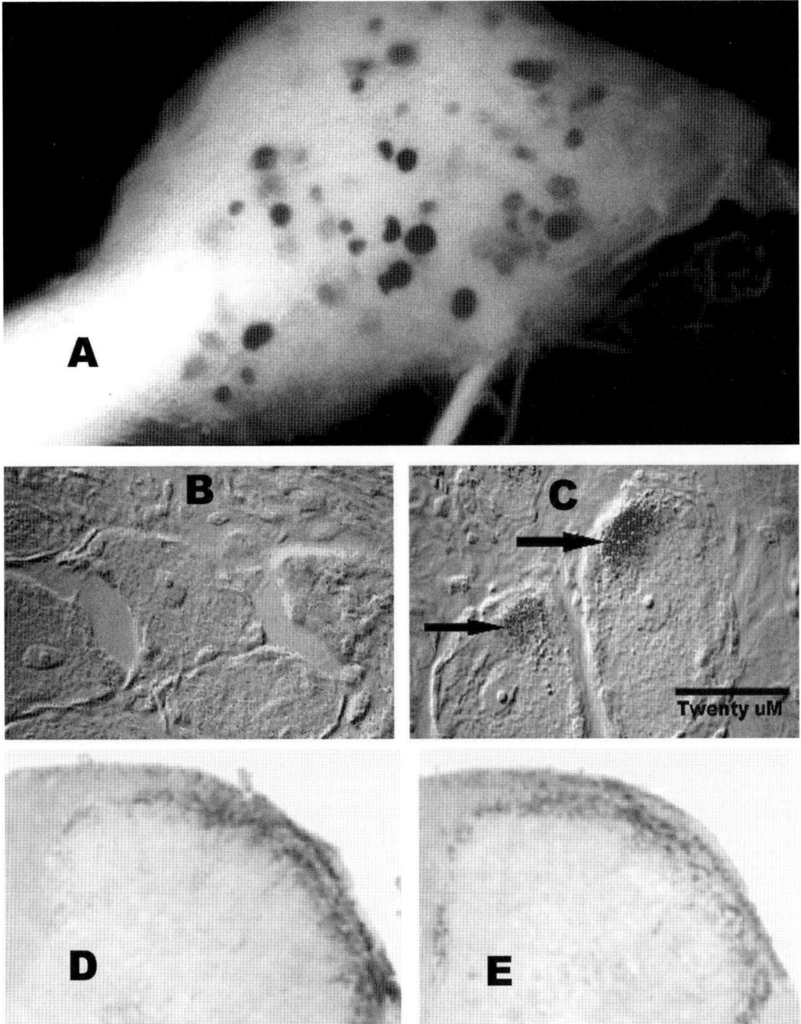

Fig. 4. Immunohistochemical demonstration of gene expression changes induced by herpes vector. (A) Whole mount of mouse dorsal root ganglia (DRG) treated with X-gal buffer 1 week after cutaneous application of a *Lac-Z* encoding herpes virus. (B) Lack of leu-enkephalin immunoreactivity in monkey DRG 4 weeks after application of *Lac-Z* encoding virus to the skin. (C) Presence of leu-enkephalin in monkey DRG after application of hPPE encoding vector. (D) Normal levels of CGRP immunoreactivity in mouse dorsal horn after application of *Lac-Z* encoding herpes to mouse skin. (E) Application of virus encoding antisense to the rat CGRP gene decreases expression by 30–40%.

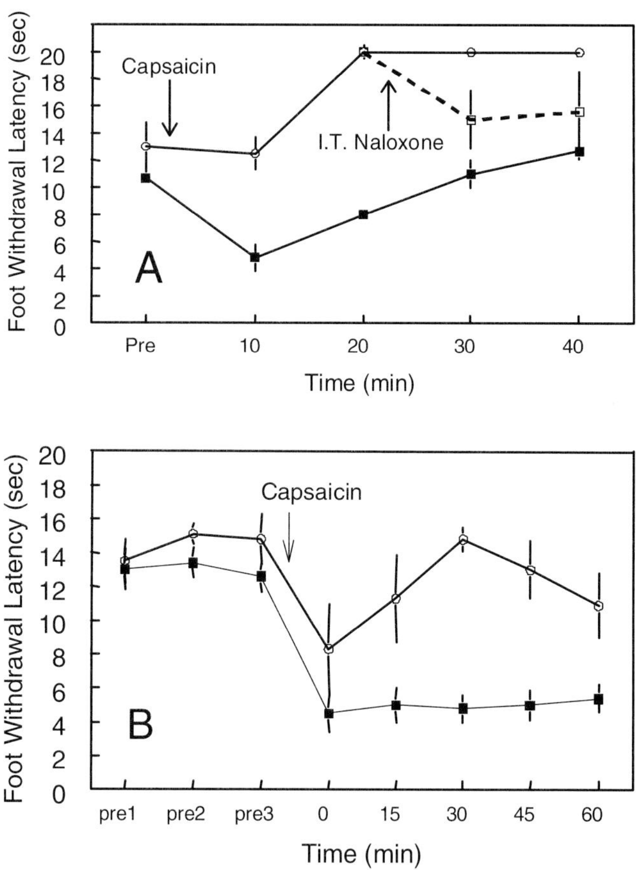

Fig. 5. Antihyperalgesic effects of cutaneous application of recombinant herpes vectors. (A) Application of hPPE (open circles), but not *Lac-Z* (filled squares) encoding herpes virus to the skin of the monkey foot blocks the thermal hyperalgesic effects of topical capsaicin application, an effect reversible by intrathecal application of naloxone (open squares and broken line). (B) Application to mouse skin of herpes vectors encoding antisense to the gene for CGRP (open circles), but not the sense sequence for *Lac-Z* (filled squares), reverses the thermal hyperalgesic effect of capsaicin application.

some monkeys strongly suggests that this effect is mediated, at least in part, by the spinal release of opioid peptides. Similarly, the introduction of the antisense sequence of CGRP by the KaCGRP vector clearly diminished, after a delay, the hyperalgesic effects of topical capsaicin in mice (Fig. 5B). The delay may be indicative of the latency of CGRP's hyperalgesic effects, and may show that the initial hyperalgesia may be primarily due to other mediators, such as substance P.

David C. Yeomans

CONCLUSIONS

With the immense and accelerating knowledge base of human genes, the number of targets that might be modified to alter neural function is constantly increasing. In this light, attempts have been made to alter the expression of a number of neuronal genes. Although the concept of gene therapy has been under investigation for perhaps three decades (Friedmann 1992), the idea of gene therapy for pain is much more recent (see Wu et al. 2001). Gene products already successfully modified include peptide neurotransmitters, enzymes, and neurotransmitter receptors.

The intention of the work detailed here is essentially preclinical. All three of these approaches, ex vivo cell transplantation, adenoviral vector application to the spinal cord, and herpes vector introduction to primary nociceptive afferents, have the potential to affect human pain syndromes. However, they are likely to have different target patient populations. Thus, although all three approaches can lead to the expression of opioid peptides in the pain system, the location and duration of expression of these peptides differs considerably between the approaches.

While protocols have been presented for government approval, much additional work remains before gene therapy can be applied to human pain patients. Careful examinations not only of analgesic efficacy and persistence of expression, but also of the potential relative safety and toxicity of these three approaches, remain to be performed. For example, testing these methods in nonhuman primates may provide a critical, predictive step in developing clinical trials. In addition, principles defined in this work are likely to be useful in other gene therapy approaches to decreasing pain sensitivity.

ACKNOWLEDGMENTS

We greatly appreciate the Neuro2A cells transfected with the POMC gene and neprilysin gene given to Dr. Saitoh by Dr. Boileau, Montreal, Canada. Dr. Mannes is supported by USPHS grant NIDA 1K08DA00422. Dr. Yeomans is supported by USPHS grants DA08256 and DA12672 and would also like to acknowledge his partner in this undertaking, Dr. Steven Wilson, at the University of South Carolina.

REFERENCES

Amalfitano A, Parks RJ. Separating fact from fiction: assessing the potential of modified adenovirus vectors for use in human gene therapy. *Curr Gene Ther* 2002; 2:111–133.

Biermann V, Volpers C, Hussmann S, et al. Targeting of high-capacity adenoviral vectors. *Hum Gene Ther* 2001; 12:1757–1769.

Bonica JJ. Cancer pain. In: Bonica JJ (Ed). *The Management of Pain.* Philadelphia: Lea & Febiger, 1990, pp 400–460.

Burton EA, Wechuck JB, Wendell SK, et al. Multiple applications for replication-defective herpes simplex virus vectors. *Stem Cells* 2001; 19:358–377.

Cleeland CS, Gonin R, Hatfield AK, et al. Pain and its treatment in outpatients with metastatic cancer. *N Engl J Med* 1994; 330:592–596.

Dmitriev IP, Kashentseva EA, Curiel DT. Engineering of adenovirus vectors containing heterologous peptide sequences in the C terminus of capsid protein IX. *J Virol* 2002; 76(14):6893–6899.

Douglas JT, Rogers BE, Rosenfeld ME, et al. Targeted gene delivery by tropism-modified adenoviral vectors. *Nat Biotechnol* 1996; 14(11):1574–1578.

Finegold AA, Mannes AJ, Iadarola MJ. A paracrine paradigm for in vivo gene therapy in the central nervous system: treatment of chronic pain. *Hum Gene Ther* 1999; 10.

Finegold AA, Perez FM, Iadarola MJ. In vivo control of NMDA receptor transcript level in motor neurons by viral transduction of a short antisense gene. *Mol Brain Res* 2001; 90:17–25.

Friedmann T. A brief history of gene therapy. *Nat Genet* 1992; 2:93–98.

Ghaddar G, Ruchon AF, Carpentier M, et al. Molecular cloning and biochemical characterization of a new mouse testis soluble-zinc-metallopeptidase of the neprilysin family. *Biochem J* 2000; 347:419–429.

Glorioso J, Bender MA, Fink D, DeLuca N. Herpes simplex virus vectors. *Mol Cell Biol Hum Dis Ser* 1995; 5:33–63.

Gossen M, Bujard H. Tight control of gene expression in mammalian cells by tetracycline-responsive promoters. *Proc Natl Acad Sci USA* 1992; 89:5547–5551.

Hagihara Y, Saitoh Y, Arita N, et al. Long-term functional assessment of encapsulated cells transfected with Tet-On system. *Cell Transplant* 1999; 8:431–434.

Hoganson DK, Sosnowski BA, Pierce GF, Doukas J. Uptake of adenoviral vectors via fibroblast growth factor receptors involves intracellular pathways that differ from the targeting ligand. *Mol Ther* 2001; 3:105–112.

Kawaja MD, Ray J, Gage FH. Employment of fibroblasts for gene transfer: applications for grafting into the central nervous system. *Genet Eng (NY)* 1991;13:205–220.

Kochanek S, Schiedner G, Volpers C. High capacity "gutless" adenoviral vectors. *Curr Opin Mol Ther* 2001; 3:454–463.

Mannes AJ, Caudle R, O'Connell, Iadarola MJ. Adenoviral transfer of LacZ to spinal cord neurons. *Brain Res* 1998; 793:1–6.

Mannes AJ, Olah Z, Caudle RM, Iadarola MJ. Gene therapy for pain: in vitro and in vivo expression of beta endorphin using a replication defective adenoassociated virus. *Anesthesiology* 1999; 91(3A):A879.

Mannes AJ, Keller J, Caudle R, Greenblatt E, Iadarola MJ. Mu-GFP, a fluorescently labeled opioid receptor. Society for Neuroscience Annual Meeting, San Diego, 2001.

Noel G, Zollinger L, Laliberté N, et al. Targeting and processing of pro-opiomelanocortin in neuronal cell lines. *J Neurochem* 1989; 52:1050–1057.

Pappas GD, Lazorthes Y, Bes JC, Tafani M, Winnie AP. Relief of intractable cancer pain by human chromaffin cell transplants: experience at two medical centers. *Neurol Res* 1997; 19(1):71–77.

Saitoh Y, Taki T, Arita N, et al. Analgesia induced by transplantation of encapsulated tumor cells secreting β-endorphin. *J Neurosurg* 1995; 82:630–634.

Saitoh Y, Eguchi Y, Hagihara Y, et al. Dose-dependent doxycycline-mediated adrenocorticotropic hormone secretion from encapsulated Tet-On proopiomelanocortin Neuro2A cells in the subarachnoid space. *Hum Gene Ther* 1998; 9:997–1002.

Thomas CE, Schiedner G, Kochanek S, Castro MG, Lowenstein PR. Peripheral infection with adenovirus causes unexpected long-term brain inflammation in animals injected intracranially with first-generation, but not with high capacity, adenovirus vectors: toward realistic long-term neurological gene therapy for chronic diseases. *Proc Natl Acad Sci USA* 2000; 97:7482–7487.

Wickham TJ. Targeting adenovirus. *Gene Ther* 2000; 7:110–114.

Wilson SP, Yeomans DC. Genetic therapy for pain management. *Curr Rev Pain* 2001; 4:445–450.

Wilson SP, Yeomans DC, Bender MA, Lu Y, Glorioso J. Antihyperalgesic effects of delivery of enkephalins to mouse nociceptive neurons by a herpes virus encoding proenkephalin. *Proc Natl Acad Sci USA* 1999; 96:3211–3216.

Wu CL, Garry MG, Zollo RA, Yang J. Gene therapy for the management of pain. Part I: Methods and strategies. *Anesthesiology* 2001; 94:1119–1132.

Yeomans DC, Proudfit HK. Nociceptive responses to high or low rates of noxious cutaneous heating are mediated by different nociceptors in the rat: electrophysiological evidence. *Pain* 1996; 68:141–150.

Yeomans DC, Cooper BY, Vierck CJ Jr. Effects of systemic morphine on responses to first or second pain sensations of primates. *Pain* 1996a; 66:253–263.

Yeomans DC, Pirec V, Proudfit HK. Nociceptive responses to high or low rates of noxious cutaneous heating are mediated by different nociceptors in the rat: behavioral evidence. *Pain* 1996b; 68:133–140.

Yeomans DC, Mannes A, Saitoh Y. Gene therapy for pain: different approaches toward a common goal. *Abstracts: 10th World Congress on Pain*. Seattle: IASP Press, 2002, p 106.

Zhang L, Hoff AO, Wimalawansa SJ, et al. Arthritic calcitonin/alpha calcitonin gene-related peptide knockout mice have reduced nociceptive hypersensitivity. *Pain* 2001; 89:265–273.

Correspondence to: David C. Yeomans, PhD, Department of Anesthesia, S268, Stanford University, 300 Pasteur Drive, Stanford, CA 94305-5117, USA. Email: dcyeomans@stanford.edu.

Proceedings of the 10th World Congress on Pain,
Progress in Pain Research and Management, Vol. 24,
edited by Jonathan O. Dostrovsky, Daniel B. Carr, and
Martin Koltzenburg, IASP Press, Seattle, © 2003.

44

Therapeutic Efficacy in Experimental Polyarthritis of Recombinant Virus-Driven Enkephalin Overproduction in Sensory Neurons

Joao Braz,[a] Alice Meunier,[b] Caroline Beaufour,[b] François Cesselin,[b] Michel Hamon,[b] and Michel Pohl[b]

[a]*W.M. Keck Foundation, University of California, San Francisco, California, USA;* [b]*INSERM, Paris, France*

Rheumatoid arthritis is a systemic autoimmune disease primarily manifested by erosive inflammation of the joints associated with intense pain (Harris 1990). Its etiology is still unknown, but significant insights into its physiopathology have been obtained from experimental animal models. Although none of these models has all the characteristics of the human disease, adjuvant-induced polyarthritis in the rat shares numerous behavioral and biochemical characteristics with rheumatoid arthritis (Calvino et al. 1987). Profound neurochemical changes in the peripheral and central nervous systems are associated with long-term alterations of pain processing and hyperalgesia in these animals (Millan et al. 1987). Thus, in polyarthritic rats, both preproenkephalin A (PA) expression and the levels of PA-derived peptides are enhanced in the dorsal horn of the spinal cord, particularly in the lumbar region that receives sensory nerves from the hindpaws (which are especially affected by the disease) (Cesselin et al. 1980). By contrast, PA expression drops in cell bodies of primary sensory neurons located in lumbar dorsal root ganglia (DRG), and the concentration of the main PA-derived peptide, met-enkephalin, is reduced in the soft tissue of ankle joints in polyarthritic rats (Pohl et al. 1994; El Hassan et al. 1998).

Recent reports are in favor of a peripheral action of opioids in the control of pain and inflammatory processes (Stein and Yassouridis 1997). At the periphery, opioid peptides are thought to originate mainly from inflammatory cells (Shäfer et al. 1994). However, the sensory neurons expressing PA (Pohl et al. 1994), with their numerous met-enkephalin-containing axons present in glabrous skin (Carlton and Coggeshall 1997) and soft tissue of joints (El Hassan et al. 1998), might represent another source of peripheral opioids also involved in the control of pain and inflammatory processes. To determine whether enkephalinergic sensory neurons could be involved in polyarthritis-related disability, we restored expression of PA in sensory neurons of the hindlimbs in polyarthritic rats using recombinant vectors derived from *Herpes Simplex* virus type 1 (HSV-1), bearing the rat PA encoding sequence. Three weeks after the rats were infected with HSVLatEnk, different tests were performed (noxious, horizontal and vertical mobility, and radiographic analyses). Then, rats were treated during 3 days with naloxone or naloxone methiodide via osmotic minipumps. Following this 3-day treatment all tests were performed once again. Polyarthritis was induced by an intradermal injection of 0.05 mL of killed *Mycobacterium butyricum* (Gouret et al. 1976) suspended (10 mg/mL) in mineral oil (Freund's adjuvant). This injection was given approximately 3 cm from the base of the tail in 6-week-old male Sprague-Dawley rats. Here we provide direct evidence for a therapeutic activity of PA overexpression in sensory neurons in polyarthritic rats.

Vectors derived from HSV-1 are particularly adapted for transgene transfer into sensory neurons (Davar et al. 1994; Goins et al. 1999), and we recently demonstrated their ability to drive PA gene expression in DRG neurons of healthy rats (Antunes-Bras et al. 1998, 2001). HSV-derived vectors used in this study, containing the rat PA cDNA (HSVLatEnk) or the β-galactosidase reporter gene (HSVLatβ-gal) under the control of a modified HSVLat promoter, were generated as described previously (Braz et al. 2001). The PA or β-galactosidase transcriptional units were inserted into the viral glycoprotein C locus. Deeply anesthetized polyarthritic rats were peripherally infected on slightly scarified hindpaws with ~5×10^6 plaque-forming units of HSVLatEnk or HSVLatβ-gal. We previously showed that recombinant HSV vector-induced increase of immunoreactive met-enkephalin-like material (MELM) concentrations in rat lumbar DRG was maximal 3 weeks after infection (Antunes-Bras et al. 1998). Because most of the polyarthritis-associated symptoms peaked 3–5 weeks after induction of the disease (Calvino et al. 1987), rats were infected with either HSVLatEnk or HSVLatβ-gal at 2 weeks after polyarthritis induction, and most experiments were performed 3 weeks later. Infection of polyarthritic rats with HSVLatβ-gal did not affect any of the parameters studied.

Peripheral inoculation of polyarthritic rats with HSVLatEnk led to a significant increase in the number of PA mRNA-expressing neurons in L4–L6 DRG, reaching ~12% of the total neuron population. PA mRNA-expressing cells were small and medium in size. Quantitative reverse transcription polymerase chain reaction (RT-PCR) performed on total RNA allowed the demonstration that PA mRNA levels in L4–L6 DRG in HSVLatEnk-infected polyarthritic rats were about eightfold higher ($P < 0.001$; $n = 5$) than in control rats. MELM concentrations in L4–L6 DRG, measured using a specific radioimmunoassay (Cesselin et al. 1980), were also significantly higher in HSVLatEnk-infected polyarthritic rats (+40%, $P < 0.01$; $n = 8$) than in paired control polyarthritic rats. On the other hand, radioimmunoassay measurement of both substance P and calcitonin gene-related peptide (CGRP) concentrations (Pohl et al. 1990) in L4–L5 DRG of control polyarthritic rats (1.6 ± 0.2 ng/mg protein and 8.3 ± 0.2 ng/mg protein, respectively, means ± SEM; $n = 8$) showed comparable levels to those in HSVLatEnk-infected rats (1.4 ± 0.1 ng/mg protein and 8.1 ± 0.4 ng/mg protein, respectively; $n = 8$), suggesting that infection per se had no effects at least on these two predominant peptides synthesized in sensory neurons.

Localization of MELM in DRG neurons of control and HSVLatEnk-infected polyarthritic rats was compared using an immunofluorescence approach with monoclonal anti-met-enkephalin antibody. No met-enkephalin-immunoreactive neurons were detected in L4–L6 DRG or corresponding dorsal roots of control polyarthritic rats. Furthermore, neuronal processes stained for MELM were only rarely detected in peripheral branches of sensory neurons originating from L4–L6 DRG in these animals. Infection of polyarthritic rats with HSVLatEnk resulted in the appearance of numerous positively stained neuronal cell bodies in the DRG. In addition, a relatively dense bundle of neuronal processes containing MELM was observed in the peripheral part of sensory neurons (peripheral output of L4–L6 DRG) in HSVLatEnk-infected rats. By contrast, few or no MELM-positively labeled nerve fibers were visualized in L4–L6 dorsal roots of these animals. Taken together, these results suggest that, in agreement with our data obtained in control healthy rats (Antunes-Bras et al. 2001), PA overexpression in DRG neurons of polyarthritic rats led to the synthesis of met-enkephalin that was preferentially transported into the peripheral part of sensory neurons.

To investigate the possible effects of met-enkephalin overproduction in lumbar DRG sensory neurons on pain-related behavior, we measured the latency of paw withdrawal evoked by noxious radiant heat (Galbraith et al. 1993) applied onto the hindpaw plantar surface in HSVLatEnk-infected versus control polyarthritic rats. Three weeks after infection with HSVLatEnk (i.e., 5 weeks after polyarthritis induction), the paw-withdrawal latency slightly but significantly increased (5.5 ± 0.2 seconds, $P < 0.001$; $n = 15$) over that measured in paired control polyarthritic rats (4.8 ± 0.2 seconds; $n = 15$) (Fig. 1A). This finding is consistent with the recently reported antihyperalgesic

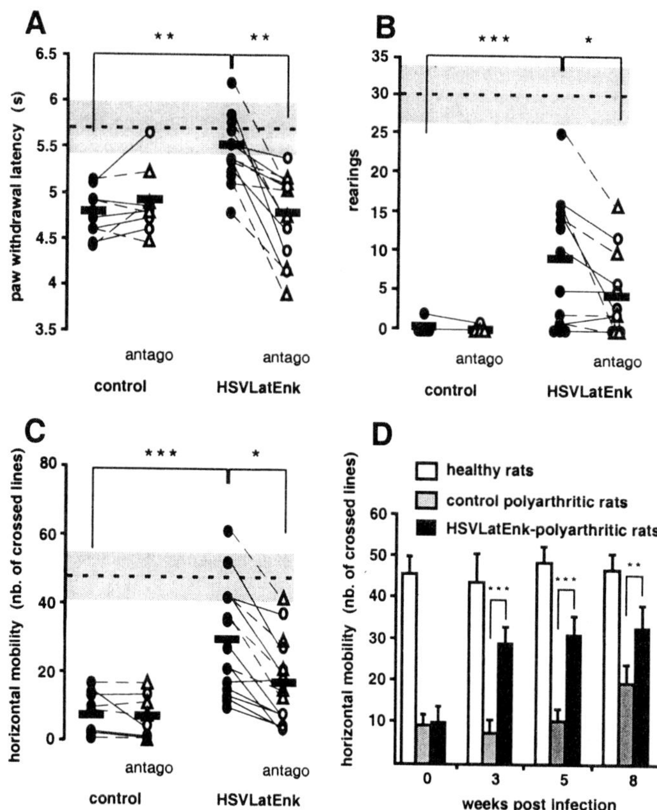

Fig. 1. HSVLatEnk-infected polyarthritic rats exhibited reduced thermal hyperalgesia and improved spontaneous locomotor activity. Response (paw-withdrawal) latencies (A) for control (n = 9) and HSVLatEnk-infected polyarthritic (n = 15) rats to radiant heating were measured 3 weeks after infection. Horizontal locomotor activity (C) and rearings (B) of control (n = 12) and HSVLatEnk-infected polyarthritic (n = 15) rats individually placed in a red-lighted open-field were monitored using a video camera and assessed every minute during a 7-minute period. Individual performances of control polyarthritic or HSVLatEnk-infected polyarthritic rats are represented (closed circles). Animals were then subcutaneously implanted for 3 days with osmotic minipumps delivering 3 mg/kg/day of either naloxone (open circles) or naloxone methiodide (triangles), and thermal hyperalgesia and locomotor activity were assessed. Long-term improvement of functional ability was estimated in additional, independent experiments (D), where locomotor activity of both control (n = 8) and HSVLatEnk-infected (n = 10) polyarthritic rats or normal healthy rats (n = 5) was also measured 5 and 8 weeks after infection. * $P < 0.05$; ** $P < 0.01$; *** $P < 0.001$ for control versus HSVLatEnk-infected polyarthritic rats (two-tailed unpaired t test) and for untreated versus naloxone/naloxone methiodide-treated animals (two-tailed paired t test).

effects of overexpressed PA in animals with experimentally induced inflammatory pain (Wilson et al. 1999; Goss et al. 2001). However, an acute painful stimulus such as radiant heat does not reflect the dimension of persistent, spontaneous pain. This statement is particularly true in polyarthritic rats, in which the most prominent behavioral change is a marked reduction of locomotion due to intense inflammatory pain and alterations of joints, especially those of the hindpaws. We therefore assessed the "functional disability" of these animals by measuring their spontaneous locomotor activity (Cain et al. 1997). Locomotor activity, both horizontal and vertical (i.e., rearings) of control healthy rats, control polyarthritic rats, and HSVLatEnk-infected polyarthritic rats were video-monitored and tape-recorded for 7 minutes in a red-lighted open-field. Five weeks after induction of the disease, both the horizontal locomotor activity (–75%, $P < 0.001$; $n = 18$) and rearings (–95%, $P < 0.001$; $n = 18$) were dramatically reduced in control polyarthritic rats. As compared with the later animals, HSVLatEnk-infected polyarthritic rats showed a remarkable improvement in both horizontal displacements (4.2× more than controls, $P < 0.001$; $n = 12$; Fig. 1C) and rearings (8× more than controls, $P < 0.001$; $n = 15$; Fig. 1B) 3 weeks after infection. This amelioration persisted during the whole observation period, for at least 8 weeks after HSVLatEnk infection (Fig. 1D).

In light of the strongly preferential transport of overproduced MELM into the peripheral fibers of sensory neurons, we assessed the involvement of opioid receptors in both the antihyperalgesic response and the improved locomotor activity of HSVLatEnk-infected polyarthritic rats by using not only naloxone, a centrally and peripherally acting opioid receptor antagonist, but also naloxone methiodide, an exclusively peripherally acting antagonist. Taking into account that PA overexpression in sensory neurons of HSVLatEnk-infected polyarthritic rats is a continuous process lasting for several weeks, we reasoned that prolonged delivery of opioid receptor antagonists might be a valuable method with which to inhibit the effects of overproduced met-enkephalin. Naloxone or naloxone methiodide was administered at a dose of 3 mg/kg/day for 3 days using subcutaneously implanted osmotic minipumps with a delivery rate of 1 μL/hour. Both compounds, which had no significant effect in control polyarthritic rats, reversed with a similar efficacy both the antihyperalgesic response ($P < 0.001$; $n = 15$; Fig. 1A) and the improved locomotor activity ($P < 0.05$; $n = 12–15$; Fig. 1B,C) in HSVLatEnk-infected polyarthritic rats. In addition, the fact that naloxone methiodide was as efficient as naloxone in suppressing the antihyperalgesic response further supports the idea that peripheral opioid receptors play a key role in opioid-induced reduction of inflammatory pain (Stein and Yassouridis 1997; Binder and Walker 1998) and in diminishing related disability in polyarthritic rats infected with HSVLatEnk.

Articular and osseous lesions, which can lead to partial or total fusion of tarsal bones, represent a prominent incapacitating symptom of polyarthritis both in humans and in animal models of the disease. As previously reported (De Castro Costa et al. 1981; Calvino et al. 1987), 2 weeks after polyarthritis induction, soft tissue swelling and increased joint diameter of hindpaws were apparent in nearly 100% of animals (bilateral hindpaw joint diameter in control polyarthritic rats: 13.3 ± 1.2 mm; n = 18 versus 9.0 ± 0.1 mm in healthy rats; n = 8; $P < 0.01$). These signs of inflammation normally worsened during the following weeks, with more hindpaw swelling and greater joint diameter (17.4 ± 1.0 mm; n = 8, $P < 0.02$) at the end of the fifth week after polyarthritis induction in control rats. By contrast, in paired HSVLatEnk-infected polyarthritic rats with reduced hyperalgesic response and improved locomotion, the hindpaw joint diameter (13.1 ± 1.0 mm; n = 8) did not enlarge from the 2nd to the 5th week after polyarthritis induction. This observation led us to evaluate the presence and severity of lesions by radiological analysis of hindlimbs, and to quantify the expression of several prominent cytokines associated with rheumatoid inflammation. In control polyarthritic rats, we observed marked lesions, including extensive erosion of bone extremities, narrowing or disappearance of joint spaces, calcification, new bone proliferation, and ankylosis (Fig. 2A). Radiogram analysis of paired HSVLatEnk-infected polyarthritic rats (Fig. 2B) revealed that the mean scores of their hindpaw joint lesions were significantly lower ($P <$ 0.005; n = 10) than those in controls (Fig. 2A). In order to more precisely analyze the individual progression of the disease, rats were radiographed 2 weeks after polyarthritis induction (Fig. 2A,B,C), just prior to their infection by either HSVLatβ-gal or HSVLatEnk. The rats were radiographed again 3 weeks later and finally after one further week following a 3-day treatment with naloxone methiodide. Despite individual variability in polyarthritis development, the hindpaw joints of 6 out of the 10 HSVLatEnk-infected polyarthritic rats examined only presented mild or medium lesions (Fig. 2B'). The other four HSVLatEnk-infected animals had extensive lesions (Fig. 2C') but never suffered the severity of joint destruction regularly observed in all control polyarthritic rats (Fig. 2A'). Naloxone methiodide treatment did not affect the lesion score in HSVLatEnk-infected polyarthritic rats, indicating that, under such conditions, a 3-day blockade of peripheral opioid receptors was unable to reverse the inhibitory action of PA overexpression on the progression of the disease. In line with the present data, several recent reports also provide evidence that opioids can modulate inflammatory processes and attenuate joint damage in polyarthritic rats (Walker et al. 1996; Binder and Walker 1998), and that opioids may modulate excessive synovial functions in patients with rheumatoid arthritis (Takeba et al. 2001).

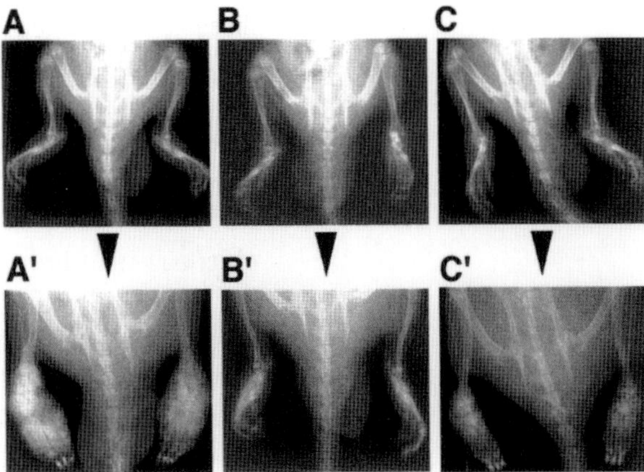

Fig. 2. Presence and severity of hindpaw joint lesions in control (A') and HSVLatEnk-infected (B', C') polyarthritic rats as examined on radiographs. At the end of the experiments (during the fourth week after infection), osseous lesions of the ankle and metatarsus were evaluated in both groups of rats (n = 8–10) using a four-degree rating scale: 0, no obvious lesions; 1, doubtful or mild lesions; 2, medium lesions with narrowing or disappearance of joint space but without extensive periostitis; 3, severe lesions with joint destruction and periostitis. Individual evolution of polyarthritis-associated joint destruction was also assessed by comparing radiograms made 2 weeks after polyarthritis induction (A, B, C), just prior to infection with either HSVLatβ-gal or HSVLatEnk, then 3 weeks later. Six out of 10 HSVLatEnk-infected rats presented mild lesions (B'), and the remaining four animals had more extensive lesions (C'), which were, however, less extensive than those of control polyarthritic rats (A').

Cytokines clearly contribute to the complex pattern of local and systemic changes associated with chronic inflammatory pain (for a review, see Dray et al. 1994; Poole et al. 1999). Numerous data support their role in the induction and perpetuation of rheumatoid inflammation (for a review, see Koch et al. 1995; Ohshima et al. 1998; de Hooge et al. 2000). Semiquantitative RT-PCR demonstrated that mRNA levels of interleukin 6 (IL-6) and interleukin-1β (IL-1-β) were approximately sixfold ($P < 0.001$; $n = 5$) and approximately twofold ($P < 0.001$; $n = 5$) higher, respectively, in hindpaw subcutaneous tissues of polyarthritic rats (5 weeks after disease induction) than in healthy control animals (Fig. 3). By contrast, in paired HSVLatEnk-infected polyarthritic rats, mRNA levels of both IL-6 and IL-1-β were significantly decreased. Concentrations of IL-6 mRNA were decreased approximately twofold ($P < 0.005$; $n = 5$), whereas IL-1-β mRNA levels were comparable to those measured in control animals. At this stage of our work it is difficult to ascertain whether decreased mRNA concentration of both cytokines represents one of the signs of reduced inflammation or whether

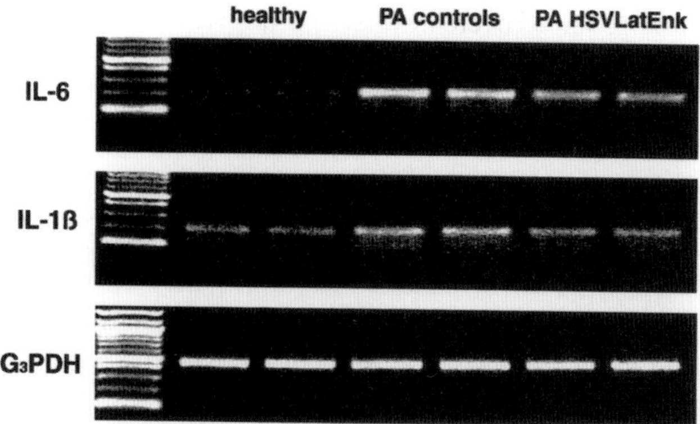

Fig. 3. Concentrations of mRNA encoding IL-6 and IL-1β were reduced in hindpaw subcutaneous tissues of HSVLatEnk-infected polyarthritic rats. Semi-quantitative RT-PCR measurement of IL-6 and IL-1β mRNA levels was performed on total RNA extracted from the subcutaneous tissues of hindpaws of healthy controls or of untreated and HSVLatEnk-treated polyarthritic rats (n = 5 for each group) 5 weeks after disease induction. 1 μg of total RNA was reverse-transcribed and amplified for 30 cycles using specific primers. The ratios of the levels (optical density measurements) of the PCR products of IL-6 or IL-1β mRNA over that of glyceraldehyde-3-phosphate dehydrogenase (G_3PDH) were compared between different groups of animals. Representative gel analyses of PCR products are shown.

overproduced PA-derived peptides directly affect the expression of these cytokines, thus helping to reduce inflammation (and probably diminishing pain-related behaviors) in HSVLatEnk-treated polyarthritic rats. However, recent data showing a direct modulatory effect of opioid peptides on excessive synthesis of several mRNA-encoding proinflammatory cytokines in cultured synovial cells from patients with rheumatoid arthritis (Takeba et al. 2001) support the idea that transgene-derived opioid peptides might also exert this activity in vivo in polyarthritic rats overproducing PA.

The present data show that restoration of PA expression in lumbar DRG neurons of polyarthritic rats, which leads to a massive transport of MELM to the peripheral processes of sensory neurons, induces mainly peripherally mediated antihyperalgesic effects and reduces disease-related functional disability in these animals. Furthermore, our studies also demonstrate the beneficial effect of PA-derived peptides on hindpaw joint lesions, given that overproduction of these opioids stopped the progression of bone erosion and periostitis. Anti-inflammatory properties of opioids in peripheral tissues might be ascribed to their immunomodulatory action, demonstrated in vitro on immunocompetent and synovial cells (Kamphuis et al. 1998; Takeba et al. 2001), as well as in relevant animal models and in clinical trials in patients (Stein and Yassouridis 1997). It is difficult to discriminate between the antihyperalgesic action of overexpressed PA-derived peptides in polyarthritic rats and the alleviation of pain that would be secondary to the reduction in the inflammatory process and in joint lesions. In any case, as in humans, polyarthritis-associated disability in rats is the consequence of both chronic pain and mechanical degradation of joints. Accordingly, the long-term amelioration in polyarthritic rats infected with HSVLatEnk probably reflects a synergic action of PA-derived peptides on both aspects of the disease.

ACKNOWLEDGMENTS

Supported by grants from INSERM, Institut UPSA de la Douleur and Bristol-Myers Squibb Foundation (Unrestricted Biomedical Research Grant).

REFERENCES

Antunes-Bras JM, Epstein AL, Bourgoin S, et al. Herpes simplex virus 1-mediated transfer of preproenkephalin A in rat dorsal root ganglia. *J Neurochem* 1998; 70:1299–1303.

Antunes-Bras JM, Becker C, Bourgoin S, et al. Met-enkephalin is preferentially transported to the peripheral processes of primary afferent fibres in both normal and proenkephalin A overexpressing rats. *Neuroscience* 2001; 103:1073–1083.

Binder W, Walker JS. Effect of the peripherally selective kappa-opioid agonist, asimadoline, on adjuvant arthritis. *Br J Pharmacol* 1998; 124:647–654.

Braz J, Beaufour C, Couteaux A, et al. Therapeutic efficacy in experimental polyarthritis of viral-driven enkephalin overproduction in sensory neurons. *J Neurosci* 2001; 21:7881–7888.

Cain CK, Francis JM, Plone MA, et al. Pain-related disability and effects of chronic morphine in the adjuvant-induced arthritis model of chronic pain. *Physiol Behav* 1997; 62:199–205.

Calvino B, Crepon-Bernard MO, Le Bars D. Parallel clinical and behavioural studies of adjuvant-induced arthritis in the rat: possible relationship with "chronic pain." *Behav Brain Res* 1987; 24:11–29.

Carlton SM, Coggeshall RE. Immunohistochemical localization of enkephalin in peripheral sensory axons in the rat. *Neurosci Lett* 1997; 221:121–124.

Cesselin F, Montastruc JL, Gros C, et al. Met-enkephalin levels and opiate receptors in the spinal cord of chronic suffering rats. *Brain Res* 1980; 191:289–293.

Davar G, Kramer MF, Garber D, et al. Comparative efficacy of expression of genes delivered to mouse sensory neurons with herpes virus vectors. *J Comp Neurol* 1994; 339:3–11.

De Castro Costa M, De Sutter P, Gybels J, et al. Adjuvant-induced arthritis in rats: a possible animal model of chronic pain. *Pain* 1981; 10:173–185.

De Hooge ASK, De Loo FAJ, Arntz AJ, et al. Involvement of IL-6, apart from its role in immunity, in mediating a chronic response during experimental arthritis. *Am J Pathol* 2000; 157:2081–2091.

Dray A, Urban L, Dickenson A. Pharmacology of chronic pain. *Trends Pharmacol Sci* 1994; 15:190–197.

El Hassan AM, Lindgren JU, Hultenby K, et al. Methionine-enkephalin in bone and joint tissues. *J Bone Miner Res* 1998; 13:88–95.

Galbraith JA, Mrosko BJ, Myers RR. A system to measure thermal nociception. *J Neurosci Meth* 1993; 49:63–68.

Goins WF, Lee KA, Cavalcoli JD, et al. Herpes simplex virus type 1 vector-mediated expression of nerve growth factor protects dorsal root ganglion neurons from peroxide toxicity. *J Virol* 1999; 73:519–532.

Goss JR, Mata M, Goins WF, et al. Antinociceptive effect of a genomic herpes simplex virus-based vector expressing human proenkephalin in rat dorsal root ganglion. *Gene Ther* 2001; 8:551–556.

Gouret C, Mocquet G, Raynaud G. Use of Freund's adjuvant arthritis test in anti-inflammatory drug screening in the rat: value of animal selection and preparation at the breeding center. *Lab Animal Sci* 1976; 26:281–287.

Harris ED. Rheumatoid arthritis. Pathophysiology and implications for therapy. *N Engl J Med* 1990; 322:1277–1289.

Kamphuis S, Eriksson F, Kavelaars A, et al. Role of endogenous pro-enkephalin A-derived peptides in human T cell proliferation and monocyte IL-6 production. *J Neuroimmunol* 1998; 84:53–60.

Koch AE, Kunkel SL, Strieter RM. Cytokines in rheumatoid arthritis. *J Investig Med* 1995; 43:28–38.

Millan MJ, Czlonkowski A, Pilcher CW, et al. A model of chronic pain in the rat: functional correlates of alterations in the activity of opioid systems. *J Neurosci* 1987; Jan 7:77–87.

Ohshima S, Saeki Y, Mima T, et al. Interleukin 6 plays a key role in the development of antigen-induced arthritis. *Proc Natl Acad Sci USA* 1998; 95:8222–8226.

Pohl M, Benoliel JJ, Bourgoin S, et al. Regional distribution of calcitonin gene-related peptide-, substance P-, cholecystokinin-, met^5-enkephalin-, and dynorphin A(1-8)-like materials in the spinal cord and dorsal root ganglia of adult rats: effects of dorsal rhizotomy and neonatal capsaicin. *J Neurochem* 1990; 55:1122–1130.

Pohl M, Collin E, Bourgoin S, et al. Expression of preproenkephalin A gene and presence of met-enkephalin in dorsal root ganglia of the adult rat. *J Neurochem* 1994; 63:1226–1234.

Poole S, de Queiraz Cunha F, Ferreira SH. Hyperalgesia from subcutaneous cytokines. In: Watkins LR, Maier SF (Eds). *Cytokines and Pain.* Basel: Birkhäuser Verlag, 1999, pp 59–87.

Schäfer M, Carter L, Stein C. Interleukin 1β and corticotropin-releasing factor inhibit pain by releasing opioids from immune cells in inflamed tissue. *Proc Natl Acad Sci USA* 1994; 91:4219–4223.

Stein C, Yassouridis A. Peripheral morphine analgesia. *Pain* 1997; 71:119–121.

Takeba Y, Suzuki N, Kaneko A, et al. Endorphin and enkephalin ameliorate excessive synovial cell functions in patients with rheumatoid arthritis. *J Rheumatol* 2001; 28:2176–2183.

Walker JS, Chandler AK, Wilson JL, et al. Effect of mu-opioids morphine and buprenorphine on the development of adjuvant arthritis in rats. *Inflamm Res* 1996; 45:557–563.

Wilson SP, Yeomans DC, Bender MA, et al. Antihyperalgesic effects of infection with a preproenkephalin-encoding herpes virus. *Proc Natl Acad Sci USA* 1999; 96:3211–3216.

Correspondence to: Michel Pohl, INSERM U288, Faculté de Médecine Pitié-Salpêtrière, 91, Boulevard de l'Hôpital, 75634 Paris Cedex 13, France. Tel: 33-1 40 77 97 09, Fax: 33-1 40 77 97 90; email: pohl@ext.jussieu.fr.

Part VII

Clinical Epidemiology

Proceedings of the 10th World Congress on Pain,
Progress in Pain Research and Management, Vol. 24,
edited by Jonathan O. Dostrovsky, Daniel B. Carr, and
Martin Koltzenburg, IASP Press, Seattle, © 2003.

45

Epidemiology of Chronic Noncancer Pain in Denmark

Marianne K. Jensen,[a] Per Sjøgren,[a] Ola Ekholm,[b] Niels K. Rasmussen,[b] and Jørgen Eriksen[a]

[a]*Multidisciplinary Pain Center, National Hospital, Copenhagen, Denmark;*
[b]*National Institute of Public Health, Copenhagen, Denmark*

In recent years several epidemiological studies have estimated the prevalence of pain in different communities to elucidate demographic characteristics and societal consequences of pain (Brattberg et al. 1989; Von Korff et al. 1990; Elliott et al. 1999; Blyth et al. 2001). Prevalence rates for chronic pain ranging from 8% to 80% have been found, primarily indicating inconsistencies in definition. However, a universal finding in the populations identified as having chronic pain was a preponderance of middle-aged women with lower socioeconomic status (Verhaak et al. 1998).

The annual incidence of chronic pain has been estimated as 1–2% (Magni et al. 1994; Waxman et al. 2000) and varies according to bodily location, with low back pain having the highest incidence of 18% (Von Korff et al. 1993). Sociodemographic factors and the presence of depression or other psychological morbidity are among the strongest predictors of chronic pain (Von Korff et al. 1993; Croft et al. 2001).

Studies on the epidemiology on pain are usually cross-sectional investigations, that is, one-time surveys. A considerable limitation of this design is that cause and effect (presumptive etiology and present pain severity or health status) are simultaneously assessed. To study the incidence, cause, and prognosis of chronic pain, cohort studies are mandatory.

The purpose of this chapter is threefold: (1) to describe how sociodemographic characteristics differ in a cohort that develops chronic pain as compared with reference groups; (2) to estimate the prevalence of chronic pain according to various sociodemographic characteristics; and (3) to identify the sociodemographic characteristics that predispose to chronic pain.

METHODS

The Danish Health and Morbidity Surveys of 1994 and 2000 are the third and fourth in a series of health surveys conducted in Denmark every sixth to seventh year (Kjøller et al. 1995, 2002). The aim of the surveys is to evaluate general health and morbidity in the Danish population in a given year, and to monitor health status over years in a cross-sectional design. The primary instrument to accomplish this evaluation is the Medical Outcomes Study 36-Item Short Form Questionnaire (SF-36), a tool that has been applied internationally for measuring health-related quality of life (Ware et al. 1994; Bjørner et al 1997).

The surveys of 1994 and 2000 used random samples that were representative of the Danish population, drawn from the government's central register. The samples for the two surveys consisted of 6,000 and 16,684 persons over 16 years of age, respectively. Data collection consisted of a face-to-face interview conducted by professional interviewers from the Danish National Institute of Social Research, as well as a postal questionnaire that included the SF-36.

Only persons who were interviewed and then completed and returned the postal questionnaire were included in the survey results. An earlier or present cancer diagnosis, indicated either by registration in the National Cancer Register or by self-report, led to exclusion.

DANISH HEALTH AND MORBIDITY SURVEY OF 1994

In the 1994 study, the question from SF-36 regarding bodily pain during the past 4 weeks was used to identify the pain and reference groups. Pain intensity is evaluated on the SF-36 using a verbal rating score (VRS) having six items: 1 = no pain; 2 = very mild; 3 = mild; 4 = moderate; 5 = severe; 6 = very severe. Persons with moderate to severe pain (rated at 4–6 points on this 1–6-point scale) were classified as a high pain group (HPG). Persons with mild (3 points), very mild (2–3 points), or no pain (1 point) were used as a reference group (RG).

DANISH HEALTH AND MORBIDITY SURVEY OF 2000

The Health and Morbidity Survey of 2000 included as an additional question: "Do you suffer from chronic/long-lasting pain lasting 6 months or more?" Based on their answer to this question, respondents were assigned to a chronic pain group (CPG) or a control group (CG). This definition of chronic pain is equivalent to the internationally accepted definition of chronic pain and in accordance with other studies using a corresponding definition (Brattberg et al. 1989; Blyth et al. 2001). We estimated the prevalence of chronic pain according to various sociodemographic characteristics. Using responses to the SF-36 question on bodily pain, dichotomized as described above, we also compared sociodemographic characteristics from the 1994 and 2000 cross-sectional surveys.

VALIDATION OF CUT-OFF SCORE

To identify the optimal cut-off score of the VRS prior to the survey of 1994, we validated the SF-36 question on bodily pain. Sensitivity, specificity, positive or negative predictive value (PV), and accuracy of possible cut-off scores were calculated using "chronic pain lasting >6 months" as the reference standard. "Accuracy" connotes how well the VRS identifies individuals with true positive and true negative "chronic pain" and "no chronic pain" in the population of interest and was considered the most important parameter. The validation data for the VRS is shown in Table I. The highest accuracy of 85% was found in Group 3, in which VRS scores were dichotomized according to the cut-off score subsequently employed in the present study. On this basis we characterized the migration of individuals into the HPG from various sociodemographic groups from 1994 to 2000.

COHORT STUDY FROM 1994–2000

In the year 2000 the participants from the 1994 survey were reinterviewed in a cohort study. According to the validation data shown in Table I, the RG

Table I
Determination of cut-off score on the SF-36 question on bodily pain, to maximize accuracy of dichotomization

Cut-off Score (VRS)			Sensitivity	Specificity			Accuracy
Group	RG	HPG	(%)	(%)	PV+	PV–	(%)
1	1	2, 3, 4, 5, 6	96	51	32	98	59
2	1, 2	3, 4, 5, 6	82	77	46	95	78
3	**1, 2, 3**	**4, 5, 6**	**51**	**92**	**62**	**89**	**85**
4	1, 2, 3, 4	5, 6	20	97	65	84	83
5	1, 2, 3, 4, 5	6	5	99	70	81	81

Abbreviations: HPG = high pain group; PV = predictive value; RG = reference group; SF-36 = Medical Outcomes Study 36-Item Short Form Questionnaire; VRS = verbal rating scale of pain intensity.
Note: The highest accuracy of 85% was found in Group 3 (boldface type), in which VRS scores were dichotomized according to the cut-off score subsequently used in the present study.

identified in 1994 was used as the baseline population that was reinvestigated 6 years later. Baseline levels of sociodemographic variables were hypothesized as determinants of migration from the RG into the HPG, and incidences were estimated for each such level.

SOCIODEMOGRAPHIC CHARACTERISTICS

Sociodemographic variables were sex, age, cohabitation status, educational status, and work-related physical strain. Age was categorized in four groups: 16–24 years, 25–44 years, 45–66 years, and 67+ years, as suggested by Kjøller et al. (2002). Cohabitation status was stratified in five groups: married, cohabiting, divorced/separated, widowed, and never married. The International Standard Classification of Education, which combines school and occupational education, was used to describe educational status (Hansen et al. 1994). This variable was categorized into three levels: <10 years, 10–12 years, and 13+ years of education.

Physical work-related strain was measured by responses to the following question: "How would you describe the physical strain of your chief occupation?" Respondents could characterize their work according to one of four categories: (1) mainly sedentary work that does not demand physical effort; (2) work that to a great extent is performed standing or walking, but otherwise does not demand physical effort; (3) standing or walking work with frequent lifting and carrying; or (4) heavy active work that is strenuous.

STATISTICAL ANALYSIS

To analyze the influence of the independent variables "sex," "age," "cohabitation status," "education," and "work-related physical strain" on the dependent variable "pain" (bodily pain during the past 4 weeks or chronic/long-lasting pain), logistic regression analysis was used. Odds ratios (OR) describe the association between pain and the independent variables. Logistic regression analysis was also used to analyze the development of pain over time, i.e., from 1994 to 2000, and to analyze the influence of the independent variables for developing pain in the following cohort. All analyses were adjusted for sex and age. The statistical analyses were performed using SAS version 8.2.

RESULTS

HEALTH AND MORBIDITY SURVEY OF 1994

In the 1994 survey, a total of 4,667 persons were interviewed (response rate 78%). Of these, 4,083 persons (87% of those interviewed and 68% of the total sample) returned the postal questionnaire. Cancer led to exclusion of 114 persons, leaving 3,969 subjects for further analysis. The investigated sample consisted of slightly more married people, slightly fewer elderly people, and fewer people with a short education, and the subjects also had poorer self-rated health status as compared with the larger sample of interviewed persons.

Analyses showed that the unequal demographic distribution among the interviewed did not influence the estimated prevalence in the entire population (Kjøller et al. 1995). The investigated sample is very similar in demographic distribution and hence the study population is considered representative of the Danish population.

The overall prevalence of moderate to high pain, by which respondents were assigned to the HPG, was 14% (16% for women and 10% for men). The prevalences of moderate to high pain according to sociodemographic variables are shown in Table II. Prevalence increased with age, peaked in the 45–66-year age group, and then declined with advancing age. Moreover, it was more likely for a person with less than 10 years of education to be in the HPG than for a person with more than 13 years. Membership in the HPG was significantly associated with having a job with light physical activity.

HEALTH AND MORBIDITY SURVEY OF 2000

In year 2000 a total of 12,333 persons were interviewed (response rate 74%), and 10,458 of them (85% of those interviewed and 63% of the total sample) returned the postal questionnaire. Of the latter, 392 persons were excluded because of cancer or procedural errors, leaving 10,066 subjects for further investigation. The study population consisted of slightly more married people and fewer elderly people compared with the original sample of 12,333 persons, and subjects also had shorter education and poorer self-rated health. The demographic distribution was very similar to that found in the 1994 survey and hence the study population was considered representative of the Danish population.

Table II
Prevalences and age- and sex-adjusted odds ratios for moderate to severe pain on the SF-36 pain question, according to sociodemographic variables; analysis of the high pain group (HPG) vs. the no- or low-pain reference group (RG)

Variable	Prevalence of Moderate to Severe Pain, % (cases)	Odds Ratio, HPG vs. RG (95% CI)
Total population	14 (563)	
Sex ($P < 0.0001$)		
Male	10 (210)	1
Female	16 (353)	1.64 (1.36–2.00)*
Age ($P = 0.01$)		
16–24 years	11 (67)	1
25–44 years	14 (214)	1.34 (1.00–1.80)*
45–66 years	16 (205)	1.65 (1.23–2.22)*
67+ years	14 (77)	1.36 (0.96–1.93)
Cohabitation status ($P = 0.02$)		
Married	14 (291)	1
Cohabiting	13 (87)	1.06 (0.80–1.40)
Divorced/separated	23 (51)	1.78 (1.27–2.50)*
Widowed	17 (42)	1.23 (0.83–1.83)
Never married	12 (92)	1.06 (0.77–1.45)
Education ($P < 0.0001$)		
<10 years	20 (180)	2.13 (1.67–2.72)*
10–12 years	14 (163)	1.38 (1.09–1.73)*
13+ years	11 (195)	1
Work-related physical strain ($P < 0.0001$)†		
Sedentary	9 (80)	1
Light activity	12 (81)	1.49 (1.08–2.06)*
Moderate	13 (91)	1.31 (0.94–1.81)
High activity	13 (10)	1.59 (0.79–3.25)

Source: Health and Morbidity Survey of 1994.
*Statistically significant; †analysis performed among those actively engaged in employment.

The prevalence of assignment to the CPG, determined by a positive response to the question: "Do you suffer from chronic/long-lasting pain lasting 6 months or more?," according to various sociodemographic characteristics, is shown in Table III. The overall prevalence of such pain was 19% (16% for men and 21% for women). The prevalence increased with age. The odds of reporting a positive response to the chronic pain question were almost two times higher for those having less than 10 years of education

Table III
Prevalences and age- and sex-adjusted odds ratios for chronic pain (>6 months), according to sociodemographic variables

Variable	Chronic Pain Prevalence, % (cases)	Odds Ratio	95% CI
Total population	19 (1871)		
Sex ($P < 0.0001$)			
Male	16 (781)	1	
Female	21 (1090)	1.40	1.26–1.55*
Age ($P < 0.0001$)			
16–24 years	9 (126)	1	
25–44 years	13 (496)	1.47	1.20–1.81*
45–66 years	23 (854)	2.96	2.43–3.62*
67+ years	29 (395)	3.90	3.13–4.85*
Cohabitation status ($P < 0.0001$)			
Married	19 (1051)	1	
Cohabiting	16 (262)	1.17	0.99–1.37
Divorced/separated	27 (147)	1.46	1.19–1.79*
Widowed	31 (188)	1.22	0.99–1.50
Never married	12 (211)	0.92	0.76–1.12
Education ($P < 0.0001$)			
<10 years	29 (77)	1.91	1.65–2.19*
10–12 years	21 (1027)	1.58	1.40–1.78*
13+ years	14 (739)	1	
Work-related physical strain ($P < 0.0001$)†			
Sedentary	12 (295)	1	
Light	14 (270)	1.13	0.93–1.36
Moderate	12 (224)	1.08	0.89–1.31
High	21 (57)	2.19	1.57–3.06*

Source: Health and Morbidity Survey of 2000.
Abbreviations: CPG = chronic pain group.
*Statistically significant; †analysis performed among those actively engaged in employment.

than for those having 13 years or more. Moreover, having a job with a high level of physical strain was statistically more likely to be associated with reporting of chronic pain than having a sedentary job.

Trends in prevalence of moderate to severe pain according to sociodemographic variables are shown in Table IV. There was no overall increase in the prevalence of moderate to severe pain. However, for the subgroups “Female” and “10–12 years of education” a statistically significant increase of reported moderate to severe pain was observed.

Table IV
Trends in prevalence of moderate to severe pain on the SF-36 pain question, according to sociodemographic variables; odds ratios are adjusted for sex and age

Variable	Prevalence of Moderate to Severe Pain, % (cases)		Odds Ratio	95% CI
	1994 Survey	2000 Survey		
Total population	14 (569)	16 (1585)	1.10	0.99–1.22
Sex				
Male	11 (215)	12 (575)	1.03	0.87–1.22
Female	17 (354)	19 (1010)	1.14	1.00–1.31*
Age				
16–24 years	11 (67)	13 (55)	1.23	0.91–1.67
25–44 years	14 (213)	14 (181)	1.07	0.90–1.26
45–66 years	17 (209)	17 (257)	1.03	0.86–1.22
67+ years	15 (80)	19 (81)	1.27	0.96–1.67
Education				
<10 years	21 (183)	21 (354)	1.02	0.83–1.25
10–12 years	14 (164)	18 (510)	1.31	1.08–1.56*
13+ years	11 (197)	13 (683)	1.15	0.97–1.38
Cohabitation status				
Married	15 (299)	15 (822)	1.05	0.91–1.22
Cohabiting	13 (86)	16 (268)	1.27	0.98–1.66
Divorced/separated	23 (50)	25 (137)	1.14	0.78–1.66
Widowed	19 (41)	19 (119)	1.09	0.73–1.62
Never married	12 (93)	13 (226)	1.05	0.81–1.36
Work-related physical strain†				
Sedentary	10 (83)	11 (267)	1.08	0.82–1.41
Light	12 (83)	12 (231)	0.91	0.69–1.20
Moderate	13 (96)	13 (245)	1.08	0.83–1.41
High	13 (11)	18 (49)	1.54	0.73–3.25

Source: Health and Morbidity Surveys of 1994 and 2000.
* Statistically significant; †analysis performed among those actively engaged in employment.

COHORT STUDY OF 1994–2000

The baseline consisted of 3,170 persons who were classified in the RG in 1994 and were obtainable for the study in 2000. At follow-up 2,294 (72%) of these persons returned the postal questionnaire. The follow-up cohort differed from the baseline population by having slightly fewer elderly persons, slightly fewer persons with an education of 10 years or less, and slightly fewer unmarried persons.

Table V shows that gender, a short education, and heavy or highly active work were risk factors for developing moderate to severe pain. The odds of developing moderate to severe pain were almost three times higher among those having a job with the highest level of physical strain than in those with a sedentary job.

Table V
Incidence of moderate to severe pain on the SF-36 pain question, according to sociodemographic variables; odds ratios are adjusted for sex and age

Variable (Baseline Level of 1994)	Incidence of Moderate to Severe Pain, % (cases)†	Odds Ratio	95% CI
Total population	11 (245)		
Sex			
Male	9 (95)	1	
Female	13 (150)	1.55	1.18–2.03*
Age			
16–24 years	10 (39)	1	
25–44 years	11 (104)	1.08	0.73–1.59
45–66 years	11 (77)	1.06	0.70–1.58
67+ years	13 (25)	1.35	0.79-2.31
Cohabitation status			
Married	11 (137)	1	
Cohabiting	10 (40)	0.95	0.63–1.43
Divorced/separated	11 (13)	0.96	0.52–1.75
Widowed	11 (9)	0.74	0.34–1.61
Never married	10 (92)	1.04	0.66–1.66
Education			
<10 years	13 (50)	1.51	1.03–2.22*
10–12 years	11 (76)	1.28	0.93–1.76
13+ years	9 (106)	1	
Work-related physical strain‡			
Sedentary	8 (48)	1	
Light activity	10 (43)	1.19	0.77–1.85
Moderate	10 (46)	1.15	0.74–1.78
High activity	20 (10)	2.74	1.19–6.31*

Source: Cohort study, 1994–2000.
*Statistically significant; †estimated as the proportion of persons developing pain over the course of 6 years; ‡analysis performed among those actively engaged in employment.

DISCUSSION

The data based on the survey of 1994 had limitations, common in studying the epidemiology of pain, of case definition and identification (Smith et al. 1996; Crombie 1997). In studies by Becker et al. (1997) and Purves et al. (1998), the bodily pain item of the SF-36 had one of the lowest scores among chronic pain sufferers, and this item was therefore chosen for identification of a pain group. Low scores on the bodily pain item correspond to high levels of pain severity. Our results indicate that high pain ratings on the VRS may identify the population most adversely affected by chronic pain.

The 2000 survey discloses a prevalence of chronic pain of 19%, which, although consistent with prevalences found in studies using a similar definition of chronic pain (Brattberg et al. 1989; Blyth et al. 2001), was higher than we would have expected. Inequalities in health are well described, and the importance of sociodemographic factors such as sex, educational level, and social status in morbidity and development of diseases has been documented (Brønum-Hansen 2000; Lissau et al. 2001). The present study reveals that such factors also influence the prevalence of chronic pain among subgroups in the population of Denmark. Moreover, our results confirm consensus findings on sociodemographic characteristics of chronic pain populations, showing an overrepresentation of middle-aged women with a lower socioeconomic background (Verhaak et al. 1998).

A major aim of epidemiology is to uncover causes of pain, and therefore longitudinal studies are mandatory. Identification of risk factors may lead to implementation of preventive strategies. The definition of pain used in the present study identified individuals with chronic pain with an accuracy of 85%. We therefore expect similar results in analyzing a more specific definition of chronic pain in a longitudinal design.

The study identifies three risk factors for chronic pain: female gender, less than 10 years of education, and a high level of work-related physical strain. Previous investigators have identified physical workload as a strong predictor for low back pain (Punnett et al. 1991; Liira et al. 1996). However, this subject is still controversial because the quality and amount of data are limited and mostly empirically based (Dionne 1999). Our present cohort data from the initially no- or low-pain group reveals that those reporting the highest level of physical strain have almost three times higher odds of reporting pain 6 years later compared with those having a sedentary job.

The purposes of epidemiological surveys on chronic pain are multiple and include the development and implementation of preventive strategies. Our intention, based on our concern about long waiting lists for the few and scattered multidisciplinary pain management centers in Denmark, was to estimate the unmet need for such treatment facilities. Further detailed analyses of the Health and Morbidity Surveys of 1994 and 2000 are now underway in order to estimate the health characteristics of those with chronic pain, the social and economic consequences of reporting chronic pain as a health-related disability, and the cost of medication and utilization of health care services.

ACKNOWLEDGMENT

The Danish Foundation of Medical Technology Assessment supported this study.

REFERENCES

Becker N, Thomsen AB, Olsen AK, et al. Pain epidemiology and health related quality of life in chronic non-malignant pain patients referred to a Danish multidisciplinary pain center. *Pain* 1997; 73:393–400.

Bjørner JB, Damsgaard MT, Watt T, et al. Dansk manual til SF-36 (Danish manual for SF-36) Etsporgeskemaon helbredsstatus (Questionnaire of health status). Copenhagen: Lagemiddelindustriforeninger, 1997.

Blyth FM, March LM, Brnabic AJM, et al. Chronic pain in Australia: a prevalence study. *Pain* 2001; 89:127–134.

Brattberg G, Thorslund M, Wikman A. The prevalence of pain in a general population. The results of a postal survey in a county of Sweden. *Pain* 1989; 37:215–222.

Brønum-Hansen H. Socioeconomic differences in health expectancy in Denmark. *Scand J Public Health* 2000; 28:194–199.

Croft PR, Lewis M, Papageorgiou AC, et al. Risk factors for neck pain: a longitudinal study in the general population. *Pain* 2001; 93:317–325.

Crombie IK. Epidemiology of persistent pain. In: Jensen TS, Turner JA, Wiesenfeld-Hallin Z (Eds). *Proceedings of the 8th World Congress on Pain,* Progress in Pain Research and Management, Vol. 8. Seattle: IASP Press, 1997, pp 53–61.

Dionne CE. Low back pain. In: Crombie IK, Croft PR, Linton SJ, LeResche L, Von Korff M (Eds). *Epidemiology of Pain.* Seattle: IASP Press, 1999, pp 283–298.

Elliott AM, Smith BH, Penny KI, Smith WC, Chambers WA. The epidemiology of chronic pain in the community. *Lancet* 1999; 354:1248–1252.

Hansen A, Kühl K. *Dansk Uddannelses Nomenklatur (Danish Educational Nomenclature).* Copenhagen: Danish Statistics and Ministry of Education, 1994.

Kjøller M, Rasmussen NK (Eds). *Danish Health and Morbidity Survey 2000 and Trends since 1987.* Copenhagen: National Institute of Public Health, 2002. Available via the Internet: www.niph.dk.

Kjøller M, Rasmussen NK, Keiding L, Petersen HC, Nielsen GA. *The Danish Health and Morbidity Survey, 1994,* 1995. Available via the Internet: www.niph.dk.

Liira JP, Shannon HS, Chambers LW, Haines TA. Long-term back problems and physical work exposures in the 1990 Ontario Health Survey. *Am J Public Health* 1996; 86:382–387.

Lissau I, Rasmussen NK, Hesse NM, Hesse U. Social differences in illness and health-related exclusion from the labour market in Denmark from 1987 to 1994. *Scand J Public Health* 2001; 29(Suppl 55):19–30.

Magni G, Moreschi C, Rigatti-Luchini S, Merskey H. Prospective study on the relationship between depressive symptoms and chronic musculoskeletal pain. *Pain* 1994; 56:289–297.

Punnett L, Fine LJ, Keyserling WM, Herrin GD, Chaffin DB. Back disorders and nonneutral trunk postures of automobile assembly workers. *Scand J Work Environ Health* 1991; 17:337–346.

Purves AL, Penny KI, Munro C, et al. Defining chronic pain for epidemiological research—assessing af subjective definition. *Pain Clinic* 1998; 10:139–147.

Smith BH, Chambers WA, Smith WC. Chronic pain: time for epidemiology. *J R Soc Med* 1996; 89:181–183.

Verhaak PFM, Kerssens JJ, Dekker J, Sorbi MJ, Bensing JM. Prevalence of chronic benign pain disorder among adults: a review of the literature. *Pain* 1998; 77:231–239.

Von Korff M, Dworkin SF, LeResche L. Graded chronic pain status: an epidemiologic evaluation. *Pain* 1990; 40:279–291.

Von Korff M, LeResche L, Dworkin SF. First onset of common pain symptoms: a prospective study of depression as a risk factor. *Pain* 1993; 55:251–258.

Ware JE, Gandek B, and the IQOLA project group. The SF-36 health survey: development and use in mental health research and IQOLA project. *Int J Ment Health* 1994, 23(2):49–73.

Waxman R, Tennant A, Helliwell P. A prospective follow-up study of low back pain in the community. *Spine* 2000; 25:2085–2090.

Correspondence to: Jørgen Eriksen, MD, Multidisciplinary Pain Center, Rigshospitalet, Dept. 7612, Blegdamsvej 9, DK-2100 Copenhagen, Denmark. Tel: 45-3545-7382; Fax: 45-3545-7349; email: jeriksen@rh.dk.

Proceedings of the 10th World Congress on Pain,
Progress in Pain Research and Management, Vol. 24,
edited by Jonathan O. Dostrovsky, Daniel B. Carr, and
Martin Koltzenburg, IASP Press, Seattle, © 2003.

46

Prevalence and Characteristics of Neuropathic Pain in 358 Patients with Leprosy

Patrick R.N.A.G. Stump,[a,b] Rosemari Baccarelli,[a] Lúcia H.S.C. Marciano,[a] José R.P. Lauris,[c] Somei Ura,[a] Manoel J. Teixeira,[b] and Marcos C.L. Virmond[a]

[a]Instituto Lauro de Souza Lima, Bauru, Brazil; [b]School of Medicine, University of São Paulo, São Paulo, Brazil; [c]School of Dentistry, University of São Paulo, Bauru, Brazil

Leprosy (Hansen's disease) is a chronic infectious disease that affects the skin and peripheral nerves. Although restricted to major endemic countries, it is the most common cause of peripheral neuropathy worldwide (Pfaltzgraff 1993; Sabin 1993). The disease is caused by Mycobacterium leprae, which has a predilection for Schwann cells. Since the introduction of an effective treatment based upon multidrug therapy (dapsone, clofazimine, and rifampin) and recommended by the World Health Organization (WHO), the prevalence of leprosy has dramatically decreased (World Health Organization 2000). However, the disease is still a public health problem in many countries, with an estimated global prevalence of nearly 600,000 cases as of the end of 2001 (World Health Organization 2002).

Damage to peripheral nerves is a key component of leprosy and, together with typical skin lesions, accounts for the major traditional clinical features of the disease. Little is known about the mechanism by which the mycobacteria infect Schwann cells, but recently some evidence has emerged. A glycoprotein (α-dystroglycan) that binds to the surface of *M. leprae* also binds to a molecule on the surface of the Schwann cell and provides a potential mechanism for internalization of the bacilli (Rambukkana 1997; Freedman 1999). In addition, it is clear that the most profoundly affected sites have distinctive common features, such as being superficial, with a low ambient temperature, and located along potentially constricting anatomical structures such as nerve sheaths.

The sensory and motor loss that follows nerve damage in leprosy is the basis for the classical features of many cases such as skin wounds, cracks, plantar ulcers, clawed hands, foot drop, and lagophthalmos (incomplete closure of the eyelids). Sensory damage includes an early loss of pain and temperature perception followed by compromise of tactile and pressure senses. The immunological status forms the basis of the Madrid classification of individual cases as indeterminate, tuberculoid, borderline, and lepromatous (Opromolla 2001), although the WHO recommends a simple operational classification as paucibacillary (PB) and multibacillary (MB) types (Dharmendra 1993). Cases with a low bacterial load or those that show no bacilli in skin smears are classified PB; these cases often show some immunological resistance to the disease. Cases with a high bacterial load or that show many bacilli in skin smears are classified MB; these cases often show poor or no resistance. The distribution and onset of nerve damage can vary according to the type of leprosy, being more disseminated and gradual in the lepromatous cases and more localized and acute in tuberculoid and borderline cases. The indeterminate type is an initial presentation of the disease in which major nerve damage has not yet developed.

One of the most remarkable aspects of leprosy to lay persons and health care workers alike is that patients are reputed to feel no pain. This widespread impression is rapidly changing as many patients who have completed their WHO multidrug therapy are now reporting complaints of stimulus-independent ongoing pain, and seeking relief. Indeed, pain in leprosy can be nociceptive due to tissue inflammation, which mostly occurs during episodes of immune activation ("reversal reaction" and "erythema nodosum leprosum") or neuropathic, due to damage or dysfunction of the nervous system.

The complex and stigmatizing burden of being diagnosed with leprosy may compel patients to focus solely upon curing their disease, which is readily achieved with the WHO drug regimen, and accept their symptoms as an inevitable concomitant or residual of the disease. However, the number of cases of leprosy with pain problems seemed to us to be substantial. The aims of this study, conducted in a country where leprosy is endemic, were to estimate the prevalence of pain in patients with leprosy and to determine the main characteristics of their pain.

METHODS

The study was conducted at the Instituto Lauro de Souza Lima, Bauru, Brazil, a national referral center for leprosy patients. Brazil has a prevalence of 77,676 cases and a high detection rate of 24.1/100,000 (41,070 new cases in 2000), which makes it the second largest endemic country for leprosy in the world after India (World Health Organization 2002).

The study included 358 patients with leprosy who presented to the Dermatological Clinic of our institute from October 1, 2001 to March 31, 2002. Among them, 215 were male (60.1%) and 143 were female (39.9%). The mean age was 54.8 years, with a range of 11–87 years (SD = 16 years).

The mean time from initial diagnosis was 18.3 years (range, 10 months to 68 years, SD = 18.5 years), and 178 (49.7%) patients were diagnosed over 10 years earlier. According to the Madrid Classification (Opromolla 2001), 207 (57.8%) were lepromatous, 92 (25.7%) borderline, 54 (15.1%) tuberculoid, and only 5 (1.4%) indeterminate. All cases were receiving treatment except for 283 (79.1%) patients who had concluded their standard course by the time of the study. Treatment regimens included the WHO multidrug therapy, dapsone plus rifampicin, or dapsone as monotherapy in some previously treated cases.

Two hundred and one (56.1%) of the patients reported past or current moderate or severe chronic neuropathic pain that interfered with activities of daily living or disturbed sleep. These cases underwent neurological examination by trained health workers, including detailed assessment focusing on the occurrence of pain, its localization, duration, pattern of symptom onset, quality, and quantity. Localization of pain refers to the anatomical distribution and trunk of the most relevant affected peripheral nerve. Duration of pain was classified according to less than or greater than the prior 6 months. The pattern of symptom onset was categorized as abrupt, insidious, or in repetitive bursts. Assessment of the quality of pain was based upon the Brazilian Portuguese version of the McGill Pain Questionnaire (Teixeira 2001). In addition, we inquired whether present pain was experienced as superficial, deep, or mixed. Pain intensity was verbally rated by patients as mild, moderate, or severe and was also rated on a graphic scale (empty to full water glass).

RESULTS

Using the day of the interview and examination as the reference point, 148 (73.6%) patients reported episodes of pain only in the past, and 53 (26.4%) had pain at present. In the 148 patients with past pain only, leprosy had been diagnosed less than 10 years earlier in 59 cases (39.8%) and more than 10 years earlier in 89 cases (60.2%). In those with present pain only 14 (26.4%) cases had been diagnosed over 10 years earlier. Pain had been present for 6 months or less in 55 cases (27.4%), whereas 141 patients (70.1%) reported pain for longer than 6 months. Only 5 patients (2.5%) could not estimate the duration of their pain. The nerve most often affected by pain was the ulnar (59.2%), followed by the tibial (30.3%), fibular (18.9%), median (4.5%), radial (2.0%), and trigeminal (1.5%). These percentages sum to greater than 100 because patients were free to indicate pain in the distribution of more than one nerve. Glove (22.4%) and stocking distributions of pain were also quite common (24.9%) (Fig. 1). The onset of episodes was reported as abrupt by 39 patients (19.4%), as insidious by 73 patients (36.3%), and as recurrent bursts by 89 patients (44.3%). The assessment of the quality of pain is shown in Fig. 2.

In the 53 patients with pain present at the time of interview, the most affected anatomical layer was deep in 30 (56.6%) patients, superficial in 8 (15.1%), and mixed in 15 (28.3%). In these patients pain was constant in 34 (64.2%) and episodic in 19 (35.8%). Verbal ratings of present pain were severe in 29 (54.7%), moderate in 17 (32.1%), and mild in only 7 patients (13.2%). On the graphic scale, 22 (41.5%) patients rated their pain as severe, 21 (39.6%) as moderate, and 10 (18.9%) as mild. These pain characteristics are summarized in Table I.

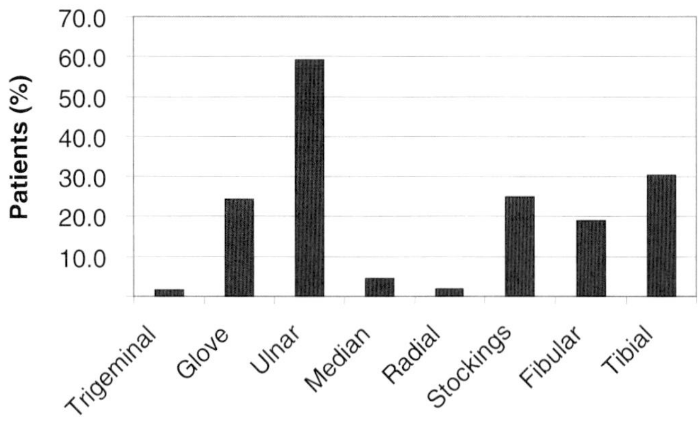

Fig. 1. Localization of pain in the 201 patients with past or present pain.

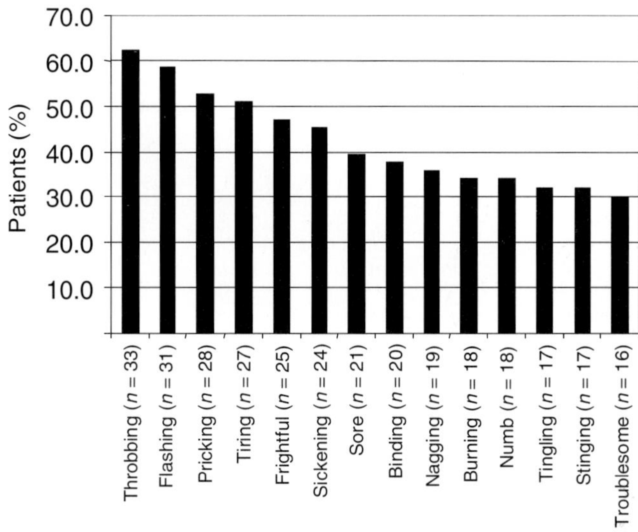

Fig. 2. Quality of pain was ascertained based on the Portuguese language version of the McGill Pain Questionnaire (cut-off = 30%).

DISCUSSION

Lack of sensation is a paradigm of leprosy, and the diagnosis of this chronic infectious disease is assured by the presence of skin lesions (usually patchy) and marked sensory loss as assessed by Semmes-Weinstein monofilaments or a ballpoint pen tip. Abnormalities include loss of touch, temperature, and pressure sensation. Although clinical consensus regards leprosy as painless, in reality nerve pain in leprosy is often present during neuritis, a feature that accompanies acute leprosy reactions. These reactive episodes frequently include entrapment of the nerve in selected sites (most often the ulnar canal at the elbow) due to edema from acute and severe inflammation of the nerve. In such a situation, activation of the nervi nervorum may be the main contributor to pain. Another possibility is that acute neural inflammation can excite and sensitize nociceptors. In some cases, there is severe destruction of nerve fibers (Garbino 1998), and the partial regeneration that follows may produce spontaneous discharges, diminution of stimulus thresholds, and exaggerated responses of nociceptors.

This study reveals that neuropathic pain that is not directly associated with an acute reactive episode may be present in a considerable proportion of patients with leprosy. In fact, out of 358 patients presenting to the outpatient dermatological clinic for other reasons, 56.1% reported prior or current episodes of neuropathic pain. Most of these patients reported that the

Table I
Characteristics of neuropathic pain among 201 cases of leprosy with past (148) or present (53) pain

	Groups	Past Pain, *N* (%)	Present Pain, *N* (%)
Clinical form	Lepromatous	94 (63.5)	26 (49.0)
	Borderline	29 (19.7)	20 (37.8)
	Tuberculoid	24 (16.2)	7 (13.2)
	Indeterminate	1 (0.6)	0 (0)
Onset	Abrupt	30 (20.3)	9 (17.0)
	Insidious	47 (31.8)	26 (49.1)
	Bursts	71 (48.0)	18 (34.0)
Duration	<6 months	49 (33.1)	6 (11.4)
	>6 months	94 (63.5)	47 (88.6)
	Not known	5 (3.4)	0 (0)
Time since leprosy diagnosis	<10 years	59 (39.8)	39 (73.6)
	>10 years	89 (60.2)	14 (26.4)
Treatment completion	Yes	130 (87.8)	40 (75.4)
	No	18 (12.2)	13 (24.6)
Pain intensity	Mild	–	10 (18.9)
	Moderate	–	21 (39.6)
	Severe	–	22 (41.5)
Verbal rating of pain intensity	Mild	–	7 (13.2)
	Moderate	–	17 (32.1)
	Severe	–	29 (54.7)
Time of worst pain	Morning	–	7 (13.3)
	Afternoon	–	9 (16.9)
	Evening	–	15 (28.3)
	Not specific	–	22 (41.5)
Anatomical layer of involvement	Superficial	–	8 (15.1)
	Deep	–	30 (56.6)
	Mixed	–	15 (28.3)
Evolution	Worsening	–	20 (42.6)
	Stable	–	24 (51.1)
	Remitting	–	9 (19.1)
Character	Episodic	–	19 (35.8)
	Constant	–	34 (64.2)

intensity was severe and sufficient to interfere with activities of daily life or with sleep.

According to the literature (Hastings 1993; Jopling 1996), the most common nerve affected in leprosy is the ulnar nerve, and we confirmed the frequency of this painful site. However, a glove and stocking distribution of pain was also frequently reported by our patients. Although involvement of nerve trunks in leprosy is common, the superficial branches and their rami may be also compromised, particularly in lepromatous and borderline cases in which dissemination of the disease is a characteristic feature.

It is important to note that, among those with present pain, 40 patients (75.4%) had completed antimicrobial treatment and, according to the present policy of leprosy control, are discharged from further followup. Such patients receive little further care. Therefore, a significant number of patients did not have ongoing access to care and could not seek assistance for relief of neuropathic pain and improvement in their quality of life. In addition, 130 patients (87.8%) with past pain had already completed treatment by the time their pain occurred. Thus, successful completion of antimicrobial treatment does not appear to prevent the occurrence of neuropathic pain. As a matter of fact, the teams caring for patients with leprosy are not generally aware of the problem of neuropathic pain. It is of utmost importance that control of neuropathic pain in leprosy be included as an issue to be dealt with by leprosy control program managers.

CONCLUSION

This study reveals a considerable prevalence of neuropathic pain among patients with leprosy and presents evidence that this common problem should be a high priority of those in charge of leprosy control programs. In fact, given the present public health policy of shorter regimens and immediate discharge of patients after completion of treatment, this problem can worsen further. Thus at present there is a strong need to review the concept of leprosy care to provide adequate attention to this disabling complication, and plenty of room for studies of new therapies to cope with this previously ignored clinical problem.

REFERENCES

Dharmendra. Classifications of leprosy. In: Hastings RC (Ed). *Leprosy*, 2nd ed. New York: Churchill Livingstone, 1993, pp 179–190.

Freedman VH, Weinstein DE, Kaplan G. How *Mycobacterium leprae* infects peripheral nerves. *Lepr Rev* 1999; 70:136–139.

Garbino JA. Manejo clínico das diferentes formas de comprometimento da neuropatia hansênica. *Hansen Int* 1998; (Special):93–99.

Jopling WH, McDougall AC (Eds). *Handbook of Leprosy,* 5th ed. New Delhi: CBS, 1996.

Hastings RC (Ed). *Leprosy,* 2nd ed. New York: Churchill Livingstone, 1993.

Opromolla DVA (Ed). *Noções de Hansenologia*. Bauru: Centro de Estudos Reynaldo Quagliatto, 2000.

Pfaltzgraff RE, Ramu G. Clinical leprosy. In: Hastings RC (Eds). *Leprosy*, 2nd ed. New York: Churchill Livingstone, 1993, pp 237–287.

Rambukkana A, Salzer JL, Yurchenco PD, Tuomanen EI. Neural targeting of *Mycobacterium leprae* mediated by the G domain of the laminin-alpha 2 chain. *Cell* 1997; 88:881–821.

Sabin TD, Swift TR, Jacobsen RR. Leprosy. In: Dyck PJ, Thomas PK, Griffin JW, Low PA, Podusco JF (Eds). *Peripheral Neuropathy*, Vol. 2. Philadelphia: Saunders, 1993, pp 1354–1379.

Teixeira MJ, Pimenta CAM. Avaliação do doente com dor. In: Teixeira JM, Figueiró JB (Eds). *Dor: epidemiologia, fisiopatologia, avaliação, síndromes dolorosas e tratamento*. São Paulo: Moreira, 2001, pp 58–68.

World Health Organization. *Guide to Eliminate Leprosy as a Public Health Problem*. Geneva: World Health Organization, 2000.

World Health Organization. *Weekly Epidemiology Report* 2002; 77(4 January).

Correspondence to: Rosemari Baccarelli, PhD, Instituto Lauro de Souza Lima Research, CP 3031, Rod. Comte Joao R. Barros Km. 225, Bauru 17.034-071, Brazil.

Proceedings of the 10th World Congress on Pain,
Progress in Pain Research and Management, Vol. 24,
edited by Jonathan O. Dostrovsky, Daniel B. Carr, and
Martin Koltzenburg, IASP Press, Seattle, © 2003.

47

The Experience of Menstrual Pain in Belgian Women

Hugues D. Malonne and Jet Van Hoek

Department of Physiology and Pharmacology, Free University of Brussels, and Pain Advisory Board, Brussels, Belgium

The aims of this observational study were to assess the prevalence of menstrual pain in the Belgian population, and to examine how Belgian women deal with this kind of pain. We polled a sample of 540 women, selected at random and therefore considered to be representative of the Belgian female population aged 15 years and older. Sixteen percent of them claimed to suffer from menstrual pain sometimes. For the great majority (89%) of those who experience menstrual pain, dysmenorrhea occurs once each month. More than three out of four women described this pain as "severe," influencing daily life by putting them in a bad mood and causing irritability. Three out of four women said that they take analgesics for their dysmenorrhea. Nearly half of the analgesics taken are low doses of ibuprofen.

METHODS

The research was conducted by means of face-to-face interviews at respondents' homes using Omnibus methodology. This method relies upon interviews of a representative sample, in which different questions are posed to individual respondents yet the aggregate sample provides comprehensive data. Dysmenorrhea was surveyed within a larger questionnaire about pain and its management in general. Answers were noted on paper questionnaires by interviewers. The data were collected in the week of 11–17 July, 2001. Confidence calculations indicate that the maximum rate of polling error is 4.2%.

RESULTS

PREVALENCE

Sixteen percent of the women questioned declared that they sometimes suffer from menstrual pain. Its prevalence is clearly much higher in younger women, affecting 42% of the 15–24 age group compared with 24% of those aged 15–50. Other factors such as social class, professional activity, language (French or Dutch), and rural or urban residence were not predictive of menstrual pain.

Women suffering from menstrual pain are more likely to report other types of pain (such as headaches and pain in muscles and joints) than are those without menstrual pain. Fifty-nine percent of the dysmenorrheic women, for example, suffer from headache at least once a month, compared with only 37% of women without dysmenorrhea. On average, dysmenorrheic women experience 1.4 other types of pain per month, compared to 0.95 for the nondysmenorrheic women.

DURATION

A large majority (89%) of the dysmenorrheic women suffer from menstrual pain at every period. In 63% these pains occur on more than one day, which corresponds with other reports (e.g., Balbi et al. 2000). On average, menstrual pains last longer than other kinds of acute pain experienced by these women: only a minority of the dysmenorrheic women said that they suffer from pain in muscles and joints (42%), backaches (35%), or toothaches (33%) that last more than one day, most of them affirming that these pains subside within a day. Headaches almost never last longer than one day (4%).

For reasons that were unclear, Dutch-speaking dysmenorrheic women complained more frequently of menstrual pains that last more than one day than did their French-speaking counterparts (71% to 52%). Younger women (15–24 years) complained less of menstrual pains lasting more than one day than did women aged between 25 and 50 (55% to 68%). Again, social class, degree of professional activity, and urban or rural residence do not seem to have any impact on the duration of these pains.

INTENSITY

Nearly four out of five dysmenorrheic women (77%) described their pain as "severe," with an average intensity of 8.0 on a scale from 0 to 11. Menstrual pains were said to be more intense than pain in muscles and joints (68% "severe"), headaches (61%), backaches (54%), and toothaches (54%).

Of the dysmenorrheic women, 18% said that their menstrual pains were moderate and 5% described them as mild.

Half of the women affected indicated that menstrual pain hinders normal daily activities, but that they can cope with it, while 39% said that it does not prevent them from living and behaving normally. Only 11% of them had the impression that it prevents them from living normally, compared to 23% for pain in muscles and joints and 62% for toothache.

Younger women (62% of those aged 15–24 years), women living in the five biggest urban areas (65%), and French-speaking women (75%) complained that menstrual pain is a hindrance for daily activities. One in five women aged between 15 and 24 considered that their menstrual pains prevent them from living and behaving normally, compared with 5% of those aged 25 to 50.

PERCEIVED SYMPTOMATOLOGY

The main perceived concomitant psychological symptoms coincide more or less with those commonly referred to in studies of primary dysmenorrhea: irritability and bad temper (70%), inability to manage day-to-day life (44%), and fatigue or lack of energy (30%) (see, e.g., Balbi et al. 2000). The influence on mood is perceived here as being almost as important as for toothache. The effects on quality of life thus are far from negligible and could have an important impact on absenteeism, as several long-term studies of young women indicate (see, e.g., Coco 1999). However, the present study did not assess absenteeism in relation to menstrual pain.

COPING BEHAVIOR

The main reaction to menstrual pain is to take an over-the-counter analgesic. Forty percent of the women affected volunteered that taking a drug is one of the main associated behaviors, and almost 74%, when asked, acknowledged use of an analgesic to ease their menstrual pain. Women aged between 15 and 25 years (85%), women living in the five biggest urban centers (89%), and French-speaking women (80%) were more eager to adopt this remedy than the average for the group as a whole (74%).

Other spontaneously associated reactions include resting (26%), taking a drug prescribed or advised by one's general practitioner (17%) or consulting him or her (10%), and trying to calm down and not to think about the pain (6–9%). Thirteen percent stated that they do nothing at all. Alternative medicine currently clearly has not made a breakthrough in this specific therapeutic area, as only a very small minority came up with solutions such as massage (2%), homeopathy and phytotherapy (1%), or ergotherapy (1%).

CHOICE OF MEDICATION

The initial choice of a specific analgesic is directed by advice from friends and family as much as by that of a doctor. Habit and what is available in the home medicine cabinet are the next most important determining factors. Drug category clearly plays a minor role in the decision process. Only a minority of the respondents spontaneously cited names such as codeine, ibuprofen, paracetamol (acetaminophen), and aspirin. Nevertheless, almost half of them apparently opt for a low-dose nonsteroidal anti-inflammatory drug (NSAID) such as ibuprofen rather than other analgesics, although many fewer recognize the names of naproxen and ibuprofen (14% and 31%, respectively) than other analgesics (53–94%).

This survey thus corroborates other available studies that show NSAIDs to be the most appropriate first-line choice of therapy in women with primary dysmenorrhea, probably because of their inhibition of the production and release of prostaglandins, which are mainly responsible for the painful uterine contractions characteristic of dysmenorrhea (Coco 1999). The preference for ibuprofen may be a rather recent phenomenon, however. The choice of ibuprofen is more likely to based on a television advertisement, or a friend's, family member's, or pharmacist's recommendation. The selection of other types of analgesics is more likely to be based on habit or what is available at home.

QUANTITY OF MEDICATION

Many more women suffering from menstrual pain take analgesic medication at least once a month than do women who are not dysmenorrheic (49% versus 20%), but when we look at overall frequency, the use of analgesics by the former group takes place within a shorter time interval than for the latter. Only 43% of dysmenorrheic women take painkillers more than once a month, compared to 58% of the unaffected women belonging to the same age category (15–50 years old), while only 8% of affected women report taking analgesics less than once per month, compared to 21% of the unaffected women. Dysmenorrheic women also differ from other women by being more likely to report that they take two doses of analgesics a month (30% compared to 18%), but on average, they do not seem to consume significantly more or fewer doses of analgesics per month (7.5 doses compared to 8.4).

This similarity in analgesic consumption is confirmed by the fact that both groups of women declare that they always have analgesics at home "just in case" (99% and 98%) and that they bring them to their workplace (51% and 47% for dysmenorrheic and nondysmenorrheic women, respectively). The only difference in attitude toward analgesics appears when we compare whether women bring analgesics along every time they leave home: 35% of the dysmenorrheic women said they prefer to have analgesics with them at all times, as compared to 25% of the unaffected group.

DISCUSSION

We found that the percentage of women who report that they suffer from menstrual pain is significantly lower than that mentioned in previous studies. Balbi and colleagues (2000), for example, cite 85% of 14–21-year-olds suffering from dysmenorrhea (compared to our result of 42% in the age category of 15–24 years), whereas Coco (1999) shows prevalence rates as high as 90%. According to Coco, primary dysmenorrhea is "so common that many women fail to report it in medical interviews, even when their daily activities are restricted." On the other hand, the women we interviewed do seem to suffer more severely than the ones in these other studies. This discrepancy could possibly be related to differences in the methodology used.

Furthermore, symptoms associated with menstruation are often subjectively and emotionally interpreted and may acquire varied meanings such as fear of being different from peers, concerns about being unwholesome, and anxiety about functioning as a normal woman (Comerci 1966). Such individual interpretations could lead to under-reporting of symptoms when data are collected via face-to-face interviews.

Finally, most of the respondents claim to adapt well to some monthly hindrance of their daily activity, which could explain why only 24% of Belgian women between 15 and 50 years old spontaneously assess their menstruation as painful.

Overall, the results of this survey on the characteristics of menstrual pain and how it is handled clearly reinforce currently available data that dysmenorrhea is a syndrome that seriously undermines the quality of life of the women affected, and thus requires a thorough therapeutic approach by health care professionals. The next phase of this study will explore in greater depth the individual variability of symptoms and their control.

REFERENCES

Balbi C, Musone R, Menditto A, et al. Influence of menstrual factors and dietary habits on menstrual pain in adolescence age. *Eur J Obstet Gynecol Reprod Biol* 2000; 91:143–148.

Coco AS. Primary dysmenorrhea. *Am Fam Physician* 1999; 60:489–496.

Comerci GD. Symptoms associated with menstruation. *Am J Obstet Gynecol* 1966; 95(7):991–996.

Correspondence to: Hugues D. Malonne, PhD, ULB-Campus Plaine, CP206-3, 1050 Brussels, Belgium. Email: hugues.malonne@ulb.ac.be.

Proceedings of the 10th World Congress on Pain,
Progress in Pain Research and Management, Vol. 24,
edited by Jonathan O. Dostrovsky, Daniel B. Carr, and
Martin Koltzenburg, IASP Press, Seattle, © 2003.

48

Pain in General Medical Patients: An Audit

Lucy Johnson, Anna Regaard, and Nina Herrington

Pain Relief Unit, King's College Hospital, London, United Kingdom

Published research suggests that general medical patients experience protracted intervals of intense pain (Bruster et al. 1994; Durieux et al. 2001). Acute pain, sleep and rest problems, stress, mood disturbances, and listlessness are common problems within this patient group (Lauri et al. 1997). While the incidence of major depression in medical inpatients is estimated to be between 5% and 10% (Silverstone et al. 1996), up to 41% may suffer with depressive symptoms (Crum et al. 1994; Creed et al. 2001), which nursing and medical staff are consistently poor at recognizing (Silverstone et al. 1996).

High levels of pain and depressive symptoms in older medical inpatients are considered strong indicators for significantly increased medical expenditure (Druss et al. 1999) and greater use of health care resources (Levenson et al. 1992; Steen et al. 2002). The growing proportion of the population over 65 years old in the United Kingdom poses serious implications for the planning of health care provision. However, evidence is scarce regarding the impact of pain on physical function and mood of hospitalized general medical patients, or concerning methods to reduce these symptoms and improve rehabilitation.

This chapter describes an audit of pain in general medical patients at our London teaching hospital where the pain team provides a service for adults and children with pain of all etiologies. An average of 158 inpatients are referred to the pain team each month. Of these, 75% are referred by surgical teams, 12% by medical specialties (e.g., diabetes, hematology, or liver), and 7% by general medical teams. Of the hospital's 950 beds, general medical patients occupy 330 beds.

STANDARD PAIN MANAGEMENT POLICY

The hospital has a seven-point pain management standard: (1) All patients should have no more than a minimal amount of pain (none to mild). (2) All patients should receive the appropriate type of analgesia specific to their type of pain. (3) All patients should receive an appropriate level of analgesia to meet their needs. (4) All patients should receive analgesia within an appropriate time frame to meet their needs. (5) No patient should be prevented from rehabilitation due to uncontrolled pain. (6) No patient should have a level of pain that impinges on his or her quality of life. (7) All patients should receive appropriate physical and behavioral therapy to meet their needs.

It was the impression of the pain team that the pain management of some medical inpatients did not meet our local standards and that these patients may find it difficult to rehabilitate and to achieve discharge criteria in a timely fashion.

OBJECTIVES

The objectives of this audit were to ascertain the prevalence of pain in general medical patients, to assess the hospital's performance regarding general medical patients with regard to local pain standards, to establish the level of mood disturbance associated with pain, and to recommend and implement changes to improve pain management for general medical patients and hence to expedite their hospital discharge.

METHODS

Two pilot studies were undertaken in an attempt to devise a survey questionnaire that would be easy to complete for this relatively elderly patient population. The final format of the questionnaire consisted of abridged elements of the Medical Outcomes Study 36-Item Short Form Questionnaire (SF-36; Ware and Sherbourne 1992), items adapted from the Brief Pain Inventory (Daut et al. 1983), and questions of our own composition.

All patients were asked whether they had experienced pain in the last week. Patients who had experienced pain were then asked 10 specific questions about their pain relating to location, intensity (on movement and rest), analgesia (timing and effect), limitation of activity, general well-being, emotional support, support with activities, and other comments. Data regarding demographics, diagnosis, use of allied medical professionals (e.g., physical therapy, occupational therapy, psychology, pain team) were also collected. Most questions were closed, although the patients and researchers could offer open-ended comments at the end of the survey.

A sample of 200 patients was sought to participate in the study. Data were collected from May to July 2002 and on "given days" all patients on the general medical wards were invited to participate. The questionnaires were administered by two of the authors (L. Johnson and A. Regaard) and were completed in their presence by each respondent. The questions were read to patients with visual impairment or reading difficulties. Standard explanations of the study purpose and instructions for completion of the questionnaire were given. This method of questionnaire administration has been suggested to improve response rate and is more easily completed by patients with poor vision, concentration, or reading and writing skills (Oppenheim 1992). An effort was made to eliminate cues that would lead respondents to answer in a particular way, as recommended by Robson (1995). The only exclusion criterion was profound confusion.

Clinical staff and managers responsible for general medical patients and the hospital's Clinical Effectiveness Department were involved from the outset. Patients were assured of anonymity and were identified by serial number only.

RESULTS

Data were collected from 200 patients. Participants' ages ranged from 24 to 97 years (mean = 70; median = 76 years). The main reasons for their hospital admissions were medical investigation or treatment (171 patients; 86%), rehabilitation (62 patients; 31%), and social problems such as inability to cope at home or homelessness (43 patients; 22%). Their main medical conditions were wide-ranging and involved falls (29 patients; 14.5%), respiratory disease (23 patients; 11.5%), and cardiovascular disease including cerebrovascular accidents (64 patients; 32%). Twelve patients (6%) were admitted for pain management.

Of the 200 patients, 126 (63%) had experienced pain during the last week and 74 (37%) had not. At rest, 25 patients (13%) had severe pain, 29 (15%) had moderate pain, 52 (25%) had mild pain, and 93 (46%) had none. During movement, 51 patients (25%) had severe pain, 47 (24%) had moderate pain, 21 (11%) had mild pain, and 79 (39%) had none.

Fig. 1 demonstrates the types of pain experienced compared with effectiveness of analgesia. Of those patients with pain, 31 (25%) had musculoskeletal or joint pain; pain relief was considered effective all or most of the

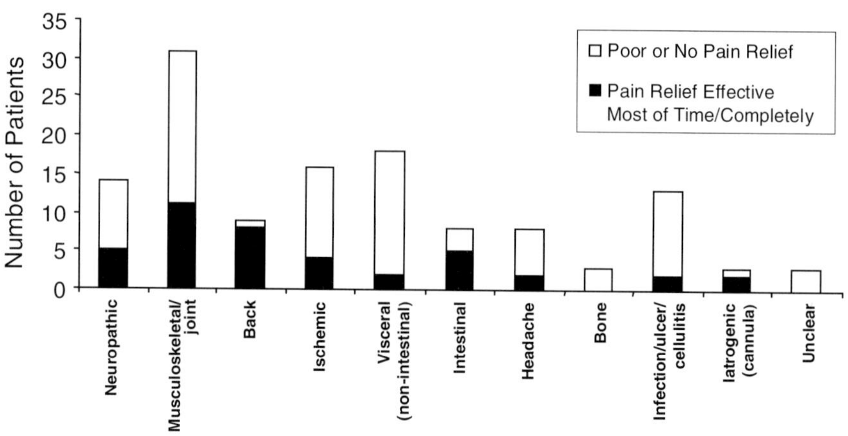

Fig. 1. Type of pain and effectiveness of pain relief.

time in 11 (35%) of these patients. Nine (29%) of these patients were not receiving their prescribed "as required" analgesic medication. Visceral pain due to hepatobiliary disease or colic occurred in 25 patients (20%); 47% of these patients indicated that their pain relief was effective all or most of the time. In 16 patients (13%) the main type of pain was ischemic, and half of these patients considered the pain to be well managed. Three of the patients with ischemic pain were not receiving their prescribed "as required" analgesia. Of the 14 patients (11%) with neuropathic pain, 36% considered their pain relief effective all or most of the time. Only three patients with neuropathic pain were prescribed antidepressant or anticonvulsant medication. Eight patients had headache, and six of these had poorly managed pain. Only one of them had received acetaminophen and codeine despite all being prescribed one or both drugs.

Of the patients who reported pain, analgesic medication was prescribed for 109 (87%), whilst 14 (11%) had no such prescription. Of patients who reported no pain, 42 (56%) were receiving analgesic medication. Fifty-three patients with pain (42%) were receiving analgesics according to a regular prescription, whilst two patients with pain were not receiving their regularly prescribed analgesics. Analgesics prescribed on an "as required" basis were being administered to 41 patients with pain (32%), but not to 32 patients (25%) who had received the same prescription.

For patients with pain, levels of physical function are shown in Fig. 2 and psychological indices are shown in Fig. 3. Verbal comments from the patients with pain emphasized the effect that pain was having on their life. Eleven patients (9%) said they were "fed up" or felt like giving up. One

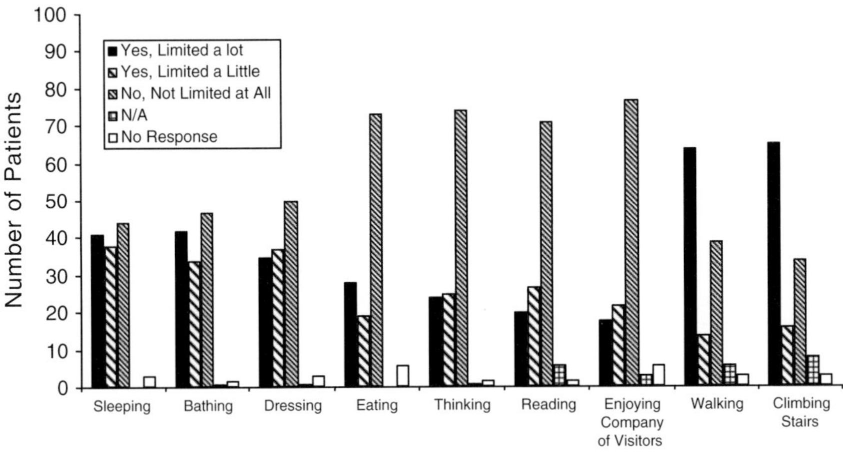

Fig. 2. Ways in which pain limits patients' activities.

patient clarified the reason as because someone took away the transcutaneous electrical nerve stimulation (TENS) machine that had been provided. One patient reported feeling too ill to think. Eight patients (6%) wrote that they were depressed or very miserable. One reported crying "because the pain killers don't help," one attributed low mood to being confined to bed for 5 months, and three complained of their lack of visitors. Eight patients (6%) made comments relating to anxiety. Anxiety was mainly attributed to housing problems or inability to cope at home. One patient expressed worry

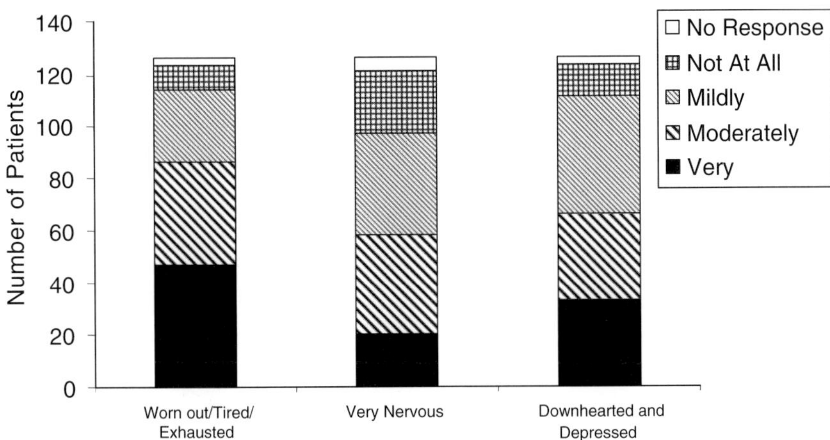

Fig. 3. General emotional status of patients.

about being a nuisance, one talked about being "scared of falling," and another claimed to have felt "paralyzed by fear."

Five patients commented that they felt well supported, while four felt unsupported. Of the latter, one patient with cancer said she had "messed the bed three times because nobody came" and another felt "nobody but God" was helping.

Three patients volunteered that they were satisfied with their pain management, saying they either felt "more relaxed than usual" or were "coping well." Ten patients (8%) said their pain killers did not help; one had not realized that it was possible to ask for analgesia "as required" and one patient, in desperation, had walked to the high street pharmacy for analgesia. In contrast, seven patients (5%) said they avoided "pain killers" because they did not like taking them. Justifications were fear of overdosing, constipation, a belief in learning to cope, and preference for homeopathy. Five patients voiced a wish to see the pain team.

Several of the patients with pain were noted either to have, or to comment upon, various long-term problems. Eight patients (6%) were physically disabled (three used wheelchairs, four were blind, and one was deaf). Of the blind patients, one also had learning difficulties and one, who spoke little English, verbalized her wish to die. Ten patients (8%) had profound psychological problems. Three patients had problems with substance misuse, and three were homeless.

Of the patients with pain, half were having regular physical therapy and a third were receiving occupational therapy. Of those receiving physiotherapy, occupational therapy, or both, 37 (60%) were greatly limited in both walking and climbing stairs. This was also the case for 27 (46%) of the patients who were not receiving physical or occupational therapy. Sleeping was limited greatly in a third of patients and not at all in another third. Eating was not limited for 60% of patients. Sleeping and eating appeared unaffected by physical or behavioral therapy. Of all the patients with pain, 77% (97) felt they were getting the support they needed with activities. This percentage increased to 89% (53) in those receiving physical therapy.

Eleven patients with pain (9%) were receiving formal behavioral support: counseling (4%), psychology (3%), and psychiatry (2%). Mood in those receiving such support was lower than the total population: 8 patients (73%) felt moderately or very worn out, tired, or exhausted; 8 (73%) felt moderately or very nervous; and 7 (63%) felt very downhearted or depressed. Of the total, 71% (89) felt they were getting the emotional support they needed. This percentage decreased to 64% (7) of the 11 receiving formal behavioral support.

Cancer was the main medical condition for 13 (7%) of the 200 patients. Six patients with cancer were experiencing pain, and four were managed by the palliative care team. In contrast, seven patients had no pain; palliative care team input had only been received by one of these patients. All cancer patients were receiving some analgesic medication (except for one of the patients with no pain), although three were not receiving either their regular or "as required" analgesia.

Twelve of the respondents (6%) had received consultation from the pain team; three also received TENS, and two had undergone neural blockade. A few patients were receiving care from a specialist clinical nurse or therapist (e.g., a dietician or behavioral therapist).

DISCUSSION

Our principal findings may be organized on a point by point basis to correspond with the hospital's pain management policy:

1) Overall, we found unacceptable levels of pain. The predominantly elderly respondents had a range of general medical conditions, with many suffering respiratory or cardiovascular disease or injuries from falls. Half of the patients experienced moderate or severe pain on movement and just less than a third experienced moderate or severe pain at rest. The data collection method may have biased the results because patients may have been reluctant to complain in front of the researcher. Further, it would have been beneficial to have recorded the number of patients who were excluded, because confused patients are particularly vulnerable to poor pain assessment and management.

2) Without detailed diagnoses and pain histories it is difficult to ascertain from our survey data whether analgesics given were specific for the type of pain. The most common types of pain were musculoskeletal and visceral; half to two thirds of such pain was poorly relieved. Ischemic pain and neuropathic pain were similarly poorly managed. Antineuralgic drugs were not usually prescribed for neuropathic pain. For headaches, suitable analgesics was prescribed but not given.

3) Pain control was acceptable for some, but unacceptable for other patients. Analgesics were prescribed for 120 respondents (60%), 42 of whom reported no pain. It could be assumed that the analgesic medication prescribed for these 42 patients was sufficient to render them pain-free. Indeed, Lauri et al. (1997) assert that three out of four medical patients suffer with acute pain. Actual pain levels and benefits of analgesia could have been determined more accurately if patients were asked whether they had pain

during the hospital stay or were taking analgesics on admission, and if the duration and dose of analgesics were recorded. Half of the patients with cancer had no pain, which may be attributed to high levels of analgesic prescription and administration, and to other forms of palliative care they were receiving.

4) Overall, patients did not receive analgesics when they needed them. Only 18 of the patients (9%) (17 with pain) had regular and "as required" analgesia both prescribed and administered. A quarter of patients with pain had not been given "as required" analgesic medication, and two had not received regularly scheduled analgesics even though these were prescribed. Failure to administer prescribed analgesics raises concerns, including nurses' competence in assessing pain. Findings of Delbanco et al. (1995) and Lauri et al. (1997) point to medical ward nurses' consistent underestimation of patients' needs and tardy response to pain. Furthermore, several respondents did not realize they had access to "as required" analgesics, or abstained due to misunderstandings about their analgesia. These misunderstandings could have limited their pain relief and might have been mitigated by better staff explanation. Poor communication, including lack of patient education and advice, has been highlighted as a major contributor to inadequate pain management in hospital patients (Bruster et al. 1994).

5) Rehabilitation was impaired due to inadequate pain management. Of the patients receiving physical therapy, 60% were significantly limited in walking and climbing stairs, which means that their pain impeded effective physical therapy.

6) Many patients with pain, including those receiving formal behavioral support, had profoundly impaired mood, with 68% feeling worn out, 52% feeling depressed, and 46% feeling nervous. Several patients volunteered that they were "fed up" or anxious, often due to social reasons. Mood, pain, fatigue, and insomnia have been demonstrated to be independent predictors of deterioration in patients' functioning (Given et al. 1994, 2001). Indeed, Bennett et al. (2002) found that pain and fatigue may be more important than medical conditions in determining whether older adults function independently. Furthermore, the presence of medical conditions in addition to these symptoms may make them perceive their function to be more limited than their performance demonstrates.

7) It is likely that patients were not receiving appropriate physical and emotional therapy to meet their needs. Whilst only a third to a half were receiving physical therapy and only 9% were receiving formal behavioral therapy, nearly three quarters of patients with pain felt they were receiving the physical and emotional support they needed. Patients tend to give high satisfaction ratings despite suboptimal clinical care (Bruster et al. 1994).

They generally underreport levels of distress and depression in clinical settings that preclude personal and emotional discussion (Peveler et al. 2002). Lack of referral to specialist therapists may be attributed to staff ineptitude in distinguishing symptoms of depression—such as sadness or loss of interest—from an appropriate response to normal life stress (Peveler et al. 2002).

RECOMMENDATIONS

Based upon our survey findings, we feel the major shortcomings identified in the assessment of pain and distress in hospitalized patients might be addressed by three broad actions:

1) Introduction of a multidisciplinary pain assessment tool.

2) Initiation of an educational program for all general medical health care professionals, involving pain assessment, analgesics appropriate for different types of pain, and accountability for monitoring and dispensing pain relievers and patient education materials.

3) Promotion of referral criteria to facilitate consultation with the pain team and counseling services, and regularly scheduled pain team rounds on the general medical wards.

Patient and clinician behavior is not generally altered simply by the provision of information. Thus, the success of these interventions should be monitored, and consideration given to the potential need for reinforcement of helpful behaviors and discouragement of unhelpful ones.

REFERENCES

Bennett J, Stewart A, Kayser-Jones J, Dale G. The mediating effect of pain and fatigue on level of functioning in older adults. *Nurs Res* 2002; 51(4):254–265.

Bruster S, Jarman B, Bosanquet N, et al. National survey of hospital patients. *BMJ* 1994; 309(6968):1542–1546.

Creed F, Morgan R, Fiddler M, et al. *Psychosomatics* 2001; 43(4):302–309.

Crum R, Cooper-Patrick L, Ford D. Depressive symptoms among general medical patients: prevalence and one year outcome. *Psychosom Med* 1994; 56(2):109–117.

Daut RL, Cleeland CS, Flanery RC. Development of the Wisconsin Brief Pain Questionnaire to assess pain in cancer and other diseases. *Pain* 1983; 17:197–210.

Delbanco TL, Stokes DM, Cleary PD, et al. Medical patients' assessments of their care during hospitalisation: insights for internists. *J Gen Intern Med* 1995; 10(12):679–685.

Druss B, Rohrbaugh R, Rosenheck R. Depressive symptoms and healthcare costs in older medical patients. *Am J Psychiatry* 1999; 156(3):477–479.

Durieux P, Bruxelle J, Savignoni A, Coste J. Prevalence and management of pain in a hospital: a cross-sectional study. *Presse Medicale* 2001; 30(12):572–576.

Given B, Given C, Stommel M. The impact of age, treatment, and symptoms on the physical and mental health of cancer patients: a longitudinal perspective. *Cancer Suppl* 1994; 74:2128–2138.

Given B, Given C, Azzouz F, Stommel M. Physical functioning of elderly cancer patients prior to diagnosis and following initial treatment. *Nursing Res* 2001; 50(4):222–232.

Lauri S, Lepisto M, Kappeli S. Patients' needs in hospital: nurses' and patients' views. *J Adv Nurs* 1997; 25(2):339–346.

Levenson J, Hamer R, Rossiter L. Psychopathology and pain in medical inpatients predict resource use during hospitalisation but not rehospitalisation. *J Psychosom Res* 1992; 36(6):585–592.

Oppenheim A. *Questionnaire Design, Interviewing and Attitude.* London: Pinter, 1992.

Peveler R, Carson A, Rodin G. Depression in medical patients. *BMJ* 2002; 325(7356):149–152.

Robson C. *Real World Research.* Oxford: Blackwell, 1995.

Silverstone P, Lemay T, Elliot J, Hsu V, Starko R. The prevalence of major depressive disorder and low self esteem in medical inpatients. *Can J Psychiatry* 1996; 41(2):65–66.

Steen H, Fink P, Frydenberg M, Oxhoj M. Use of health services, mental illness, and self-rated disability and health in medical inpatients. *Psychosom Med* 2002; 64(4):668–675.

Ware J, Sherbourne C. The SF-36 short-form health status survey 1, conceptual framework and item selection. *Med Care* 1992; 30:473–483.

Correspondence to: Lucy Johnson, MSc, Pain Relief Unit, King's College Hospital, Denmark Hill, London SE5 9RS, United Kingdom. Email: Lucy.Johnson@kingsch.nhs.uk.

Part VIII

Pain Assessment: Quantitative and Qualitative

Proceedings of the 10th World Congress on Pain,
Progress in Pain Research and Management, Vol. 24,
edited by Jonathan O. Dostrovsky, Daniel B. Carr, and
Martin Koltzenburg, IASP Press, Seattle, © 2003.

49

Quantitative Sensory Testing: Clinical Considerations and New Methods[1]

Richard H. Gracely,[a] Eli Eliav,[b] and Per Hansson[c]

[a]Departments of Medicine/Rheumatology and Neurology, University of Michigan Health System and Veterans Affairs Medical Center, Ann Arbor, Michigan, USA; [b]Oral Sensory Changes, Department of Oral Diagnosis, Oral Medicine and Radiology, Hadassah School of Dental Medicine, Jerusalem, Israel; [c]Department of Surgical Sciences, Section of Clinical Pain Research and Neurogenic Pain Unit, Multidisciplinary Pain Center, and Department of Rehabilitation Medicine, Karolinska Institute/Hospital, Stockholm, Sweden

Quantitative sensory testing (QST) refers to a set of methods that extend the traditional neurological examination of sensory function. QST uses psychophysical procedures and an array of stimulus modalities to assess the functional capacity of primary afferent fibers as well as to gain information about spinal processing and the sensory projection system. The general approach to the assessment of primary afferent function is shown in Table I, which describes tests for the large-diameter, thickly myelinated Aβ fibers that under normal conditions mediate nonpainful tactile sensations, and for the thinly myelinated Aδ and unmyelinated C fibers that mediate both painful and nonpainful sensations.

Reviews of these methods emphasize that considerable information can be gained by verbal reports and simple bedside tests that use minimal equipment (Gracely et al. 1996). This chapter describes important clinical considerations for the use of QST in the evaluation of neuropathic pain arising from nerve injury, and illustrates a new method for QST that uses electrical stimuli to identify inflammatory processes that are accompanied by minimal, if any, mechanical injury.

---

[1] Based on a Congress workshop.

Table I
Quantitative sensory testing (QST) of primary afferent function

Aβ Fibers	Aδ Fibers	C Fibers
Myelination		
Thick	Thin	None
Tests		
Stroking	Cold threshold	Warm threshold
Gauze	Pinprick*	Painful heat
Brush	Painful heat	Slow ramp in hairy skin
Cotton applicator	Electrical pain threshold	Glabrous skin pain threshold
Calibrated monofilament		Suppressed Aδ fibers†
Vibration		Pressure pain threshold
Tuning fork		
Vibrameter		
Electrical detection threshold		

* Pricking pain threshold in hairy, nonfacial skin.
† In hairy skin first exposed to painful heat to suppress Aδ nociceptors.

CLINICAL ASPECTS OF SOMATOSENSORY EXAMINATION IN NEUROPATHIC PAIN

A comprehensive examination of patients with neuropathic pain should assess sensory, motor, and autonomic signs to confirm or reject the suspected anatomical site of the lesion as inferred from a careful history. Because nociception is mediated by the somatosensory system, the diagnosis of painful neuropathy rests heavily on the demonstration of sensory abnormalities in the area corresponding to the territory of the damaged nerve, plexus, root, or central pathway. A careful bedside examination of somatosensory functions using an array of simple instruments (a paintbrush for the sensation of touch, a warm and cold object, and a pin) to explore the entire spectrum range of fibers and pathways is a crucial starting strategy because sensory aberrations may be confined to single or few modalities (Hansson 1994). To avoid a chaotic exploration of somatosensory function a tentative diagnosis should guide the sensory examination. Therefore, the sensory examination should optimally be performed at the end of the diagnostic work-up when information collected up to that point has been evaluated. The bedside examination generally offers a sufficient basis for adequate diagnosis and clinical management. The array of sensory aberrations found in patients with neuropathic pain includes hypo- and hyperesthesia as well as qualitative and spatiotemporal alterations, all equally important to evaluate (Table II) (Hansson and Kinnman 1996). Because the distribution of sensory abnormalities matches the territory innervated by the damaged nervous structure, the borders of the area of sensory dysfunction should be carefully

Table II
Common sensory abnormalities in neuropathic pain

Quantitative	Qualitative	Spatial	Temporal
Hypoesthesia	Allodynia	Dyslocalization	Aftersensation
Hyperesthesia	Dysesthesia	Extraterritorial spread	Abnormal latency
Hypoalgesia	Paresthesia	Radiation	
Hyperalgesia			

identified using different modalities (Hansson et al. 2001). If the examination is started within the area of dysfunction and is directed toward the normal surrounding area, the area of abnormality will appear larger than when testing from outside in. The reason for this discrepancy is the inherent reaction time to perception and subsequent verbal communication. In clinical practice we recommend going from the inside out to explore an area of sensory deficit and from the outside in to explore a territory with positive sensory phenomena, such as mechanical or thermal allodynia or hyperalgesia. The latter technique will minimize the duration of painful stimulation during the examination.

From detailed studies in patients with central pain due to stroke or multiple sclerosis, the common denominator regarding signs on somatosensory examination seems to be involvement of the spino- (or trigemino) thalamocortical system resulting in altered sensibility to temperature and/or noxious stimuli (Leijon et al. 1989; Osterberg et al. 1994; Boivie 1999). The painful condition seems to be unrelated to alterations in other somatosensory pathways or motor systems. No common anatomical denominator has been identified in peripheral neuropathic pain states.

Extraterritorial spread of pain and/or sensory dysfunction, as a symptom or sign of central sensitization or disinhibition, should be accepted only after carefully excluding non-neurological conditions such as musculoskeletal pain. This phenomenon exists only occasionally, and usually evolves after a period of proper distribution of symptoms and signs, and may in some cases also be interpreted as individual variations in the innervation territories of nerves or roots (Tal and Bennett 1994; Sotgiu and Biella 1995; Lacerenza et al. 1996). The extent of extraterritorial spread may vary over time and is difficult to distinguish from psychogenic amplification.

To further explore somatosensory function, psychophysical QST techniques may be added to standard clinical neurophysiological methods, which fall short in demonstrating pathology of the small-fiber system as well as positive phenomena such as dynamic mechanical allodynia (Hansson 1994). QST techniques provide modality-specific, graded assessment of both deficits and positive phenomena in terms of altered perception threshold and/or the stimulus-response relationship of different somatosensory modalities (Hansson and Lindblom 1993). For each stimulus mode there is a variety of increasingly complex test procedures. The type and number of tests to be applied must be chosen with due consideration of both the duration and discomfort of testing, and their appropriateness for each patient. The most common somatosensory modalities examined clinically when pain due to neuropathy is suspected are touch, vibration, and temperature, the latter including noxious heat and cold. Techniques to quantify such modalities include von Frey filaments, vibrometry, and Peltier element-based heating and cooling devices for assessment of the four different thermal percepts (warmth, coolness, heat pain, and cold pain) (Hansson and Lindblom 1993). Detection of an abnormality may be made based upon historical comparison with standard control values, although concurrent comparison to a contralateral unaffected site, when available, may be the best approach (Kemler et al. 2000).

Importantly, signs of sensory aberrations are not equivalent to neuropathy. Sensory alterations were originally described in the context of neuropathic pain, but recent findings have indicated that subgroups of patients with nociceptive pain, e.g., musculoskeletal pain, may report similar but transitory and variable sensory disturbances, including a distribution that lacks distinct borders, in the painful area and/or in remote sites of referred symptoms (Leffler et al. 2000a,b). On somatosensory examination, specific findings are characteristic of true neuropathic conditions in that modality profile and distinct borders of abnormalities are reproducible during one examination (with the exception of dynamic mechanical allodynia; see above). The physiological basis for the abnormal somatosensory findings in nociceptive pain states is unknown, but the phenomenon clearly indicates that the presence of sensory abnormalities in pain states is not pathognomonic for neuropathic pain. In addition, patients with psychogenic pain conditions, such as conversion hysteria, frequently report sensory abnormalities, indicating prominent interactions between the psyche and the soma. Again, the crucial part of the sensory examination in such cases is to titrate carefully the distribution of the sensory abnormalities using bedside tools in an effort to evaluate a suspected neuroanatomical locus deduced from the history. Given that sensory alterations are not restricted to neuropathic pain states, the outcome of sensory examinations, especially in the hands of clinicians lacking experience in detailed sensory examination, may be confusion and possible diagnostic error.

In summary, the diagnosis of peripheral or central neuropathic pain should be made only when the history and signs indicate neuropathy in conjunction with a neuroanatomically correlated distribution of pain characteristics and sensory abnormalities. Although its role in everyday clinical diagnostic work is limited, QST eventually may become a powerful tool to unravel pathophysiological mechanisms underlying a specific pain condition. A prerequisite for such a possibility is extensive and meticulous collaboration between preclinical and clinical scientists and practitioners, to link specific somatosensory signs and mechanisms. Such information is crucial in developing a mechanism-based classification and appropriate treatment of pain.

ELECTRICAL DETECTION THRESHOLDS IDENTIFY CLINICAL INFLAMMATION

A new QST method uses detection of nonpainful sensations evoked by electrical stimuli as a measure of neural inflammation. This method is based on the concept that inflammatory processes invade the sheaths of nerves in passage and that the resulting neuritis is associated with increased mechanical sensitivity at the distal terminus of the nerve in the target tissue (Eliav and Gracely 1998; Eliav et al. 1999, 2001). Studies in animals indicate that an inflammatory milieu produced by an experimental neuritis leads to behavioral signs of increased sensitivity to stimulation of Aβ mechanoreceptors, and physical evidence at the light microscopic level of endoneuronal infiltration of granulocytes and other leukocytes accompanied by minimal or no neural degeneration (Eliav et al. 1999).

The clinical application of neuritis-induced mechanical sensitivity has been validated in an oral surgery model (Eliav and Gracely 1998). Postsurgical inflammation peaks 2 days after surgery (Troullos et al. 1990), and the inflammation associated with extraction of a lower third molar tooth occurs in the vicinity of the inferior alveolar and lingual nerves. Patients scheduled for an extraction of a lower-third molar were evaluated by QST examination before, and 2 and 8 days after, the extraction. The sensory tests were performed in the nerve target organs (anterior two-thirds of the tongue for the lingual nerve, lower lip and chin for the inferior alveolar nerve) and in a control site (below the eye, in the infraorbital nerve territory). In the inferior alveolar and lingual nerve territories there was increased sensitivity to mechanical and electrical stimulation 2 days after surgery that returned to normal 8 days after surgery. There were no changes in thermal sensitivity (cold, warm, heat pain) at these locations and no changes of any kind at the control site below the eye. A subsequent study replicated this effect and also observed that preoperative treatment with 8 mg dexamethasone reduced signs of inflammation and blocked the hypersensitivity effect, while acetaminophen, a commonly used analgesic with minimal anti-inflammatory properties, had no effect on the postoperative increase in mechanical and electrical sensitivity (R. Baron et al., unpublished observations).

Under normal conditions, detection of light touch evoked by a nylon filament or similar tactile stimulus is mediated by the large-diameter, rapidly conducting Aβ mechanoceptors. The involvement of these Aβ afferents in the increased mechanical sensitivity is confirmed by the concomitant increased sensitivity to electrical stimuli, which at detection levels bypass the mechanoceptor (and any receptor processes such as suppression or sensitization) to directly activate the axons of the Aβ primary afferents. The lack of any effect on extensive thermal testing suggests that the sensitivity of smaller primary afferent fibers, the thinly myelinated Aδ and unmyelinated C fibers, is not altered by the neural inflammation.

USE OF ELECTRICAL DETECTION IN TEMPOROMANDIBULAR DIAGNOSIS

Pain in the temporomandibular region can be derived from a muscular problem, articular problem (internal derangements or inflammatory process within the joint), or combined pathology, and the appropriate diagnosis can be difficult. The signs and symptoms of temporomandibular disorder (TMD) include jaw and facial pain, limited mouth opening, changes in jaw relationship, a variety of joint sounds, and degenerative changes in the joint itself. The most common complaint is pain accompanied by difficulty in opening the mouth wide and made worse by any activity requiring significant jaw movement (Griffith 1983; Stegenga et al. 1989; Bell 1990; Fricton 1991; Mohl and Dixon 1994; Okeson 1996; Sharav 1999; Greene 2001; Svensson 2001). It is useful to divide TMDs into broad categories of articular or masticatory muscle disorders. Articular disorders (arthralgias) are a group of conditions arising from and causing pain in the joint, including internal derangements, osteoarthritis, and inflammatory joint disease. Masticatory muscle disorders are characterized by pain arising from the surrounding muscles (myalgia, myofascial pain). TMDs can be subclassified as functional disorders of the muscles, pathology of the joint, or a combination (Eversole and Machado 1985; Benoliel and Sharav 1998). Primary pain in the joint or muscle may also lead to secondary changes in another site that becomes a further source of pain and functional impairment (Parker 1990; Okeson 1996; Benoliel and Sharav 1998; Sharav 1999).

An inflammatory process in the joint usually accompanies articular disorders, whereas the etiology of masticatory muscle pain is not considered to involve inflammation (Reid et al. 1994; Stegenga 2001). The auriculotemporal branch of the trigeminal nerve innervates both the joint and the overlying skin (Last 1978). In the presence of an inflammatory process within the joint, the nerve may develop neuritis. It is possible to assess the degree of inflammation within the joint by means of QST on the skin overlying the joint.

Teich and colleagues (2001) performed extensive sensory testing in 72 patients with painful TMD in three trigeminal nerve sites: auriculotemporal (AUT), buccal (BUC), and mental (MNT). Detection threshold ratios were calculated by dividing the electrical threshold on the affected side by that on the control side; thus, ratios of less than 1 indicate hypersensitivity of the affected side. The results are shown in Fig. 1. In 10 control subjects these ratios did not vary significantly from the expected value of 1. In 44 patients diagnosed with arthralgia by a second clinician, the mean ratio obtained for the AUT territory (0.63) was significantly lower than those for the MNT (1.02) and BUC (0.96) territories ($P < 0.0001$ for both comparisons) and significantly lower ($P < 0.0001$) compared to the AUT ratios in subjects

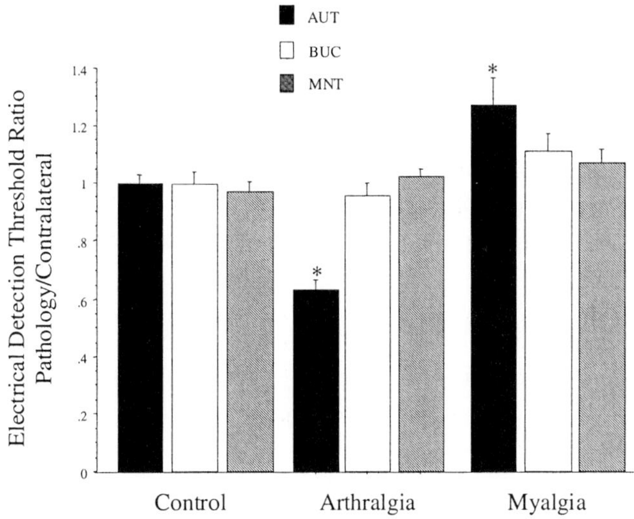

Fig. 1. Electrical detection threshold ratios (pathology detection threshold divided by contralateral detection threshold) are presented for the arthralgia and myalgia patients and for the control group. The sensory tests were assessed in three nerve sites: auriculotemporal (AUT), buccal (BUC), and mental (MNT). The electrical detection threshold ratios in the AUT territory were significantly lower in arthralgia patients than in those with myalgia or in the control group. In the myalgia group the electrical detection threshold ratio in the AUT territory was significantly higher than in the other groups, but not significantly different from other sites within the group (mean ± SEM: AUT territory, arthralgia patients: 0.633 ± 0.031, myalgia patients: 1.355 ± 0.109, control subjects: 1.001 ± 0.088, ANOVA $F_{2,79} = 33.533$, $P < 0.0001$). No significant differences in detection threshold ratios were detected in the BUC and MNT nerve territories.

with myalgia (1.27) or controls (1). The elevated electrical detection threshold ratio within the AUT territory of the myalgia group was also significantly greater than that of control subjects (Dunnett test, $P < 0.05$).

NORMALIZATION AFTER TREATMENT FOR INFLAMMATION

Joint lavage was performed in 10 arthralgia patients suffering from severe pain and with limited mouth opening. Following the procedure, the mean electrical detection threshold ratio in the AUT territory was significantly elevated from 0.64 to 0.99, indicating resolution of the hypersensitivity (paired t test: $P < 0.001$). This normalization suggests that the joint lavage ameliorated the inflammatory environment (Nitzan et al. 1991), reducing nerve inflammation and sensory changes.

These preliminary data lead to three conclusions: (1) large myelinated fiber hypersensitivity is found in the skin overlying painful TMDs with clinical pathology but is not found in controls or in patients with muscle-related facial pain. This hypersensitivity is not unique to the skin overlying an orofacial joint, having been observed also for osteoarthritis of the hand (Farrell et al. 2000). (2) Cutaneous hypersensitivity associated with underlying joint inflammation is abolished after treatment of the joint inflammation. (3) The opposite effect of large-fiber hyposensitivity was observed for patients with tonic muscular pain, consistent with recent observations of bilaterally elevated monofilament pressure detection thresholds to unilateral muscle pain and suggesting involvement of central mechanisms (Stohler et al. 2001).

SENSORY CHANGES AND ORAL MALIGNANCIES

The inflammatory milieu produced by malignant processes (Anneroth et al. 1986) infects the trunks of nerves passing through this environment. This neural involvement results in both pain and altered sensory function in the target organs of the nerve, such as the trigeminal nerve territory (Burt et al. 1992; Lossos et al. 1992; Bar Ziv and Slasky 1997; Portenoy and Lesage 1999; Shotts et al. 1999).

The use of electrical detection thresholds to identify neuritis induced by malignant processes was evaluated in 23 patients referred to the maxillofacial surgery department, Barzilai Medical Center, Ashkelon, Israel, and the Department of Oral Diagnosis, Oral Medicine, and Radiology, Hadassah School of Dental Medicine, Jerusalem, Israel, for the evaluation of oral lesions (Eliav et al. 2002). All lesions were classified as within, near, or outside the tested nerve territory. The sensitivity of Aβ primary afferents was assessed by the determination of electrical detection thresholds bilaterally at regions innervated by the three peripheral branches of the trigeminal nerve. Electrical detection threshold ratios between the affected and unaffected side were correlated with the results of physical examination, radiographic imaging, and biopsy. Biopsy showed that the lesions in 10 of these 12 patients with asymmetrical thresholds were malignant. No malignancy was found in the remaining 11 patients. Fig. 2 shows that in all cases in which biopsy confirmed malignancy, the electrical detection threshold in the affected nerve was lowered by 20% or more compared to the contralateral side (mean ratio: 0.61 for nerves with a lesion within their territory, 0.78 for nerves with lesions near their territory, and 1.01 for nerves with no lesion in their territory). Two cases gave false-positive results. In the first case the ratio was 0.37, and biopsy revealed some atypical cells but no malignant lesion. In the second case the ratio in the nerve territory was 0.62, and the biopsy revealed solar keratosis. The ratio for electrical detection threshold of nerves that were near but not in the region of the lesions was reduced by at least 20% in 5 of the 10 malignant lesions, suggesting an extraterritorial effect due to central sensitization (Tal and Bennett 1994; Chacur et al. 2001). In contrast, the detection thresholds for nerves in the territory of benign lesions did not differ from those in the contralateral side (mean ratio: 0.96 for nerves with

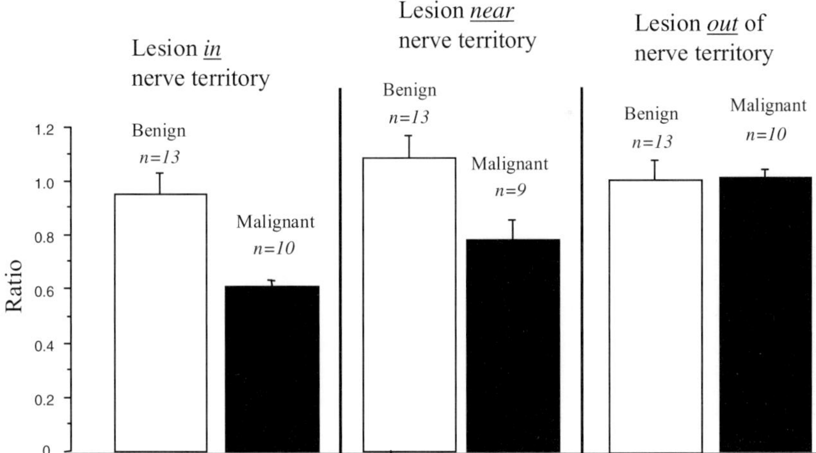

Fig. 2. Electrical detection threshold ratios according to location of lesion in benign and malignant conditions. The results are presented as the ratio of detection thresholds on the side of the lesion divided by the detection ratio on the contralateral side. Ten lesions were diagnosed as malignant by biopsy. In all cases in which malignancy was confirmed, the electrical detection threshold in the affected nerve was lowered by 20% or more compared to the contralateral side (mean ± SEM: 0.607 ± 0.025 for lesion in the nerve territory, 0.781 ± 0.072 for lesion near the nerve territory, and 1.012 ± 0.032 for lesion outside the nerve territory).

lesions in their territory, 1.09 for nerves with lesions near their territory, and 1.01 for nerves with no lesions in their territory).

These results suggest that psychophysical detection of Aβ primary afferent hypersensitivity is a sensitive and specific indicator of soft tissue malignancy located along the course of the nerve and that this method may aid in early detection of malignancies.

CURRENT STATUS OF QST

While studies of the efferent, motor nervous system rely on the measurement of physical movement and movement-related activity, studies of the afferent, sensory nervous system must rely on subjective descriptions of experience. QST provides a systematic analysis of sensory function. The information obtained by such testing aids diagnosis and promises to be increasingly useful for the disparate goals of individual clinical decision making (diagnosis, choice of treatment, monitoring treatment efficacy, medicolegal evaluation) and basic investigations of underlying mechanisms. The present utility of QST is limited by insufficient knowledge of mechanisms and by the paucity of available treatments. Its utility will increase in parallel with our understanding of the mechanisms that initiate and maintain chronic pain conditions. Similarly, the utility of QST for guiding choice of treatment and monitoring treatment efficacy will increase once there are more specific and efficacious treatments from which to choose.

REFERENCES

Anneroth G, Hansen LS, Silverman Jr. S. Malignancy grading in oral squamous cell carcinoma. I. Squamous cell carcinoma of the tongue and floor of the mouth: histologic grading in clinical evaluation. *J Oral Pathol* 1986; 15:162–168.

Bar-Ziv J, Slasky BS. CT imaging of mental nerve neuropathy: the numb chin syndrome. *Am J Roentgenol* 1997; 168:371–376.

Bell WE. *Temporomandibular Disorders, Classification, Diagnosis and Management,* 3rd ed. Chicago: Yearbook, 1990, pp 299–301.

Benoliel R, Sharav Y. Craniofacial pain of myofascial origin: temporomandibular pain and tension-type headache. *Compendium* 1998; 19:701–722.

Boivie J. Central pain. In: Wall PD, Melzack R (Eds). *Textbook of Pain.* Edinburgh: Churchill Livingstone, 1999, pp 879–914.

Burt RK, Sharfman WH, Karp BL, Wilson WH. Mental neuropathy (numb chin syndrome): a harbinger of tumor progression or relapse. *Cancer* 1992; 70:877–881.

Chacur M, Milligan ED, Gazda LS, et al. A new model of sciatic inflammatory neuritis (SIN): induction of unilateral and bilateral mechanical allodynia following acute unilateral perisciatic immune activation in rats. *Pain* 2001; 94:231–244.

Eliav E, Gracely RH. Sensory changes in the territory of the lingual and inferior alveolar nerves following lower third molar extraction. *Pain* 1998; 77:191–199.

Eliav E, Herzberg U, Ruda MA, Bennett GJ. Neuropathic pain from an experimental neuritis of the rat sciatic nerve. *Pain* 1999; 83:169–182.

Eliav E, Benoliel R, Tal M. Inflammation with no axonal damage of the rat saphenous nerve trunk induces ectopic discharge and mechanosensitivity in myelinated axons. *Neurosci Lett* 2001; 311:49–52.

Eliav E, Teich S, Benoliel R, et al. Large myelinated nerve fiber hypersensitivity in oral malignancy. *Oral Surg Oral Med Oral Pathol Oral Radiol Endod* 2002; 94:45–50.

Eversole LR, Machado L. Temporomandibular joint internal derangement and associate neuromuscular disorders. *J Am Dent Assoc* 1985; 110:69–75.

Farrell MJ, Gibson SJ, McMeeken JM, Helme RD. Increased movement pain in osteoarthritis of the hands is associated with Aβ mediated cutaneous mechanical sensitivity. *J Pain* 2000; 1(3):229–242.

Fricton JR. Clinical care for myofascial pain. *Dent Clin North Am* 1991; 122:25–32.

Gracely RH, Price DD, Roberts WJ, Bennett GJ. Quantitative sensory testing in patients with CRPS-I and II. In: Jänig W, Stanton-Hicks M (Eds). *Reflex Sympathetic Dystrophy—A Reappraisal,* Progress in Pain Research and Management, Vol. 6. Seattle: IASP Press, 1996, pp 151–172.

Greene CS. The etiology of temporomandibular disorders: implication for treatment. *J Orofac Pain* 2001; 15:93–105.

Griffith RH. Report of the president's conference on examination, diagnosis and management of temporomandibular disorders. *J Am Dent Assoc* 1983; 106:75–77.

Hansson P. Possibilities and potential pitfalls of combined bedside and quantitative somatosensory analysis in pain patients. In: Boivie J, Hansson P, Lindblom U (Eds). *Touch, Temperature, and Pain in Health and Disease: Mechanisms and Assessments*, Progress in Pain Research and Management, Vol. 3. Seattle: IASP Press, 1994, pp 113–132.

Hansson P, Kinnman E. Unmasking of neuropathic pain mechanisms in a clinical perspective. *Pain Rev* 1996, 3:272–292.

Hansson P, Lindblom U. Assessment of somatosensory dysfunction in neuropathic pain. *Pain Digest* 1993, 3:36–42.

Hansson P, Lacerenza M, Marchettini P. Aspects of clinical and experimental neuropathic pain: the clinical perspective. In: Hansson PT, Fields HL, Hill RG, Marchettini P (Eds). *Neuropathic Pain: Pathophysiology and Treatment*, Progress in Pain Research and Management, Vol. 21. Seattle: IASP Press, 2001, pp 1–18.

Kemler MA, Schouten HJA, Gracely RH. Diagnosing sensory abnormalities with either normal values or from contralateral skin: comparison of two approaches in Complex Regional Pain Syndrome I. *Anesthesiology* 2000; 93:18–27.

Lacerenza M, Marchettini P, Formaglio F, et al. Extra-territorial mechanical hyperalgesia in patients with proven nerve damage involves adjacent undamaged nerves. *Abstracts: 8th World Congress on Pain.* Seattle: IASP Press, 1996, p 37.

Last RJ. *Anatomy Regional and Applied,* 6th ed. Edinburgh: Churchill Livingstone, 1978, pp 392–446.

Leffler AS, Kosek E, Hansson P. The influence of pain intensity on somatosensory perception in patients suffering from subacute/chronic lateral epicondylalgia. *Eur J Pain* 2000a; 4:57–71.

Leffler AS, Kosek E, Hansson P. Injection of hypertonic saline into musculus infraspinatus resulted in referred pain and sensory disturbances in the ipsilateral upper arm. *Eur J Pain* 2000b; 4:73–82.

Leijon G, Boivie J, Johansson I. Central post-stroke pain—neurological symptoms and pain characteristics. *Pain* 1989; 36:13–25.

Lossos A, Siegal T. Numb chin syndrome in cancer patients: etiology, response to treatment and prognostic significance. *Neurology* 1992; 42:1181–1884.

Mohl ND, Dixon DC. Current status of diagnostic procedures for temporomandibular disorders. *J Am Dent Assoc* 1994; 125:56–64.

Okeson JP. *Orofacial Pain, Guidelines for Assessment, Diagnosis and Management.* Quintessence, 1996, pp 113–158.

Osterberg A, Boivie J, Holmgren H, Thuomas K-Å, Johansson I. The clinical characteristics and sensory abnormalities of patients with central pain caused by multiple sclerosis. In: Gebhart GF, Hammond DL, Jensen TS (Eds). *Proceedings of the 7th World Congress on Pain,* Progress in Pain Research and Management, Vol. 2. Seattle: IASP Press, 1994, pp 789–796.

Parker MW. A dynamic model of etiology in temporomandibular disorders. *J Am Dent Assoc* 1990; 120:283–289.

Portenoy RK, Lesage P. Management of cancer pain. *Lancet* 1999; 353:1695–1700.

Reid KI, Gracely RH, Dubner RA. The influence of time, facial side and location on pain-pressure thresholds in chronic myogenous temporomandibular disorders. *J Orofac Pain* 1994; 8:258–265.

Sharav Y. Orofacial pain. In: Wall PD, Melzack R (Eds). *Textbook of Pain,* 4th ed. London: Churchill Livingstone, 1999, pp 711–738.

Shotts RH, Porter SR, Kumar N, Scully C. Longstanding trigeminal sensory neuropathy of nontraumatic cause. *Oral Surg Oral Med Oral Pathol Oral Radiol Endod* 1999; 87:572–576.

Sotgiu ML, Biella G. Spinal expansion of saphenous afferents after sciatic nerve constriction. *Neuroreport* 1995, 6:2305–2308.

Stegenga B. Osteoarthritis of the temporomandibular joint organ and its relationship to disc displacement. *J Orofac Pain* 2001; 15:193–205.

Stegenga B, De Bont LG, Boering G. A proposed classification of temporomandibular disorders based on synovial joint pathology. *Cranio* 1989; 7(2):107–118.

Stohler SS, Kowalski CJ, Lund JP. Muscle pain inhibits cutaneous touch perception *Pain* 2001; 92:327–333.

Svensson P, Graven-Nielsen T. Craniofacial muscle pain: review of mechanisms and clinical manifestations. *J Orofac Pain* 2001; 15:117–142.

Tal M, Bennett GJ. Extra-territorial pain in rats with a peripheral mononeuropathy: mechano-hyperalgesia and mechano-allodynia in the territory of an uninjured nerve. *Pain* 1994; 57:375–382.

Teich S, Benoliel R, Eliav E. Neurophysiologic parameters in the diagnosis of TMD pathologies. *Abstracts: Annual Meeting of the Israel Pain Association.* Israel, 2001.

Troullos ES, Hargraves KM, Butler DP, Dionne RA. Comparison of non-steroidal anti-inflammatory drugs, ibuprofen and flurbiprofen, with methylprednisolone and placebo for acute pain, swelling, and trismus. *J Oral Maxillofac Surg* 1990; 48:945–952.

Correspondence to: Richard H. Gracely, PhD, Department of Medicine, Division of Rheumatology, University of Michigan, 7B19 300 North Engals, Ann Arbor, MI 48109, USA. Tel: 734-763-0907; Fax: 734-615-5467; email: rgracely@umich.edu.

Proceedings of the 10th World Congress on Pain,
Progress in Pain Research and Management, Vol. 24,
edited by Jonathan O. Dostrovsky, Daniel B. Carr, and
Martin Koltzenburg, IASP Press, Seattle, © 2003.

50

What Decline in Pain Intensity Is Meaningful to Patients with Acute Pain?

M. Soledad Cepeda,[a] Juan M. Africano,[a]
Rodolfo Polo,[a] Ramiro Alcala,[a] and Daniel B. Carr[b]

[a]Department of Anesthesia, San Ignacio Hospital and Javeriana University School of Medicine, Bogota, Colombia; [b]Departments of Anesthesia and Medicine, Tufts-New England Medical Center and Tufts University School of Medicine, Boston, Massachusetts, USA

The most salient (Turk and Melzack 2001) and most commonly reported (Carr et al. 2002) dimension of the experience of pain is its intensity. The 0–10 verbal numeric rating scale (NRS) and the 0–10 visual analogue scale (VAS) of pain intensity are commonly used for this purpose. However, little is known about the significance from the patient's point of view of changes in the NRS or VAS.

To establish the clinical significance of any change in a symptom scale score, it is necessary to compare it with a change in a global measure of improvement (Jaeschke et al. 1989). In pain studies, a key global measure of improvement is the degree of pain relief reported by the patient. In order to determine the meaning of a decrease in pain intensity, one must ask the patient to report pain intensity on two or more occasions, and also to indicate the pain relief experienced from the first to the second time (Max et al. 1991). In this context, a decline in pain intensity may be considered to be clinically meaningful to patients if it leads them to report "much," "very much," or "complete" pain relief as opposed to "none" or "minimal" pain relief.

Efforts have been made to determine the clinical meaning of a decrease in the NRS or VAS in children and adults. In a small study of children with acute pain (N = 73), the "minimal" decline in VAS rating discernible to patients was found to be 10 mm on a 0–100 mm scale (Powell et al. 2001). Two other studies have evaluated, respectively, the meaning of changes in pain intensity in adult patients with cancer pain (Farrar et al. 2000) or adults with chronic noncancer pain (Farrar et al. 2001). These latter two studies were retrospective analyses of randomized controlled trials (RCTs) that had not been designed for the purpose of determining the clinical meaning of a decrease in pain intensity, and hence are susceptible to measurement error. We have identified no studies to date that evaluate the meaning of changes in the NRS in an adult population with acute postoperative pain. The clinical meaning of a change in the NRS in patients with cancer pain or chronic noncancer pain may differ from that in patients with acute pain (Carr et al. 1992) because the latter two types of pain have distinct effects on coping abilities and mood (Jacox et al. 1994; Turk and Flor 1999), and thereby may influence patients' interpretation of decrements in pain intensity.

The proportion of subjects with specific percentage reductions in pain intensity is increasingly employed as a measure of treatment efficacy. For example, the threshold of a 50% decline in the NRS or VAS is used to dichotomize outcomes of pain treatment so as to calculate the number-needed-to-treat (NNT) in meta-analyses of RCTs (Moore et al. 1996, 1997a,b). Although a 50% decline in pain intensity correlates well with other measures of pain intensity and pain relief (Moore et al. 1996, 1997a,b), the clinical meaning to patients of specific percentage reductions in pain intensity in patients with acute pain is unknown.

This chapter describes a study intended to characterize the clinical meaning of absolute and relative (i.e., percentage) declines in the NRS in patients with acute postoperative pain during initial treatment in the post-anesthesia care unit (PACU).

METHODS

This study was approved by the Institutional Review Board of San Ignacio Hospital. We enrolled 720 patients, all of whom completed the study. According to the hospital's standard of care for patients admitted to the PACU after surgical procedures, patients were asked to rate their baseline pain on a 0–10 NRS (0, "no pain"; 10, "worst pain imaginable"). We recruited patients with pain intensity greater than 4/10 on the NRS and asked them to describe their pain intensity on a four-point verbal rating scale (VRS) as "none," "mild," "moderate," or "severe." After initial pain assessment, all patients received intravenous opioids. To guide ongoing analgesic titration, patients rated their pain intensity on the NRS every 10 minutes, at which times they also indicated the degree of pain relief on a five-point Likert scale (PRLS). The choices on the PRLS were "no improvement," "minimal improvement," "much improvement," "very much improvement," or "complete pain relief." According to the standard of care in the institution, all patients received analgesics until their pain intensity was 4 or less on the NRS.

The opioids employed for customary treatment of postoperative pain were morphine, hydromorphone, or fentanyl. Patients younger than 65 years received a loading dose of 2.5 mg of morphine; the dose for hydromorphone was 0.5 mg, and that for fentanyl was 25 µg. For patients aged 65 years or older, each loading dose was decreased by 40%. To assess and compare the doses of these three opioids we converted them into equipotent doses of morphine. We considered 1 mg of parenteral morphine equivalent to 0.2 mg of parenteral hydromorphone and to 0.01 mg of parenteral fentanyl (Janssen 1984; Carr et al. 1992; Woodhouse et al. 1999).

STATISTICAL METHODS

For the analysis of continuous variables, we estimated means and standard deviations. For discrete variables, we calculated percentages. We used box plots to present the distribution of the changes in NRS values and percentage pain reduction according to pain relief category.

To determine the decrement in the NRS that corresponded to each category of pain relief on the PRLS, we used a linear regression model. For this purpose we estimated the decline from baseline pain intensity at each subsequent assessment. We included the baseline VRS (moderate or severe pain), and the interaction between the VRS and three categories of the PRLS (minimal, much, and very much improvement) in the model. We did not include the "complete" pain relief category of the PRLS in our statistical model because few patients experienced complete pain relief. In the regression model, the dependent variable was the difference in the pain intensity, and the independent variables were the categories of the PRLS, the categories of VRS, and the interaction terms.

Each patient had multiple pain evaluations (until the NRS reached 4/10 or less), and these measures were not independent. To take this lack of independence into consideration, we employed an analysis of repeated measures using generalized estimating equations (GEE) to adjust the standard errors (White 1982; Zeger et al. 1988).

To determine the meaning of a percentage pain reduction in the NRS and the impact of baseline VRS and NRS values upon the meaning of a percentage pain reduction, we followed a procedure similar to that described above. We calculated the percentage of reduction in NRS pain intensity from baseline as 100*([baseline NRS – subsequent NRS]/baseline NRS).

P values less than 0.05 were considered significant. 95% confidence intervals (CI) were also estimated. All statistical calculations were performed with STATA statistical software, version 7.0 SE.

RESULTS

The characteristics of the subjects included in the study, the intensity of their baseline pain, the type of opioid and dose received, and the percentages of patients with each category of pain relief are listed in Table I.

In terms of baseline pain intensity, we found that a median value of 6 on the NRS corresponded to moderate pain on the VRS, and a median value of 8 on the NRS corresponded to severe pain on the VRS.

Table I
Characteristics of the subjects included in the study, intensity of baseline pain, type of opioid and dose received, and degree of pain relief

Number of patients	720
Mean number of observations per patient	5
Age	
Mean (years) ± SD	40.9 ± 15.1
Range (years)	16–88
Percentage of women	62.2
Weight (kg) ± SD	65.2 ± 11.8
Baseline pain intensity	
Patients with moderate pain (%)	43.7
Patients with severe pain (%)	56.3
Etiologic factor	
Surgical pain (%)	96.9
Trauma pain (%)	3.1
Type of analgesic	
Morphine (%)	93.4
Hydromorphone (%)	6.2
Fentanyl (%)	0.4
Average cumulative morphine equivalent dose per patient (mg) ± SD (see Methods for calculation of morphine equivalents)	5.1 ± 3.1
Range of cumulative morphine equivalent doses per patient (mg)	1.5–17.5
Pain relief	
Much improvement (%)	55.7
Very much improvement (%)	40.8
Complete pain relief (%)	3.5

MEANING OF AN ABSOLUTE CHANGE IN THE NRS

Exploratory analysis showed that larger absolute declines in the NRS correspond to greater degrees of patient-reported pain relief on the PRLS (data not shown). Linear regression analysis reveals that when baseline pain is severe, larger changes ($P = 0.001$) in the NRS are necessary to achieve similar degrees of pain relief to when baseline pain is moderate. The interactions between pain relief and baseline pain intensity are statistically significant ($P = 0.001$ for both). Thus, when baseline pain is severe, even larger decreases in the NRS are required for "much" or "very much" improvement than those necessary to obtain "minimal" improvement. The meaning of changes in the NRS according to baseline pain intensity can be seen in Table II.

MEANING OF A PERCENTAGE CHANGE IN THE NRS

Exploratory analysis showed that greater percentage reductions in pain intensity occur with greater magnitudes of patient-reported pain relief (Fig. 1).

Linear regression analysis showed that the percentage reduction in the NRS necessary for patients to discern "minimal" improvement is similar for baseline pain of moderate or severe intensity ($P = 0.5$). However, the interactions between pain relief and baseline pain are statistically significant ($P =$ 0001 for both). In other words, when baseline pain is severe, greater percentage pain reductions are necessary to obtain "much" or "very much" improvement than those necessary to produce "minimal" improvement. The meaning of percentage pain reductions stratified according to baseline pain intensity can be seen in Table II.

Table II
Meaning to patients of absolute and percentage declines in pain intensity on the 0–10 numeric rating scale (NRS), for patients having moderate or severe baseline pain

	Moderate Baseline Pain		Severe Baseline Pain	
	Change in NRS	Change in NRS (%)	Change in NRS	Change in NRS (%)
Minimal improvement	1.3 (1.2–1.4)	20.1 (18.1–22.2)	1.8 (1.7–1.9)	20.3 (19.0–21.6)
Much improvement	2.4 (2.2–2.6)	34.7 (32.7–36.8)	4.0 (3.9–4.1)	44.4 (43.2–45.6)
Very much improvement	3.5 (3.3–3.8)	45.0 (43.1–46.8)	5.2 (5–5.4)	56.1 (53.9–58.4)

Note: Numbers in parentheses denote 95% confidence intervals.

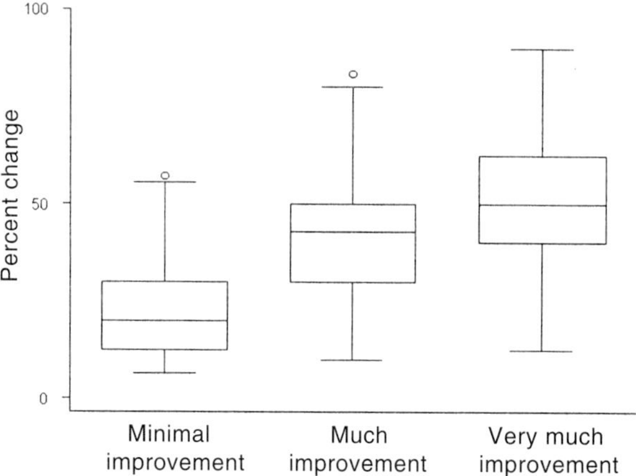

Fig. 1. Box plots of percentage changes in the 0–10 numerical rating scale of pain intensity (NRS) corresponding to three categories of patient-rated pain relief. The three diagrams illustrate the percentage changes in the NRS pain score corresponding to each of three patient-reported categories of pain relief. The horizontal line in the middle of each box represents the median. The lower and upper edges of the box represent the 25th and 75th percentiles, respectively, and the interior of the box is the interquartile range (IQR). The lines extending upwards and downwards from the box are "whiskers" that extend to the next highest or lowest adjacent values. The upper adjacent value is the data point less than or equal to the percentile 75 + 1.5*IQR. The lower adjacent value is the smallest data point greater or equal to the percentile 25 – 1.5*IQR. Observed points more extreme than the adjacent values are plotted as circles. Larger changes in the NRS pain score occur with increasing degrees of pain relief.

DISCUSSION

Pain evaluation is a crucial step toward adequate control of acute postoperative pain (Carr et al. 1992; Carr and Goudas 1999). An understanding of the meaning of changes in the NRS or percentage pain reduction is indispensable to appreciating the impact of pain treatment from the patient's point of view. We found that in patients with acute pain, the meanings of absolute changes as well as percentage reductions in the NRS depend upon baseline pain intensity.

In children, the equivalent of a one-unit decrement in the NRS has been reported as the threshold for clinical significance (Powell et al. 2001). Our study in adults supports this finding: we found that a change of 1.3 units on the NRS is the threshold for minimal pain relief when the baseline pain intensity is moderate. However, the authors of the pediatric study did not evaluate the effect of baseline pain intensity upon the meaning of changes in pain intensity. We found in adults that when baseline pain is severe, the minimum clinically significant decrease in the NRS is 1.8 units.

Although it is important to identify the minimal change in the NRS that is discernible to patients, identification of this threshold is only one part of characterizing the response to analgesics. We found that a decline in the NRS must be 2.4 units or more to be identified with "much" improvement in patients whose baseline pain is "moderate" on the VRS. Other researchers have reported similar results for patients with cancer pain, but baseline pain intensity was not considered in their analysis (Farrar et al. 2000). We found that if baseline pain is "severe" on the VRS, the change in the NRS must be 4.0 units for patients to experience "much" improvement. Farrar et al. (2001), in a study of patients with chronic noncancer pain, considered the effect of baseline pain intensity and found, as did we, that the meaning of a change in the NRS depends upon initial pain intensity.

It is not surprising that the relationships between decrements in pain intensity and corresponding degrees of patient-reported pain relief vary according to initial pain intensity. Lasagna, in a classic paper (1962), found that initial pain intensity was a predictor of pain relief after morphine administration. Patients with more intense initial pain were less likely to experience complete pain relief.

As for the clinical meaning of percentage pain reduction, we found that independent of baseline pain severity, the minimum discernible change in the NRS (i.e., identified by patients as barely "minimal" improvement on the PRLS) is 20%. The American College of Rheumatologists (ACR) has defined improvement as a 20% decrease in pain; pain alleviation is one of five core parameters used to decide treatment effectiveness (Felson et al. 1995, 1998). In the present study, to achieve greater than "minimal" pain relief the percentage reduction must be 35% if baseline pain is "moderate" or 44% if it is "severe." Recent studies in patients with chronic noncancer and cancer pain that employed somewhat different methodologies found that a 30–33% decline in VAS was judged to be clinically important by patients (Farrar et al. 2000, 2001). The Oxford Pain Research Group uses a cutoff of 50% to dichotomize pain intensity outcomes in their calculation of NNTs within meta-analyses of RCTs (Moore et al. 1996). Our present results suggest that this cutoff may be too stringent.

In summary, the declines in the NRS that patients judge to be meaningful, as determined from their PRLS reports of "much" or "very much" pain relief, depend upon the severity of baseline pain. For moderate baseline pain, a decrease of 2.4 units (35%) on the NRS is required for clinically meaningful pain relief. Patients with severe initial pain require larger decreases in the NRS and greater percentage pain reductions to obtain corresponding degrees of pain relief. The findings of this study support and extend other emerging research designed to help clinicians and researchers interpret patient-based estimates of pain treatment efficacy. The present findings are applicable in the clinical setting to refine pain treatment algorithms, and in the research arena to interpret treatment efficacy.

ACKNOWLEDGMENT

Supported in part by the Department of Anesthesia, San Ignacio Hospital, Javeriana University School of Medicine; by Colciencias; and by the Saltonstall and Armington Funds for Pain Research. Grünenthal-Colombia provided support for the research nurses who collected patient data.

REFERENCES

Carr DB, Goudas LC. Acute pain. *Lancet* 1999; 353:2051–2058.

Carr DB, Jacox AK, Chapman CR, et al. *Acute Pain Management: Operative or Medical Procedures and Trauma.* Clinical Practice Guideline. AHCPR Publication No. 92-0032. Rockville, MD: Agency for Health Care Policy and Research, 1992.

Carr DB, Goudas L, Lawrence D, et al. *Management of Cancer Symptoms: Pain, Depression and Fatigue.* Evidence Report/Technology Assessment No. 61. AHRQ Publication No. 02-E032. Rockville, MD: Agency for Healthcare Research and Quality, 2002.

Farrar JT, Portenoy RK, Berlin JA, Kinman JL, Strom BL. Defining the clinically important difference in pain outcome measures. *Pain* 2000; 88:287–294.

Farrar JT, Young JP, LaMoreaux L, Werth JL, Poole RM. Clinical importance of changes in chronic pain intensity measured on an 11-point numerical pain rating scale. *Pain* 2001; 94:149–158.

Felson DT, Anderson JJ, Boers M, et al. American College of Rheumatology. Preliminary definition of improvement in rheumatoid arthritis. *Arthritis Rheum* 1995; 38:727–735.

Felson DT, Anderson JJ, Lange ML, Wells G, LaValley MP. Should improvement in rheumatoid arthritis clinical trials be defined as fifty percent or seventy percent improvement in core set measures, rather than twenty percent? *Arthritis Rheum* 1998; 41:1564–1570.

Jacox AK, Carr DB, Payne R, et al. *Management of Cancer Pain.* Clinical Practice Guideline No. 9. Rockville, MD: Agency for Health Care Policy and Research, 1994.

Jaeschke R, Singer J, Guyatt GH. Measurement of health status. Ascertaining the minimal clinically important difference. *Control Clin Trials* 1989; 10:407–415.

Janssen PA. The development of new synthetic narcotics. In: Estafanous FG (Ed). *Opioids in Anesthesia.* Boston: Butterworth, 1984, pp 37–44.

Lasagna L. The psychophysics of clinical pain. *Lancet* 1962; 2:572–575.

Max MB, Laska EM. Single-dose analgesic comparisons. In: Max MB, Portenoy RK, Laska EM (Eds). *The Design of Analgesic Clinical Trials.* New York: Raven Press, 1991, pp 55–96.

Moore A, McQuay H, Gavaghan D. Deriving dichotomous outcome measures from continuous data in randomised controlled trials of analgesics. *Pain* 1996; 66:229–237.

Moore A, Moore O, McQuay H, Gavaghan D. Deriving dichotomous outcome measures from continuous data in randomised controlled trials of analgesics: use of pain intensity and visual analogue scales. *Pain* 1997a; 69:311–315.

Moore A, McQuay H, Gavaghan D. Deriving dichotomous outcome measures from continuous data in randomised controlled trials of analgesics: verification from independent data. *Pain* 1997b; 69:127–130.

Powell CV, Kelly AM, Williams A. Determining the minimum clinically significant difference in visual analog pain score for children. *Ann Emerg Med* 2001; 37:28–31.

Turk DC, Flor H. Chronic pain: a biobehavioral perspective. In: Gatchel RJ, Turk DC (Eds). *Psychosocial Factors in Pain: Critical Perspectives.* New York: Guilford Press, 1999, pp 18–34.

Turk DC, Melzack R. The measurement of pain and the assessment of people experiencing pain. In: Turk DC, Melzack R (Eds). *Handbook of Pain Assessment,* 2nd ed. New York: Guilford Press, 2001, pp 3–11.

White H. Maximum likelihood estimation of misspecified models. *Econometrica* 1982; 50:1–25.

Woodhouse A, Ward ME, Mather LE. Intra-subject variability in post-operative patient-controlled analgesia (PCA): is the patient equally satisfied with morphine, pethidine and fentanyl? *Pain* 1999; 80:545–553.

Zeger SL, Liang KY, Albert PS. Models for longitudinal data: a generalized estimating equation approach. *Biometrics* 1988; 44:1049–1060.

Correspondence to: Daniel B. Carr, MD, Saltonstall Professor of Pain Research, Department of Anesthesia, #298, Tufts-New England Medical Center, 750 Washington Street, Boston, MA 02111, USA. Tel: 617-636-9710; Fax: 617-636-9709; email: daniel.carr@tufts.edu.

Proceedings of the 10th World Congress on Pain,
Progress in Pain Research and Management, Vol. 24,
edited by Jonathan O. Dostrovsky, Daniel B. Carr, and
Martin Koltzenburg, IASP Press, Seattle, © 2003.

51

Should We Measure Depression, Anxiety, and Anger as Distinct Mood States in Chronic Pain Patients?

Stephen J. Gibson,[a,b,c] Kathryn Garland,[a] Pauline Gardner,[a] Carolyn Arnold,[a] and George Mendelson[a]

[a]*Caulfield Pain Management and Research Centre, Caulfield, Victoria, Australia;* [b]*National Ageing Research Institute, Parkville, Victoria, Australia;* [c]*Department of Medicine, University of Melbourne, Parkville, Victoria, Australia*

Mood disturbance is common in chronic pain. Within multidisciplinary pain management programs it is now routine clinical practice to assess the levels of depression and anxiety as well as other mood states, such as fear, anger, and frustration. Depression and anxiety are usually conceptualized as distinct entities (Izard 1977; McNair et al. 1981; Schulz et al. 1994), although there is a very high concurrence of anxious and depressive disorders within clinical populations (Mountjoy and Roth 1982; Zimmerman et al. 2002). Moreover, strong correlations (>0.6) between self-rated measures of anxiety and depression have been consistently noted, and there is considerable symptom overlap between these constructs (Tanaka-Matsumi and Kameoka 1986; Watson and Clark 1992; Castern et al. 1995; Lovibond and Lovibond 1995; Gibson 1997). An alternative theoretical model of the phenomenological dimensions of mood emphasizes the concept of positive-negative emotion or generalized affective distress, particularly when dealing with populations that lack underlying psychiatric disease (Watson and Tellegen 1985; Schulz et al. 1994). However, the adequacy of this conceptual model for the study of mood disturbance in patients with chronic pain has yet to be fully examined.

Nelson and Novy (1997) documented a high degree of convergence in symptom presentation when using the Beck Depression Inventory (BDI) and the Spielberger State-Trait Anxiety Inventory (STAI) in patients attending a multidisciplinary pain management clinic. While it was possible to distinguish between different dimensions of anxiety and symptoms of depression, several items were misclassified or showed substantial cross-loadings on more than one dimension of mood. A second-order factor analysis also yielded only one primary construct, namely, negative affect. These findings raise important questions about the underlying structure of mood and the discriminative validity of standard psychometric measures when used in patients with chronic pain. However, it remains unclear whether such problems reflect imperfect psychometric measures (BDI, STAI) or a more fundamental issue with the phenomenological clarity of specific mood states. The other major concern with current research is the reliance on comparing measures of depression and anxiety to the exclusion of other mood states. If the notion of general affective distress is a more parsimonious characterization of mood disturbance in patients with chronic pain, then one might expect other mood states, such as anger or frustration, to display a similar convergence in symptom presentation. We are not aware of any previous attempts to investigate this issue in chronic pain patients. This chapter describes a study designed to examine the underlying dimensions of mood state and the extent to which different psychometric measures of depression, anxiety, and anger covary. Two different pain management clinics were studied as an indication that the findings could be generalized across different psychometric measures and across different samples of chronic pain patients.

METHODS

A convenience sample of 456 patients (mean age ± standard deviation = 45.9 + 14.7 years, 57% female) completed several different psychometric measures of depression, anxiety, and anger on admission to the Caulfield Pain Management and Research Centre, Melbourne, Australia. All patients completed the questionnaires by themselves at a special interview session prior to having the standard clinical assessment by the multidisciplinary team. Depression was measured using the 20-item Zung Self-Rating Depression Scale (ZDS, Zung 1965), the 21-item Beck Depression Inventory (BDI, Beck et al 1996) and a 10-cm visual analogue scale (VAS) of depressed mood anchored with "not at all depressed" at the extreme left and "very depressed" at the extreme right. Anxiety was monitored using the State-Trait Anxiety Inventory (STAI), which comprises two 20-item scales designed to assess transient (state) and more stable (trait) symptoms of anxiety (Spielberger 1983). All participants also completed a 10-cm VAS ranging from "not anxious" to "very anxious." Feelings of anger and hostility were assessed using three separate VAS scales. Participants were asked to place a mark on a 10-cm line spanning "not angry" to "very angry." A similar procedure was used for feelings of frustration and irritability. All measures have demonstrated reliability and validity for use with chronic pain patients.

A second sample of 469 older patients (mean age ± standard deviation = 72.5 + 10.1 years, 69% female) attending the Melbourne Extended Care/National Ageing Research Institute (MECRS/NARI) Geriatric Pain Centre also completed a battery of psychometric measures on admission. The 30-item Geriatric Depression Scale (Yesavage et al. 1983) and the depression subscale of the Profile of Mood States (POMS) questionnaire (McNair et al. 1981) were used to assess symptoms of depression. Anxiety was measured on the STAI and the POMS tension subscale, while anger was monitored via the POMS anger subscale and on a 10-cm VAS, anchored with "not at all angry" at the left extreme and "very angry" at the right. All measures have been shown to be valid and reliable for use in older chronic pain patients (Gibson 1997; Gibson and Helme 2000). The size of print was enlarged to make it easier for the older adults to read. All patients completed the questionnaires by themselves, although a research nurse was available to provide assistance if required.

RESULTS

A scatterplot of the BDI and STAI (state version) scores in the Caulfield sample is presented in Fig. 1 as an illustrative example of the very tight relationship between differing constructs of mood. Univariate Pearson correlations between the various psychometric measures of depression, anxiety, and anger are shown in Table I for the Caulfield sample and in Table II for the geriatric chronic pain patients. As might be expected, highly significant ($P < 0.0001$) correlations were observed between complementary measures of depression, as well as between common measures of anxiety or anger, regardless of which sample was examined. Perhaps more surprising is the extremely high degree of association between measures of putatively different mood states. The magnitude of relationship was at least comparable and often exceeded the relationship between complementary measures of the same construct (see Tables I and II). For instance, the maximum correlation for like measures of anxiety was 0.721, whereas the correlation between the STAI trait version and the Zung depression score was 0.782 (see Table I). Similarly, the correlation between psychometric measures of anger was 0.482, yet the POMS anger subscale correlated 0.710 with the POMS depression score (see Table II). In general, the absolute magnitude of correlation was

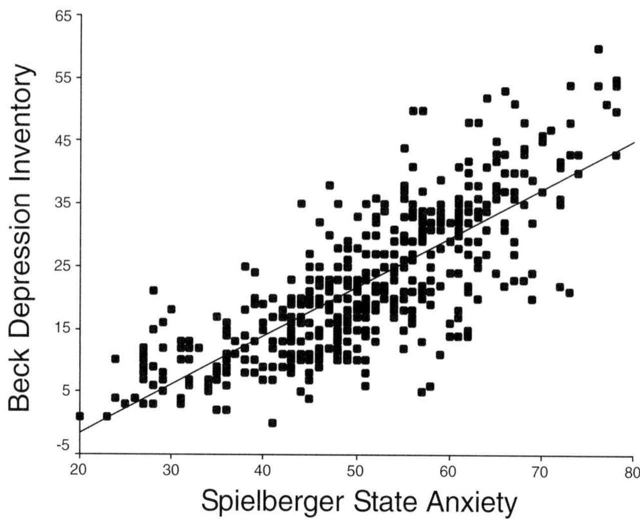

Fig. 1. Scatterplot of the relationship between the Beck Depression Inventory and the Spielberger State-Trait Anxiety Inventory (state version) in chronic pain patients attending the Caulfield Pain Management and Research Centre.

somewhat lower between VAS scales than for multi-item questionnaires of the same construct.

An iterative principal components analysis (PCA) was applied to the 9 × 9 intermeasure correlation matrix taken from the entire Caulfield sample. The Kaiser criterion of the number of eigenvalues greater than 1.0, an examination of the scree plot, and the percentage of variance accounted for by each factor (>5% of total variance) all suggested a simple one-factor solution, accounting for 73.65% of the variance in patient scores across all measures. Given that only one factor was extracted, the solution could not be rotated. The factor loadings of the different measures all exceeded 0.75, thereby emphasizing a single homogeneous dimension of mood being monitored by the nine different psychometric questionnaires. The highest factor loadings were found for the STAI trait version (0.856), the VAS for depression (0.838), and the BDI (0.816). A similar PCA undertaken on the 7 × 7 intermeasure correlation matrix from the MECRS/NARI geriatric sample also revealed one underlying factor of general mood state as the most parsimonious solution. This solution incorporated all measures of depression, anxiety, and anger, accounting for more than 83% of the variance in patient scores. Substantial factor loadings in excess of 0.88 were found for all measures, with the highest loadings being for the STAI trait anxiety score (0.948) and the POMS depression subscale (0.931).

Table I
Pearson correlations between different measures of mood in chronic pain patients attending the Caulfield Pain Management and Research Centre ($n = 456$)

	BDI	VAS-dep	STAI-state	STAI-trait	VAS-anx	VAS-ang	VAS-irrit	VAS-frust
ZDS	.765*	.591*	.766*	.782*	.540*	.517*	.547*	.544*
BDI		.581*	.761*	.722*	.497*	.536*	.557*	.518*
VAS-dep			.595*	.557*	.687*	.702*	.711*	.727*
STAI-state				.721*	.580*	.492*	.528*	.514*
STAI-trait					.590*	.597*	.587*	.568*
VAS-anx						.653*	.656*	..694*
VAS-ang							.694*	.653*
VAS-irrit								.698*

Abbreviations: BDI = Beck Depression Inventory; STAI = State-Trait Anxiety Inventory; VAS-ang = visual analogue scale for anger; VAS-anx = VAS for anxiety; VAS-frust = VAS for frustration; VAS-irrit = VAS for irritability; VAS-dep = VAS for depression; ZDS = Zung Self-Rating Depression Scale. Asterisks (*) denote statistical significance ($P < 0.0001$).

DISCUSSION

The present findings demonstrate a strong association between psychometric measures of different mood states in patients suffering from chronic pain. Indeed, there is a remarkable degree of concordance between self-rated depression, anxiety, and anger, regardless of the type of measurement scale used to monitor these constructs. The magnitude of correlation between different mood states was at least comparable and often exceeded the relationship between complementary measures of the same construct. Moreover, a PCA

Table II
Pearson correlations between psychometric measures of mood in older chronic pain patients attending the MECRS/NARI Pain Management Centre ($n = 469$)

	POMS-dep	STAI-state	STAI-trait	POMS-anx	POMS-ang	VAS-ang
GDS	.799*	.762*	.753*	.742*	.499*	.594*
POMS-dep		.721*	.835*	.779*	.710*	.602*
STAI-state			.795*	.712*	.556*	.456*
STAI-trait				.788*	.573*	.472*
POMS-anx					.601*	.521*
POMS-ang						.482*

Abbreviations: GDS = Geriatric Depression Scale; MECRS/NARI = Melbourne Extended Care/National Ageing Research Institute; POMS-ang = Profile of Mood States for anger; POMS-anx = Profile of Mood States for anxiety; STAI = State-Trait Anxiety Inventory; VAS-ang = visual analogue scale for anger. Asterisks (*) denote statistical significance ($P < 0.0001$).

of the several different psychometric measures of anger, depression, and anxiety confirmed only one underlying dimension of mood. This analysis is consistent with previous reports of the frequent convergence in symptoms of depression and anxiety (Tanaka-Matsumi and Kameoka 1986; Watson and Clark 1992; Lovibond and Lovibond 1995; Zimmerman et al. 2002) and extends this observation to include measures of anger. On the basis of these findings, it seems likely that many of the mood symptoms as described by chronic pain patients may be best understood as a type of generalized affective distress.

In explaining the high degree of association between measures, one can consider the extent of overlap in symptom content between the various psychometric questionnaires. For instance, items such as, "blue," "feel like crying," "can't put disappointments behind me," and "wish I could be as happy as others," taken from the STAI, might be considered by some as more appropriate symptoms of depressed affect. In a similar fashion, items including "irritable" and "restless" from the ZDS and "agitation" and "irritability" from the BDI share a considerable conceptual overlap with other measures of anxiety and anger. To some extent this overlap reflects a taxonomic problem because symptoms of restlessness and irritability are included in the diagnostic criteria for both generalized anxiety disorder and major depression. However, symptom overlap does not offer a full explanation for the strong association between measures, which persists even after elimination of the shared item content (Clark and Watson 1992). Moreover, while the magnitude of correlation was generally higher between multi-item questionnaires, VAS ratings of depression, anxiety, and anger also displayed significant interscale correlations, often in excess of 0.6 or 0.7. VAS measures have no shared item content or apparent conceptual overlap and are usually considered as simple, quantitative, unidimensional measures of a specified mood state.

A common cause of differing negative mood states, including depression, anxiety, and anger may reside in the environmental situation faced by the individual patient (Lovibond and Lovibond 1995). Dealing with a persistent pain complaint may have wide-ranging psychological impacts. It has been argued that the longer pain persists, the greater is the chance that the individual will become withdrawn, anxious, and depressed. Anger, frustration, and irritability also may result as the individual tries and fails with a variety of medical and alternative treatments. Individual patients are known to differ widely in the extent of pain impact on mood, yet it is not unreasonable to expect that a disturbance in any one aspect of mood will be accompanied by concomitant change in other negative mood states. Another potential reason for the strong association is that certain cognitive schema are common to the generation of different mood states. Catastrophic thinking has been documented as a frequent cognitive appraisal in many patients with chronic pain, particularly when conventional medical treatments have failed (Keefe et al. 2001). Catastrophizing represents a nonspecific subjective distress that incorporates elements of helplessness, fear, and low self-efficacy in response to ongoing demands (Turner and Aaron 2001). These elements have been identified as important cognitive components of depressed affect, anxiety, and anger (Beck et al. 1979), which may help account for at least some of the shared variance between differing mood states. This view also reinforces the likelihood of a nonspecific mood disturbance or general affective distress in patients with chronic pain and may provide a clear cognitive basis for the strong underlying relationship between measures of depression, anxiety, and anger.

Overall, there appears to be an almost inseparable concordance between self-rated measures of depression, anxiety, and anger in patients with chronic pain, regardless of the type of sample or measurement instrument used to monitor these constructs. This wide-ranging and pervasive mood disturbance might be best characterized as a type of generalized affective distress rather than as separate diagnostic entities of specific psychopathological states. In addition, one may question the need to monitor individual mood states. Perhaps some composite measure of affective distress might better represent the emotional suffering seen in patients with unremitting, bothersome pain. However, it should be acknowledged that the present study only examined the relationship between total psychometric scores and not individual symptoms of depression, anxiety, and anger. Previous item-based analyses of psychometric measures of depression and anxiety have yielded separate, identifiable constructs and even subdimensions of anxiety and depressive affect (Lovibond and Lovibond 1995, Nelson and Novy 1997). Future work should investigate whether similar findings can be obtained with an item-level analysis of anger scales considered together with measures of depression and anxiety. Such work should ultimately lead to a more comprehensive understanding of the nature and phenomenology of emotional suffering experienced by patients with chronic pain.

REFERENCES

Beck AT, Rush AJ, Shaw BF, Emery G. *Cognitive Therapy.* New York: Guilford Press, 1979.

Beck AT, Steer RA, Brown GK. *Beck Depression Inventory,* 2nd ed. San Antonio, TX: Psychological Corporation, 1996.

Castern RJ, Parmelee PA, Kleban MH, Powel-Lawton M, Katz IR. The relationships among anxiety, depression, pain in a geriatric institutionalised sample. *Pain* 1995; 61:271–276.

Gibson SJ. The measurement of mood states in older adults. *J Gerontol B Psychol Sci Soc Sci* 1997; 52B:167–174.

Gibson SJ, Helme RD. Cognitive factors and the experience of pain and suffering in older persons. *Pain* 2000; 85:375–383.

Izard CE. *Human Emotions*. New York: Plenum Press, 1977.

Keefe FJ, Lumley M, Anderson T, Lynch T, Carson KL. Pain and emotion: new research directions. *J Clin Psychol* 2001; 57:587–607.

Lovibond PF, Lovibond SH. The structure of negative emotional states: comparison of the depression anxiety stress scales (DASS) with the Beck depression and anxiety inventories. *Behav Res Ther* 1995; 33:335–343.

McNair DM, Lorr M, Droppelmann LF. Edits manual: *Profile of Mood States*. San Diego, CA: Educational and Industrial Testing Service, 1981.

Mountjoy CQ, Roth M. Studies in the relationship between depressive disorders and anxiety states. *J Affect Disord* 1982; 4:127–147.

Nelson DV, Novy DM. Self-report differentiation of anxiety and depression in chronic pain. *J Pers Assess* 1997; 69:392–407.

Schulz R, O'Brien AT, Tompkins CA. The measurement of affect in the elderly. *Annu Rev Gerontol Geriatr* 1994; 14:210–233.

Spielberger CD. *Manual for the State-Trait Anxiety Inventory*. Palo Alto, CA: Consulting Psychologists Press, 1983.

Tanaka-Matsumi J, Kameoka VA. Reliabilities and concurrent validities of popular self-report measures of depression, anxiety and social desirability. *J Consult Clin Psychol* 1986; 54:328–333.

Turner JA, LA. Pain-related catastrophizing: what is it? *Clin J Pain* 2001; 17:65–71.

Watson D, Clark LA. Affects separable and inseparable: on the hierarchical arrangement of the negative affects. *J Pers Soc Psychol* 1992; 62:489–505.

Watson D, Tellegen A. Towards a consensual structure of mood. *Psychol Bull* 1985; 98:219–235.

Yesavage JA, Brink TL, Rose TK, et al. Development and validation of a geriatric depression screening scale: a preliminary report. *J Psychol Res* 1983; 17:37–49.

Zimmerman M, Chelminski I, McDermut W. Major depressive disorder and axis 1 diagnostic comorbidity. *J Clin Psychiatry* 2002; 63;187–193.

Zung WWK. A self-rating depression scale. *Arch Gen Psychiatry* 1965; 12:63–70.

Correspondence to: Stephen J. Gibson, PhD, National Ageing Research Institute, P.O. Box 31, Parkville, VIC 3052, Australia. Email: s.gibson@nari.unimelb.edu.au.

Proceedings of the 10th World Congress on Pain,
Progress in Pain Research and Management, Vol. 24,
edited by Jonathan O. Dostrovsky, Daniel B. Carr, and
Martin Koltzenburg, IASP Press, Seattle, © 2003.

52

How Stories Remake What Pain Unmakes[1]

Arthur W. Frank

Department of Sociology, University of Calgary, Calgary, Alberta, Canada

My theme is the power of stories. This chapter is constructed around three stories. The first describes a patient's need to have her story heard and witnessed. The second story both presents an allegory of pain and demonstrates the centrality of story in the human project. The third story is the author's own pain narrative, and it suggests how a change in perception of how pain is integrated into the world can affect the patient's response to pain.

Later in this chapter I will distinguish between narrative and story, but to begin, let me tell you a *story* that introduces the kind of ill person I am talking about and the problems such a person confronts.

A couple of weeks ago I received a phone message from a woman I will call Mary. She was calling from another city. She wanted to know if I was the author of the books that she named. So I called back. Mary has breast cancer, and she began to tell me what was shaping up as a long story. As much as this chapter advocates clinicians listening to patients, let me be clear at the outset that I am willing to set limits. I interrupted Mary, told her I was going to be in her city the next week, and said that I had a time slot when we could meet. So we did meet, in a pleasant sort of half coffee bar

---

[1] *Editor's Note:* The three presentations within the workshop, "Subjectivity Affirmed: How Qualitative Research Helps Us to Understand Pain and Suffering" were quite different from each other. Their distinctiveness precluded merging of their content. This chapter, based solely upon Dr. Frank's presentation, was selected by the presenters and moderator of the workshop to exemplify the insight and strength that narrative and textual analysis can achieve. The tone of Dr. Frank's oral presentation is retained in the written version, in part to underscore his argument that stories are *addressed* to specific listeners.

half gift shop. Mary is undergoing radiation and is bald. I admired her for not wearing anything on her head; that requires poise for a woman, even by today's fashion standards. Mary is not lacking in poise.

Mary began our conversation by saying that her "sense of integrity as a person is nonexistent." She is careful with words and she meant *integrity* in a structural sense: she is not holding together; she is not, literally, integral. Cancer has upset the fragile balance that her life was, and she cannot see how she will ever put the pieces back together again. During much of the time we were together she was close to tears, and she had several good cries. I mean they were *good.* She told me, and this is important to tell you, that she never cries when she is at the cancer center. I wish her physicians and nurses there could have seen our conversation. I wish they could see Mary as I doubt they have seen her. She speaks very highly of the professionals who care for her, but when she is with them, she holds back an important part of herself. My belief is that if Mary could cry in her clinic, it would help her to regain some measure of integrity. The complementary part of this belief is that if that clinic were the sort of place where patients could cry, physicians and nurses would enhance their integrity.

I want to tell you two more things about Mary. The first is that she not only *told* me that her integrity as a person was lost, but also *showed* me her unraveled life in her speech. Mary became silent at regular intervals while we talked. She did not *lapse* into silence; that conventional phrase is wrong. There was nothing *lapsed* about her silences. She *descended* into silence. Silence seemed to be where she went when words could no longer describe who she was and what she was going through. Her silences expressed the *beyond* that she is on the edge of. Mary showed me how integrity of self and the self's capacity for language get lost together. Mary's loss of integrity as a person is part and parcel of her inability to tell a cohesive, uninterrupted narrative of her life.

The last thing I want to mention about Mary is that I think she will be all right, at some point down a difficult road. There is much rhetoric in the culture of cancer support groups about becoming better-than-well, or some such phrase, as a result of having cancer. I believe that because Mary has let herself unravel, and because she is such a keen observer of her own unraveling, she can reassemble herself to be more durable, more useful, and finer than she was before she became ill. This new integrity has nothing to do with how long she lives. The best way I can express it is that at some point, I think she will feel that she has "gotten it right."

I have written about Mary at such length because her story introduces some important ideas about narrative and medicine, and she introduces the kind of ill person I am talking about. For pain specialists, the patients for whom narrative is most important are those like Mary, who are falling apart. These are the patients for whom whatever you are trying medically is not working, or maybe you think it is working but your patient still wants something *more,* and you cannot figure out what.

Let me approach this troublesome and crucial *more* by writing about how stories work in our personal lives and our collective lives. Again I will proceed by telling a story, this time a very old one that I have adapted from a version by the novelist John Gardner (1978).

> In ancient days, the god Thor made a circle around middle earth, in order to hold at bay the chaos that hates the world of gods and humans. But the gods grew older and the circle weakened; chaos encroached. Then Wotan, the god of wisdom, caught the king of the trolls. He held him in an arm lock and asked the question: "How can the light and order triumph over darkness and chaos?"
>
> The Troll King, who seems pretty cool under the circumstances, said: "Give me your left eye, then I'll tell you."
>
> Wotan plucked out his left eye and gave it to him. "Now tell me."
>
> "The secret," said the Troll King, "is, *Watch with both eyes.*" (adapted from Gardner 1978)

I tell you this old story for several reasons. First, and this does have clinical relevance, I hope you enjoyed the story. The literary critic Anatole Broyard (1992), when he was dying of prostate cancer, gave a grand rounds presentation at the University of Chicago, and one of the things he told the assembled clinicians was that he would like a doctor who *enjoyed* him; that choice of words is worth thinking about, because enjoying each other is not often depicted as essential to the clinician-patient relationship. Broyard continues: "I want to be a good story for him." As I understand Broyard, he equates being recognized as a "good story" with being recognized as human.

Second, I hope you can recognize Wotan as a sort of patient. Every patient who is in pain would like to grab his or her physician in an arm lock and demand to know how to protect his or her life from the chaos of pain that is breaching the circle that we all draw around our lives. The patient is asking, as David Morris put it in his presentation: "Will I get better?" This is Wotan's question: Can I keep out the chaos? The physician fears being held in that arm lock, because she or he cannot answer the question. And the patient feels that fear and fears all the more him or herself. Thus too often in the clinic, fear encounters fear.

Third, the story does not speak explicitly about pain, but when Wotan plucked out his eye, it cannot have merely tickled. One level of the story is about how pain is endurable when it is part of some purpose. But notice something crucial about narrative. Purposes only become purposes within a story; until then, they are only abstract possibilities, without much interest. Possibilities become meaningful when they matter to some character in a story; the story *creates* the stakes on what becomes the purpose. Wotan's gaining of wisdom is a purpose that holds our interest for at least two reasons. The first is that Wotan's sacrifice of his eye sets the stakes high. The second reason is that in stories before this one—because stories never travel alone—we have heard something about the monsters inside the chaos that threatens the world of gods and humans, and the story has taught us that what is outside the circle is worth fearing. Wotan's purpose, like the hero's purpose in any good story, becomes the listeners' purpose. What the hero seeks to become, in questing for that purpose, is an ideal that elevates our sights as we hear the story. That is what Gardner (1978) meant by *moral* fiction: fiction that offers its readers ideals for their lives. My interest is in moral medicine.

The last idea that I want to draw from the story of Wotan's eye is that people tell stories not to express who they already are. People tell stories to *become* who they are. Wotan becomes the god of wisdom when he plucks out his eye. Until he is defined by his action in that story, he lacks character, in both the literary and the moral sense. Patients need to tell stories to become the persons the new circumstances of illness are requiring them to be. Patients often do not yet know what questions to ask, because they are unsure of what life is the ground of asking. Like Mary in my first story, such patients descend into silence. They fear being there alone.

A story as old as the tale of Wotan's eye reminds us of the crucial part that stories play in the human enterprise: I mean that word, *enterprise*; humanity is an undertaking, a project. Stories restore and enhance humans' sense of what their project is. The Canadian anthropologist Julie Cruikshank spent years in the Yukon interviewing native elders, five women who were master storytellers (Cruikshank 1998). She reports that in the interviews, these women "kept redirecting our work away from secular history and toward stories about how the world began and was transformed to be suitable for human beings." The story of Wotan's eye is about how the world became suitable for human beings, and graphically evokes the work that humans must keep doing—in the absence of the gods—to sustain that suitability.

For the people of the Yukon, as for the northern Europeans, the human world is always coming apart: the trolls and frost giants are always unmaking it. Elaine Scarry, in her influential study, *The Body in Pain* (1985), writes about pain as *unmaking* a person's world. Northern stories reflect people who felt unmaking in their bones; that unmaking was the wolf always at the door. Pain patients live with a wolf at the door. Clinicians work to support patients as their worlds are being unmade; this work seeks to keep the patient's world and the larger world suitable for human beings.

Cruikshank's experience interviewing Yukon elders also mirrors how medicine starts off wanting to *use* narrative as a technique for its established purposes, and how physicians and nurses can be redirected by stories. Cruikshank reports that at least in her early interviews, she kept trying to get the women to talk about what she calls secular history, which is the social scientific equivalent of medical talk about symptoms and treatments. This is what our respective professions are expected to talk about: what we are ostensibly trained for and paid to do. Cruikshank's interview respondents, these Yukon elders, would have none of it. To tell her who they were, they had to tell her their stories, the stories about how ancient heroes transformed the world into a place suitable for human beings. These elders were teaching Cruikshank that she could only understand the contemporary lives and conflicts of the native people if she could think *with* those stories.

Thinking *with* stories means having more than a literary or scholarly knowledge of the stories. I discuss thinking *with* stories in *The Wounded Storyteller* (Frank 1995); Morris (2001) elaborates the need for clinicians to think *with* stories. To turn Cruikshank into a fully human anthropologist, these generous women had to teach her to allow their stories to organize the patterns she used to know the world. As Cruikshank came to realize, the elders thought *with* stories about the contemporary issues their people faced. The stories organized and made sense of these issues, suggesting appropriate responses. The elders, I emphasize, did not just tell traditional stories as something they did, among other things they might do. They *were* the stories; they embodied these stories in the sense that the stories, like habitually repeated patterns of using the body, had become their internal representational schema, near to what cognitive scientists call the body schema, that organizes both their perceptions of the world and their expressions of these perceptions.

A storyteller in a traditional community, Cruikshank tells us, is a kind of moral orchestrator, whose art consists not only in knowing the story's words, but in having the judgment to be able to tell the *right* story—the story that can, in a specific situation, move particular people to think in new ways about who they are and what they are called to do. Applying this concept to medicine takes as little time as adding, at the end of a patient's story, some tag line such as: "I think what you've just said is very important," or, "That story you've told gives me a new way to understand you." But the simplicity of the words is deceptive. Just *saying* those sorts of things is like only knowing the names of the characters and the plot of the traditional story.

The moral competence of the native elder is recognizing when a person or group needs a particular story. The judgment and moral imagination of the clinician lies in knowing *when* and *how* to say something in response to the patient's story. Again, what is said may be simple—simple is often best—but its effect depends on the clinician already having communicated, in the quality of *attention* to the patient's story, that the comment afterwards is not merely another technique picked up in a continuing medical education workshop. You have to be *caught up,* which is an act of surrender that is difficult for professionals.

Stories told in clinics are not myths and legends; they are more along the lines of "a funny thing happened to me today." Stories seem to report on events that the teller has experienced, seen, or heard about second-hand, but as I have been suggesting, stories do more than report. Stories are *addressed* to someone: I am not telling my story to the air, I am telling it to *you.* I am claiming that this story should matter to you, and that claim is part of the larger claim that I, the storyteller, should matter to you. My capacity to tell the story shows you why I should matter. Think again of Anatole Broyard's desire to be a good story for his physician.

Thus beyond stories' reporting function, stories also have a relationship function. The Russian literary critic and moral philosopher, Mikhail Bakhtin (1984), described stories as *double voiced*: they both represent reports of past events and create the present, evolving relationship between teller and listener. Most observers of stories notice the same duality: report and relationship. Thus we who listen need to echo the Troll King's advice to Wotan: *listen with both ears.* Unfortunately, the generally depressing literature on medical training suggests that somewhere in the process of becoming a doctor, many people make a version of Wotan's bargain: they trade that second ear for professionalism, and later they find they cannot be wise without what they have traded away. But happily, the trade was not for keeps.

Professionalism in the sciences likes reports that it calls *objective*; ideal reports can be quantified, as when pain is rated on a scale. I do not dispute the utility of scales, but the student of narrative is skeptical that one version of objectivity will end up reifying a number, treating it as if it were meaningful in itself. Stories cannot be forced into being single voiced. The attempt is doomed: however much the listener wants to efface himself or herself from the storytelling scene, the storyteller will put the listener back in. The number on the pain rating scale is addressed to a presumed listener for whom it is a message: what number is chosen remains intractably a comment on the relationship between teller and listener, and this comment requires interpretation. A low score may not mean low pain, but rather be an expression of the patient's trust that the physician will recognize what is not being explicitly claimed, and value the claim more highly for its understatement. A high score may be a way of opening a dialogue about something else that the patient wants the clinician to hear. This something else may not affect treatment, but it is part of what the patient needs the clinician to know, in order for the patient to *be known,* because relationships are an end in themselves.

This limitation of objectivity should not distress anyone. On the contrary, the relationship level is where physicians and nurses can use themselves (their life experiences and their physical presence). Another of my beliefs affirms the frequently rehearsed argument that medicine's enormous technological advances of the last half-century plus have seduced physicians especially, nurses less, into giving up on their healing presence and touch as the most important treatment intervention. So many great physicians and nurses have emphasized this personal presence, yet it is constantly subordinated to other interventions. A shared trust in the healing potential of personal presence was key to the workshop on which this chapter was based.

My core argument is that, as important as any pain specialist's medicine cabinet is, all the interventions that treat the body as an object, and that consequently understand pain as something inside the body, will never be enough for many patients. We are again faced with that troublesome and crucial quality of *more.* Sooner or later, what affects pain is the relationship between the patient and the clinician, and this relationship is a story. A patient like Mary is literally crying out for relationships.

The importance of human relationships, mediated by stories, for the treatment of pain is not news. Palliative care has probably put forward the argument most carefully. Listen to a physician, Anna Towers, who practices in Montreal. Towers often admits patients to her unit because they are in pain that other hospital units are unable to treat. Her unit probably is more sophisticated in the medications they administer, but she emphasizes that what counts is whether patients experience "a shift in perception"; that's her phrase, "a shift in perception." "The pain would still be there," Towers writes—and I think of Wotan's empty eye socket—"but it would be experienced differently, and the suffering reduced. The patient would reach a deeper level of understanding, almost as if the suffering had been given new meaning" (Barnard et al. 2000).

This word *meaning* is one of our densest. I understand Towers using this word to point toward ways that suffering is given a place in stories that make sense of who the patient is. The patient may not *want* to be who they are—most of Towers' patients would rather not have terminal diseases—but who they are becomes all right, because it is part of a story that rings true.

What Elizabeth Kübler-Ross (1969) made famous as dying people's stage of "acceptance" is, for me, being able to put one's death into a story where it fits.

Here I reach the distinction promised earlier between story and narrative. These terms need to be distinguished from each other, even though they overlap and often are used as synonyms. I have written, as have others, that people tell *stories* and only academics study *narrative.* A child would never ask her parent to "tell me a narrative." Narratives are collections of words in which analysts locate certain properties: semantic properties, contextual properties. The analysis of these properties is useful in the same way that dissection is useful. But by the time we get to narrative, the story is already as dead as a butterfly pinned in a collector's box. Stories are face to face; again, they are *addressed* by one person to another. The storyteller *calls upon* her audience: a good storyteller makes her audience feel *chosen.* A wise and clever patient can make her clinician feel chosen; a wise clinician knows to feel chosen, even when her patient is not such a good storyteller. The chosen one is called, summoned, by another person, and being chosen is a responsibility.

Lest that responsibility sound ominous, I add quickly that the call is not necessarily to *do* something. The call is to be part of a relationship. It is a call that physicians, so far as I can tell, are taught next to nothing about in medical schools, and a call that becomes increasingly difficult for nurses to attend to, in the conditions of their work. The call is to *be* someone in relation to another. That, again, is not so difficult. The genius of how we humans work, as storytelling animals, is that the very telling of a story can change the experience of what the story reports. When the ancient Norse, huddled in their hovels, told the story about Thor's circle, they felt protected; their sense of vulnerability shifted. When the aboriginal people of the Yukon told their creation stories, their unrelenting environment became a place where people could live a *human* life. Pain patients are wired the same way these people were and are. To return to Anna Towers' phrase, the pain is experienced differently and the patient experiences a shift in perception.

What is this shift in perception that Towers claims her patients experience? It is seeing what happens as events in a different sort of story, a story with a different *purpose.* The classic testimony to the reality of this shift in perception is the Holocaust memoir of the psychiatrist Victor Frankl (1959), who popularized the idea that survival becomes possible when pain is given meaning. Again that tricky word *meaning.* What Frankl points to is not some abstract propositional meaning, as in "the meaning of," but rather meaning as living *gesture*: the starving prisoner sharing his last crust of bread is one of his examples. The gestures that are so moving in Frankl's memoir are the small acts through which people redraw Thor's circle around themselves, if only momentarily. They are the acts through which people in the most dehumanizing circumstances resist the unmaking and sustain some corner of the world as temporarily habitable for human beings.

Frankl's message has rung true for literally millions of suffering people; its reception is its truth, because he has shifted people's perceptions. Frankl promises that if you can understand yourself as part of a story in which you are playing some part in keeping the world suitable for human beings, then your suffering becomes bearable. Maybe you will survive in a physical sense, as Frankl claimed Nazi camp survivors did, and maybe you will not, as Anna Towers' patients do not. The ancient wisdom that palliative care has renewed is that we should not be surprised or offended by death. What counts is the story that one feels a part of as one dies, and what story the dying person makes others feel they are part of. The real work of palliative care is helping people to make a good story of their deaths, and I think that is a paradigm for any medical specialization in pain.

Frankl's emphasis on the importance of people's beliefs about their proper role places him as one contemporary successor to the ancient tradition of Stoicism. The Roman Stoic philosopher, Marcus Aurelius (2002), sounds like a contemporary psychologist when he offers advice on responding to one's own chronic pain: he counsels "that pain is neither unbearable nor unending, as long as you keep in mind its limits and don't magnify them in your imagination." Imagination can be the medium through which physical pain unmakes a person's world. It can also be Thor's hammer: the means of beating back the chaos. The clinical task is helping people to use their imaginations well. Let me tell my last story about using imagination.

When I had testicular cancer in the mid-1980s, I went through a long period of misdiagnosis; my best estimate from different studies is that about half the men so diagnosed experience such delay. Tumors from testicular cancer grow rapidly, so I truly was, to use a phrase that offends some people, full of cancer. Tumors were wrapped around my renal arteries and were cutting off my kidneys. The pain was not only the sharp jabs of being pounded in the mid-back; I was suffocating. Pain was beyond this or that hurting here or there; explosions turned into implosions. My physician was blinded by the normal results of basic blood, urine, and x-ray tests and didn't get his hands on me carefully enough to feel the tumors. So he treated my pain as an overuse injury from sports. I had experienced such injuries, and I knew something completely different was sweeping through my body.

Without any medical anchor, my imagination was unleashed to magnify my pain. I was living in that condition describable only by the medical oxymoron, *chronic acute pain.* That bit of twisted language suggests how the narrative ordering of my life had broken down. I was being unmade. Unmaking is a condition in which the terror of dissolution is felt; it becomes the body's experience. I had no language for this experience. The dissolution of unmaking leaves no capacity for metaphors. It is only later, in trying to account for it, that Thor and all the creatures that he seeks to keep outside his circle—the frost giants and trolls and serpents—become metaphors.

Then I had my own version of the experience that Anna Towers describes: the perception of pain shifted, and the suffering acquired some meaning. I wrote about this shift in my first book, *At the Will of the Body* (Frank 1991), and here I will tell the shortest version of the story. The pain I was living with was worst at night, after I had tried to lie down, so I spent my nights wandering about the house. Both because I was too exhausted to tolerate light and because I hoped not to disturb my wife, I wandered about in the dark. One night I was sitting on the landing on our staircase, and I discovered an image that had materialized on a large window. The window was lightly frosted—it was early fall—and a tree just outside the window was backlit by a street lamp beyond the tree. The window had become a perfectly etched sculpture of a tree. The sight captured me in its transient, contingent perfection. I had to become caught up in it, because there was no way to catch the image and make it permanent for later contemplation. I knew I had to be *there,* just *then,* to see it. No one else would ever see it. The image had chosen me as its witness, and pain had allowed me to be this witness.

At that moment I realized two things. The first was that I had actually forgotten pain for a moment. I had not thought that was possible. Realizing that pain could be forgotten, however briefly, broke its hold. The second realization was that the story of having to be there to see the window had, for a moment, trumped the story that pain only prevented me from doing what I wanted, which was, most of all, to be back in bed asleep. Here is the shift of perception, in which the sufferer crosses the boundary from unmaking to remaking. Pain, suddenly and decisively, *made* something possible. Instead of unmaking my world, it made a world.

Even before chemotherapy began the pain did go away, and I could sleep again. I cannot credit that welcome relief to the power of narrative. The coda of my story is that the memory of pain remained, for me, the truth of cancer; in pain I saw cancer face to face. Maybe I like the Wotan story so much because it provides a metaphor in which plucking out a testicle is a good bargain for a kind of wisdom.

If you as clinicians think *with* my window story—do not make it an object of analysis but just let it affect what you make of your other thoughts—you might hear your patients differently, and you might experience yourself differently, as you hear them. All this about narrative and story is ultimately simple: *can you help people in pain to find their moment in front of their version of my window*? The window could have been anything; the seeds of perception are scattered all around us.

Helping people see the stories that they are living, and that could change their lives, depends on seeing those stories yourself as they float by, as yet unformed as narratives. You begin to imagine how some story that the patient is living but cannot yet tell could matter to the patient, if it could be told. You are not feeling what the patient feels—it is not that sense of empathy. Rather, you imagine how this story matters for this other person, given who they are and what they face. Listening and responding to patients' stories is a skill, but not a technique. This skill may be best described as a moral commitment that becomes a habit, as much who you are as what you do.

Thor's hammer may be too militant a metaphor for this moral commitment, and Wotan plucking out his eye may be too sacrificial. Each metaphor is imperfect, but stories continue to emerge that do the work of keeping the world suitable for human beings.

ACKNOWLEDGMENT

My thanks to my co-presenters, David Morris and Alan Radley, for generously allowing my paper to represent our workshop. Thanks also to Daniel Carr for proposing the topic ("Subjectivity Affirmed") in which this presentation took place, and for securing support from the Saltonstall and Armington Funds to make it possible.

REFERENCES

Bakhtin M. *Problems of Dostoevsky's Poetics.* Minneapolis: University of Minnesota Press, 1984.

Barnard D, Towers A, Boston P, Lambrinidou Y. *Crossing Over: Narratives of Palliative Care.* New York: Oxford University Press, 2000, p 189.

Broyard A. *Intoxicated by My Illness: And Other Writings on Life and Death.* New York: Clarkson Potter, 1992, p 45.

Cruikshank J. *The Social Life of Stories: Narrative and Knowledge in the Yukon Territory.* Lincoln: University of Nebraska Press, 1998.

Frank AW. *The Wounded Storyteller: Body, Illness, and Ethics.* Chicago: University of Chicago Press, 1995.

Frank AW. *At the Will of the Body: Reflections on Illness.* Boston: Houghton Mifflin, 1991.

Frankl VE. *Man's Search for Meaning.* New York: Washington Square, 1959.

Gardner J. *On Moral Fiction.* New York: Basic Books, 1978, p 3.
Kübler-Ross E. *On Death and Dying.* New York: Macmillan, 1969.
Marcus Aurelius. *Meditations,* book VII, verse 64. Gregory Hays, translator. New York: Modern Library, 2002.
Morris DB. Narrative, Ethics, and Pain: Thinking *with* Stories." *Narrative* 2001, 9:55–77.
Scarry E. *The Body in Pain: The Making and Unmaking of the World.* New York: Oxford University Press, 1985.

Correspondence to: Arthur W. Frank, PhD, Department of Sociology, University of Calgary, Calgary, AB, Canada T2N 1N4. Email: frank@ucalgary.ca.

Proceedings of the 10th World Congress on Pain,
Progress in Pain Research and Management, Vol. 24,
edited by Jonathan O. Dostrovsky, Daniel B. Carr, and
Martin Koltzenburg, IASP Press, Seattle, © 2003.

53

Fear in Musculoskeletal Pain

Johan W.S. Vlaeyen

Department of Medical, Clinical, and Experimental Psychology, Maastricht University, Maastricht, The Netherlands

HOW DOES FEAR RELATE TO PAIN?

Pain is a universal experience that leads to the urge to escape the situation in which it occurs. As such, pain can best be conceptualized as an emotional experience, as emotions are believed to drive action. In acute injury, escape from the harmful situation and the associated withdrawal behavior promote the healing process. In most cases, healing occurs in within a couple of weeks and the pain subsides quickly. However, in some individuals with pain, the immediate withdrawal behaviors do not lead to the anticipated reduction of pain, which than is interpreted as a signal of a continuous threat to the integrity of the body. A mismatch then occurs between what the patient expects (a quick decrease of pain) and what actually happens (increasing or lasting pain). Such a negative interpretation may not always reflect a true threat, and in such cases catastrophic misinterpretations of benign physical sensations may occur. Sometimes these may be fueled by external information such as unfavorable pain histories of relatives or acquaintances, or verbal or visual information provided by health care providers that suggests the probability of a serious illness causing the pain complaints. Catastrophic interpretations, and fear reactions in particular, always increase the individual's distress level. In pain patients, interpretational errors such as catastrophizing inevitably result in pain-related fear: fear of pain, fear of injury, or fear of physical activity, depending on the anticipated source of threat. Evidence is accumulating that these misinterpretations and the associated pain-related fear are likely to cause a cascade of psychological and physical events including hypervigilance, muscular reactivity, avoidance and guarding behaviors, and physical disuse, which in turn perpetuate the pain problem.

In the late 20th century, several pain researchers studying the clinical differences between acute and chronic back pain observed that pain of recent onset was associated with a pattern of physiological responses seen in fear and anxiety states. In contrast, chronic pain was better characterized by a habituation of autonomic responses and by a pattern of signs seen in depressive disorders. Only recently have fear responses in musculoskeletal pain been subject to study. A Medline search shows that scientific interest in the role of fear and anxiety in chronic pain states indeed lags behind interest in depression, although it has received increasing attention in the last decade (Fig. 1).

This chapter presents the current state of the art regarding the role of pain-related fear in musculoskeletal pain. We will review existing data on the impact of pain-related fear on pain and pain disability, focusing on escape and avoidance behaviors and attentional processes. In addition, we will critically appraise the available data relevant to assessment methods and novel interventions for fear reduction in chronic musculoskeletal pain. Finally, we will provide some directions for future research.

SOME DEFINITIONS

Anxiety and fear are negative affects that are so closely related that the terms are often used interchangeably. They commonly share several characteristics. They are future-oriented, and refer to the anticipation of danger or

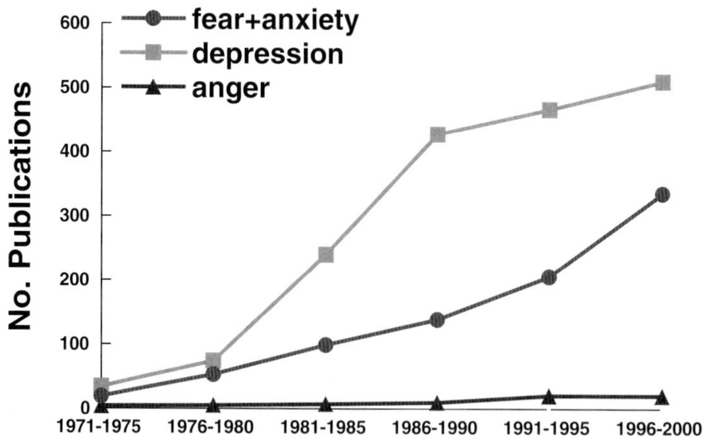

Fig. 1. Numbers of publications on chronic pain and fear and anxiety, depression, and anger from a search of Medline (1971–2000).

discomfort with tense apprehensiveness. They also are both accompanied by heightened arousal and increased awareness of bodily sensations. Although it is not always easy to make the distinction between fear and anxiety in clinical practice, this distinction is theoretically based on the source of threat. In fear it is rather specific, while in anxiety it is more elusive (Rachman 1998). The term "fear" is used when there is a identifiable threat, such as a poisonous snake. Fear may be rational or irrational. Intense, but irrational fears are called "phobias." "Panic" is probably one of the purest expressions of fear. Patients experiencing a panic attack report extreme fear and terror, thoughts of dying, and an overwhelming urge to escape or "get out of here."

In describing the clinical differences between acute and chronic pain, Sternbach (1974) observed that pain of recent onset was associated with a pattern of responses similar to anxiety, while chronic pain was characterized by signs seen in depressive disorders. More recently, behavioral theorists have challenged the assumption that anxiety is only of importance in acute pain states. For example, a psychological analysis of patients with acute back pain revealed that acute pain reactions were comparable with those in chronic pain groups. A follow-up of the sample showed a surprisingly small decline of typical acute pain reactions over time, in contrast to the impact of pain and disability, which had a more marked decline (Philips and Grant 1991). Fear has become the focus of research with growing evidence for the idea that in a substantial number of chronic pain patients "fear of the evil is worse than the evil itself" (Arntz et al. 1990). Recent evidence has shown that when attempting movements that they fear will cause pain, patients with chronic low back pain typically show behavioral (escape and avoidance), cognitive (worry), and psychophysiological responses, rendering support for the idea that chronic pain and chronic fear share important characteristics (Philips 1987; Asmundson et al. 1999; Vlaeyen and Linton 2000).

In relation to pain, both the terms "pain anxiety" (McCracken et al. 1998) and "pain-related fear" (Vlaeyen et al. 1995a; Crombez et al. 1999) have been used interchangeably, although given the presence of an identifiable threat of pain or (re)injury in most anxious patients with musculoskeletal pain, the term "pain-related fear" might be preferable. The term "fear-avoidance" was introduced by Lethem et al. (1983), pointing to the detrimental consequences of the avoidance behaviors that are so typical of fear reactions. Some authors have gone so far as to consider the anxiety often reported by chronic pain patients an irrational fear or phobia, because the clinician often does not recognize the rationality of the threat. For example, the term "kinesiophobia" was introduced for the condition in which a patient experiences "an excessive, irrational, and debilitating fear of physical movement and activity resulting from a feeling of vulnerability to painful injury or reinjury" (Kori et al. 1990). There is some question whether indeed pain-related fear can be regarded as a phobia. Comparing kinesiophobia with criteria for specific phobias listed in the *Diagnostic and Statistical Manual of Mental Disorders* (DSM-IV; American Psychiatric Association 2000), there is at least one difference. In phobic patients, the person recognizes that the fear is excessive or unreasonable. In contrast, most back pain patients are convinced that certain movements are harmful for them. The other DSM-IV criteria of specific phobias seem to match the concept of kinesiophobia quite well (Vlaeyen et al. 2002c). Evidence suggests that during physical examination, chronic pain patients experience substantial anxiety with intensity comparable to that found in patients with panic disorder (Hadjistavropoulos and LaChapelle 2000).

MODERN THEORIES OF EMOTION

Emotions are currently conceptualized by most theorists as fundamental action tendencies whose purpose is to motivate behavior related to successful survival. Some of these behaviors include preparing for, avoiding, and escaping potentially dangerous life-threatening events, which are at the heart of the emotions of fear and anxiety (Barlow 2002). One of the most prominent theories of emotion is the bio-informational theory put forward by Lang (Lang 1979; Lang et al. 1998). This theory conceptualizes emotions as networks of action tendencies stored in memory along three levels: a perceptual level, a response level, and a semantic level. The theory predicts that events that match elements of the network can activate the whole network. The better the match, the stronger the emotion. In other words, fear and anxiety are behavior programs (much like computer programs) comprising stimulus, response, and meaning structures (data files). Data at the stimulus level will prompt action and define the function and direction of the act. Response propositions are data in the form of response components of the emotion. Finally, meaning propositions contain information that helps interpret the stimulus information and response propositions. Consider the following situation of a fearful patient with back pain: "I am cleaning the house. When picking up a book from the table, I hear a crack in my back and feel a shooting pain. The slightest movement is painful. I keep thinking how bad the pain is. There might be something wrong. I'd better stay still, otherwise I might be in danger of re-injuring myself."

In this situation, stimulus information is the recognition of the frightening object (bodily sensations such as shooting pain). Response propositions are relevant responses, such as avoiding movement. The meaning propositions tie these two together. For example, they may include the following statement: "In this situation, these pain sensations are unpredictable and dangerous, and I need to be careful."

THREE BASIC FEARS

Some researchers propose that most fears stem from three basic fears or "sensitivities": fear of anxiety symptoms (anxiety sensitivity), fear of negative evaluation (social evaluation sensitivity), and fear of illness or injury (illness/injury sensitivity) (Reiss 1987). The remainder of this chapter will focus on pain-related fear as being more closely linked to the illness/injury sensitivity concept. The reason is that pain is often linked with injury, and one of the most salient fears in patients with chronic pain is the fear that pain is a sign of (impending) injury or illness. Again, in musculoskeletal pain syndromes such as back pain, fear of movement/(re)injury (kinesiophobia) has received most attention in recent years (Vlaeyen and Linton 2000). Indeed, a recent epidemiological study examining pain-related fear in 437 individuals reporting current back pain, randomly drawn from the open population in The Netherlands, revealed a high percentage of participants who endorsed beliefs that back pain is harmful (Picavet et al. 2002). For example, 68.6% of participants agreed or strongly agreed with the following statement: "Simply being careful not to make unnecessary movements is the safest thing I can do to prevent back pain," and 48.8% agreed or strongly agreed with "Back pain always means that the body is injured." Similar findings have been reported in the United States (Von Korff and Moore 2001).

PAIN CATASTROPHIZING

"An ache beneath the sternum, in connoting the possibility of sudden death from heart failure, can be a wholly unsettling experience, whereas the same intensity and duration of ache in a finger is a trivial annoyance easily disregarded." With this statement, Henry Beecher (1956, p 159) emphasized the importance of cognitive processes in the pain experience (Beecher 1959) and gave an early example of what is now called a catastrophic (mis)interpretation of bodily sensations. Pain catastrophizing is considered an exaggerated negative orientation toward noxious stimuli, and has been shown to mediate distress reactions to painful stimulation (Sullivan et al. 1995). In further support of this idea, Crombez and colleagues (1998a) found that pain-free volunteers with a high frequency of catastrophic thinking about pain become more fearful when threatened with the possibility of intense pain than do students with a low frequency of catastrophic thinking.

In sum, evidence indicates that catastrophizing thoughts are strongly associated with fearful responding and might be considered a precursor of pain-related fear.

WHAT IS THE IMPACT OF PAIN-RELATED FEAR?

FEAR CREATES THE URGE TO AVOID OR ESCAPE

One of the main features of fear and anxiety is the tendency to avoid and escape from the perceived threat. Although chronic pain in itself cannot always be avoided, the activities assumed to increase pain or (re)injury may be. A consequence, however, is that daily activity levels decrease, possibly resulting in functional incapacity. A number of studies have investigated the association between pain-related fear and physical performance, including range of motion as measured with a flexometer (McCracken et al. 1993), weight lifting (Vlaeyen et al. 1995a; Van den Hout et al. 2001), knee-extension-flexion (Crombez et al. 1998b, 1999), lumbar extension (Al-Obaidi et al. 2000), and lifting and carrying objects (Burns et al. 2000). Inducing pain anticipation (by instruction) led to significantly lower levels of behavioral performance as well as increased pain intensity and fear during a physical performance test (Pfingsten et al. 2002). In a large Swedish general population study, pain-related fear was strongly related to the performance of activities of daily living (highest quartile: odds ratio [OR] = 2.5; Buer and Linton 2002). Interestingly, these avoidance behaviors appear to generalize to increased functional disability (Waddell et al. 1993; Crombez et al. 1999; Fritz et al. 2001). A Dutch study showed that individuals with back pain who reported pain-related fear (highest third) had an increased risk for being disabled due to back pain 6 months later (OR = 4.6, 95% confidence interval [CI] = 2.6–8.0) (Picavet et al. 2002).

Based on these and other studies, a cognitive-behavioral model has been developed that postulates two opposing behavioral responses of confrontation and avoidance. This model presents possible pathways by which injured patients can become trapped in a downward spiral of increasing avoidance, disability, and pain (see Fig. 2). The model, which is based on previous work (Lethem et al. 1983; Philips 1987; Waddell et al. 1993), predicts several ways in which pain-related fear can lead to disability: (1) Negative appraisals about pain and its consequences, such as catastrophic thinking, are considered a potential precursor of pain-related fear. (2) Fear is characterized by escape and avoidance behaviors, of which the immediate consequence is that daily activities expected to produce pain are no longer undertaken. Avoidance of daily activities results in functional disability. (3) Because

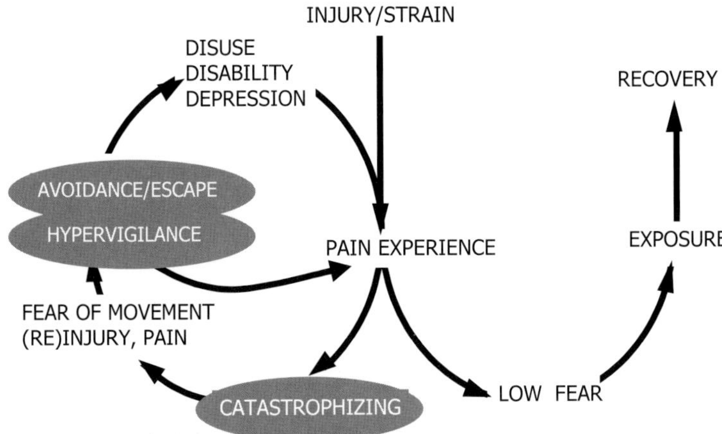

Fig. 2. A cognitive-behavioral model of pain-related fear. If pain, possibly caused by an injury or strain, is interpreted as threatening (pain catastrophizing), pain-related fear evolves. This fear leads to avoidance and escape, followed by disability, disuse, and depression. The latter will maintain the pain experiences, thereby fueling the vicious circle of increasing fear and avoidance. A more direct causal link between pain-related fear and pain is assumed to be mediated by hypervigilance. In noncatastrophizing patients, pain-related fear is minimal and rapid resumption daily activities is likely to occur, accelerating recovery. Based on Vlaeyen et al. (1995a).

avoidance behaviors occur in anticipation of pain rather than as a response to pain, these behaviors may persist because there are fewer opportunities to correct the (wrongful) expectancies and beliefs about pain as a signal of threat of physical integrity. In this case, fearful beliefs may become dissociated from actual pain experiences. (4) Longstanding avoidance and physical inactivity have a detrimental impact on the musculoskeletal and cardiovascular systems, leading to "disuse syndrome" (Bortz 1984), which may further worsen the pain problem. In addition, avoidance also means withdrawal from essential reinforcers, leading to mood disturbances such as irritability, frustration, and depression. Both depression and disuse are known to be associated with decreased pain tolerance (Romano and Turner 1985; McQuade et al. 1988), and hence they might promote the painful experience.

FEAR DIRECTS ATTENTIONAL FOCUS

The most important function of anxiety is probably to facilitate the early detection of potentially threatening situations. In other words, highly anxious individuals demonstrate hypervigilance, both generally and specifically. General hypervigilance (or distractibility) refers to the propensity to attend to any irrelevant stimuli being presented. Specific hypervigilance involves the inclination to attend selectively to threat-related rather than to neutral stimuli. Laboratory studies with healthy subjects and experimentally induced pain stimuli have shown that the effect of anxiety upon pain perception is mediated by attentional processes (Arntz et al. 1994; Eccleston and Crombez 1999; Keogh et al. 2001). Very little research has directly examined hypervigilance in pain patients who report pain-related fear (Asmundson et al. 1997). Eccleston et al. (1997) and Crombez et al. (1996a) used a primary task paradigm in which subjects are requested to direct the attentional focus toward a mental task while receiving painful stimuli. Degradation of mental task performance is also taken as an index of attentional interference due to body hypervigilance. These researchers found that disruption of attentional performance was most pronounced in chronic pain patients who reported pain-related fear, somatic awareness, and high pain intensity. Using a more direct paradigm of body scanning reaction time, in which subjects were asked to respond as quickly as possible to stimuli by pressing a button corresponding to the correct body site, we found that the latency to detect non-noxious electrical stimuli at various body sites was predicted by pain-related fear in both fibromyalgia (Peters et al. 2000) and chronic low back pain (Peters et al. 2002). Other methods that have been utilized, such as the dot-probe paradigm , showed similar results (Keogh et al. 2001). Brain imaging studies provide further support for the mediating role of attentional processes in enhancing pain perception (e.g., Bantick et al. 2002).

ASSESSMENT OF PAIN-RELATED FEAR

Measuring pain-related fear is an important, but sometimes a difficult, task in clinical and research settings. A basic question that may be asked is: What the patient is afraid of? In other words: What is the nature of the perceived threat? The most common answer would be pain. Nevertheless, the relationship between avoidance behavior and specific fears appears to be more complex than the answer to this question may imply. Patients for example, may not view their problem as involving fear at all and may simply see difficulty in performing certain movements or activities. Other patients may fear not so much *current* pain, but pain that will be experienced at a later time, for example the day after physical exercise. Finally, patients may not fear pain itself, but the impending (re)injury that it is supposed to indicate. The literature reflects this lack of clarity by discussing measures for the assessment of fear of pain, fear of work and physical activity, and fear of (re)injury as a result of movement. Overall, these pain-specific measures of pain-related fear are better predictors of pain, disability, and pain behavior than are more general anxiety measures or measures of negative affect (McCracken et al. 1996).

FEAR OF PAIN

An early attempt to quantitate chronic pain patients' attitudes concerning activity and pain was the Pain and Impairment Relationship Scale (PAIRS) (Riley et al. 1988). This scale, which has 15 items, each rated on a 7-point Likert scale, has satisfactory psychometric characteristics. The Pain Anxiety Symptoms Scale (PASS) was developed to measure cognitive anxiety symptoms, escape and avoidance responses, fearful appraisals of pain, and physiological anxiety symptoms related to pain (McCracken et al. 1992). The validity of the PASS has been supported by positive correlations with measures of anxiety, cognitive errors, depression, and disability (McCracken et al. 1996). Recently a short version has been developed (McCracken and Dhingra 2002).

FEAR OF WORK-RELATED ACTIVITIES

The Fear-Avoidance Beliefs Questionnaire (FABQ) focuses on the patient's beliefs about how work and physical activity affect his or her low back pain (Waddell et al. 1993). The FABQ consists of two scales, fear-avoidance beliefs about physical activity and fear-avoidance beliefs about work. The authors found that fear-avoidance beliefs about work are strongly correlated with disability in daily living and work lost in the past year, more so than biomedical variables such as anatomical pattern of pain, time pattern, and severity of pain.

FEAR OF MOVEMENT AND (RE)INJURY

The Survey of Pain Attitudes (SOPA) was developed to assess patients' attitudes toward five dimensions of the chronic pain experience: pain control, pain-related disability, medical cures for pain, solicitude of others, and medication for pain (Jensen and Karoly 1992). Because of the authors' clinical observation of an association between chronic pain patients' hesitancy to exercise and the expressed fear of possible injury, a new scale (harm) was added to the original instrument (Jensen et al. 1994). As did the disability and control scales, the harm scale independently predicted levels of dysfunction. The Tampa Scale for Kinesiophobia (TSK) is a 17-item questionnaire to assess fear of (re)injury due to movement (R.P. Miller et al., unpublished manuscript). Each item is provided with a Likert scale with scoring alternatives ranging from "strongly agree" to "strongly disagree." Most psychometric research has been conducted with the Dutch version of the TSK (Goubert et al. 2000). The TSK appears to be sufficiently reliable and valid in predicting activity intolerance and disability. Modest but significant correlations were found with measures of pain intensity, catastrophizing, impact of pain on daily life activities, and generalized fear. Regression analyses revealed that levels of disability were best predicted by pain-related fear, and that the latter was best predicted by catastrophizing. Pain intensity levels and biomedical findings were significantly less predictive of both pain-related fear and disability levels (Vlaeyen et al. 1995b). Moreover, the TSK discriminated well between avoiders and confronters during a behavioral performance task (Vlaeyen et al. 1995a; Crombez et al. 1999).

COMPLEMENTARY MEASURES

Questionnaires for the assessment of pain-related fear are now available, although the validity of some of them requires further exploration. For clinical purposes, these seem suitable for screening patients to identify those with excessive pain-related fear. However, the questionnaires do not tell us precisely what it is that causes the individual to be fearful. To identify the idiosyncratic aspects of fear and the essential fear-provoking stimuli in a particular patient, the Photograph Series of Daily Activities (PHODA) was developed (Kugler et al. 1999). PHODA uses 100 photographs representing various physical daily life activities including lifting, bending, walking, and bicycling. Patients are presented with these photographs and are requested to place each along a fear thermometer scale. This scale consists of a vertical line with 11 anchor points (ranging from 0 to 100) printed on a 60 × 40 cm hardboard. The fear thermometer is placed vertically on a table in front of the patient along with the following instructions: "Please watch each photograph carefully, and try to imagine yourself performing the same movement. Place the photograph on the thermometer according to the extent in which you feel that this movement is harmful to your back." In our experience, abrupt changes in movement (e.g., suddenly being hit) or activities consisting of repetitive spinal compressions (riding a bicycle on a bumpy road) are frequently mentioned stimuli in chronic back pain patients who score high on the pain-related fear measures. These situations are feared because of beliefs about the causes of pain, such as ruptured or severely damaged nerves ("If I lift heavy weights, the nerves in my back might be damaged."). PHODA appears to be a practical tool to establish graded fear hierarchies.

FEAR REDUCTION IN MUSCULOSKELETAL PAIN

What treatment implications can be derived from the pain-related fear model? Peter Lang's bio-informational theory of fear predicts that there are two main prerequisites to reducing fear: (1) the fear network must be activated, and (2) new information must be available that discredits the fear expectations that are inherent to the fear memory. In clinical practice, several techniques aimed at reducing fears in patients with chronic pain have been applied, with mixed success: verbal reassurance, education, physical exercise or graded activity, and exposure to movement in the form of behavioral experiments (see Table I).

VERBAL REASSURANCE

Verbal reassurance generally consists of two classes of verbal cues: verbal statements intended to emotionally reassure patients directly, such as "I wouldn't worry if I were you," and verbal statements that indicate the absence of a medically relevant diseases, such as: "There is nothing wrong with your back" (Coia and Morley 1998). Doctors can tell their patients that they do not have the particular disease they fear, often supporting their assertions by showing them negative test results, and sometimes by providing an alternative nondisease explanation such as stress, muscle pain, or physical overuse. The major problem with verbal reassurance is its inherent ambiguity: "How can it be that there is nothing wrong with my back and yet I still feel pain?" A surprisingly small number of studies have examined the effects of verbal reassurance, and their overall conclusion is that it does not reduce fears and can even have paradoxical effects. In the long run, reassurance can increase fear in a number of patients (McDonald et al. 1996; Donovan and Blake 2000). These results are not surprising, as verbal reassurance does not activate the fear network (but rather attenuates it), and

Table I
Four fear-reduction techniques, differing in their power to reduce fear according to the extent to which they activate the fear network and to which they disconfirm the fear expectations that are inherent to the fear memory

Fear Reduction	Activation	Disconfirmation
Reassurance	–	–
Education	–	+
Exercise/graded activity	+	+/–
Exposure to movement	++	++

neither does it provide new information that refutes previous beliefs. What moderately fearful patients may need is a credible explanation of their symptoms that provides a better account of the current situation than does the disease model. In order to achieve this goal in the area of chronic musculoskeletal pain, several researchers have developed education materials aiming at modifying beliefs about hurt and harm (Burton et al. 1999).

EDUCATION

Another way of reducing levels of fear is to provide new information about the irrationality of the feared consequences. Patients can be educated in such a way that they view their pain as a common condition that can be self-managed, rather than as a serious disease or a condition that needs careful protection. A major goal of such education is to increase the willingness of patients to re-engage in activities they have avoided for a long time. The aim is to correct the misinterpretations and misconceptions that have occurred early on during the development of the pain-related fear. One study evaluated a booklet (known as "the back book") especially designed for lay people in a group of patients consulting their family physician with a new pain episode (Burton et al. 1999). Although there were no differences in pain intensity, patients receiving the experimental booklet showed significantly greater early improvement in beliefs, and this was maintained at 1 year. Thus, a greater proportion of patients with an initially high pain-related fear who received the experimental booklet had clinically important reductions in pain-related fear at 2 weeks, followed by a clinically important improvement in their disability levels. Moore et al. (2000) examined the effects of a two-session group educational intervention for back pain patients seen in primary care. Besides a group meeting, patients received one individual meeting and a telephone conversation with the group leader and with a psychologist experienced in chronic pain management. The intervention was supplemented by educational materials (a book and videos) supporting active management of back pain. A control group received usual care supplemented by a book on back pain care. Participants assigned to the self-care intervention showed significantly greater reductions in back-related worry and fear-avoidance beliefs than did the control group (Moore et al. 2000). A population-based public health prevention program was carried out in Victoria, Australia (Buchbinder et al. 2001). The program consisted of a large media campaign using television and radio commercials, printed advertisements, outdoor billboards, seminars, workplace visits, and publicity articles using positive messages of back pain. Positive results for this unique project were found for back pain beliefs both among patients and among doctors, and a decline occurred in number of claims for back pain, rates of days compensated, and medical payments for claims for back pain. Evidence also suggests that subchronic low back pain may be managed successfully with an approach that includes clinical examination combined with information for patients about the nature of the problem, provided in a manner designed to reduce fear and motivate patients to resume light activity (Indahl et al. 1998).

EXERCISE/GRADED ACTIVITY

Although most exercise and graded activity programs are not designed primarily to reduce pain-related fear, but rather to increase activity levels despite pain, these programs may have fear-reducing effects. Mannion et al. (1999) compared three active treatments: (1) active physical therapy, (2) muscle reconditioning on training devices, and (3) low-impact aerobics. After therapy, significant reductions were observed in pain intensity, frequency, pain disability, pain catastrophizing, and pain-related fear. These effects were maintained over the subsequent 6 months, except in patients receiving physical therapy, who increased their levels of pain-related fear and disability. A subsequent study suggested that the improvements are a result of the positive experience of completing the prescribed exercises without undue harm (Mannion et al. 2001). Similar long-term benefit has been observed for an operant-graded activity program (Van den Hout et al., in press).

EXPOSURE IN VIVO

Philips (1987) was one of the first to argue for the systematic application of graded exposure in order to uncouple ("discomfirm") expectations of pain and harm and the actual pain and other adverse consequences of activity. She further suggested: "These disconfirmations can be made more obvious to the sufferer by helping to clarify the expectations he/she is working with, and by delineating the conditions or stimuli which he feels are likely to fulfil his expectations. Repeated, graded, and controlled exposures to such situations under optimal conditions are likely to produce the largest and most powerful disconfirmations" (Philips 1987, p 279). Experimental support for this idea is provided by the match/mismatch model of pain, which states that people initially tend to overpredict how much pain they will experience, but after some exposures these predictions tend to be corrected to match the actual experience (Rachman and Arntz 1991). A similar pattern was found in a sample of patients with chronic low back pain who were requested to perform four sets of exercises (two with each leg) at maximal force (Crombez et al. 1996b). During each set baseline pain, expected pain, and experienced pain were recorded. As predicted, the patients initially overpredicted pain, but after repetition of the set of exercises they readily corrected the overprediction. The expectancy did not seem to generalize to the set of exercises with the other leg, because a small increase in pain expectancy re-emerged. But again, expectancies were immediately corrected after another performance. Recently, these findings were replicated with two other physical activities: forward bending and straight leg raising (Goubert et al. 2002).

In analogy with the treatment of phobias, graded exposure to back-stressing movements has been evaluated as a treatment for back pain patients reporting substantial fear of movement and (re)injury. A detailed description of the experimental protocol can be found in Vlaeyen et al. (2002c). In a replicated single-case crossover experiment, four consecutive patients with chronic low back pain who were referred for outpatient behavioral rehabilitation, and who reported substantial fear of movement and (re)injury (TSK score > 40), were randomly assigned to receive one of two sequences of interventions (Vlaeyen et al. 2001). One group of patients received the exposure to back-stressing movements first, followed by operant graded activity. In the second group, the sequence of treatment modalities was reversed. Daily measures of pain-related cognitions and fears were recorded with visual analogue scales. Using time series analysis, we found that improvements only occurred during the exposure, and not during the graded activity, irrespective of the treatment order. Analysis of pretreatment and post-treatment differences also revealed that decreases in pain-related fear paralleled decreases in pain catastrophizing and pain disability and, in half of the cases, an increase in pain control.

In a subsequent study patients carried an ambulatory activity monitor at home for 1 week after each treatment module (Vlaeyen et al. 2002a). Analyses revealed that decreases in pain-related fear again occurred at the introduction of the exposure module only. Additionally, these improvements coincided with decreases in pain disability, pain vigilance, and an increase in physical activity. In both studies, the exposure treatment was embedded in a multidisciplinary treatment program, which may have confounded the results. In two further studies, one of which was carried out in a different country (Sweden) , exposure to back-stressing movements was the sole treatment. Again, similar effects were found (Linton et al. 2002a; Vlaeyen et al. 2002b). Because fear reductions occurred rapidly at the very beginning of the exposure treatment during which education was also provided, a subsequent study was designed to disentangle the effects of education, graded activity, and graded exposure (de Jong et al. 2002). After a 3-week no-treatment baseline measurement period, all the patients attended an education session in which it was explained that their pain was not a serious disease or a condition requiring careful protection. This education session was followed by another 3-week no-treatment period. Patients were then randomly assigned to receive either 3-week exposure or 3-week graded activity. In all patients, the education session reduced the report of pain-related fear. Fear was further reduced during exposure, but not during graded activity. Furthermore, perceived disability was not influenced by the educational session, and only changed during the exposure condition. These results suggest that education may reduce distress, but does not change patients' behaviors. Taken together, this emerging evidence indicates that graded exposure to movement can be an effective treatment in patients with musculoskeletal pain who report substantial pain-related fear.

CHALLENGES AND FUTURE DIRECTIONS

What are the origins of catastrophic beliefs about pain and pain-related fear in patients with chronic musculoskeletal pain? Fears can originate from traumatic experience. Chronic low back pain patients who retrospectively reported a sudden traumatic pain onset scored higher on the TSK than did patients with a gradual onset of pain (Vlaeyen et al. 1995a). Additionally, a large percentage of people with chronic musculoskeletal pain meet DSM-IV criteria for post-traumatic stress disorder (Asmundson et al. 1998). Fearful appraisals about pain may be fueled by intense, unexpected, and novel bodily sensations. Pain-related fear may also be influenced by external information from the social environment. Significant others, including health care providers, may verbally and nonverbally convey the message that there might be something dangerously wrong with the back. It is likely that this threatening information will be incorporated into the individual's personal beliefs and convictions. Rainville conjectured that "Patients' attitudes and beliefs (and thereby patients' disability levels) may be derived from the projected attitudes and beliefs of health care providers" (Rainville et al. 1995). Empirical studies seem to support this idea. A recent study showed that therapists with a biomechanical view on back pain scored daily physical activities as more harmful and were less likely to recommend return to daily life activities as compared to the more behaviorally oriented therapists. This finding suggests that some health care providers are also fearful about their patients' vulnerability to re-injury (Houben et al., in press). Health care providers with higher levels of such fears also have an increased risk for believing sick leave to be a good treatment, for not providing good information about activities, and for being uncertain about identifying patients at risk for developing persistent pain problems (Linton et al. 2002b).

SUMMARY AND CONCLUSIONS

Pain-related fear can best be considered a normal response to unusual threatening information from inside or outside the body. The accumulating evidence that pain-related fear may be more disabling than pain itself refutes the early notion that the lowered ability to accomplish tasks of daily living in chronic pain patients is merely the consequence of pain severity. Possible mechanisms of pain-related fear include: (1) catastrophic misinterpretations of bodily sensations, possibly influenced by health care providers' orientation towards pain; (2) avoidance and escape behaviors as major action tendencies associated with fear; and (3) hypervigilance that in itself may amplify the pain experience. These mechanisms have important clinical implications. Assessment of pain-related fear and of patients' current concerns is warranted. Reliable and well-validated measures are now available, and presentation of visual materials such as pictures of back-stressing activities and movements appear quite helpful in establishing a hierarchy of idiosyncratic fear stimuli. Fear-reduction techniques, of which exposure to back-stressing movements appears the most powerful, may help customizing cognitive-behavioral interventions for chronic musculoskeletal pain. A number of unresolved issues merit future research attention. These include the origins of pain-related fear, the role of illness information and feedback from medical specialists and therapists about diagnostic test results, the early identification of individuals with pain-related fear, the relationship between pain-related fear and aspects of muscular disuse and reactivation, and finally, the evaluation of the long-term effects of fear reduction techniques in patients with chronic pain who suffer from pain-related fear.

REFERENCES

Al-Obaidi SM, Nelson RM, Al-Awadhi S, Al-Shuwaie N. The role of anticipation and fear of pain in the persistence of avoidance behavior in patients with chronic low back pain. *Spine* 2000; 25:1126–1131.

American Psychiatric Association. *Diagnostic and Statistical Manual of Mental Disorders,* 4th ed. Washington, DC: American Psychiatric Association, 2000.

Arntz A, van Eck M, Heijmans M. Predictions of dental pain: the fear of any expected evil, is worse than the evil itself. *Behav Res Ther* 1990; 28:29–41.

Arntz A, Dreessen L, De Jong P. The influence of anxiety on pain: attentional and attributional mediators. *Pain* 1994; 56:307–314.

Asmundson GJ, Kuperos JL, Norton GR. Do patients with chronic pain selectively attend to pain-related information? Preliminary evidence for the mediating role of fear. *Pain* 1997; 72:27–32.

Asmundson GJ, Norton GR, Allerdings MD, Norton PJ, Larsen DK. Posttraumatic stress disorder and work-related injury. *J Anxiety Disord* 1998; 12:57–69.

Asmundson GJ, Norton PJ, Norton GR. Beyond pain: the role of fear and avoidance in chronicity. *Clin Psychol Rev* 1999; 19:97–119.

Bantick SJ, Wise RG, Ploghaus A, et al. Imaging how attention modulates pain in humans using functional MRI. *Brain* 2002; 125:310–319.

Barlow DH. *Anxiety and its Disorders: The Nature and Treatment of Anxiety and Panic.* New York: Guilford Press, 2002.

Beecher HK. *Measurement of Subjective Responses: Quantitative Effects of Drugs.* New York: Oxford University Press, 1959.

Bortz WM. The disuse syndrome. *West J Med* 1984; 141:691–694.

Buchbinder R, Jolley D, Wyatt M. 2001 Volvo award winner in clinical studies: effects of a media campaign on back pain beliefs and its potential influence on management of low back pain in general practice. *Spine* 2001; 26:2535–2542.

Buer N, Linton SJ. Fear-avoidance beliefs and catastrophizing: occurrence and risk factor in back pain and ADL in the general population. *Pain* 2002; 99:485–491.

Burns JW, Mullen JT, Higdon LJ, Wei JM, Lansky D. Validity of the pain anxiety symptoms scale (PASS): prediction of physical capacity variables. *Pain* 2000; 84:247–252.

Burton AK, Waddell G, Tillotson KM, Summerton N. Information and advice to patients with back pain can have a positive effect. A randomized controlled trial of a novel educational booklet in primary care. *Spine* 1999; 24:2484–2491.

Coia P, Morley S. Medical reassurance and patients' responses. *J Psychosom Res* 1998; 45:377–386.

Crombez G, Eccleston C, Baeyens F, Eelen P. The disruptive nature of pain: an experimental investigation. *Behav Res Ther* 1996a; 34:911–918.

Crombez G, Vervaet L, Baeyens F, Lysens R, Eelen P. Do pain expectancies cause pain in chronic low back patients? A clinical investigation. *Behav Res Ther* 1996b; 34:919–925.

Crombez G, Eccleston C, Baeyens F, Eelen P. When somatic information threatens, catastrophic thinking enhances attentional interference. *Pain* 1998a; 75:187–198.

Crombez G, Vervaet L, Lysens R, Baeyens F, Eelen P. Avoidance and confrontation of painful, back-straining movements in chronic back pain patients. *Behav Modif* 1998b; 22:62–77.

Crombez G, Vlaeyen JW, Heuts PH, Lysens R. Pain-related fear is more disabling than pain itself: evidence on the role of pain-related fear in chronic back pain disability. *Pain* 1999; 80:329–339.

de Jong J, Vlaeyen J, Geilen M, Heuts P. Fear of movement/(re)injury in chronic low back pain: education or exposure in vivo as mediator to fear reduction? *Abstracts: 10th World Congress on Pain.* Seattle: IASP Press, 2002, p 71.

Donovan JL, Blake DR. Qualitative study of interpretation of reassurance among patients attending rheumatology clinics: "just a touch of arthritis, doctor?" *BMJ* 2000; 320:541–544.

Eccleston C, Crombez G. Pain demands attention: a cognitive-affective model of the interruptive function of pain. *Psychol Bull* 1999; 125:356–366.

Eccleston C, Crombez G, Aldrich S, Stannard C. Attention and somatic awareness in chronic pain. *Pain* 1997; 72:209–215.

Fritz JM, George SZ, Delitto A. The role of fear-avoidance beliefs in acute low back pain: relationships with current and future disability and work status. *Pain* 2001; 94:7–15.

Goubert L, Crombez G, Vlaeyen JWS, et al. De Tampa schaal voor kinesiofobie: psychometrische karakteristieken en normering [The Tampa scale for kinesiophobia: psychometric properties and norms]. *Gedrag en Gezondheid* 2000; 28:54–62.

Goubert L, Francken G, Crombez G, Vansteenwegen D, Lysens R. Exposure to physical movement in chronic back pain patients: no evidence for generalization across different movements. *Behav Res Ther* 2002; 40:415–429.

Hadjistavropoulos HD, LaChapelle DL. Extent and nature of anxiety experienced during physical examination of chronic low back pain. *Behav Res Ther* 2000; 38:13–29.

Houben RMA, Vlaeyen JWS, Peters ML, et al. Health care providers' attitudes and beliefs towards common low back pain. Factor structure and psychometric properties of the HC-PAIRS. *Clin J Pain;* in press.

Indahl A, Haldorsen EH, Holm S, Reikeras O, Ursin H. Five-year follow-up study of a controlled clinical trial using light mobilization and an informative approach to low back pain. *Spine* 1998; 23:2625–2630.

Jensen MP, Karoly P. Pain-specific beliefs, perceived symptom severity, and adjustment to chronic pain. *Clin J Pain* 1992; 8:123–130.

Jensen MP, Turner JA, Romano JM, Lawler BK. Relationship of pain-specific beliefs to chronic pain adjustment. *Pain* 1994; 57:301–309.

Keogh E, Ellery D, Hunt C, Hannent I. Selective attentional bias for pain-related stimuli amongst pain fearful individuals. *Pain* 2001; 91:91–100.

Kori SH, Miller RP, Todd DD. Kinesiophobia: a new view of chronic pain behavior. *Pain Manage* 1990; Jan/Feb:35–43.

Kugler K, Wijn J, Geilen M, de Jong J, Vlaeyen JWS. *The Photograph Series of Daily Activities (PHODA).* CD-Rom version 1.0. Heerlen: Institute for Rehabilitation Research and School for Physiotherapy, 1999. Available from phoda@hszuyd.nl.

Lang PJ. Presidential address, 1978. A bio-informational theory of emotional imagery. *Psychophysiology* 1979; 16:495–512.

Lang PJ, Bradley MM, Cuthbert BN. Emotion and motivation: measuring affective perception. *J Clin Neurophysiol* 1998; 15:397–408.

Lethem J, Slade PD, Troup JD, Bentley G. Outline of a fear-avoidance model of exaggerated pain perception. *Behav Res Ther* 1983; 21:401–408.

Linton SJ, Overmeer T, Janson M, Vlaeyen JWS, de Jong JR. Graded in vivo exposure treatment for fear-avoidant pain patients with functional disability: a case study. *Cog Behav Ther* 2002a; 31:49–58.

Linton SJ, Vlaeyen J, Ostelo R. The back pain beliefs of health care providers: are we fear-avoidant? *J Occup Rehabil* 2002b; 12:223–232.

Mannion AF, Muntener M, Taimela S, Dvorak J. A randomized clinical trial of three active therapies for chronic low back pain. *Spine* 1999; 24:2435–2448.

Mannion AF, Junge A, Taimela S, et al. Active therapy for chronic low back pain: part 3. Factors influencing self-rated disability and its change following therapy. *Spine* 2001; 26:920–929.

McCracken LM, Dhingra L. A short version of the Pain Anxiety Symptoms Scale (PASS-20): preliminary development and validity. *Pain Res Manage* 2002; 7:45–50.

McCracken LM, Zayfert C, Gross RT. The Pain Anxiety Symptoms Scale: development and validation of a scale to measure fear of pain. *Pain* 1992; 50:67–73.

McCracken LM, Gross RT, Sorg PJ, Edmands TA. Prediction of pain in patients with chronic low back pain: effects of inaccurate prediction and pain-related anxiety. *Behav Res Ther* 1993; 31:647–652.

McCracken LM, Gross RT, Aikens J, Carnrike Jr CL. The assessment of anxiety and fear in persons with chronic pain: a comparison of instruments. *Behav Res Ther* 1996; 34:927–933.

McCracken LM, Faber SD, Janeck AS. Pain-related anxiety predicts non-specific physical complaints in persons with chronic pain. *Behav Res Ther* 1998; 32:621–630.

McDonald IG, Daly J, Jelinek VM, Panetta F, Gutman JM. Opening Pandora's box: the unpredictability of reassurance by a normal test result. *BMJ* 1996; 313:329–332.

McQuade KJ, Turner JA, Buchner DM. Physical fitness and chronic low back pain: an analysis of the relationships among fitness, functional limitations, and depression. *Clin Orthop* 1988; 233:198–204.

Moore JE, Von Korff M, Cherkin D, Saunders K, Lorig K. A randomized trial of a cognitive-behavioral program for enhancing back pain self care in a primary care setting. *Pain* 2000; 88:145–153.

Peters ML, Vlaeyen JW, van Drunen C. Do fibromyalgia patients display hypervigilance for innocuous somatosensory stimuli? Application of a body scanning reaction time paradigm. *Pain* 2000; 86:283–292.

Peters ML, Vlaeyen JW, Kunnen AM. Is pain-related fear a predictor of somatosensory hypervigilance in chronic low back pain patients? *Behav Res Ther* 2002; 40:85–103.

Pfingsten M, Leibing E, Harter W. Fear-avoidance behavior and anticipation of pain in patients with chronic low back pain: a randomized controlled study. *Pain Med* 2002; 2:259–266.

Philips HC. Avoidance behaviour and its role in sustaining chronic pain. *Behav Res Ther* 1987; 25:273–279.

Philips HC, Grant L. The evolution of chronic back pain problems: a longitudinal study. *Behav Res Ther* 1991; 29:435–441.

Picavet SJ, Vlaeyen JWS, Schouten J. Pain catastrophizing and kinesiophobia: predictors of chronic low back pain. *Am J Epidemiol* 2002; 156:1028–1034.

Rachman S. *Anxiety.* Hove: Psychology Press, 1998.

Rachman S, Arntz AR. The overprediction and underprediction of pain. *Clin Psychol Rev* 1991; 11:339–355.

Rainville J, Bagnall D, Phalen L. Health care providers' attitudes and beliefs about functional impairments and chronic back pain. *Clin J Pain* 1995; 11:287–295.

Reiss S. Theoretical perspectives on the fear of anxiety. *Clin Psychol Rev* 1987; 7:585–596.

Riley JF, Ahern DK, Follick MJ. Chronic pain and functional impairment: assessing beliefs about their relationship. *Arch Phys Med Rehabil* 1988; 69:579–582.

Romano JM, Turner JA. Chronic pain and depression: does the evidence support a relationship? *Psychol Bull* 1985; 97:18–34.

Sternbach RA. *Pain Patients: Traits and Treatment.* New York: Academic Press, 1974.

Sullivan MJL, Bishop SR, Pivik J. The pain catastrophizing scale: development and validation. *Psychol Assess* 1995; 7:524–532.

Van den Hout JH, Vlaeyen JW, Houben RM, Soeters AP, Peters ML. The effects of failure feedback and pain-related fear on pain report, pain tolerance, and pain avoidance in chronic low back pain patients. *Pain* 2001; 92:247–257.

Van den Hout JHC, Vlaeyen JWS, Heuts PH, Zijlema JHL, Wijnen JAG. Secondary prevention of work-related disability in non-specific low back pain: a randomized clinical trial, evaluating problem solving therapy when added to behavioral graded activity. *Clin J Pain;* in press.

Vlaeyen JW, Linton SJ. Fear-avoidance and its consequences in chronic musculoskeletal pain: a state of the art. *Pain* 2000; 85:317–332.

Vlaeyen JW, Kole-Snijders AM, Boeren RG, van Eek H. Fear of movement/(re)injury in chronic low back pain and its relation to behavioral performance. *Pain* 1995a; 62:363–372.

Vlaeyen JW, Kole-Snijders AMJ, Rotteveel AM, Ruesink R, et al. The role of fear of movement/(re)injury in pain disability. *J Occup Rehabil* 1995b; 5:235–252.

Vlaeyen JW, de Jong J, Geilen M, Heuts PH; van Breukelen G. Graded exposure in vivo in the treatment of pain-related fear: a replicated single-case experimental design in four patients with chronic low back pain. *Behav Res Ther* 2001; 39:151–166.

Vlaeyen JW, De Jong J, Geilen M, Heuts PH, Van Breukelen G. The treatment of fear of movement/(re)injury in chronic low back pain: further evidence on the effectiveness of exposure in vivo. *Clin J Pain* 2002a; 18:251–261.

Vlaeyen JW, de Jong JR, Onghena P, Kerckhoffs-Hanssen M, Kole-Snijders AMJ. Can pain-related fear be reduced? The application of cognitive-behavioral exposure in vivo. *Pain Res Manage* 2002b; 7:144–153.

Vlaeyen JW, de Jong JR, Sieben JM, Crombez G. Graded exposure in vivo for pain-related fear. In: Turk DC, Gatchel RJ (Eds). *Psychological Approaches to Pain Management. A Practitioner's Handbook.* New York: Guilford, 2002c, pp 210–233.

Von Korff M, Moore JC. Stepped care for back pain: activating approaches for primary care. *Ann Intern Med* 2001; 134:911–917.

Waddell G, Newton M, Henderson I, Somerville D, Main CJ. A Fear-Avoidance Beliefs Questionnaire (FABQ) and the role of fear-avoidance beliefs in chronic low back pain and disability. *Pain* 1993; 52:157–168.

Correspondence to: Johan W.S. Vlaeyen, PhD, Department of Medical, Clinical, and Experimental Psychology, Maastricht University, P.O.Box 616, 6200 MD Maastricht, The Netherlands. Email: j.vlaeyen@dep.unimaas.nl.

Proceedings of the 10th World Congress on Pain,
Progress in Pain Research and Management, Vol. 24,
edited by Jonathan O. Dostrovsky, Daniel B. Carr, and
Martin Koltzenburg, IASP Press, Seattle, © 2003.

54

Self, Identity, and Acceptance in Chronic Pain[1]

Geert Crombez,[a] Stephen Morley,[b] Lance McCracken,[c] Tom Sensky,[d,e] and Tamar Pincus[f]

[a]Department of Experimental Clinical and Health Psychology, Faculty of Psychology and Educational Sciences, Ghent University, Ghent, Belgium; [b]Department of Clinical Psychology, School of Medicine, University of Leeds, Leeds, United Kingdom; [c]Pain Management Unit, Royal National Hospital for Rheumatic Disease, University of Bath, Bath, United Kingdom; [d]Department of Psychological Medicine, Imperial College, London, United Kingdom; [e]West Middlesex University Hospital, Isleworth, Middlesex, United Kingdom; [f]Department of Psychology, Royal Holloway Hospital, University of London, Egham, United Kingdom

Chronic pain is associated with suffering and disability. Although the terms *pain, suffering,* and *disability* are often used interchangeably, they are not synonymous. *Suffering* occurs when the person perceives impending harm (Cassell 1982). It continues until the threat of harm has passed or until the integrity of the person can be restored in some other manner. *Disability* is the difficulty experienced in accomplishing tasks of daily living. The person most often values these tasks because they relate to core beliefs, expectations, aspirations, and life goals. Therefore, chronic pain is more than a simple threat to physical integrity and a cause of disability. It is a threat to self and identity: pain threatens "who I am" and "who I want to be" and places restrictions on "what I might become."

To cope with the threat to self, patients try to solve the problem of pain by seeking curative treatment and analgesia. When chronic pain cannot be managed in these ways, patients sometimes resort to self-management and must learn additional strategies to cope with pain. Active coping strategies, such as problem solving and attentional control over pain, are often considered

[1] Based on a Congress workshop.

superior to other forms of coping. In chronic pain, the efficacy of most of these coping techniques is temporary and limited. Ongoing unsuccessful attempts to control the pain may fuel further feelings of frustration and distress, which become part of the problem of chronic pain. Aldrich et al. (2000) have argued that an exclusive and unsuccessful search for a medical solution may be conceptualized as misdirected problem-solving and may result in more suffering and a poorer quality of life. It has been proposed that coping should be redirected at accepting pain and changing the self instead of the pain (e.g., Schmitz et al. 1996).

Despite the clear importance of self in chronic pain, hardly any systematic research had addressed this issue (but see Large 1985; Large and Strong 1997). In psychology, however, the study of self is not new. Issues related to self were central early on in psychology, and the concept of self is at the core of traditional views of personality. At the broadest level, the self consists of attributes or characteristics that are consciously acknowledged by the individual through language. It is the answer to the open-ended question "Who am I?" Surely, the answer will not be simple, and will consist of a set of attributes reflecting the sense of adequacy across diverse domains such as cognitive competence (e.g., "I am smart"), athletic competence (e.g., "I'm good at swimming), and social competence (e.g., "I'm a caring parent"). The aims of this chapter are therefore to introduce and summarize a new area in the study of chronic pain. First, we introduce different ways to understand the self. Second, we discuss the implications of these concepts for the process of therapeutic change and possibilities for research.

THEORETICAL APPROACHES TO SELF

A SOCIAL-COGNITIVE VIEW

Markus (1977) has stressed the dynamic, social, and multifaceted nature of the self. The self continually changes as it regulates behavior in a reciprocal process of social interaction. There is not one self, but many selves. Selves may be positive or negative (competent or incompetent), and may exist in the past, present, and future. Markus discussed possible selves as important motivators and bridges between the present and the future. Building upon these ideas, Higgins (1987) developed a theoretical model in which experienced discomfort and suffering are linked to the presence of discrepancies between selves. Self is defined not only in terms of the individual's actual attributes and characteristics (the "actual self"), but also according to those features a person would like to possess or to which he or she aspires (the "ideal self"), and the features a person considers he or she ought to have (the "ought self"). According to Higgins, people are motivated to reduce discrepancies between their actual and ideal selves, and between their actual and ought selves as they give rise to distress (Higgins et al. 1994). Furthermore, the type of discrepancy determines the kind of distress experienced and also influences perception and memory.

The concept of self-discrepancy is of importance in pain research. Indeed, qualitative research by sociologists (e.g., Charmaz 1999) has revealed that chronic pain pushes the actual self away from the expected trajectory of normal development and further distances the actual self from the ideal self. In these studies patients with chronic pain consistently report striving to avoid unwanted aspects of their actual self and to regain their former self. The emotional consequences of failing to achieve this goal are often considerable. One way of regaining positive affect may therefore be the reduction of self-discrepancies by redefining the contents of the ideal self and the ought self.

A BEHAVIORAL VIEW

The behavioral view of self rejects the notion of self as an inner agent or as the essence of who the person is (Skinner 1953). The sense of self is based on self-knowledge or self-awareness, which in turn is a product of language and social circumstances. Hayes and Gregg (2001) propose a contemporary view of self. They suggest a distinction between different senses of self, including a "conceptualized self" and an "observing self."

The "conceptualized self" is similar to common usage of the term. It includes the notions we retain about our personal characteristics and attributes, and our story of who we are by virtue of our life history. Importantly, we are expected and expect ourselves to act consistently in relation to these self-descriptive attributes. Otherwise we may be accused of "not being our self" (Hayes et al. 1999). A problem may arise when people overidentify with their "conceptualized self" (Hayes and Gregg 2001).

The behavioral processes involved in overidentification with the conceptualized self are beyond the scope of this short description (see Hayes et al. 1999; Hayes and Gregg 2001). Suffice it to say that the conceptualized self is then sensed as the essence of who the person is, or as a living person. Naturally, any threats to the attributes of the conceptualized self will feel like a fundamental threat to the living person. The person may rigidly defend any threats to the contents of the conceptualized self, including denying or avoiding reality, and generally resisting change (Hayes et al. 1999). Obviously, chronic pain leads to significant changes in behavior, thinking, and feeling: the cherished self-descriptions can no longer be true to the same extent and in the same way as before the presence of chronic pain. The conceptualized self becomes discrepant with reality and impossible to maintain.

The "observing self" described by Hayes and Gregg (2001) is what gives the person the ability to respond to his or her own responding. It allows awareness of thoughts and feelings as the material of personal identity without preoccupation with their content (Hayes et al. 1999). The observing self is therefore distinct from the conceptualized self, but provides the ability to report on events relevant to the conceptualized self. The sense of an observing self is incorporated into many other traditions and therapy approaches such as Zen Buddhism, Mindfulness Meditation approaches (Kabat-Zinn 1990), and Metacognitive Awareness (Teasdale et al. 1995). The usefulness of the observing self is that it allows the person to recognize and experience a sense of self separate from the content of one's thoughts and feelings about one's identity. This ability makes threats to that content less threatening to the functioning of the person.

IMPLICATIONS AND APPLICATIONS FOR CHRONIC PAIN

The two described approaches to self have not been fully developed within the field of pain, although we believe that the study of self in pain is an emerging area. This chapter describes advances in the theoretical understanding of self in chronic pain, introduces tools to assess self in chronic pain for both research and practice, and discusses the clinical implications for the process of therapeutic change.

ENMESHMENT

In the field of social cognition and abnormal psychology, experimental tasks have been developed to investigate how individuals bias the processing of information with reference to the self (e.g., Gemar et al. 2001). In a typical memory bias paradigm (e.g., Pincus et al. 1995), participants are presented with a series of words that might be used to describe personal characteristics. Words are representative of various domains, such as pain, health, and affective state. The task is to indicate whether or not the word belongs to the self, or to another person such as one's best friend. Finally, the participant is asked to recall as many words as possible. The presence of a memory bias is indicated by the increased recall of the words from one or more particular domains. The main finding of the study by Pincus et al. (1995) was that patients with pain and elevated depression scores showed a bias toward negative pain words but not toward negative depression words.

Recently, Pincus and Morley (2001) reviewed the evidence for information processing biases in chronic pain. They suggested that the pattern of results could be best understood as the consequence of the interaction of three relatively stable sets of interconnected knowledge, attributes, or characteristics, labeled as the self schema, the pain schema, and the illness/health schema. According to the model, chronic pain patients with poor psychological adjustment show a pattern of "enmeshment," so that information about the pain schema and the illness schema is essentially interconnected with more fundamental negatively charged information about the self. In contrast to this situation, patients who are better adjusted are able to maintain a separation between core attributes of the self-schema and characteristics relating to the pain schema and the illness schema.

DEVELOPING ASSESSMENTS FOR RESEARCH AND CLINICAL USE

The enmeshment model suggests that pain patients who are "enmeshed" and therefore distressed show a closer interconnection between characteristics of the self-schema and the pain schema. Morley and his colleagues (Barton and Morley 1999) have begun to explore this idea. They have developed a stem-completion task to test hypotheses concerning the specificity of cognitive content in depression. Patients are asked to complete short sentence stems in their own words. The completions are then coded for their degree of affective "valence" and content. Persons with a diagnosis of depression are more likely to make negative completions related to self, others, and the future, as predicted by Beck's model of depression (Beck et al. 1979). Preliminary studies of persons with chronic pain with and without depression (Clyde et al. 2002) show that this methodology can tap into the cognitive content of pain patients. As predicted, the number of negative completions made by pain sufferers is proportional to the severity of their depression. However, the content of the completions did not map onto the domains predicted by Beck's model of depression. As predicted by the enmeshment model, the self was negatively related to characteristics of the illness schema and the pain schema.

Morley and his colleagues (2003) have also used a modified measure of self-discrepancy in which patients with chronic pain generated descriptions of their actual self, their "hoped-for" self (a combination of attributes of the ought and ideal selves), and the "feared-for" self (the representation of attributes and characteristics they wish to avoid). Participants made judgments of whether their hoped-for and feared-for selves were contingent on the presence and absence of pain, respectively. This latter judgment is considered an assessment of the extent to which the self-schema is enmeshed with the pain schema. This experiment revealed that depressive mood was best predicted by the discrepancy between the actual self and the hoped-for self and by the extent of enmeshment, more than could be accounted for by demographic variables, pain severity, and disability.

It is clear from the above that increased focus on the self by researchers and clinicians can improve understanding of suffering in chronic pain. Although references to suffering are ubiquitous in the pain literature, there is very little published work on how to quantify it. Büchi and colleagues (1998) have developed a tool called PRISM (Pictorial Representation of Self and Illness Measure) as a quantitative measure of suffering (Büchi et al. 2002). In essence, the patient is presented with a white A4-sized board with a 6-cm yellow circle in one corner. The patient is asked to imagine that the board represents his or her life as it is currently, and the yellow disk represents the self. The patient is then handed a red disk, 4 cm in diameter, and asked to imagine that it represents the illness. The patient is asked: "Where would you put the illness disk to show its importance in your life at the moment?" The quantitative measure derived from PRISM is the distance between the self disk and the illness disk. This index is inversely related to pain intensity as well as to the magnitude of depressive symptoms, and appears to reflect the intrusiveness of the illness in the person's life (Büchi et al. 1998, 2002). PRISM can be useful clinically in understanding the relationships between the patient, his or her illness, and other facets of the person's life (Büchi and Sensky 1999). Used in this way, PRISM is an aid to better understand the individual's suffering in the context of his or her illness narrative.

ACCEPTANCE AS A FOCUS FOR TREATMENT

In the behavioral view on self, we have argued that people might overidentify with their conceptualized self. If so, they will tend to see the content of the conceptualized self as the essence of who they are, and not simply as thoughts and feelings. Chronic pain is likely to be an extremely distressing experience when this is the case. People will compare their selves before and after the onset of pain and wish to reclaim their old selves. As mentioned, they may avoid the threat that confronts them, seek additional cures for pain despite repeated failure to find one, and suffer from avoidance of life circumstances that could provide different but satisfying opportunities.

The behavioral senses of self described above are integrated into a therapy approach called Acceptance and Commitment Therapy (Hayes et al. 1999). This approach aims to reduce overidentification with the cognitive and emotional content of the conceptualized self, to reduce attempts to control unwanted thoughts and feelings, and to increase healthy behavior. It neutralizes threats to the conceptualized self by showing that they need not be relevant to healthy functioning. The sense of the observing self can be enhanced in therapy to provide the person with a stable sense of self, aware of but less influenced by threatening emotional circumstances. When one is seeing one's experience from the perspective of an observer in this way, private experiences are no longer as threatening. People need not act fully consistently with how they think or feel; they are free to act in the way that works best for them according to their important goals (Hayes et al. 1999).

Acceptance of unwanted experience is increasingly considered a useful solution for behavior problems where efforts to control the problem fail. This notion has been applied to chronic pain with encouraging initial results. Acceptance of chronic pain is defined simply as living with pain, experiencing it without reaction, disapproval, or the need to change it (McCracken 1999; Risdon et al. 2003). McCracken (1998) showed that acceptance of chronic pain is associated with lower pain intensity, less pain-related anxiety and avoidance, less depression, less disability, more daily activity, and better work status. Acceptance is better than pain severity or depression at discriminating dysfunctional chronic pain sufferers from adaptive copers (McCracken et al. 1999). Preliminary analyses from a sample of 70 chronic pain sufferers attending an interdisciplinary pain management center show that increased acceptance during the course of treatment substantially predicts improved disability and mood and decreased anxiety and avoidance (McCracken et al. 2002).

CONCLUSIONS

The experience of chronic illness in general and of pain in particular inevitably leads a person to reappraise his or her self. This chapter has introduced different theoretical accounts of the self and outlined their implications for theory, research, and practice. The concepts outlined offer a framework for better understanding of self and identity in chronic pain. Models derived from social psychology and abnormal psychology focus upon the emotional consequences of self-discrepancies and the devastating effects of enmeshment of the self with pain and illness. The behavioral model stresses that these self-discrepancies arise from an overidentification with the conceptualized self. These models have divergent implications for treatment. The social/abnormal psychology model might involve a redefinition of possible selves (the ideal self, ought self, and hoped-for self). It is clear that such a redefinition will not be a single act, but an endpoint of negotiation within the social niche. According to the behavioral model, the conceptualized self may be redefined as self-descriptions, i.e., thoughts and feelings that should have less impact on the individual. Despite their differences the models show a remarkable degree of overlap. For example, with a well-developed observing self and in the presence of acceptance, enmeshment is less likely, and suffering is reduced. Not only can these models inform clinical practice, but they also generate testable hypotheses to pursue in further research.

In keeping with the cognitive-social model, the models described here view the self as the product of interactions between the person, his or her history, the illness, and the wider context. This multidimensionality is helpful when compared with trait models of the self that take no account of illness or social context. However, these new models also highlight how much more work is required to develop an adequate understanding of self and pain. In particular, almost all the research cited has been conducted in Western societies, and there are prominent cultural components of the response to illness (Sensky 1996) as well as of perceptions of self (Kanagawa et al. 2001).

REFERENCES

Aldrich S, Eccleston C, Crombez G. Worrying about chronic pain: vigilance to threat and misdirected problem solving. *Behav Res Ther* 2000; 38:457–470.

Barton SB, Morley S. Specificity of reference patterns in depressive thinking: agency and object roles in self-representation. *J Abnorm Psychol* 1999; 108:655–661.

Beck AT, Rush AJ, Shaw BF, Emery G. *Cognitive Therapy of Depression*. Chichester: John Wiley & Sons, 1979.

Büchi S, Sensky T. PRISM: Pictorial Representation of Illness and Self Measure. A brief nonverbal measure of illness impact and therapeutic aid in psychosomatic medicine. *Psychosomatics* 1999; 40:14–320.

Büchi S, Sensky T, Sharpe L. Timberlake N. Graphic representation of illness: a novel method of measuring patients' perceptions of the impact of illness. *Psychother Psychosom* 1998; 67:222–225.

Büchi S, Buddeberg C, Klaghofer R, et al. Preliminary validation of PRISM (Pictorial Representation of Illness and Self Measure)—a brief method to assess suffering. *Psychother Psychosom* 2002; 71:333–341.

Cassell EJ. The nature of suffering and the goals of medicine. *N Engl J Med* 1982; 306:639–645.

Charmaz K. From the "sick role" to stories of self: understanding the self in illness. In Contrada RJ, Ashmore RD (Eds). *Self, Social Identity, and Physical Health,* Vol. 2. Oxford: Oxford University Press, 1999, pp 209–239.

Clyde Z, Barton SB, Morley S. Sentence completion for depression—an alternative method of measuring depression in chronic pain patients. *Abstracts: 10th World Congress on Pain*. Seattle: IASP Press, 2002, p 575.

Gemar MC, Segal ZV, Sagrati S, Kennedy SJ. Mood-induced changes on the implicit association test in recovered depressed patients. *J Abnorm Psychol* 2001; 110:282–289.

Hayes SC, Gregg J. Functional contextualism and the self. In: Muran JC (Ed). *Self-Relations in the Psychotherapy Process*. Washington, DC: American Psychological Association, 2001, pp 291–307.

Hayes SC, Strosahl KD, Wilson KG. *Acceptance and Commitment Therapy: An Experiential Approach to Behavior Change*. New York: Guilford Press, 1999.

Higgins ET. Self-discrepancy: a theory relating self and affect. *Psychol Rev* 1987; 94:319–340.

Higgins ET, Roney CJ, Crowe E, Hymes C. Ideal versus ought predictions for approach and avoidance: distinct self-regulatory systems. *J Pers Soc Psychol* 1994; 66:276–286.

Kabat-Zinn J. *Full Catastrophe Living*. New York: Delta/Dell Publishing, 1990.

Kanagawa C, Cross SE, Markus HR. "Who am I?" The cultural psychology of the conceptual self. *Pers Soc Psychol Bull* 2001; 27:90–103.

Large R. Self-concepts and illness attitudes in chronic pain: a repertory grid study of a pain management programme. *Pain* 1985; 23:113–119.

Large R, Strong J. The personal constructs of coping with chronic low back pain: is coping a necessary evil? *Pain* 1997; 73:245–252.

Markus H. Self-schemata and processing information about the self. *J Pers Soc Psychol* 1997; 35:63–78.

McCracken LM. Learning to live with the pain: acceptance of pain predicts adjustment in persons with chronic pain. *Pain* 1998; 74:21–27.

McCracken LM. Behavioral constituents of chronic pain acceptance: results from factor analysis of the Chronic Pain Acceptance Questionnaire. *J Back Musculoskeletal Rehab* 1999; 13:93–100.

McCracken LM, Spertus IL, Janeck AS, Sinclair D, Wetzel FT. Behavioral dimensions of adjustment in persons with chronic pain: pain-related anxiety and acceptance. *Pain* 1999; 80:283–289.

McCracken LM, Eccleston C, Bell L. Change in self-management behavior in treatment for chronic pain: the role of reduced struggling with pain. *Abstracts: 10th World Congress on Pain*. Seattle: IASP Press, 2002, p 70.

Morley S, Davies C, Barton SB. "Future possible selves": conditionality and adjustment in chronic pain. *Abstracts: Annual Meeting of the British Pain Society*, Glasgow, 2003.

Pincus T, Morley S. Cognitive processing bias in chronic pain: a review and integration. *Psychol Bull* 2001; 127:599–617.

Pincus T, Pearce S, McClelland A. Endorsement and memory bias of self-referential pain stimuli in pain patients. *Br J Clin Psychol* 1995; 34:267–277.

Risdon A, Eccleston C, Crombez G, McCracken LM. How can we learn to live with pain? A Q-Methodological analysis of the diverse understandings of acceptance of chronic pain. *Soc Sci Med* 2003; 56:375–386.

Schmitz U, Saile H, Nilges P. Coping with chronic pain: flexible goal adjustment as an interactive buffer against pain-related distress. *Pain* 1996; 67:41–51.

Sensky T. Eliciting lay beliefs across cultures: principles and methodology, *Br J Cancer* 1996; 74(Suppl XXIX):S63–S65.

Skinner BF. *Science and Human Behavior*. New York: Free Press, 1953.

Teasdale JD, Segal ZV, Williams JMG. How does cognitive therapy prevent depressive relapse and why should attentional control (mindfulness) help? *Behav Res Ther* 1995; 33:25–39.

Correspondence to: Geert Crombez, PhD, Department of Experimental Clinical and Health Psychology, Faculty of Psychology and Educational Sciences, Ghent University, Henri Dunantlaan 2, 9000 Ghent, Belgium. Email: geert.crombez@rug.ac.be.

Part IX

Specific Clinical Syndromes and Settings

Proceedings of the 10th World Congress on Pain,
Progress in Pain Research and Management, Vol. 24,
edited by Jonathan O. Dostrovsky, Daniel B. Carr, and
Martin Koltzenburg, IASP Press, Seattle, © 2003.

55

Molecular Mechanisms That Generate and Maintain Cancer Pain

Patrick W. Mantyh, Christopher D. Nelson, Molly A. Sevcik, Nancy M. Luger, and Mary Ann C. Sabino

Neurosystems Center and Departments of Preventive Sciences, Psychiatry, Neuroscience, and Cancer Center, University of Minnesota, Minneapolis, Minnesota, USA; and Veterans Affairs Medical Center, Minneapolis, Minnesota, USA

The negative impact that cancer pain has on quality of life cannot be overestimated. As advances in cancer detection and therapy are extending the life expectancy of cancer patients, there is increasing focus on improving their quality of life. Many patients present with pain as the first sign of cancer, and 30–50% of all cancer patients will experience moderate to severe pain (Mercadante 1997; Mercadante and Arcuri 1998; Portenoy and Lesage 1999; Portenoy et al. 1999). Cancer-associated pain can occur at any time during the evolution of the disease, but the frequency and intensity of this pain tend to increase with advancing stages of cancer. Of patients with metastatic or advanced cancer, 75–95% will experience significant, life-altering cancer-induced pain (Mercadante 1997; Mercadante and Arcuri 1998; Portenoy and Lesage 1999; Portenoy et al. 1999).

The treatment of cancer pain can involve a variety of modalities. Therapies targeted at decreasing tumor size are often effective and include radiation, chemotherapy, and surgery. However, these treatments can be burdensome to administer and are accompanied by significant negative side effects. Medications targeted at decreasing inflammation and pain, such as nonsteroidal anti-inflammatory drugs or opiates, can also be very useful, but these too are accompanied by unwanted side effects.

The relative ineffectiveness of current treatments reflects the fact that therapies have not changed for decades (Coyle et al. 1990; Payne 1997; Payne et al. 1998; Hoskin 2000). Largely because of treatment-associated side effects, 45% of cancer patients have inadequate and undermanaged pain control (de Wit et al. 2001; Meuser et al. 2001). A formidable obstacle to the development of new therapies is the fact that the current neurobiological basis for pharmacological treatments is largely empirical, and is based on scientific advances in painful conditions other than those induced by cancer.

Recently, the first animal models of cancer pain have been developed. In the mouse femur model, bone cancer pain is induced by injecting murine osteolytic sarcoma cells into the intramedullary space of the mouse femur (Fig. 1) (Schwei et al. 1999). Critical to this model is ensuring that the tumor cells are confined within the marrow space of the injected femur and that they do not invade adjacent soft tissues, which would directly affect the joints of the muscle, making behavioral analysis problematic (Schwei et al. 1999; Honore et al. 2000a; Luger et al. 2001). Following injection the tumor cells proliferate, and ongoing, movement-evoked, and mechanically evoked pain-related behaviors develop that increase in severity with time (Table I). These pain behaviors correlate with the progressive tumor-induced bone destruction that ensues, which appears to mimic the condition in patients with primary or metastatic bone cancer. These models have allowed us to gain mechanistic insights into how cancer pain is generated and how the sensory information it initiates is processed as it moves from sense organ to the cerebral cortex under a constantly changing molecular architecture. As detailed below, these insights promise to fundamentally change the way cancer pain is controlled.

PRIMARY AFFERENT SENSORY NEURONS

Primary afferent sensory neurons are the gateway by which sensory information from peripheral tissues is transmitted to the spinal cord and brain (Fig. 2), and these neurons innervate the skin and every internal organ of the body, including mineralized bone, marrow, and periosteum. The cell bodies of sensory fibers that innervate the head and body are housed in the trigeminal and dorsal root ganglia, respectively, and can be divided into two major categories: myelinated A fibers and smaller-diameter unmyelinated C fibers. Nearly all large-diameter myelinated Aβ fibers normally conduct non-noxious stimuli applied to the skin, joints, and muscles, and thus these large sensory neurons usually do not conduct noxious stimuli (Djouhri et al. 1998). In contrast, most small-diameter sensory fibers—unmyelinated C fibers and finely myelinated A fibers—are specialized sensory neurons known as nociceptors, whose major function is to detect environmental stimuli that are perceived as harmful and convert them into electrochemical signals that

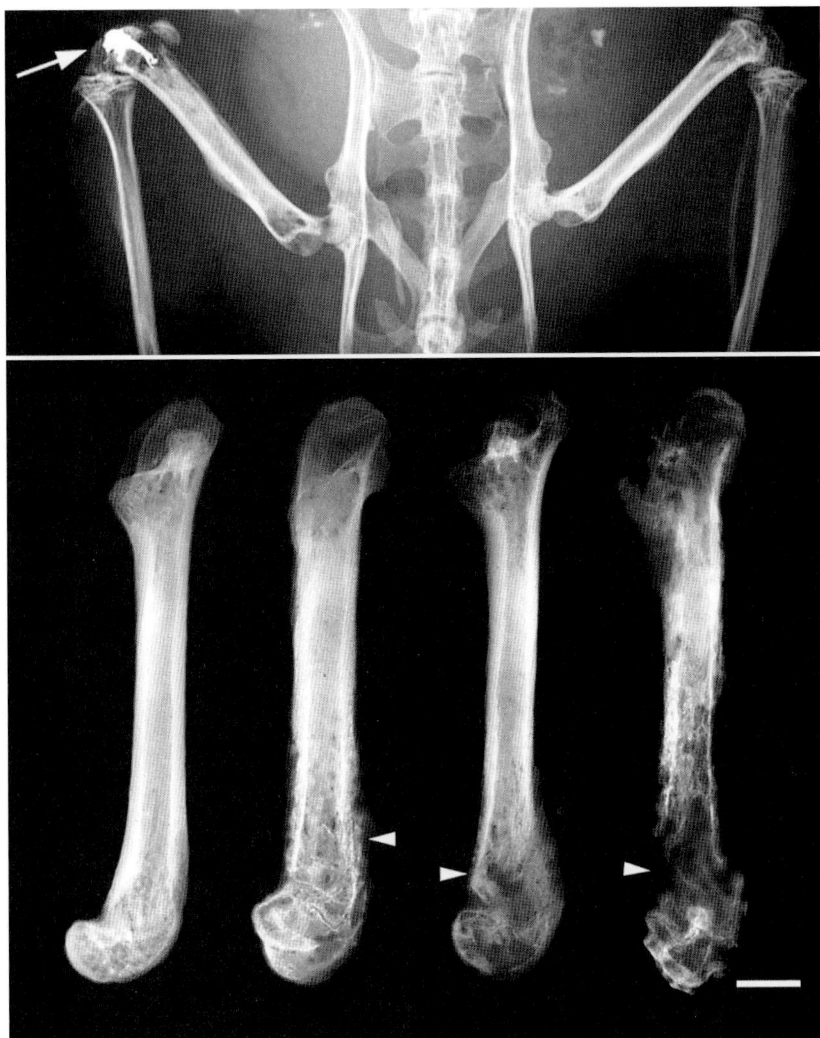

Fig. 1. Progressive destruction of mineralized bone in mice with bone cancer. (A) Low-power anterior-posterior radiograph of mouse pelvis and hindlimbs after a unilateral injection of sarcoma cells into the distal part of the femur and closure of the injection site with an amalgam plug (arrow), which prevents the tumor cells from growing outside the bone (Honore et al. 2000c). Radiographs of murine femora (B) show the progressive loss of mineralized bone caused by tumor growth. These images are representative of the stages of bone destruction in the murine femur. At week 1 there is a minor loss of bone near the distal head (arrow); at week 2, substantial loss of mineralized bone at both the proximal and distal (arrow) heads; and at week 3, loss of mineralized bone throughout the entire femur and fracture of distal head (arrow). Scale bar: 2 mm. Modified from Schwei et al. (1999).

Table I
Development of chronic pain in mice with bone cancer

Pain Behavior	Naive	Sham	Sarcoma Day 6	Sarcoma Day 10	Sarcoma Day 14
I. Ongoing Pain					
Guarding (seconds) over 2-minute observation period	0.4 ± 0.2	1.4 ± 0.5	2.1 ± 0.5	4.3* ± 0.8	15.2* ± 3.3
No. flinches over 2-minute observation period	1.7 ± 0.7	3.1 ± 0.7	7.7 ± 1.6	13.0* ± 2.0	24.5* ± 3.8
II. Movement-evoked Pain					
A. Ambulatory Pain					
Forced ambulation on rotarod: 5 (normal) to 0 (impaired)	4.7 ± 0.3	4.4 ± 0.3	3.8 ± 0.4	2.5* ± 0.3	2.3* ± 0.3
Limb use during normal ambulation: 4 (normal) to 0 (impaired)	4.0 ± 0.0	3.9 ± 0.1	3.7 ± 0.2	3.5* ± 0.3	2.7* ± 0.3
B. Palpation-evoked Pain (over 2-minute period)					
Guarding (seconds) following nonpainful palpation	0.4 ± 0.4	1.4 ± 0.5	1.9 ± 0.6	7.1* ± 0.6	18.1* ± 4.0
No. flinches following nonpainful palpation	2.0 ± 1.2	3.1 ± 0.7	7.0 ± 2.1	19.0* ± 1.1	30.5* ± 5.1

Note: The development of pain behaviors closely follows the time course of tumor growth and tumor-induced bone remodeling seen in Fig. 1. Data are presented as means ± SEM; asterisks (*) denote $P < 0.05$ vs. sham.

are then transmitted to the central nervous system (CNS). Unlike primary sensory neurons involved in vision or olfaction, which are required to detect only one type of sensory stimulus (light or chemical odorants, respectively), individual primary sensory neurons of the pain pathway have the remarkable ability to detect a wide range of stimulus modalities, including those of physical and chemical nature (Basbaum and Jessel 2000; Julius and Basbaum 2001). To accomplish this, nociceptors express an extremely diverse repertoire of transduction molecules that can sense forms of noxious stimulation (thermal, mechanical, and chemical), albeit with varying degrees of sensitivity.

The past few years have seen remarkable progress toward understanding the signaling mechanisms and specific molecules that nociceptors use to detect noxious stimuli. For example, the vanilloid receptor TRPV1 (formerly known as VR1), which is expressed by most nociceptors, detects heat (Kirschstein et al. 1999) and also appears to detect extracellular protons (Bevan and Geppetti 1994; Caterina et al. 2000; Welch et al. 2000) and lipid metabolites (Tominaga et al. 1998; Nagy and Rang 1999). In order to detect noxious mechanical stimuli, nociceptors express mechanically gated channels

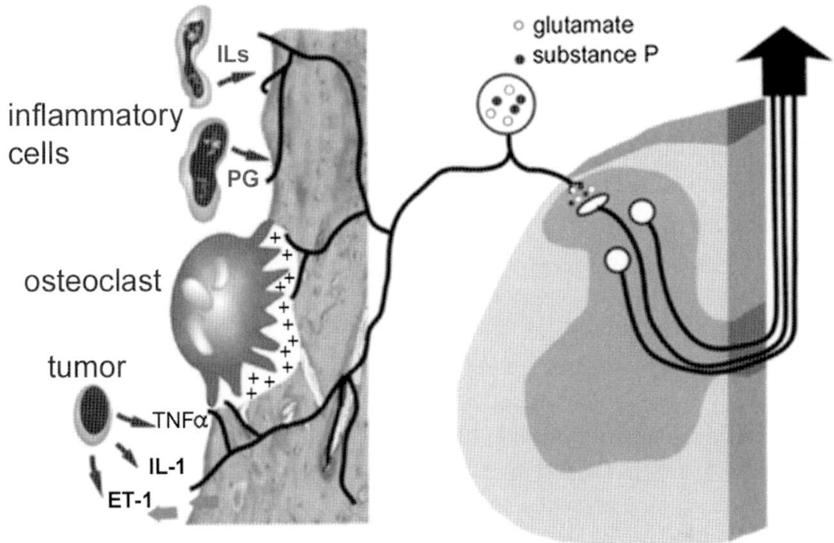

Fig. 2. Sensory neurons and detection of noxious stimuli due to tumor cells. Nociceptors use a diversity of signal-transduction mechanisms to detect noxious physiological stimuli, and many of these mechanisms may be involved in driving cancer pain. Thus, when nociceptors are exposed to products of tumor cells, tissue injury, or inflammation, their excitability is altered and this nociceptive information is relayed to the spinal cord and then to higher centers of the brain. Some of the mechanisms that appear to be involved in generating and maintaining cancer pain include activation of nociceptors by factors such as extracellular protons (+), endothelin-1 (ET-1), interleukins (ILs), prostaglandins (PG), and tumor necrosis factor α (TNF-α).

that initiate a signaling cascade upon excessive stretch (Price et al. 2001). The cells also express several purinergic receptors capable of sensing adenosine triphosphate (ATP), which may be released from cells upon excessive mechanical stimulation (Krishtal et al. 1988; Xu and Huang 2002).

To sense noxious chemical stimuli, nociceptors express a complex array of receptors capable of detecting inflammation-associated factors released from damaged tissue. These factors include protons (Bevan and Geppetti 1994; Caterina et al. 2000), endothelins (Nelson and Carducci 2000), prostaglandins (Alvarez and Fyffe 2000), bradykinin (Alvarez and Fyffe 2000), and nerve growth factor (McMahon 1996). Aside from providing promising targets for the development of more selective analgesics, identification of receptors expressed on the nociceptor surface has increased our understanding of how different tumors generate cancer pain in the peripheral tissues they invade and destroy.

In addition to expressing channels and receptors that detect tissue injury, sensory neurons are highly "plastic," in that they can change their phenotype in the face of a sustained peripheral injury. Following tissue injury, sensory neuron subpopulations alter patterns of signaling peptide and growth factor expression (Woolf and Salter 2000). This change in phenotype of the sensory neuron in part underlies peripheral sensitization, whereby the activation threshold of nociceptors is lowered so that a stimulus that would normally be perceived as mildly noxious is perceived as highly noxious (hyperalgesia). Damage to a peripheral tissue also activates previously "silent" or "sleeping" nociceptors, which then become highly responsive both to normally non-noxious stimuli (allodynia) and to noxious stimuli (hyperalgesia).

There are several examples of nociceptors that undergo peripheral sensitization in experimental cancer models (Schwei et al. 1999; Honore et al. 2000a,c,d; Luger et al. 2001). In normal mice, the neurotransmitter substance P is synthesized by nociceptors and released in the spinal cord in response to a noxious, but not to a non-noxious, palpation of the femur. In mice with bone cancer, normally nonpainful palpation of the affected femur induces the release of substance P from primary afferent fibers that terminate in the spinal cord. Substance P in turn binds to and activates the neurokinin-1 receptor that is expressed by a subset of spinal cord neurons (Mantyh et al. 1995a,b; Hunt and Mantyh 2001). Similarly, normally non-noxious palpation of tumor-bearing limbs of mice with bone cancer also induces the expression of c-Fos protein in spinal cord neurons. In normal animals that do not have cancer, only noxious stimuli will induce the expression of c-Fos in the spinal cord (Hunt et al. 1987). Thus, peripheral sensitization of nociceptors appears to be involved in the generation and maintenance of bone cancer pain.

PROPERTIES OF TUMORS THAT EXCITE NOCICEPTORS

Tumor cells and tumor-associated cells that include macrophages, neutrophils, and T-lymphocytes secrete a wide variety of factors that sensitize or directly excite primary afferent neurons (Fig. 2). These include prostaglandins (Nielsen et al. 1991; Galasko 1995), endothelins (Nelson and Carducci 2000; Davar 2001), interleukins 1 and 6 (Watkins et al. 1995; Leskovar et al. 2000; Opree and Kress 2000), epidermal growth factor (Stoscheck and King 1986), transforming growth factor (Poon et al. 2001; Roman et al. 2001), and platelet-derived growth factor (Daughaday and Deuel 1991; Radinsky 1991; Silver 1992). Receptors for many of these factors are expressed by primary afferent neurons. Each of these factors may play an important role in generating pain in particular forms of cancer, and therapies that block two of these factors, prostaglandins and endothelins, are currently approved for use in patients with other painful, nonmalignant indications.

Prostaglandins are pro-inflammatory lipids that are formed from arachidonic acid by the action of cyclooxygenase (COX) and other downstream synthetases. There are two distinct forms of the COX enzyme, COX-1 and COX-2. Prostaglandins are involved in the sensitization or direct excitation of nociceptors by binding to several prostanoid receptors (Vasko 1995). Several tumor cells and tumor-associated macrophages express high levels of COX-2 and produce large amounts of prostaglandins (Dubois et al. 1996; Molina et al. 1999; Kundu et al. 2001; Ohno et al. 2001; Shappell et al. 2001).

The COX enzymes are a major target of current medications, and nonselective COX inhibitors such as aspirin or ibuprofen are commonly administered for reducing both inflammation and pain. A major problem with using nonselective COX inhibitors to block cancer pain is that these compounds inhibit both COX-1 and COX-2, and inhibition of the constitutively expressed COX-1 can cause gastrointestinal bleeding and ulcers. In contrast, the new selective COX-2 inhibitors, or coxibs, preferentially inhibit COX-2 and avoid many of the side effects of COX-1 inhibition, which may allow their use in treating cancer pain. Other experiments have suggested that COX-2 is involved in angiogenesis and tumor growth (Masferrer et al. 2000; Moore and Simmons 2000), so in cancer patients, in addition to blocking cancer pain, COX-2 inhibitors may have the added advantage of reducing the growth and metastasis of the tumor. COX-2 inhibitors show significant promise for alleviating at least some aspects of cancer pain, although clearly more research is required to fully define the actions of COX-2 in different types of cancer.

A second pharmacological target for treating cancer pain is the peptide endothelin-1. Several tumors, including prostate cancer, express high levels of endothelins (Shankar et al. 1998; Kurbel et al. 1999; Nelson and Carducci 2000), and clinical studies have reported a correlation between the severity of the pain in patients with prostate cancer and plasma levels of endothelins (Nelson et al. 1995). Endothelins could contribute to cancer pain by directly sensitizing or exciting nociceptors, given that a subset of small unmyelinated primary afferent neurons express receptors for endothelin (Pomonis et al. 2001). Direct application of endothelin to peripheral nerves activates primary afferent fibers and induces pain behaviors (Davar et al. 1998). Like prostaglandins, endothelins that are released from tumor cells are also thought be involved in regulating angiogenesis (Dawas et al. 1999) and tumor growth (Asham et al. 1998), suggesting again that endothelin antagonists may be useful not only in inhibiting cancer pain but in reducing the growth and metastasis of the tumor.

TUMOR-INDUCED RELEASE OF PROTONS AND ACIDOSIS

Tumor cells become ischemic and undergo apoptosis as the tumor burden exceeds its vascular supply (Helmlinger et al. 2002). Local acidosis, a state where an accumulation of acid metabolites is present, is a hallmark of tissue injury (Reeh and Steen 1996; Julius and Basbaum 2001). In the past few years the concept that sensory neurons can be directly excited by protons or acidosis has generated intense research and clinical interest. Studies have shown that subsets of sensory neurons express different acid-sensing ion channels (Olson et al. 1998; Julius and Basbaum 2001). The two major classes of acid-sensing ion channels expressed by nociceptors are TRPV1 (Caterina et al. 1997; Tominaga et al. 1998) and the acid-sensing ion channel-3 (ASIC-3) (Bassilana et al. 1997; Olson et al. 1998; Sutherland et al. 2000). Both of these channels are sensitized and excited by a decrease in pH. More specifically, TRPV1 is activated when the pH falls below 6.0, while the pH that activates ASIC-3 appears to be highly dependent on the coexpression of other ASIC channels in the same nociceptor (Lingueglia et al. 1997).

There are several mechanisms by which a decrease in pH could be involved in generating and maintaining cancer pain. As tumors grow, tumor-associated inflammatory cells invade the neoplastic tissue and release protons that generate local acidosis (Helmlinger et al. 2002). A second mechanism by which acidosis may occur is apoptosis of the tumor cells. Release of intracellular ions may generate an acidic environment that activates signaling by acid-sensing channels expressed by nociceptors.

Tumor-induced release of protons and acidosis may be particularly important in the generation of bone cancer pain. In both osteolytic (bone-destroying) and osteoblastic (bone-forming) cancers there is a significant proliferation and hypertrophy of osteoclasts (Clohisy et al. 2000a,b, 2001). Osteoclasts are terminally differentiated, multinucleated cells of the monocyte lineage that are uniquely designed to resorb bone by maintaining an extracellular microenvironment of acidic pH (4.0–5.0) at the interface between osteoclast and mineralized bone (Delaisse and Vaes 1992). Studies have shown significant expression of ASIC (Olson et al. 1998) and TRPV1 (Tominaga et al. 1998; Guo et al. 1999) in peptidergic afferent fibers, and we have localized peptidergic fibers in bone marrow and cortical bone (Mach et al. 2002). This evidence suggests that exposure of these sensory fibers to the osteoclast's acidic extracellular microenvironment could activate resident proton-sensitive ion channels, stimulating pain sensation. Recent experiments in a murine model of bone cancer pain reported that osteoclasts play an essential role in cancer-induced bone loss, and that osteoclasts contribute to the etiology of bone cancer pain (Honore et al. 2000a; Luger et al.

2001). Recent work has shown that osteoprotegerin (Honore et al. 2000a) and a bisphosphonate (Fulfaro et al. 1998; Mannix et al. 2000), both of which are known to induce osteoclast apoptosis, are effective in decreasing osteoclast-induced bone cancer pain. Similarly, TRPV1 or ASIC antagonists may be used to reduce pain in patients with soft-tissue tumors or bone cancer by blocking excitation of the acid-sensitive channels on sensory neurons.

RELEASE OF GROWTH FACTORS BY TUMOR CELLS

One of the most important discoveries in the past decade has been the demonstration that the biochemical and physiological status of sensory neurons is maintained and modified by factors derived from the innervated tissue. Changes in the periphery associated with inflammation, nerve injury, or tissue injury are mirrored by changes in the phenotype of sensory neurons (Honore et al. 2000a,b,c). After peripheral nerve injury, expression of a subset of neurotransmitters and receptors by damaged sensory neurons is altered in a highly predictable fashion. These changes are caused, in part, by a change in the tissue level of several growth factors released from the environment local to the injury site, including nerve growth factors (NGF) (Fu and Gordon 1997; Koltzenburg 1999; Fukuoka et al. 2001) and glial-derived neurotrophic factor (GDNF) (Boucher and McMahon 2001; Hoke et al. 2002). These neurochemical changes can be reversed in a receptor-specific fashion by intrathecal or peripheral application of NGF or GDNF (Verge et al. 1995; Bennett et al. 1996, 1998; Boucher et al. 2000; Ramer et al. 2000).

While it has been reported that the level of NGF expression correlates with the extent of pain in pancreatic cancer (Zhu et al. 1999; Schneider et al. 2001), relatively little is known about how other tumors affect the synthesis and release of growth factors. However, one certainty is that the repertoire of growth factors to which the sensory neuron is exposed will change as the developing tumor invades the peripheral tissue that the neuron innervates. Thus, in addition to a disruption of the growth factors normally released by the intact peripheral tissue, one can expect release of a variety of additional growth factors by tumor cells as well as by tumor-infiltrating leukocytes, which can comprise up to 80% of the total tumor mass (Zhang et al. 2002). Activated leukocytes synthesize and release high levels of several growth factors (Stoscheck and King 1986; Daughaday and Deuel 1991; Radinsky 1991; Silver 1992; Leon et al. 1994; Caroleo et al. 2001; Poon et al. 2001; Roman et al. 2001), and thus one would expect a significant change in the phenotype and response characteristics of the sensory neurons following tumor invasion of a peripheral organ.

While tumor presence alters the invaded tissue, it is also clear that the affected tissue also influences the phenotype of the invading tumor (Mundy 2002). Because the local environment can influence the type of molecules that tumor cells express and release, it follows that the same tumor in the same individual may be painful at one site of metastasis but not at another. Clinical observations reveal that pain from cancer can be quite perplexing because the size, location, or type of cancer tumor does not necessarily predict symptoms. Different patients with the same cancer may have vastly different symptoms. Renal cancer may be painful in one person and asymptomatic in another. Metastases to multiple bones within the same patient may result in pain in one bone, but not in the others. Small cancer deposits in bone may be very painful, while large soft-tissue cancers may be painless (Mantyh et al. 2002). Important areas for future research include identification of tissue-specific mechanisms of cancer pain, comparing soft tissue with bone, as well as site-specific mechanisms, comparing intramembranous bones (ribs) with endochondral bones (femurs). It will also be of interest to determine patient-specific factors that influence disease progression and its relationship to pain perception.

TUMOR-INDUCED DISTENSION AND DESTRUCTION OF SENSORY FIBERS

In general, previous reports have suggested that tumors are not highly innervated by sensory or sympathetic neurons (O'Connell et al. 1998; Seifert and Spitznas 2001; Terada and Matsunaga 2001). However, in many cancers, rapid tumor growth frequently entraps and injures nerves, causing mechanical injury, compression, ischemia, or direct proteolysis (Mercadante 1997). Proteolytic enzymes produced by the tumor can also injure sensory and sympathetic fibers, causing neuropathic pain.

The capacity of a tumor to injure and destroy peripheral nerve fibers has been directly observed in an experimental model of bone cancer. Following injection and containment of lytic murine sarcoma cells in the intramedullary of the mouse femur, tumor cells grow in the marrow space and disrupt innervating sensory fibers. As the tumor cells grow they first compress and then destroy both the hematopoietic cells of the marrow and the sensory fibers that normally innervate the marrow, mineralized bone, and periosteum (Schwei et al. 1999).

While the mechanisms by which any neuropathic pain is generated and maintained are still not well understood, several therapies that have proven useful in the control of other types of neuropathic pain may also be useful in treating tumor-induced neuropathic pain. For example, gabapentin, which was originally developed as an anticonvulsant but whose mechanism of action remains unknown, is effective in treating several forms of neuropathic pain and may also be useful in treating cancer-induced neuropathic pain (Ripamonti and Dickerson 2001).

CENTRAL SENSITIZATION IN CANCER PAIN

A critical question is whether the spinal cord and forebrain also undergo significant neurochemical changes as a chronic cancer pain state develops. The murine cancer pain model revealed extensive neurochemical reorganization within spinal cord segments that receive input from primary afferent neurons innervating the cancerous bone (Honore et al. 2000a,c; Luger et al. 2001). These changes included astrocyte hypertrophy (Fig. 3) and upregulation of the prohyperalgesic peptide dynorphin. Spinal cord neurons that normally would only be activated by noxious stimuli were activated by normally non-noxious stimuli. These spinal cord changes were attenuated by blocking the tumor-induced tissue destruction and pain (Honore et al. 2000a; Luger et al. 2001). Together, these neurochemical changes suggest that cancer pain induces and is at least partially maintained by a state of central sensitization, in which an increased transmission of nociceptive information allows normally non-noxious input to be amplified and perceived as noxious stimuli.

Once nociceptive information has been transmitted to the spinal cord by primary afferent neurons, it can travel via multiple ascending "pain" pathways that project from the spinal cord to higher centers of the brain. Classically, the main emphasis in examining the ascending conduction of pain has been placed on spinothalamic tract neurons. However, data from recent clinical studies have necessitated a reassessment of this position by showing significant attenuation of some forms of difficult-to-control visceral cancer pain following lesion of the axons of nonspinothalamic tract neurons (Willis et al. 1999; Nauta et al. 2000). Together these data suggest that one reason that cancer pain is frequently perceived as such an intense and disturbing pain is that it ascends to higher centers of the brain via multiple parallel neuronal pathways. Importantly for cancer patients, many of whom frequently experience anxiety or depression, it is clear that higher centers of the brain can modulate the ascending conduction of pain. Descending pathways that modulate the ascending conduction of cancer pain may play an important role in either enhancing or inhibiting the patient's perception of pain. The general mood and attention of the patient thus may be significant factors in determining the pain's intensity and degree of unpleasantness.

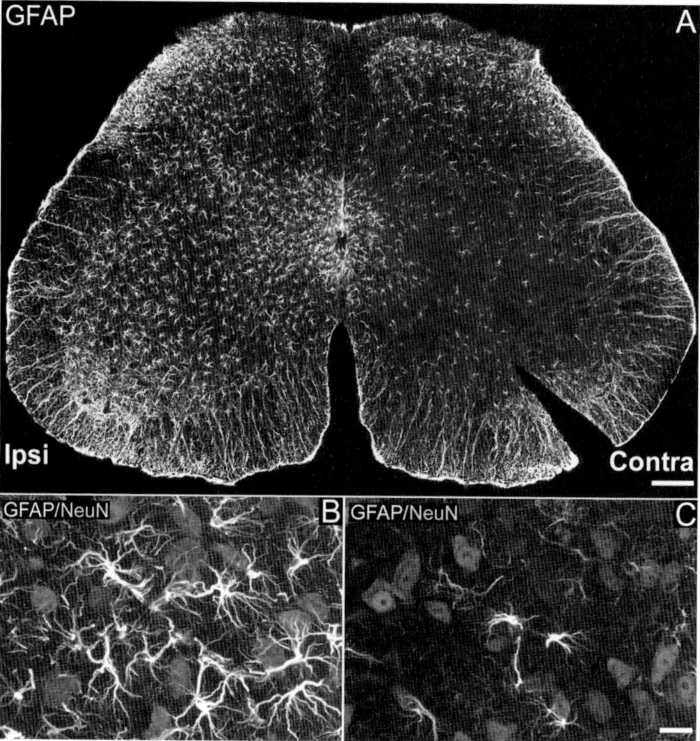

Fig. 3. Cancer-induced reorganization of the CNS. Chronic cancer pain not only sensitizes peripheral nociceptors, but also can induce significant neurochemical reorganization of the spinal cord. This reorganization may participate in the phenomenon of central sensitization, i.e., an increased responsiveness of spinal cord neurons involved in transmission of pain. (A) Confocal image of a coronal section of the mouse L4 spinal cord showing glial fibrillary acidic protein (GFAP)-positive astrocytes (white) which have undergone hypertrophy on the side ipsilateral to the tumor-bearing bone. Panels B and C show higher magnification of the ipsilateral and contralateral dorsal horn seen in panel A, with colocalization of the neuron-specific antibody NeuN. Note that while the astrocytes (spindle-shaped cells) have undergone a massive hypertrophy, there does not appear to be any significant loss of Neu-N positive neurons. Scale bars: A, 200 μm; B and C, 30 μm. Modified from Schwei et al. (1999).

A CHANGING SET OF FACTORS MAY DRIVE CANCER PAIN AS THE DISEASE PROGRESSES

Cancer pain frequently becomes more severe as the disease progresses, and adequate control of cancer pain becomes more difficult to achieve without encountering significant unwanted side effects (Payne 1998; Foley 1999; Portenoy and Lesage 1999). While tolerance may contribute to the escalation of the dose of analgesics required to control cancer pain, a compatible possibility is that with the progression of the disease, different factors assume a greater importance in driving cancer pain. For example, in the mouse model of bone cancer, as tumor cells first begin to proliferate, pain-related behaviors start to occur long before any significant bone destruction is evident. This pain may be due to prohyperalgesic factors such as prostaglandins and endothelin that are released by the growing tumor cells and subsequently activate nociceptors in the marrow. Pain at this stage might be attenuated by COX-2 inhibitors and endothelin antagonists. As the tumor continues to grow, sensory neurons innervating the marrow are compressed and destroyed, causing a neuropathic pain to develop that may best respond to treatment with drugs such as gabapentin that are known to attenuate noncancer-induced neuropathic pain. When the tumor begins to induce proliferation and hypertrophy of osteoclasts, the pain due to excessive osteoclast activity might be largely blocked by anti-osteoclastogenic drugs such as bisphosphonates or osteoprotegerin (Fig. 4). As the tumor cells completely fill the intramedullary space, tumor cells begin to die, generating an acidic environment; antagonists to TRPV1 or ASICs may attenuate the pain induced by this acidosis. Finally, as bone destruction compromises the mechanical strength of the bone, antagonists that block the mechanically gated channels and/or ATP receptors in the richly innervated periosteum may attenuate movement-evoked pain.

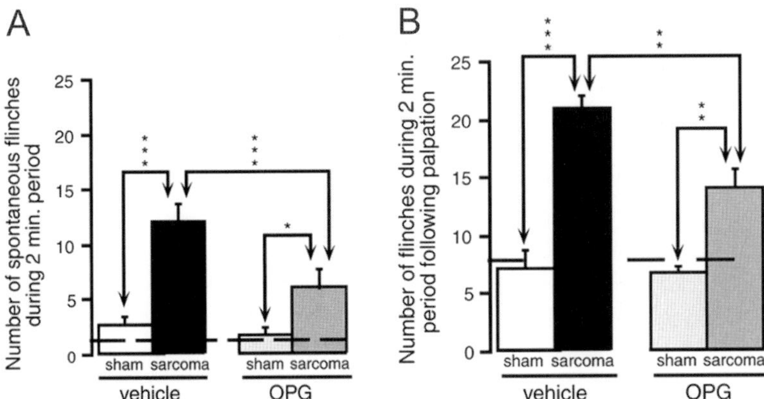

Fig. 4. Attenuation of bone cancer pain by osteoprotegerin (OPG). Histograms show that administration of OPG beginning 6 days after tumor implantation attenuated both (A) spontaneous and (B) palpation-evoked pain in mice at day 17 following tumor implantation (modified from Honore et al. 2000). OPG is a naturally occurring protein that is a secreted decoy receptor that inhibits osteoclast differentiation, proliferation, and hypertrophy, resulting in reduced osteoclast activity and bone resorption. $*P < 0.05$; $**P < 0.01$; $***P < 0.001$.

While the above pattern of tumor-induced tissue destruction and nociceptor activation may be unique to bone cancer, an evolving set of nociceptive events probably occurs in other cancers. This complex pattern may in part explain why cancer pain is frequently difficult to treat and why it is so heterogeneous in nature and severity. Changes in tumor-induced tissue injury, in nociceptor activation, and in the CNS areas involved in transmitting these nociceptive signals as the disease progresses suggest that different therapies will be efficacious at particular stages of the disease. Understanding how tumor cells differentially excite nociceptors at different stages of the disease, and how the phenotype of nociceptors and CNS neurons involved in nociceptive transmission change as the disease progresses, should allow a mechanistic approach to designing more effective therapies to treat cancer pain.

FUTURE DIRECTIONS

For the first time, animal models of cancer pain are now available that mirror the picture of patients with cancer pain. Information generated from these models should help elucidate the mechanisms that generate and maintain different types of cancer pain. Many of these cancer models have been developed using murine and rat neoplasms, but implantation of human tumors in immunocompromised rodent strains should allow examination of the pain that different human tumors generate. These animal models may also offer insight into one of the major conundrums of cancer pain: that the severity of cancer pain is so variable from patient to patient, from tumor to tumor, and even from site to site. Newer molecular techniques using microarrays and proteomics should reveal which specific features of different tumors are important in inducing cancer pain. Once we have determined the mechanisms by which the different types of cancer induce pain, we can identify molecular targets and develop mechanism-based therapies. Ultimately, the key will be to integrate information about tumor biology and the host's response to neoplasia with our understanding of how chronic pain is generated and maintained. These studies should improve the quality of life of all those who suffer from cancer pain.

ACKNOWLEDGMENTS

This work was supported by NIH grants NINDS NS23970, NIDA 11986, NIDCR Training Grants DEO7288, DE00270 (M.C.S.), and by a Merit Review from the Vererans Administration.

REFERENCES

Alvarez FJ, Fyffe RE. Nociceptors for the 21st century. *Curr Rev Pain* 2000; 4(6):451–458.

Asham EH, Loizidou M, Taylor I. Endothelin-1 and tumour development. *Eur J Surg Oncol* 1998; 24(1):57–60.

Basbaum AI, Jessel TM. The perception of pain. In: Kandel ER, Schwartz JH, Jessell TM (Eds). *Principles of Neural Science.* New York: McGraw-Hill, 2000, pp 472–490.

Bassilana F, Champigny G, Waldmann R, et al. The acid-sensitive ionic channel subunit ASIC and the mammalian degenerin MDEG form a heteromultimeric H^+-gated Na^+ channel with novel properties. *J Biol Chem* 1997; 272(46):28819–28822.

Bennett DL, French J, Priestley JV, McMahon SB. NGF but not NT-3 or BDNF prevents the A fiber sprouting into lamina II of the spinal cord that occurs following axotomy. *Mol Cell Neurosci* 1996; 8(4):211–220.

Bennett DL, Michael GJ, Ramachandran N, et al. A distinct subgroup of small DRG cells express GDNF receptor components and GDNF is protective for these neurons after nerve injury. *J Neurosci* 1998; 18(8):3059–3072.

Bevan S, Geppetti P. Protons: small stimulants of capsaicin-sensitive sensory nerves. *Trends Neurosci* 1994; 17(12):509–512.

Boucher TJ, McMahon SB. Neurotrophic factors and neuropathic pain. *Curr Opin Pharmacol* 2001; 1(1):66–72.

Boucher TJ, Okuse K, Bennett DL, et al. Potent analgesic effects of GDNF in neuropathic pain states. *Science* 2000; 290(5489):124–127.

Caroleo MC, Costa N, Bracci-Laudiero L, Aloe L. Human monocyte/macrophages activate by exposure to LPS overexpress NGF and NGF receptors. *J Neuroimmunol* 2001; 113(2):193–201.

Caterina MJ, Schumacher MA, Tominaga M, et al. The capsaicin receptor: a heat-activated ion channel in the pain pathway. *Nature* 1997; 389(6653):816–824.

Caterina MJ, Leffler A, Malmberg AB, et al. Impaired nociception and pain sensation in mice lacking the capsaicin receptor. *Science* 2000; 288(5464):306–313.

Clohisy DR, Perkins SL, Ramnaraine ML. Review of cellular mechanisms of tumor osteolysis. *Clin Orthop Res* 2000a; (373):104–114.

Clohisy DR, Ramnaraine ML, Scully S, et al. Osteoprotegerin inhibits tumor-induced osteoclastogenesis and bone growth in osteopetrotic mice. *J Orthop Res* 2000b; 18(6):967–976.

Clohisy DR, O'Keefe PF, Ramnaraine ML. Pamidronate decreases tumor-induced osteoclastogenesis in mice. *J Orthop Res* 2001; 19(4):554–558.

Coyle NJ, Adelhardt KM, Foley KM, Portenoy RK. Character of terminal illness in the advanced cancer patient: pain and other symptoms during the last four weeks of life. *J Pain Symptom Manage* 1990; 5(2):83–93.

Daughaday WH, Deuel TF. Tumor secretion of growth factors. *Endocrinol Metab Clin North Am* 1991; 20(3):539–563.

Davar G. Endothelin-1 and metastatic cancer pain. *Pain Med* 2001; 2(1):24–27.

Davar G, Hans G, Fareed MU, et al. Behavioral signs of acute pain produced by application of endothelin-1 to rat sciatic nerve. *Neuroreport* 1998; 9(10):2279–2283.

Dawas K, Laizidou M, Shankar A, et al. Angiogenesis in cancer: the role of endothelin-1. *Ann R Coll Surg Engl* 1999; 81:306–310.

Delaisse J-M, Vaes G. Mechanism of mineral solubilization and matrix degradation in osteoclastic bone resorption. In: Rifkin BR, Gay CV (Ed). *Biology and Physiology of the Osteoclast.* Ann Arbor: CRC, 1992, pp 289–314.

de Wit R, van Dam F, Loonstra S, et al. The Amsterdam Pain Management Index compared to eight frequently used outcome measures to evaluate the adequacy of pain treatment in cancer patients with chronic pain. *Pain* 2001; 91(3):339–349.

Djouhri L, Bleazard L, Lawson SN. Association of somatic action potential shape with sensory receptive properties in guinea-pig dorsal root ganglion neurones. *J Physiol* 1998; 513(Pt 3):857–872.

Dubois RN, Radhika A, Reddy BS, Entingh AJ. Increased cyclooxygenase-2 levels in carcinogen-induced rat colonic tumors. *Gastroenterology* 1996; 110(4):1259–1262.

Foley KM. Advances in cancer pain. *Arch Neurol* 1999; 56(4):413–417.

Fu SY, Gordon T. The cellular and molecular basis of peripheral nerve regeneration. *Mol Neurobiol* 1997; 14(1-2):67–116.

Fukuoka T, Kondo E, Dai Y, et al. Brain-derived neurotrophic factor increases in the uninjured dorsal root ganglion neurons in selective spinal nerve ligation model. *J Neurosci* 2001; 21(13):4891–4900.

Fulfaro F, Casuccio A, Ticozzi C, Ripamonti C. The role of bisphosphonates in the treatment of painful metastatic bone disease: a review of phase III trials. *Pain* 1998; 78(3):157–169.

Galasko CS. Diagnosis of skeletal metastases and assessment of response to treatment. *Clin Orthop* 1995; (312):64–75.

Guo A, Vulchanova L, Wang J, et al. Immunocytochemical localization of the vanilloid receptor 1 (VR1): relationship to neuropeptides, the P2X3 purinoceptor and IB4 binding sites. *Eur J Neurosci* 1999; 11(3):946–958.

Helmlinger G, Sckell A, Dellian M, et al. Acid production in glycolysis-impaired tumors provides new insights into tumor metabolism. *Clin Cancer Res* 2002; 8(4):1284–1291.

Hoke A, Gordon T, Zochodne DW, Sulaiman OA. A decline in glial cell-line-derived neurotrophic factor expression is associated with impaired regeneration after long-term Schwann cell denervation. *Exp Neurol* 2002; 173(1):77–85.

Honore P, Luger NM, Sabino MA, et al. Osteoprotegerin blocks bone cancer-induced skeletal destruction, skeletal pain and pain-related neurochemical reorganization of the spinal cord. *Nat Med* 2000a; 6(5):521–528.

Honore P, Menning PM, Rogers SD, et al. Neurochemical plasticity in persistent inflammatory pain. *Prog Brain Res* 2000b; 129:357-363.

Honore P, Rogers SD, Schwei MJ, et al. Murine models of inflammatory, neuropathic and cancer pain each generates a unique set of neurochemical changes in the spinal cord and sensory neurons. *Neuroscience* 2000c; 98(3):585–598.

Honore P, Schwei J, Rogers SD, et al. Cellular and neurochemical remodeling of the spinal cord in bone cancer pain. *Prog Brain Res* 2000d; 129:389–397.

Hoskin P. In: Body J-J (Ed). *Radiotherapy, Tumor Bone Diseases and Osteoporosis in Cancer Patients.* New York: Marcel Dekker, 2000, pp 263–286.

Hunt SP, Mantyh PW. The molecular dynamics of pain control. *Nat Rev Neurosci* 2001; 2(2):83–91.

Hunt SP, Pini A, Evan G. Induction of c-fos-like protein in spinal cord neurons following sensory stimulation. *Nature* 1987; 328(6131):632–634.

Julius D, Basbaum AI. Molecular mechanisms of nociception. *Nature* 2001; 413(6852):203–210.

Kirschstein T, Greffrath W, Busselberg D, Treede RD. Inhibition of rapid heat responses in nociceptive primary sensory of rats by vanilloid receptor antagonists. *J Neurophysiol* 1999; 82(6):2853–2860.

Koltzenburg M. The changing sensitivity in the life of the nociceptor. *Pain* 1999; (Suppl 6):S93–102.

Krishtal OA, Marchenko SM, Obukhov AG. Cationic channels activated by extracellular ATP in rat sensory neurons. *Neuroscience* 1988; 27(3):995–1000.

Kundu N, Yang QY, Dorsey R, Fulton AM. Increased cyclooxygenase-2 (COX-2) expression and activity in a murine model of metastatic breast cancer. *Int J Cancer* 2001; 93(5):681–686.

Kurbel S, Kurbel B, Kovacic D, et al. Endothelin-secreting tumors and the idea of the pseudoectopic hormone secretion in tumors. *Med Hypotheses* 1999; 52(4):329–333.

Leon A, Buriani A, Dal Toso R, et al. Mast cells synthesize, store, and release nerve growth factor. *Proc Natl Acad Sci USA* 1994; 91:3739–3743.

Leskovar A, Moriarty LJ, Turek JJ, et al. The macrophage in acute neural injury: changes in cell numbers over time and levels of cytokine production in mammalian central and peripheral nervous systems. *J Exp Biol* 2000; 203:1783–1795.

Linguеglia E, Weille JR, Bassilana F, et al. A modulatory subunit of acid sensing ion channels in brain and dorsal root ganglion cells. *J Biol Chem* 1997; 272:29778–29783.

Luger NM, Honore P, Sabino MAC, et al. Osteoprotegerin diminishes advanced bone cancer pain. *Cancer Res* 2001; 61(10):4038–4047.

Mach DB, Rogers SD, Sabino MC, et al. Origins of skeletal pain: sensory and sympathetic innervation of the mouse femur. *J Neurosci* 2002; 113(1):155–166.

Mannix K, Ahmedazai SH, Anderson H, et al. Using bisphosphonates to control the pain of bone metastases: evidence based guidelines for palliative care. *Palliat Med* 2000; 14:455–461.

Mantyh PW, DeMaster E, Malhotra A, et al. Receptor endocytosis and dendrite reshaping in spinal neurons after somatosensory stimulation. *Science* 1995a; 268(5217):1629–1632.

Mantyh PW, Allen CJ, Ghilardi JR, et al. Rapid endocytosis of a G protein-coupled receptor: substance P evoked internalization of its receptor in the rat striatum in vivo. *Proc Natl Acad Sci USA* 1995b; 92(7):2622–2626.

Mantyh PW, Clohisy DR, Koltzenburg M, Hunt SP. Molecular mechanisms of cancer pain. *Nature Rev Cancer* 2002; 2(3):201–209.

Masferrer JL, Leahy KM, Koki AT, et al. Antiangiogenic and antitumor activities of cyclooxygenase-2 inhibitors. *Cancer Res* 2000; 60(5):1306–1311.

McMahon SB. NGF as a mediator of inflammatory pain. *Philos Trans R Soc Lond B Biol Sci* 1996; 351(1338):431–440.

Mercadante S. Malignant bone pain: pathophysiology and treatment. *Pain* 1997; 69(1-2):1–18.

Mercadante S, Arcuri E. Breakthrough pain in cancer patients: pathophysiology and treatment. *Cancer Treat Rev* 1998; 24(6):425–432.

Meuser T, Pietruck C, Radbruch L, et al. Symptoms during cancer pain treatment following WHO guidelines: a longitudinal follow-up study of symptom prevalence, severity and etiology. *Pain* 2001; 93(3):247–257.

Molina MA, Sitja-Arnau M, Lemoine MG, et al. Increased cyclooxygenase-2 expression in human pancreatic carcinomas and cell lines: Growth inhibition by nonsteroidal anti-inflammatory drugs. *Cancer Res* 1999; 59(17):4356–4362.

Moore BC, Simmons DL. COX-2 inhibition, apoptosis, and chemoprevention by nonsteroidal anti-inflammatory drugs. *Curr Med Chem* 2000; 7(11):1131–1144.

Mundy GR. Metastases to bone: causes, consequences, and therapeutic opportunities. *Nature Rev Cancer* 2002; 2:584–593.

Nagy I, Rang H. Noxious heat activates all capsaicin-sensitive and also a sub-population of capsaicin-insensitive dorsal root ganglion neurons. *Neuroscience* 1999; 88(4):995–997.

Nauta HJW, Soukup VM, Fabian RH, et al. Punctate midline myelotomy for the relief of visceral cancer pain. *J Neurosurg* 2000; 92(Suppl 2S):125–130.

Nelson JB, Carducci MA. The role of endothelin-1 and endothelin receptor antagonists in prostate cancer. *BJU Int* 2000; 85(Suppl 2):45–48.

Nelson JB, Hedican SP, George DJ, et al. Identification of endothelin-1 in the pathophysiology of metastatic adenocarcinoma of the prostate. *Nat Med* 1995; 1(9):944–999.

Nielsen OS, Munro AJ, Tannock IF. Bone metastases: pathophysiology and management policy. *J Clin Oncol* 1991; 9(3):509–524.

O'Connell JX, Nanthakumar SS, Nielsen GP, Rosenberg AE. Osteoid osteoma: the uniquely innervated bone tumor. *Modern Pathol 1*998; 11(2):175–180.

Ohno R, Yoshinaga K, Fujita T, et al. Depth of invasion parallels increased cyclooxygenase-2 levels in patients with gastric carcinoma. *Cancer* 2001; 91(10):1876–1881.

Olson TH, Riedl MS, Vulchanova L, et al. An acid sensing ion channel (ASIC) localizes to small primary afferent neurons in rats. *Neuroreport* 1998; 9(6):1109–1113.

Opree A, Kress M. Involvement of the proinflammatory cytokines tumor necrosis factor-alpha, IL-1 beta, and IL-6 but not IL-8 in the development of heat hyperalgesia: effects on heat-evoked calcitonin gene-related peptide release from rat skin. *J Neurosci* 2000; 20(16):6289–6293.

Payne R. Mechanisms and management of bone pain. *Cancer* 1997; 80(Suppl 8):1608–1613.

Payne R. Practice guidelines for cancer pain therapy. Issues pertinent to the revision of national guidelines. *Oncology* 1998; 12(11A):169–175.

Payne R, Mathias SD, Pasta DJ, et al. Quality of life and cancer pain: satisfaction and side effects with transdermal fentanyl versus oral morphine. *J Clin Oncol* 1998; 16(4):1588–1593.

Pomonis JD, Rogers SD, Peters CM, et al. Expression and localization of endothelin receptors: implication for the involvement of peripheral glia in nociception. *J Neurosci* 2001; 21(3):999–1006.

Poon RT, Fan ST, Wong J. Clinical implications of circulating angiogenic factors in cancer patients. *J Clin Oncol* 2001; 19(4):1207–1225.

Portenoy RK, Lesage P. Management of cancer pain. *Lancet* 1999; 353(9165):1695–1700.

Portenoy RKD, Payne D, Jacobsen P. Breakthrough pain: characteristics and impact in patients with cancer pain. *Pain* 1999; 81(1-2):129–134.

Price MP, McIlwrath SL, Xie JH, et al. The DRASIC cation channel contributes to the detection of cutaneous touch and acid stimuli in mice. *Neuron* 2001; 32(6):1071–1083.

Radinsky R. Growth factors and their receptors in metastasis. *Semin Cancer Biol* 1991; 2(3):169–177.

Ramer MS, Priestley JV, McMahon SB. Functional regeneration of sensory axons into the adult spinal cord. *Nature* 2000; 403(6767):312–316.

Reeh PW, Steen KH. Tissue acidosis in nociception and pain. *Prog Brain Res* 1996; 113:143–151.

Ripamonti C, Dickerson ED. Strategies for the treatment of cancer pain in the new millennium. *Drugs* 2001; 61(7):955–977.

Roman C, Saha D, Beauchamp R. TGF-beta and colorectal carcinogenesis. *Microsc Res Tech* 2001; 52(4):450–457.

Schneider MB, Standop J, Ulrich A, et al. Expression of nerve growth factors in pancreatic neural tissue and pancreatic cancer. *J Histochem Cytochem* 2001; 49(10):1205–1210.

Schwei MJ, Honore P, Rogers SD, et al. Neurochemical and cellular reorganization of the spinal cord in a murine model of bone cancer pain. *J Neurosci* 1999; 19(24):10886–10897.

Seifert P, Spitznas M. Tumours may be innervated. *Virchows Archiv* 2001; 438(3):228–231.

Shankar A, Loizidou M, Aliev G, et al. Raised endothelin 1 levels in patients with colorectal liver metastases. *Br J Surg* 1998; 85(4):502–506.

Shappell SB, Manning S, Boeglin WE, et al. Alterations in lipoxygenase and cyclooxygenase-2 catalytic activity and mRNA expression in prostate carcinoma. *Neoplasia* 2001; 3(4):287–303.

Silver BJ. Platelet-derived growth factor in human malignancy. *Biofactors* 1992; 3(4):217–227.

Stoscheck CM, King Jr LE. Role of epidermal growth factor in carcinogenesis. *Cancer Res* 1986; 46(3):1030–1037.

Sutherland S, Cook S, Ew M. Chemical mediators of pain due to tissue damage and ischemia. *Prog Brain Res* 2000; 129:21–38.

Terada T, Matsunaga Y. S-100-positive nerve fibers in hepatocellular carcinoma and intrahepatic cholangiocarcinoma: an immunohistochemical study. *Pathol Int* 2001; 51(2):89–93.

Tominaga M, Caterina MJ, Malmberg AB, et al. The cloned capsaicin receptor integrates multiple pain-producing stimuli. *Neuron* 1998; 21(3):531–543.

Vasko MR. Prostaglandin-induced neuropeptide release from spinal cord. *Prog Brain Res* 1995; 104:367–380.

Verge VM, Richardson PM, Wiesenfeld-Hallin Z, et al. Differential influence of nerve growth factor on neuropeptide expression in vivo: a novel role in peptide expression in adult sensory neurons. *J Neurosci* 1995; 15(3):2081–2096.

Watkins LR, Goehler LE, Relton J, et al. Mechanisms of tumor necrosis factor-alpha (TNF-alpha) hyperalgesia. *Brain Res* 1995; 692(1–2):244–250.

Welch JM, Simon SA, Reinhart PH. The activation mechanism of rat vanilloid receptor 1 by capsaicin involves the pore domain and differs from the activation by either or heat. *Proc Natl Acad Sci USA* 2000; 97(25):13889–13894.

Willis WD, Al-Chaer ED, Quast MJ, Westlund KN. A visceral pain pathway in the dorsal column of the spinal cord. *Proc Natl Acad Sci USA* 1999; 96(14):7675–7679.

Woolf CJ, Salter MW. Neuronal plasticity: increasing the gain in pain. *Science* 2000; 288(5472):1765–1769.

Xu GY, Huang LYM. Peripheral inflammation sensitizes P2X receptor-mediated responses in dorsal root ganglion neurons. *J Neurosci* 2002; 22(1):93–102.

Zhang F, Lu W, Dong Z. Tumor-infiltrating macrophages are involved in suppressing growth and metastasis of human prostate cancer cells by INF-beta gene therapy in nude mice. PG-2942-51. *Clin Cancer Res* 2002; 8(9).

Zhu ZW, Friess H, diMola FF, et al. Nerve growth factor expression correlates with perineural invasion and pain in human pancreatic cancer. *J Clin Oncol* 1999; 17(8):2419–2428.

Correspondence to: Patrick W. Mantyh, PhD, Neurosystems Laboratory, University of Minnesota, 18-154 Moos Tower, 515 Delaware Street, Minneapolis, MN 55455, USA. Email: manty001@umn.edu.

Proceedings of the 10th World Congress on Pain,
Progress in Pain Research and Management, Vol. 24,
edited by Jonathan O. Dostrovsky, Daniel B. Carr, and
Martin Koltzenburg, IASP Press, Seattle, © 2003.

56

Pathophysiology and Treatment of Complex Regional Pain Syndromes

Ralf Baron, Andreas Binder, Jörn Schattschneider, and Gunnar Wasner

Neurology Clinic, Christian-Albrechts University, Kiel, Germany

Insight into the pathophysiological mechanisms underlying complex regional pain syndrome (CRPS) has progressed dramatically over the last few years (Harden et al. 2001). It has become obvious that multiple mechanisms may occur in different individual patterns. These consist of somatosensory dysfunctions (including pain) that interact with changes related to the sympathetic nervous system, with peripheral inflammatory reactions, and with changes in the somatomotor system. All of these abnormalities, which can be triggered by various events, may be the consequence of alterations in the brain.

The publication of standardized diagnostic criteria for CRPS was a major advance in the classification of regional pain disorders associated with vasomotor or sudomotor abnormalities (Stanton-Hicks et al. 1995). Based on these criteria, clinical research on mechanisms was performed on a much more homogeneous group of patients and was therefore comparable for the first time. However, the criteria were based on the consensus opinion of a small group of expert clinicians. While this was an appropriate first step, it is important to continuously improve these initial criteria by validating and if necessary modifying them according to the results of systematic research. The current diagnostic criteria are adequately sensitive in that they rarely miss a case of CRPS. However, both internal and external validation research suggests that the syndrome is overdiagnosed (Bruehl et al. 1999). The inclusion of motor and trophic signs and symptoms could improve specificity without losing sensitivity (Bruehl et al. 2002). The establishment of modified diagnostic criteria could greatly improve the quality of studies on pathophysiological mechanisms and therapy. A diversified research strategy and an ongoing consensus process on CRPS including diagnostics, mechanisms, and therapy provide a glimmer of hope that we will ultimately be able to intervene successfully against this cruel disease.

CLINICAL CHARACTERISTICS

CRPS TYPE I

Characteristically, patients with CRPS-I (formerly known as reflex sympathetic dystrophy) develop asymmetrical distal extremity pain and swelling after a trauma without presenting an overt nerve lesion. Precipitating events include fracture or minor soft tissue trauma, as well as stroke and myocardial infarction. The swelling and pain often develop at a site *remote* from the inciting injury, and there may be no obvious local tissue-damaging process at the site of pain and swelling (Wasner et al. 1998). CRPS-I patients often report a *burning spontaneous pain* felt in the distal part of the affected extremity. Characteristically, the pain is disproportionate in intensity to the inciting event. The pain usually increases when the extremity is in a dependent position. Stimulus-evoked pains are a striking clinical feature; they include mechanical and thermal allodynia and hyperalgesia. These sensory abnormalities often appear early, are most pronounced distally, and have no consistent spatial relationship to individual nerve territories or to the site of the inciting lesion. Typically pain can be elicited by movements and pressure at the joints (deep somatic allodynia), even if the joints are not directly affected by the inciting lesion. *Autonomic abnormalities* include swelling, changes in sweating, and altered blood flow to the skin. In the acute stages of CRPS-I, the affected limb is often warmer than the contralateral limb. Sweating abnormalities, either hypohidrosis or, more frequently, hyperhidrosis, are present in nearly all CRPS-I patients. The acute distal swelling of the affected limb depends critically on aggravating stimuli. *Trophic changes* such as abnormal nail growth, increased or decreased hair growth, fibrosis, thin glossy skin, and osteoporosis may occur, particularly in chronic stages. Restrictions of passive movement are often present in long-standing cases and may be related to both functional motor disturbances and trophic changes of joints and tendons. *Weakness* often affects all muscles of the affected distal extremity. Small accurate movements are characteristically impaired. Nerve conduction and electromyography studies are normal, except in patients at advanced stages of the disorder. About half of patients have a postural or action tremor that represents increased physiological tremor. About 10% of cases involve dystonia of the affected hand or foot.

CRPS TYPE II

Causalgia was originally described as a burning pain that develops in the distal extremity following traumatic partial peripheral nerve injury. In addition to spontaneous pain, patients report exquisite hypersensitivity of the skin to light mechanical stimulation. Furthermore, movement, loud noises, or strong emotions can trigger their pain. Distal extremity swelling, smoothness and mottling of the skin, and in some cases, acute arthritis may be present. In most cases the affected limb is cold and sweaty. The sensory and trophic abnormalities spread beyond the innervation territory of the injured peripheral nerve and often occur *remote* from the site of injury. Because these symptoms show many similarities to those of CRPS-I, this syndrome is now called CRPS-II.

PATHOPHYSIOLOGICAL MECHANISMS

SENSORY ABNORMALITIES AND PAIN

Numerous animal experimental findings suggest that spontaneous pain and various forms of hyperalgesia at the distal extremity (Sieweke et al. 1999; Maleki et al. 2000) are generated by processes of peripheral and central sensitization of the nociceptive system. In addition, up to 50% of patients with chronic CRPS-I develop hypoesthesia and hypoalgesia throughout the affected half of the body or in the upper quadrant ipsilateral to the affected extremity. Systematic quantitative sensory testing has shown that patients with these generalized hypoesthesias have increased thresholds to mechanical, cold, warm, and heat stimuli compared with the responses generated from the healthy body side. Patients with these extended sensory deficits have a longer disease duration, greater pain intensity, a higher frequency of mechanical allodynia, and a higher tendency to develop changes in the somatomotor system than do patients with spatially restricted sensory deficits (Rommel et al. 2001).

These changed somatosensory perceptions are most likely due to changes in the central representation of somatosensory sensations in the thalamus and cortex (Maleki et al. 2000). Accordingly, positron emission tomography (PET) studies have demonstrated adaptive changes in the thalamus during the course of the disease (Fukumoto et al. 1999). Furthermore, a recent magnetoencephalogram (MEG) study demonstrated a shortened distance between little finger and thumb representations in the primary somatosensory (S1) cortex on the painful side. The MEG S1 responses were increased on that side, indicating processes of central sensitization (Juottonen et al. 2002; see also Baron et al. 2000) (Fig. 1).

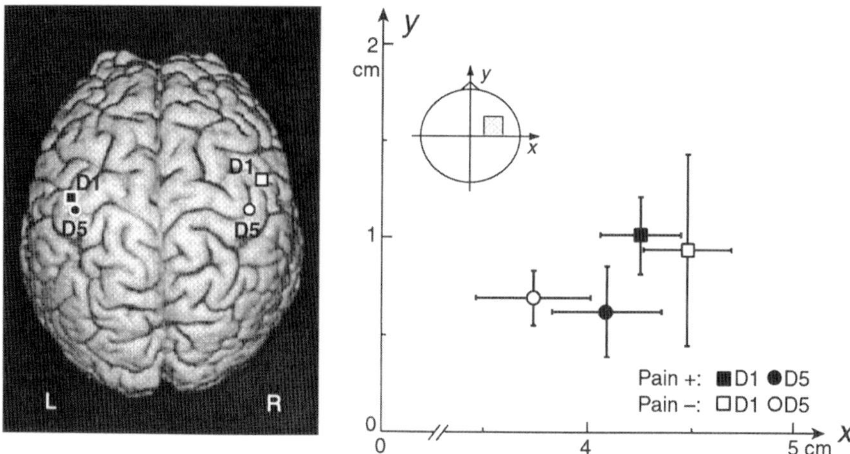

Fig. 1. Left: sources of cortical responses to tactile stimuli of the healthy (open symbols) and painful (filled symbols) sides applied to digits one (squares) and five (circles) in a CRPS patient. Right: the mean (± SEM) source locations in the S1 region. The insert illustrates the coordinate system where the x axis goes from the left to the right preauricular point and the y axis from inion to nasion. From Juottonen et al. (2002), with permission.

We do not know whether these central changes depend on continuous nociceptive input from the affected extremity or whether they are specific to the disease.

AUTONOMIC SYMPTOMS CAUSED BY CENTRAL ABNORMALITIES

Sympathetic denervation and denervation hypersensitivity, found *within the territory of the lesioned nerve* in CRPS-II, cannot completely account for all vasomotor and sudomotor abnormalities observed in CRPS. First, in CRPS-I there is *no overt nerve lesion* (Goldstein et al. 2000), and second, in CRPS-II the autonomic symptoms spread *beyond the territory of the lesioned nerve*. In fact, there is direct evidence for a reorganization of central autonomic control in these syndromes.

Hyperhidrosis, as mentioned above, is found in many CRPS patients. Resting sweat output, as well as thermoregulatory and axon reflex sweating, is increased in CRPS-I patients (Chelimsky et al. 1995; Birklein et al. 1997). Increased sweat production cannot be explained by a peripheral mechanism because, unlike blood vessels, sweat glands do not develop denervation supersensitivity.

To study cutaneous sympathetic vasoconstrictor innervation in CRPS-I patients, we analyzed central sympathetic reflexes induced by thermoregulatory (whole-body warming or cooling) and respiratory stimuli (Wasner et al. 1999, 2001). We measured sympathetic effector organ function, i.e., skin temperature and skin blood flow, bilaterally at the extremities by infrared thermometry and laser Doppler flowmetry. Under normal conditions these reflexes show no differences between the two sides of the body. In CRPS patients, three distinct vascular regulation patterns were identified that related to the duration of the disorder (Fig. 2). In the "warm regulation type" (found at the acute stage, less than 6 months after onset of CRPS), the affected limb was warmer and skin perfusion values were higher than contralaterally during the entire spectrum of sympathetic activity. Even significant body cooling failed to activate sympathetic vasoconstrictor neurons (Wasner et al. 1999). Consistently, direct measurements of norepinephrine levels from the venous effluent above the area of pain showed a *reduction* in the affected extremity (Wasner et al. 1999). In the "intermediate type," temperature and perfusion were either warmer or colder, depending on the degree of sympathetic activity. In the "cold regulation type" (found at the chronic stage), temperature and perfusion were lower on the affected side during the entire thermoregulatory cycle. Norepinephrine levels, however, were still lower on the affected side (Wasner et al. 2001). These data support the idea that CRPS-I is associated with a pathological unilateral inhibition of cutaneous sympathetic vasoconstrictor neurons, leading to a warmer affected limb in the acute stage (Baron and Maier 1996; Birklein et al. 1998). The locus of pathophysiological changes underlying such disturbed reflex activity must be in the central nervous system. Secondary changes in the neurovascular transmission may induce severe vasoconstriction and cold skin in chronic CRPS (Goldstein et al. 2000). Accordingly, α-adrenoceptor density was increased in skin biopsies of patients with CRPS-I (Drummond et al. 1996). Furthermore, skin lactate was increased in CRPS patients, indicating an enhanced anaerobic glycolysis, probably as a result of vasoconstriction and chronic tissue hypoxia (Birklein et al. 2000).

However, the few microneurographic studies of small sympathetic nerve fascicles that have been conducted so far in patients with CRPS have not confirmed reflex abnormalities. The average skin sympathetic activity (a combination of vasoconstrictor and sudomotor activity) was the same on both sides of the body (Casale and Elam 1992).

NEUROGENIC INFLAMMATION

Some of the clinical features of CRPS, particularly in its early phase, could be explained by an inflammatory process (Leitha et al. 1996; van der Laan and Goris 1997; Calder et al. 1998). Increasing evidence indicates that a localized *neurogenic inflammation* might be involved in the generation of

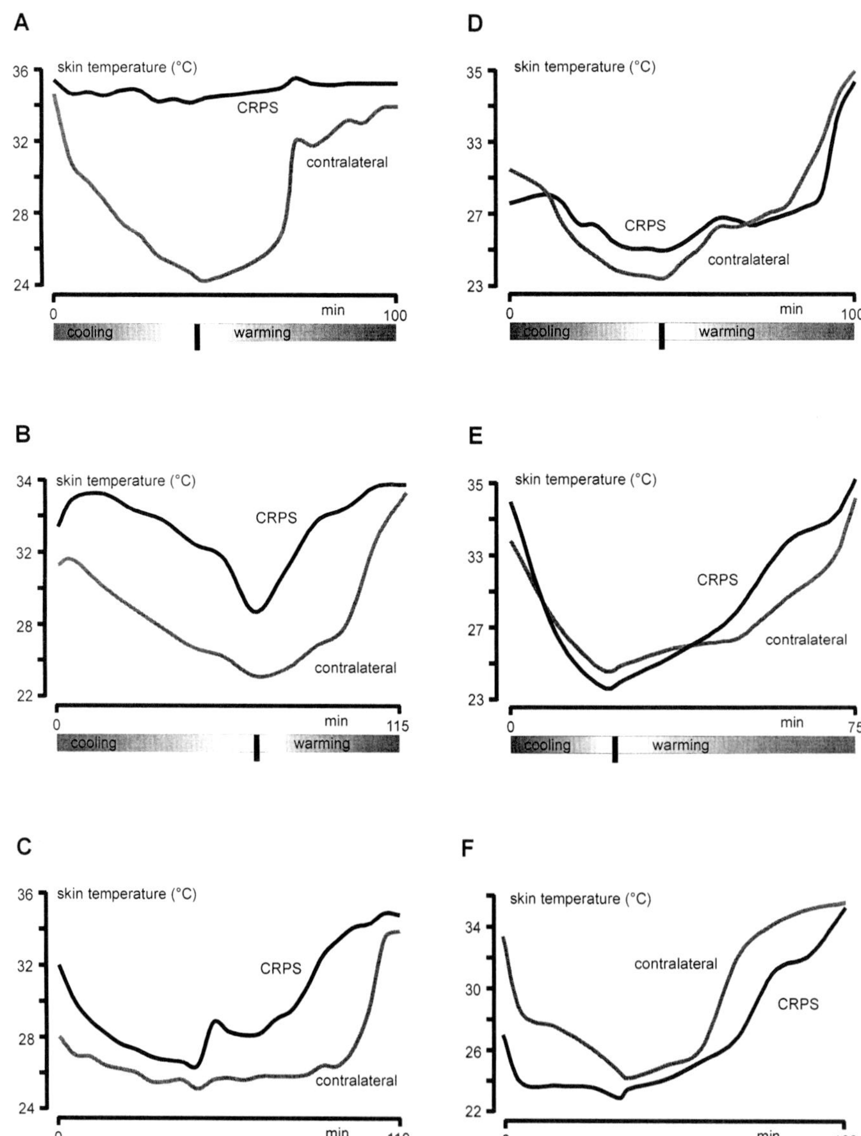

acute edema, vasodilatation, and increased sweating. Scintigraphic investigations with radiolabeled immunoglobulins show extensive plasma extravasation in patients with acute CRPS-I (Oyen et al. 1993). Analysis of joint fluid and synovial biopsies in CRPS patients have shown an increase in protein concentration and synovial hypervascularity (Renier et al. 1983). Furthermore, synovial effusion is enhanced in affected joints as measured with magnetic resonance imaging (MRI), which seems to be a valuable additional diagnostic tool (Graif et al. 1998). In patients with acute untreated CRPS-I, axon reflex activation in nociceptive fibers (neurogenic inflammation) was elicited by strong transcutaneous electrical stimulation via intradermal microdialysis capillaries. Protein extravasation that was simultaneously assessed by the microdialysis system was provoked only in the affected extremity. The time course of electrically induced protein extravasation in these patients resembled that observed following application of exogenous substance P (Weber et al. 2001). As further support of a neurogenic inflammatory process, axon reflex vasodilatation as measured by laser Doppler flowmetry was significantly increased after C-fiber stimulation on the affected side. Accordingly, systemic calcitonin gene-related peptide (CGRP) levels were increased during the acute stage of CRPS but not in chronic stages (Birklein et al. 2001). In the fluid of artificially produced skin blisters, levels of interleukin-6 (IL-6) and tumor necrosis factor α (TNF-α) were significantly higher in the involved extremity as compared with the normal extremity (Huygen et al. 2002). The production of nitric oxide in peripheral

---

← **Fig. 2.** Characteristics of skin temperature as a measure of cutaneous sympathetic vasoconstrictor activity at the fingers or toes of both hands or feet in patients with CRPS during a controlled thermoregulatory cycle (controlled alteration in cutaneous sympathetic activity). Controlled thermoregulatory changes (whole-body cooling and warming) were applied by means of a thermal suit to change environmental temperature in a standardized way and reflexively alter skin sympathetic vasoconstrictor activity. The subject was lying in a suit supplied by tubes, in which running water at an inflow temperature of 12°C or 50°C was used to cool or warm the whole body. During the experiment, the skin temperature of the fingers of both hands was monitored at regular intervals. Three distinct vascular regulation patterns could be identified. (A–C) Patients with a "warm" regulation type showed higher cutaneous temperature and perfusion values at the affected limb than at the contralateral limb during the whole thermoregulatory cycle (the entire spectrum of physiological sympathetic vasoconstrictor activity). (D, E) In patients with an "intermediate" type, the direction of the temperature difference between sides changed during the thermoregulatory cycle. In some patients the affected side was warmer when sympathetic activity was high and colder during inhibition of sympathetic activity (D). Vasoconstriction during cooling and vasodilatation during warming were less intense on the affected limb than on the contralateral limb. In other patients the affected side was colder during high sympathetic activity and warmer during inhibition of sympathetic outflow (E). (F) Patients with a "cold" regulation type had lower skin temperature and perfusion values on the affected side during the entire spectrum. From Wasner et al. (2001), with permission.

blood monocytes was significantly increased after stimulation with interferon-γ in CRPS patients compared with controls (Hartrick 2002). Also, increased axon reflex sweating could be explained by release of CGRP during neurogenic inflammation from nociceptive terminals that act on peripheral sweat glands (Birklein et al. 2001).

Thus, the preponderance of evidence indicates that neurogenic inflammatory processes are involved in the pathogenesis of early CRPS. However, the exact mechanisms of initiation and maintenance of these inflammatory reactions are unclear. One central issue is whether the sympathetic nervous system may contribute to the early inflammatory state. Animal studies have demonstrated that the sympathetic nervous system can influence the intensity of an inflammatory process (Levine et al. 1986), and clinical studies indicate that sympatholytic procedures can ameliorate both pain and inflammation. However, this concept has yet to be proven in patients with CRPS.

MOTOR ABNORMALITIES

About 50% of patients with CRPS show a decrease in active range of motion, an increase in physiological tremor, and a reduction in active motor force in the affected extremity (Schwartzman and Kerrigan 1990; Deuschl et al. 1991). In about 10% of cases, mostly chronic cases, dystonia develops in the affected hand or foot (Marsden et al. 1984; Bhatia et al. 1993). It is unlikely that these motor changes are related to a peripheral process such as the influence of the sympathetic nervous system on neuromuscular transmission or contractility of skeletal muscle. These somatomotor changes are more likely to be generated by changes in central sensorimotor integration. In support of this view, a neglect-like syndrome was clinically described as responsible for the disuse of the extremity (Galer et al. 1995). Furthermore, we used kinematic analysis of target reaching as well as grip force analysis to quantitatively assess motor deficits in CRPS patients (Schattschneider et al. 2001). Pathological sensorimotor integration in the parietal cortex may induce abnormal central programming and processing of motor tasks. MEG-based cortical rhythm analysis demonstrated altered reactivity of the motor cortex oscillation to tactile stimulation, suggesting a sustained inhibition of the motor cortex in CRPS patients (Juottonen et al. 2002).

SYMPATHETICALLY MAINTAINED PAIN

Definition. Based on experience and recent clinical studies, the term *sympathetically maintained pain* (SMP) has been redefined. Neuropathic pain patients presenting with similar clinical signs and symptoms can be divided into two groups according to whether selective sympathetic blockade has no effect or a positive effect. The pain component that is relieved by specific sympatholytic procedures is considered to be sympathetically maintained. Thus, SMP is now defined to be a *symptom* or the underlying *mechanism* in a subset of patients with neuropathic disorders and *not a clinical entity*. The positive effect of a sympathetic blockade is *not essential* to diagnosis of CRPS (Stanton-Hicks et al. 1995; Schurmann et al. 2001).

Animal studies. After experimental nerve injury in animals, surviving cutaneous afferents, including those in continuity with their peripheral targets, may develop noradrenergic sensitivity (Fig. 3A,B). Furthermore, a novel pattern of sympathetic skin innervation occurs after a mental nerve injury in the rat (Ruocco et al. 2000), with dopamine-β-hydroxylase-positive fibers sprouting into the upper dermis, a region usually devoid of such fibers. Ectopic innervation of the superficial dermis by sympathetic fibers may play an important role in the interactions between the sympathetic and regenerating sensory fibers containing substance P.

In addition to the peripheral interaction, coupling of sympathetic and afferent neurons may also occur within the dorsal root ganglion (DRG, Fig. 3A). Sympathetic postganglionic fibers that normally innervate blood vessels within the DRG sprout to form basket-like terminals around large primary afferent somata that project into the injured nerve. However, the relationship of such sprouting to pain is uncertain. Sprouting of sympathetic postganglionic terminals largely occurs around the somata of larger, presumably non-nociceptive primary afferents. Activation of afferent neurons to sympathetic stimulation tends to occur in the first 20 days after the lesion, but later on, depression of afferent activity is predominant. Catecholaminergic baskets form around DRG cells in the same nerve lesion model after 30 days.

Animal studies demonstrate that catecholamines can also activate *intact primary afferent C-nociceptors after tissue inflammation* (thermal and chemical sensitization). This concept is of particular interest because of the evidence that, in its early phase, CRPS-I might have an inflammatory component. Sensitization of nociceptive primary afferents by proinflammatory mediators as bradykinin and nerve growth factor (NGF) depends on an intact sympathetic nervous system rather than on sympathetic activity or norepinephrine release. Bradykinin and norepinephrine may act indirectly on nociceptor terminals by inducing the release of prostaglandins from sympathetic fibers (Fig. 3C).

Knowledge about the subtypes of α-adrenoreceptor(s) involved in sympathetic-afferent coupling is important for an understanding of the underlying neural mechanism, and may be useful in the design of more specific treatment modalities for neuropathic pain conditions involving sympathetic

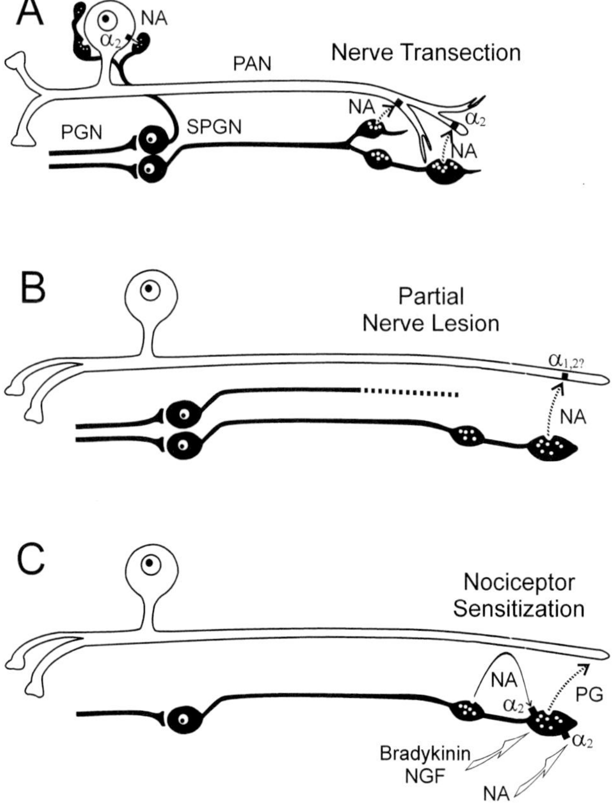

Fig. 3. Influence of sympathetic activity and catecholamines on primary afferent neurons. (A) Complete nerve lesion. The sympathetic-afferent interaction is located in the neuroma and in the dorsal root ganglion. It is mediated by norepinephrine (NA) released from postganglionic neurons and α-adrenoreceptors expressed at the plasma membrane of afferent fibers. (B) Partial nerve lesion. Partial nerve injury is followed by a decrease of the sympathetic innervation density (stippled postganglionic neuron). This event induces an upregulation of functional α_2-adrenoceptors at the membrane of intact nociceptive fibers. (C) After tissue inflammation, intact but sensitized primary afferents acquire norepinephrine sensitivity. Norepinephrine does not act directly on afferents but induces the release of prostaglandins (PG) from sympathetic terminals that sensitize the afferents. In accordance, nociceptor sensitization induced by bradykinin and nerve growth factor (NGF) is also mediated by PG release from postganglionic fibers. From Baron et al. (1999), with permission.

efferent activity. Adrenergic sensitization of polymodal nociceptors is largely mediated by α_2-adrenoceptors, whereas sympathetic-sensory coupling after nerve injury uses both α_1- and α_2-adrenoceptors. In the latter case, mRNA for α_{2A}-adrenoceptors is clearly upregulated in DRG neurons. For a review of pertinent results from animal studies, see Baron et al. (1999).

Clinical studies support the idea that nociceptors develop catecholamine sensitivity after complete or partial nerve lesions. In amputees, perineuronal administration of physiological doses of norepinephrine induced more pain than did saline injections (Raja et al. 1998). Furthermore, intraoperative stimulation of the sympathetic chain increased spontaneous pain in patients with causalgia (CRPS-II), but not in patients with hyperhidrosis (White and Sweet 1969). In CRPS-II and post-traumatic neuralgias, intradermal norepinephrine, in physiologically relevant doses, evoked greater pain in the affected regions of patients with SMP than in the contralateral unaffected limb and in control subjects (Torebjörk et al. 1995; Ali et al. 2000).

We performed a study in patients with CRPS using physiological stimuli of the sympathetic nervous system (Baron et al. 2002). Cutaneous sympathetic vasoconstrictor outflow to the painful extremity was experimentally activated to the highest possible physiological degree by whole-body cooling. During the thermal challenge the affected extremity was maintained at 35°C in order to avoid thermal effects at the nociceptor level. The intensity as well as area of spontaneous pain and mechanical hyperalgesia (dynamic and punctate) increased significantly in patients who had been classified as having SMP by positive sympathetic blocks but not in patients with sympathetically independent pain (SIP) (Fig. 4). The experimental setup we used selectively alters sympathetic cutaneous vasoconstrictor activity without influencing other sympathetic systems innervating the extremities, i.e., the piloerector, sudomotor, and muscle vasoconstrictor neurons. Therefore, the interaction of sympathetic and afferent neurons we measured is likely to be located within the skin, as predicted by the pain-enhancing effect of intracutaneous norepinephrine injections. Interestingly, the relief of spontaneous pain after sympathetic blockade was more pronounced than were changes in spontaneous pain that could be induced experimentally by sympathetic activation. One explanation for this discrepancy might be that a complete sympathetic block affects all sympathetic outflow channels projecting to the affected extremity. It is very likely that in addition to a coupling in the skin, a sympathetic-afferent interaction may also occur in other tissues, in particular in the deep somatic domain such as the bones, muscles, or joints. Supporting this view, these structures are extremely painful in some cases of CRPS (Baron and Wasner 2001). Furthermore, some patients may be characterized by a selective or predominant sympathetic-afferent interaction in deep somatic tissues sparing the skin (Wasner et al. 1999).

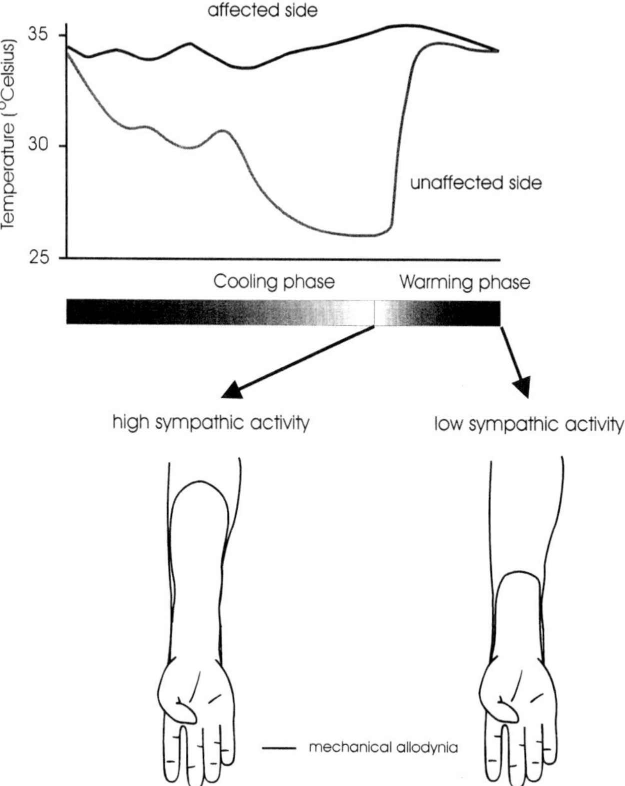

Fig. 4. Influence of cutaneous sympathetic vasoconstrictor activity on pain in a patient with chronic CRPS-I and SMP. Thermal stimuli were applied that induce changes of activity in sympathetic vasoconstrictor neurons innervating the skin and also modulate norepinephrine release. The patient was lying in a thermal suit (see above) to cool or warm the whole body. Cooling induces a massive tonic activation of cutaneous vasoconstrictor neurons, whereas warming leads to a decrease of their activity. In this way sympathetic activity was switched on and off in a controlled manner during simultaneous measurement of pain sensation (measurement of area of mechanical allodynia to phasic light touch exerted by gently moving a cotton swab over the skin). High sympathetic activity during cooling induces a decrease of skin temperature due to vasoconstriction (unaffected side; monitoring the effect of whole-body cooling and warming). During the experiment the forearm temperature on the affected side was kept at 35°C by a feedback-controlled heat lamp to exclude temperature effects on the sensory receptors (upper record). Activation of cutaneous vasoconstrictor neurons increased the area of allodynia in this patient, indicating that in CRPS with SMP a pathological coupling between sympathetic and nociceptive neurons does exist. This functional coupling is absent in CRPS patients without SMP. Modified from Baron et al. (2002), with permission.

DIAGNOSTIC TESTS THAT AID THE DIAGNOSIS OF CRPS

At present the diagnosis of CRPS is based on the clinical criteria described above. However, several tests and procedures are valuable diagnostic tools.

Bone scintigraphy can provide information about vascular bone changes (Kozin et al. 1981), but this test is only positive for significant changes during the subacute period (up to 1 year). The specificity and sensitivity of this method are unknown, as is the case for any other test for CRPS, because there is no known standard against which to compare it. Plain radiographs can be used to evaluate the status of mineralization, but these are only positive in chronic stages. Quantitative sensory testing (QST) provides information about the sensory symptom profile (function or dysfunction of unmyelinated and myelinated afferent fibers) using psychophysical testing of thermal threshold, thermal pain threshold, and vibratory threshold. However, there is no specific sensory profile for CRPS. Autonomic testing with the quantitative sudomotor axon reflex test (QSART) measures the function of sudomotor reflex loops (Chelimsky et al. 1995). Swelling can be quantified by measuring water displacement. Autonomic vascular function can be tested by using laser Doppler flowmetry (Birklein et al. 1998; Wasner et al. 1999, 2001) and infrared thermography (Gulevich et al. 1997).

Skin temperature assessment is an easy measure of vascular function that may be particularly helpful in the diagnosis of CRPS. We performed a study using controlled thermoregulation (whole-body warming and cooling) to change cutaneous sympathetic vasoconstrictor activity (Wasner et al. 2002). Skin temperature in the affected and unaffected limbs was measured by infrared thermometry under resting conditions (before temperature challenge in the office at room temperature) and was continuously monitored during controlled modulation of sympathetic activity. Asymmetries in skin temperature between limbs were minor under resting conditions in most patients. However, during controlled thermoregulation, temperature differences between both sides increased dynamically and were most prominent at a high to medium level of vasoconstrictor activity. In patients suffering from painful limbs of other origin and in healthy volunteers, there were only minor differences in temperature between both sides, both at rest and during thermoregulatory changes of sympathetic activity. When comparing the diagnostic value of skin temperature asymmetries in CRPS, we found that sensitivity was only 32% under resting conditions, but increased up to 76% during controlled alteration of sympathetic activity. Specificity was 100% at rest and 93% during controlled thermoregulation (Fig. 5).

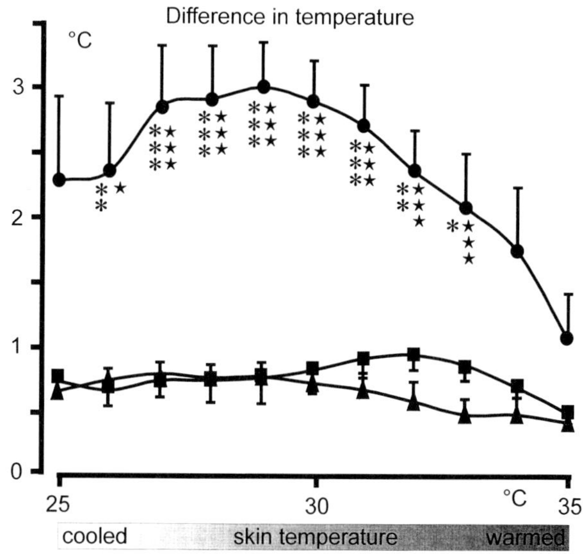

Fig. 5. Average absolute differences between sides in skin temperature of the fingers or toes of the hands or feet in 25 patients with CRPS (circles), in 20 healthy controls (squares), and in 15 control patients with extremity pain of other origin (triangles) during a controlled thermoregulatory cycle (controlled alteration in cutaneous sympathetic activity). The level of overall cutaneous sympathetic vasoconstrictor activity was estimated indirectly by using the skin temperature on the unaffected side (or right side in healthy controls) as a reference value. A skin temperature on the healthy side of 25°C indicates a high level, a temperature of 30°C an intermediate level, and a temperature of 35°C a complete inhibition of sympathetic vasoconstrictor activity to the skin. Data are presented as mean ± SEM. Asterisks (*) denote significant difference between CRPS patients compared with healthy controls, and compared with patients with extremity pain of other origin. One symbol, $P < 0.05$; two symbols, $P < 0.01$; three symbols, $P < 0.001$. From Wasner et al. (2001), with permission.

In conclusion, the degree of unilateral vascular disturbances in CRPS and the temperature differences between the affected and unaffected side depend critically on environmental temperature and spontaneous sympathetic activity. However, the maximal skin temperature difference that occurs during the thermoregulatory cycle distinguishes CRPS from other extremity pain syndromes with high sensitivity and specificity.

THERAPY FOR CRPS

Poor understanding of the underlying pathophysiological abnormalities and the lack of objective diagnostic criteria have resulted in inherent difficulties in conducting clinical therapy trials. Therefore, few evidence-based treatment regimens for CRPS are available so far. In fact, two literature reviews of outcome studies find discouragingly little consistent information regarding pharmacological agents and methods of treatment for CRPS (Kingery 1997; Perez et al. 2001). In the absence of more specific information about pathophysiological mechanisms and treatment, we must rely on outcomes from treatment studies for other neuropathic pain syndromes. Furthermore, the still hypothetical concept of mechanism-based treatment must be transferred from ideas derived from animal experiments using peripheral nerve lesions to the situation in CRPS patients.

GENERAL RULES

Treatment should be immediate, and most importantly, must be directed toward restoration of full function of the extremity. This objective is best attained in a comprehensive interdisciplinary setting with particular emphasis on pain management and functional restoration (for a treatment algorithm see Stanton-Hicks et al. 1998). The pain team should include neurologists, anesthetists, orthopedic specialists, physical therapists, and psychologists.

The general principles of pharmacological treatment are the individualization of therapy and the titration of a given pharmacological agent, balancing desired effects with side effects. A drug should be considered to elicit no response only when a sufficient period of time has passed to judge its efficacy. Destructive surgery on the peripheral or central afferent nervous system in cases of CRPS always increases the risk for persistent deafferentation pain.

PHARMACOLOGICAL THERAPY

Nonsteroidal anti-inflammatory drugs can be used to relieve mild to moderate pain. Opioids strongly inhibit central nociceptive neurons, mainly through their interaction with μ-opioid receptors. Although opioids have not been studied in CRPS, in other neuropathic pain syndromes they are clearly analgesic when compared to placebo. However, there are no long-term studies of the use of oral opioids in treating chronic neuropathic pain, including CRPS. Even without solid scientific evidence, the expert opinion of pain clinicians is that opioids could be part of a comprehensive pain treatment program for CRPS. Tricyclic antidepressants have shown analgesic effect in several neuropathic pain states and should be tested in CRPS. Sodium channel-blocking agents, lidocaine, mexiletine, and tocainide, and the anticonvulsant carbamazepine relieve neuropathic pain. Intravenous lidocaine may be effective in CRPS (Wallace et al. 2000). The mechanism of action of gabapentin has not yet been completely resolved, but it probably includes an inhibition of central calcium channels. In a recent study, gabapentin had a promising effect on CRPS (Mellick et al. 1995). Glucocorticoids taken orally have clearly demonstrated efficacy in controlled trials (Christensen et al. 1982). There is no evidence that other immune-modulating therapies, notably intravenous immunoglobulins or immunosuppressive drugs, have a place in the treatment of CRPS. Transdermal application of the α_2-adrenoceptor agonist clonidine, which is thought to prevent the release of catecholamines by a presynaptic action, may be helpful when small areas of hyperalgesia are present (Davis et al. 1991). Intravenous bisphosphonates (alendronate, clodronate) have significantly reduced pain and swelling and have improved movement of the affected limb (Adami et al. 1997; Varenna et al. 2000).

INTERVENTIONAL THERAPY AT THE SYMPATHETIC NERVOUS SYSTEM

Currently, two therapeutic techniques are used to block sympathetic nerves: (1) injections of a local anesthetic around sympathetic paravertebral ganglia that project to the affected body part (sympathetic ganglion blocks); and (2) regional intravenous application of guanethidine, bretylium, or reserpine (which all deplete norepinephrine in the postganglionic axon) to an isolated extremity blocked with a tourniquet (intravenous regional sympatholysis).

Although sympatholytic therapy frequently results in substantial or even complete pain relief, blockade of sympathetic activity is ineffective in some patients. Nonetheless, there is compelling historical, basic, and clinical scientific evidence that an adequate sympatholytic trial should be performed by a qualified clinician in an attempt to differentiate between SMP and SIP. Symptoms other than pain may also improve after sympathetic blocks.

Many uncontrolled surveys have reviewed the effect of sympathetic interventions in CRPS and post-traumatic neuralgias. In CRPS, about 85% of patients report a positive acute effect, but fewer patients experience long-term relief (60% with sympathetic block and 30% with intravenous regional sympatholysis). In post-traumatic neuralgias, sympatholytic interventions are clearly less effective. One controlled study in patients with CRPS-I has shown that sympathetic block with local anesthetic has the same immediate effect on pain as a control injection with saline (Price et al. 1998). However, after 24 hours, patients in the local anesthetic group were much better, indicating that nonspecific effects are important initially and that efficacy of sympatholytic interventions can best be evaluated after 24 hours. Interestingly, one prospective study showed that perioperative stellate ganglion blocks in patients with a history of CRPS can significantly reduce the recurrence rate of this disease (Reuben et al. 2000). Overall, controlled studies using guanethidine intravenous regional sympatholysis have not shown a beneficial effect (Blanchard et al. 1990; Jadad et al. 1995; Ramamurthy and Hoffman 1995).

There is a desperate need for controlled studies that assess the acute as well as the long-term effect of sympathetic blockade on pain and other CRPS symptoms, in particular motor function. Adequate sympathetic ganglion blocks should be performed rather than intravenous regional sympatholysis.

STIMULATION TECHNIQUES AND SPINAL DRUG APPLICATION

Transcutaneous electrical nerve stimulation (TENS) may be effective in some cases and has minimal side effects. Epidural spinal cord stimulation has shown efficacy in one randomized study in selected chronic CRPS patients (Kemler et al. 2000a) and may be a promising treatment for this group of patients. Interestingly, because these patients had undergone previous unsuccessful surgical sympathectomy, the pain-relieving effect was not associated with peripheral vasodilatation and sympathetic blockade (Kemler et al. 2000b). Central disinhibition processes were more likely involved. Other stimulation techniques, namely peripheral nerve stimulation with implanted electrodes and deep brain stimulation (of the sensory thalamus and medial lemniscus), have been effective in selected cases of CRPS (Hassenbusch et al. 1996).

In selected patients with severe refractory CRPS, epidural administration of the *N*-methyl D-aspartate (NMDA) antagonist ketamine as well as the adrenoceptor agonist clonidine induced analgesia associated with marked side effects such as sedation and hypotension (Rauck et al. 1993; Takahashi et al. 1998). Intrathecal baclofen demonstrated a positive outcome in CRPS patients with severe dystonia (van Hilten et al. 2000).

PHYSICAL THERAPY

Clinical experience clearly indicates that physical therapy is of the utmost importance in achieving recovery of function and rehabilitation (Sherry et al. 1999). However, few clinical trials have been conducted to demonstrate the efficacy of physical therapy or its effect on the natural course of the disease (Oerlemans et al. 1999). At the acute stage of CRPS, when patients still suffer from severe pain, it is usually impossible to carry out intensive active therapy. Painful interventions and in particular aggressive physical therapy at this stage lead to deterioration. Therefore, immobilization and careful contralateral physical therapy should be the acute treatment of choice. Later, when pain subsides, passive physical therapy and active isometric training followed by active isotonic training should be performed in combination with sensory desensitization programs.

FUTURE PERSPECTIVES

One of the most distressing symptoms in CRPS is undoubtedly the pain. However, unlike most other human pain states, CRPS is not just a pain disease. The typical clinical symptom constellation also includes severe somatomotor and autonomic abnormalities as well as trophic changes of the skin and deep somatic tissues. These features may lead to chronic disability of the extremity if early treatment and rehabilitation fail.

Animal models for neuropathic pain that are available so far do not mimic this variety of symptoms. Therefore, we must intensify our research on patients who suffer from CRPS to gather more insight into the pathophysiological mechanisms of this extremely complex symptomatology. Such an approach is likely to confirm that important components of the pathophysiology of CRPS are located within the central nervous system. This will include not only the autonomic, sensory, and motor systems, but also most likely centers for the processing of cognitive and affective information.

One of the unsolved features of this chronic pain disorder is the fact that only a small minority of persons who experience the same kinds of trauma go on to develop it. In contrast, after experimental nerve lesions almost all animals develop neuropathic pain behavior. Gene technology will provide modern tools to characterize the distinct genetic pattern of patients who are at risk of developing CRPS.

ACKNOWLEDGMENTS

This work was supported by the Deutsche Forschungsgemeinschaft (DFG Ba 1921/1-1) and the BMBF Network "Neuropathic Pain."

REFERENCES

Adami S, Fossaluzza V, Gatti D, Fracassi E, Braga V. Bisphosphonate therapy of reflex sympathetic dystrophy syndrome. *Ann Rheum Dis* 1997; 56:201–204.

Ali Z, Raja SN, Wesselmann U, et al. Intradermal injection of norepinephrine evokes pain in patients with sympathetically maintained pain. *Pain* 2000; 88:161–168.

Baron R, Maier C. Reflex sympathetic dystrophy: skin blood flow, sympathetic vasoconstrictor reflexes and pain before and after surgical sympathectomy. *Pain* 1996; 67:317–326.

Baron R, Wasner G. Complex regional pain syndromes. *Curr Pain Headache Rep* 2001; 5:114–123.

Baron R, Levine JD, Fields HL. Causalgia and reflex sympathetic dystrophy: does the sympathetic nervous system contribute to the generation of pain? *Muscle Nerve* 1999; 22:678–695.

Baron R, Baron Y, Disbrow E, Roberts TP. Activation of the somatosensory cortex during A-beta-fiber mediated hyperalgesia, a MSI study. *Brain Res* 2000; 871:75–82.

Baron R, Schattschneider J, Binder A, Siebrecht D, Wasner G. Relation between sympathetic vasoconstrictor activity and pain and hyperalgesia in complex regional pain syndromes: a case-control study. *Lancet* 2002; 359:1655–1660.

Bhatia KP, Bhatt MH, Marsden CD. The causalgia-dystonia syndrome. *Brain* 1993; 116:843–851.

Birklein F, Sittle R, Spitzer A, et al. Sudomotor function in sympathetic reflex dystrophy. *Pain* 1997; 69:49–54.

Birklein F, Riedl B, Neundörfer B, Handwerker HO. Sympathetic vasoconstrictor reflex pattern in patients with complex regional pain syndrome. *Pain* 1998; 75:93–100.

Birklein F, Weber M, Neundorfer B. Increased skin lactate in complex regional pain syndrome: evidence for tissue hypoxia? *Neurology* 2000; 55:1213–1215.

Birklein F, Schmelz M, Schifter S, Weber M. The important role of neuropeptides in complex regional pain syndrome. *Neurology* 2001; 57:2179–2184.

Blanchard J, Ramamurthy S, Walsh N, Hoffman J, Schoenfeld L. Intravenous regional sympatholysis: a double-blind comparison of guanethidine, reserpine, and normal saline. *J Pain Symptom Manage* 1990; 5:357–361.

Bruehl S, Harden RN, Galer BS, et al. External validation of IASP diagnostic criteria for complex regional pain syndrome and proposed research diagnostic criteria. *Pain* 1999; 81:147–154.

Bruehl S, Harden RN, Galer BS, et al. Complex regional pain syndrome: are there distinct subtypes and sequential stages of the syndrome? *Pain* 2002; 95:119–124.

Calder JS, Holten I, McAllister RM. Evidence for immune system involvement in reflex sympathetic dystrophy. *J Hand Surg (Br)* 1998; 23:147–150.

Casale R, Elam M. Normal sympathetic nerve activity in a reflex sympathetic dystrophy with marked skin vasoconstriction. *J Auton Nerv Syst* 1992; 41:215–219.

Chelimsky TC, Low PA, Naessens JM, et al. Value of autonomic testing in reflex sympathetic dystrophy. *Mayo Clin Proc* 1995; 70:1029–1040.

Christensen K, Jensen EM, Noer I. The reflex dystrophy syndrome response to treatment with systemic corticosteroids. *Acta Chir Scand* 1982; 148:653–655.

Davis KD, Treede RD, Raja SN, Meyer RA, Campbell JN. Topical application of clonidine relieves hyperalgesia in patients with sympathetically maintained pain. *Pain* 1991; 47:309–317.

Deuschl G, Blumberg H, Lücking CH. Tremor in reflex sympathetic dystrophy. *Arch Neurol* 1991; 48:1247–1252.

Drummond PD, Skipworth S, Finch PM. Alpha 1-adrenoceptors in normal and hyperalgesic human skin. *Clin Sci (Colch)* 1996; 91:73–77.

Fukumoto M, Ushida T, Zinchuk VS, Yamamoto H, Yoshida S. Contralateral thalamic perfusion in patients with reflex sympathetic dystrophy syndrome. *Lancet* 1999; 354:1790–1791.

Galer BS, Butler S, Jensen MP. Case reports and hypothesis: a neglect-like syndrome may be responsible for the motor disturbance in reflex sympathetic dystrophy (Complex Regional Pain Syndrome-1). *J Pain Symptom Manage* 1995; 10:385–391.

Goldstein DS, Tack C, Li ST. Sympathetic innervation and function in reflex sympathetic dystrophy. *Ann Neurol* 2000; 48:49–59.

Graif M, Schweitzer ME, Marks B, Matteucci T, Mandel S. Synovial effusion in reflex sympathetic dystrophy: an additional sign for diagnosis and staging. *Skeletal Radiol* 1998; 27:262–265.

Gulevich SJ, Conwell TD, Lane J, et al. Stress infrared telethermography is useful in the diagnosis of complex regional pain syndrome, type I (formerly reflex sympathetic dystrophy). *Clin J Pain* 1997; 13:50–59.

Harden RN, Baron R, Jänig W. *Complex Regional Pain Syndrome*, Progress in Pain Research and Management, Vol. 22. Seattle: IASP Press, 2001.

Hartrick CT. Increased production of nitric oxide stimulated by interferon-gamma from peripheral blood monocytes in patients with complex regional pain syndrome. *Neurosci Lett* 2002; 323:75–77.

Hassenbusch SJ, Stanton-Hicks M, Schoppa D, Walsh JG, Covington EC. Long-term results of peripheral nerve stimulation for reflex sympathetic dystrophy. *J Neurosurg* 1996; 84:415–423.

Huygen FJ, De Bruijn AG, De Bruin MT, et al. Evidence for local inflammation in complex regional pain syndrome type 1. *Mediators Inflamm* 2002; 11:47–51.

Jadad AR, Carroll D, Glynn CJ, McQuay HJ. Intravenous regional sympathetic blockade for pain relief in reflex sympathetic dystrophy: a systematic review and a randomized, double-blind crossover study. *J Pain Symptom Manage* 1995; 10:13–20.

Juottonen K, Gockel M, Silen T, et al. Altered central sensorimotor processing in patients with complex regional pain syndrome. *Pain* 2002; 98:315–323.

Kemler MA, Barendse GA, van Kleef M, et al. Spinal cord stimulation in patients with chronic reflex sympathetic dystrophy. *N Engl J Med* 2000a; 343:618–624.

Kemler MA, Barendse GA, van Kleef M, Egbrink MG. Pain relief in complex regional pain syndrome due to spinal cord stimulation does not depend on vasodilation. *Anesthesiology* 2000b; 92:1653–1660.

Kingery WS. A critical review of controlled clinical trials for peripheral neuropathic pain and complex regional pain syndromes. *Pain* 1997; 73:123–139.

Kozin F, Soin JS, Ryan LM, Carrera GF, Wortmann RL. Bone scintigraphy in the reflex sympathetic dystrophy syndrome. *Radiology* 1981; 138:437–443.

Leitha T, Korpan M, Staudenherz A, Wunderbaldinger P, Fialka V. Five phase bone scintigraphy supports the pathophysiological concept of a subclinical inflammatory process in reflex sympathetic dystrophy. *Q J Nucl Med* 1996; 40:188–193.

Levine JD, Taiwo YO, Collins SD, Tam JK. Noradrenaline hyperalgesia is mediated through interaction with sympathetic postganglionic neurone terminals rather than activation of primary afferent nociceptors. *Nature* 1986; 323:158–160.

Maleki J, LeBel AA, Bennett GJ, Schwartzman RJ. Patterns of spread in complex regional pain syndrome, type I (reflex sympathetic dystrophy). *Pain* 2000; 88:259–266.

Marsden CD, Obeso JA, Traub MM, et al. Muscle spasms associated with Sudeck's atrophy after injury. *BMJ (Clin Res Ed)* 1984; 288:173–176.

Mellick GA, Mellicy LB, Mellick LB. Gabapentin in the management of reflex sympathetic dystrophy. *J Pain Symptom Manage* 1995; 10:265–266.

Oerlemans HM, Oostendoorp RA, de Boo T, Goris RJ. Pain and reduced mobility in complex regional pain syndrome I: outcome of a prospective randomised controlled trial of adjuvant therapy versus occupational therapy. *Pain* 1999; 83:77–83.

Oyen WJ, Arntz IE, Claessens RM, et al. Reflex sympathetic dystrophy of the hand: an excessive inflammatory response? *Pain* 1993; 55:151–157.

Perez RS, Kwakkel G, Zuurmond WW, de Lange JJ. Treatment of reflex sympathetic dystrophy (CRPS type 1): a research synthesis of 21 randomized clinical trials. *J Pain Symptom Manage* 2001; 21:511–526.

Price DD, Long S, Wilsey B, Rafii A. Analysis of peak magnitude and duration of analgesia produced by local anesthetics injected into sympathetic ganglia of complex regional syndrome patients. *Clin J Pain* 1998; 14:216–226.

Raja SN, Abatzis V, Frank SM. Role of a-adrenoceptors in neuroma pain in amputees. *Anesthesiology* 1998; 89:A1083.

Ramamurthy S, Hoffman J. Intravenous regional guanethidine in the treatment of reflex sympathetic dystrophy/causalgia: a randomized, double-blind study. Guanethidine Study Group. *Anesth Analg* 1995; 81:718–723.

Rauck RL, Eisenach JC, Jackson K, Young LD, Southern J. Epidural clonidine treatment for refractory reflex sympathetic dystrophy. *Anesthesiology* 1993; 79:1163–1169.

Renier JC, Arlet J, Bregeon C, et al. The joint in algodystrophy. Joint fluid, synovium, cartilage. *Rev Rhum Mal Osteoartic* 1983; 50:255–260.

Reuben SS, Rosenthal EA, Steinberg RB. Surgery on the affected upper extremity of patients with a history of complex regional pain syndrome: a retrospective study of 100 patients. *J Hand Surg (Am)* 2000; 25:1147–1151.

Rommel O, Malin JP, Zenz M, Jänig W. Quantitative sensory testing, neurophysiological and psychological examination in patients with complex regional pain syndrome and hemisensory deficits. *Pain* 2001; 93:279–293.

Ruocco I, Cuello AC, Ribeiro-Da-Silva A. Peripheral nerve injury leads to the establishment of a novel pattern of sympathetic fibre innervation in the rat skin. *J Comp Neurol* 2000; 422:287–296.

Schattschneider J, Wenzelburger R, Deuschl G, Baron R. Kinematic analysis of the upper extremity in CRPS. In: Harden RN, Baron R, Jänig W (Eds). *Complex Regional Pain Syndrome,* Progress in Pain Research and Management, Vol. 22. Seattle: IASP Press, 2001, pp 119–128.

Schurmann M, Gradl G, Wizgal I, et al. Clinical and physiologic evaluation of stellate ganglion blockade for complex regional pain syndrome type I. *Clin J Pain* 2001; 17:94–100.

Schwartzman RJ, Kerrigan J. The movement disorder of reflex sympathetic dystrophy. *Neurology* 1990; 40:57–61.

Sherry DD, Wallace CA, Kelley C, Kidder M, Sapp L. Short- and long-term outcomes of children with complex regional pain syndrome type I treated with exercise therapy. *Clin J Pain* 1999; 15:218–223.

Sieweke N, Birklein F, Riedl B, Neundorfer B, Handwerker HO. Patterns of hyperalgesia in complex regional pain syndrome. *Pain* 1999; 80:171–177.

Stanton-Hicks M, Jänig W, Hassenbusch S, et al. Reflex sympathetic dystrophy: changing concepts and taxonomy. *Pain* 1995; 63:127–133.

Stanton-Hicks M, Baron R, Boas R, et al. Complex regional pain syndromes: guidelines for therapy. *Clin J Pain* 1998; 14:155–166.

Takahashi H, Miyazaki M, Nanbu T, Yanagida H, Morita S. The NMDA-receptor antagonist ketamine abolishes neuropathic pain after epidural administration in a clinical case. *Pain* 1998; 75:391–394.

Torebjörk E, Wahren L, Wallin G, Hallin R, Koltzenburg M. Noradrenaline-evoked pain in neuralgia. *Pain* 1995; 63:11–20.

van der Laan L, Goris RJ. Reflex sympathetic dystrophy. An exaggerated regional inflammatory response? *Hand Clin* 1997; 13:373–385.

van Hilten BJ, van de Beek WJ, Hoff JI, Voormolen JH, Delhaas EM. Intrathecal baclofen for the treatment of dystonia in patients with reflex sympathetic dystrophy. *N Engl J Med* 2000; 343:625–630.

Varenna M, Zucchi F, Ghiringhelli D, et al. Intravenous clodronate in the treatment of reflex sympathetic dystrophy syndrome. A randomized, double blind, placebo controlled study. *J Rheumatol* 2000; 27:1477–1483.

Wallace MS, Ridgeway BM, Leung AY, Gerayli A, Yaksh TL. Concentration-effect relationship of intravenous lidocaine on the allodynia of complex regional pain syndrome types I and II. *Anesthesiology* 2000; 92:75–83.

Wasner G, Backonja MM, Baron R. Traumatic neuralgias: complex regional pain syndromes (reflex sympathetic dystrophy and causalgia): clinical characteristics, pathophysiological mechanisms and therapy. *Neurol Clin* 1998; 16:851–868.

Wasner G, Heckmann K, Maier C, Baron R. Vascular abnormalities in acute reflex sympathetic dystrophy (CRPS I)—complete inhibition of sympathetic nerve activity with recovery. *Arch Neurol* 1999; 56:613–620.

Wasner G, Schattschneider J, Heckmann K, Maier C, Baron R. Vascular abnormalities in reflex sympathetic dystrophy (CRPS I): mechanisms and diagnostic value. *Brain* 2001; 124:587–599.

Wasner G, Schattschneider J, Baron R. Skin temperature side differences—a diagnostic tool for CRPS? *Pain* 2002; 98:19–26.

Weber M, Birklein F, Neundorfer B, Schmelz M. Facilitated neurogenic inflammation in complex regional pain syndrome. *Pain* 2001; 91:251–257.

White JC, Sweet WH. *Pain and the Neurosurgeon.* Springfield, IL: Charles C. Thomas, 1969.

Correspondence to: Prof. Ralf Baron, Dr. med., Klinik für Neurologie, Christian-Albrechts-Universität Kiel, Niemannsweg 147, 24105 Kiel, Germany. Tel: 49-431-597-2633; Fax: 49-431-597-2712; email: r.baron@neurologie.uni-kiel.de.

Proceedings of the 10th World Congress on Pain,
Progress in Pain Research and Management, Vol. 24,
edited by Jonathan O. Dostrovsky, Daniel B. Carr,
and Martin Koltzenburg, IASP Press, Seattle, © 2003.

57

Pain in Individuals with Developmental Disabilities: Challenges for the Future[1]

Tim F. Oberlander,[a] Frank Symons,[b] Katinka van Dongen,[c] and Huda Huijer Abu-Saad[c]

[a]*Division of Developmental Pediatrics, University of British Columbia and Centre for Community Child Health Research, Children's and Women's Health Centre of British Columbia, Vancouver, British Columbia, Canada;* [b]*Department of Educational Psychology, University of Minnesota, Minneapolis, Minnesota, USA;* [c]*Center for Nursing Research, Maastricht University, Maastricht, The Netherlands*

Until recently pain in people with disabilities received very little scientific attention. Individuals with disabilities have been systematically excluded from most research studies on pain. Expression of pain by these individuals is frequently variable and ambiguous, and its recognition by caregivers is idiosyncratic. These uncertainties present a tremendous challenge for clinicians and researchers alike. Even when pain-specific behaviors are present, such behaviors may be altered, blunted, or confused with other sources of generalized arousal. There is no reason to believe that pain is any less frequent in someone with a developmental or acquired disability, or that such an individual would be insensitive or indifferent to pain. Numerous functional limitations as well as the underlying neurological condition itself frequently confound the presentation of pain. Regardless of the degree of the disability, pain is often a part of daily life.

How can pain be assessed and managed when typical means of verbal or nonverbal communication or cognition are altered or absent? In the absence of easily recognized verbal or motor-dependent forms of communication, it remains uncertain whether the pain experience itself is different or whether only its expressive manifestations are altered. Indeed, in the absence of easily recognizable means of communication or motor skills, pain may remain

[1] Based on a Congress workshop.

under-recognized or undertreated. In spite of the potential for altered nociception and pain expression, there is no evidence that cognitively or motor-impaired individuals are spared any of the miseries of a noxious experience. In this chapter we review recent progress and a number of key challenges facing this field. These include the epidemiology and functional impact of pain in persons with a developmental disability, pain in individuals with self-injurious behaviors, and the difficulties of assessing pain in children with severe intellectual and communicative disabilities. Many fundamental questions about how the pain system functions when its underlying neural substrate is altered remain unanswered, thus limiting our understanding of how to assess and manage pain in individuals with disabilities. It is hoped that the topics raised in this chapter will serve to stimulate future research and clinical work.

PROGRESS AND CHALLENGES

Recognition is growing that the study of pain in individuals with a developmental disability is an opportunity to reexamine our understanding of what constitutes the universal but highly personal human experience of pain. Typically the "afferent component" of pain is perceived or experienced before "efferent responses" such as self-report or behavioral changes occur (Anand et al. 1997). Feeling and reporting pain are often parallel and related phenomena, but self-report, nonverbal expression, and evidence of tissue damage can be highly discordant (Craig 1992; Manne et al. 1992), particularly among individuals with disabilities (Porter et al. 1996; Oberlander et al. 1999; Hadjistavropoulos et al. 2000). Many disabilities are associated with painful conditions that require recurrent noxious and invasive procedures, resulting in frequent pain during daily life. The situation is compounded by difficulties in communicating distress and impairments in motor skills needed to solicit help, which in turn may lead to increased incidence, severity, and duration of pain.

The past 10 years have seen exponential growth in research activity in this field spanning from preterm infants (Oberlander et al. 2002), to children with cognitive and communication impairments (McGrath et al. 1998), to adults with cerebral palsy (Turk et al. 1997; Schwartz et al. 1999; Stallard et al. 2001, 2002a; Engel et al. 2002), to the frail elderly with dementia (Farrell et al. 1996; Hadjistavropoulos et al. 2000) (Fig. 1). Using the key words *brain injury, communication impairment, self-injurious behavior, cognitive impairment/mental retardation,* and *cerebral palsy,* a search of Medline, Pubmed, and PsychLit databases yielded 492 articles dating from 1966 to

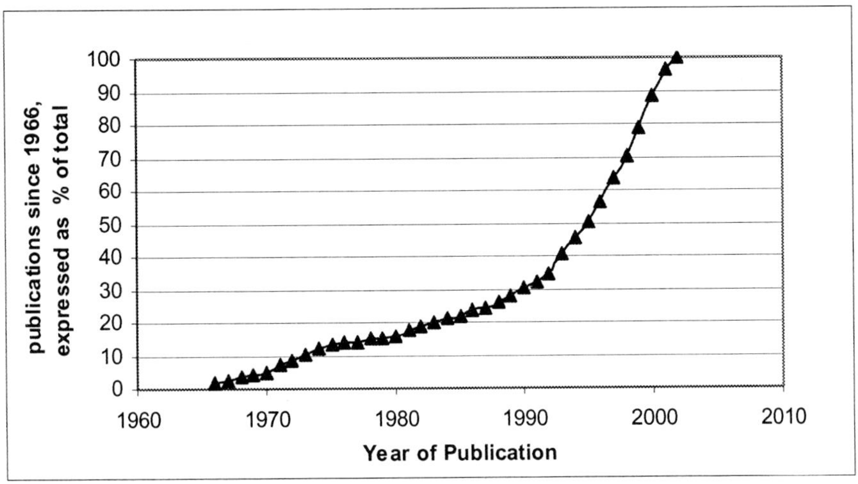

Fig. 1. Number of publications per year since 1966 citing pain in individuals with disabilities.

2002. Early papers identified in this search, while containing one or more of these key words, typically were case reports describing individuals undergoing orthopedic surgery where the term "pain" was used to describe the reason for the procedure or was used as a nonspecific outcome measure. More recently, reports have explored the epidemiology of pain (Hodgkinson et al. 2001; Engel et al. 2002), biobehavioral reactivity to vaccine-related pain in adolescents with cerebral palsy (Oberlander et al. 1999), and response to pain in the elderly with dementia (Porter et al. 1996). Empirical studies have yielded important inventories of behaviors considered to be related to pain among children and adults with significant neurological impairments (Stallard et al. 2002b; Tyler et al. 2002). Validity and reliability of a number of multidimensional instruments to assess pain in children and adults with communication and cognitive impairments have recently been established (McGrath et al. 1998; Breau et al. 2000, 2001, 2002a; Collignon and Giusiano 2001; Hunt et al. 2002), and work to understand the clinical utility of these tools is pending. Studies of novel treatment strategies are still lacking. While the absolute number of publications in this field remains small, the recent growth in this field parallels similar trends in pain-related pediatric research presented at Pediatric Academic Societies Annual Meetings, World Congresses on Pain presented by the International Association for the Study of Pain (IASP), and published papers in the pediatric literature since the 1970s (Schechter 1987). The impact this research will have on changes in the recognition, assessment, and management of pain in individuals with disabilities remains to be defined.

Recently, IASP has made a substantial change to the definition of pain itself, further highlighting the increasing attention to this field. IASP refers to pain as "an unpleasant sensory and emotional experience associated with actual or potential tissue damage, or described in terms of such damage" (Merskey 1986). Characterization of the experience of pain as an unpleasant sensory and emotional experience with actual or potential tissue damage should be applicable to anyone regardless of a disability. However, emphasis on self-report assumes a capacity for effective verbal communication of this highly personal subjective experience. Recently, the definition of pain has been supplemented to recognize that "the inability to communicate in no way negates the possibility that an individual is experiencing pain and is in need of appropriate pain-relieving treatment" (www.iasp-pain.org). While this addition acknowledges the needs of an individual with a disability and the importance of communication limitations in diverse populations, it characterizes such an individual as being unable to communicate. In accepting this definition, one must keep in mind that persons who are impaired in verbal self-report are still able to communicate very effectively via nonverbal behavior (K.D. Craig, personal communication). It is important to recognize that the IASP addendum does not specify or restrict the form of communication that may be impaired. If signals of acute distress in individuals with communication impairments are dismissed or ignored because of a lack of a capacity for self-report, pain may remain poorly treated (Anand and McGrath 1993; Walco et al. 1994; Anand and Craig 1996). All features of the behavioral response to pain need to be accepted as evidence of its presence and should not be discounted as a "surrogate measure" of pain (Anand and Craig 1996). However limited the behavioral and physiological repertoire that is available to the individual, an expression of distress during nociception should be taken as the pain measure.

EPIDEMIOLOGY

Our incomplete understanding of the epidemiology of pain across the spectrum of disabilities continues to limit research and clinical care. What is known suggests that pain is common and poorly treated among adults and children with disabilities. Turk et al. (1997) found that 84% of women with cerebral palsy (CP) report experiencing pain secondary to their condition. Schwartz et al. (1999) report that over two-thirds of adults with CP report one or more areas of pain of 3 months' duration or longer. Similar levels of pain have been reported by Engels et al. (2002) among adults with CP who reported that they frequently did not have access to health care providers to manage their pain; even when interventions were available they were only moderately helpful.

Limited reports suggest that pain is also under-recognized and under-treated among children with CP and brain injury (Oberlander and O'Donnell 2001). There is good reason to believe that pain is much more a part of the daily lives of most of these children than for those without developmental disabilities (McGrath et al. 1998). At present, there are no satisfactory epidemiological data regarding the incidence or prevalence of chronic or acute pain in populations of children with developmental disabilities. Estimates of the extent of pain in these children might be derived using indirect measures from what we know about pain in children in general. Given that 30–40% of children experience a recurrent pain (headaches, abdominal pain, or musculoskeletal pain) (Mikkelsson et al. 1997) at least once a week (Sillanpaa 1983; McGrath 1990; Abu-Arefeh and Russell 1994; Kristjansdottir 1997; Lee and Olness 1997) and that the prevalence of weekly episodes of stomach pain and back pain may be as high as 15–20% of school-age children (Borge et al. 1994), there is no reason to believe that children with developmental disabilities do not have similar levels of chronic recurrent pain. An estimated 15–20% of all children (Boyle et al. 1994) have some level of developmental disability that may be associated with either difficulty in communicating distress or an increased incidence of pain, or both. While the etiology of the underlying conditions varies, the additive effects of pain in the presence of a disability are common to all conditions. Therefore, even by crude indirect methods it might be reasonable to estimate that pain is more common in children with developmental disabilities than among children in general, highlighting the urgency for future study in this area.

FUNCTIONAL IMPACT OF PAIN

Efforts to understand pain in this setting also requires an evaluation of the functional impact of the pain, its role in quality of life, and its interaction with the disability itself. Studies of pain typically focus on describing the symptoms, duration, and intensity of pain without accounting for the functional consequences of the symptom, even though these are likely to have a major impact on the individual. The measurement of functional disability related to pain in adults has received considerable attention because of issues related to employment status, cost of care, and disability payments. However, work on pain-related functional disability in pediatric populations is limited. Recently, systematic work has characterized functional impairment associated with various childhood disabilities (Nagi 1991; World Health Organization 1980; Butler and Campbell 2000). Palermo (2000) has reviewed work characterizing the deleterious impact of pain on child and family functioning.

Nagi (1991) and Butler and Campbell (2000) have proposed multidimensional models that define the disabling processes consistent with the five dimensions of the World Health Organization's system of impairment and disability (Table I). Using this schema, the impact of CP can be described (Table II). Taking this one step further, using the Butler framework one can assess the functional impact of pain in an adolescent with CP (Table III). Based on this model the *pathophysiology* of the disability would be the central lesions (presumably prenatal ischemic neurological injury), as well as a chronic headache, which may or may not be related to factors associated with the disease (e.g., hydrocephalus/shunt malfunction or a concurrent migraine disorder). Here the disease and pain together receive consideration as potentially interrelated but separate pathophysiological entities. The *impairment* would include the neuromotor impairment (spasticity) and frequency and intensity of the symptom (head pain), regardless of the etiology. Compounding the impairment are the cognitive and communication limitations that also result from central impairment. The *functional limitations* that follow may be a consequence of motor, cognitive, and communication limitations as well as the effect of the pain on activities of daily living (e.g., sleep, self-care, and the adolescent's relationship with his or her family and peers). An individual's *disability* may be difficulty in carrying on life as an adolescent attending school or in age-appropriate social relationships. Finally, the *societal limitations* are those barriers placed by society that limit classroom participation, even in a modified setting, because teachers may

Table I
Model of disability and chronic pain: five dimensions of human functioning

Dimension	Description
Pathophysiology	Interruption or interference of normal physiology and developmental processes or structures
Impairment	Loss or abnormality of body structure or body function
Functional limitation	Restriction of ability to perform activities
Disability	Inability to participate in typical societal role functions
Societal limitation	Barriers to full participation in society that result from attitudes, architectural barriers, and social policies

Source: Adapted from Butler (2000) and Oberlander et al. (2003).

Table II
Examples of selected effects of cerebral palsy on dimensions of human functioning

Dimension	Examples
Pathophysiology	Cystic lesions and white matter loss as a result of periventricular leukomalacia of the premature infant's brain
Impairment	Spasticity, contractures, low endurance, perceptual dysfunction
Functional limitation	Awkward walking with fatigue, difficulty dressing, poor concentration and sustained listening, reading problems
Disability	Learning delays, education in restricted environment, limited sports participation, interference with dating and sexuality, not able to take communion at church, cannot participate in family activity by doing chores at home, unable to achieve independent living
Societal limitation	Exclusion from school/city team sports, denial of medical treatment or equipment by insurer, government action that blocks the building of independent living units for people with disabilities, failure of voters to support funding of wheelchair lifts for public buses

have difficulty understanding, managing, and coping with a student's pain. An individual may also be denied appropriate and timely pain management because caregivers may not accept that the pain is "real" when the ability to express it with discrete words and motor movements is limited.

This model of compounding disabling processes has important implications for understanding pain in the individual with intellectual impairment. It identifies the functional consequences of pain, suggests its optimal assessment (frequency, duration, and intensity), and indicates measurements of functional limitations that might be related to the underlying neurological condition. It also helps distinguish between individuals who experience pain with few or no functional limitations from those who are more severely restricted in function. While the former individuals may be separate from the latter in an etiological sense, pain assessment and management in this setting are invariably influenced by the functional limitations (i.e., a limited capacity to communicate pain) associated with the neurological impairment. The model illustrates the potential for an additive effect of chronic pain on the underlying disability and the role of the context in which the individual lives. Further work is needed to develop measures to quantify the impact of chronic and acute pain and its influence on quality of life. This model also needs to include ways to assess the impact of social and family supports on daily pain.

Table III
Examples of selected effects of pain on dimensions of human functioning in a child with cerebral palsy

Dimension	Examples
Pathophysiology	Altered pain system function (neurotransmitters, reduced descending inhibition, increased excitatory neurochemicals)
Impairment	Technological assistive devices (G-tube, intrathecal pumps), spasticity, contractures, low endurance, perceptual dysfunction
Functional limitation	Increased incidence of pain-related invasive procedures, awkward walking/seating/communication, difficulty in activities of daily living
Disability	Headaches prevent/limit attendance or performance at school
Societal limitation	Exclusion from school, denial of appropriate pain management (others might assume that the individual is not in pain because of difficulty in communicating distress)

THE CHALLENGES OF PAIN AND SELF-INJURY IN DEVELOPMENTAL DISABILITIES

Self-injurious behavior (SIB) is among the most prevalent and destructive forms of severe behavior disorder seen in persons with neurodevelopmental disorders (Schroeder et al. 2001). Approximately 30% of persons with autism and 50% of persons with severe to profound mental retardation display clinically significant SIB (Luiselli et al. 1992; Thompson et al. 1995; Schroeder et al. 1997). Chronic self-injury that occurs at high rates over long time periods can also result in irreversible tissue damage, sensory impairment, or brain injury. Given this potential for such severe injury, it is reasonable to consider whether mechanisms for perceiving and responding to pain may be abnormal in persons with SIB.

Models and mechanisms. In behavioral models of SIB, if no consistent pattern of discernible environmental variables correlates with self-injury, it is often proposed that the behavior is not socially mediated and may be maintained by sensory consequences arising from self-inflicted stimulation. Direct evidence linking nonsocial SIB to sensory variables is scant, however, and the mechanisms regulating sensory behavior and their relation to biological variables have not been delineated. In one model of pain and SIB, self-injury may signal the presence of pain from a source of acute discomfort associated with an unidentified but specific medical problem (e.g., an ear infection) that the individual cannot otherwise control because of deficits in adaptive behavior or communicative competency (Carr and Smith 1995). Pediatricians have widely observed that developing infants typically tug and poke at their ears and slap or scratch the side of their face and head when they have ear infections. Presumably this behavior serves a social function, enabling primary caregivers to comfort the infant and treat the infection causing the pain. Thus, the person with developmental disabilities who has menstrual discomfort (Carr et al. 1993), ear-ache (O'Reilly 1997), or allergies (Kennedy and Meyer 1996), or is experiencing other sources of acute pain and discomfort that may not be obvious to an outside observer may engage in SIB as a social or communicative act. In this model, the sensory and expressive components of pain would be intact.

Alternatively, in a different model of pain and SIB, some persons with chronic SIB and developmental disabilities may have reduced pain-related capacities in the form of altered pain sensory thresholds or impairments in pain expression and regulation due to a congenital condition or acquired trauma. In this model, the self-inflicted stimulation associated with SIB and the ensuing cascade of peripheral and neurochemical events may be highly resistant to change. From this perspective, for a subset of individuals, SIB that occurs independently of external environmental variables and that is not directly related to an acute medical problem may be considered a form of sensory disorder that results in part from dysfunctional peripheral and central mechanisms regulating sensory and pain function. This conceptualization of SIB does not directly address etiology but does provide a framework to consider the role of internal consequences that maintain severe, persistent self-injury with limited behavioral components. A more basic biological function of SIB, then, may be the self-regulation of pain by activation of the body's endogenous pain and analgesia regulatory mechanisms. Support for the involvement of endogenous opioids in self-injury has come from studies that have demonstrated altered β-endorphin levels in persons with SIB (Sandman et al. 1991) and from controlled treatment trials of the opioid antagonist naltrexone (Buzan et al. 1995; Symons et al. 1998; Sandman et al. 1999).

Pain sensitivity and expression. The largest single risk factor for the development of self-injury is mental retardation, with the prevalence of SIB rising rapidly from mild/moderate to severe/profound mental retardation (Rojahn 1994). Given this epidemiology, it is of interest that many people with mental retardation appear to demonstrate remarkable insensitivity to pain. For instance, people with developmental disabilities do not always grimace, wince, or cry out following an injury or the discomfort often associated with medical care (Roy and Simon 1987; Biersdorff 1994). A consistent failure to display pain behaviors might suggest that the experience of pain may be absent or substantially altered. In other nonverbal or similarly compromised populations (e.g., neonates, infants, and the medically frail elderly), objective measurement strategies have been used to identify pain based on facial coding of expression during known painful events such as vaccination, blood draw, or minor invasive procedures (Izard et al. 1980; Grunau and Craig 1987, 1990). This work draws upon the large body of empirical evidence for objective, nonverbal signs of emotional expression based on changes in facial action (Eckman and Friesen 1978). Work with facial action coding has identified reliable configurations of facial muscles that correspond to discrete emotional states and includes a "pain face" configuration of facial action units (Craig et al. 1992). In studies of individuals with developmental disorders, facial action coding has been used to identify painful experiences during invasive procedures (LaChapelle et al. 1999; Oberlander et al. 1999). Facial actions associated with acute vaccine- and venipuncture-related pain among nonverbal individuals with developmental disabilities corresponded to the timing of the injection. Importantly, these studies showed that it is impossible to quantitate the magnitude of pain expression in nonverbal persons with severe cognitive disabilities. These studies have consistently shown that while the sensitivity to painful stimuli may be lower in persons with mental retardation, painful events do reliably elicit the same types of nonverbal pain expression seen in persons without developmental disabilities. The application of facial action coding technology to patients with chronic SIB is an important next step, and preliminary work suggests the feasibility of doing so (see Figs. 1, 2).

Self-injury, pain, and sensory function. In many syndromes associated with developmental disorders, empirical evidence for altered sensory function and diminished sensitivity to painful stimuli is scarce despite years of anecdotal reports. In autism and related pervasive developmental disorders, for example, it has long been recognized that many individuals have reduced sensation or responses to nociceptive stimuli (Ornitz 1976). This observation takes on added significance considering an estimated prevalence of self-injury as high as 40–50% in persons with autism (Bartak and Rutter 1976). In Prader-Willi syndrome (PWS), individuals have a remarkable tendency for repeated persistent skin picking accompanied by little apparent pain response. Brandt and Rosen (1998) documented sensory abnormalities in patients with PWS compared with matched controls. Overall, there appear to be subgroups of individuals with syndromes of developmental disability,

Fig. 2. Coders, trained to the criteria in the Facial Action Coding Scale (FACS), coded videotaped segments to determine the frequency of pain-related Facial Action Units (FAUs) and were blind to whether the segments were taped before or after periods of self-injurious behavior (SIB). (A) Results suggested that, when several individuals were examined as a group ($N = 10$), there was a significant elevation in pain expression from pre- to post-SIB periods. (B) This group trend was due to the fact that a majority (60%) of the SIB cases tended to exhibit this pain expression pattern following a bout of severe SIB. (C) One-third of subjects exhibited no apparent increase in pain expression following SIB incidents. ⟶

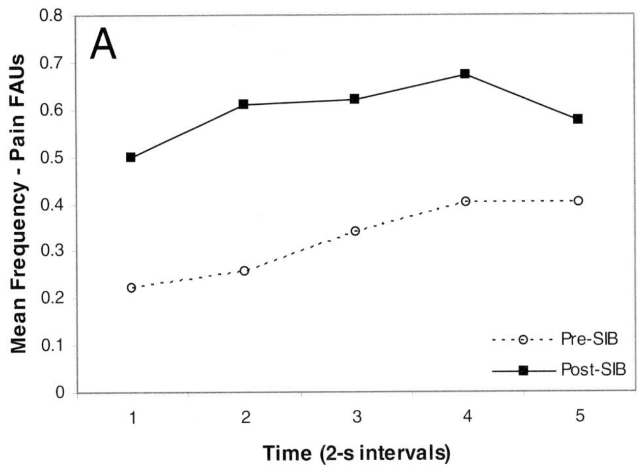
A
Mean Frequency - Pain FAUs
0.8
0.7
0.6
0.5
0.4
0.3
0.2
0.1
0
1
2
3
4
5
Time (2-s intervals)
Pre-SIB
Post-SIB

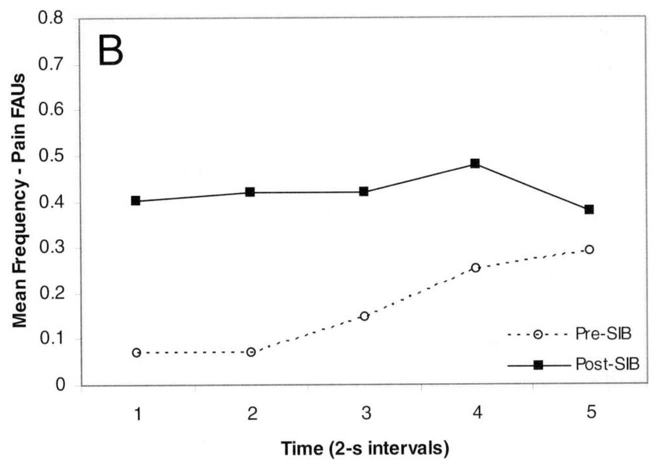
B
Mean Frequency - Pain FAUs
0.8
0.7
0.6
0.5
0.4
0.3
0.2
0.1
0
1
2
3
4
5
Time (2-s intervals)
Pre-SIB
Post-SIB

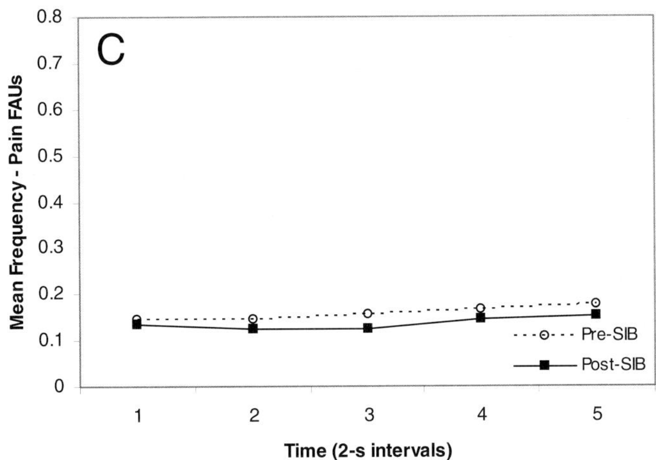
C
Mean Frequency - Pain FAUs
0.8
0.7
0.6
0.5
0.4
0.3
0.2
0.1
0
1
2
3
4
5
Time (2-s intervals)
Pre-SIB
Post-SIB

such as Lesch-Nyhan syndrome and Cornelia de Lange syndrome, in which pain transmission is impaired and SIB is highly prevalent (Symons and Thompson 1997). Most recently, Nolano et al (2000) documented the absence of skin innervation (C and Aδ fibers) as the morphological basis underlying pain insensitivity in a single case study of a young girl with mental retardation and chronic SIB. Further work on peripheral pain mechanisms in SIB appears warranted.

In summary, clinical observations suggest that some individuals with developmental disabilities who persistently self-injure are insensitive to nociceptive stimuli, yet the role of biological factors related to pain in individuals with SIB has received little systematic study. Considerable evidence from both clinical and preclinical studies of chronic pain and its behavioral sequelae supports the hypothesis that some forms of chronic SIB may be mediated by altered pain mechanisms, consistent with the notion of an injury-induced sensory disorder (Symons 2002). From this perspective, a number of issues specific to pain and self-injury remain to be systematically examined in patients with SIB.

THE CHALLENGES OF CREATING PAIN ASSESSMENT TOOLS FOR DEVELOPMENTAL DISABILITIES

Despite the inevitability of painful procedures in the life of most children with severe intellectual disability, a review of the literature on pain in this pediatric population in 1997 revealed a paucity of pain assessment tools for this population (Huijer Abu-Saad 1997). Fortunately, this situation is changing rapidly. As described above, several authors have recently suggested that intellectually disabled children are likely to process information and communicate distress differently than normal children (Gilbert-MacLeod et al. 2000; Breau et al. 2001). Oberlander et al. (1999b) and Stallard et al. (2001) reported that although parents and caregivers have observed that these children have altered pain behaviors, there is no conclusive evidence to suggest that they are insensitive or indifferent to pain. Recent evidence points to intact pain sensitivity in at least a substantial proportion of intellectually disabled children (Gilbert-MacLeod et al. 2000; Malviya et al. 2001). Additionally, a number of instruments to assess pain in such children have recently been reported (Giusiano et al. 1995; Collignon et al. 1997; Breau et al. 2000, 2002a,b; Collignon and Giusiano 2001; Hadden and von Baeyer 2002; Hunt et al. 2002; Stallard et al. 2002c). Several studies (Breau et al. 2000; Collignon and Giusiano 2001; Hunt et al. 2002; Stallard et al. 2002c) identified possible multidimensional pain cues in children with cognitive impairment. These include vocalizations (e.g., crying, screaming, moaning), facial expression, increased or decreased movement, altered muscle tone, guarding or protection of the painful area, changes in social interaction, and changes in eating and sleeping. Physiological changes such as changes in skin color, shivering, and sweating were only described by Breau et al. (2001). Developing an instrument to assess pain in this heterogeneous population, however, remains a challenge. Below we report on the results of a series of studies aimed at developing an instrument to assess medically related acute pain in the child with severe intellectual and communicative disabilities. This series of studies addressed two questions: How do severely intellectually disabled children express their pain, and how do impairments that limit the expression of pain influence the development of a valid and reliable pain assessment tool? This project involved collaboration between the Center for Nursing Research, Maastricht University, and Sophia Children's Hospital and Erasmus University, Rotterdam.

Study I: Item devising. Items for the scale were devised by conducting a qualitative study. The purpose of this study was to gain insight into nonverbal pain expressions that caregivers and clinicians use to identify pain in children and adolescents with severe intellectual and communicative disabilities (K. van Dongen et al., unpublished manuscript). Data were collected by observing 32 children in situations likely to be associated with procedural pain (e.g., vaccinations against influenza, physical therapy, and dental procedures) and in unstructured interviews with a sample of 29 caregivers including parents, nurses, physicians, physical therapists, a dentist, a dental hygienist, a psychologist, and an orthopedic specialist. Analyses addressed whether the identified expressions were comparable with measurement scale items (n = 138) taken from the literature on pain assessment in various nonverbal populations. Initially, seven dimensions of pain were postulated: Facial, Vocal, Motor, Physiological, Social-Emotional, Activities of Daily Living, and Injured Body Part. Altogether, an item bank of 209 expressions was compiled comprising pain cues from the literature and from our own interviews and observations. Forty-two measurement scale items taken from the literature were not replicated in our observations. We concluded that nonverbal pain expressions are diverse and depend on the individuals' functional abilities and behavioral repertoires, and so a child's "normal" behavior must be taken into account when diagnosing pain. This study documents the large number of indicators used to assess pain and hence demonstrates the difficulty in accurately assessing pain in this patient population. The challenge of reducing the large number of obtained indicators to a short clinically relevant scale became the focus of the next studies.

Study II: Pain expressions used by nurses: content validity, face validity, and interpretability. A second cross-sectional study sought to understand the type and relative importance of nonverbal expressions observed by nurses working with persons with severe or profound intellectual disability. Nurses (n = 109) (M.G. Zwakhalen et al., unpublished manuscript) were presented with 158 indicators of pain based on findings from Study I, described above, and on existing tools developed for assessment in a similar setting (Giusiano et al. 1995; Collignon et al. 1997; McGrath et al. 1998). Nurses were asked to rate each indicator on a scale of 1 to 10, with 1 representing "not at all important" and 10 "extremely important" to indicate pain. In total, the nurses chose all 158 indicators as being important to indicate pain. The highest mean scores were given to the indicators reflecting "painful expression during manipulation" (mean ± SD = 9.43 ± 1.80) and "crying during manipulation" (9.30 ± 2.11). Nurses caring for individuals with severe intellectual disability use many more indicators to assess pain than do nurses caring for profoundly intellectually disabled individuals. This finding stresses the importance of functional abilities as determinants of pain expression. We concluded that behaviors relating directly to the situation in which they occur are regarded as most important for diagnosing pain. These findings underline the difficulty of pain assessment when no obvious cause is present. Furthermore, nurses regard physical signs suggestive of pain, such as swelling, as important for labeling behavior as pain behavior. Finally, while this study supported the content validity of the expressions of pain collected in the qualitative study, it was not useful in reducing the number of items in the tool.

Study III: Pain expressions used by parents: initial item reduction. The first two studies generated a large number of items and provided evidence for interpretability and face and content validity. This left us with many more items than we could ultimately include in the scale. Due to the heterogeneity of the sample we decided to limit further item reduction and tool testing to profoundly intellectually disabled nonverbal children, comprising a somewhat more homogenous population. Because parents are an important source of information for health professionals, the third study focused on parental judgments about the occurrence of the behavioral items collected (Van Dongen et al. 2003). Parents (n = 99) were asked to complete a questionnaire based on the expressions in the scale described above and to choose the items indicative of pain in their children. All items with valid percentage scores over 75% on the option "never present" when the child is in pain (i.e., a child *never* uses a particular behavior to express pain) were discarded from the draft scale. Twenty-eight expressions from the draft scale were removed as a result, mostly relating to the Injured Body Part dimension (e.g., "Hunching, pushing injured body part") and items relating to self-injurious and aggressive behavior (e.g., "Head banging," "Destructive behavior"). The 10 items indicated by parents as most frequently occurring were: "Restless movements," "Facial tension," "Restlessness," "Facial restlessness," "Seeking comfort or physical closeness," "Looking sad," "Looking anxious," "High muscle tone," "Grimacing," and "Tears." Of the 141 items initially used, 113 were retained (Hunt et al. 2002). This study provided further evidence of the content validity of the indicators and was useful in slightly reducing the total number of items. This reduction was insufficient to render the scale clinically useable, and further reductions were considered necessary.

Study IV: Clinical observations: psychometric evaluation. The aim of this study was to select pain-specific items for inclusion in an instrument to assess procedure-related pain. Children aged 3–19 years (n = 52) with profound intellectual disabilities admitted to Sophia Children's Hospital for medical procedures under general anesthesia were included in this study. Patients were observed and videotaped for 6-minute periods on seven occasions: before hospitalization, at specific time periods during and after painful procedures during hospitalization, and at home after discharge (van Dongen et al. 2003). A distinction was made between three episodes relating to postoperative pain and one episode most likely causing brief spells of acute pain. A pain intensity score on a 0–4-point VAS was derived from clinical observations and from the video recordings of the different episodes. This continuous scale was anchored at either end by the phrases "no, not present" and "yes, continuously present." We identified a group of shared pain expressions, 40 of which comprised a potentially valid and internally consistent selection. Facial and vocal/physiological items generally had the best psychometric properties for diagnosing procedure-related pain in children with profound intellectual and communicative disabilities. This study resulted in the final version of the scale, the Kids with Intellectual Disabilities Pain Assessment Instrument for Nonverbal Signals (KIDPAINS). Acute nonsurgical pain might involve conceptually different types of behavior in comparison with postoperative pain, but this possibility needs further investigation. KIDSPAINS is being further developed and tested.

CONCLUSIONS

Efforts to understand pain in individuals with intellectual impairment have increased substantially during the past decade. Despite extensive work to characterize pain behavior and assess, quantify, and manage pain in diverse populations of individuals with disabilities across the age spectrum, numerous questions remain. At a very basic level our understanding of relationships between altered neurological function and the pain system remain incomplete. Similarly, research needs to address questions about how social and cognitive impairments influence the expression of pain, and how best to take these impairments into consideration when devising strategies to reduce suffering in intellectually disabled individuals subject to repetitive painful procedures. Further attention must be directed toward understanding the impact of family and social and cultural influences on the pain experience of these individuals. Finally we need to seek ways to translate research findings into meaningful clinical and public health policies for populations of individuals with intellectual impairment.

ACKNOWLEDGMENTS

Support for this work was received from the National Organization for Scientific Research in The Netherlands (to H.H. Abu-Saad and K. von Dongen). We are very grateful to Victoria Nethercot for her thoughtful work in editing this manuscript.

REFERENCES

Abu-Arefeh I, Russell G. Prevalence of headache and migraine in schoolchildren. *BMJ* 1994; 309:765–769.

Anand KJS, McGrath PA. An overview of current issues and their historical background. In: Anand KJS, McGrath PA. *Pain in Neonates*. Amsterdam: Elsevier, 1993; pp 1–18.

Anand KJ, Craig KD. New perspectives on the definition of pain. *Pain* 1996; 67:3–6.

Anand KS, Grunau RE, Oberlander TF. Developmental character and long-term consequences of pain in infants and children. *Child Adolesc Psychiatr Clin N Am* 1997; 6:703–724.

Bartak L, Rutter M. Differences between mentally retarded and normally intelligent autistic children. *J Autism Child Schizophr* 1976; 6:109–120.

Biersdorff KK. Incidence of significantly altered pain experience among individuals with developmental disabilities. *Am J Ment Retard* 1994; 98:619–631.

Borge AI, Nordhagen R, Moe B, Botten G, Bakketeig LS. Prevalence and persistence of stomach ache and headache among children: follow-up of a cohort of Norwegian children from 4 to 10 years of age. *Acta Paediatr* 1994; 83:433–437.

Boyle CA, Decoufle P, Yeargin-Allsopp M. Prevalence and health impact of developmental disabilities in US children. *Pediatrics* 1994; 93:399–403.

Brandt BR, Rosen I. Impaired peripheral somatosensory function in children with Prader-Willi syndrome. *Neuropediatrics* 1998; 29:124–126.

Breau LM, McGrath PJ, Camfield C, Rosmus C, Finley GA. Preliminary validation of an observational pain checklist for persons with cognitive impairments and inability to communicate verbally. *Dev Med Child Neurol* 2000; 42:609–616.

Breau LM, Camfield C, McGrath PJ, Rosmus C, Finley GA. Measuring pain accurately in children with cognitive impairments: refinement of a caregiver scale. *J Pediatr* 2001; 138:721–727.

Breau LM, Finley GA, McGrath PJ, Camfield CS. Validation of the Non-communicating Children's Pain Checklist–Postoperative Version. *Anesthesiology* 2002a; 96:528–535.

Breau LM, McGrath PJ, Camfield CS, Finley GA. Psychometric properties of the Non-Communicating Children's Pain Checklist–Revised. *Pain* 2002b; 99:349–357.

Butler C, Campbell S. Evidence of the effects of intrathecal baclofen for spastic and dystonic cerebral palsy. AACPDM Treatment Outcomes Committee Review Panel. *Dev Med Child Neurol* 2000; 42:634–645.

Buzan RD, Thomas M, Dubovksy SL, Treadway J. The use of opiate antagonists for recurrent self-injurious behavior. *J Neuropsychiatry Clin Neurosci* 1995; 7:437-444.

Carr EG, Smith CE. Biological setting events for self-injury. In: *Ment Retard Dev Disabil Res Rev* 1995; 1:94–98.

Carr EG, Smith CE, Magito-McLaughlin D, et al. Moon, menses, and meaning: complex determinants of problem behavior. Chicago: Annual Meeting of the Assocation for Behavior Analysis, 1993.

Collignon P, Giusiano B. Validation of a pain evaluation scale for patients with severe cerebral palsy. *Eur J Pain* 2001; 5:433–442.

Collignon P, Biusiano B, Boutin AM, Combes JC. Utilisation d'une échelle d'hétéroévaluation de la douleur chez le sujet sévérement polyhandicapé. *Douleur Analgesique* 1997; 1:27–32.

Craig KD. The facial expression of pain: better than a thousand words? *Am Pain Soc J* 1992; 1:153–162.

Craig KD, Prkachin KM, Grunau RE. The facial expression of pain. In: Turk MA, Melzack R (Eds). *Handbook of Pain Assessment*. New York: Guilford Press, 1992, pp 257–276.

Eckman P, Friesen WV. *Investigator's Guide to the Facial Action Coding System*. Palo Alto: Consulting Psychologists Press, 1978.

Engel JM, Kartin D, Jensen MP. Pain treatment in persons with cerebral palsy: frequency and helpfulness. *Am J Phys Med Rehabil* 2002; 81:291–296.

Farrell MJ, Katz B, Helme RD. The impact of dementia on the pain experience. *Pain* 1996; 67:7–15.

Gilbert-MacLeod CA, Craig KD, Rocha EM, Mathias MD. Everyday pain responses in children with and without developmental delays. *J Pediatr Psychol* 2000; 25:301–308.

Giusiano B, Jimeno MT, Collignon P, Chau Y. Utilization of neural network in the elaboration of an evaluation scale for pain in cerebral palsy. *Methods Inf Med* 1995; 34:498–502.

Grunau RV, Craig KD. Pain expression in neonates: facial action and cry. *Pain* 1987; 28:395–410.

Grunau RVE, Craig KD. Facial activity as a measure of neonatal pain expression. In: Tyler DC, Krane EJ (Eds). *Advances in Pain Research and Therapy*. New York: Raven Press, 1990, pp 147–155.

Hadden KL, von Baeyer CL. Pain in children with cerebral palsy: common triggers and expressive behaviors. *Pain* 2002; 99:281–288.

Hadjistavropoulos T, LaChapelle DL, MacLeod FK, Snider B, Craig KD. Measuring movement-exacerbated pain in cognitively impaired frail elders. *Clin J Pain* 2000; 16:54–63.

Hodgkinson I, Jindrich ML, Duhaut P, et al. Hip pain in 234 non-ambulatory adolescents and young adults with cerebral palsy: a cross-sectional multicentre study. *Dev Med Child Neurol* 2001; 43:806–808.

Huijer Abu-Saad H. Pijn en verstandelijke handicap: een verkening (Pain and mental retardation: a survey). In: *Handboek Mogelijkheden*, Vol. III. Utrecht: De Tijdstroom, 1997, pp 8.1–8.16.

Hunt A, Goldman A, Seers K, et al. Validation of the paediatric pain profile, a behaviour rating scale to assess pain in children with severe neurological impairment. *Abstracts: 10th World Congress on Pain*. Seattle: IASP Press, 2002, pp 559–560.

Izard CE, Huebner RR, Risser D, McGinnes GC, Dougherty LM. The young infant's ability to produce discrete emotional expressions. *Dev Psychol* 1980; 16:132–140.

Kennedy CH, Meyer KA. Sleep deprivation, allergy symptoms, and negatively reinforced problem behavior. *J Appl Behav Anal* 1996; 29:133–135.

Kristjansdottir G. Prevalence of pain combinations and overall pain: a study of headache, stomach pain and back pain among school-children. *Scand J Soc Med* 1997; 25:58–63.

LaChapelle DL, Hadjistavropoulos T, Craig KD. Pain measurement in persons with intellectual disabilities. *Clin J Pain* 1999; 15:13–23.

Lee LH, Olness KN. Clinical and demographic characteristics of migraine in urban children. *Headache* 1997; 37:269–276.

Luiselli JK, Matson JL, Singh NN. *Self-Injurious Behavior: Analysis, Assessment, and Treatment*. New York: Springer-Verlag, 1992.

Malviya S, Voepel-Lewis T, Tait AR, et al. Pain management in children with and without cognitive impairment following spine fusion surgery. *Paediatr Anaesth* 2001; 11:453–458.

Manne SL, Jacobsen PB, Redd WH. Assessment of acute pediatric pain: do child self-report, parent ratings, and nurse ratings measure the same phenomenon? *Pain* 1992; 48:45–52.

McGrath PA. *Pain in Children: Nature, Assessment, and Treatment.* New York: Guilford Press, 1990.

McGrath PJ, Rosmus C, Canfield C, Campbell MA, Hennigar A. Behaviours caregivers use to determine pain in non-verbal, cognitively impaired individuals. *Dev Med Child Neurol* 1998; 40:340–343.

Merskey HE. Classification of chronic pain: descriptions of chronic pain syndromes and definitions of pain terms. *Pain* 1986; (Suppl 3):51.

Mikkelsson M, Salminen JJ, Kautiainen H. Non-specific musculoskeletal pain in preadolescents: Prevalence and 1-year persistence. *Pain* 1997; 73:29–35.

Nagi S. Concepts Revisited: implications for prevention. In: Pope A, Taylor A (Eds). *Disability in America: Toward a National Agenda for Prevention.* Washington, DC: National Academy Press, 1991; 309–327.

O'Reilly MF. Functional analysis of episodic self-injury correlated with recurrent otitis media. *J Appl Behav Anal* 1997; 30:165–167.

Oberlander TF, Craig KD. Pain and the child with a developmental disability. In: Schechter NL, Berde CB, Yaster M (Eds). Pain in Infants, Children and Adolescents, 2nd ed. Baltimore: Lippincott, Williams and Wilkins, 2003.

Oberlander TF, O'Donnell ME. Beliefs about pain among professionals working with children with significant neurologic impairment. *Dev Med Child Neurol* 2001; 43:138–140.

Oberlander TF, Gilbert CA, Chambers CT, O'Donnell ME, Craig KD. Biobehavioral responses to acute pain in adolescents with a significant neurologic impairment. *Clin J Pain* 1999; 15:201–209.

Oberlander TF, Grunau RE, Whitfield MF, Fitzgerald C, Lee S. Does parenchymal brain injury affect biobehavioral pain responses in VLBW infants at 32 wks post conceptional age? *Pediatrics* 2002; 110:570–576.

Ornitz EM. The modulation of sensory input and motor output in autistic children. In: Schopler E, Reichler RJ (Eds). *Psychopathology and Child Development*. New York: Plenum Press, 1976, pp 115–133.

Porter FL, Malhotra KM, Wolf CM, et al. Dementia and response to pain in the elderly. *Pain* 1996; 68:413–421.

Rojahn J. Epidemiology and topographic taxonomy of self-injurious behavior. In: Thompson T, Gray DB (Eds). *Destructive Behavior in Developmental Disabilities: Diagnosis and Treatment.* Thousand Oaks: Sage Publications, 1994, pp 49–67.

Roy A, Simon GB. Intestinal obstruction as a cause of death in the mentally handicapped. *J Ment Defic Res* 1987; 31 (Pt 2):193–197.

Sandman CA, Barron JL, Chicz-DeMet A, DeMet EM. Plasma β-endorphin levels in patients with self-injurious behavior and stereotypy. *Am J Ment Retard* 1991; 95:84-92.

Sandman CA, Spence MA, Smith M. Proopiomelanocortin (POMC) dysregulation and response to opiate blockers. *Ment Retard Dev Disabil Res Rev* 1999; 5:314-321.

Schechter NL. The status of pediatric pain control: pain management in children. *Child Adolesc Psychiatr Clin N Am* 1987; 6:687–702.

Schroeder SR, Oster-Granite ML, Berkson G, Loupe PS, Stodgell CJ. Severe behavior problems among people with developmental disabilities. In: MacLean WE Jr (Ed). *Ellis' Handbook of Mental Deficiency, Psychological Theory, and Research.* Mahwah: Lawrence Erlbaum, 1997, pp 439–464.

Schroeder SR, Oster-Granite ML, Berkson G, et al. Self-injurious behavior: gene-brain-behavior relationships. *Ment Retard Dev Disabil Res Rev* 2001; 7:3–12.

Schwartz L, Engel JM, Jensen MP. Pain in persons with cerebral palsy. *Arch Phys Med Rehabil* 1999; 80:1243–1246.

Sillanpaa M. Prevalence of headache in prepuberty. *Headache* 1983; 23:10–14.

Stallard P, Williams L, Lenton S, Velleman R. Pain in cognitively impaired, non-communicating children. *Arch Dis Child* 2001; 85:460–462.

Stallard P, Williams L, Velleman R, Lenton S, McGrath PJ. Brief report: behaviors identified by caregivers to detect pain in noncommunicating children. *J Pediatr Psychol* 2002a; 27:209–214.

Stallard P, Williams L, Velleman R, Lenton S, McGrath PJ. Intervening factors in caregivers' assessments of pain in non-communicating children. *Dev Med Child Neurol* 2002b; 44:213–214.

Stallard P, Williams L, Velleman R, et al. The development and evaluation of the pain indicator for communicatively impaired children (PICIC). *Pain* 2002c; 98:145–149.

Symons F. Pain and self-injury: mechanisms and models. In: Schroeder SR, Thompson T, Oster-Granite ML (Eds). *Self-Injurious Behavior: Genes, Brain, And Behavior.* Washington, DC: American Psychological Association, 2002, pp 223–234.

Symons F, Thompson T. A review of self-injurious behavior and pain in persons with developmental disabilities. *Int Rev Res Ment Retard* 1997; 21:69–111.

Symons FJ, Fox ND, Thompson T. Functional communication training and naltrexone treatment of self-injurious behavior: an experimental case report. *J Appl Res Intellect Disabil* 1998; 11:273-292.

Thompson T, Schroeder S. Self-injury in developmental disabilities: neurobiological and environmental mechanisms. In: Thompson T, Schroeder SR (Eds). *Ment Retard Dev Disabil Res Rev* 1995; 1(2):87–89.

Turk MA, Geremski CA, Rosenbaum PF, Weber RJ. The health status of women with cerebral palsy. *Arch Phys Med Rehabil* 1997; 78:S10–S17.

Tyler EJ, Jensen MP, Engel JM, Schwartz L. The reliability and validity of pain interference measures in persons with cerebral palsy. *Arch Phys Med Rehabil* 2002; 83:236–239.

van Dongen KAJ, Huijer Abu-Saad H, Hamers JPH, Zwakhalen MG. Pain assessment in the intellectually disabled child: the challenges of tool development. *Suffering Child* 2003; in press.

Walco GA, Cassidy R C, Schechter NL. Pain, hurt, and harm: the ethics of pain control in infants and children. *N Engl J Med* 1994; 331:541–544.

World Health Organization. *International Classification of Impairments, Disabilities and Handicaps.* Geneva: World Health Organization, 1980.

Correspondence to: Tim F. Oberlander, MD, FRCPC, Division of Developmental Pediatrics, University of British Columbia, Centre for Community Child Health Research, 4480 Oak Street, Vancouver, BC, Canada V6N 2H4. Tel: 604-875-3570; Fax: 604-875-3569; email: toberlander@cw.bc.ca.

Proceedings of the 10th World Congress on Pain,
Progress in Pain Research and Management, Vol. 24,
edited by Jonathan O. Dostrovsky, Daniel B. Carr, and
Martin Koltzenburg, IASP Press, Seattle, © 2003.

58

Phantom Limb Pain: Causes and Cures[1]

Herta Flor,[a] Marshall Devor,[b] and Troels S. Jensen[c]

[a]Department of Clinical and Cognitive Neuroscience at the University of Heidelberg, Central Institute of Mental Health, Mannheim, Germany; [b]Department of Cell and Animal Biology, Institute of Life Sciences, Hebrew University of Jerusalem, Jerusalem, Israel; [c]Department of Neurology and Danish Pain Research Center, Aarhus University Hospital, Aarhus, Denmark

Phantom limb pain is a frequent sequel of amputation. Peripheral factors such as local changes in the residual limb and alterations in severed nerves and associated dorsal root ganglia (DRG), as well as central changes such as synaptic reorganization at spinal, brainstem, thalamic, and cortical levels all contribute to phantom pain. To date, few mechanism-based treatments for phantom limb pain have been proposed and so most of the literature on treatment is based on anecdotes. Interventions targeting central and peripheral changes hold out some promise. Attempts to prevent phantom limb pain by peripheral analgesia have not yielded consistent results, but other approaches to the reversal or prevention of pain memory formation may be effective.

The amputation of a limb is usually followed by the sensation that the deafferented body part is still present. Nonpainful phantom sensations may include a specific position, shape, or movement of the missing limb, and feelings of warmth or cold, itching, tingling, or electric sensations, and other paresthesias. "Phantom limb pain" is pain in a body part that is no longer present. Phantom pain occurs to some degree in 50–80% of all amputees (Jensen and Nikolajsen 1999; Kooijman et al. 2000; Nikolajsen and Jensen 2001). It may be perceived along with a certain position or movement of the phantom, and may be elicited or exacerbated by a range of physical factors (e.g., changes in weather or pressure on the residual limb) and psychological

[1] Based on a Congress workshop.

factors (e.g., emotional stress). It seems to be more intense in the distal portions of the phantom and may have a number of different qualities such as stabbing, throbbing, burning, or cramping (Hill 1999).

CLINICAL CHARACTERISTICS

Phantom limb pain, as a neuropathic pain syndrome, is assumed to reflect damage to the axons of peripheral neurons and secondary changes induced in central neurons. Phantom body pain may also occur following spinal cord injury. Phantom limb pain is infrequent if amputation occurs at a very young age. However, older children exhibit as high an incidence of phantom limb pain as adults (Krane and Heller 1995). Phantom sensations occur occasionally in congenital amputees (i.e., those born without a limb), but phantom limb pain seems to be very rare under these circumstances (Flor et al. 1998). The long-term course of phantom limb pain is unclear: some authors report a slight decline in pain prevalence over several years, but others describe high prevalence rates in long-term amputees.

Sometimes pain in the phantom is similar to the limb pain prior to amputation. The reported likelihood of such persistence ranges from 10% to 79%, depending upon the type and time of assessment (for reviews see Katz and Melzack 1990; Jensen et al. 1985). Nikolajsen et al. (1997b) point out that variations in assessment methods and potential biases of retrospective studies underlie variations in estimates of the incidence of these "pain memories." Whether phantom limb pain is more frequent in female amputees is controversial (Ehde et al. 2000).

MECHANISMS

Both peripheral and central factors have been described as determinants of phantom limb pain. Psychological factors do not seem to be a primary cause, but they may well affect the course and severity of the pain (Sherman et al. 1987). The current consensus is that changes throughout the neuraxis contribute to the experience of phantom limb pain.

PERIPHERAL FACTORS

The importance of nociceptive input from the residual limb as a determinant of phantom limb pain is supported by the moderately high correlation between pain in the residual limb (stump) and phantom limb pain (Jensen and Nikolajsen 1999). Ectopic discharge from stump neuromas has been postulated as a potential source of such nociceptive input (Nyström and Hagbarth 1981). When peripheral nerves are cut or injured, terminal swelling and regenerative sprouting of the injured axon end occur. In this process neuromas form in the residual limb. The disorganized endings of C fibers and demyelinated A fibers in neuromas have increased excitability and often show spontaneous impulse activity. Mechanical, chemical, and thermal stimulation may further exacerbate this ectopic discharge. The increased excitability and ectopic discharge in injured nerves seem to result from upregulation or novel expression, and altered kinetics, of molecules that mediate neuronal excitability, such as voltage-sensitive sodium channels (Devor et al. 1993; Devor and Seltzer 1999). In addition, abnormal connections between injured axons, such as ephapses, may contribute to the spontaneous ectopic activity. Phantom limb pain is often present very soon after amputation, before a palpable neuroma could have formed. Yet ectopic discharge also appears rapidly, apparently first in the swollen endbulbs of the divided axon rather than in outgrowing sprouts.

Local anesthesia of the stump does not uniformly suppress phantom limb pain (Birbaumer et al. 1997), a negative finding that motivated a search for other peripheral sources of ectopic input. One important source is the DRG. Ectopic impulses originating in the DRG can summate with other impulses coming from neuromas in the stump. Indeed, processes such as cross-excitation can lead to the depolarization and activation of neighboring neurons, augmenting the overall afferent barrage (Devor and Seltzer 1999; see Fig. 1). In experimental preparations and in humans, local anesthetic block of neuromas eliminates spontaneous and stimulation-induced nerve activity from the stump, but not ectopic activity originating in the DRG (Nyström and Hagbarth 1981).

Interestingly, genetic factors affect the predisposition to develop ectopy from neuromas and DRG, and to experience neuropathic pain. For example, Seltzer and colleagues (2001) recently presented evidence in the mouse that one or more genes on chromosome 15 predispose the animal to the pain behavior that follows peripheral neurectomy. This neuroma model of neuropathic pain has been considered to be a valid animal surrogate of phantom limb pain in humans (see also Devor and Raber 1990).

Sympathetic nervous system activation may account for the frequent exacerbation of phantom pain at times of emotional distress. Increased sympathetic nerve activity, as well as elevated levels of circulating epinephrine, can trigger and exacerbate ectopic neuronal activity from neuromas (Devor et al. 1994). In addition to occurring at the level of the neuroma, this sympathetic-sensory coupling also happens in the DRG (Devor and Seltzer 1999). Additional factors such as limb temperature, oxygenation level, and local

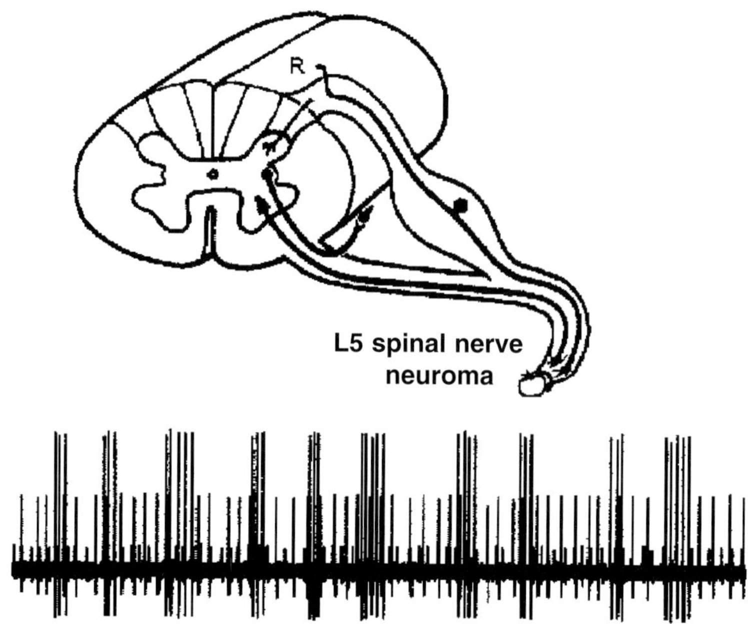

Fig. 1. High levels of ectopic afferent discharge are recorded from dorsal roots following transection of sensory axons distal to the dorsal root ganglion. In the situation shown, about 80% of the activity originates within the ganglion, the remaining 20% originating in the nerve end neuroma. The trace shows three afferent axons, distinguishable by spike height and discharge pattern, recorded simultaneously in a microfilament (R) teased from the L5 dorsal root in a nerve-injured rat (adapted from Liu et al. 2000).

inflammation within neuromas and associated DRG may also account for fluctuations in phantom limb pain intensity.

The sympathetic maintenance of phantom limb pain in some patients is supported by evidence that systemic adrenergic blocking agents, or targeted chemical or surgical blockade of sympathetic nerves and ganglia, may reduce phantom limb pain. Likewise, injections of epinephrine into stump neuromas increase phantom limb pain and paresthesias in some amputees (Chabal et al. 1992). Although sympathetically maintained pain does not necessarily covary with regional sympathetic abnormalities, in some patients sympathetic dysregulation in the residual limb is apparent. Reduced surface blood flow has been implicated as a predictor of burning phantom limb pain (Sherman and Bruno 1987). In addition, the onset and intensity of cramping and squeezing phantom pain sensations have been related to muscle tension in the residual limb (Sherman et al. 1992). Physiological correlates have not yet been identified for any other descriptors of phantom pain.

CENTRAL FACTORS

Ectopic neuroma and DRG discharge originating in injured peripheral nerves, although primary causes of phantom limb pain, are unlikely to be the only contributors. Central factors must also play a role. It is likely that different subgroups of patients have a different balance of peripheral and central factors, with distinct and differentiable pathologies (Sherman 1997). Anecdotal evidence in human amputees suggests that spinal mechanisms may play a role in phantom limb pain. For example, during spinal anesthesia, phantom pains have been reported to occur in patients who never previously experienced phantom pain (for a review, see Jensen and Nikolajsen 1999). Experimental data in human amputees are lacking, but increasing evidence from animal models of nerve injury is becoming available.

Increased activity in peripheral nociceptors leads to persistent changes in the synaptic responsiveness of neurons in the dorsal horn of the spinal cord, a process termed *central sensitization* (Doubell et al. 1999). Central sensitization may also follow nerve injury such as occurs during amputation, either as the result of increased (ectopic) activity in the periphery, or due to specific central effects of axotomy. Spinal changes associated with nerve injury include increased firing rates of dorsal horn neurons, structural changes at the central endings of primary sensory neurons, and reduced inhibitory processes. Inhibitory GABAergic and glycinergic interneurons in the spinal cord may be destroyed by rapid ectopic discharge or other effects of axotomy, contributing to a hyperexcitable spinal cord.

The cascade of biological events that take place in the spinal cord after peripheral nerve damage, including central sensitization, amplifies the ectopic impulse barrage entering the spinal cord from the periphery and may also trigger abnormal firing of spinal origin. Part of this sensitization is due to facilitation of the response of NMDA receptors to the primary afferent neurotransmitter glutamate (Sandkühler 2000). A remarkable effect of the spinal changes evoked by nerve injury is that low-threshold afferents may become coupled to ascending spinal projection neurons that carry nociceptive information. When this happens, normally innocuous A-fiber input from residual intact low-threshold peripheral afferents and ectopic input both may contribute to phantom pain sensation.

A number of additional central processes are thought to contribute to the hyperexcitability of spinal cord circuitry following major nerve damage. For example, there may be a downregulation of opioid receptors, both on primary afferent endings and on intrinsic spinal neurons. This downregulation is expected to exaggerate the disinhibition due to reduction of GABAergic and glycinergic activity. In addition, cholecystokinin, an endogenous peptide antagonist of the opioid system, is upregulated in injured tissue (for a review, see Woolf and Mannion 1999). Another interesting example of altered gene expression after axotomy is the appearance of the neuropeptide substance P in low-threshold Aβ neurons. Substance P is normally expressed only by Aδ and C afferents, most of which are nociceptors. The injury-triggered expression of substance P by Aβ fibers may render them more like nociceptors, and may allow ectopic or normal activity in Aβ fibers to trigger and maintain central sensitization. Such changes in gene expression in injured afferents (and in some postsynaptic spinal neurons) that alter their functioning (i.e., their "phenotype") are referred to as "phenotypic switches." Recent work based on gene chip technology indicates that hundreds of genes are up- or downregulated in DRG and spinal neurons after peripheral nerve injury (Costigan et al. 2002; Xiao et al. 2002).

Following peripheral nerve injury, some sensory neurons of the DRG die, leading to the degeneration of their central projection axons. Massive loss of afferent fibers (deafferentation) occurs when dorsal roots are injured or are avulsed from the spinal cord. Deafferentation may act hand-in-hand with the central effects of peripheral denervation to bring about the plethora of changes that contribute to spinal hyperexcitability.

A mechanism that may be of special relevance to phantom phenomena is the invasion of regions of the spinal cord that have been vacated by injured afferents. For example, in the neuroma model in rats and cats, there is an expansion of neuronal receptive fields in skin adjacent to the denervated part of the limb, and a shift of activity from these adjacent areas into regions of the spinal cord that previously served the now-denervated portion of the limb (Devor and Wall 1978). Such reorganization of the spinal map of the limb, probably due to unmasking of previously silent connections, is also reflected in brainstem and cortical remapping.

Supraspinal changes related to phantom limb pain involve the brainstem, thalamus, and cerebral cortex (for a review, see Flor 2000). New insights into phantom limb pain have come from studies demonstrating changes in the functional and structural architecture of primary somatosensory cortex subsequent to amputation and deafferentation in adult monkeys. Amputation of digits in an adult owl monkey led to an invasion of adjacent areas into the representation zone of the deafferented fingers (for a review, see Kaas 2000). Several imaging studies (e.g., Flor et al. 1995; Grüsser et al. 2001) have reported that upper-extremity amputees show a shift of the mouth into the hand representation in the primary somatosensory cortex (see Fig. 2). Flor et al. (1995) provided evidence that these cortical changes are less related to referred sensations (such as the elicitation of phantom sensation in the amputated portion of the arm subsequent to stimulation of the face, as suggested

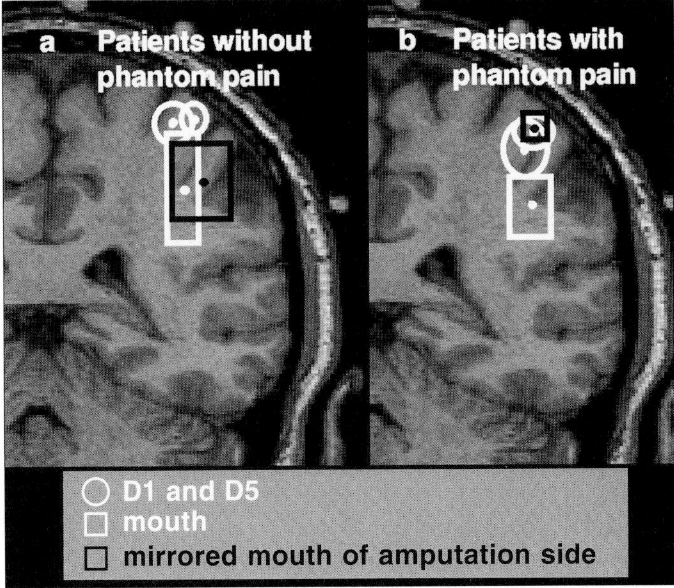

Fig. 2. (a) Means (dots) and standard deviations (rectangles or circles) of the localization of the digits (circles) and the mouth (rectangles) in patients without phantom limb pain. The localization of the mouth is clearly separated from the digits, and the mouth representations of both hemispheres are symmetrical. (b) The same representations for a group of upper-extremity amputees with phantom limb pain. Here, the mouth representation of the amputation side has moved into the cortical hand region.

by Ramachandran et al. [1992]) than to the presence of phantom limb pain. The more pronounced the shift of the mouth representation into the zone that formerly represented the now-amputated hand and arm, the more severe the phantom limb pain.

These cortical changes can be reversed by eliminating peripheral input from the amputation stump using brachial plexus anesthesia. In one study, peripheral anesthesia completely eliminated cortical reorganization and phantom limb pain in half of the subjects. In the others, both cortical reorganization and phantom limb pain remained unchanged (Birbaumer et al. 1997). This result suggests that in some amputees, cortical reorganization and phantom limb pain may be maintained by peripheral input, whereas in others central, potentially intracortical, changes are more important.

It was recently shown that axonal sprouting in cortex underlies sensory cortical reorganization observed in amputated monkeys (Florence et al. 1998). Cortical reorganization can also be found in the motor cortex. In patients with phantom limb pain but not in pain-free amputees, lip movements activated the area of the motor cortex where the amputated hand and arm were formerly represented (Lotze et al. 1999). The extent to which spinal changes contribute to these supraspinal alterations is unknown.

Thalamic stimulation and recordings in human amputees reveal that reorganization also occurs at the thalamic level and is closely related to the perception of phantom limbs and phantom limb pain (Davis et al. 1998). Studies in animals have shown that these changes may be relayed from the spinal cord and brainstem (Florence and Kaas 1995). However, changes at subcortical levels may also originate in the cortex, which has strong efferent connections to the thalamus and lower structures (Ergenzinger et al. 1998).

Pain memories established prior to the amputation may be powerful elicitors of phantom limb pain (Katz and Melzack 1990; Flor 2002). The original assumption of a "somatosensory pain memory" as noted by Katz and Melzack (1990) was based on findings that amputees often report phantom limb pain that is similar in both quality and location to pain experienced before the amputation. However, Jensen and his colleagues (Jensen and Nikolajsen 1999; Jensen et al. 1985; Nikolajsen at al. 1997b) have noted that explicit memories of preamputation pain are relatively rare in chronic phantom limb pain. Pain memories are, however, more likely to be implicit and not readily accessible to conscious recall. The term "implicit pain memory" refers to central changes produced by nociceptive input, which alter somatosensory processing yet do not require changes in the conscious component of the pain experience (Flor 2002). In patients with back pain, increasing chronicity is correlated with an expansion of the representation zone of the back in the primary somatosensory cortex (Flor et al. 1997). Acute pain likewise alters the body representation in the primary somatosensory cortex (Soros et al. 2001). These data suggest that long-lasting noxious input may lead to long-term central changes, especially at the cortical level. The primary somatosensory cortex is well recognized to participate in the processing of pain, and may be important for the sensory-discriminative aspects of the pain experience. There have also been reports that phantom limb pain is abolished after surgical excision of portions of the primary somatosensory cortex and that stimulation of the somatosensory cortex evokes phantom limb pain (Appenzeller and Bicknell 1969). If a somatosensory pain memory has been established with an important neural correlate in spinal and supraspinal structures, such as the primary somatosensory cortex, subsequent deafferentation and invasion of the amputation zone by neighboring input may preferentially activate cortical neurons coding for pain. The cortical area coding input from the periphery seems to stay assigned to the original zone of input, so activation of the cortical zone representing the amputated limb is referred to this limb and is interpreted as phantom sensation and phantom limb pain. Reorganization is likely not only in areas involved in sensory-discriminative aspects of pain, but also in areas that mediate affective-motivational aspects of pain such as the insula and the anterior cingulate cortex. Plastic changes in these areas may contribute to the experience of phantom pain (Wei and Zhuo 2001). The importance of sensitization prior to amputation was confirmed by a study by Nikolajsen et al. (2000b), who reported a close association between mechanical sensitivity prior to amputation and early phantom limb pain. However, the authors only tested pain thresholds and not sensitization. Further research is needed to better clarify these relationships.

TREATMENT

Several studies, including large surveys of amputees, have shown that most treatments for phantom limb pain are ineffective and are not mechanism-based (Sindrup and Jensen 1999). Most such studies are uncontrolled short-term assessments of small numbers of patients. The maximum decrease in pain intensity reported from a host of treatments such as local anesthesia, sympathectomy, dorsal root entry zone lesions, cordotomy and rhizotomy, neurostimulation, or pharmacological interventions such as anticonvulsants, barbiturates, antidepressants, neuroleptics, and muscle relaxants seems to be around 30%. This benefit does not exceed the placebo effect reported in other studies.

Pharmacological interventions include a host of agents. Although tricyclic antidepressants and sodium channel blockers have been described as treatments of choice for neuropathic pain (Sindrup and Jensen 1999), there are no controlled studies of their use in phantom limb pain. Controlled studies have only been conducted for opioids (Huse et al. 2001), calcitonin (Jaeger and Maier 1992), and ketamine (Nikolajsen et al. 1996), all of which decreased phantom limb pain. Memantine, like ketamine an NMDA-receptor antagonist, was, however, ineffective (Nikolajsen et al. 2000a), even though animal studies suggest that cortical reorganization can be prevented and reversed by NMDA-receptor antagonists or GABA agonists (see Jones 2000 for a review). In one controlled study, transcutaneous nerve stimulation (TENS) yielded a small benefit on phantom limb pain (Katz and Melzack 1991).

Reports of mechanism-based treatments consist of a few small, mostly uncontrolled studies. Lidocaine reduced phantom limb pain in patients with neuromas in two small-sample controlled, blinded, randomized trials (Chabal et al. 1989, 1992). Biofeedback treatment that results in vasodilatation or decreased muscle tension in the residual limb reduces phantom limb pain and thus may benefit patients in whom peripheral factors contribute to the pain (Sherman 1989). Based on findings from neuroelectric and neuromagnetic source imaging, changes in cortical reorganization might influence phantom limb pain. Animal work on stimulation-induced plasticity suggests that extensive, behaviorally relevant (but not passive) stimulation of a body part leads to an expansion of its cortical representation zone. For example, recent work found that intensive use of a myoelectric prosthesis was positively correlated with both reduced phantom limb pain and reduced cortical reorganization (Lotze et al. 1999). When the contribution of cortical reorganization was factored out, the relationship between prosthesis use and reduced phantom limb pain was no longer significant, suggesting that cortical reorganization mediates this relationship. An alternative approach in patients where prosthesis use is not viable is the application of behaviorally relevant stimulation. Two weeks of discrimination training consisted of application of electric stimuli to the stump for 2 hours per day while patients tried to discriminate their frequency or the location of application and received feedback. This intervention led to significant improvements in phantom limb pain and a significant reversal of cortical reorganization (Flor et al. 2001). A control group of patients who received standard medical treatment and general psychological counseling did not show any changes in cortical reorganization or in their phantom limb pain. The goal of treatment was to provide input into the amputation zone and thus undo the reorganization provoked by amputation.

In summary, controlled trials to determine the efficacy of treatments for phantom limb pain are rare. Treatments that have been efficacious in controlled trials include opioids, calcitonin, ketamine, TENS, and sensory discrimination training. Uncontrolled studies report decreased phantom limb pain with lidocaine, biofeedback, prosthesis training, and motor cortex stimulation. In light of the paucity of controlled studies, it seems reasonable to base the treatment of phantom pain on recommendations for neuropathic pain in general, such as antidepressant medication and calcium channel blockers including carbamazepine. In addition, opioids, calcitonin, ketamine, TENS, or sensory discrimination training might be applied.

PREVENTION

As noted above, Katz and Melzack (1990) emphasize that somatosensory pain memories may be revived after an amputation and may lead to phantom limb pain. They note that implicit and explicit memory components can be differentiated, and that both contribute to the experience of phantom limbs and phantom limb pain. They therefore suggest that both memory components must be targeted in trials of interventions to prevent phantom limb pain, i.e., that both general and spinal anesthesia are needed.

Preemptive analgesia refers to the attempt to prevent chronic pain by intervention prior to acute pain, e.g., before and during surgery. Based on preclinical data that document sensitization of spinal neurons by an afferent barrage, it has been suggested that general anesthesia should be supplemented by peripheral anesthesia that prevents peripheral nociceptive input from reaching the spinal cord and higher centers. However, preemptive analgesia that includes both general and spinal anesthesia has not consistently been efficacious in preventing phantom limb pain (for a review, see Jensen and Nikolajsen 2000). Whereas several studies reported a reduction of the incidence of phantom limb pain when additional epidural anesthesia was used in the pre- and perioperative stages, one recent controlled study failed to find a beneficial effect on the development of phantom limb pain (Nikolajsen et al. 1997a). A preexisting pain memory that has already led to central and especially cortical changes would not necessarily be affected by short-term interruption of the afferent barrage. Thus it is possible that peripheral analgesia in the perioperative phase might eliminate new but not preexisting central changes. In addition, brief peripheral blockade is inadequate to prevent discharges from severed peripheral nerves from reaching the central nervous system Here, NMDA antagonists as well as GABA agonists might be beneficial to prevent both central reorganization and phantom limb pain. A recent study (Wiech et al. 2001) used brachial plexus anesthesia and either the NMDA-receptor antagonist memantine or placebo in patients undergoing surgical amputation of individual fingers or a hand. In this placebo-controlled, double-blind randomized trial, memantine significantly reduced the incidence of phantom limb pain 1 year after the surgery from 72% to 20%, whereas placebo failed to show a similar effect.

THE FUTURE

Both peripheral and central factors and their interaction must be examined more closely, in animal models of amputation-related pain as well as in human amputees. The role of spinal mechanisms has not yet been sufficiently elucidated. The detection of genes relevant to the development of phantom pain-like behaviors in animal is an important step that may help researchers to identify predisposing factors for phantom limb pain and to develop new therapies. Evaluation of improved treatments for phantom limb pain requires prospective, randomized, double-blinded, placebo-controlled treatment trials that employ clear and uniform outcome measures. Only then will effective, evidence-based interventions become available.

ACKNOWLEDGMENTS

The preparation of this chapter was supported by grants from the Deutsche Forschungsgemeinschaft (H. Flor), the U.S.-Israel Binational Science Foundation (M. Devor), and the Karen Elise Jensens Foundation (T.S. Jensen).

REFERENCES

Appenzeller O, Bicknell JM. Effects of nervous system lesion on phantom experience in amputees. *Neurology* 1969; 19:141–146.

Birbaumer N, Lutzenberger W, Montoya P, et al. Effects of regional anesthesia on phantom limb pain are mirrored in changes in cortical reorganization. *J Neurosci* 1997; 17:5503–5508.

Chabal C, Jacobson, L, Russell LC, Burchiel KJ. Pain responses to perineuromal injection of normal saline, gallamine, and lidocaine in humans. *Pain* 1989; 36:321–325.

Chabal C, Jacobson L, Russell LC, Burchiel KJ. Pain response to perineuromal injection of normal saline, epinephrine, and lidocaine in humans. *Pain* 1992; 49:9–12.

Costigan M, Befort K, Karchewski L, et al. Replicate high-density rat genome oligonucleotide microarrays reveal hundreds of regulated genes in the dorsal root ganglion after peripheral nerve injury. *Bio Med Central Neurosci* 2002; 3:16.

Davis KD, Kiss ZHT, Luo L, et al. Phantom sensations generated by thalamic microstimulation. *Nature* 1998; 391:385–387.

Devor M, Raber P. Heritability of symptoms in an experimental model of neuropathic pain. *Pain* 1990; 42:51–67.

Devor M, Seltzer Z. Pathophysiology of damaged nerves in relation to chronic pain. In: Wall PD, Melzack RA (Eds). *Textbook of Pain*. New York: Churchill-Livingstone, 1999, pp 128–164.

Devor M, Wall PD. Reorganization of the spinal cord sensory map after peripheral nerve injury. *Nature* 1978; 276:76.

Devor M, Govrin-Lippman R, Angelides K. Na^+ channel immunolocalization in peripheral mammalian axons and changes following nerve injury and neuroma formation. *J Neurosci* 1993; 13:1976–1992.

Devor M, Jänig W, Michaelis M. Modulation of activity in dorsal root ganglion neurones by sympathetic activation in nerve-injured rats. *J Neurophysiol* 1994; 71:38–47.

Doubell TP, Mannion RJ, Woolf CJ. The dorsal horn: state-dependent sensory processing, plasticity and the generation of pain. In Wall PD, Melzack RA (Eds). *Textbook of Pain,* 4th ed. Edinburgh: Churchill Livingstone, 1999, pp 165–181.

Ehde DM, Czerniecki JM, Smith DG, et al. Chronic phantom sensations, phantom pain, residual limb pain, and other regional pain after lower limb amputation. *Arch Phys Med Rehab* 2000; 8:1039–1044.

Ergenzinger ER, Glasier MM, Hahm JO, Pons TP. Cortically induced thalamic plasticity in the primate somatosensory system. *Nature Neurosci* 1998; 1:226–229.

Flor H. The functional organization of the brain in pain. *Prog Brain Res* 2000; 129:313–322.

Flor H. Phantom limb pain: characteristics, aetiology and treatment. *Lancet Neurol* 2002; 3:182–189.

Flor H, Elbert T, Knecht S, et al. Phantom limb pain as a perceptual correlate of cortical reorganization following arm amputation. *Nature* 1995; 357:482–484.

Flor H, Braun C, Elbert T, Birbaumer N. Extensive reorganization of primary somatosensory cortex in chronic back pain patients. *Neurosci Lett* 1997; 224:5–8.

Flor H, Elbert T, Mühlnickel W, et al. Cortical reorganization and phantom phenomena in congenital and traumatic upper-extremity amputees. *Exp Brain Res* 1998; 119:205–212.

Flor H, Denke C, Schaefer M, Grüsser S. Sensory discrimination training alters both cortical reorganization and phantom limb pain. *Lancet* 2001; 357:1763–1764.

Florence SL, Kaas JH. Large-scale reorganization at multiple levels of the somatosensory pathway following therapeutic amputation of the hand in monkey. *J Neurosci* 1995; 15:8083–8095.

Florence SL, Taub HB, Kaas JH. Large-scale sprouting of cortical connections after peripheral injury in adult macaque monkeys. *Science* 1998; 282:1117–1120.

Grüsser S, Winter C, Mühlnickel W, et al. The relationship of perceptual phenomena and cortical reorganization in upper extremity amputees. *Neuroscience* 2001; 102:263–272.

Hill A. Phantom limb pain: a review of the literature on attributes and potential mechanisms. *J Pain Symptom Manage* 1999; 17:125–142.

Huse E, Larbig W, Flor H, Birbaumer N. The effect of opioids on phantom limb pain and cortical reorganization. *Pain* 2001; 90:47–55.

Jaeger H, Maier C. Calcitonin in phantom limb pain: a double-blind study. *Pain* 1992; 48:21–27.

Jensen TS, Krebs B, Nielsen J, Rasmussen P. Immediate and long-term phantom limb pain in amputees: incidence, clinical characteristics and relationship to pre-amputation pain. *Pain* 1985; 21:267–278.

Jensen TS, Nikolajsen L. Phantom pain and other phenomena after amputation. In: Wall PD, Melzack RA (Eds). *Textbook of Pain*, 4th ed. Edinburgh: Churchill Livingston, 1999, pp 799–814.

Jensen TS, Nikolajsen L. Pre-emptive analgesia in postamputation pain: an update. *Prog Brain Res* 2000; 129:493–503.

Jensen TS, Krebs B, Nielsen J, Rasmussen P. Immediate and long-term phantom limb pain in amputees: incidence, clinical characteristics and relationship to pre-amputation pain. *Pain* 1985; 21:267–278.

Jones EG. Cortical and subcortical contributions to activity-dependent plasticity in primate somatosensory cortex. *Annu Rev Neurosci* 2000; 23:1–37.

Kaas JH. The reorganization of sensory and motor maps after injury in adult mammals. In: Gazzaniga MS (Ed). *The New Cognitive Neurosciences.* Cambridge, MA: MIT Press, 2000, 223–236.

Katz J, Melzack R. Pain 'memories' in phantom limbs: review and clinical observations. *Pain* 1990; 43:319–336.

Katz J, Melzack RA. Auricular transcutaneous electrical nerve stimulation (TENS) reduces phantom limb pain. *J Pain Symptom Manage* 1991; 6:77–83.

Kooijman CM, Dijkstra PU, Geertzen JHB, Elzinga A, van der Schans CP. Phantom pain and phantom sensations in upper limb amputees: an epidemiological study. *Pain* 2000; 87:33–41.

Krane EJ, Heller LB. The prevalence of phantom sensation and pain in pediatric amputees. *J Pain Symptom Manage* 1995;10:21–29.

Lotze M, Grodd W, Birbaumer N, et al. Does use of a myoelectric prosthesis prevent cortical reorganization and phantom limb pain? *Nat Neurosci* 1999; 2:501–502.

Nikolajsen L, Jensen TS. Phantom limb pain. *Br J Anaesth* 2001; 87:107–116.

Nikolajsen L, Hansen CL, Nielsen J, et al. The effect of ketamine on phantom limb pain: a central neuropathic disorder maintained by peripheral input. *Pain* 1996; 67:69–77.

Nikolajsen L, Ilkjaer S, Christensen JH, Kroner K, Jensen TS. Randomised trials of epidural bupivacaine and morphine in prevention of stump and phantom pain in lower-limb amputation. *Lancet* 1997a; 350:1353–1357.

Nikolajsen L, Ilkjaer S, Kroner K, Christensen JH, Jensen TS. The influence of preamputation pain on postamputation stump and phantom pain. *Pain* 1997b; 72:393–405.

Nikolajsen L, Gottrup H, Kristensen AG, Jensen TS. Memantine (a *N*-methyl-D-aspartate receptor antagonist) in the treatment of neuropathic pain after amputation or surgery: a randomized, double-blinded, cross-over study. *Anesth Analg* 2000a; 91:960–966.

Nikolajsen L, Ilkjaer S, Jensen TS. Relationship between mechanical sensitivity and postamputation pain: a perspective study. *Eur J Pain* 2000b; 4:327–334.

Nyström B, Hagbarth KE. Microelectrode recordings from transected nerves in amputees with phantom limb pain. *Neurosci Lett* 1981; 27:211–216.

Ramachandran VS, Rogers-Ramachandran D, Stewart M. Perceptual correlates of massive cortical reorganization. *Science* 1999; 258:1159–1160.

Sandkühler J. Learning and memory in pain pathways. *Pain* 2000; 88:113–118.

Seltzer Z, Wu T, Max MB, Diehl SR. Mapping a gene for neuropathic pain-related behavior following peripheral neurectomy in the mouse. *Pain* 2001; 93:101–106.

Sherman RA. Stump and phantom limb pain. *Neurol Clin* 1989; 7:249–264.

Sherman RA (Ed). *Phantom Limb Pain*. New York: Plenum, 1997.

Sherman RA, Bruno GM. Concurrent variation of burning phantom limb and stump pain with near surface blood flow in the stump. *Orthopedics* 1987; 10:1395–1402.

Sherman RA, Sherman CJ, Bruno GM. Psychological factors influencing chronic phantom limb pain: an analysis of the literature. *Pain* 1987; 28:285–295.

Sherman RA, Griffin VD, Evans CB, Grana AS. Temporal relationships between changes in phantom limb pain intensity and changes in surface electromyogram of the residual limb. *Int J Psychophysiol* 1992; 13:71–77.

Sindrup SH, Jensen TS. Efficacy of pharmacological treatments of neuropathic pain: an update and effect related to mechanism of drug action. *Pain* 1999; 83:389–400.

Soros P, Knecht S, Bantel C, et al. Functional reorganization of the human primary somatosensory cortex after acute pain demonstrated by magnetoencephalography. *Neurosci Lett* 2001; 298:195–198.

Wei F, Zhuo M. Potentiation of sensory responses in the anterior cingulate cortex following digit amputation in the anaesthetised rat. *J Physiol* 2001; 532:823–833.

Wiech K, Preissl H, Kiefer T, et al. Prevention of phantom limb pain and cortical reorganization in the early phase after amputation in humans. *Soc Neurosci Abstr* 2001; 28:163–169.

Woolf CJ, Mannion RJ. Neuropathic pain: aetiology, symptoms, mechanisms, and management. *Lancet* 1999; 353:1959–1964.

Xiao H-S, Huang Q-H, Zhang F-X, et al. Identification of gene expression profile of dorsal root ganglion in the rat peripheral axotomy model of neuropathic pain. *Proc Natl Acad Sci USA* 2002; 99:8360–8365.

Correspondence to: Herta Flor, PhD, Department of Clinical and Cognitive Neuroscience at the University of Heidelberg, Central Institute of Mental Health, J5, D-68159 Mannheim, Germany. Tel: 49-621-170322; Fax: 49-621-1703932; email: flor@zi-mannheim.de.

Proceedings of the 10th World Congress on Pain, Progress in Pain Research and Management, Vol. 24, edited by Jonathan O. Dostrovsky, Daniel B. Carr, and Martin Koltzenburg, IASP Press, Seattle, © 2003.

59

Acute Pain Management in the Chronic Pain Sufferer[1]

Stephen E. Abram

Department of Anesthesiology, University of New Mexico School of Medicine, Albuquerque, New Mexico, USA

Managing acute postsurgical or post-traumatic pain in patients with chronic painful conditions represents a major challenge to the medical and nursing communities. This group of patients is often undertreated, for a variety of reasons. Patients with chronic pain who are treated with long-term opioids are often considered to be "addicted" or "drug seeking" by physicians or nurses. It is not uncommon to find that doses of opioids ordered for postsurgical pain are lower than the doses patients were taking for their daily preoperative pain management. Physicians may assume that a patient's chronic daily opioid intake is sufficient to "cover" their postoperative pain. Tolerance is a significant issue for most patients on chronic opioid medication. Dose requirements to satisfactorily control their acute postsurgical pain may be several-fold higher than those appropriate for opioid-naive patients. Chronic pain patients often have developed considerable sensitization of nociceptive systems because of *N*-methyl D-aspartate (NMDA)-mediated hyperalgesia induced either by repeated nociceptor activation (Woolf and Thompson 1991) or by chronic opioid administration.

In many situations acute pain is superimposed upon chronic pain. Cancer pain is one such example, as surgical interventions are commonly performed on patients with severe preoperative cancer-related pain. Patients with complex regional pain syndrome occasionally undergo procedures involving the affected limb; adequate pain control is essential to prevent exacerbation of pain from postsurgical nociceptive inputs. Patients with chronic back pain are frequently subjected to repeated spine operations, often with catastrophic increases in pain in the perioperative period. Numerous medical conditions

[1] Based on a Congress workshop.

are typified by chronic pain with superimposed acute exacerbations, such as sickle cell disease, migraine, and chronic pancreatitis. Management of episodic pain in individuals with chronic pain between the acute episodes is particularly difficult.

Several strategies may be used to address the management of acute pain in the chronic pain sufferer. One scheme, often overlooked, is to consider elective tapering and discontinuation of chronically administered opioids for certain chronic pain patients in advance of their next acute pain episode, particularly in patients identified as having opioid-induced hyperalgesia. By converting their daily regimen to one that does not include opioids, clinicians can reserve opioids for episodes of acute pain. This strategy is most likely to be appropriate for conditions such as sickle cell disease or chronic pancreatitis, in which acute painful episodes are common. One of the most effective strategies is to employ regional anesthetic techniques in the post-operative or post-trauma patient. If the noxious stimulus can be effectively blocked from activating spinal cord neurons, the patient should require only maintenance drug doses. Another common strategy is to utilize non-opioid analgesics, such as nonsteroidal anti-inflammatory drugs. In animal models a number of drugs, particularly NMDA-receptor antagonists, prevent or reduce tolerance to opioids and augment their analgesic effect (Mao et al. 1995). Some of these drugs have preemptive analgesic effects when administered prior to surgical incision (Fu et al. 1997). NMDA antagonists also block opioid-induced hyperalgesia (Laulin et al. 2002). Finally, rotation of opioids may overcome opioid tolerance or diminish nociceptive responses to high levels of input.

Although several animal models can guide management of acute pain in the chronic pain patient, few clinical studies have addressed this issue. Almost no information exists on the efficacy of systemic opioids or on dose requirements for postoperative pain in opioid-tolerant patients, and we lack publications documenting the efficacy of regional anesthetic techniques for these patients. Therefore, many of the recommendations regarding therapy expressed in this chapter are opinions based on theoretical considerations. Clinical research is greatly needed to guide practice in this area.

OPIOID THERAPY

Systemic opioids are likely to be ineffective for managing acute pain in patients chronically treated with high doses of opioids. This inadequacy will be particularly apparent in patients who have developed centrally mediated hyperalgesia associated with neuropathy, persistent nociceptive pain, or chronic opioid use. The development of tolerance is extremely variable. Some patients are able to maintain a satisfactory degree of opioid analgesia for long periods of time, while others require rapid dose escalation to maintain adequate analgesia. Individuals maintained on methadone for substance abuse treatment are likely to have marked tolerance to the analgesic effect of μ-opioids, while patients receiving opioid analgesics for painful conditions appear to maintain much more effective analgesia (Doverty et al. 2001).

The mechanisms that underlie the enhanced sensitivity of spinal neurons that are activated by painful stimuli are well documented (Mayer et al. 1999). Brief activation of a peripheral nociceptor produces depolarization of the postsynaptic spinal neuron, mediated through release of excitatory amino acids (EAAs) such as glutamate, which leads to opening of the α-amino-3-hydroxy-5-methyl-4-isoxazole propionate (AMPA) receptor and entry of Na^+ into the cell. Persistent and/or intense activation of peripheral nociceptors causes prolonged release of EAAs, resulting in activation of the NMDA receptor, which allows Ca^{2+} entry into the cell, stimulating increased production of NO, prostaglandins, dynorphin, and other mediators of the hyperalgesic state. These reactions, as well as those mediated by EAA activation of the metabotropic NMDA receptor, lead to an increased activation and translocation of protein kinase C (PKC) from the cytosol to the cell membrane, resulting in phosphorylation and sensitization of the NMDA receptor and other excitotoxic consequences.

Prolonged activation of postsynaptic opioid receptors also can produce sensitization. In addition to activation of G-protein-coupled K^+ channels, there is activation/translocation of PKC, which, in addition to its enhancement of NMDA-receptor responsiveness, can modulate or uncouple G-protein-activated K^+ channels, reducing the efficacy of both exogenous and endogenous opioids. Likewise, elevation of intracellular PKC levels associated with prolonged noxious stimulation has the same inhibitory effect on the μ-opioid receptor. Thus, prolonged opioid administration can produce both tolerance and hyperalgesia, while prolonged intense noxious stimulation can cause decreased responsiveness to opioids.

In animal models, NMDA antagonists are capable of blocking central sensitization associated with persistent noxious stimulation (Woolf and Thompson 1991; Yamamoto and Yaksh 1992a), with experimental mononeuropathy (Yamamoto and Yaksh 1992b), and with chronic opioid administration (Mao et al. 1994; Laulin et al. 2002). NMDA antagonists also are capable of blocking the development of opioid tolerance (Mao et al. 1994; Dunbar et al. 1998). It would seem logical, therefore, to use NMDA antagonists in the perioperative period in an effort to reverse established tolerance and to avert augmentation of spinal sensitization by surgical stimulation.

Both ketamine (Fu et al. 1997) and dextromethorphan (Helmy and Baly 2001), when administered preoperatively, improve postoperative analgesia and reduce opioid requirements in opioid-naive patients. Such studies have not been conducted in patients who are chronically treated with opioids, or who have chronic pain but are not taking opioids.

Ketamine, in addition to its NMDA-antagonist effects, has substantial analgesic effects that are not mediated through the μ-opioid receptor. It has been used as a rescue analgesic in patients with severe cancer pain that could not be managed by opioids alone (Clark and Kalan 1995). Intravenous bolus administration of 10–30 mg of ketamine can provide substantial analgesic effects without significant psychotomimetic effects. The drug may be coadministered with opioids by continuous infusion or using patient-controlled analgesia (PCA). While there has been no formal study of the use of intravenous (i.v.) ketamine for acute pain in patients with chronic pain, I have found it helpful in this situation, particularly in the early postoperative period for patients who have been unresponsive to very large doses of opioids.

Some opioids have intrinsic NMDA-antagonist effects (Ebert et al. 1998). These include methadone, ketobemidone, and propoxyphene. Of these, methadone would seem to be the most useful in the management of severe acute pain. Both the *d*- and *l*-isomers have noncompetitive NMDA-antagonist effects (Gorman et al. 1997). The clinically available form of the drug is the *dl*-isomer. In opioid-naive patients, an effective protocol is to administer 10 mg methadone i.v. prior to induction of anesthesia, and to titrate up to 10 mg more in the early postoperative period. Patients usually require little additional opioid in the next 24 hours because of the long half-life of methadone. While there is little experience in using this technique to manage acute pain in opioid-tolerant patients, a similar approach would seem reasonable, perhaps using higher doses chosen according to the patient's preoperative opioid consumption. This drug must be administered cautiously, however, particularly in older patients, again because of its long duration and its tendency to accumulate during repeated dosage. While methadone's NMDA-antagonist effect may be theoretically beneficial, there are few clinical data to indicate that this mechanism is important in either acute or chronic pain management (Ebert et al. 1998), and the extreme opioid tolerance evident in patients on methadone maintenance tends to discount this theory.

Considerable experimental evidence indicates that certain opioids are more efficacious than others, and that drugs with greater efficacy are better able to achieve effective analgesia when the noxious stimulus is intense or when the organism has developed tolerance to opioids. More efficacious drugs are said to have a higher intrinsic activity, i.e., they produce a given analgesic effect at a lower fractional receptor occupancy than do drugs with a lower intrinsic activity. For instance, sufentanil might produce complete analgesia to a given painful stimulus with occupation of 10% of the available opioid receptors, while meperidine might require 70% receptor occupancy to achieve the same effect. As the stimulus intensity is increased, a small increase in the dose of sufentanil would be sufficient to maintain analgesia, while a substantial increase in the meperidine dose would be required. As the intensity is further increased, meperidine might become ineffective at any dose, while sufentanil would still remain effective at a moderately increased dose. Similarly, those drugs with a high intrinsic activity would require small increases in the dose to produce effective antinociception in an animal made tolerant to opioids, while a substantial increase in the dose of meperidine (which has a low intrinsic activity) would be required. These effects can be evaluated by comparing dose-response curves for various opioids in animals subjected to increasingly intense noxious stimuli or made opioid tolerant.

Paronis and Holzman (1992) studied the effect of opioid tolerance on dose-response curves for a number of drugs, using the rat tail-flick model. In morphine-tolerant animals, dose-response curves for systemically administered fentanyl and methadone showed very little rightward shift, morphine exhibited a moderate rightward shift, and meperidine showed a substantial increase in dose requirements. Buprenorphine, an agonist-antagonist drug, was essentially ineffective in opioid-tolerant animals. Interestingly, when animals were made tolerant to meperidine rather than morphine, there was a greater rightward shift in dose-response curves for all drugs tested. On the other hand, in animals made tolerant to fentanyl, a drug with a high intrinsic activity, there was a much smaller increase in dose requirements for all drugs tested. These data suggest that fentanyl and sufentanil might be rational choices for PCA or i.v. infusion in managing postoperative or post-traumatic pain in opioid-tolerant patients. They also suggest that tolerance may be less of a problem when opioids with a high intrinsic activity are used chronically. One must realize, however, that findings in animals rendered tolerant to opioids over a several-day period may not generalize to the situation of chronic clinical opioid administration.

Abram et al. (1997) studied the ability of several systemically administered opioids to produce antinociception to a noxious radiant heat stimulus as the stimulus intensity was increased. They utilized a radiant heat source directed toward the plantar surface of the hindpaw of rats confined in Plexiglas cages on a glass surface (Hargreaves et al. 1988). They established dose-response curves for a standard level of heat intensity, then repeated the experiment using a higher stimulus intensity on the opposite limb. They found that fentanyl and sufentanil exhibited substantially less of a rightward shift in their dose-responses curve for the high-intensity stimulus than did meperidine or morphine. The ratios of the ED_{50}s for the high-intensity versus low-intensity stimuli were as follows: meperidine 11.8, morphine 6.1, hydromorphone 2.6, fentanyl 2.3, and sufentanil 1.8.

Few studies have assessed the merits of using opioids with high intrinsic activity in patients with chronic pain. Paix et al. (1995) evaluated the benefit of initiating a subcutaneous infusion of fentanyl in patients who had developed intolerable side effects to morphine. Nine patients had been treated with subcutaneous morphine infusions, one with oral morphine, and one with epidural morphine. Six of 11 patients experienced complete resolution of side effects, and the remaining 5 had partial resolution. Five of the 11 patients had improvement in their analgesia. Two patients were subsequently switched to sufentanil because of the high fluid volumes of fentanyl that were required. The mean relative potency of fentanyl to morphine was 68:1. Watanabe et al. (1998) reported 17 patients with cancer pain who were switched to subcutaneous fentanyl infusion from morphine or hydromorphone because of intolerable side effects. Ten of these patients experienced satisfactory analgesia with improvement in side effects. The ratio of morphine to fentanyl doses was 85:1, while the ratio of hydromorphone to fentanyl doses was 23:1.

de Leon-Casasola and Lema (1994) evaluated the benefits of sufentanil as a rescue drug for managing postoperative pain in patients with cancer pain who used opioids chronically. They used a combination of epidural bupivacaine and morphine as their primary analgesic technique for patients undergoing abdominal surgery for tumor resection. Twenty patients who experienced inadequate analgesia with this regimen (with pain intensity ratings of 7–10 on a visual analogue scale [VAS] of 0–10) were switched to a regimen of epidural bupivacaine plus sufentanil. VAS scores during the latter therapy ranged from 0 to 3/10, and supplemental i.v. PCA morphine requirements dropped significantly.

A previously unpublished case report of a patient I have treated illustrates the benefit of changing to an opioid with a higher intrinsic activity. A 24-year-old male with an osteosarcoma of the thoracic spine was treated at home with sustained-release morphine at a dose of 240 mg t.i.d. He was somnolent much of the time, with inadequate pain control when awake. He was admitted for tumor resection and spinal fusion from T6 to T8. He underwent thoracotomy and exposure of the tumor, but tumor resection and spine stabilization were impossible because of the extent of tumor spread. The pain service was consulted on the second postoperative day because of inadequate pain control. The patient was then receiving 240 mg sustained-release morphine t.i.d. plus PCA morphine bolus doses of 4 mg i.v. with

10-minute lockout, plus 2 mg/hour continuous infusion. He was using 12–20 mg/hour of morphine. He was either in severe pain (verbal rating 9–10/10) or somnolent, and was unable to communicate with family and hospital personnel. He was placed on transdermal fentanyl 100 μg/hour; the i.v. PCA and morphine infusion were continued, and the oral morphine was discontinued. Twelve hours later, his pain rating was 3–4/10, and he could communicate easily with friends and family. He was discharged home on the seventh postoperative day on 150 μg/hour transdermal fentanyl and had a pain score of 2–4/10.

Another strategy to provide adequate analgesia is to employ intrathecal or epidural opioid administration. Experimental evidence from studies using high- versus low-intensity noxious thermal stimulation shows that intrathecal morphine has a higher intrinsic activity than does systemic morphine (Abram et al. 1997). The ratio of analgesic ED_{50}s for high- to low-intensity stimulation for systemic morphine was 6.1:1, while the ratio for intrathecal morphine was 2.1:1. On the other hand, there was little difference in intrinsic activity between systemic and spinal administration of either fentanyl or sufentanil. Considerable clinical evidence attests that epidural and intrathecal morphine are more efficacious than systemic morphine in the management of acute pain (Bromage et al. 1980), chronic pain (Winkelmuller and Winkelmuller 1996), and cancer pain (Hogan et al. 1991). On the other hand, de Leon-Casasola's study showed a high incidence of inadequate analgesia during postoperative use of epidural morphine plus bupivacaine in a group of patients with cancer undergoing abdominal surgery (de Leon-Casasola and Lema 1994).

NON-OPIOID MEDICATIONS

Clonidine provides analgesia for postoperative pain when administered either intravenously (Marinangeli et al. 2002), epidurally (Armand et al. 1998), or intrathecally (Dahl and Raeder 2000). Administered by any route, it causes dose-related sedation and a reduction in heart rate and blood pressure, side effects that limit its utility. A dose-finding study of intravenous clonidine showed that 5 μg/kg provided better analgesia than 2 or 3 μg/kg, but produced severe hypotension and sedation (Marinangeli et al. 2002). Postoperative pain studies have shown epidural clonidine to be up to twice as potent as intravenous clonidine (Armand et al. 1998). A study of the effects of epidural and intrathecal clonidine on experimental pain found that intrathecal clonidine was two to six times as potent as epidural clonidine. A study of intrathecal clonidine for postoperative pain after cesarean section reported 4 to 6 hours of satisfactory analgesia following a 150-μg dose (Dahl and Raeder 2000). Because of its high incidence of side effects, clonidine is mainly used in conjunction with opioids. No studies were found that assessed its efficacy at providing analgesia for acute pain in chronic pain sufferers.

Nonsteroidal anti-inflammatory drugs (NSAIDs) should theoretically provide adequate analgesia in opioid-tolerant patients. However, NSAIDs may have suboptimal effects in patients with spinal sensitization associated with chronic painful conditions. Mack et al. (2001) examined the effects of a single dose of i.v. ketorolac on postoperative morphine requirements in patients undergoing microsurgical lumbar discectomy. Many of these patients had significant pain preoperatively. In their study, ketorolac failed to reduce postoperative PCA morphine requirements. There was a significant correlation between preoperative pain severity and postoperative morphine utilization ($r = 0.46$, $P < 0.01$). Interestingly, there was no correlation between preoperative and postoperative opioid use.

The use of NSAIDs postoperatively is limited by their effects on platelet function. Selective cyclooxygenase-2 (COX-2) inhibitors, which have minimal effects on platelet function, have significant analgesic and opioid-sparing effects in the perioperative period (Katz 2002). Oral valdecoxib at doses of 20 and 40 mg has comparable efficacy and longer duration than oxycodone 10 mg in combination with acetaminophen 1000 mg following dental surgery (Barton et al. 2002). Valdecoxib improved analgesia and reduced opioid requirements in patients undergoing hip arthroplasty (Daniels et al. 2002). In that study, the drug was given preoperatively and twice daily for 48 hours postoperatively. Parecoxib is an injectable prodrug of valdecoxib that has been tested for its postoperative analgesic effects. Single i.v. doses of 20 and 40 mg parecoxib were comparable to 30 mg ketorolac and superior to 4 mg i.v. morphine on the first postoperative day following hysterectomy or myomectomy (Camu et al. 2002).

REGIONAL ANESTHESIA

Regional anesthetic techniques, continued into the postoperative period, are a logical choice for acute pain control in patients with chronic pain. Intrathecal local anesthetics are capable of blocking spinal sensitization in the rat formalin test (Coderre et al. 1990). One would anticipate that fairly dense neuraxial conduction blockade would be required in patients with sensitization of nociceptive pathways, and that when mixtures of local anesthetic and opioid are given spinally, opioid requirements would be high. de Leon-Casasola et al. (1993) compared postoperative medication requirements in opioid-naive cancer patients versus those chronically taking opioids. The latter had been taking opioids for at least 3 months prior to operation, and had a mean oral morphine usage of 183 mg/day. Epidural infusion of 0.1% bupivacaine plus 0.01% morphine was started postoperatively. Infusion rates were increased and supplemental i.v. morphine was administered in order to maintain VAS pain scores below 4/10. Patients using opioids preoperatively required three times the dose of epidural medications and five times the dose of i.v. morphine to maintain pain scores below 4. Epidural analgesia could be weaned in the opioid-naive group after 3 days, but the group using opioids preoperatively had to be maintained on the epidural infusion for a mean of 9 days in order to maintain their pain intensity below 4.

CONCLUSIONS

There is little information from clinical trials to guide the treatment of acute pain for patients with preexisting chronic pain. It is not clear whether the difficulties in managing such patients are related to opioid tolerance or to sensitization of pain projection systems by chronic painful conditions or opioid administration. Animal data and the little clinical information available suggest that a variety of techniques may be helpful. These include the use of opioids with high efficacy (high intrinsic activity), the use of NMDA antagonists, spinal or epidural opioid administration, the use of non-opioid analgesics in patients on chronic opioid treatment, and the use of continuous regional anesthetic techniques. The management of acute pain in patients with chronic pain is a common problem, yet one that is extremely challenging to physicians and distressing to patients. It would greatly benefit from careful, extensive clinical investigation.

REFERENCES

Abram SE, Mampilly GA, Milosavljevic D. Assessment of the potency and intrinsic activity of systemic versus intrathecal opioids in rats. *Anesthesiology* 1997; 87:127–134.

Armand S, Langlade A, Boutros A, et al. Meta-analysis of the efficacy of extradural clonidine to relieve postoperative pain: an impossible task. *Br J Anaesth* 1998; 81:126–134.

Barton SF, Langeland FF, Snabes MC, et al. Efficacy and safety of intravenous parecoxib sodium in relieving acute postoperative pain following gynecologic laparotomy surgery. *Anesthesiology* 2002; 97:306–314.

Bromage PR, Camporesi E, Chestnut D. Epidural narcotics for postoperative analgesia. *Anesth Analg* 1980; 59:473–479.

Camu F, Beecher T, Recker DP, Verburg KM. Valdecoxib, a Cox-2 specific inhibitor, is an efficacious opioid-sparing analgesic in patients undergoing hip arthroplasty. *Am J Ther* 2002; 9:43–51.

Clark JL, Kalan GE. Effective treatment of severe cancer pain of the head using low-dose ketamine in an opioid tolerant patient. *J Pain Symptom Manage* 1995; 10:310–314.

Coderre TJ, Vaccarino AL, Melzack R. Central nervous system plasticity in the tonic pain response to subcutaneous formalin injection. *Brain Res* 1990; 535:155–158.

Dahl V, Raeder JC. Non-opioid postoperative analgesia. *Acta Anaesth Scand* 2000; 44:1191–1203.

Daniels SE, Desjardins PJ, Talwalker S, et al. The analgesic efficacy of valdecoxib vs. oxycodone/acetaminophen after oral surgery. *J Am Dental Assoc* 2002; 133:611–621.

de Leon-Casasola OA, Myers DP, Donaparthi S, et al. A comparison of postoperative epidural analgesia between patients with chronic cancer taking high doses of oral opioids versus opioid-naive patients. *Anesth Analg* 1993; 76:302–307.

de Leon-Casasola OA, Lema MJ. Epidural bupivacaine/sufentanil therapy for postoperative pain control in patients tolerant to opioid and unresponsive to epidural bupivacaine/morphine. *Anesthesiology* 1994; 80:303–309.

Doverty M, Somogyi AA, White JM, et al. Methadone maintenance patients are cross-tolerant to the antinociceptive effects of morphine. *Pain* 2001; 93:155–163.

Dunbar SA, Yaksh TL. Concurrent spinal infusion of MK-801 blocks spinal tolerance and dependence induced by chronic intrathecal morphine in the rat. *Anesthesiology* 1996; 84:1177–1188.

Ebert B, Thorkildsen C, Andersen S, et al. Opioid analgesics as non-competitive *N*-methyl-D-aspartate (NMDA) antagonists. *Biochem Pharmacol* 1998; 56:553–559.

Fu ES, Miguel R, Scharf FE. Preemptive ketamine decreases postoperative narcotic requirements in patients undergoing abdominal surgery. *Anesth Analg* 1997; 84:1086–1090.

Gorman AL, Elliott KJ, Inturrisi CE. The d- and l- isomers of methadone bind to the non-competitive site on the *N*-methyl-D-aspartate (NMDA) receptor in the rat forebrain and spinal cord. *Neurosci Lett* 1997; 223:5–8.

Hargreaves K, Dubner R, Brown F, Flores C, Joris J. A new and sensitive method for measuring thermal nociception in cutaneous hyperalgesia. *Pain* 1988; 32:77–88.

Helmy SAK, Baly A. The effect of the preemptive use of the NMDA antagonist dextromethorphan on postoperative analgesic requirements. *Anesth Analg* 2001; 92:739–744.

Hogan QH, Haddox JD, Abram SE, et al. Epidural opiates and local anesthetics for the management of cancer pain. *Pain* 1991; 46:271–279.

Katz WA. Cyclooxygenase-2-selective inhibitors in the management of acute and perioperative pain. *Cleve Clin J Med* 2002; 69(Suppl 1):S165–175.

Laulin JP, Maurette P, Corcuff JB, et al. The role of ketamine in preventing fentanyl-induced hyperalgesia and subsequent acute morphine tolerance. *Anesth Analg* 2002; 94:1263–1269.

Mack PG, Hass D, Lavayne MH. Postoperative narcotic requirement after microscopic lumbar discectomy is not affected by intraoperative ketorolac or bupivacaine. *Spine* 2001; 26:658–661.

Mao J, Price DD, Mayer DJ. Thermal hyperalgesia in association with the development of morphine tolerance in rats: roles of excitatory amino acid receptors and protein kinase C. *J Neurosci* 1994; 14:1201–2312.

Mao J, Price DD, Mayer DJ. Mechanisms of hyperalgesia and morphine tolerance: a current view of their possible interactions. *Pain* 1995; 62:259–274.

Marinangeli F, Ciccozzi A, Donatelli F, et al. Clonidine for postoperative pain: a dose finding study. *Eur J Pain* 2002; 6:35–42

Mayer DJ, Mao J, Holt J, Price DD. Cellular mechanisms of neuropathic pain, morphine tolerance, and their interactions. *Proc Natl Acad Sci USA* 1999; 96:7731–7736.

Paix A, Coleman A, Lees J, et al. Subcutaneous fentanyl and sufentanil infusion substitution for morphine intolerance in cancer pain management. *Pain* 1995; 63:263–269.

Paronis CA, Holtzman SG. Development of tolerance to the analgesic activity of mu agonists after continuous infusion of morphine, meperidine or fentanyl in rats. *J Pharmacol Exp Ther* 1992; 262:1–9.

Watanabe S, Pareira J, Hanson J, Bruera E. Fentanyl by continuous subcutaneous infusion for the management of cancer pain: a retrospective study. *J Pain Symptom Manage* 1998; 16:323–326.

Winkelmuller M, Winkelmuller W. Long-term effects of continuous intrathecal opioid treatment in chronic pain of nonmalignant etiology. *J Neurosurg* 1996; 85:458–467.

Woolf CJ, Thompson SWN. The induction and maintenance of central sensitization is dependent on *N*-methyl-D-aspartic acid receptor activation: implications for the treatment of post-injury pain hypersensitivity states. *Pain* 1991; 44:293–299.

Yamamoto T, Yaksh TL. Comparison of the antinociceptive effects of pre- and posttreatment with MK-801, an NMDA antagonist, on the formalin test in the rat. *Anesthesiology* 1992a; 77:757–763.

Yamamoto T, Yaksh TL. Studies on the spinal interaction of morphine and the NMDA antagonist MK-801 on the hyperesthesia observed in a rat model of sciatic mononeuropathy. *Neurosci Lett* 1992b; 135:67–70.

Correspondence to: Stephen E. Abram, MD, Department of Anesthesiology, School of Medicine, University of New Mexico, Surge Building, 2701 Frontier NE, Albuquerque, NM 87131-5216, USA. Email: sabram@salud.unm.edu.

Proceedings of the 10th World Congress on Pain,
Progress in Pain Research and Management, Vol. 24,
edited by Jonathan O. Dostrovsky, Daniel B. Carr, and
Martin Koltzenburg, IASP Press, Seattle, © 2003.

60

Opioids for Chronic Noncancer Pain

Eija Kalso

*Pain Clinic, Department of Anesthesia and Intensive Care Medicine,
Helsinki University Central Hospital, Helsinki, Finland*

WHY ARE OPIOIDS SO SPECIAL?

Opioids have a special place in pain medicine. They are among the most powerful analgesics in clinical use. The remarkable advances that have been made in the management of cancer-related pain are mainly due to the widely accepted use of strong opioids as advocated by the World Health Organization (1996). Why did it take so long for opioids to gain acceptance in the management of cancer pain, and why is the threshold so high for the use of opioids in chronic noncancer pain?

To try to answer this question, let us compare opioids with two other major groups of analgesics, nonsteroidal anti-inflammatory drugs (NSAIDs) and tricyclic antidepressants (TCAs). NSAIDs are widely used for nociceptive pain. They are effective, but can cause serious adverse effects (allergy, renal failure, gastric ulcers, and heart failure) as described by McQuay and Moore (this volume). In neuropathic pain TCAs are the standard. Their adverse effect profile resembles that of opioids—sedation, dizziness, dry mouth, and constipation. Analgesic tolerance is seen with opioids, and long-term follow-up studies are required to find out whether tolerance limits their usefulness for chronic pain. However, all randomized and controlled studies on antidepressants and anticonvulsants are of 3–6 weeks' duration (McQuay et al. 1996). Because plasticity is a typical phenomenon in the central nervous system, one could argue that there is no reason why tolerance should not also develop to the analgesic effects of antidepressants. Respiratory depression is a serious complication related to opioids. However, if the opioid dose is titrated against pain and adjusted carefully, respiratory depression should not be a problem.

Both antidepressants and opioids have psychoactive effects. However, opioids are unique in being able to produce significant euphoria by activating the reward system that mediates opioid craving. Thus, addiction potential and the potential for drug diversion are major barriers to prescribing opioids for chronic noncancer pain.

Genetic vulnerability (Laakso et al. 2002), chronic exposure to the drug, and unfavorable psychosocial factors are all needed for addiction to occur. Patients with chronic noncancer pain may have major psychosocial and economic risk factors and may, indeed, be at a higher risk for addictive behavior. The available data suggest that drug abuse or addiction may occur in 3.2–18.9% of patients with chronic noncancer pain (Fishbain et al. 1992). This important issue, however, must be researched more carefully.

When assessing the efficacy and safety of opioids during long-term treatment it is important to remember that the endogenous opioid system is involved in many physiological functions in addition to pain perception and affective behavior. It is a key element in neuroendocrine physiology and in immune and autonomic functions such as respiration, blood pressure, thermoregulation, and gastrointestinal motility.

HOW DO OPIOIDS PRODUCE ANALGESIA?

Opioids mediate analgesia in the spinal cord by activating opioid receptors that are located mainly on presynaptic C and Aδ fibers but also postsynaptically on projection neurons and interneurons. Supraspinal sites for opioid analgesia include the periaqueductal grey, where opioid receptor activation leads to activation of descending inhibition via serotonin and norepinephrine pathways to the spinal cord. This "simple" system is responsible for sensory analgesia. Opioids have also important effects on the affective modulation of pain. Brain imaging studies have shown that areas like the anterior cingulate cortex are involved in the affective elements of opioid analgesia (Rainville et al. 2000). Opioids also modulate other neurotransmitter systems such as cholinergic, noradrenergic, and dopaminergic circuits. And last but not least, opioids can produce analgesia in the periphery, where their receptors are newly expressed during inflammation (Stein et al. 1989).

Can sensory and affective analgesia be separated? In theory, pure sensory analgesia should be achievable through segmental spinal opioid analgesia. In practice this is not possible because subarachnoidally administered opioids will eventually migrate to supraspinal sites. In the clinic, spinal opioids are rarely used in chronic pain. Systemic opioids will activate both sensory and affective components of analgesia, two aspects of pain modulation that are closely tied.

Affective analgesia should be separated from anxiolysis, which is another important effect of opioids, as is their antidepressant effect. Modern theories of depression suggest that the opioid network could be involved in the anhedonic form of depression (Nestler et al. 2002). Indeed, case reports suggest that opioids may have marked antidepressant effects in patients who have severe and refractory major depression (Stoll and Rueter 1999). On the other hand, some patients report depression as an adverse effect of opioids. These mood-modifying effects are important, and their role in the effects of opioids when treating chronic pain should not be ignored.

CAN OPIOIDS ALLEVIATE ALL PAINS?

Case reports and uncontrolled studies argue that different types of pain show variable responses to opioids. Nociceptive pains have been thought to be responsive to opioids, whereas neuropathic pains were claimed to be nonresponsive (Arnér and Meyerson 1988). Animal studies and controlled studies soon questioned these opinions. This important issue was also the topic of the first International Association for the Study of Pain (IASP) Research Symposium, held in Helsinki, Finland, in December 1998 (Kalso et al. 1999a). At that time it was obvious that we were fairly well informed about the basic mechanisms of opioid sensitivity, but that only a couple of controlled clinical studies were available to guide our clinical practice. Fortunately, the intervening years have produced more controlled clinical studies, and in 2002 we are much more knowledgeable than in 1998. However, the really tough questions still remain to be answered.

WHAT HAVE ANIMAL MODELS OF NOCICEPTION TAUGHT US ABOUT OPIOID SENSITIVITY?

Mechanisms of neuropathic pain have been intensely investigated. Animal studies suggest that opioids are effective for most neuropathic pains. The spinal nerve ligation model seems to be the least responsive, and even high doses of intrathecal (i.t.) morphine do not reverse tactile allodynia in this model (Bian et al. 1995; Lee et al. 1995). Individual components of neuropathic pain models appear to have distinct responses to opioids. Dynamic allodynia seems to be particularly nonresponsive to morphine, but shows a good response to pregabalin (Field et al. 1999). This selectivity of opioid responsiveness is understandable in that dynamic allodynia is mediated through Aβ fibers that normally do not express opioid receptors (Taddese et al. 1995). Several other factors have been suggested to reduce the antinociceptive effects of opioids (Table I). Opioid receptors are predominantly located presynaptically. Dorsal rhizotomy results in a loss of spinal δ- and μ-opioid receptors, which could explain poor opioid sensitivity in deafferentation pain states (Besse et al. 1990). Disrupted synergy between the supraspinal and spinal opioid mechanisms, possibly mediated by dynorphin and the *N*-methyl D-aspartate (NMDA) receptor, has been suggested as another mechanism of decreased opioid efficacy in neuropathic pain (Bian et al. 1999). Various endogenous "anti-opioid" peptides have been found to antagonize antinociceptive effects of opioids (Cesselin 1995). Most evidence supports a critical role of cholecystokinin (Xu et al. 1993; Nichols et al. 1995). Rat models of visceral pain have suggested that analgesics acting through the κ-opioid receptor, directly or indirectly, may be more effective than μ- and δ-opioid receptor agonists (Burton and Gebhart 1998).

Tolerance is a complicated phenomenon in the rat, and even more so in patients with chronic pain. In the intact rat, tolerance to the analgesic effects of opioids develops rapidly and reliably (Yu et al. 1997). Opioid tolerance may share some cellular mechanisms involved in central sensitization in models of chronic neuropathic pain (Mayer et al. 1999).

Rodents manifest gender differences in the antinociceptive activity of μ-opioid agonists (Cicero et al. 1996, 2002), and these differences depend on genotype (Mogil et al. 2000). Bergeson et al. (2001) mapped four important quantitative trait loci (QTL) that influence the magnitude of opioid antinociception to chromosome 1 (females only), proximal chromosome 9 (females only), mid-chromosome 9, and proximal chromosome 10. Interestingly, the chromosome

Table I
Factors that reduce opioid antinociception*

Loss of opioid receptors
Disrupted synergy between supraspinal and spinal opioid systems
Anti-opioid peptides
Non-opioid mechanisms (NMDA)
Tolerance
Aβ-fiber-mediated allodynia

* Several of these factors are due to plastic changes in the nervous system and may share cellular mechanisms or anatomical circuits.

10 QTL comaps to the same region as the μ-opioid-receptor gene, and chromosome 1 QTL comaps with the κ-opioid receptor gene.

MULTIPLE FACTORS CAN AFFECT OPIOID SENSITIVITY IN THE CLINIC

In chronic noncancer pain the effectiveness of opioids depends on many factors, particularly the type of pain (Table II). Opioid sensitivity also depends on the outcome chosen to indicate analgesia. Differences in the responses to various opioids may reflect characteristics such as distinct pharmacokinetics. Adverse effects may significantly restrict dose escalation of opioids, and tolerance may diminish their analgesic effect in the long run. Genetic variability of opioid receptor expression, of other neurotransmitter systems that mediate opioid effects, and in the metabolism and interactions of different opioids may explain a significant part of the variability in response to these agents. Recently, gender differences have been under intense clinical study. Although the results are conflicting, women appear to have greater responsiveness to κ-opioid agonists than do men (Gear et al. 1996).

Table II
Factors that affect opioid sensitivity in the clinic

Type of pain
nociceptive, neuropathic
mechanism based
Outcome
30% pain relief
50% pain relief
global improvement
quality of life
function
Opioid pharmacokinetics
bioavailability
polymorphic drug metabolism
drug interactions (methadone, oxycodone)
P-glycoprotein
Adverse effects
nausea, vomiting
constipation
sedation
Tolerance
Genetic variability
Gender
Age

Elderly patients have a greater analgesic response to opioids than do young or middle-aged patients (Gordon and Preiksaitis 1988).

ALL OPIOIDS ARE NOT ALIKE

All WHO (1996) step 3 opioids that are clinically relevant (fentanyl, hydromorphone, morphine, and oxycodone) are selective μ-opioid agonists (Magnan et al. 1982; Raynor et al. 1994, 1995; Monory et al. 1999). However, these closely related drugs have pharmacokinetic differences. Fentanyl has a very low oral bioavailability (<2%) and is therefore administered transdermally in chronic pain. Oral bioavailability is highest for methadone, intermediate for oxycodone, and lowest and most variable for morphine and hydromorphone.

Interestingly, individuals may vary significantly in their response to different opioids (Heiskanen and Kalso 1997). This variability can be explained, at least partly, by differences in renal or hepatic elimination. Morphine is mainly glucuronated, and its metabolism and pharmacokinetic interactions are straightforward compared with oxycodone and methadone, which are metabolized through the CYP (cytochrome P) 450 system. Oxycodone is metabolized to an active metabolite (oxymorphone) via the CYP 2D6 isoenzyme. The latter isoenzyme is not inducible but is genetically controlled, and likely to be inhibited by other drugs. The metabolism of methadone is complicated, involving at least three CYP isoenzymes (1A2, 2D6, and 3A4). The 3A4 isoenzyme is inducible, and drug interactions can lead to serious complications during methadone therapy (Herrlin et al. 2000). Finally, P-glycoprotein, the "multidrug resistance protein" may act to limit the entry of some opioids (morphine, fentanyl, methadone) into the brain (Thompson et al. 2000; Wandel et al. 2002). Drugs that inhibit P-glycoprotein may increase the central effects of these opioids.

Opioids may have effects on other, non-opioid systems relevant to pain modulation. The NMDA receptor complex is important for central sensitization, and antagonists at this receptor have been shown to abolish wind-up. Accordingly, the combination of an opioid with an NMDA-receptor antagonist provides profound antinociception (Chapman and Dickenson 1992). In addition, NMDA antagonism may delay or even reverse the development of analgesic tolerance to morphine (Elliott et al. 1994). In the rat, methadone has been shown to be a noncompetitive NMDA receptor antagonist with activity equivalent to that of dextromethorphan (Ebert et al. 1995). The clinical relevance of this observation remains to be investigated. For a more thorough review on differences between opioids, see Gourlay (1999).

HOW EFFECTIVE ARE OPIOIDS IN CHRONIC NONCANCER PAIN? A SYSTEMATIC REVIEW SUGGESTS SOME ANSWERS

Full reports of randomized controlled trials (RCTs) of WHO step 3 opioids (fentanyl, hydromorphone, methadone, morphine, oxycodone, and oxymorphone) were sought systematically. A broad free-text search was conducted of the following databases: Medline (1966 to May 2002), EMBASE (1980 to May 2002), the Cochrane Library (on line May 2002), and the Oxford Pain Relief Database (1950 to 1994) (Jadad et al. 1996). There was no restriction on language of publication. Reference lists of retrieved reports and reviews were searched for additional trials.

Thirteen randomized and placebo-controlled trials were found. Four were on intravenous opioid testing (Rowbotham et al. 1991; Dellemijn et al. 1997; Attal et al. 2002; Wu et al. 2002). Two of these trials either included (Attal et al. 2002) or reported in a separate paper (Dellemijn et al. 1998) the results of an open-label follow-up study. All four trials were crossover studies in neuropathic pain (postherpetic neuralgia, mixed neuropathic pains, central pain, and phantom pain) (Fig. 1). When either pain intensity difference or pain relief was used as the endpoint, all four studies reported a mean of 30–55% pain relief. The placebo response varied from an increase of pain by 5% to a decrease of pain by 25% (Fig. 1). In the open-label follow-up studies, the respective daily oral/transdermal doses of the opioid were lower and the response during the 1–3 months' follow-up was less than during acute intravenous testing lasting from 80 minutes to 5 hours.

Nine studies compared oral opioids during a period ranging from 4 days to 8 weeks (Fig. 2). Four studies were of neuropathic pain (Watson et al. 1998; Harke et al. 2001; Huse et al. 2001; Raja et al. 2002), four were of musculoskeletal pain (Moulin et al. 1996; Caldwell et al. 1999, 2002; Roth et al. 2000), and one was of mixed pains (Maier et al. 2002). Roth et al. (2000) compared two doses of daily oxycodone (20 mg and 40 mg) with placebo. In all studies of neuropathic pain and Roth's study of osteoarthritis pain (at the higher dose of oxycodone), mean pain relief was at least 30%, whereas in the other studies on osteoarthritis or other musculoskeletal pain it was less than 30%.

Magnetoencephalography of three patients showed initial evidence for reversal of cortical reorganization concurrent with oral morphine treatment and reduction in pain intensity (Huse et al. 2001).

It can be concluded that opioids relieve chronic neuropathic pains at least as well as chronic musculoskeletal pains if a decrease in pain intensity or pain relief is used as the outcome measure. Most of these studies also used other measures (functional status, mood, and quality of life), which

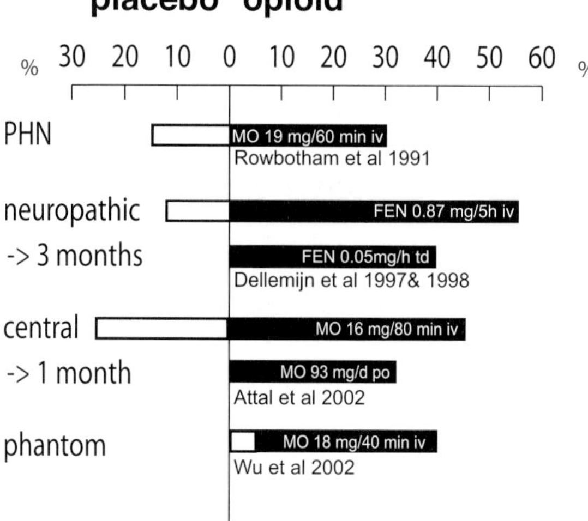

Fig. 1. The mean percentage decrease in pain intensity is shown following the intravenous (i.v.) administration of morphine (MO) or fentanyl (FEN) in neuropathic pain. The left-hand bar indicates the response after placebo and the right-hand bar the effect after the opioid. The pain condition is given on the left (PHN = postherpetic neuralgia). The dose and duration of the infusions are given in the right-hand bars. The results for an open-label follow-up study with transdermal (t.d.) fentanyl (Dellemijn et al. 1998) and oral morphine (p.o.) (Attal et al. 2002) are also shown. All i.v. studies used a crossover design.

will be reported in the full version of this systematic review (E. Kalso et al., unpublished manuscript).

These randomized and controlled studies leave open many important questions, particularly regarding addiction liability and the outcome in complicated cases with behavioral or medical comorbidities. Patients with addictive behavior were uniformly excluded from these trials, which enrolled subjects who were "ideal" candidates for opioid treatment. A good example is the MONTAS study (Maier et al. 2002). Out of nearly 1,000 patients screened, only about 5% were eventually included in the study.

ADVERSE EFFECTS ARE AN ISSUE

In the studies included in the systematic review, adverse effects are a major reason for discontinuation of treatment. Constipation and nausea are the most common adverse effects and also lead to dropouts in controlled trials. Both constipation and nausea occurred significantly more often with opioid therapy compared with treatment with tricyclic antidepressants in the

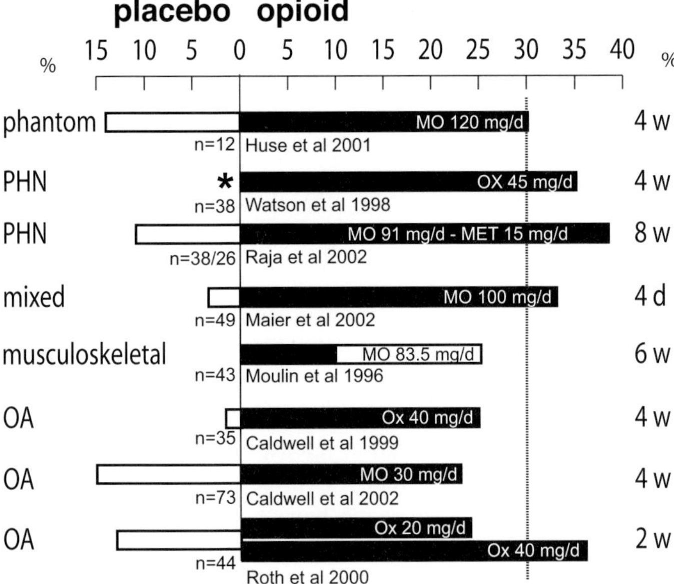

Fig. 2. The mean percentage decrease in pain intensity is shown in the right-hand bars following oral administration of morphine (MO) or oxycodone (OX) and in the left-hand bars after placebo. The pain condition is indicated on the left and the duration of the study on the right (w = week; d = day). The open bar in Moulin et al.'s study indicates the mean decrease in pain intensity when morphine was given as the first drug, and the filled bar indicates the response to morphine when it was given in the second period following placebo. Placebo had no analgesic effect in this study. An asterisk (*) to the left shows that this bar indicates mean pain relief (VAS) as the study did not report baseline pain intensities. The mean pain relief with placebo was 21/100. The study by Raja et al. (2002) had three arms in the crossover design: placebo, an opioid, and a tricyclic antidepressant. Thirty-eight patients were on a mean daily dose of 91 mg of morphine, whereas 26 patients were on a mean daily dose of 15 mg of methadone (MET). Forty-six patients were on a mean daily dose of 89 mg of nortriptyline, and 13 patients were on a mean daily dose of 63 mg of desipramine. Mean pain relief was 38% for the opioids, 32% for the antidepressants, and 11% for placebo. All studies except those of Caldwell et al. (1999 and 2002) and Roth et al. (2000) used a crossover design. It was not possible to extract data for pain intensity differences from Harke et al. (2001). The dotted vertical line indicates the 30% decrease in pain intensity that has been suggested to represent the mean clinically important difference in pain relief in chronic pain (Farrar et al. 2000).

only study that compared these two treatments with placebo in postherpetic neuralgia (Raja et al. 2002). Other frequent adverse effects of opioids include drowsiness, pruritus, dizziness, dry mouth and dizziness. Dellemijn et al. (1998) reported high incidences of sweating, anorexia, and clouded vision. Their study also assessed the severity of the adverse effects and found that the mean intensity of adverse effects, particularly that of sedation, decreased gradually over 2–3 months. Tolerance does not seem to develop to the constipating effect of opioids, and so should be treated early and effectively.

Two of the nine RCTs on oral opioids reported withdrawal symptoms that occurred in 1–2% of the patients (Roth et al. 2000; Maier et al. 2002). After the treatment period, drug craving was reported by 8.7% of patients on morphine compared with 4.3% on placebo (Moulin et al. 1996).

IS TOLERANCE AN ISSUE?

Analgesic tolerance is a well-researched adaptive response to opioids. All the long-term changes originate from μ-opioid receptor activation, and multiple genes influence this adaptation at the genetic level (Kieffer and Evans 2002). Receptor desensitization upon prolonged exposure to agonists is a common phenomenon for many G-protein-coupled receptors such as opioid receptors. Several mechanisms have been suggested to explain the desensitization (Beaumont and Henderson 1999). The behavioral correlate (analgesic tolerance) is even more complex as it may depend on environment (Siegel 1976) and on the type of pain (Christensen and Kayser 2000).

In the clinic, opioid tolerance is seen either as a decrease in pain relief when the opioid dose is stable or as a need to increase the dose (and often, frequency) in order to maintain pain relief. Clinicians often report a "honeymoon" effect, meaning that after the first few weeks of good pain relief, pain intensity levels begin to rise. This effect was clearly seen in the study by Moulin et al. (1996) and also to some extent in that by Caldwell et al. (1999). Whether the delayed increases in pain intensity reflect tolerance or the fact that the patients were initially able to move more and therefore developed more pain, is unclear. Forty-eight of the 50 patients who participated in the intravenous fentanyl study by Dellemijn et al. (1997) continued to the transdermal open-label follow-up (Dellemijn et al. 1998). After two years, nine (19%) were still using transdermal fentanyl. Pain relief was substantial in four, moderate in two, and negligible in three patients.

Tolerance, whatever its mechanisms, can be a clinical problem. The open-label follow-up studies would indicate that even though the initial response to opioid therapy may be good, only a minority of patients will benefit from long-term opioid treatment.

HOW TO CHOOSE THE RIGHT PATIENTS FOR OPIOID TREATMENT: ARE GUIDELINES NEEDED?

The basic principle in medicine is not to harm the patient. This simple goal should assist the physician in choosing the right patients for chronic opioid treatment. Therapy should enhance pain relief and quality of life without compromising the patient's autonomy.

The balance between opioid efficacy and adverse effects has been discussed above. Setting a goal before treatment begins and assessing how this goal is achieved in a predefined trial period should help both the patient and the physician. Chronic opioid treatment often is straightforward. In some cases, because of the unclear nature of the pain condition and multiple psychosocial complicating factors, much effort and wisdom is needed to achieve the goal of improving the patient's quality of life and functional status without causing harm. The patient and the physician can make a formal agreement (a contract) for opioid treatment. This agreement can also inform the patient about the possible benefits and harms of the planned treatment. For centuries the medical use of opioids has raised political and societal concerns. A few therapeutic disasters may have long-lasting consequences on a clinician or community of clinicians, and may prevent patients in true need from getting this treatment.

Many parties are involved in the use of opioids for chronic noncancer pain: the patient, the physician and other health care professionals, pharmacies, the pharmaceutical industry, and political decision-makers. Several guidelines have been proposed and can be modified for national needs (American Academy of Pain Medicine 1996; Kalso et al. 1999b; Perrot et al. 1999; National Agency for Medicines, Sweden 2002). Adherence to a shared guideline should assist all parties in achieving the common goal: not to harm the patient. An outline of some of the major issues that these guidelines address is shown in Table III.

WHAT DOES THE FUTURE HAVE IN STORE?

Controlled long-term studies are needed to answer simple but important questions on treatment adherence, safety, and tolerance. RCTs with active control medications would be helpful in assessing the effectiveness of opioids in comparison with the alternative treatments. RCTs are urgently needed on the efficacy of methadone in chronic pain management. The usefulness of

Table III
Core guidelines for using opioids in chronic noncancer pain

1) The management of chronic pain should be directed by the underlying cause of the pain. Whatever the cause, the primary goal of patient care should be symptom control.
2) Opioid treatment should be considered for both neuropathic and nociceptive pain if other reasonable therapies fail to provide adequate analgesia within a reasonable time frame.
3) The aims of opioid treatment are to relieve pain and improve the patient's quality of life. Both of these aims should be assessed during a trial period.
4) The prescribing physician should be familiar with the patient's psychosocial status.
5) The use of sustained-release opioids administered at regular intervals is recommended.
6) Treatment should be monitored regarding aspects such as pain relief, functional status, quality of life, adverse effects, changes in treatment, and opioid dosage.
7) A contract setting out the patient's rights and responsibilities may help to emphasize the importance of patient involvement.
8) Opioid treatment should not be considered a lifelong treatment.

Source: Adapted from Kalso et al. (in press).

opioid rotation, combinations of different opioids, and addition of adjuvant therapies such as NMDA antagonists, cholecystokinin antagonists, and gabapentin should also be explored. The utility of peripheral opioid receptor agonists, δ-opioid agonists, and enzyme inhibitors to increase the effectiveness of endogenous opioid systems are further possibilities for future study.

ACKNOWLEDGMENTS

I am grateful for many stimulating discussions with various friends and colleagues, particularly Amanda C. de C. Williams, Henry McQuay, Andrew Moore, Jayne Edwards, Phil Wiffen, and Vesa Kontinen. Jayne and Phil also helped with the searching of the literature and Vesa with the drawing of the figures.

REFERENCES

American Academy of Pain Medicine. *The Use of Opioids for the Treatment of Chronic Pain,* 1996. Available via the Internet: www.painmed.org/productpub/statements/opioidstmt.html.

American Academy of Pain Medicine. *Long-term Controlled Substances Therapy for Chronic Pain: Sample Agreement,* 2001. Available via the Internet: www.painmed.org/productpub/statements/sample.html.

American Academy of Pain Medicine. *Consent for Chronic Opioid Therapy,* 2002. Available via the Internet: www.painmed.org/productpub/statements/opioidconsent.html.

Arnér S, Meyerson BA. Lack of analgesic effect of opioids on neuropathic and idiopathic forms of pain. *Pain* 1988; 33:11–23.

Attal NA, Guirimand F, Brasseur L, et al. Effects of IV morphine in central pain. A randomized placebo-controlled study. *Neurology* 2002; 58:554–563.

Beaumont V, Henderson G. Relevance of proposed mechanisms of G-protein-coupled receptor desensitization to opioid receptors. In: Kalso E, McQuay HJ, Wiesenfeld-Hallin Z (Eds). *Opioid Sensitivity of Chronic Noncancer Pain,* Progress in Pain Research and Management, Vol. 14. Seattle: IASP Press, 1999.

Bergeson SE, Helms ML, O'Toole LA, et al. Quantitative trait loci influencing morphine antinociception in the four mapping populations. *Mamm Genome* 2001; 12:546–553.

Besse D, Lombard MC, Zajac JM, Roques BP, Besson JM. Pre- and postsynaptic distribution of m, d and k opioid receptors in the superficial layers of the cervical dorsal horn of the rat spinal cord. *Brain Res* 1990; 521:15–22.

Bian D, Nichols ML, Ossipov MH, Lai J, Porreca F. Characterization of the antiallodynic efficacy of morphine in a model of neuropathic pain in rats. *Neuroreport* 1995; 6:1981–1984.

Bian D, Ossipov MH, Ibrahim M, et al. Loss of antiallodynic and antinociceptive spinal/supraspinal morphine synergy in nerve-injured rats: restoration by MK-801 or dynorphin antiserum. *Brain Res* 1999; 831:55–63.

Burton MB, Gebhart GF. Effects of kappa-opioid receptor agonists on responses to colonorectal distension in rats with and without acute colonic inflammation. *J Pharmacol Exp Ther* 1998; 285:707–715.

Caldwell JR, Hale ME, Boyd RE, et al. Treatment of osteoarthritis pain with controlled release oxycodone or fixed combination oxycodone plus acetaminophen added to nonsteroidal antiinflammatory drugs: a double blind, randomized, multicenter, placebo controlled trial. *J Rheumatol* 1999; 26:862–869.

Caldwell JR, Rapoport RJ, Davis JC, et al. Efficacy and safety of a once-daily morphine formulation in chronic, moderate-to-severe osteoarthritis pain: results from a randomized, placebo-controlled, double-blind trial and an open-label extension trial. *J Pain Symptom Manage* 2002; 23:278–291.

Cesselin F. Opioid and anti-opioid peptides. *Fundam Clin Pharmacol* 1995; 9:409–433.

Chapman V, Dickenson AH. The combination of NMDA antagonism and morphine produces profound antinociception in the rat dorsal horn. *Brain Res* 1992; 573:321–323.

Christensen D, Kayser V. The development of pain-related behaviour and opioid tolerance after neuropathy-inducing surgery and sham surgery. *Pain* 2000; 88:231–238.

Cicero TJ, Nock B, Meyer ER. Gender-related differences in the antinociceptive properties of morphine. *J Pharmacol Exp Ther* 1996; 279:767–773.

Cicero TJ, Nock B, O'Connor L, Meyer ER. Role of steroids in sex differences in morphine-induced analgesia: activational and organizational effects. *J Pharmacol Exp Ther* 2002; 300:695–701.

Dellemijn PLI, Vanneste JAL. Randomised double-blind active-placebo-controlled crossover trial of intravenous fentanyl in neuropathic pain. *Lancet* 1997; 349:753–758.

Dellemijn PLI, van Duijn H, Vanneste JAL. Prolonged treatment with transdermal fentanyl in neuropathic pain. *J Pain Symptom Manage* 1998; 16:220–229.

Ebert B, Andersen S, Krogsgaard-Larsen P. Ketobemidone, methadone and pethidine are non-competitive N-methyl-D-aspartate (NMDA) antagonists in the rat cortex and spinal cord. *Neurosci Lett* 1995; 187:165–168.

Elliott KJ, Hynansky A, Inturrisi CE. Dextromethorphan attenuates and reverses analgesic tolerance to morphine. *Pain* 1994; 59:361–368.

Farrar JT, Portenoy RK, Berlin JA, Kinman JL, Strom BL. Defining the clinically important difference in pain outcome measures. *Pain* 2000; 88:287–294.

Field MJ, Bramwell S, Hughes J, Singh L. Detection of static and dynamic components of mechanical allodynia in rat models of neuropathic pain: are they signalled by distinct primary sensory neurones. *Pain* 1999; 83:303–311.

Fishbain DA, Rosomoff HL, Rosomoff RS. Drug abuse, dependence, and addiction in chronic pain patients. *Clin J Pain* 1992; 8:77–85.

Gear RW, Miaskowski C, Gordon NC, et al. Kappa-opioids produce significantly greater analgesia in women than in men. *Nature Med* 1996; 2:1248–1250.

Gordon M, Preiksaitis HG. Drugs and the aging brain. *Geriatrics* 1988; 43:69–78.

Gourlay GK. Different opioids—same actions? In: Kalso E, McQuay HJ, Wiesenfeld-Hallin Z (Eds). *Opioid Sensitivity of Chronic Noncancer Pain,* Progress in Pain Research and Management, Vol. 14. Seattle: IASP Press, 1999, pp 97–115.

Harke H, Gretenkort P, Ladleif HU, Rahman S, Harke O. The response of neuropathic pain and pain in Complex Regional Pain Syndrome I to carbamazepine and sustained-release morphine in patients pretreated with spinal cord stimulation: a double-blinded randomized study. *Anesth Analg* 2001; 92:488–495.

Heiskanen T, Kalso E. Controlled-release oxycodone and morphine in cancer related pain. *Pain* 1997; 73:37–45.

Herrlin K, Segerdahl M, Gustafsson LL, Kalso E. Methadone, ciprofloxacin, and adverse drug reactions. *Lancet* 2000; 356:2069–2070.

Huse E, Larbig W, Flor H, Birbaumer N. The effect of opioids on phantom limb pain and cortical reorganization. *Pain* 2001; 90:47–55.

Jadad AR, Carroll D, Moore A, McQuay H. Developing a database of published reports of randomised clinical trials in pain research. *Pain* 1996; 66:239–246.

Kalso E, McQuay HJ, Wiesenfeld-Hallin Z (Eds). *Opioid Sensitivity of Chronic Noncancer Pain,* Progress in Pain Research and Management, Vol. 14. Seattle: IASP Press, 1999a.

Kalso E, Paakkari P, Stenberg I (Eds). *Opioids in Chronic Non-Cancer Pain, Situation and Guidelines in Nordic Countries.* Helsinki: National Agency for Medicines, Finland, 1999b.

Kalso E, Allan L, Dellemijn PLI, et al. Recommendations for using opioids in chronic non-cancer pain. *Eur J Pain*; in press.

Kieffer BL, Evans CJ. Opioid tolerance—in search of the holy grail. *Cell* 2002; 108:587–590.

Laakso A, Mohn AR, Gainetdinov RR, Caron MG. *Neuron* 2002; 36:213–228.

Lee Y-W, Chaplan SR, Yaksh TL. Systemic and supraspinal but not spinal opiates suppress allodynia in a rat neuropathic pain model. *Neurosci Lett* 1995; 199:111–114.

Magnan J, Paterson SJ, Tavani A, Kosterlitz HW. The binding spectrum of narcotic analgesics with different agonist and antagonist properties. *Naunyn-Schmiedebergs Arch Pharmacol* 1982; 319:197–205.

Maier C, Hildebrandt J, Klinger R, et al. Morphine responsiveness, efficacy and tolerability in patients with chronic non-tumor associated pain—results of a double-blind placebo-controlled trial (MONTAS). *Pain* 2002; 7:223–233.

Mayer DJ, Mao J, Holt J, Price DD. Cellular mechanisms of neuropathic pain, morphine tolerance, and their interactions. *Proc Natl Acad Sci USA* 1999; 96:7731–7736.

McQuay HJ, Tramèr M, Nye BA, et al. A systematic review of antidepressants in neuropathic pain. *Pain* 1996; 68:217–227.

Medical Products Agency. *Use of Opioids for Chronic Non-cancer Related Pain: Recommendations.* Läkemedelsverket: Medical Products Agency, Sweden, 2002; 13:12–75.

Mogil JS, Chesler EJ, Wilson SG, Juraska JM, Sternberg WF. Sex differences in thermal nociception and morphine antinociception in rodents depend on genotype. *Neurosci Biobehav Rev* 2000; 24:375–389.

Monory K, Greiner E, Sartania N, et al. Opioid binding profiles of new hydrazone, oxime, carbazone and semicarbazone derivatives of 14-alkoxymorphinans. *Life Sci* 1999; 64:2011–2020.

Moulin DE, Iezzi A, Amireh R, et al. Randomised trial of oral morphine for chronic non-cancer pain. *Lancet* 1996; 347:143–147.

Nestler EJ, Barrot M, DiLeone RJ, et al. Neurobiology of depression. *Neuron* 2002; 34:13–25.

Nichols ML, Bian D, Ossipov MH, Porreca F. Evidence for regulation of opioid activity by CCK in a model of neuropathic pain. *J Pharmacol Exp Ther* 1995; 275:1337–1345.

Perrot S, Bannwarth B, Bertin P, et al. Use of morphine in nonmalignant joint pain: the Limoges recommendations. The French Society for Rheumatology. *Rev Rhum Engl Ed* 1999; 66:571–576.

Rainville P, Bushnell MC, Duncan GH. PET studies of the subjective experience of pain. In: Casey KL, Bushnell MC (Eds). *Pain Imaging,* Progress in Pain Research and Management, Vol. 18. Seattle: IASP Press, 2000.

Raja SN, Haythornwaite JA, Pappagallo M, et al. Opioids versus antidepressants in postherpetic neuralgia: a randomized placebo-controlled trial. *Neurology* 2002; 59:1015–1021.

Raynor K, Kong H, Chen Y, et al. Pharmacological characterization of the cloned kappa-, delta-, and mu-opioid receptors. *Mol Pharmacol* 1994; 45:330–334.

Raynor K, Kong H, Mestek A, et al. Characterization of the cloned human mu opioid receptor. *J Pharmacol Exp Ther* 1995; 272:423–428.

Roth SH, Fleischmann RM, Burch FX, et al. Around-the-clock, controlled-release oxycodone therapy for osteoarthritis-related pain. *Arch Intern Med* 2000; 160:853–860.

Rowbotham MC, Reisner-Keller LA, Fields HL. Both intravenous lidocaine and morphine reduce the pain of postherpetic neuralgia. *Neurology* 1991; 41:1024–1028.

Siegel S. Morphine analgesic tolerance: its situation specificity supports a Pavlovian conditioning model. *Science* 1976; 193:323–325.

Stein C, Millan MJ, Shippenberg TS, Peter K, Herz A. Peripheral opioid receptors mediating antinociception in inflammation: evidence for involvement of mu, delta and kappa receptors. *J Pharmacol Exp Ther* 1989; 248:1269–1275.

Stoll AL, Rueter SBA. Treatment augmentation with opiates in severe and refractory major depression. *Am J Psychiatry* 1999; 156:2017.

Taddese A, Nah S-Y, McCleskey EW. Selective opioid inhibition of small nociceptive neurons. *Science* 1995; 270:1366–1369.

Thompson SJ, Koszdin K, Bernards CM. Opiate-induced analgesia is increased and prolonged in mice lacking P-glycoprotein. *Anesthesiology* 2000; 92:1392–1399.

Wandel C, Kim R, Wood M, Wood A. Interaction of morphine, fentanyl, sufentanil, alfentanil and loperamide with the efflux drug transporter P-glycoprotein. *Anesthesiology* 2002; 96:913–920.

Watson CPN, Babul N. Efficacy of oxycodone in neuropathic pain. A randomized trial in postherpetic neuralgia. *Neurology* 1998; 50:1837–1841.

World Health Organization. *Cancer Pain Relief,* 2nd ed. Geneva: World Health Organization, 1996.

Wu CL, Tella P, Staats PS, et al. Analgesic effects of intravenous lidocaine and morphine on postamputation pain. *Anesthesiology* 2002; 96:841–848.

Xu X-J, Puke MJC, Verge VMK, et al. Up-regulation of cholecystokinin in primary sensory neurons is associated with morphine insensitivity in experimental neuropathic pain. *Neurosci Lett* 1993; 152:129–132.

Yu W, Hao J-X, Xu X-J, Wiesenfeld-Hallin Z. The development of morphine tolerance and dependence in rats with chronic pain. *Brain Res* 1997; 756:141–146.

Correspondence to: Eija Kalso, MD, DMedSci, Pain Clinic, Department of Anesthesia and Intensive Care Medicine, Helsinki University Central Hospital, P.O. Box 340, FIN-00029 HUS, Finland. Tel: 358-9-47175885; Fax: 358-9-47175641; email: eija.kalso@helsinki.fi.

Proceedings of the 10th World Congress on Pain,
Progress in Pain Research and Management, Vol. 24,
edited by Jonathan O. Dostrovsky, Daniel B. Carr, and
Martin Koltzenburg, IASP Press, Seattle, © 2003.

61

Pain and Aging: The Pain Experience over the Adult Life Span

Stephen J. Gibson

National Ageing Research Institute, Parkville, Victoria; Department of Medicine, University of Melbourne, Melbourne, Victoria; Caulfield Pain Management and Research Centre, Caulfield, Victoria, Australia

The aging of the world's population is one of the great social and medical achievements of this century. In most developed countries where data are available, life expectancy has almost doubled over the past 100 years. By 2050 approximately 23% of the world's population will be over 60 years old, a proportion that climbs to 30–40% in certain Asian and European countries (U.S. Bureau of the Census 2002). While the global increase in life expectancy has resulted mainly from a reduction in the mortality rate during childhood and early adulthood, the influence of an extension to maximum life expectancy has also been recently acknowledged (Vaupel 1997). The past 30 years have seen a dramatic drop in the mortality rate for individuals over 80 years of age. The number of centenarians is increasing at about 8% per year, and death rates have fallen by one-third among centenarians in recent years. This remarkable improvement in the survival of the oldest old has started to challenge our traditional views on the upper limits of longevity, although the extent of increase that might be possible remains unknown (the oldest verified case, Jeanne Calment, died at 122 years, 5 months, and an unverified case in Malaysia is said to have died at 141 years). In any event it is clear that in the years to come there will be a massive increase in the number of older persons surviving into their eighth, ninth, and tenth decade and beyond.

Advancing age is known to be associated with a much greater prevalence of persistent pain, ranging from approximately 25% to 65% in community-dwelling older persons and up to 80% for those in residential care or a nursing home (Helme and Gibson 2001). Many reasons could explain the wide variation in absolute prevalence figures between different studies, including the nature of the survey method (telephone, postal, or interview), the population under study, and the operational definition of persistent pain. However, a consensus view would suggest that at least 50% of the older population suffers from at least one persistent and bothersome pain complaint at any point in time. With such a high prevalence of pain, the massive demographic shift in the age distribution of the worlds' population will provide both challenges and opportunities for pain clinicians and the pain research community alike.

POSSIBLE PAIN-RELATED IMPLICATIONS OF AN AGING SOCIETY

The sheer number of older persons who will be seeking help with pain management will place an enormous burden on existing health care services (Lloyd-Sherlock 2000). Current models of pain treatment also may require some revision in order to meet the special needs of older persons. For instance, outpatient multidisciplinary pain management clinics may be less accessible to frail older adults, and treatment protocols are likely to require modification (Gibson et al. 1996; Helme et al. 1996; Gagliese and Melzack 1997a). It may be necessary to undertake a more comprehensive and time-consuming assessment as well as to include the primary caregiver in all aspects of pain assessment and management. This inclusion can often improve adherence to a treatment plan, particularly when communication problems are at issue. There should be greater attention to issues of polypharmacy and comorbidity and more specific expertise in painful pathologies common in old age, such as osteoarthritis, postherpetic neuralgia, osteoporosis, diabetic peripheral neuropathy, and post-stroke pain syndromes. Given that many frail older persons have difficulties with transportation or reside in institutions, the innovative clinician will have an opportunity to help move the essential features of multidisciplinary treatment into a more home-based service and thereby improve access to care for this disadvantaged group (Kung et al. 2000).

The other major area of challenge and opportunity relates to the current lack of knowledge and scarcity of research on pain and aging. Inclusion of older persons into mainstream pain research endeavors could generate insights and contribute to a better understanding of nociceptive processes, pain, and suffering. By way of example, the study of pain in demented older adults gives us the rather unique opportunity to explore the role of cognition in shaping the overall pain experience. Is depression still a feature of chronic pain when there is no memory of long-term suffering? As another example, most neurophysiological systems are known to change as a function of age. In particular, neural plasticity and mechanisms of neuronal regeneration and repair are impaired in the very old (Verdu et al. 2000). By assessing groups of varied ages it should be possible to conduct natural experiments on the underlying mechanisms of healing and normal resolution of painful pathology.

The lack of current research on pain and aging also provides an urgent challenge. To date, there has not been a single randomized control trial of outpatient multidisciplinary pain treatment for older adults. Only in the last 5 years have studies begun to systematically examine the reliability and validity of common pain assessment tools when used in older persons (Herr and Garand 2001). Information is scarce on how to assess and manage pain in special older populations, such as those with dementia (Hadjistavropoulos and Craig 2002) or those in nursing home care (Ferrell et al. 2000). Possible age differences in the functional and psychological impacts of persistent pain also are understudied (Gibson et al. 1994a). Historically, there has been almost no professional education on pain management in older persons, even within the geriatric components of the medical curriculum (Weiner 2002). While all these issues are of vital importance, perhaps the most fundamental question that must be answered relates to age differences in pain perception and report. Given that a patient's description of pain and discomfort greatly influences the assessment and diagnosis of most medical conditions, such information is essential to guide clinical practice and to develop more rational, age-appropriate pain management strategies. In the past, two main lines of evidence have been used to examine age differences: laboratory investigations using experimentally controlled levels of noxious stimulation, and retrospective reviews of medical records to study age-related variations in the clinical presentation of painful disease.

CLINICAL STUDIES OF AGE DIFFERENCES IN PAIN

Several recent reports have examined age differences in pain as a presenting symptom of medical complaints that are typically painful. Most of these studies have focused on visceral pain complaints, particularly abdominal pain associated with acute infection or different forms of malignancy, and chest pain from myocardial infarction or ischemia. Abdominal complaints such as peritonitis, peptic ulcer, and intestinal obstruction show an age-related change in pain symptoms and presentation. About 45% of older adults with appendicitis do not have lower right quadrant pain as a presenting symptom compared to fewer than 5% of younger adults (Wroblewski and Mikulowski 1991). Pain not only becomes more occult in patients over 60 but in marked contrast to young adults, the group of clinical symptoms (nausea, fever, and tachycardia) with the highest diagnostic accuracy for appendicitis for this age group does not even include abdominal pain (Albano 1975; Wroblewski and Mikulowski 1991). With regard to pain associated with various types of malignancy, a retrospective review of 1,500 cases revealed a marked difference in the incidence of pain between younger adults (55% with pain), middle-aged adults (35% with pain), and older adults (26% with pain) (Cherng et al. 1991). With one exception (Vigano et al. 1998), most observational studies also note a significant decline in the intensity of cancer pain symptoms in adults of advanced age (70 years or older) (Brescia et al. 1992; Caraceni and Portenoy 1999).

Variations in the classic presentation of "crushing" myocardial pain in the chest, left arm, and jaw are known to be widespread in older adults. Retrospective studies show that approximately 35–42% of adults over the age of 65 years experience an apparently silent or painless heart attack (MacDonald et al. 1983). Quantitative and experimentally controlled studies of myocardial pain in patients with coronary artery disease often employ strenuous physical exercise to induce myocardial ischemia as indexed by a 1-mm drop in the ST segment of the electrocardiogram. By comparing the onset and degree of exertion-induced ischemia with subjective pain report, it is possible to provide an experimentally controlled evaluation of myocardial pain across the adult life span. Several studies have documented a significant age-related delay between the onset of ischemia and the report of chest pain (Miller et al. 1990; Ambepitiya et al. 1994). Adults over 70 years old take almost three times as long as young adults to first report the presence of pain (Ambepitiya et al. 1994). Moreover, the pain is less severe in older subjects, even in studies that control for variations in the extent of ischemia. Collectively, these findings provide strong support for the view that myocardial pain may be muted in adults of advanced age.

An atypical presentation of pain symptoms has also been documented for pneumonia, pneumothorax, and postoperative and arthritic pains. For instance, several studies suggest that older adults report a lower intensity of pain in the postoperative recovery period, even after matching for the type of surgical procedure and the extent of tissue damage (Meier et al. 1996; Thomas et al. 1998). This change is thought to be clinically significant and is in the order of a 10–20% reduction per decade after the age of 60 years (Meier et al. 1996; Thomas et al. 1998). The findings for chronic musculoskeletal pain are equivocal, with reports of increased arthritic pain in older adults (Wilkieson et al. 1993; Harkins et al. 1994), decreased pain severity

(Lichtenberg et al. 1984; Parker et al. 1988), or no change (Yunus et al. 1988; Gagliese and Melzack 1997a). Studies on patients with musculoskeletal pain attending multidisciplinary pain management clinics show similarly mixed findings. The findings may depend on the type of pain assessment scale used because studies with a unidimensional measure such as a visual analogue scale or word descriptor have typically found no age difference (Middaugh et al. 1988; Sorkin et al. 1990; Corran et al. 1994; Benbow et al. 1996; Riley et al. 2000). In contrast, reports based on multidimensional measures have reported an age-related decline in pain intensity and unpleasantness (Turk et al. 1995; Corran et al. 1997; Gagliese and Melzack 1997a; Gibson and Helme 2001). This apparent disparity may arise because visual analogue scales are less appropriate for use in older persons, or it could be that only the quality of chronic pain sensation changes rather than the intensity (Gagliese and Melzack 1997a).

In summary, there is strong evidence for a clinically significant reduction in the frequency and intensity of pain symptoms with advancing age. It is tempting to conclude that old age is associated with a general decline in the perceived severity of most types of clinical pain, although one must exercise caution due to methodological weakness in many of these studies. Methodological limitations include use of a retrospective review of medical records to evaluate pain symptoms rather than patient self-report, the often unmeasured impact of comorbidity and drug effects in many older patients, as well as selection bias often associated with convenience sampling techniques. Another major problem with most clinical studies is that one can seldom control for the severity of disease. As a result it remains somewhat unclear as to whether the observed aging effects reflect an age-related difference in disease severity, a difference in willingness to report pain as a symptom, or a true age-related change in the pain experience. To overcome these uncertainties, many investigators have turned to psychophysical studies and use experimentally controlled levels of noxious input to anchor the subjective experience against a stimulus of known intensity, thereby providing a quantitative comparison of pain sensitivity between different age groups.

PSYCHOPHYSICAL STUDIES OF AGE DIFFERENCES IN PAIN

Over 50 studies and several recent reviews have reported age differences in the sensitivity to experimentally induced pain (Harkins 1996; Walco and Harkins 1999; Gibson and Helme 2001; Gibson and Farrell 2003). The vast majority of studies have focused on pain threshold: the minimum amount of noxious stimulation required to first elicit the report of pain. Unfortunately, the results have been somewhat mixed. Twenty-one studies report an increase in pain threshold with advancing age (Chapman and Jones 1944; Hall and Stride 1954; Schuldermann and Zubek 1962; Sherman and Robillard 1964; Procacci et al. 1970; Clark and Mehl 1971; Dyck et al. 1984; Neri and Agazzani 1984; Tucker et al. 1989; Gibson et al. 1991a; Lautenbacher and Strian 1991; Horch et al. 1992; Jensen et al. 1992; Tremblay et al. 1993; Chakour et al. 1996; Heft et al. 1996; Lasch et al. 1997; Mertz et al. 1998; Meliala et al. 1999; Scudds and Scudds 1999; Helme et al. 2002). Three studies report a decrease in pain threshold with age (Edwards and Fillingim 2001a; Lautenbacher et al. 2002; Pickering et al. 2002) and 17 studies report that it remains unchanged (Schumacher et al. 1940; Mumford 1965; Collins and Stone 1966; Notermans 1966; Harkins and Chapman 1976, 1977; Laitinen and Eriksson 1985; Kenshalo 1986; Meh and Denislic 1994; Yarnitsky et al. 1995; Lucantoni et al. 1997; Liou et al. 1999; Meliala et al. 1999; Zheng et al. 2000; Edwards and Fillingim 2001a; Lautenbacher et al. 2002; Pickering et al. 2002). Given that a slightly higher proportion of studies report a significant age difference, the weight of evidence might suggest a slight increase in pain threshold, or in other words a decrease in sensitivity to experimental pain. However, simply to count studies finding a significant age-related difference is not particularly edifying because this approach fails to reveal reasons for the conflicting results. Differences in methodology, sample size, and the types of experimental noxious stimulation make between-study comparisons difficult. Moreover, we have no indication about the size of differences between age groups, yet this consideration is important to understanding age-related change in pain sensitivity. To overcome such problems, meta-analysis has become an increasingly popular tool for the review and quantitative synthesis of information from several related but independent studies.

Fig. 1 summarizes the results of a meta-analysis undertaken on all available pain threshold studies with sufficient information to calculate an effect size for age differences in pain sensitivity. As can be seen, the vast majority of studies document a higher pain threshold in older adults even though in some cases the 95% confidence interval includes zero, thereby indicating that the observed age difference fails to reach statistical significance. The age-related increase in pain threshold appears most obvious for studies using noxious heat, although similar findings also occur for electrical stimulation, but with a reduced effect size for the difference between age groups. Studies using mechanical stimuli, particularly those conducted more recently, show mixed results. Combining all pain threshold studies into a single quantitative estimate of overall effect size indicates a highly significant ($P < 0.0005$) age difference of approximately 0.74 effect size. This estimate combines data

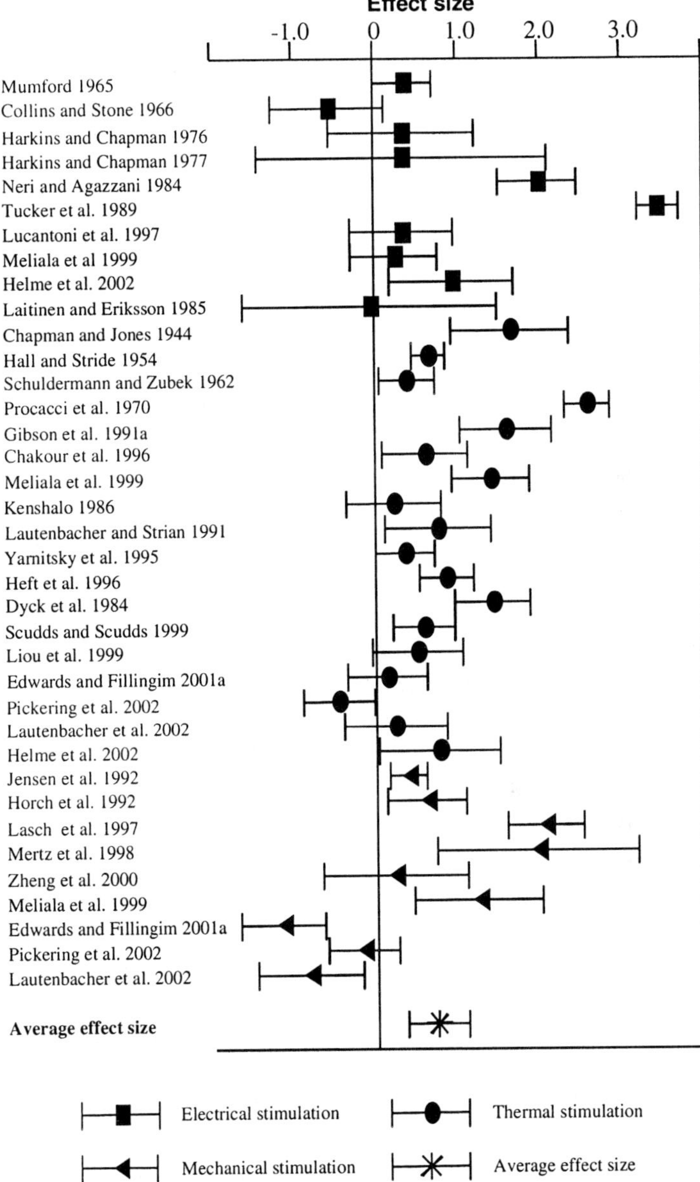

Fig. 1. Meta-analysis of all available studies on age differences in pain threshold. Values refer to the effect size of age difference ± 1.96 SEM. Studies not included due to lack of sufficient information to calculate an effect size include Schumacher et al. (1940), Clarke and Mehl (1971), Notermans (1966), Tremblay et al. (1993), Meh and Denislic (1994), and Scudds and Scudds (1999). Studies not included due to heterogeneity of effect size include Sherman and Robillard (1960, 1964).

from over 4,000 subjects across 37 studies and provides very strong support for a true age-related increase in pain threshold, despite the somewhat variable findings of individual studies. An effect size of 0.74 is considered by most to be quite large (Cohen 1988) and in practical terms would equate to a 2°–3°C increase in the temperature required by older persons to first report the presence of pain. The clinical implications of an increased pain threshold remain controversial because clinical pain always occurs well above threshold intensity and, typically, for a much longer duration. Nonetheless, these findings may indicate some impairment in the early warning functions of pain, because if pain threshold is raised then the gap between the recognition of an injurious stimulus and the onset of consequent tissue damage may be reduced.

If advancing age is associated with a decreased sensitivity to pain across the entire stimulus-response function, then one might expect older persons to be at increased risk of injury and undiagnosed disease. Although studies of clinical pain as a presenting symptom provide some support for this view, few experimental studies have examined age differences in pain sensitivity to suprathreshold stimuli, and their findings have been mixed (Harkins et al. 1986; Gibson et al. 1991a; Tremblay et al. 1993). Another convenient limit in the stimulus-response function is pain tolerance, usually defined as the intensity at which a person seeks to withdraw from any further noxious stimulation. In some ways pain tolerance can be considered as the highest ethically permissible point on the experimental stimulus-response function for pain. To date, there have been 10 age-related comparisons of pain tolerance in response to a variety of noxious stimuli including heat, cold, mechanical pressure, ischemic pain, and noxious electrical stimulation (Collins and Stone 1966; Woodrow et al. 1972; Neri and Agazzani 1984; Walsh et al. 1989; Washington et al. 2000; Edwards and Fillingim 2001a,b; Pickering et al. 2002). While most studies on pain sensitivity suggest a modest increase in pain threshold in later life, a meta-analysis of all available pain tolerance studies suggests an age-related decline in the ability or willingness to endure very strong pain (see Fig. 2). The consistency of age-related decreases in pain tolerance for differing types of noxious stimuli adds some confidence to the finding, and the pooled effect size is highly significant ($P < 0.001$) at –0.45. The reduced ability to tolerate or endure strong pain might result in a greater vulnerability to, or a greater impact of, severe pain states in older persons. These findings also highlight the intensity-dependent nature of age-related changes in pain sensitivity in which older adults have a reduced sensitivity to mild pain, but an apparent increased susceptibility to severe pain. When attempting to explain the differential effects of aging on pain

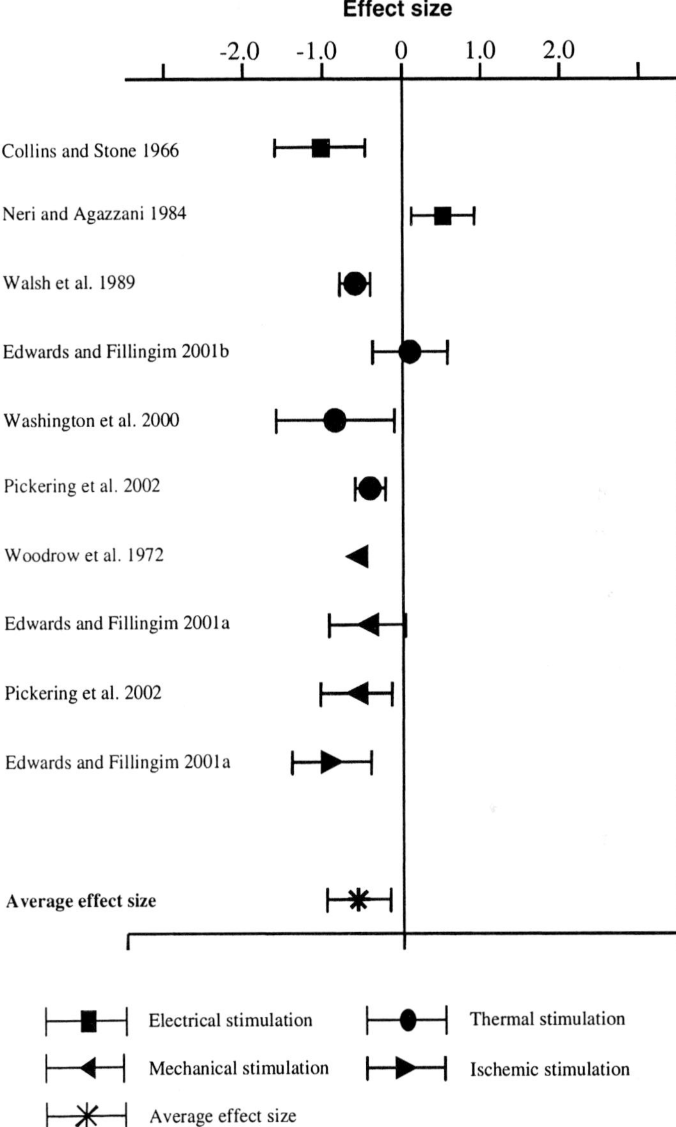

Fig. 2. Meta-analysis of all available studies on age differences in pain tolerance. Values refer to the effect size of age difference ± 1.96 SEM.

sensitivity, one might consider age differences in the neurophysiological processes related to nociception, altered psychological processes including belief structures and coping mechanisms, and secondary age-associated changes in health and social and economic circumstances.

AGE DIFFERENCES IN NOCICEPTIVE NEUROPHYSIOLOGY

Animal and human studies have documented structural, biochemical, and functional changes in the peripheral nervous system of aged subjects (Verdu et al. 2000; Gibson and Farrell 2003). The density of unmyelinated and myelinated fibers decreases by up to 50% in very old age (Ochoa and Mair 1969; Verdu et al. 2000). Signs of neuronal damage or degeneration (e.g., axonal involution, Wallerian degeneration) increase with advancing age (Drac et al. 1991), and there is a marked reduction in the content and turnover of neurotransmitter systems known to be involved in nociception (e.g., substance P, calcitonin gene-related peptide [CGRP], and somatostatin) (Khalil et al. 1994; Bergman et al. 1996). In terms of function, peripheral nerve conduction velocity slows down (Kakigi 1987), and the observed age difference in pain sensitivity has been suggested as a likely consequence of neuronal damage and loss over the life span (Verdu et al. 2000). A study by Chakour et al. (1996) has also noted a differential age-related change in nociceptive Aδ-fiber, but not C-fiber, function. Because myelinated Aδ fibers are involved in rapid stimulus recognition and slow conducting unmyelinated C fibers signal ongoing, poorly localized pain, these findings may show a selective impairment in the early warning functions of nociceptive primary afferent neurons (Gibson and Farrell 2003).

Comparable degenerative changes have been noted in the aged central nervous system (CNS). There is a loss of myelin, evidence of axonal involution, and altered neurochemistry in spinal dorsal horn neurons. Substance P and CGRP content are reduced, and there is a progressive loss of serotonergic and noradrenergic neurons in lamina I leading to a possible impairment in the descending pain inhibitory systems (Bergman et al. 1996; Laporte et al. 1996; Iwata et al. 2002). At supraspinal levels, there is reduced neurotransmitter content and expression, decreased metabolic turnover, and a loss of neurons and dendritic connections throughout the cerebral cortex, midbrain, and brainstem (Wong et al. 1984; Pakkenberg and Gundersen 1997; Barili et al. 1998). Such changes are widespread throughout all areas of the CNS, including areas known to be involved in processing of nociceptive information, such as the prefrontal cortex, primary and secondary somatosensory cortex, hippocampus, anterior cingulate, insula, and thalamus.

Given the enormous physiological reserve of the CNS, it is important to be able to demonstrate some functional consequences of the age-dependent changes in neuronal density, structure, and neurochemistry. Two early studies of cerebral evoked potentials in response to noxious laser stimulation demonstrate a reduced amplitude of response, an increase in response latency, and a wider topographic spread of cortical activation in aged subjects

(Gibson et al. 1991a, 1993). These findings have the potential to indicate age-related slowing in the cognitive processing of noxious information and a wider recruitment of CNS neurons during the cortical processing of noxious input. However, more recent neuroimaging techniques, with better temporal and spatial resolution, are required to confirm this suggestion. Several studies have also started to investigate age-related differences in CNS neurophysiological processes involved in the onset or maintenance of clinical pain states, including mechanisms of secondary hyperalgesia, temporal summation, and endogenous inhibitory systems.

A recent study has examined age differences in the time course of capsaicin-induced hyperalgesia (Zheng et al. 2000). Older adults took slightly longer to first report pain following administration of capsaicin, but there was no age difference in the magnitude or size of heat-induced or mechanically induced hyperalgesia. The area of heat hyperalgesia rapidly decreased over time in both age groups. In marked contrast, the area of mechanical hyperalgesia or tenderness persisted for the duration of the study (3 hours) in older adults but resolved fully in less than an hour in the younger participants. As capsaicin-induced mechanical hyperalgesia is known to be mediated by sensitized dorsal horn neurons, these findings may indicate age differences in the plasticity of spinal cord neurons following an acute injury. The slow resolution of mechanical hyperalgesia may reflect a reduced capacity of the aged CNS to reverse the sensitization process once it has been initiated.

Temporal summation, the progressive enhancement of pain during repeated stimulation, is another process that depends on CNS nociceptive function. It is thought to result from a hyperexcitable state of spinal dorsal horn neurons and may play a role in at least some aspects of central sensitization. Harkins and colleagues (1996) were the first to document a 21% increase in reported pain intensity of young adults over the course of four successive heat stimulations to the hand about 2.5 seconds apart, compared to an 83% increase in older persons. This result has since been confirmed by others (Edwards and Fillingim 2001b; Gibson et al. 2002) and suggests that the aged CNS may be more prone to upregulation and sensitization upon repeated stimulation. More recently our group has examined age-related changes in temporal summation at different frequencies of repeated stimulation (Gibson et al. 2002). Regardless of stimulation frequency, older persons showed a greater percentage increase in self-rated pain intensity by the fifth stimulus repetition when compared to younger adults (see Fig. 3). Consistent with earlier findings (Price et al. 1977), temporal summation failed to occur when repeated stimuli were delivered longer than 3 seconds apart in the young adult group. However, older adults showed obvious temporal

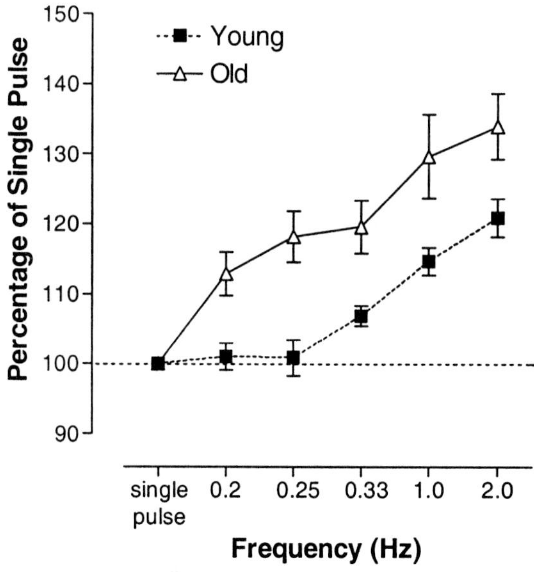

Fig. 3. The effect of age on temporal summation at different frequencies of stimulus repetition. Values refer to the percentage increase (mean ± SD) in self-rated pain intensity when compared to a single noxious stimulus of the same intensity.

summation even when the repetition rate of stimulation was considerably slower at 5 seconds apart (see Fig. 3). These findings might suggest that the young adult's nervous system manages to recover much faster between successive stimulations and can reverse the hyperexcitable state of dorsal horn neurons at stimulation rates longer than once every 3 seconds. In contrast, older persons appear to maintain this post-stimulation hyperexcitable state for a much longer period, thereby allowing for summation to occur even when the stimulus repetition rate is relatively slow. Consistent with the findings on capsaicin-induced hyperalgesia (Zheng et al. 2000), these results add further evidence of reduced plasticity in the aged CNS and demonstrate the much longer time required for the system to recover from perturbation.

Another example of an age-related change in nociceptive neurophysiological function relates to the endogenous pain inhibitory system. Descending modulation is known to mediate endogenous analgesia and is important in shaping the clinical pain experience. Several animal studies over the past 15–20 years have documented a decline in the descending opioid and non-opioid analgesic systems with advancing age (see Gibson and Helme 1995 for review). Washington et al. (2000) have examined age-related differences in the magnitude of endogenous analgesia in human volunteers. A comparison was made of pain threshold intensity in response to noxious electrical stimulation before, immediately after, and 1 hour after repeated immersion of the hand in ice-cold water until pain tolerance was reached. Ice-water immersion was used as a conditioning stimulus of strong ongoing pain in order to activate the endogenous pain inhibitory system. Regardless of age, pain threshold increased immediately after the conditioning stimulus (indicative of analgesia), but this effect was relatively transient and returned to baseline within 1 hour. Of perhaps greater interest, the magnitude of analgesic response was lower in persons of advanced age (a 40% increase in pain threshold) when compared to younger adults (a 150% increase in pain threshold) (Washington et al. 2000). These findings indicate an age-related reduction in the efficacy of endogenous analgesic mechanisms and are consistent with the preclinical literature. A reduction in descending control is likely to make it more difficult for older persons to cope with severe pain states and may help to explain some of the reported age variation in pain tolerance.

Documented alterations in nociceptive neurophysiology help us to understand intensity-dependent changes in pain perception and report across the age spectrum. At threshold levels of noxious stimulation, deficits in primary afferent function and CNS transmission may result in a decrease in pain sensitivity. With more intense levels of stimulation or during pathophysiological pain states such as hyperalgesia, age-associated deficits in neuronal plasticity and endogenous analgesia may predispose to greater vulnerability.

AGE DIFFERENCES IN PAIN-RELATED PSYCHOLOGICAL FACTORS

The second major area in which age may influence pain perception and report relates to psychological factors. Pain is a complex perceptual experience. The context in which noxious information is processed, the cognitive beliefs of the individual, and the meanings attributed to pain symptoms are important factors in shaping this experience. Older adults may perceive pain as something to be expected—just a normal part of old age (Hofland 1992). With some exceptions (Gagliese and Melzack 1997b; McCracken 1998), recent empirical studies of pain appraisals and aging provide clear support for this view (Stoller 1993; Liddell and Locker 1997; Ruzicka 1998; Weiner and Rudy 2002). For instance, a large community study by Stoller (1993) demonstrated that 43% of older persons attribute mild joint pain to part of the normal aging process, while only 21% thought that pain was a sign of disease. Such misattribution has important implications because older people appear to feel less threatened by mild pain symptoms and are less likely to seek treatment. However, this misattribution only occurs for mild aches and pains; if pain is severe, older persons are more likely to interpret the experience as a sign of serious illness and are more likely to seek rapid medical care than their younger counterparts (Leventhal and Prohaska 1986; Stoller 1993).

Clinical research has begun to focus on age differences in other types of pain beliefs, such as stoicism, control over pain, and beliefs in finding a cure. The conviction that organic issues are important in determining pain experience has been reported to be similar in younger and older chronic pain patients (Gagliese and Melzack 1997b), although older patients are less inclined to acknowledge that pain leads to emotional disturbance (Cook et al. 1999). In addition, older patients have a lower cognitive risk of helplessness, less self-blame, and a greater desire for finding a breakthrough treatment (Cook et al. 1999). The locus of control scale has been used to examine age differences in cognitive factors related to control over pain. Older patients with chronic pain have a greater belief in pain severity being dictated by chance or fate (Gibson and Helme 2000) compared to younger pain patients, who are more likely to endorse their own behaviors and actions as the strongest determinant of pain severity. Belief in chance factors was shown to be associated with increased pain, depression, functional impact, and the choice of maladaptive coping strategies. Using a revised version of the pain attitudes questionnaire (Yong et al. 2001), our group has recently found that older patients with chronic pain express more stoic fortitude and greater cautious self-doubt (see Table I). This finding is consistent with other studies of stoic attitudes in older pain patients (Machin and Williams 1998) and provides strong empirical support for the widely held view that older cohorts are generally more stoic in response to pain. Also shown in Table I is a comparison of pain beliefs as measured on the Survey of Pain Attitudes questionnaire. Older adults appear to endorse a higher conviction in finding a medical cure for pain and have greater control as well as a lesser belief that persistent pain is disabling (see Table I).

Patients with persistent pain develop a variety of coping strategies in order to deal with its negative impact on quality of life. Self-perceived confidence in being able to use coping methods to successfully manage pain does not appear to change with advancing age (Keefe and Williams 1990; Keefe et al. 1991; Corran et al. 1994; Gagliese et al. 2000). The literature on age differences in use of coping strategies continues to expand, although the results are mixed. Studies by Keefe and colleagues have shown no age differences in the frequency of coping strategy use, although there was a strong trend for older adults to use more praying and hoping than the young (Keefe and Williams 1990; Keefe et al. 1991). Conversely, older people

Table I

An age-based comparison of pain attitudes and beliefs using the Pain Attitudes Questionnaire and the Survey of Pain Attitudes Inventory in chronic pain patients

	Age Group (years)				
Pain Beliefs	<40 ($n = 105$)	41–59 ($n = 115$)	60–79 ($n = 90$)	80+ ($n = 31$)	Significance
PAQ-R					
Stoic-fortitude	2.914 ± 0.704	3.149 ± 0.821	3.240 ± 0.722	3.538 ± 0.878	***, 1 < 2 = 3 < 4
Stoic-concealment	3.377 ± 0.847	3.432 ± 0.792	3.238 ± 0.772	3.560 ± 0.852	ns
Stoic-superiority	2.992 ± 0.693	3.042 ± 0.623	2.941 ± 0.621	3.126 ± 0.698	ns
Cautious-self-doubt	2.099 ± 0.765	2.003 ± 0.737	2.290 ± 0.735	2.235 ± 0.853	*, 1 = 2 < 3 = 4
Cautious-reluctance	3.468 ± 0.993	3.432 ± 0.988	3.393 ± 0.801	3.500 ± 0.823	ns
SOPA-B					
Control	2.682 ± 0.873	2.942 ± 0.960	2.950 ± 0.784	3.085 ± 0.772	*, 1 < 2 = 3 = 4
Disability	4.120 ± 0.896	3.828 ± 0.857	3.756 ± 1.029	3.789 ± 1.070	*, 1 > 2 = 3 = 4
Harm	3.337 ± 0.917	3.073 ± 0.889	3.227 ± 0.864	3.068 ± 0.870	ns
Emotion	3.342 ± 1.244	3.260 ± 1.149	3.250 ± 1.159	2.801 ± 1.227	ns
Medication	3.469 ± 1.022	3.620 ± 1.010	3.610 ± 1.035	3.862 ± 1.059	ns
Solicitude	2.504 ± 1.048	2.357 ± 0.917	2.665 ± 0.988	2.236 ± 0.947	ns
Cure	2.807 ± 1.000	3.055 ± 0.842	2.811 ± 0.864	3.169 ± 1.017	*, 1 = 3 < 2 = 4

Note: PAQ-R = Pain Attitudes Questionnaire-Revised; SOPA-B = Survey of Pain Attitudes-Brief; data are means ± SD; $N = 341$, * $P < 0.05$; *** $P < 0.001$; ns = not significant.

with chronic pain report fewer cognitive coping strategies and an increased use of physical methods of pain control compared to young adults (Sorkin et al. 1990). Corran et al. (1994) examined a large sample of outpatients attending a multidisciplinary pain treatment center and found a significantly higher use of praying and hoping as well as less frequent use of ignoring pain in adults over 60 years old. A recent study may help reconcile the disparity between Keefe's findings and the work of others (Sorkin et al. 1990; Corran et al. 1994; McCracken 1998). Based on the fact that coping efforts are very dependent on the specific nature of the problem, Watkins et al. (1999) conducted a study of mild versus severe pain in young (34–50-year-old), middle-aged (51–65-year-old), and older (66–85-year-old) patients with rheumatoid arthritis. Age differences were clear for patients in mild pain, with middle-aged and older adults reporting more catastrophizing and praying and hoping, but fewer self-coping statements than younger adults. However, when pain was severe, the tendency to utilize such coping strategies was similar for all age groups. Thus, it would appear that even clearly identified age differences in coping might depend on the specific situation and the intensity of the pain problem.

Overall, there do appear to be age differences in pain beliefs, coping, attributional style, and attitudes toward pain. If a pain symptom is mild or transient in older adults, it is likely to be attributed to the normal aging process, to be more readily accepted, and to be accompanied by a different choice of coping strategies. These factors are likely to diminish the importance of mild aches and pains and even alter the meaning of pain symptoms. More stoic attitudes to mild pain and a stronger belief in chance factors as the major determinant of pain severity are likely to lead to the under-report of mild pain symptoms by older adults. However, many of the age differences in coping, misattribution, and beliefs disappear if pain is persistent or severe.

THE EFFECT OF SECONDARY AGE-ASSOCIATED INFLUENCES ON PAIN

The last area of explanation for age differences in pain perception relates to more indirect or secondary age-associated changes in health and social and economic circumstances. This topic has received almost no systematic empirical investigation, yet these types of influence could explain many of the observed age related differences in pain. Prominent among these factors are the increased level of comorbid disease and the concomitant increase in medication use during later stages of life. The typical 70-year-old living in the community has on average 3.6 medical conditions and takes an average of seven different medications. This age-associated increase in comorbidity could account for much of the observed age-related difference in pain. For instance, at least some patients with silent myocardial infarction were unable to provide a reliable history due to the presence of dementia or a lack of consciousness (MacDonald et al. 1983). A study on the absence of pain in pneumonia noted a much higher prevalence of concurrent disease in the oldest patients, particularly coronary artery disease, and a higher use of NSAIDs, hypnotic drugs, and sedative medications (Esposito 1984). A majority of older persons suffer from arthritis of the weight-bearing joints, and while such problems are usually mild, studies have shown an increased pain threshold in those with pre-existing clinical pain (Gracely 1984; Gibson et al. 1991b, 1994b). Similarly, there is a well-documented relationship between hypertension and reduced sensitivity to pain. A higher systolic blood pressure is associated with a significantly higher pain threshold (Guasti et al. 1995; D'Antono et al. 1999). Given that more than 60% of the older adult population have a systolic reading above 140 mmHg (Fagard 2002), this single factor alone could account for much of the observed age-related increase in pain threshold. Of course, the increased level of comorbid disease could be a double-edged sword. Conditions like hypertension, diabetes, neurological disease, and arthritis could raise pain threshold and thereby impair the early warning functions of pain onset. On the other hand, as the weight of comorbid pathology increases, it may contribute to a worsening of pain severity and impact. The prevalence and severity of comorbid disease were very high in a sample of older patients attending a multidisciplinary treatment center (Helme and Gibson 1997). Comorbidity is associated with a 30% increase in self-rated pain intensity and increased levels of mood disturbance and functional impairment. It appears that a certain critical burden of disease is required, as comorbidity affecting fewer than three organ systems had no effect on the clinical presentation of older patients (Farrell et al. 1995; Neufeld et al. 2002). These findings emphasize the need to examine comorbid disease burden as part of the routine clinical assessment of older patients with chronic pain, and highlights the importance of this issue as a potential explanation for age-related variations in the experience of pain.

The major changes that occur in social circumstances throughout the adult life span might be expected to influence pain and its expression. Various stages of social functioning have been described, including leaving the family unit during young adulthood and preparing for independent life through academic and vocational training. During the third to fifth decades of life individuals may begin their own nuclear family, consolidate career choices, and develop new social networks. Middle age is often characterized by a reassessment of life goals, achieving independence from offspring, attaining relative financial comfort, and preparing for retirement. During old age, there is typically a greater freedom to pursue personal life interests and pastimes and reduced societal and vocational responsibility. Very advanced age may also be associated with an increased burden of chronic ailments, economic constraints, death of one's spouse and friends, and consequent social isolation. It is clear that loneliness and bereavement affect mood state and thereby pain. Bradbeer and colleagues (2003) have found that widowhood is associated with an increased risk of pain in older persons living in the community, and widows with mood disturbance are more likely to experience pain that is moderate to severe. It has been suggested that older persons may be more likely to complain of pain in order to receive social contact that would otherwise be unavailable (Fordyce 1978). A study of older patients with chronic pain has shown increasing levels of pain with increasing social support (Helme et al. 1996). Others, however, have reported that social factors such as income, residential status, and frequency of social contact were similar in older adults with and without chronic pain (Roy and Thomas 1987). Moreover, viewed within the context of multiple health problems, loss of loved ones, and the foreboding prospect of institutional care, mild aches and pains may be considered unimportant. Some older persons must cope with decreasing economic resources during retirement, which could reduce access to appropriate health care including pain management and thereby reduce the ability to cope with persistent pain states. Studies of comorbidity and social and economic change should be considered as a priority for future research because this information is vital for a more comprehensive understanding of age differences in the pain experience.

CONCLUDING REMARKS

The rapid aging of the world's population has led to a clear need for comprehensive information about the pain experience over the adult lifespan. Studies of clinical and experimental pain to date reveal age-related differences in pain perception and report. The response to mild pain may be somewhat less in older adults, but they are more susceptible to severe pain. These intensity-dependent, age-related changes may be conceptualized as a reduced capacity in the functional reserve of the pain system at both extremes of the pain intensity spectrum. The increase in pain threshold may indicate some deficit in the early warning function of pain and could lead to delays in diagnosis and poorer recovery. Conversely, decreased pain tolerance highlights the greater vulnerability of older persons and suggests their greater difficulty in being able to endure or cope with more severe pain. There are many reasons for observed age-related changes in pain, including physiological, psychological, and social influences, but our current knowledge remains incomplete. Given the progressive shift in the age distribution of our society, the time for action is now. Future efforts must be directed specifically toward the older segments of the population, in terms of more research, better professional education, and the development of pain management strategies that better meet the needs of older persons who suffer from distressing pain.

ACKNOWLEDGMENTS

The work presented in the manuscript represents a team effort and my thanks go to Dr. Mike Farrell, Dr. Benny Katz, Professor Robert Helme, Dr. Trevor Corran, Max Neufeld, Professor Zeinab Khalil, the other members of the NARI/MECRS pain management team, and the many Honors and PhD students who have contributed to this work. My thanks also go to the National Health and Medical Research Council of Australia for ongoing project grant support (#9533911, 9634540, 9835608, and 2139291).

REFERENCES

Albano W, Zielinski, CM, Organ CH. Is appendicitis in the aged really different? *Geriatrics* 1975; 30:81–88.

Ambepitiya G, Roberts M, Ranjadayalan K, Tallis R. Silent exertional myocardial ischemia in the elderly: a quantitative analysis of anginal perceptual threshold and the influence of autonomic function. *J Am Geriatr Soc* 1994; 42:732–737.

Barili P, De Carolis G, Zaccheo D, Amenta F. Sensitivity to ageing of the limbic dopaminergic system: a review. *Mech Ageing Dev* 1998; 106:57–92.

Benbow S, Cossins L, Wiles JR. A comparative study of disability, depression and pain severity in young and elderly chronic pain patients. In: *Abstracts: 8th World Congress on Pain.* Seattle: IASP Press, 1996, p 289.

Bergman E, Johnson H, Zhang X, Hokfelt T, Ulfhake B. Neuropeptides and neurotrophin receptor mRNAs in primary sensory neurons of aged rats. *J Comp Neurol* 1996; 375:303–319.

Bradbeer M, Hyong HH, Kendg HL, Helme RD, Gibson SJ. Widowhood and other demographic associations of pain in independent older people. *Clin J Pain* 2003; in press.

Brescia FJ, Portenoy RK, Ryan M, Krasnoff L, Gray G. Pain, opioid use, and survival in hospitalized patients with advanced cancer. *J Clin Oncol* 1992; 10:149–155.

Caraceni A, Portenoy RK. An international survey of cancer pain characteristics and syndromes. IASP Task Force on Cancer Pain. *Pain* 1999; 82:263–274.

Chakour M, Gibson SJ, Bradbeer M, Helme RD. The effect of age on A delta and C fibre thermal pain perception. *Pain* 1996; 64:143–152.

Chapman BW, Jones CM. Variations in cutaneous and visceral pain sensitivity in normal subjects. *J Clin Invest* 1944; 23:81–91.

Cherng CH, Ho ST, Kao SJ, Ger LP. The study of cancer pain and its correlates. *Ma-Tsui-Hsueh-Tsa-Chi* 1991; 29:653–657.

Clark WC, Mehl L. Thermal pain: a sensory decision theory analysis of the effect of age and sex on d', various response criteria, and 50% pain threshold. *J Abnorm Psychol* 1971; 78:202–212.

Cohen J. *Statistical Power Analysis for the Behavioral Sciences.* Hillsdale, NJ: Lawrence Erlbaum, 1988.

Collins LG, Stone LA. Pain sensitivity, age and activity level in chronic schizophrenics and in normals. *Br J Psychiatry* 1966; 112:33–35.

Cook AJ, DeGood DE, Chastain DC. Age differences in pain beliefs. *Abstracts: 9th World Congress on Pain.* Seattle: IASP Press, 1999, p 557.

Corran TM, Gibson SJ, Farrell MJ, Helme RD. Comparison of chronic pain experience between young and elderly patients. In: Gebhart GF, Hammond DL, Jensen TS (Eds). *Proceedings of the 7th World Congress on Pain,* Progress in Pain Research and Management, Vol. 2. Seattle: IASP Press, 1994, pp 895–906.

Corran TM, Farrell MJ, Helme RD, Gibson SJ. The classification of patients with chronic pain: age as a contributing factor. *Clin J Pain* 1997; 13:207–214.

D'Antono B, Ditto B, Rios N, Moskowitz DS. Risk for hypertension and diminished pain sensitivity in women: autonomic and daily correlates. *Int J Psychophysiol* 1999; 31:175–187.

Drac H, Babiuch M, Wisniewska W. Morphological and biochemical changes in peripheral nerves with aging. *Neuropathologia Polska* 1991; 29:49–67.

Dyck PJ, Karnes J, O'Brien PC, Zimmermann IR. Detection thresholds of cutaneous sensation. In: Dyck PJ, Thomas PK, Lambert EH, Bunge R (Eds). *Peripheral Neuropathy.* Philadelphia: W.B. Saunders, 1984, pp 1103–1138.

Edwards RR, Fillingim RB. Age-associated differences in responses to noxious stimuli. *J Gerontol A Biol Sci Med Sci* 2001a; 56:M180–185.

Edwards RR, Fillingim RB. The effects of age on temporal summation and habituation of thermal pain: clinical relevance in healthy older and younger adults. *J Pain* 2001b; 6:307–317.

Esposito AL. Community-acquired bacteremic pneumococcal pneumonia: effect of age on manifestations and outcome. *Arch Int Med* 1984; 144:945–948.

Fagard RH. Epidemiology of hypertension in the elderly. *Am J Geriatr Cardiol* 2002; 11:23–28.

Farrell MJ, Gibson SJ, Helme RD. The effect of medical status on the activity level of elderly pain clinic patients. *J Am Geriatr Soc* 1995; 43:102–107.

Ferrell BA, Stein WM, Beck JC. The Geriatric Pain Measure: validity, reliability and factor analysis. *J Am Geriatr Soc* 2000; 48:1669–1673.

Fordyce WE. Evaluating and managing chronic pain. *Geriatrics* 1978; 33:59–62.

Gagliese L, Melzack R. Age differences in the quality of chronic pain: a preliminary study. *Pain Res Manage* 1997a; 2:157–162.

Gagliese L, Melzack R. Lack of evidence for age differences in pain beliefs. *Pain Res Manage* 1997b; 2:19–28.

Gagliese L, Jackson M, Ritvo P, Wowk A, Katz J. Age is not an impediment to effective use of patient-controlled analgesia by surgical patients. *Anesthesiology* 2000; 93:601–610.

Gibson SJ, Farrell MJ. A review of age differences in the neurophysiology of nociception and the perceptual experience of pain. *Clin J Pain* 2003; in press.

Gibson SJ, Helme RD. Age differences in pain perception and report: a review of physiological, psychological laboratory and clinical studies. *Pain Rev* 1995; 2:111–137.

Gibson SJ, Helme RD. Cognitive factors and the experience of pain and suffering in older persons. *Pain* 2000; 85:375–383.

Gibson SJ, Helme RD. Age-related differences in pain perception and report. *Clin Geriatr Med* 2001; 17:433-456.

Gibson SJ, Gorman MM, Helme RD. Assessment of pain in the elderly using event-related cerebral potentials. In: Bond MR, Charlton JE, Woolf CJ (Eds). *Proceedings of the VIth World Congress on Pain,* Pain Research and Clinical Management, Vol. 4. Amsterdam: Elsevier, 1991a, pp 523–529.

Gibson SJ, LeVasseur SA, Helme RD. Cerebral event-related responses induced by CO_2 laser stimulation in subjects suffering from cervicobrachial syndrome. *Pain* 1991b; 47:173–182.

Gibson SJ, Helme RD, Gorman MM. Age related changes in the scalp topography of cerebral event related potentials following noxious CO_2 laser stimulation. *Abstracts: 7th World Congress on Pain*. Seattle: IASP, 1993, p 159.

Gibson SJ, Katz B, Corran TM, Farrell MJ, Helme RD. Pain in older persons. *Disabil Rehabil* 1994a; 16:127–139.

Gibson SJ, Littlejohn GO, Gorman MM, Helme RD, Granges G. Altered heat pain thresholds and cerebral event-related potentials following painful CO_2 laser stimulation in subjects with fibromyalgia syndrome. *Pain* 1994b; 58:185–193.

Gibson SJ, Farrell MJ, Katz B, Helme RD. Multidisciplinary management of chronic non-malignant pain in older adults. In: Ferrell B, Ferrell B (Eds). *Pain in the Elderly.* Seattle: IASP Press, 1996, pp 91–100.

Gibson SJ, Chang W, Farrell MJ. Age interacts with frequency in the temporal summation of painful electrical stimuli. *Abstracts: 10th World Congress on Pain.* Seattle: IASP Press, 2002, p 906.

Gracely RH. Subjective quantification of pain perception. In: Bromm B (Ed). *Neurophysiological Correlates of Pain.* Amsterdam: Elsevier, 1984, pp 371–387.

Guasti L, Cattaneo R, Rinaldi O, et al. Twenty-four-hour noninvasive blood pressure monitoring and pain perception. *Hypertension* 1995; 25:1301–1305.

Hadjistavropoulos T, Craig KD. A theoretical framework for understanding self-report and observational measures of pain: a communications model. *Behav Res Ther* 2002; 40:551–570.

Hall KRL, Stride E. The varying response to pain in psychiatric disorders: a study in abnormal psychology. *Br J Med Psychol* 1954; 27:48–60.

Harkins SW. Geriatric pain. Pain perceptions in the old. *Clin Geriatr Med* 1996; 12:435–459.

Harkins SW, Chapman CR. Detection and decision factors in pain perception in young and elderly men. *Pain* 1976; 2:253–264.

Harkins SW, Chapman CR. The perception of induced dental pain in young and elderly women. *J Gerontol* 1977; 32:428–435.

Harkins SW, Price DD, Martelli M. Effects of age on pain perception: thermonociception. *J Gerontol* 1986; 41:58–63.

Harkins SW, Price DD, Bush FM, Small RE. Geriatric pain. In: Wall PD, Melzack R (Eds). *Textbook of Pain.* New York: Churchill Livingstone, 1994, pp 769–784.

Harkins SW, Davis MD, Bush FM, Kasberger J. Suppression of first pain and slow temporal summation of second pain in relation to age. *J Gerontol A Biol Sci Med Sci* 1996; 51:M260–265.

Heft MW, Cooper BY, O'Brien KK, Hemp E, O'Brien R. Aging effects on the perception of noxious and non-noxious thermal stimuli applied to the face. *Aging: Clin Exp Res* 1996; 8:35–41.

Helme RD, Gibson SJ. Pain in the elderly. In: Jensen TS, Turner JA, Wiesenfeld-Hallin Z (Eds). *Proceedings of the 8th World Congress on Pain,* Progress in Pain Research and Management, Vol. 8. Seattle: IASP Press, 1997, pp 919–944.

Helme RD, Gibson SJ. The epidemiology of pain in elderly people. *Clin Geriatr Med* 2001; 17:417–431.

Helme RD, Katz B, Gibson SJ, et al. Multidisciplinary pain clinics for older people. Do they have a role? *Clin Geriatr Med* 1996; 12:563–582.

Helme RD, Farrell M, Meliala A, Gibson SJ. Decreasing stimulus duration accentuates ageing differences in pain threshold. *Abstracts: 10th World Congress on Pain.* Seattle: IASP Press, 2002, p 911.

Herr KA, Garand L. Assessment and measurement of pain in older adults. *Clin Geriatr Med* 2001; 17:457–478.

Hofland SL. Elder beliefs: blocks to pain management. *J Geriatr Nurs* 1992; 18:19–24.

Horch K, Hardy M, Jimenez S, Jabaley M. An Automated Tactile Tester for evaluation of cutaneous sensibility. *J Hand Surg (Am)* 1992; 17:829–837.

Iwata K, Fukuoka T, Kondo E, et al. Plastic changes in nociceptive transmission of the rat spinal cord with advancing age. *J Neurophysiol* 2002; 87:1086–1093.

Jensen R, Rasmussen BK, Pedersen B, Lous I, Olesen J. Cephalic muscle tenderness and pressure pain threshold in a general population. *Pain* 1992; 48:197–203.

Kakigi R. The effect of aging on somatosensory evoked potentials following stimulation of the posterior tibial nerve in man. *EEG Clin Neurophysiol* 1987; 68:227–286.

Keefe FJ, Caldwell DS, Martinez S, et al. Analyzing pain in rheumatoid arthritis patients: pain coping strategies in patients who have had knee replacement surgery. *Pain* 1991; 46:153–160.

Kenshalo DR. Somesthetic sensitivity in young and elderly humans. *J Gerontol* 1986; 41:M732–742.

Khalil Z, Ralevic V, Bassirat M, Dusting GJ, Helme RD. Effects of ageing on sensory nerve function in rat skin. *Brain Res* 1994; 641:265–272.

Kung F, Gibson SJ, Helme RD. A community-based program that provides free choice of intervention for older people with chronic pain. *J Pain* 2000; 1:293–308.

Laitinen LV, Eriksson AT. Electrical stimulation in the measurement of cutaneous sensibility. *Pain* 1985; 22:139–150.

Laporte AM, Doyen C, Nevo IT, et al. Autoradiographic mapping of serotonin 5-HT1A, 5-HT1D, 5-HT2A and 5-HT3 receptors in the aged human spinal cord. *J Chem Neuroanat* 1996; 11:67–75.

Lasch H, Castell DO, Castell JA. Evidence for diminished visceral pain with aging: studies using graded intraesophageal balloon distension. *Am J Physiol* 1997; 272:g1–g3.

Lautenbacher S, Strian F. Similarities in age differences in heat pain perception and thermal sensitivity. *Funct Neurol* 1991; 6:129–135.

Lautenbacher S, Nielsen J, Bar S, Strate P, Arendt-Nielsen L. Pain processing and somatosensation in young and elderly individuals. *Abstracts: 10th World Congress on Pain.* Seattle: IASP Press, 2002, p 913.

Leventhal EA, Prohaska TR. Age, symptom interpretation, and behavior. *J Am Geriatr Soc* 1986; 34:185–191.

Lichtenberg PA, Skehan MW, Swensen CH. The role of personality, recent life stress and arthritic severity in predicting pain. *J Psychosom Res* 1984; 28:231–236.

Liddell A, Locker D. Gender and age differences in attitudes to dental pain and dental control. *Community Dent Oral Epidemiol* 1997; 25:314–318.

Liou JT, Lui PW, Lo YL, et al. Normative data of quantitative thermal and vibratory thresholds in normal subjects in Taiwan: gender and age effect. *Zhonghua Yi Xue Za Zhi (Taipei)* 1999; 62:431–437.

Lloyd-Sherlock P. Population ageing in developed and developing regions: implications for health policy. *Soc Sci Med* 2000; 51:887–895.

Lucantoni C, Marinelli S, Refe A, Tomassini F, Gaetti R. Course of pain sensitivity in aging: pathological aspects of silent cardiopathy. *Arch Gerontol Geriatr* 1997; 24:281–286.

MacDonald JB, Ballie J, Williams BO, Ballantyne D. Coronary care in the elderly. *Age Ageing* 1983; 12:17–20.

Machin P, Williams AC de C. Stiff upper lip: coping strategies of World War II veterans with phantom limb pain. *Clin J Pain* 1998; 14:290–294.

McCracken LM. Learning to live with the pain: acceptance of pain predicts adjustment in persons with chronic pain. *Pain* 1998; 74:21–27.

Meh D, Denislic M. Quantitative assessment of thermal and pain sensitivity. *J Neurol Sci* 1994; 127:164–169.

Meier DE, Morrison RS, Ahronheim JC. Quantifying pain and discomfort from procedures in hospitalized patients: validation of a new tool. *Proceedings of the American Geriatric Society*. Atlanta: American Geriatric Society, 1996, p 127.

Meliala A, Gibson SJ, Helme RD. The effect of stimulation site on the detection and pain thresholds in young and older adults. *Abstracts: 9th World Congress on Pain*. Seattle: IASP Press, 1999, p 559.

Mertz H, Fullerton S, Naliboff B, Mayer EA. Symptoms and visceral perception in severe functional and organic dyspepsia. *Gut* 1998; 42:814–822.

Middaugh SJ, Levin RB, Kee WG, Barchiesi FD, Roberts JM. Chronic pain: its treatment in geriatric and younger patients. *Arch Phys Med Rehabil* 1988; 69:1021–1026.

Miller PF, Sheps DS, Bragdon EE, et al. Aging and pain perception in ischemic heart disease. *Am Heart J* 1990; 120:22–30.

Mumford JM. Pain perception threshold and adaptation of normal human teeth. *Arch Oral Biol* 1965; 10:957–968.

Neri M, Agazzani E. Aging and right-left asymmetry in experimental pain measurement. *Pain* 1984; 19:43–48.

Neufeld M, Katz B, Farrell MJ, Gibson SJ. The influence of comorbid disease on clinical presentation of older chronic pain patients. *Abstracts: 10th World Congress on Pain*. Seattle: IASP Press, 2002, p 909.

Notermans SLH. Measurement of pain threshold determined by electrical stimulation and its clinical application. Part I. Method and factors possibly influencing the pain threshold. *Neurology* 1966; 16:1071–1086.

Ochoa J, Mair WGP. The normal sural nerve in man. II. Changes in the axon and Schwann cells due to ageing. *Acta Neuropathol (Berl)* 1969; 13:217–239.

Pakkenberg B, Gundersen HJ. Neocortical neuron number in humans: effect of sex and age. *J Comp Neurol* 1997; 384:312–320.

Parker J, Frank R, Beck N, et al. Pain in rheumatoid arthritis: relationship to demographic, medical, and psychological factors. *J Rheumatol* 1988; 15:433–437.

Pickering G, Jourdan D, Eschalier A, Dubray C. Impact of age, gender and cognitive functioning on pain perception. *Gerontology* 2002; 48:112–118.

Price DD, Hu JW, Dubner R, Gracely RH. Peripheral suppression of first pain and central summation of second pain evoked by noxious heat pulses. *Pain* 1977; 3:57–68.

Procacci P, Bozza G, Buzzelli G, Della Corte M. The cutaneous pricking pain threshold in old age. *Gerontologia Clin* 1970; 12:213–218.

Riley JL, Wade JB, Robinson ME, Price DD. The stage of pain processing across the adult lifespan. *J Pain* 2000; 1:162–170.

Roy R, Thomas MR. Elderly persons with and without pain: a comparative study. *Clin J Pain* 1987; 3:102–106.

Ruzicka SA. Pain beliefs. What do elders believe? *J Holist Nurs* 1998; 16:369–382.

Schuldermann E, Zubek JP. Effect of age on pain sensitivity. *Percept Motor Skills* 1962; 14:295–301.

Schumacher GA, Goodell H, Hardy JD, Wolff HG. Uniformity of the pain threshold in man. *Science* 1940; 92:110–112.

Scudds RJ, Scudds RA. A comparison of hot and cold pain thresholds between young subjects and young-elderly, middle-elderly and old-elderly subjects. *Abstracts: 9th World Congress on Pain*. Seattle: IASP Press, 1999, p 560.

Sherman ED, Robillard E. Sensitivity to pain in relationship to age. *J Am Geriatr Soc* 1964; 12:1037–1044.

Sorkin BA, Rudy TE, Hanlon RB, Turk DC, Steig RL. Chronic pain in old and young patients: differences appear less important than similarities. *J Gerontol* 1990; 45:P64–68.

Stoller EP. Interpretations of symptoms by older people. *J Aging Health* 1993; 5:58–81.

Stoller EP, Forster LE, Portugal S. Self care responses to symptoms by older people. *Med Care* 1993; 31:24–42.

Thomas T, Robinson C, Champion D, McKell M, Pell M. Prediction and assessment of the severity of post-operative pain and of satisfaction with management. *Pain* 1998; 75:177–185.

Tremblay N, Allard N, Veillette Y. Effect of age on pain perception: preliminary results. *Abstracts: 7th World Congress on Pain*. Seattle: IASP, 1993, p 1998.

Tucker MA, Andrew MF, Ogle SJ, Davison JG. Age-associated change in pain threshold measured by transcutaneous neuronal electrical stimulation. *Age Ageing* 1989; 18:241–246.

Turk DC, Okifuji A, Scharff L. Chronic pain and depression: role of perceived impact and perceived control in different age cohorts. *Pain* 1995; 61:93–101.

U.S. Bureau of the Census. *International Data Base,* Vol. 2002. U.S. Bureau of the Census, 2002.

Vaupel JW. The remarkable improvements in survival at older ages. *Philos Trans R Soc Lond B Biol Sci* 1997; 352:1799–1804.

Verdu E, Ceballos D, Vilches JJ, Navarro X. Influence of aging on peripheral nerve function and regeneration. *J Peripher Nerv Syst* 2000; 5:191–208.

Vigano A, Bruera E, Suarez-Almazor ME. Age, pain intensity, and opioid dose in patients with advanced cancer. *Cancer* 1998; 83:1244–1250.

Walco GA, Harkins SW. Lifespan developmental approaches to pain. In: Gatchel RJ, Turk DC (Eds). *Psychosocial Factors in Pain: Critical Perspectives.* New York: Guilford Press, 1999, pp 107–117.

Walsh NE, Schoenfeld L, Ramamurthy S, Hoffman J. Normative model for cold pressor test. *Am J Phys Med Rehabil* 1989; 68:6–11.

Washington LL, Gibson SJ, Helme RD. Age-related differences in the endogenous analgesic response to repeated cold water immersion in human volunteers. *Pain* 2000; 89:89–96.

Watkins KW, Shifren K, Park DC, Morrell RW. Age, pain, and coping with rheumatoid arthritis. *Pain* 1999; 82:217–228.

Weiner DK. Improving pain management for older adults: an urgent agenda for the educator, investigator, and practitioner. *Pain* 2002; 97:1–4.

Weiner DK, Rudy TE. Attitudinal barriers to effective treatment of persistent pain in nursing home residents. *J Am Geriatr Soc* 2002; 50:2035–2040.

Wilkieson CA, Madhok R, Hunter JA, Capell HA. Toleration, side-effects and efficacy of sulphasalazine in rheumatoid arthritis patients of different ages. *Q J Med* 1993; 86:501–505.

Wong DF, Wagner HNJ, Dannals RF, et al. Effects of age on dopamine and serotonin receptors measured by positron tomography in the living human brain. *Science* 1984; 226:1393–1396.

Woodrow KM, Friedman GD, Siegelaub AB, Collen MF. Pain tolerance: differences according to age, sex and race. *Psychosom Med* 1972; 34:548–556.

Wroblewski M, Mikulowski P. Peritonitis in geriatric inpatients. *Age Ageing* 1991; 20:90–94.

Yarnitsky D, Sprecher E, Zaslansky R, Hemli JA. Heat pain thresholds: normative data and repeatability. *Pain* 1995; 60:329–332.

Yong HH, Gibson SJ, Horne DJ, Helme RD. Development of a pain attitudes questionnaire to assess stoicism and cautiousness for possible age differences. *J Gerontol B Psychol Sci Soc Sci* 2001; 56:P279–284.

Yunus MB, Holt GS, Masi AT, Aldag JC. Fibromyalgia syndrome among the elderly: comparison with younger patients. *J Am Geriatr Soc* 1988; 36:987–995.

Zheng Z, Gibson SJ, Khalil Z, Helme RD, McMeeken JM. Age-related differences in the time course of capsaicin-induced hyperalgesia. *Pain* 2000; 85:51–58.

Correspondence to: Stephen J. Gibson, PhD, National Ageing Research Institute, P.O. Box 31, Parkville, VIC 3052, Australia. Email: s.gibson@nari.unimelb.edu.au.

Proceedings of the 10th World Congress on Pain,
Progress in Pain Research and Management, Vol. 24,
edited by Jonathan O. Dostrovsky, Daniel B. Carr, and
Martin Koltzenburg, IASP Press, Seattle, © 2003.

62

Pain in Survivors of Torture and Organized Violence[1]

Amanda C. de C. Williams,[a] Kirstine Amris,[b] and Jannie Van Der Merwe[a]

[a]INPUT Pain Management Unit, St. Thomas Hospital, London, United Kingdom; [b]International Rehabilitation Council for Torture Victims, Copenhagen, Denmark

"Pain is one of the most frequent complaints of torture survivors, and even though psychological complications are no doubt a major problem, most of the patients experience and present their symptoms as somatic diseases. Overemphasizing the importance of the psychological aspects may result in insufficient somatic pain diagnoses and treatment" (Thomsen et al. 2000, p 156).

Torture is variously defined, but the most widely used definition is that of the United Nations Convention against Torture (www.unhchr.ch):

> [A]ny act by which severe pain or suffering, whether physical or mental, is intentionally inflicted on a person for such purposes as obtaining from him or a third person information or a confession, punishing him for an act that he has committed or is suspected of having committed, or intimidating or coercing him or a third person, or for any reason based on discrimination of any kind, when such pain or suffering is inflicted by or at the instigation of or with the consent or acquiescence of a public official or other person acting in an official capacity.

According to this definition, torture takes place in more than half of the countries in the world, whether or not they have ratified the convention. The International Rehabilitation Council for Torture Victims (IRCT; www.irct.org) provides a rough estimate of the prevalence of primary torture victims worldwide

[1] Based on a Congress workshop.

of between 10 and 100 millions. Torture is now most often used as an "oppressive instrument ... in the preservation of power" (Maio 2001), aiming to destroy people physically and psychologically. Many people die under torture, so those we see are literally survivors. Since the end of the cold war, victims are not predominantly political prisoners but poor people, minorities, immigrants, criminals, and suspects, often women and children, and many torturers are military or paramilitary personnel or police. Torture occurs across the continents, not only in conflict zones or under clearly oppressive regimes. For instance, several first world democracies, including the United States, show an increase in the use of electrical devices, including so-called "sublethal" weapons, to control prisoners (Wright 2001).

RECOGNITION AND PREVALENCE

Few medical or psychological studies have examined the health consequences of torture and other forms of organized violence. Both physical and psychological methods can leave physical and psychological effects. What is written about the long-lasting physical and psychological after-effects of torture is often descriptive, based on a selected population, and closely connected to the particular context and setting of that population. Clinical studies are limited by a lack of descriptive or diagnostic criteria applicable across populations and settings, and the choice of comparison populations and assessment instruments is complex.

Under-reporting and underdetection of the effects of torture make it hard to estimate prevalence. Many torture survivors go unrecognized in health systems in their country of residence. Prevalence estimates among refugees run from 5% to 35%; one estimate for the United States suggests 400,000 torture survivors living there (Piwowarczyk et al. 2000). A study in an urban U.S. internal medicine outpatient clinic (Eisenman et al. 2000) of patients born elsewhere found 6.6% who reported torture, none of whom had previously disclosed this to medical staff. A Danish study of refugees from the Middle East found that 55% of male and 12% of female refugees had been tortured (Thomsen et al. 2000). In the United Kingdom in 1999, 8.4% of asylum seekers reported torture, certainly an underestimate (Burnett and Peel 2001). A large-scale study of Bhutanese refugees in camps in Nepal (Van Ommeren et al. 2001) found that those who had been tortured (compared with nontortured refugees) were more likely to meet ICD-10 criteria (World Health Organization 1992) for persistent somatoform pain disorder (51% versus 28%).

SIGNS AND SYMPTOMS

The most important point to make is that very few methods of torture leave long-term signs that could not have arisen from injury without torture. All that the clinician can do is comment on the likelihood that any observable signs and symptoms are consistent with the effects of torture. However, this course is complicated by a number of factors. In many countries, torturers aim to leave as little evidence as possible on the body of the victim to confound attempts to document torture. Further, we know very little about what some of these abuses, particularly when prolonged, do to the human body, as their effects cannot be deduced from any research methods, even with cadavers. In some cases the victim cannot recall or be clear on what was done to him or her, particularly when he or she was unconscious at the time or sustained head injury. Most often, years have elapsed since the torture was inflicted, and the survivor may have undergone other privations and health insults in the interim. The most common complaints in long-term survivors of torture are headache, musculoskeletal pain, and abdominal pain (Eisenmann et al. 2000; Burnett and Peel 2001).

There are two major reasons for medical and psychological examination of the torture survivor: to document the torture and its effects, and to deliver health care. It is therefore helpful for clinicians to be cognizant of torture methods, as listed in Table I and illustrated in Figs. 1 to 4.

In a small but detailed study of 18 male torture survivors with pain (Thomsen et al. 2000), neuropathic pain was associated with hanging from retroflexed arms (which can cause partial or full brachial plexus injury), beating of the soles of the feet (falanga/falaka), beating and kicking of the head, and positional torture generating back pain and injury including disk herniation. Amris and Prip (2000b) emphasized the likelihood of multiple pain mechanisms, including fibromyalgic diffuse chronic pain, and noted (as do Burnett and Peel 2001) that poor conditions in prison complicate health problems and healing. Rape and sexual assault, which are often particularly difficult for the male or female victim to disclose, leave few signs (Lawson 1999; Peel et al. 2000; Burnett and Peel 2001). Lawson (1999, p. 267) concluded that "[o]ften physical stigmata of mistreatment understated the full extent of the pain and suffering inflicted upon the victims."

Studies to detect skeletal lesions (such as from beating) include bone scintigraphy (Mirzaei et al. 1998; Tunca and Lök 1998); plain X-rays to assess changes in periosteal appearance from falanga and palmatoria (beating on the shins) (Vogel, cited in Bonner 2001); and magnetic resonance imaging (MRI) to show thickened plantar aponeurosis from falanga (Savnik et al. 2000) and axonal-myelin degeneration in the brachial plexus from hanging by the arms (Öge et al. 1997). There is some debate about the utility of such special tests. They are of obvious benefit in documenting torture and supporting claims of survivors in whom they are found, but their absence does not necessarily disprove the claim, although such suggestions have been made (Forrest 1999). Research in this area enables us to gain knowledge about the etiology of torture-induced lesions, which is necessary for appropriate diagnosis and treatment. For instance, it is common for hanging by the arms (Fig. 1) to cause pain in the shoulder region and shoulder dysfunction, but pain might originate from any or all of partial lesions of the

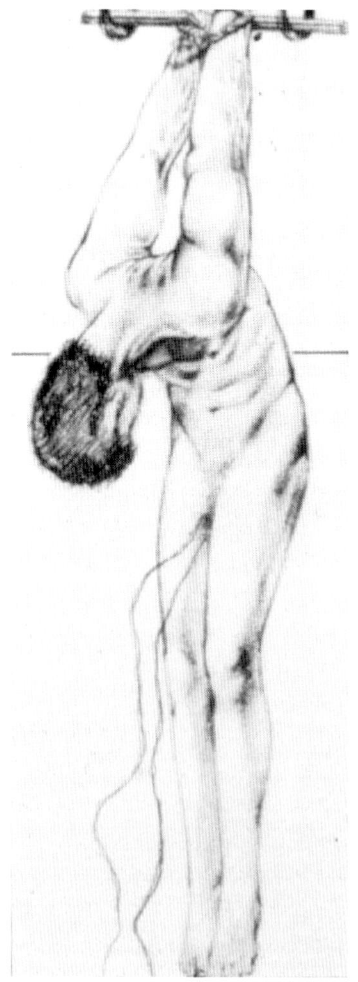

Fig. 1. Hanging with retroflexed arms with electrical torture. Printed with the permission of IRCT.

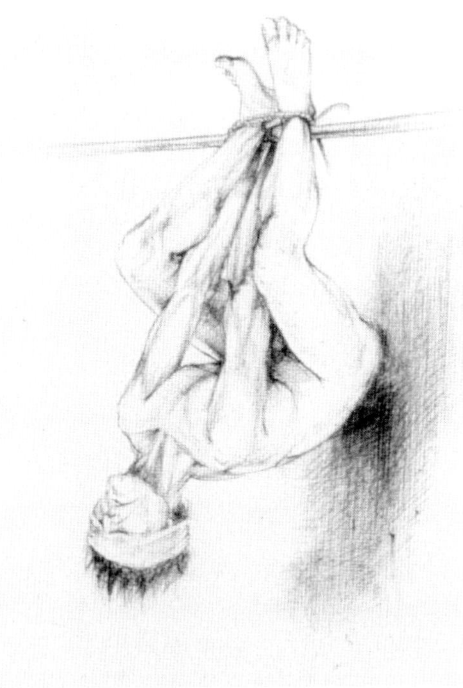

Fig. 2. Suspension by arms and legs. Printed with the permission of IRCT.

brachial plexus, damage to cartilaginous joint structures, or overload injuries to soft tissue structures secondary to joint distortion or dislocation.

Full discussion of psychological symptoms associated with torture is beyond the remit of this chapter, but it is necessary to raise several important issues. It is very common for torture survivors to present with predominantly physical or somatic symptoms: pain, fatigue, weakness, and sleep problems. There is no consensus on the extent to which these symptoms are best addressed as medical/physical problems and extensively investigated, or assumed to be the presentation of psychological disturbance such as depression, chronic anxiety, and post-traumatic stress disorder (PTSD) or other trauma-related problems. Both chronic pain and PTSD need to be seen as the result of a complex interrelationship among psychological, biological, and social processes. The meaning of the trauma, physiological response and physical sequelae, pre-existing personality and experience, and the extent of social support are all critical factors in a person's eventual presentation. In addition, PTSD may be associated with increased pain (Geisser et al. 1996), and pain can trigger flashbacks (Asmundson et al. 1998). Further,

Table I
Ten most common physical methods of torture reported by survivors in Denmark, 1996–1997

Physical Torture Methods	Frequency (%)
Widespread beating	100
Suspension by arms or legs, including hanging by retroflexed arms (see Figs. 1 and 2)	80
Falanga/falaka: beating soles of feet (see Fig. 4)	80
Electric torture: electrodes applied to vulnerable areas (see Fig. 1)	44
Tying arms, legs, and/or neck	39
Sexual torture, including rape, of males or females	37
Burning or mutilation	29
Telephono: direct blow to both ears	27
Restraint or forced positions for long periods (see Fig. 3)	24
Submersion: immersion of airways, drowning	24

these terms may not be applicable to people whose cultures do not divide the physical and psychological domains, for whom psychological disorder is seriously stigmatized, and/or for whom there is no "folk psychology" of normal disturbance after abnormal events (see Holtz 1998; Van Ommeren et al. 2001). The application of translated forms of Western-developed diagnostic questionnaires falls far short of proper description of torture survivors' experience and problems. There is a considerable risk of chronic pain being assigned the status of a symptom of PTSD but not addressed in its own right. On the other hand, chronic pain may complicate the recognition of PTSD (Kulich et al. 2000).

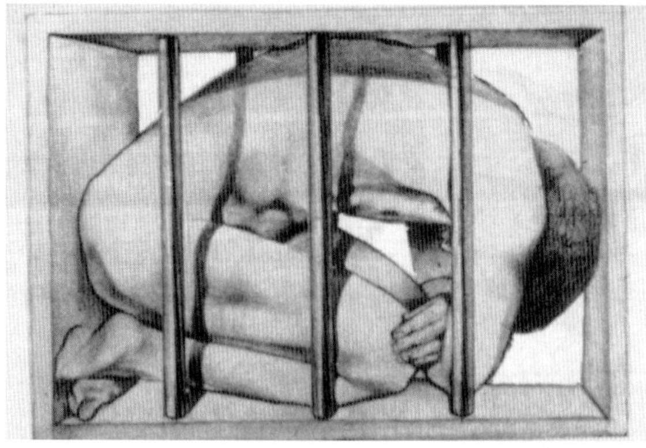

Fig. 3. Forced position. Printed with the permission of IRCT.

Table II
Services offered to torture survivors by responding projects in different regions

Region	*N*	Medical Services	Pain Service	Physical Therapy	Psychol. Services	Compl. Therapy
India and Southeast Asia	5	5	0	1	5	1
Australia and New Zealand	4	2	2	2	3	2
Middle East	2	2	0	2	1	1
Europe	20	12	3	7	13	4
North America	7	5	1	2	7	2
Africa	3	2	0	1	2	1
Worldwide	41	28	6	15	31	11

There is controversy over the utility of the diagnosis of PTSD and about the inevitability and specificity of longstanding psychological trauma from torture, for which evidence is lacking, although the assumption is widespread (Turner and Gorst-Unsworth 1990; Mollica and Caspi-Yavin 1991; Basoglu et al. 1994a,b; de Vries 1998; Summerfield 1998a,b). Studies across diverse populations have identified some protective factors for long-term mental health, such as commitment to the cause that occasioned the torture, good social support, and preparedness (lacking in those who are victimized randomly or for involuntary membership in a racial or religious group). Factors that appear to prolong depression and trauma-related symptoms in exiles after torture include poor emotional support, separation from family, isolation from ethnic or religious community, racial attacks in exile, poverty, and poor general health (Basoglu et al. 1994a,b; Hauff and Vaglum 1995; Gorst-Unsworth and Goldenberg 1998; Holtz 1998; Mollica et al. 1999).

TREATMENT OF PHYSICAL AND PSYCHOLOGICAL PROBLEMS

There are no prospective studies of treatment, although there are some very useful accounts (Amris and Prip 2000a,b). That is not to say that we have no idea what treatment is effective, but a more rigorous approach would be to diagnose or formulate problems and then to apply evidence-based treatments. We do know that it can be therapeutic for a torture survivor to provide an account to a sympathetic health professional, who documents the testimony and normalizes symptoms as a reaction to an extreme abnormal experience (Pope and Garcia-Peltoniemi 1991). Access to good treatment facilities and social support, even in refugee settlements, is associated with less psychological disturbance (Holtz 1998; Van Ommeren et al 2001).

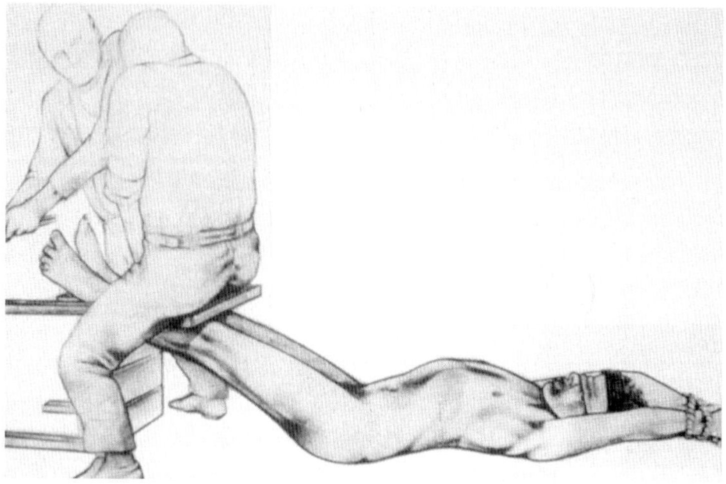

Fig. 4. Beating of the soles of the feet (falanga). Printed with the permission of IRCT.

But it is not necessarily straightforward to direct torture survivors with pain into mainstream services, for several reasons. Because of their experiences of torture and imprisonment, many are uncomfortable, for instance, with figures of authority or with being physically handled by strangers. Some survivors do not speak the language of the host country sufficiently to communicate their needs, and health care systems may be poorly provided with trained interpreters. Many clinicians feel daunted by treating torture survivors and prefer to refer them to specialist projects, most of which are outside mainstream health care systems and have limited resources and treatment options. In addition, many patients who are refugees present other significant welfare problems such as lack of housing, and need for financial or social support. Symptom relief may not be the highest priority among victims themselves.

Thus, while there are risks of overemphasizing pain problems and treatment, pain treatment is arguably more often neglected through being interpreted in purely psychological terms by health workers unfamiliar with pain diagnosis and treatment.

SURVEY OF PAIN PROBLEMS AND THEIR TREATMENT BY TORTURE SURVIVOR ORGANIZATIONS WORLDWIDE

In order to determine the extent to which pain was identified and treated in torture survivors, the following questions were e-mailed or mailed to all relevant projects listed in the IRCT directory: (1) In the survivors of torture whom you see, how common is pain as a problem? (2) What help can you offer for pain?, and (3) If you would like to offer more help for pain than you do at present, what resources would you need?

In all, 154 projects were contacted, of which 41 (27%) replied, with the highest response rate from projects in India and Southeast Asia (5/11, 45%), and the lowest in Africa (3/16, 19%), excluding Central and South American projects, which require recontacting when the materials have been translated. Although the response rate is somewhat disappointing, some projects work under extremely difficult conditions and many are under-resourced. All projects in North America, India and Southeast Asia, Africa, and Australia and New Zealand, one in the Middle East, and several (11/20) in Europe described pain as common, very common, universal, or present in ≥80% of survivors seen; one in the Middle East and two in Europe described it as uncommon, or present in ≤20% of survivors. Although not requested to do so, the majority of projects in Europe, the Middle East, and Africa distinguished in their replies between "physical" and "psychological" pain; few did so in North America. Some centers, particularly in Europe, had an entirely psychogenic model of pain.

Few responding projects (two in Australia and New Zealand, three in Europe, and one in North America) offered access to a pain service, although 60–100% of projects in all continents had some access to general medical services (which often prescribed widely used analgesics such as nonsteroidal anti-inflammatory drugs and antidepressants); see Table II. Physical therapy was the most common physical treatment mentioned. Most projects also had psychological, psychiatric, or counseling provision; fewer had complementary therapies, and a very few provided only complementary therapy. The wish list for extra resources ranged from peace in order to be able to work, to social welfare resources, translated materials, and money for uninsured patients to fill analgesic prescriptions. Eleven projects specifically identified the need for further pain education and six for contact with other torture survivor treatment projects.

WHAT CAN PAIN CLINICIANS DO?

It is easy for those who work with pain to feel bewildered by the complex problems, in health and welfare generally, that are presented by torture survivors, often without a common language. In addition, it is easy to slip into feeling that torture survivors "must have done something to deserve it" by political activity, or that they are making false claims in order to gain resident status in a first world country (Basoglu 1993; Nathanson 2001). Blaming the victim in this fashion risks doing a grave injustice to those who have suffered dreadfully in the cause of freedoms and rights that most of us are fortunate enough to take for granted. A paper by Pope and Garcia-Peltoniemi (1991) describes the difficulties that face health professionals working with torture survivors, and notes the virtual silence on torture in mainstream medical, psychiatric, and psychological journals and publications, which has started to change in the intervening years.

Pain clinicians can usefully consider the following actions: (1) Recognize signs of torture in patients in their practice; be aware of prevalence, likely signs, and conditions that enable torture survivors to disclose their experiences. (2) Assess and document torture injuries and lasting effects, such as pain. There are some internationally agreed guidelines for assessment: the Istanbul Protocol (Iacopino et al. 1999; United Nations Convention on Human Rights), to which health professionals made the major contribution, concerns effective investigation and documentation for torture and alleged torture and how to report it. Some projects have also produced useful guidelines. Assessment for clinical practice is rather different from assessment for documentation. (3) Attempt to provide the best possible evidence-based treatment for torture survivors, with attention to conditions under which treatment is carried out, which may require adaptation in order to prevent further distress. IRCT is currently attempting to implement minimum standards in multidisciplinary rehabilitation of torture survivors provided at affiliated centers worldwide; input from pain specialists would be very welcome. (4) Offer clinical services, consultancy, and training, paid or unpaid, to torture survivor organizations. (5) Be aware of the social and political context of torture in survivors' home countries, and of the social and political system of the host country from the point of view of the refugee. (6) Raise awareness about the health effects of torture in professional bodies and promote lobbying of governments for humane treatment, particularly in those countries that are signatories to the U.N. Convention against Torture. There is an increasing tendency toward detention of refugees and asylum seekers in some countries while their status is resolved. Detention in implicitly punitive centers, which often lack adequate health care resources, can retraumatize refugees (see Nathanson 2001). Even in countries where torture is a routine act of an oppressive regime, international public awareness can have a surprisingly powerful influence (Basoglu 1993). (7) Be aware of the potential for the use of methods to control persons in state custody, including the use of "nonlethal weapons," to meet the definition of torture (as did certain methods used on republican Irish prisoners by the British government in the 1980s). (8) Be alert to the involvement of doctors and other health professionals, wittingly or unwittingly, voluntarily or coerced, in torture procedures, as detailed in the Declaration of Tokyo adopted by the World Medical Association in 1975, and by Physicians for Human Rights (Salinsky 1998; Bateman 2001; see also Maio 2001). (9) Conduct and support local and international research and clinical case studies of the assessment and treatment of torture survivors, at the same time remaining aware that there is a small risk that some research findings can be used to refine torture.

ACKNOWLEDGMENTS

We are grateful to Drs. Philippe Lacoux and Patricia Roche, who along with the authors were panel members in the workshop on this topic at the 10th World Congress on Pain; to Kate McGuire of Medicins sans Frontières for discussion of many ideas addressed here; and to all those who responded to the survey of torture survivor treatment projects.

REFERENCES

Amris K, Prip K. Physiotherapy for torture victims (I). *Torture* 2000a; 10:73–76.

Amris K, Prip K. Physiotherapy for torture victims (II). *Torture* 2000b; 10:112–116.

Asmundson GJG, Norton GR, Allerdings BA, Larsen DK. Posttraumatic stress disorder and work-related injury. *J Anxiety Disord* 1998; 12:57–69.

Basoglu M. Prevention of torture and care of survivors. *JAMA* 1993; 151:76–81.

Basoglu M, Paker M, Paker O, et al. Psychological effects of torture: a comparison of tortured with nontortured political activists in Turkey. *Am J Psychiatry* 1994a; 270:606–611.

Basoglu M, Paker M, Paker O, et al. Factors related to long-term traumatic stress responses in survivors of torture in Turkey. *Am J Psychiatry* 1994b; 272:357–363.

Bateman C. Ongoing human rights abuses. *S Afr Med J* 2001; 91:624–625.

Bonner J. On the trail of the torturers. *New Scientist* 2001; May:46–49.

Burnett A, Peel M. The health of survivors of torture and organised violence. *BMJ* 2001; 322:606–609.

Eisenman DP, Keller AS, Kim G. Survivors of torture in a general medical setting: how often have patients been tortured, and how often is it missed? *West J Med* 2000; 172:301–304.

Forrest DM. Examination for the late physical after effects of torture. *J Clin Forensic Med* 1999; 6:4–13.

Geisser ME, Roth RS, Bachman JE, Eckert TA. The relationship between symptoms of post-traumatic stress disorder and pain, affective disturbance and disability among patients with accident and non-accident related pain. *Pain* 1996; 66:207–214.

Gorst-Unsworth C, Goldenberg E. Psychological sequela of torture and organised violence suffered by refugees from Iraq. *Br J Psychiatry* 1998; 172:90–94.

Hauff E, Vaglum P. Organised violence and the stress of exile. *Br J Psychiatry* 1995; 166:360–367.

Holtz TH. Refugee trauma versus torture trauma: a retrospective controlled cohort study of Tibetan refugees. *J Nerv Ment Dis* 1998; 186:24–34.

Iacopino V, Özkalipçi Ö, Schlar C. The Istanbul Protocol: international standards for the effective investigation and documentation of torture and ill treatment. *Lancet* 1999; 354:1117.

Kulich RJ, Mencher P, Bertrand MA, Maciewicz MD. Comorbidity of post-traumatic stress disorder and chronic pain: implications for clinical and forensic assessment. *Curr Rev Pain* 2000; 4:36–48.

Lawson M. Recent medical evidence for torture and human rights abuse in Sierra Leone: a report for the Medical Foundation for the Victims of Torture. *Med Confl Surviv* 1999; 15:255–270.

Maio G. History of medical involvement in torture—then and now. *Lancet* 2001; 357:1609–1611.

Mirzaei S, Knoll P, Lipp RW, et al. Bone scintigraphy in screening of torture survivors. *Lancet* 1998; 352:949–951.

Mollica RF, Caspi-Yavin Y. Measuring torture and torture-related symptoms. *J Cons Clin Psychol* 1991; 3:581–587.

Mollica RF, McInnes K, Sarajlic N, et al. Disability associated with psychiatric comorbidity and health status in Bosnian refugees living in Croatia. *JAMA* 1999; 282:433–439.

Nathanson V. Editorial: Doctors and torture. *Brit Med J* 2001; 319:397–398.

Öge AE, Boyaciyan A, Gürvitt H. Magnetic nerve root stimulation in two types of brachial plexus injury: segmental demyelination and axonal degeneration. *Muscle Nerve* 1997; 20:823–832.

Peel M, Mahtani A, Hinshelwood G, Forrest D. The sexual abuse of men in detention in Sri Lanka. *Lancet* 2000; 355:2069–2070.

Piwowarczyk L, Moreno A, Grodin M. Health care of torture survivors. *JAMA* 2000; 284:539–541.

Pope KS, Garcia-Peltoniemi RE. Responding to victims of torture: clinical issues, professional responsibilities, and useful resources. *Prof Psychol Res Pract* 1991; 22:269–276

Salinsky M. Torture continues in Turkey: findings of a new report. *Lancet* 1998; 352:1854.

Savnik A, Amris K, Røgind H, et al. MRI of the plantar structures of the foot after falanga torture. *Eur Radiol* 2000; 10:1655–1659.

Summerfield DA. "Trauma" and the experience of war: a reply. *Lancet* 1998a; 351:1580–1581.

Summerfield DA. Letter: trauma, post-traumatic stress disorder, and war. *Lancet* 1998b; 352:911.

Thomsen AB, Eriksen J, Smidt-Nielsen K. Chronic pain in torture survivors. *Forensic Science Int* 2000; 108:155–163.

Tunca M, Lök V. Bone scintigraphy in screening of torture survivors. *Lancet* 1998; 352:1859.

Turner S, Gorst-Unsworth C. Psychological sequelae of torture: a descriptive model. *Br J Psychiatry* 1990; 157:475–480.

United Nations Convention on Human Rights. Available via the Internet at: www.unchr.ch.

Van Ommeren M, de Jong JTVM, Sharma B, et al. Psychiatric disorders among tortured Bhutanese refugees in Nepal. *Arch Gen Psychiat* 2001; 58:475–482.

de Vries F. To make a drama out of a trauma is fully justified. *Lancet* 1998; 351:1579–1580.

World Health Organization. *International Statistical Classification of Disease and Related Health Problems,* 10th rev. Geneva: World Health Organization, 1992.

Wright S. The role of sub-lethal weapons in human rights abuse. *Med Conflict Survival* 2001; 17:221–233.

Correspondence to: Amanda C. de C. Williams, PhD, INPUT Pain Management Unit, St. Thomas Hospital, Lambeth Palace Road, London SE1 7EH, United Kingdom. Email: amanda.williams@kcl.ac.uk.

Proceedings of the 10th World Congress on Pain,
Progress in Pain Research and Management, Vol. 24,
edited by Jonathan O. Dostrovsky, Daniel B. Carr, and
Martin Koltzenburg, IASP Press, Seattle, © 2003.

63

Legal Aspects of End of Life Treatment in Australia, Canada, the United States, the United Kingdom, Poland, France, Germany, Japan, and The Netherlands[1]

Danuta Mendelson,[a] Timothy Stoltzfus Jost,[b]
and Michael Ashby[c]

[a]School of Law, Deakin University, Burwood, Victoria, Australia; [b]School of Law, Washington and Lee University, Lexington, Virginia, United States; [c]Monash Medical Centre, Clayton, Victoria, Australia

Analysis of the legal and ethical issues pertaining to end of life care involves interdisciplinary approaches encompassing medicine, law, and ethics. From a legal point of view matters are complicated by the fact that criminal law, the law of battery and negligence, as well as constitutional and international law are implicated. Moreover, the response to these problems in each country is shaped by its juridical system, social structure, history, religion, culture, and international conventions that have been incorporated into the law of the respective countries.

Poland, the United Kingdom, The Netherlands, Japan, and France are unitary systems, whereas Canada, Germany, the United States, and Australia are federations in which the legislatures of constituent provinces or states have the power to regulate locally the practice of medicine and the conduct of medical practitioners. The United Kingdom, Canada, the United States, and Australia have common law systems in which the law is based on judge-ordered precedents as well as legislation. The legal systems of Poland, France, Germany, Japan, and The Netherlands are based primarily on national civil and criminal codes, although their appellate courts do make authoritative rulings on the law. This chapter will examine the common law countries together, as

[1] Based on a Congress workshop.

they share a common legal tradition and common precedents, while the civil law systems, which are more diverse, will be discussed separately.

To add to the complexity, national laws of members of the European Union, including the United Kingdom, Germany, The Netherlands, and France, are subject to the *European Convention on Human Rights and Fundamental Freedoms* (entered into in Rome on 4 November 1950), as interpreted by the European Court of Human Rights in Strasbourg. Poland, as an aspiring member of the European Union, is adapting its laws to fit in with the European Union's jurisprudence. We will highlight a selection of the major similarities, differences, and problems raised by these issues.

Anxieties about responsibility for causing death permeate practice and debate related to death and dying. Analysis of causation is central to any determination of the moral character and legality of medical decisions or palliative interventions at the end of life. However, difficulties with semantics, evidence, and legal arguments require elucidation for an analysis of causation to be accomplished (Ashby 1997a, 1998). The term *causation* is usually employed in medicine and science in a narrow empirical sense to mean the facts or data pertaining to a given situation, and their relationship to one another (Ashby 1997b). In a legal sense, causation encompasses the facts and is a factor in determining legal liability (Freckelton and Mendelson 2002). It can be argued that narrow empirical causality applied in the setting of terminal care cannot alone account for the distinction between accepted palliative care practice and euthanasia.

In the experience of caring and being cared for, intention, honesty, and respect for the patient and the life that is ending are decisive. Palliative care must be clear about its intentions, and accept that there are some occasions when the process of death is hastened, either unknowingly or knowingly. It may be that the concept of "natural death," generally understood in terms of human agency in death causation, should also embrace non-obstruction of the dying process (Ashby and Mendelson 2003).

CONSENT AND REFUSAL OF TREATMENT

As a general rule, all common law and most civil law jurisdictions presume every adult to have the mental capacity to consent to or to refuse any medical intervention, including life-saving or life-sustaining treatment, unless and until that presumption is rebutted. It is irrelevant that the refusal may not be in the best interests of the patient, or may even entail the risk of death. The refusal must, however, be unequivocal, and often must be recorded in writing. The right to refuse medical treatment is based on the principle of personal autonomy and was upheld in *Pretty v the United Kingdom* (European Court of Human Rights [Fourth Section], Strasbourg, 29 April 2002), which noted that the right to refuse treatment conforms with the privacy guarantees contained in Article 8 of the *European Convention on Human Rights.* This article states that "Everyone has the right to respect for his private and family life" and that "There shall be no interference by a public authority with the exercise of this right except such as is in accordance with the law and is necessary in a democratic society."

COMMON LAW COUNTRIES

In general, the common law countries have adopted similar philosophical and juridical approaches toward end of life treatment. This is true with respect to palliative care, withholding and termination of life-sustaining treatment, assisted suicide, and euthanasia.

ADVANCE DIRECTIVES

All common law countries have either statutory or common law provisions enabling adults of sound mind to execute advance directives such as "living wills," "right to die" statements (called an "individual instruction" under the *Uniform Health Care Decisions Act* in the United States), and refusal of treatment certificates. Adults may appoint an agent or guardian with the power to refuse medical treatment, including life-saving treatment and continuing administration of life support systems, once they become incompetent. Except in the United States, guardianship (conservator) boards and courts have the power to review advance directives and decisions by agents with medical powers of attorney. Given the grave consequences that follow refusal of life-saving treatment, courts and tribunals tend to demand strict compliance with the statutory requirements for valid execution of refusal documents. Some jurisdictions exclude palliative care from the statutory right to refuse medical treatment.

PALLIATIVE CARE

The law sees a sharp distinction between appropriate palliative care, offered with an intention to ease a patient's pain and suffering, and actions specifically aimed at ending the patient's life. In Canada, the Ontario Coroner has laid down four conditions which must generally be satisfied for palliative care interventions to be legal in his jurisdiction, and would find widespread support amongst palliative care practitioners everywhere. They are (1) the care must be intended solely to relieve suffering; (2) it must be administered in response to suffering or signs of suffering; (3) it must be commensurate with that suffering; and (4) it cannot be a deliberate infliction of death. Documentation is required, and the doses of opioids must be increased progressively (Parliament of Canada 1995; Lavery and Singer 1997).

The most controversial legal issue with respect to palliative care in the countries under consideration has been the use of opioids to alleviate suffering of patients in their final stages of life, particularly when the drugs prescribed for this purpose are suspected of causing death. The United States Federation of State Medical Boards adopted in 1998 the "Model Guidelines for the Use of Controlled Substances for the Treatment of Pain." The common law courts have stated that a physician: "is entitled to do all that is proper and necessary to relieve pain and suffering, even if the measures he takes may incidentally shorten life" (*R v Adams* [1957]; Devlin 1986, p. 71). Under this doctrine, sometimes called the doctrine of double effect, the cause of death of patients who die while receiving appropriate pain treatment will be attributed to the underlying disease in situations where the patient's pain and other discomforts were controlled through properly calibrated titration of dosages, even if the dosages were high (Wilson 1992). Though the legal principle is sound, it is based on expert medical evidence of 40 years ago. In fact, there is no clinical evidence that morphine causes death, if used with appropriate skill to palliate symptoms. In particular, the respiratory depressant effects have been shown to be minimal in opioid-tolerant patients; furthermore, pain acts as antagonist to respiratory depression and to the sedative effects of opioids (DuBose and Berde 1997). However, as is true for any class of drugs, opioids are dangerous if used inappropriately.

There is now a substantial body of clinical experience in palliative care about safe standards of practice, with particular regard to initial doses for opioid-naive patients and subsequent dose titration according to the person's pain or symptom reporting. It is widely assumed that the morphine (or other opioid) dosage per se is the main determinant of whether the drug causes or hastens death, but in reality there is no such determinative or threshold dose. It is the size of the initial dose and the rate of subsequent incremental dose increases that are important. Gradual dose escalation is usual practice, and rapid dose escalation in response to inadequate pain control is typically well tolerated by patients who have already been treated with opioids for some time, that is, who are no longer "opioid-naive." The issue of terminal sedation is controversial because although sedation does not kill, death is clearly expected. Sedative drugs are commonly used in terminal care (when death is believed to be imminent), in order to maintain comfort and dignity by alleviation of agitation, anxiety, and so-called "terminal restlessness." They are used proportionately to the patient's distress, and not to bring about death (Ashby 1997b; Mendelson 1997).

Palliative care practitioners rarely use morphine for its sedative properties at any stage of an illness, especially when patients are trying to function as normally as possible, and sedation is usually unwelcome. In terminal care, sedative drugs (usually benzodiazepines) are titrated against agitation and distress, but occasionally also against another symptom (e.g., pain or shortness of breath) where other measures have failed and the patient may wish to be less aware of what he or she is experiencing. If patients are conscious and competent they are asked if they wish to be more sedated, but they are often unable to give this consent due to incompetence. Patients are frequently unconscious and/or cognitively impaired, and therefore incompetent, in the terminal stages of their illness, that is, the last few hours or days of life. It is clearly not possible to state categorically that sedation in this context has no effect on time of survival.

The precise timing of death is unpredictable, and determination of the relative causal contributions of disease-related, physiological, and pharmacological factors is not usually measurable. Nevertheless, in common law countries, terminal sedation is recognized as an aspect of palliative treatment. Outside the setting of terminal care, so-called "pharmacological oblivion" is not part of accepted palliative care practice.

WITHDRAWAL AND WITHHOLDING OF MEDICAL TREATMENT FROM INCOMPETENT OR UNCONSCIOUS PATIENTS FOR WHOM THERE IS NO ADVANCE DIRECTIVE

Nonconsensual medical treatment violates the principle of personal autonomy. Incompetent patients, whose wishes cannot be ascertained, may be treated nonvoluntarily under the doctrine of necessity, where their best interests require that necessary treatment be administered for the protection of their health and, possibly, (sapient) life. However, the duty to medically intervene ceases once it becomes clear that "all hope of a return to an even partial exercise of human life is irreparably lost" (*In re Quinlan* [1976]).

In the United States, when determining how to evaluate requests to terminate life-sustaining treatment for incompetent patients, courts have often articulated the principle that "it is best to err, if at all, in favor of preserving life" (*In re Conroy* [1985]). The U.S. Supreme Court has noted the constitutionality of incorporating such a principle in state law (*Cruzan v Director, Missouri Dept. of Health* [1990]). Effectively, many courts have set the continuation of life (and thus the continuation of treatment) as the default position; unless substantial evidence supports the position that the patient had elected the termination of treatment, it is presumed that the patient would elect to have treatment continued.

In England, Wales, and Northern Ireland, but not in Scotland (*Law Hospital NHS Trust v Lord Advocate* [1996]), the discontinuance of artificial nutrition and hydration for an incompetent patient in a vegetative state who has not executed a valid direction requires a prior sanction of the High Court of England by way of a declaration based on the best interests test (*Airedale NHS Trust v Bland* [1993]). Following the enactment of the *Human Rights Act* (1998) by the United Kingdom Parliament, previous English decisions, such as that in the *Bland* case, became subject to the *European Convention on Human Rights and Fundamental Freedoms*. Under the *Human Rights Act*, public authorities can be liable for their omissions as well as their actions. Consequently, in *NHS Trust A v M; NHS Trust B v H* [2001] the reasoning in *Bland* was re-examined. The High Court of England determined that withdrawal of artificial nutrition and hydration from patients in a permanent vegetative state did not constitute an intentional deprivation of life within the meaning of Article 2 of the *European Convention on Human Rights and Fundamental Freedoms*, which provides that: "everyone's right to life shall be protected by law. No one shall be deprived of his life intentionally." The Court interpreted this clause as a prohibition of deliberate acts resulting in deprivation of life by someone acting on behalf of the state (most hospitals in England are run by the National Health Service Trust).

Under the best interests doctrine, treatment necessary for protection of health and (sapient) life can be administered to patients who are incompetent and thus incapable of expressing consent. However, once it becomes clear that the patient is permanently comatose or in a permanent vegetative state, then although, on the one hand, termination of life supports does not further the incompetent person's best interests, on the other hand, his or her interests in being kept alive also cease, taking with them the justification for the nonconsensual medical treatment. In such circumstances, there is no longer a duty to provide life-sustaining treatment, and therefore a responsible decision by doctors not to provide it is an omission. In such cases, the death of the patient is the result of the illness or injury from which he or she suffered, and that cannot be described as a deprivation. The court also found that Article 2 did not impose a positive obligation to provide life-sustaining treatment in cases where such treatment is not in the best interest of the patient.

In Australia, the legal situation regarding withdrawal and withholding of life-saving or life-sustaining treatment is unclear. In 1992, the High Court of Australia determined that where persons are disabled by age or mental incapacity from giving valid consent, an order or directive must be sought from the Family Court or Guardianship Board for authorization of nontherapeutic procedures (*Secretary, Department of Health and Community Services (NT) v JWB and SMB* [1992]). Because discontinuance of life-sustaining treatment is nontherapeutic, it might be prudent for doctors to seek similar directives. The South Australian *Consent to Medical Treatment and Palliative Care Act* (1995, section 17) may serve as a model for the common law rule. This act provides that in cases where there is no valid prior direction to the contrary, a medical practitioner responsible for the treatment or care of a patient in the terminal phase of a terminal illness is "under no duty to use, or to continue to use, life sustaining measures in treating the patient if the effect of doing so would be merely to prolong life in a moribund state without any real prospect of recovery or in a persistent vegetative state." In such cases, "the non-application or discontinuance of life sustaining measures … does not constitute an intervening cause of death." In Canada the law is not dissimilar to Australia.

ASSISTED SUICIDE AND EUTHANASIA

In no common law jurisdiction is suicide now considered a crime. However, with the exception of the state of Oregon in the United States, all common law countries prohibit aiding or assisting the suicide of another. The law distinguishes between a physician's conduct in letting a patient die from an underlying disease and conduct that makes the patient die. It is the intention to bring about the death of another that forms the basis of the commission of the crime of assisted suicide and that of murder. The majority of the Supreme Court of Canada, in *Rodriguez v British Columbia* (1993), determined that the long-standing blanket statutory prohibition against assisted suicide fulfills the government's objective of safeguarding the vulnerable, is grounded in the state interest in protecting life, and reflects the policy of the state that human life should not be depreciated by allowing life to be taken. In 1995, in its *Of Life and Death: Report,* the Canadian Senate Special Committee on Euthanasia and Assisted Suicide recommended that the prohibition of assisted suicide remain intact.

Likewise in the United Kingdom, the House of Lords in *R (Pretty) v the DPP* (2001), determined, and the European Court of Human Rights affirmed (unanimously dismissing Mrs. Pretty's appeal in *Pretty v the United Kingdom*, the European Court of Human Rights [Fourth Section], Strasbourg, 29 April 2002), that there is no right to assisted suicide under common law or statute, and that no such right is guaranteed by the *European Convention on Human Rights.* The European Court of Human Rights declared that Article

2, which safeguards the right to life, cannot be interpreted as "conferring the diametrically opposite right, namely a right to die; nor can it create a right to self-determination in the sense of conferring on an individual the entitlement to choose death rather than life."

Both the House of Lords and the European Court of Justice, in the case of *Pretty,* adopted the reasoning of the majority in *Rodriguez v British Columbia* that the long-standing blanket statutory prohibition against assisted suicide fulfills the government's objective of protecting the vulnerable, is grounded in the state interest in protecting life, and reflects the policy of the state that human life should not be depreciated by allowing life to be taken. It is the vulnerability of the class of those who might seek assisted suicide that provides the rationale for the law against it.

There have been no appellate decisions regarding assisted suicide in Australia. In 1995, the Northern Territory's unicameral parliament enacted the *Rights of the Terminally Ill Act* (RTIA), which decriminalized physician-assisted suicide and euthanasia by designating such conduct as legitimate "medical treatment." However in 1996, the Federal Parliament preempted RTIA by enacting *The Euthanasia Laws Act* (1997) under its plenary powers to make laws for territories.

The Supreme Court of the United States in the cases of *Vacco v Quill* (1997) and *Washington v Glucksberg* (1997) decided that statutes prohibiting physician-assisted suicide are constitutionally valid. In *Washington v Glucksberg*, Justice Rehnquist, writing for the court, announced that the Due Process Clause protects those rights and liberties that are "deeply rooted in this nation's history and tradition." The court then concluded that neither suicide nor assisted suicide has been well accepted in this society, and that it could not meet this "deeply rooted" test.

Only one state, Oregon, has legalized assisted suicide. The *Oregon Death with Dignity Act* (1995) allows a physician to prescribe a lethal dose of medication to a competent, adult patient, although the patient must then take the medication himself or herself. The act prohibits a physician from directly acting in a way that would end the patient's life, thus prohibiting active euthanasia. Two physicians are required to diagnose the patient as suffering with a terminal illness that will lead to death within 6 months. In November of 2001, U.S. Attorney General John Ashcroft ruled that the federal controlled substances laws prohibit Oregon physicians from prescribing controlled drugs for the purposes of assisting suicides. This ruling, if it stands, would expose Oregon doctors who comply with the statute to federal civil and criminal sanctions, and to losing their license to prescribe controlled substances. As of this writing, its implementation has been blocked by a temporary injunction.

Euthanasia or mercy killing is a crime in the United States, Australia, Canada, and the United Kingdom. In 2001, the Supreme Court of Canada in *R v Latimer* (2001) determined that mercy killing motivated by the "necessity" of eliminating pain amounts to murder, stating that: "Killing a person—in order to relieve the suffering produced by a medically manageable physical or mental condition—is not a proportionate response to the harm represented by the non-life-threatening suffering resulting from that condition."

CIVIL LAW COUNTRIES

POLAND

Medical practice in Poland is governed by several statutes and by the *Code of Medical Ethics* (*Kodeks Etyki Lekarskiej* [1993]) (CME), which is not a legal statute, and as such is not a source of law. The CME includes provisions relating specifically to treatment of patients at the end of life, and the Polish Constitutional Tribunal in its opinion of 7 October 1992 determined that although norms set out in the CME have the character of ethical obligations rather than legal rules, they can be used to define more precisely the content of legal principles. Medical practitioners, therefore, are under a legal obligation to adhere to the ethical norms of the CME (Zielonka 2001; Zelichowski 2002). This general rule, however, is subject to qualification in cases where there is conflict between the norms of the CME and substantive (statutory) law. According to the Polish Constitutional Tribunal's Opinion of 17 March 1993, a medical practitioner cannot be penalized for practicing medicine in accordance with the law, even if such conduct is contrary to a principle of professional ethics. Conversely, medical practitioners will be punished if they infringe the law, but not the CME, or if they act contrary to both the law and the CME.

The conflict between legal rules and ethical norms is particularly acute in the case of withdrawal and withholding of life-saving treatment from incompetent terminally ill patients. Polish law does not recognize instruments such as advance directives or refusal of treatment certificates (Zelichowski 1999). Article 38 of Chapter 5 headed "Principles of Medical Practice" in the *Medical Profession Act* (*Ustawa o zawodzie lekarza* [2002]) provides that: "a physician may decide to discontinue or not institute a treatment (unless prompt medical intervention is necessary), but is obliged to inform the patient before doing so and suggest other factual opportunities for obtaining medical treatment." The clause in parentheses refers to the duty to rescue provision contained in Article 30 of the *Medical Profession Act,* which imposes upon medical practitioners a duty to always save human life when a delay would result in death or serious physical or mental injury, or in other cases of emergency. In turn, the positive duty to act to save human life is in line with "the duty to rescue" expressed in Article 162.1 of the Polish *Penal Code* (*Kodeks karny* [1997]), whereby a failure to help a person who is in an immediate danger of death or serious injury, where rendering of such help is possible without the risk of death or serious injury to oneself is a punishable offense (*Penal Code* Article 162.2).

It is difficult to reconcile Article 162 of the *Penal Code* and Article 30 of the *Medical Profession Act* with Article 32(1) of the CME, which states that "In terminal states the physician does not have the duty to undertake and continue resuscitation or persistent treatment, nor to resort to extraordinary measures," and Article 32(2), which vests in the medical practitioner the right to discontinue resuscitation based on assessment of the likely therapeutic success. Yet, unless the conflict between the substantive civil and criminal law and the CME can be resolved, substantive law, that is the duty to rescue, will prevail over deontological and ethical principles (Zelichowski 1999).

Under Article 150 of the Polish *Penal Code*, mercy killing is prohibited by law, but may or may not incur a jail term. Article 31 of the CME prohibits the practice of euthanasia. According to the Constitutional Tribunal's Opinion of 17 March 1993, medical practitioners who practice euthanasia—conduct that is contrary to the substantive law (the *Constitution of the Polish Republic,* 1997, Article 38), and medical ethics—will be held legally responsible for the patient's death.

FRANCE

Following the draft recommendation by the Council of Europe of May 1999, encouraging member states to give incurable and dying patients the right to palliative care, the French Parliament enacted the law of 9 June, 1999, directed at guaranteeing access to palliative care for anyone "whose state of ill health requires it." Article L-711-4 of the *Code of Public Health* requires that "health care establishments give preventive, curative, or palliative care to patients as required by their state of health and ensure the continuity of such care once they are discharged." The law of 9 June 1999 reinforces Article 38 of the *Code of Medical Deontology* (*Code de Déontologie Médicale* [1995]), which, unlike the Polish *Code of Medical Ethics*, has statutory force, and is thus legally binding. The *Code of Medical Deontology* (CMD) mandates that: "a dying person must be attended until the last, and given appropriate care and suitable support to preserve the quality of the life which is ending. A patient's dignity should be protected, and his or her entourage comforted." The first clause of Article 37 of the CMD states: "In any circumstances, the physician should do his utmost to alleviate the sufferings of his patient, and give him moral solace."

Though the emphasis is on alleviation of "sufferings" (*les souffrances*), and on the preservation of the dying person's quality of life, the law provides statutory encouragement for doctors to treat their patients with adequate doses of analgesic medication. The care provided must be "conscientious and accord with the scientific data" (CMD, Article 32).

Article 37 of the CMD cautions medical practitioners to "avoid any unreasonable obstinacy in pursuing investigations and treatments." In the context of the provision, the reference is presumably to avoidance of "aggressive" or "futile" treatment (Duguet 2001, p. 114), that may or may not encompass withdrawal or withholding of life-sustaining treatment. The burden of proving consent to treatment is on the doctor (Cour de Cassation, 25 February 1997; Nys 1999, p. 221). It is unclear whether the right to refuse treatment extends to death choices. However, it is arguable that a number of earlier decisions denying the patient's right to refuse life-saving treatment and imposing sanctions on physicians who complied with such refusals may have to be reconsidered in the light of the law of 9 June 1999.

France has neither statutory rules nor medico-ethical guidelines (Ferrand 2001) governing the withholding and withdrawal of life-sustaining treatments from incompetent patients. French law grants relatives the right to be "notified and informed," but they cannot consent to care on behalf of an incompetent relative (CMD, Article 36). Indeed, the legal position relating to withholding and withdrawal of life-sustaining treatment is complex. Just as in Poland, the well-entrenched positive duty to rescue a person in danger embodied in Article 223-6(2) of the 1992 French *Criminal Code* (*Code Penal*) makes failure to rescue an offense: "Any person who willfully fails to render or to obtain assistance to an endangered person when such was possible without danger to himself or others, shall be subject to like punishments." The medical duty to assist is expressed in a mandatory form in Article 9 of the CMD: "Every doctor who is in the presence of a patient or of a wounded person in danger, or is informed that a patient or a wounded person is in danger, must provide assistance or make sure that that person receives the necessary care."

The crime of failure to rescue belongs to the category of "endangering behavior" offenses (Dadamo 1997, p. 212), which also includes that of deliberately exposing a person to possible death or injury (Article 223-1 of the 1992 *Criminal Code*). Decisions to discontinue vasopressive drugs, undertake terminal weaning from ventilation, or withhold cardiopulmonary resuscitation and mechanical ventilation from a patient would fall within these categories of offense (Nys 1999, p. 225). This approach is in harmony with the second clause of Article 38 of the CMD, which mandates that a physician "has no right to deliberately bring about death."

Inciting another to commit suicide is a crime under Article 223-13 of the *Criminal Code* punishable by 3 years' imprisonment. Providing drugs, lethal substances, or mechanical devices designed to enable a patient to commit suicide would come within the scope of this offense. Encouragement and advertising of methods to commit suicide is an offense against the person under Article 223-14 of the *Criminal Code*. However, with the advent of the World Wide Web, this law may be difficult to police.

With regard to euthanasia, Article 221-1 of the *Criminal Code* states that "the fact of voluntarily killing another constitutes murder." The offense of homicide must be a positive intentional act rather than an abstention that causes death. Killing another person on request will fulfill the requirement. Article 121-3(1) provides that intention is an essential element of major crimes. Article 221-5 of the *Criminal Code* includes a specific offense of poisoning defined as "attacking the life of another through the use or administration of substances that cause death," which is punishable by 30 years' imprisonment. In prosecuting the employees of the French National Blood Transfusion Center for knowingly placing on the market unheated blood products infected with HIV, the Cour de Cassation (Criminal Chamber, 22 June 1994), did not exclude the possibility that the offense of poisoning could be made out without the specific intention to kill.

GERMANY

As in the common law countries, a competent dying patient in Germany has the right to refuse treatment intended to extend life (decision by the German Supreme Court [*Bundesgerichtshof*], 28 November 1957). This right is referred to as *passive Sterbehilfe* and is generally accepted.

Suicide is not illegal in Germany, but the law prohibits euthanasia, which is killing another at that person's request (judgment of the German Federal Court of Justice of 7 February 2001). Killing another at that person's "express and serious request" is a lesser offense than murder or manslaughter, and is punishable by 6 months to 5 years in prison. In a 2001 case, however, the German Supreme Court held that a leader of an assisted suicide group who aided an elderly woman suffering from multiple sclerosis and other infirmities to commit suicide by supplying a deadly drug was not guilty of causing the death. The court accepted that the patient herself was responsible for her own death, and that the defendant, who assisted her by supplying the means of the death, was not responsible. The court, however, affirmed a conviction of the defendant for violating the controlled substances laws in supplying the drug, and rejected a defense of necessity put forward by the defendant to that charge.

The assistance of a patient by a doctor in committing suicide can collide with a well recognized duty of rescue imposed upon doctors by German law. In the 1984 *Wittig* case, the German Supreme Court held that a doctor who does not try to forestall the consequences of an attempted suicide may be criminally liable (Nys 1991, p. 232). In the 1988 *Hackethal* case, however, the Supreme Court suggested that the doctor may be freed from the obligation to rescue the patient if the patient experienced his life as torture and wanted to escape it (Nys 1999, p. 233), and in the 2001 case noted above, the court held that the duty of rescue did not apply because the patient, upon taking the drug, became rapidly unconscious and beyond help.

The right of self-determination recognized in these cases does not end when the patient becomes incompetent. In its judgment of 13 September 1994, the Supreme Court explicitly recognized that the patient's right to self-determination encompasses a right to refuse life-sustaining treatment, and that this right could be exercised on behalf of incompetents where sufficient evidence exists, based on the patient's written or oral statements, religious views, and value system indicating that the person would have declined treatment.

The German law recognizes living wills (*Patientverfügungen*), though they do not seem to have the force that they have in the United States, but are rather a datum to consider in making end of life determinations. Patients may also grant another person a power of attorney to make medical decisions (*Vorsorgevollmachten*) in the future event of incapacity, and/or nominate a guardian for the guardianship court to appoint in the event of incapacity. Under the guardianship law, the guardianship court must approve any medical decisions made by a guardian or power of attorney that threaten death or long-lasting threats to health.

Where no living will or person holding a power of attorney or guardian exists, the attending physician must attempt to determine what the incompetent patient would have wanted done in the situation. This should be discerned by considering the patient's earlier statements, religious convictions, and attitude toward pain, as well as from the seriousness of the patient's current condition. If it is impossible to determine the patient's presumed will, the doctor should decide in the patient's best interest.

Although German law places a heavy emphasis on the patient's right of self-determination, it also emphasizes the obligations of physicians to dying patients. In particular, the doctor has an obligation to protect the patient from pain. In several cases, health care professionals have been found civilly or criminally liable for causing unnecessary pain to patients by failing to provide adequate pain therapy (Kutzer 2001a). Moreover, a doctor who does attempt to protect a patient from pain can expect the protection of the law. In a 1996 case, the German Supreme Court held that a doctor did not break the law by providing a dying patient with medically indicated pain medication in accordance with the expressed or presumed wishes of the patient, just because the pain medication may have hastened the patient's death (decision of 15 November 1996; Nys 1991, p. 232; Kutzer 2001b, p. 2). This process is referred to in the German literature as *indirekte Sterbehilfe*.

Nevertheless, some critics have charged that German doctors are reluctant to provide adequate pain therapy. A recent article by Klaus Kutzer, a justice of the German Supreme Court, quotes Professor Dr. Zenz as stating that prescribing of opiates in Germany for pain treatment lags 10 years behind that of other European countries (Kutzer 2001a). Kutzer suggested that this might in part be due to restrictive interpretations of the German controlled substances regulations. Despite a commitment to palliative care as an alternative to euthanasia, palliative care still seems underdeveloped in Germany (Csef 2001; Sohn 2001).

JAPAN

The law respecting end of life decisions seems somewhat less developed in Japan than in the other countries in this survey (Scherer and Simon 1999). No statutory scheme has emerged for dealing with end of life decisions, and only a handful of judicial precedents give guidance. There is also little legal authority on pain management.

Patient autonomy is not as firmly established in Japan as in other countries. Japanese doctors are reluctant to disclose (and patients perhaps reluctant to receive) a terminal diagnosis, especially one of cancer (Leflar 1996), apparently believing that the patient will give up trying to survive in the face of such a diagnosis. Japanese doctors are more likely to disclose the diagnosis to the family, and work with them to deceive the patient (Kimura 1998).

Article 202 of the Japanese *Criminal Code* prohibits assistance in suicide or killing another on request. Physicians rely on this statute in refusing requests for termination of end of life treatment. On the other hand, once doctors decide that further treatment is not indicated, they can rely on Article 35 of the Criminal Code, which offers a defense of justification for acts done "in the course of legitimate business." However, in a recent decision, the Japanese Supreme Court unanimously concluded that doctors who transfused a Jehovah's Witness against her express instructions had infringed on her personal rights, and awarded damages for emotional distress (*Takeda v State,* 2000).

Two reported court decisions involving euthanasia are the primary sources of end of life decision-making law in Japan. Kimura (1998, p. 192) has described a 1962 case in which the Nagoya High Court countenanced the legal possibility of euthanasia. In this case a son was charged with "ascendant homicide" (the aggravated crime of killing one's ancestor) for poisoning his terminally ill father, who was suffering great pain, allegedly at the father's request. The court identified six conditions that had to be present before it could be accepted: (1) the patient must be suffering from an incurable and imminently terminal condition, (2) the patient must be suffering unbearable and unrelievable pain, (3) the patient must be killed with the intention of alleviating the pain, (4) the act should be done only at the patient's explicit request, (5) the euthanasia should normally be carried out by a physician, and (6) the euthanasia must be carried out through ethically acceptable means. The court held that the final two conditions had not been met in a case of a son's euthanasia of a parent· and thus convicted the son. He was sentenced to 4 years in prison, with 3 years suspended. In four subsequent cases of euthanasia by relatives, various courts found one or more criteria to be lacking and thus found guilt, but in each the defendant was sentenced to a relatively light sentence.

A 1995 case from the Yokohama District Court involved a criminal prosecution of a doctor who had, in response to a patient's family's insistent and incessant requests, first terminated nutrition and hydration, then injected the patient with high doses of analgesics, and finally injected the patient with verapamil (a calcium channel blocker used for high blood pressure and irregular heart beat) and potassium chloride, causing the patient's death. The court convicted the doctor of murder (Yamazaki 1997; Hoshio 1997; Jost 2000) but only sentenced him to 2 years in prison.

The court held that treatment of patients may be terminated if death is unavoidable and the patient is in the final stages of an incurable disease. The court suggested that more than one doctor should make the judgment of the impossibility of recovery. The patient should make an informed expression of a desire that treatment should cease. If the patient is unable to consent, the family should be given accurate information about the patient's condition and then be allowed to state the patient's "inferred intent," based on their knowledge of the patient's character and values. Having expressed its hope that patients would in the future have living wills, the court noted that if a living will was vague or remote in time it might not be of much use. The court concluded that life support measures (including artificial nutrition and hydration) could be terminated, but that the decision of which treatments to terminate and when was a medical judgment, presumably primarily for doctors to make.

With respect to euthanasia, the court distinguished between passive euthanasia (the cessation of life-sustaining treatment), indirect euthanasia (terminal sedation), and active euthanasia. The court stated that euthanasia is only appropriate if: (1) physical pain is difficult to bear (mental suffering does not suffice), (2) the time of unavoidable death is near, (3) methods of eliminating the pain are exhausted, and (4) there is a clear expression of intent to accept death. Active euthanasia can only be imposed if death is imminent, but indirect euthanasia can be used to hasten death. Active euthanasia is also only permissible if there is a clear expression of the patient's intent—substituted judgment does not suffice. Passive euthanasia, on the other hand, can be based on medical judgment as to futility and on the family's statement of intent, based on the patient's inferred intent, as noted above.

In the 1995 case, the Yokohama District Court held that active euthanasia was inappropriate because there was no informed consent on the part of the patient (who had not been told he was dying of cancer), the patient was unconscious and therefore not experiencing pain, and the family had not been told that the patient was not in pain. The court also faulted the doctor for relying on the family's judgment, as he had only known them a short time, and for buckling under to the son's insistence on euthanasia, given the doctor's "higher status and position."

The law that emerges from these cases contrasts with the law of common law countries in that it is more open to euthanasia, but more reticent to accept withdrawal of treatment (which is, effectively treated as a form of euthanasia). The two court decisions, for example, would not seem to countenance withdrawal of life-sustaining treatment for a nonterminal patient in a persistent vegetative state. Advance directives have no particular legal status in Japan, though several organizations offer advance directive forms and encourage their use.

Japan has a very strict narcotic law, and medical use of narcotics is limited. One expert states "Such a rigid and complicated system of justifying the use of narcotics has forced many cancer patients with treatable pain to suffer compared with other advanced countries" (Kimura 1998, p. 189). Physicians seem to fear that use of narcotics to control pain might lead to addiction or shorten the patient's life.

THE NETHERLANDS

The Netherlands was until recently the only nation in the world to have legalized euthanasia (it was joined in 2002 by Belgium). The Dutch *Criminal Code*, like the German and Japanese, prohibits taking the life of another person "at the other person's express and earnest request" (Article 293), and also prohibits murder (Article 289), manslaughter (Article 287), and assisted suicide (Article 294). However, since the *Schoonheim* decision (Nederlandse Jurisprudentie 1985, no. 106) and through the mid-1900s, Dutch prosecutors have refrained from prosecuting doctors who committed euthanasia when the doctors conformed with certain substantive and procedural requirements established by the Supreme Court (Griffiths et al. 1998). The court based these requirements on its interpretation of Article 40 of the Criminal Code, which literally provides that "A person who commits an offense as a result of a force that he could not be expected to resist is not criminally liable." In the 1984 *Schoonheim* case—in which a general practitioner was prosecuted for killing a 93-year-old woman who was near the end of her life and had requested euthanasia—the court accepted the argument that the killing was justified because the doctor had resolved in a responsible way a conflict between the professional duty to preserve life and the duty to spare a patient from suffering and thus met the defense of necessity recognized by Article 40.

In April of 2001, the Dutch parliament adopted the *Termination of Life on Request and Assisted Suicide (Review Procedures) Act* (TLRASA), which also amended the *Criminal Code* and the *Burial and Cremation Act*. This statute, which went into effect in 2002, legalizes the practice of euthanasia and of assistance in suicide by physicians when specific substantive and procedural requirements are met (Kimsma and van Leeuwen 2001). The TLRASA amends Articles 293 and 294 of the *Criminal Code*, which prohibit killing on request and assistance in suicide, to provide that those acts are not illegal "if committed by a physician who fulfills the due care criteria" of the TLRASA, "and if the physician notifies the municipal pathologist" in accordance with section 7(2) of the *Burial and Cremation Act*. The "due care" criteria of section 2 of the TLRASA require that the physician: "a. holds the conviction that the request by the patient was voluntary and well-considered; b. holds the conviction that the patient's suffering was lasting and unbearable. c. has informed the patient about the situation he was in and about his prospects; d. and the patient holds the conviction that there was no other reasonable solution for the situation he was in; e. has consulted at least one other, independent physician who has seen the patient and has given his written opinion on the requirements of due care, referred to in parts a–d, and f. has terminated a life or assisted in a suicide with due care."

Section 10 of the TLRASA further requires that a doctor who performs euthanasia or assists with suicide under the statute must notify the local coroner of the death, providing the coroner with a detailed report on compliance with the due care requirements. The coroner must in turn notify a regional review committee established under the act for reviewing euthanasia cases. The coroner may also notify the prosecutor, who may in turn inform the coroner and regional review committee if he objects to the burial or cremation of the patient. Section 8 provides for a regional review committee, which must include at least one legally trained member (the chair), one physician, and one ethicist, that reviews the report and decides whether the doctor has complied with the due care criteria. By virtue of section 9, the committee may inform the prosecutor or the regional health care inspector if it concludes that the statutory procedure has not been complied with (in general, the committee must inform the physician of its decision within 6 weeks). Under the new procedure, the committees will have the power to shield physicians reporting cases of euthanasia or assisted suicide to the local coroner from the threat of prosecution.

Under sections 2(3) and 2(4) of the *Burial and Cremation Act,* a physician may terminate the life of a child aged 16 to 18 or assist with his or her suicide at the child's request after consulting the child's parents. If the child is between 12 and 16, the attending physician may only honor a request for euthanasia or assistance in suicide if the child's parent or guardian agrees. With regard to persons who are incompetent, but prior to becoming incompetent had executed an advance directive requesting that their lives be terminated upon reaching some future state of deterioration, the physician may honor this request, if otherwise in compliance with the due care criteria.

The statute does not require that the patient be in a terminal condition. It does not even require that the suffering be physical. In the *Chabot* case (Nederlandse Jurisprudentie 1994, no. 656; reproduced in Griffiths et al. 1998, p. 329), the Supreme Court of The Netherlands recognized that the patient's "unbearable and hopeless suffering" could be mental rather than physical, although it upheld the conviction of the psychiatrist in the particular case for violating other requirements in euthanizing an inconsolably grieving woman at her request. Every year a handful of psychiatric patients are euthanized or assisted in suicide.

The statute does not address the practices of withdrawal of medical treatment or of terminal sedation. Dutch law permits competent patients to request that life-sustaining treatments (including artificial nutrition and hydration) be withdrawn or withheld (Nys 1999). Written advance directives, executed by a patient while competent and refusing treatment under specified circumstances, are also recognized under Article 450(3) of the *Medical Contracts Act,* though the statute also permits doctors to override the refusal if there are "well founded reasons for doing so" (Nys 1991). Physicians may also withdraw or withhold treatment that they regard as "futile" (Nys 1991, pp 234–235). Finally, doctors are permitted to administer drugs as necessary to relieve pain, even though the pain medication may hasten death (Nys

1991). These practices are regarded as "normal medical practice," and deaths resulting from them are regarded as natural deaths. They account for far more deaths than declared euthanasia or assisted suicide, 38.5% versus 2.7%, according to Griffiths et al. (1998).

Another issue not resolved by the new act is the treatment of severely defective newborns. A high percentage of deaths of seriously defective newborns (62%) result from acts that hasten death, including simple withdrawal or withholding of life-sustaining treatments (23%), terminal sedation (27%), or the administration of drugs to hasten death (9%) (Griffiths et al. 1998). Two courts have exonerated doctors prosecuted for murder for terminating the life of severely defective newborns in cases in which life-prolonging treatment was withdrawn, with the parents' agreement, and the baby continued to suffer (Griffiths et al. 1998).

Finally, the statute does not address the situation of patients in a persistent vegetative state (except insofar as they have earlier executed an advance directive). A recent case found a general practitioner guilty of murder for killing an 84-year-old dying patient who was in a coma, but the court imposed only a suspended fine as a sanction (Sheldon 2001). Because the patient was incapable of voluntarily requesting euthanasia, the case was not covered by the statute. Surveys, however, show that the killing of patients in the absence of a voluntary request is not uncommon (perhaps about 1,000 cases a year), and might in some cases be justified under the Dutch defense of necessity (Griffiths et al. 1998).

The practice of euthanasia in The Netherlands has been widely condemned by external commentators, and is not universally accepted within The Netherlands. The new Conservative government elected in the summer of 2002 has pledged itself to review the practice of euthanasia. A significant majority of the Dutch population, however, seems to have accepted the current practice. Dutch commentators also often claim that other countries permit very similar medical practices, but simply do not admit to doing so. Without joining this debate, we consider that The Netherlands holds down the most extreme position in its end of life law of all countries in our survey.

REFERENCES

Ashby M. Life and death: the Canadian and Australian Senates on palliative care and euthanasia. *J Law Med* 1997a; 5:40–51.

Ashby M. The fallacies of death causation in palliative care. *Med J Aust* 1997b; 166:176–177.

Ashby M. Palliative care, death causation, public policy and the law. *Prog Palliative Care* 1998; 693:69–77.

Ashby M, Mendelson D. Natural death in 2003: are we slipping backwards? *J Law Med* 2003; 10(3):260–265.

Csef H. Euthanasia as an ethical problem. In: Sohn W, Zenz M (Eds). *Euthanasia in Europe*. Stuttgart: Schattauer, 2001, pp 71–80.

Dadamo C, Farran S. *French Substantive Law: Key Elements*. London: Sweet & Maxwell, 1997.

Devlin P. *Easing the Passing: The Trial of Dr. John Bodkin Adams*. London: Faber and Faber, 1986.

DuBose R, Berde CB. Respiratory effects of opioids. *IASP Newsletter* 1997:3–5.

Duguet AM. Euthanasia and assistance to end of life legislation in France. *Eur J Health Law* 2001; 8:109–123.

Ferrand E, Ingrand RP, Lemaire F. Withholding and withdrawal of life support in intensive-care units in France: a prospective survey. *Lancet* 2001; 357(9249):9–14.

Freckelton I, Mendelson D (Eds). *Causation in Law and Medicine*, The International Library of Medicine, Ethics and Law Series. Aldershott: Ashgate Dartmouth, 2002.

Griffiths J, Bood A, Weyers H. *Euthanasia and the Law in the Netherlands*. Amsterdam: Amsterdam University Press, 1998.

Gutierrez E. Debate on euthanasia encouraged in Japan. *Lancet* 1997; 349:409.

Jost TS (Ed). *Readings in Comparative Law and Bioethics*. Durham, NC: Carolina Academic Press, 2000.

Kimura R. Death dying, and advance directives in Japan. In: Sass H-M, Veatch RM, Kimura R (Eds). *Advance Directives and Surrogate Decision Making in Health Care*. Baltimore: Johns Hopkins University Press, 1998, pp 136–198.

Kimsma G, van Leeuwen E. The new Dutch law on legalizing physician-assisted death. *Camb Q Healthc Ethics* 2001; 10:445.

Kutzer K. Rechtliche Aspekte der Behandlung Schwerstkranker bei irreversiblen Schädigungen. *Europäische Akademie Newsletter* 2001a:June.

Kutzer K. Pain therapy from the legal perspective, Saarland. *Pain Forum* 2001b:20.

Lavery JV, Singer P. The 'Supremes' decide on assisted suicide: what should a doctor do? *CMAJ* 1997:157:405–406.

Leflar RB. Informed consent and patients' rights in Japan. *Houston Law Rev* 1996; 33:1–112.

Mendelson D. *Quill*, *Glucksberg* and palliative care: does alleviation of pain necessarily hasten death? *J Law Med* 1997; 5:110–113.

Nys H. Physician involvement in a patient's death: a continental European perspective. *Med Law Rev* 1999; 7:208–246.

Parliament of Canada. *Of Life and Death: Report of Special Senate Committee on Euthanasia and Assisted Suicide*. Ottawa: Parliament of Canada, 1995, pp 26–27.

Scherer JM, Simon RJ. *Euthanasia and the Right to Die: A Comparative View*. Lanham: Rowman and Littlefield, 1999.

Sheldon T. Dutch GP found guilty of murder faces no penalty. *BMJ* 2001; 322:509.

Sohn W. Care for the dying between the right to self-determination and the obligation to provide treatment. In: Sohn W, Zenz M (Eds). *Euthanasia in Europe*. Stuttgart: Schattauer, 2001, pp 67–70.

Wilson WC, et al. Ordering and administration of sedatives and analgesics during the withholding and withdrawal of life support from clinically ill patients. *JAMA* 1992; 267:949–953.

Yamazaki F. A thought on terminal care in Japan. In: Hoshio K (Ed). *Japanese and Western Bioethics*. Dordrecht: Kluwer Academic, 1997.

Zielonka TM. Na marginesie Kodeksu Etyki Lekarskiej. *Gazeta Lekarska* 2001; 10.

Zelichowski M. Kodeks Etyki Lekarskiej. *Medycyna Praktyczna* 2002: 28 March. Available via the Internet at: http://mp.pl/ (visited Jan. 25, 2003).

Zelichowski M. Bez zgody pacjenta. Rzeczpospolita 1999: 4 November. Available via the Internet at: http://www.mp.pl/ (visited Jan. 25, 2003).

Correspondence to: Danuta Mendelson, PhD, LLM, School of Law, Deakin University, Burwood Highway, Burwood, VIC 3125, Australia. Email: dmendel@deakin.edu.au.

Part X

Nonpharmacological Treatments and Outcomes Assessment

Proceedings of the 10th World Congress on Pain,
Progress in Pain Research and Management, Vol. 24,
edited by Jonathan O. Dostrovsky, Daniel B. Carr, and
Martin Koltzenburg, IASP Press, Seattle, © 2003.

64

Cognitive Behavioral Treatment

Amanda C. de C. Williams

INPUT Pain Management Unit, St. Thomas Hospital,
London, United Kingdom

This chapter addresses the place of cognitive behavioral treatment (CBT) for chronic pain, and examines the most important sources of variance in outcome of CBT. Consideration of how CBT can become more effective leads to a "normal psychology of pain" and reflection on the next generation of treatment and treatment studies.

CBT is still largely delivered only after all other interventions have failed, to those whose pain problem persists despite addressing its cause where identified, and after various medical and physical analgesic interventions. Is this its only and proper place, or might psychological problems be addressed alongside treatment of the cause of pain and of pain itself? We know that psychological problems are not simply the consequence of persistent pain. Distress measured during acute pain predicts the likelihood of persistent pain and disability, as well as long-term distress, far more accurately than do biological measures, pain intensity, or extent of disability during the acute stage. Those data come from an important systematic review of prospective studies of low back pain in primary care by Pincus et al. (2002). Distress in these studies is largely measured by catastrophizing, but is likely also to comprise fear of persistent pain and bodily harm, which will doubtless be studied further in the next 10 years. Fear is clearly associated with disability because it generates avoidance (of feared activities and physical demands), and avoidance constitutes functional shortcomings that cannot be attributed directly to physical impairment or pain. The literature on pain and fear is best summarized in a state of the art review by Vlaeyen and Linton (2000), and is discussed by Vlaeyen in this volume.

Catastrophizing is a robust and key concept for psychological work in pain, originating with Keefe in the early 1980s (Rosenstiel and Keefe 1983), and most recently critically reviewed by Sullivan et al. (2001). It comprises three elements (Keefe et al. 2000): a focus on threatening information, internal or external ("I can feel my neck click whenever I move"); an overestimate of the extent of threat ("The bones are crumbling and I'll become paralyzed"); and an underestimate of personal and broader resources to mitigate the danger and disastrous consequences ("Nobody understands how to fix the problem, and I just can't bear any more pain"). During the last decade, "catastrophizing has risen to the status of one of the most important psychological predictors of the pain experience" (Sullivan et al. 2001, p. 53). Catastrophizing predicts pain intensity ratings, disability, use of health care and of drugs, and is even an important variable in research in pain-free subjects undergoing experimental pain tasks.

Seven published systematic reviews and meta-analyses in adults address the efficacy of CBT for chronic pain (see Table I), and at least one update is in preparation. There are also two meta-analyses of psychological work for people with rheumatoid arthritis (Superio-Cabuslay et al. 1996; Astin et al. 2002), but because some included treatments are no more than general education those meta-analyses are not discussed here. However, arthritis trials and arthritis patients are appropriately included among the meta-analyses of CBT for chronic pain. A systematic review and meta-analysis of CBT for chronic pain in children and adolescents (Eccleston et al. 2002) is not covered in this chapter.

Table I
Systematic reviews and meta-analyses of CBT for chronic pain

Reference	Search*	RCTs?	Control†	Trial *N*	Patient *N*	Pain Type
Malone and Strube 1988	1984	no	no	48	?	mixed, dental and head
Cutler et al. 1994	1991	no	no	37	3418	mixed
Flor et al. 1992	1990	no	alt.	65	3089	mixed, not head
Turner 1996	1994	yes	alt.	4	227	low back
Morley et al. 1999	1996	yes	no/alt.	25	1672	mixed, not head
Van Tulder et al. 2000	1999	yes	no/alt.	7 & 6	419 & 345	low back
Guzmán et al. 2001	1998	yes	alt.	10	1964	low back
Morley et al., in prep.	2002	yes	alt.	32	2968	mixed, not head

* Last year included in literature search.
† No = no treatment control group (e.g., waiting list); alt. = alternative treatment control group (e.g., treatment as usual, physical therapy, prescribed drugs).

The four trials comparing CBT with no treatment (Malone and Strube 1988; Cutler et al. 1994, using nonrandomized studies; Morley et al. 1999; Van Tulder et al. 2000, using randomized controlled trials [RCTs]) showed a clear benefit of CBT in a range of outcomes described below. The five that compared CBT with treatment as usual (Flor et al. 1992, using randomized and nonrandomized studies; Turner 1996; Morley et al. 1999; Van Tulder et al. 2000; Guzmán et al. 2001 using RCTs) also showed a benefit of CBT over alternatives across a range of outcomes, but less conclusively than trials with no-treatment controls. Some of the most important outcomes among the diverse ones assessed are shown in Fig. 1. Data in this figure are from the meta-analysis by Morley et al. that compared CBT with no treatment. The results are presented in terms of effect size for the post-treatment difference between groups treated with CBT and untreated controls, expressed in units of standard deviation. In this metric, 0.5 (the dotted line) is considered moderate improvement. It is evident that most mean differences achieve about that level and that none of the confidence intervals cross the zero line, which would indicate no difference between treatment and control.

Substantial evidence thus supports CBT as the treatment of choice. But to determine how outcomes could be better, CBT and its delivery require some elaboration. CBT is based on learning theory, whose tenets are that behavior is largely learned, consciously or not; that it can be changed by directed learning, consciously mediated or not; and that ways of thinking and beliefs can also be learned, consciously or not, and can also be changed. CBT draws on rich theoretical and empirical work. Its application to pain

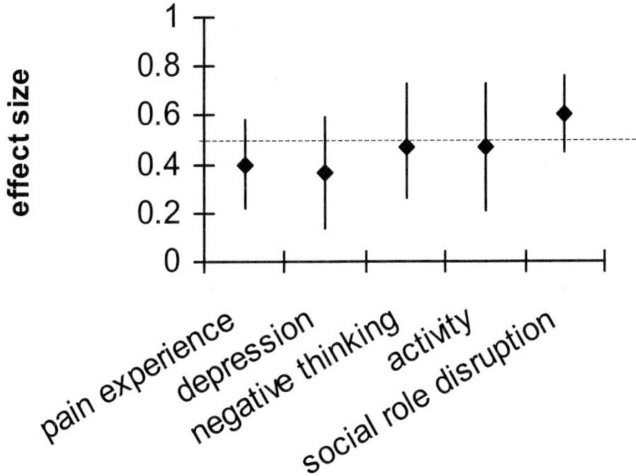

Fig. 1. Effect sizes for cognitive behavioral treatment (CBT) versus untreated waiting-list controls.

patients is largely extrapolated from well-established work in treatment of psychological problems (Roth and Fonagy 1996). However, CBT is not generally the treatment of choice from the patient's point of view because patients formulate their problems differently than research psychologists (Radley and Billig 1996; Reitsma and Meijler 1997). Rather than seeking help for pain behavior, secondary gain, or overdependence on welfare payments, patients instead hope for pain relief. In the psychological domain, patients' main psychological complaint is of frustration (Price 1999), but we have no psychology of frustration. Patients' preference for attempts at curative treatment is one of the factors that maintain CBT as an "end of the line" treatment.

If patients are to select psychological treatments, we need to be able to provide them with information in a form that we lack at present. We must be able not only to describe the treatment, but also to compare the same outcomes of alternative treatments using the same categories and metrics. Medical and physical treatments, many now summarized in systematic reviews and meta-analyses (see the Cochrane and Bandolier Web sites, www.cochrane.org and www.jr2.ox.ac.uk/bandolier, respectively; McQuay and Moore 1998), often set the criterion of 50% pain relief as their major outcome, although this is perhaps unduly stringent for chronic pain (Farrar et al. 2000). Studies of these treatments also present data on adverse effects, which is important information for patients. These strengths are not shared by studies of psychological treatment, which express pain reduction in terms of mean differences between groups, data that cannot be applied to individual cases and in which statistical significance is often substituted for clinical meaning (Turk et al. 2000). They also fail to describe adverse effects or worsening attributable to treatment. On the other hand, a wider range of outcomes are assessed in studies of psychological treatments than in those of medical and physical treatments. Outcomes assessed in psychological treatment trials usually include function and mood, of major importance to patients, and sometimes include subsequent independence in health care, of importance to health care providers and funders. The follow-up interval, of particular relevance for chronic problems, is usually longer than in medical and physical studies. Given these differences, comparison of medical and psychological treatments for chronic pain is problematic.

Nevertheless, Fig. 2 shows an attempt at such a comparison. Data for the two medical treatments, antidepressants for peripheral diabetic neuropathy and anticonvulsants for trigeminal neuralgia, are taken from the Bandolier Web site, and that for CBT versus untreated waiting list controls from a study that generalized the results of an RCT to nonrandomized patients (Williams et al. 1996, 1999). The data are expressed in terms of numbers

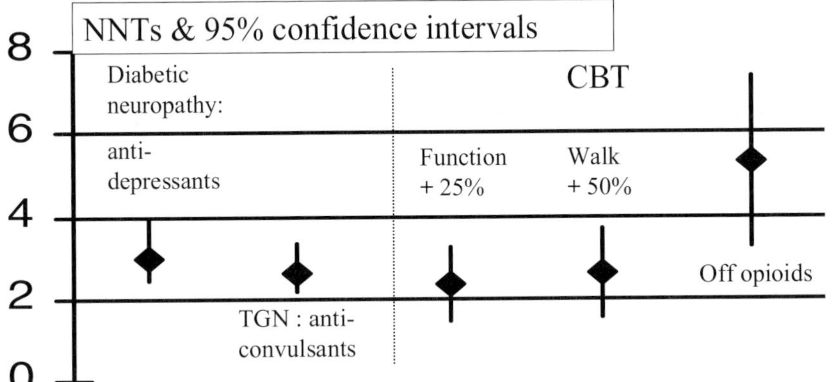

Fig. 2. Numbers needed to treat (NNTs) for medical treatments versus CBT.

needed to treat (NNTs), a metric used more commonly in medical rather than psychological studies but of particular use clinically. The NNT is the number of patients who must be treated for one to improve in the treatment group who would not have done so in the control group; so, the lower the NNT, the better. An NNT of two, for example, means either that both patients in the treatment group improved, compared to only one of two in the control group; or that one of two in the treatment group improved but neither of those in the control group. It does not tell one the fate of those who did not improve: they may have worsened, not changed, or dropped out.

Although these results attest that CBT is a powerful intervention, we are still some way from being able to specify with confidence what constitutes best practice. In addition, results across a range of outcomes vary considerably. For these reasons it is worth examining the sources of variance in some detail. These will be described in three categories: patients, treatment content, and treatment process.

First, the issue of attributing outcome variance to patient characteristics remains unresolved (Morley and Williams 2002). Despite much searching among individual, demographic, and medical variables, no consistent predictors have emerged. Much of the searching lacks a theoretical basis or draws on inappropriate psychiatric models rooted in dualistic thinking about pain, and where positive findings emerge they are likely to represent chance features of the sample population that are not borne out by studies in other centers. More consistent data are emerging from examination of baseline cognitive content (beliefs, including fears) and processing (such as catastrophizing), mood, and function. These data, which arise from hypothesis testing, together suggest that predictors should reflect immediate characteristics of the patient, rather than group characteristics such as age, educational status, or site of pain.

Second, treatment content can be described in terms of behavior change and cognitive change. Aims in the area of behavior change are to increase range and level of activity including work; to increase independence in health care and decrease dependence on family, friends, or societal resources for help in daily life and for health care; and in some CBT programs, to reduce pain. The methods employed toward these aims are behavioral activation, including goal setting and pacing of progress toward goals; manipulation of cues for and consequences of behaviors to promote change; behavioral experimentation in areas of unnecessary fear; application of relaxation during activity and at rest; adoption of a fitness routine; and reduction of analgesic and/or psychotropic drugs that have proved ineffective. Aims in the area of cognitive and emotional change are to reduce distress associated with pain, depression, or depressed mood; to lessen fear about pain and about damage; to reduce frustration and increase control; to decrease health care use; and (not universally) to decrease pain. The relevant methods are education about pain, damage, and health; challenging thought content and thinking biases associated with unwanted emotions and behaviors; thought experiment; and attention control techniques.

Many studies have attempted to identify the unique contribution of single or combined behavioral or cognitive methods by "component dismantling" designs, in which the outcome of complete CBT is compared with the outcome of complete CBT minus one component (such as cognitive intervention). Although these studies provide a wealth of data, they would only be able to quantify the contribution of that component if certain assumptions were true. These assumptions are that each component of CBT affects only one outcome, and is unique in its effects, and that therapeutic components combine additively. Unfortunately, these assumptions cannot be sustained: each component affects multiple outcomes, and by design, effects are much more likely to be synergistic than additive and independent (Morley and Williams 2002). Clinically, some patients grasp explanations of their pain such that its meaning changes and they are freed to become more active without anxiety or self-imposed limitations. Other patients only overcome those barriers through steady exposure and discovery that what they avoided is safe and rewarding; reflection on this experience helps them to change their mistaken assumptions about the meaning of pain. Many patients seem to require both explanation and personal experience, and some seem to respond to neither.

Given that component dismantling is not going to provide the recipe for best content of a CBT program, how should its content be decided? The best option is to use a constructive approach drawing on evidence showing what works in pain patients (for instance, Vlaeyen's work on fears). In the absence of specific evidence for pain control, one may (as with several behavior change methods) extrapolate when effectiveness is proven in related fields. Concepts pertinent to the development and maintenance of chronic pain that are adapted from related fields can provide robust working hypotheses. Lacking either specific evidence or plausibly generalized concepts, reference to theory and testing hypotheses derived from that theory are preferable to an ad hoc approach to choosing treatment techniques based upon their face validity. There is a risk of harm to patients when hopes are raised unrealistically and underpowered treatment is offered.

Treatment processes may be located in patients (therapeutic alliance with, investment in, or engagement with treatment staff and with fellow patients if treated in a group; expectations of outcome from treatment; and adherence to treatment methods); in treatment staff (therapeutic alliance, skills, and competence; expectations of success or allegiance to a therapeutic school; and adherence to treatment methods); and in the context and method of delivery (patient selection and group factors, integration with patients' own social contexts, time and length of treatment, and setting). There are certain analogies for these variables in medical settings: for instance, the quality of a drug or equipment, or the skills of staff in delivering an "epidural" injection epidurally, and so on, but in psychological work far less can be taken for granted (like drug purity), and most skills are interpersonal ones that are subtle and complex.

Work at my program has identified up to 15% of variance in outcome attributable to time and length of treatment, and a consistent 1–4% variance due to patients' expectations of success, after adjustment for baseline differences and other relevant variables. Evaluation of the impact of therapeutic alliance upon outcomes of pain treatment is in its early stages, although such alliance accounts for up to 30% of variance in outcome of individual psychological therapy (Roth and Fonagy 1996). Emerging evidence identifies both patient-to-patient group and patient-to-staff alliance as influential in outcome. The most notable is the greater immediate reduction, continued on 1-month follow-up, of catastrophizing among those with a higher therapeutic alliance to staff, compared to smaller short-term and absent long-term treatment benefits in those with lower therapeutic alliance.

Adherence to treatment methods is not widely measured, and when it is, it is often expressed in terms of frequency. However, for some treatment methods, appropriateness of use may be a more relevant distinction than frequency because we cannot, for example, specify on empirical grounds a "good enough" frequency of using relaxation. In a sample of over 2,000 patients treated with CBT for chronic pain, those who challenged thoughts as a daily habit or when they felt depressed were less depressed at 1 and 9 months after treatment than were those who used the method of challenging thoughts when their pain was bad. Those who challenged thoughts daily also catastrophized less.

During the 9 months after CBT, 32% of patients (N = 1382) had no further medical or physical health care (nor any prescription analgesic use), 30% had one episode of care or analgesic use, and the remainder received no more than five. Receipt of further health care was unrelated to adherence to treatment methods or to personal or pain characteristics, nor to any baseline measure: the only predictor in a logistic regression was poorer self-efficacy (confidence in managing various activities despite pain; Nicholas et al. 1992) at 1-month follow-up.

The major findings were on length of treatment. Outcomes of three CBT programs, taught by the same staff in the same setting, were compared in 1,977 patients treated over 10 years. The longer and more intensive program was used for patients who were more disabled and distressed—patients were assigned deliberately to each program, not randomized. Retrospective data examination showed these differences to be substantial and also indicated that patients in this longer program were using greater quantities of drugs at the time of enrollment, although this was not a criterion used to assign them to this program. The two shorter programs, both the same total number of days, were run either intensively or over an extended time period. Patients made clinically and statistically significant gains in all three programs, with the largest amount of variance accounted for by their baseline data. Treatment differences added up to 15% of variance. Although their poor baseline status would predict the worst outcomes for those assigned to the longest treatment, the longer, more intensive treatment enabled patients to equal those who completed the shorter programs in improvement of depressed mood, self-efficacy, and walking performance, and to surpass them in reductions in catastrophizing and achieving and maintaining abstinence analgesic and psychotropic drugs.

These observations suggest a dose-response effect supported by findings of other studies, although no significant correlation has been shown between length and efficacy of treatment (Flor et al. 1992). The failure to observe a linear correlation might be accounted for by a sigmoid relationship between treatment duration and response. Early CBT programs were longer than any that are now in use: Flor et al. (1992) provided a mean of 96 hours (range 4–264) and Morley et al. (1999) calculated a median of 16 hours, (range 6–90), reduced further to 12 hours in the update in progress. The shortening of CBT programs between the two reviews appears to have taken place without obvious loss of efficacy. Some of the shortest programs, however, now are not only rather disappointing in terms of efficacy, but are often shorter than comparable treatments for distressed patients without pain. The capacity of such brief programs to effect the necessary changes can only be a matter of conjecture until demonstrated empirically. Attempts to change behavior without addressing the beliefs that underpin it, to bring about cognitive change in problem areas by general advice, to provide treatment so brief and unfocused that patients neither make a therapeutic alliance with treatment staff nor feel that they have been heard and understood, are compromises that shorten CBT but at the cost of making lasting or even short-term change. Selection of the least disabled and distressed patients for such brief treatment is only a partial solution.

In summary, in the search for sources of variance in outcomes of CBT and for ways to improve them, patient characteristics have been overestimated as a source, and treatment content and process underestimated. When models and hypotheses concerning these are better developed, interactions of all three can be examined. This is entirely consistent with a normal psychology of pain, that recognizes pain as a biological and psychological threat to an individual's integrity which those individuals manage with varying short and long term effectiveness. Within this framework, people with chronic pain could be considered not necessarily to be in some way vulnerable to pain, or weak or deficient before the onset of pain, but to be a cross-section of the psychologically robust and less robust. Pain presents specific challenges and patients have both biological and psychological reasons for their behavior in the face of those challenges.

To the detriment of both, the biological and psychological models remain largely unintegrated. From the astounding advances made in neuroscience since the proposal of the gate control model we know much more about the biology of pain, but this knowledge is largely restricted to peripheral and spinal mechanisms of acute pain in animals. Apart from recent imaging studies defining areas of cortical activity, most exciting findings but not always straightforward to interpret, psychologists work with the conscious and voluntarily reported experiences of humans, often with clinical and persistent pain. Models connecting these levels are largely lacking, not least because of the proliferation of overlapping concepts in psychology used to characterize patient-reported experiences and behavior. Yet we lack a comprehensive model (such as exists in neurophysiology, for example) to test these concepts against one another. We do not yet know how to parse the cognitive domain. Frameworks that offer some systematic principles for doing so, such as evolutionary psychology's approach to the function of behavior and emotion (Barkow et al. 1992), are almost universally neglected in pain. Evolutionary psychology proposes that attention and emotion are controlled by an organism's priorities, of which the threat of pain is a major component, and that many responses are initiated without a conscious decision. Conscious control, with which psychologists and others work in pain management, provides checks and redirection of behavior compatible with further priorities of the individual. On reflection, it is surprising that so much change can be effected by psychologists working with patients' conscious and voluntary report of their behavior.

I venture to propose, in the absence of other guiding principles, four core concepts in the normal psychology of pain. First is attention, in which the understanding of pain as an interruption by virtue of its being a biological threat is key(and persistent pain as a persistent interruption) (Eccleston and Crombez 1999). Second is catastrophizing (described at the beginning of this chapter) and processing the content of attention in negative ways that amplify the threat. Third is avoidance, behavior logically related to the predictions generated by catastrophizing and by fears of pain and of (re)injury (Vlaeyen and Linton 2000). The concepts of fear, avoidance, and catastrophizing are better grounded in theory and are more empirically supported than are processes of "somatization" to account for patients' anxious preoccupation with pain and related symptoms (Sharpe and Williams 2002). Fourth is depression, now undergoing reevaluation in chronic pain to characterize the extent to which pain is processed in a self-denigratory way as a threat to identity and self-worth (Pincus and Morley 2001; Clyde and Williams 2002; Morley and Williams 2002). Some patients, while clearly distressed by pain and its impact on their lives, assert that they are doing as well as possible under the circumstances. Thus, their limitations are attributable to pain and not to personal deficiencies; the process of acceptance (McCracken 1998) is related to the issue of depression. This list differs radically from one that might have been made 10 years ago, in which distraction, behavioral contingencies, and coping strategies would have been prominent.

Treatment that reflects this view will aim for an endpoint not of freedom from symptoms but of maximum freedom from the negative impact of pain; that is, changing the individual's relationship to the pain, and its meaning for him or her. Key tasks in treatment, therefore, will be to develop these core concepts in relation to the prediction of observable behaviors, to work toward their integration with neurophysiological models of pain, and to extend cognitive concepts into interpersonal behavior (as is already occurring with some concepts such as catastrophizing). Further advances in treatment will result from the application of specific cognitive and behavioral techniques to well-identified behavioral and psychological problems in pain patients engaged in medical and physical treatments. Such advances will include extending CBT methods into populations with primary pathologies such as arthritis (see Astin et al. 2002), cancer (Turk and Fernandez 1990; Syrjala et al. 1995; Turk et al. 1998), spinal cord injury (Turner et al. 2002), and sickle cell disease (Thomas et al. 2001). The next generation of treatment studies must draw upon more explicit models to inform design of intervention and choice of outcomes, and must focus on understanding mechanisms as well as on quantifying effects. Such progress promises to consolidate and extend the effectiveness of treatment, its accurate targeting, its acceptability to patients, and its ease of integration with medical and physical therapies.

ACKNOWLEDGMENTS

Many of the ideas in this paper have been developed in collaboration with Chris Eccleston and Stephen Morley; I am also indebted to Chris Main, Frank Keefe, and the late Patrick Wall, mentors over many years, and to Eija Kalso and the Oxford pain research group with whom I have worked on reviews of evidence.

REFERENCES

Astin JA, Beckner W, Soeken K, Hochberg MC, Berman B. Psychological interventions for rheumatoid arthritis: a meta-analysis of randomized controlled trials. *Arthritis Rheum* 2002; 47:291–302.

Barkow JH, Cosmides L, Tooby J (Eds). *The Adapted Mind.* Oxford: Oxford University Press, 1992.

Clyde Z, Williams ACdeC. Depression and mood. In: Linton SJ (Ed). *New Avenues for the Prevention of Chronic Musculoskeletal Pain and Disability*, Pain Research and Clinical Management, Vol. 12. Amsterdam: Elsevier Science, 2002, pp 105–121.

Cutler RB, Fishbain DA, Rosomoff HL, et al. Does nonsurgical pain center treatment of chronic pain return patients to work? *Spine* 1994; 19:643–652.

Eccleston C, Crombez G. Pain demands attention: a cognitive-affective model of the interruptive function of pain. *Psychol Bull* 1999; 125:356–366.

Eccleston C, Morley S, Williams ACdeC, Yorke L, Mastroyannopoulou K. Systematic review of randomised controlled trials of psychological therapy for chronic pain in children and adolescents, with a subset meta-analysis. *Pain* 2002; 99:157–165.

Farrar JT, Portenoy RK, Berlin JA, Kinman JL, Strom BL. Defining the clinically important difference in pain outcome measures. *Pain* 2000; 88:287–294.

Flor H, Fydrich T, Turk DC. Efficacy of multidisciplinary pain treatment centers: a meta-analytic review. *Pain* 1992; 49:221–230.

Guzmán J, Esmail R, Karjalainen K, Irvin E, Bombadier C. Multidisciplinary rehabilitation for chronic low back pain: systematic review. *BMJ* 2001; 322:511–516.

Keefe FJ, Lefebvre JC, Egert JR, et al. The relationship of gender to pain, pain behavior, and disability in osteoarthritis patients: the role of catastrophizing. *Pain* 2000; 87:325–334.

Malone MD, Strube MJ. Meta-analysis of non-medical treatments for chronic pain. *Pain* 1988; 34:231–244.

McCracken LM. Learning to live with the pain: acceptance of pain predicts adjustment in persons with chronic pain. *Pain* 1998; 74:21–27.

McQuay H, Moore A. *An Evidence-based Resource for Pain Relief.* Oxford: Oxford University Press, 1998.

Morley S, Williams ACdeC. Conducting and evaluating treatment outcome studies. In: Turk DC, Gatchel RJ (Eds). *Psychological Approaches to Pain Management: A Practitioners Handbook,* 2nd ed. New York: Guilford Press, 2002, pp 52–68.

Morley SJ, Eccleston C, Williams ACdeC. Systematic review and meta-analysis of randomised controlled trials of cognitive behaviour therapy and behaviour therapy for chronic pain in adults, excluding headache. *Pain* 1999; 80:1–13.

Nicholas MK, Wilson PH, Goyen J. Comparison of cognitive-behavioral group treatment and an alternative non-psychological treatment for chronic low back pain. *Pain* 1992; 48:339–347.

Pincus T, Morley S. Cognitive processing bias in chronic pain: a review and integration. *Psychol Bull* 2001; 127:599–617.

Pincus T, Burton AK, Vogel S, Field AP. A systematic review of psychological factors as predictors of chronicity/disability in prospective cohorts of low back pain. *Spine* 2002; 27:E109–E120.

Price DD. *Psychological Mechanisms of Pain and Analgesia,* Progress in Pain Research and Management, Vol. 15. Seattle: IASP Press, 1996.

Radley A, Billig M. Accounts of health and illness: dilemmas and representations. *Social Health Illness* 1996; 18:220–240.

Reitsma B, Meijler WJ. Pain and patienthood. *Clin J Pain* 1997; 13:9–21.

Rosenstiel AK, Keefe FJ. The use of coping strategies in chronic low back pain patients: relationship to patient characteristics and current adjustment. *Pain* 1983; 17:33–44.

Roth A, Fonagy P. *What Works for Whom? A Critical Review of Psychotherapy Research.* New York: Guilford Press, 1996.

Sharpe M, Williams ACdeC. Treating patients with somatoform pain disorder and hypochondriasis. In: Turk DC, Gatchel R (Eds). *Psychological Approaches to Pain Management: A Practitioners Handbook,* 2nd ed. New York: Guilford Press, 2002, pp 515–533.

Sullivan MJL, Thorn B, Haythornthwaite JA, et al. Theoretical perspectives on the relation between catastrophizing and pain. *Clin J Pain* 2001; 17:53–61.

Superio-Cabuslay E, Ward MM, Lorig KR. Patient education interventions in osteoarthritis and rheumatoid arthritis: a meta-analytic comparison with nonsteroidal antiinflammatory drug treatment. *Arthritis Care Res* 1996; 9:292–301.

Syrjala KL, Donaldson GW, Davis MW, Kippes ME, Carr JE. Relaxation and imagery and cognitive-behavioral training reduce pain during cancer treatment: a controlled clinical trial. *Pain* 1995; 63:189–198.

Thomas VJ, Gruen R, Shu S. Cognitive-behavioural therapy for the management of sickle cell disease pain: identification and assessment of costs. *Ethn Health* 2001; 6:59–67.

Turk DC. Statistical significance and clinical significance are not synonyms! *Clin J Pain* 2000; 16:185–187.

Turk DC, Fernandez E. On the putative uniqueness of cancer pain: do psychological principles apply? *Behav Res Ther* 1990; 28:1–13.

Turk DC, Sist T, Okifuji A, et al. Adaptation to metastatic cancer pain, regional/local cancer pain and non-cancer pain: role of psychological and behavioral factors. *Pain* 1998; 74:247–256.

Turner JA. Educational and behavioral interventions for back pain in primary care. *Spine* 1996; 21:2851–2857.

Turner JA, Jensen MP, Warms CA, Cardenas DD. Catastrophizing is associated with pain intensity, psychological distress, and pain-related disability among individuals with chronic pain after spinal cord injury. *Pain* 2002; 98:127–134.

Van Tulder MW, Ostelo R, Vlaeyen JWS, et al. Behavioral treatment of for chronic low back pain: a systematic review within the framework of the Cochrane Back Review Group. *Spine* 2000; 25:2688–2699.

Vlaeyen JWS, Linton SJ. Fear-avoidance and its consequences in chronic musculoskeletal pain: a state of the art. *Pain* 2000; 85:317–332.

Williams ACdeC, Richardson PH, Nicholas MK, et al. Inpatient vs. outpatient pain management: results of a randomised controlled trial. *Pain* 1996; 66:13–22.

Williams ACdeC, Nicholas MK, Richardson PH, Pither CE, Fernandes J. Generalizing from a controlled trial: the effects of patient preference versus randomization on the outcome of inpatient versus outpatient chronic pain management. *Pain* 1999; 83:57–65.

Correspondence to: Amanda C. de C. Williams, PhD, INPUT Pain Management Unit, St. Thomas Hospital, London SE1 7EH, United Kingdom. Email: amanda.williams@kcl.ac.uk.

Proceedings of the 10th World Congress on Pain,
Progress in Pain Research and Management, Vol. 24,
edited by Jonathan O. Dostrovsky, Daniel B. Carr, and
Martin Koltzenburg, IASP Press, Seattle, © 2003.

65

Hypnotic Analgesia and Its Applications in Pain Management[1]

Robert G. Large,[a] Donald D. Price,[b] and Russell Hawkins[c,d]

[a]*The Auckland Regional Pain Service, Auckland District Health Board, Auckland, New Zealand;* [b]*Departments of Oral and Maxillofacial Surgery and Neuroscience, University of Florida, Gainesville, Florida, USA;* [c]*School of Psychology, University of South Australia, Adelaide, Australia;* [d]*Flinders Medical Centre, Pain Management Unit, Adelaide, Australia*

Hypnotic analgesia has been described in anecdotal terms for centuries. Recent research has built on a modern understanding of hypnosis using psychometric, neurophysiological, and imaging techniques. We now have a better understanding of the psychological and neurophysiological mechanisms that underpin this phenomenon. At the same time, clinical trials testing the efficacy of hypnosis in acute and chronic pain management have been growing in number. This chapter surveys current knowledge of the mechanisms of hypnotic analgesia and the efficacy of hypnosis in acute and chronic pain management.

MECHANISMS OF HYPNOTIC ANALGESIA

WHAT IS A HYPNOTIC STATE AND HOW DOES IT FACILITATE SUGGESTIONS FOR ANALGESIA?

In an experiential-phenomenological study of the common elements that comprise the experience of a hypnotic state (Price and Barrell 1990), graduate students and faculty experienced several hypnotic inductions. A group consensus regarding the common elements that were necessary or sufficient

---

[1] Based on a Congress workshop.

for a hypnotic state was then determined. The consensus elements included: (1) A feeling of mental relaxation (a letting go of tensions or becoming at ease, not necessarily physical relaxation); (2) an absorbed and sustained focus of attention on one or few targets; (3) a relative absence of judging, monitoring, and censoring; (4) a suspension of one's usual orientation toward time, location, and/or sense of self; and (5) an experience of one's own responses as automatic (i.e., without deliberation and/or effort).

It was also evident from descriptions of the observers' direct experiences of the hypnotic state that interrelationships existed among these elements. Thus, element 1 ("relaxation, becoming at ease") and element 2 ("absorbed and sustained focus") appeared to provide a supportive general background for elements 3 ("absence of judging, monitoring, censoring") and 4 ("suspension of usual orientation toward time and location"). The latter two elements, in turn, appeared to maintain element 5 ("automaticity"). Finally, all observers agreed that elements 4 ("suspension") and 5 ("automaticity") directly contributed to perceived hypnotic depth. In a separate study (Price 1996), subjects then rated these factors during conditions of normal waking baseline and hypnotic state. Path analysis of these ratings provided a preliminary confirmation of these interactions. The experiential and conceptual basis for these common experiential dimensions is generally supported by the work of others (Bowers 1978; Pekula and Kumar 1984).

Because a hypnotic state facilitates incorporation of suggestions, such as those for analgesia, this model implicitly provides a basis for an intervention that is unique and distinguishable from other types of psychologically mediated increases in responsiveness to suggestion (e.g., placebo). This basis is evident in the phenomenology of the interrelationships between the common dimensions of this model and may be recognized in the following description.

A hypnotic state begins with a relaxed condition of mental (and often physical) ease in combination with an absorbed and sustained focus on an object or objects of attention (Hilgard 1977). Thus, initial suggestions for induction of this state are almost always directed toward these two dimensions. However, this state can occur naturally during fascination, watching an absorbing movie, or watching ripples in a stream. It captures us. At first, it can be effortful, but with time one proceeds from an *active* form of concentration to a relaxed, *passive* form. There is often an inhibition or reduction in the peripheral range of one's experience. At the same time, this relaxation and reduction in range of attention support a *lack* of monitoring and censoring of that which is allowed into experience. Hence, inconsistencies are now more tolerable. Contradictory statements, which once arrested attention and caused confusion or disturbance, now no longer do so. The uncensored acceptance of what is being said by the hypnotist is not checked against one's own associations. Consequently, one no longer chooses or validates the correctness of incoming statements. This lack of censorship allows thinking and meaning-in-itself to be disconnected from active reflection. From this way of experiencing, there emerges the sense of *automaticity,* wherein thinking does not precede an action but action precedes thought (Bowers 1978). Thus, if the hypnotist suggests a bodily action, a sensation, or a lack of sensation (e.g., pain), there is no experience of deliberation or effort on the part of the subject. The subject simply and automatically identifies with the suggested action, sensation, or lack of sensation, as it is suggested. In this way, a hypnotic state *facilitates* the incorporation of suggestions, such as analgesia.

It may well be that what is unique about hypnotic suggestions is not the end result of the suggestions themselves, such as pain relief, but the way in which the suggestions implicitly or explicitly refer to the source of experiential change—it is both internal and automatic. The nature of hypnotic suggestions for analgesia refers to an innate and *self-directed* capacity to alter one's own experience, often with the effect that one can experience sensations differently (Barber and Adrian 1982). The source of experiential change is perceived as occurring automatically and from within.

DO ASSOCIATIONS EXIST BETWEEN DIMENSIONS OF HYPNOTIC STATE AND NEURAL ACTIVITY IN SPECIFIC BRAIN REGIONS?

Rainville et al. (1999) used positron emission tomography (PET) to show differences in brain activity between normal waking and hypnotic states. In comparison to normal baseline, hypnotic states displayed higher neural activity (measured by regional cerebral blood flow) in occipital cortical areas as well as in anterior cingulate regions. In a subsequent study Rainville et al. (2002) showed significant associations between ratings of absorption and mental relaxation and activity in brain areas critically involved in the regulation of consciousness. In the case of absorption, these areas included the pontomesencephalic brainstem, medial thalamus, and rostral anterior cingulate cortex. These areas involve a distributed brain network that is part of an attentional system. In the case of mental relaxation, increases in occipital cortical activity were most likely related to decreased arousal that occurs in the face of increased focus on one or few objects of attention. Interestingly, both studies were conducted on the same subjects that exhibited decreased pain responses as a result of hypnotic suggestions. Thus, taken together, both self-ratings and changes in activity within brain structures involved in regulation of conscious states provide evidence that subjects undergoing hypnotic analgesia do indeed develop a hypnotic state during hypnotic analgesia. This interpretation is supported further by the results that self-ratings of absorption, relaxation, and brain activity were all significantly correlated with hypnotic susceptibility scores and by the finding that the degree of analgesia was also significantly correlated with hypnotic susceptibility scores.

IS HYPNOTIC ANALGESIA ACCOMPANIED BY CHANGES IN NEURAL ACTIVITY IN PAIN-RELATED AREAS OF THE CENTRAL NERVOUS SYSTEM?

Subjects in the studies described above by Rainville et al. (1999, 2002) also were participants in two brain imaging studies of hypnotic analgesia. In both studies, subjects rated pain sensation intensity and pain unpleasantness of moderately painful immersion of the left hand in a 47°C water bath. Two experimental conditions of the first study included one in which hypnotic suggestions were given to *enhance* pain unpleasantness and another in which suggestions were given to *decrease* pain unpleasantness. Suggestions also were given in both conditions to the effect that, unlike pain unpleasantness, pain sensation would not change. Suggestions for enhancement of unpleasantness increased the magnitude of both pain-unpleasantness ratings and neural activity in the anterior cingulate cortex (ACC, area 24) in comparison to the condition wherein suggestions for decreased unpleasantness were given. Neural activity in the primary (S1) somatosensory cortex, and subjects' mean ratings of pain sensation intensity, were not statistically different across the two experimental conditions. A second study used hypnotic suggestions to modify the intensity of pain sensation. In this experiment, the suggestions were effective in producing parallel changes in ratings of pain sensation intensity and neural activity in the S1 somatosensory cortex (Hofbauer et al. 2001).

Brain-imaging studies of hypnotic analgesia are complemented by studies that question whether hypnotic analgesia involves descending brain-to-spinal cord inhibitory mechanisms. An example of this approach is a study by Kiernan et al. (1995), who examined changes in the R-III, a nociceptive spinal reflex, during hypnotic reduction of pain sensation and unpleasantness. The R-III was measured in 15 healthy volunteers who gave sensory and affective ratings on a visual analogue scale of an electrical stimulus during conditions of resting wakefulness without suggestions and during hypnosis with suggestions for hypnotic analgesia. A critically important feature of this study was that subjects were blind to the physiological index being measured and, when later informed that measurements were being made of the R-III flexion reflex, were unable to intentionally reduce the magnitude of this reflex. Hypnotic sensory analgesia was partially yet reliably related to reduction in the R-III ($R^2 = 0.51$, $P < 0.003$), suggesting that it is at least partly mediated by descending antinociceptive mechanisms that exert control at spinal levels.

TOP-DOWN MODULATION OF PAIN SENSATION AND PAIN AFFECT BY COGNITIVE FACTORS

Current knowledge about the brain mechanisms of pain modulation by hypnosis is consistent with other studies of neural circuits that provide top-down modulation of pain experience. Central neural mechanisms associated with such phenomena as placebo/nocebo, hypnotic suggestion, attention, distraction, and even ongoing emotions are now thought to modulate pain by decreasing or increasing neural activity within many of the brain structures involved in pain. This modulation includes endogenous pain-inhibitory and pain-facilitatory pathways and circuitry.

Porro and colleagues (2002) used functional magnetic resonance imaging (fMRI) to study activity in cortical nociceptive brain regions of healthy volunteers while they expected the nociceptive stimulation of one foot, which might be stimulated with painful subcutaneous injection of ascorbic acid. Mean fMRI signal intensity increased over baseline values during both actual nociceptive stimulation and anticipation of pain in the absence of stimulation. These increases occurred in precisely the same cortical areas, including the contralateral S1, and bilaterally in the ACC, insular cortex, and medial prefrontal cortex. In all of these areas, changes in signal intensity during anticipation of pain were in the same direction as during pain itself but about 30–40% as large. These results provide evidence for top-down mechanisms involved in sensory and affective dimensions of pain, even in the absence of actual nociceptive stimulation. Thus, the cortical networks involved in pain may be directly influenced by cognitive factors. These are likely to include not only anticipation of the presence of pain, but also anticipation of its reduction, as in the case of placebo or hypnotic analgesia.

DONALD D. PRICE

HYPNOSIS IN CHRONIC PAIN MANAGEMENT: EFFICACY TRIALS

The persistent or relapsing nature of chronic pain challenges the therapist to develop strategies that will endure beyond the therapy session, or that can be utilized by the patient as self-management techniques. The literature is extensive on the use of hypnosis for clinical pain. Most published accounts are anecdotal and uncontrolled, but are particularly useful in gleaning techniques and approaches. Generally, the techniques described are highly individualized and do not tend to involve standardized scripts.

CONTROLLED CLINICAL TRIALS

Melzack and Perry (1975) compared alpha EEG feedback with hypnosis in the form of a modified Hartland ego-strengthening tape in 24 patients with established chronic pain syndrome. Six patients had alpha feedback, 6 had hypnosis, and 12 the combination. The combination was the most effective, and hypnosis was superior to alpha feedback. Elton et al (1980) compared hypnosis with placebo tablets and "behavioral psychotherapy" in 30 patients with chronic pain syndrome. The hypnosis group had the best outcomes. Hypnosis was individualized to patient needs; this study was one of the few controlled trials to do so. James et al. (1989) selected five highly hypnotizable subjects with chronic pain and used a multiple baseline design to track treatment effects. Hypnosis was individualized, and each patient developed self-hypnosis exercises. Two patients had long-term resolution, two continued to use self-hypnosis effectively, and one patient showed no change. Edelson and Fitzpatrick (1989) randomized 27 patients with chronic pain to three groups: hypnosis, cognitive-behavioral therapy, and a control condition. The hypnosis and cognitive-behavioral therapy components were identical except for the use of an induction procedure in hypnosis. The cognitive-behavioral therapy group showed increased activity and decreased pain, while the hypnosis group showed a reduction in pain intensity only.

McCauley et al. (1983) randomized 17 patients with low back pain to undergo self-hypnosis or relaxation. Both groups reported significant decreases in pain scores at 3 months. Self-hypnosis patients reported less time to sleep onset, and physicians rated their use of medications as less problematic.

Whorwell et al. (1984) compared hypnosis in the form of general relaxation and ego-strengthening suggestions to "supportive psychotherapy" in a controlled trial of 30 patients with irritable bowel syndrome. The hypnosis group reported reductions in pain experience and abdominal distension, with no change in the supportive psychotherapy group.

Following hypnosis, Prior et al. (1990) found a reduction in rectal sensitivity assessed by balloon manometry in 15 patients with irritable bowel syndrome. In contrast, Haanen et al. (1991), in 40 patients with fibromyalgia, found that hypnosis diminished pain and fatigue and improved sleep compared with physical therapy, but did not reduce tender point sensitivity. In another study on irritable bowel syndrome, Houghton et al. (1996) compared 25 patients treated with hypnosis to 25 patients attending clinics but not receiving hypnosis. Hypnosis-treated patients reported less severe pain, bloating, nausea, flatulence, urinary symptoms, lethargy, backache, and dyspareunia. Psychic well-being, mood, locus of control, physical well-being, and work attitude were improved. Work adherence was improved in the hypnosis group.

Galovski and Blanchard (1998) conducted an American replication of the U.K. studies of irritable bowel syndrome (Whorwell et al. 1984; Prior et al. 1990; Houghton et al. 1996). Six pairs of patients matched for disease severity were randomized in a multiple baseline study. Improvements were noted in pain, constipation, and flatulence. Forbes et al. (2000) compared hypnosis by a hypnotherapist with a therapeutic audiotape in irritable bowel syndrome. Seventy-six percent improved with hypnotherapy, and the tape was effective for 59%. In 54 patients with complete data, symptom scores were reduced significantly ($P < 0.05$) with hypnotherapy, compared with the tape.

Lu et al. (2001) compared acupuncture with hypnosis for facial, head, and neck pain. Acupuncture was best for acute pain but hypnosis was best for what the authors termed "psychogenic pain." Gay et al. (2002) compared Ericksonian hypnosis (a method emphasizing indirect and permissive suggestions) with Jacobson relaxation (a method using alternate tensing and relaxing of sequential muscle groups) in osteoarthritis. They found decreased pain and reduced analgesic use in both treatment groups compared with controls. Langenfeld et al. (2002) investigated the use of hypnosis in HIV/AIDS-related pain using an A-B time series analysis in five patients over 12 weeks. All five patients showed significant decreases in at least one of the three dependent measures: severity of pain, time spent in pain, and amount of p.r.n. medication taken.

Olness et al. (1987) studied 28 children with classic migraine. Children experienced a significant decline in headache frequency after learning self-hypnosis compared with using propranolol, which was no better than placebo. Van Dyck et al. (1991) studied 55 patients with tension headache, comparing autogenic training (a relaxation technique employing suggestions of warmth and heaviness) with future-oriented hypnotic imagery. The treatments were equally effective. Ter Kuile et al. (1994) compared autogenic training and cognitive self-hypnosis (which explicitly attempts to change appraisal and cognitive coping processes) in recurrent headache. There were no differences between treatment conditions. Subjects who were more easily hypnotized did better in both treatments.

SUMMARY OF EFFICACY TRIALS

The results of studies looking at the efficacy of hypnosis in chronic noncancer pain are promising. However, hypnosis has not been shown to be superior to relaxation or other psychological interventions. Rigorous experimental methodology generates studies that use standardized hypnotic approaches, while the more sophisticated, individualized techniques are more often applied in case reports or small group designs. There is still a need for rigorous evaluation of the more sophisticated hypnotic interventions and this is more likely to be met by the accumulation of good single subject and small group studies than by randomized controlled trials. Ideally, it might be possible to combine the advantages of both types of approaches.

ROBERT G. LARGE

HYPNOSIS IN PAIN MANAGEMENT: LITERATURE REVIEWS

Turner and Chapman (1982) reported finding no controlled studies comparing hypnosis with a credible placebo for the control of chronic pain. They concluded that "the clinical research in this area is sparse, appallingly poor, and has failed to convincingly demonstrate that hypnosis has more than a placebo effect in relieving chronic pain" (Turner and Chapman 1982, p. 30). This section will consider literature syntheses published since that time in order to determine whether any alternative conclusion is now justified.

ASSESSMENT OF THE QUALITY OF INTEGRATIVE LITERATURE

McQuay and Moore (1998) warn that reviews of inadequate quality may be worse than none, because faulty decisions may be made with unjustified confidence. Oxman and Guyatt (1991) have provided a method of assessing the quality of a review, which will be used herein.

Searches for reviews of hypnosis and clinical pain (not primary trials) were conducted using multiple electronic databases (search terms and inclusion criteria are available from R. Hawkins), and a prominent Internet discussion list on hypnosis was used to appeal for additional information about hypnosis and pain (hypnosis-request@maelstrom.stjohns.edu). Hard copies of all potentially eligible reviews were obtained and assessed for their quality. Quality scores ranged from 0 to 8 on a 9-point scale. The median score was 1 (mean = 2.9, mode = 1). Reviews were categorized according to the type of pain considered (a full reference list is available from R. Hawkins).

DESCRIPTIONS OF THE INCLUDED REVIEWS

In the interest of brevity only a few illustrative studies will be presented. A more detailed account is available elsewhere (Hawkins 2001).

Various types of pain in aggregate. Montgomery et al. (2000) produced the only meta-analysis of the effects of hypnosis on pain found in the literature. They restricted inclusion to studies that used hypnosis to attempt to reduce pain, studies that included a no-treatment or standard-treatment control group, and studies that presented sufficient data to allow the calculation of effect sizes. This approach resulted in the inclusion of 18 studies and the calculation of 27 effect sizes. Overall the results indicated a moderate to large effect size (d = 0.74). Based upon combined analyses from more than 900 participants, the authors concluded that hypnotic suggestion is effective for analgesia. They found that for 75% of the aggregate study population, hypnosis provided substantial pain relief.

Pediatric oncology. Liossi (2000) reviewed applications of clinical hypnosis in pediatric oncology, including pain control during invasive procedures. She reviewed eight studies using hypnosis. In all the studies considered, hypnosis was associated with reduced pain. Hypnotic effects were typically equivalent to the control interventions when the latter were used.

Burns. Everett et al. (1993) compared four randomly assigned groups (hypnosis, lorazepam, hypnosis and lorazepam, or opioid medication alone). All groups showed decreases in pain reports, but no treatment group was superior to the others. A subsequent study (Patterson and Ptacek 1997) demonstrated that when baseline pain was not considered, the experimental group (hypnosis) did not differ from the control group, but when patients with high initial pain scores were considered separately, there was a significant difference between groups in favor of the hypnosis group. Patterson et al. (1997) concluded that there was "compelling evidence" for the analgesic effect of hypnosis in burn patients.

Gastrointestinal pain/irritable bowel syndrome. Talley et al. (1996) reviewed psychological treatments, including hypnosis, for the treatment of irritable bowel syndrome. They required that in order to qualify a study as methodologically acceptable it would have to achieve six out of eight quality criteria. The only report to achieve this a priori standard was a hypnotherapy study (Whorwell et al. 1984). This study showed that irritable bowel syndrome patients improved significantly more than did controls. Talley et al. (1996) were nonetheless critical of the Whorwell study because it utilized nonconsecutive volunteers and largely excluded subjects over 50 years old. Given that the Whorwell study achieved the a priori quality score, it is surprising that Talley et al. (1996, p. 285) concluded that "no trial to date has produced unequivocal evidence that psychological treatment is efficacious in irritable bowel syndrome."

Childbirth. Baram (1995) reported that there were only two well-designed randomized studies of hypnosis in labor and delivery. The first of these (Freeman et al. 1986) showed no advantage of hypnosis over psychoprophylaxis. The second (Harmon et al. 1990) initially trained women to control experimentally induced ischemic pain before applying this newly developed skill to labor. This study also assessed hypnotic susceptibility. Hypnosis resulted in shorter stage one labor, less medication requested, a greater proportion of spontaneous deliveries, higher Apgar scores, and less pain. Women who were highly susceptible and hypnotized had less postpartum depression.

Headache. Spinhoven (1988) reviewed hypnosis for headache control. A comparison of hypnosis with other psychological treatments (biofeedback, relaxation training, autogenic training) showed that while all treatments achieved some success in reducing headache, none of these procedures consistently showed superior results than the others.

SUMMARY OF LITERATURE REVIEWS

"Best available evidence" has come to be understood in terms of level, quality, relevance, and strength (National Health and Medical Research Council 1998). *Level* refers to the study design used in attempts to minimize bias, *quality* refers to attempts to minimize bias within a study, *relevance* refers to the extent to which the findings from a study might be applied in other clinical settings to different patients, and *strength* refers to the magnitude of effect sizes or to other statistical measures such as statistical and clinical effectiveness and the width of confidence levels.

Level of evidence. If an arbitrary cut-off quality score of 7/9 or above is used to assess reviews, it can be concluded that Level I evidence (evidence from a systematic review of all relevant trials) exists for the efficacy of hypnotic analgesia in the form of the meta-analysis conducted by Montgomery et al. (2000). Level I evidence also exists for the effects of hypnosis on pain specifically related to cancer and invasive medical procedures (Sellick and Zaza 1998; Pan et al. 2000) and for its effects on pain in gastrointestinal disease and irritable bowel syndrome (Talley et al. 1996). There is a conspicuous lack of Level I evidence (at the quality level nominated) for the application of hypnosis in the treatment of such prevalent forms of pain as low back pain, headache, childbirth, and burn pain.

Quality. Although there are some notable exceptions (e.g., Patterson's studies of burn patients and the Whorwell group's studies of irritable bowel syndrome), poor methodological quality remains pervasive in the hypnosis and pain literature. In particular, there remains a heavy reliance on case reports or uncontrolled studies, and high-quality randomized controlled trials are notably lacking in specific areas (e.g., chronic pain, including low back pain). Some studies may have been well designed but are not well reported; for example, it is not always clear from the publications whether random allocation to groups has occurred. Multiple other threats to internal validity exist, including a failure to include a credible placebo control condition.

Relevance. The pain of invasive medical procedures in children suffering from cancer has been often enough studied for generalization to be possible. Remarkably, the same cannot be said for various other types of pain, including chronic pain types typically treated in multidisciplinary pain clinics. The general failure to utilize or present detailed treatment protocols renders replication difficult. The extent to which generalization is possible is unknown. Threats to external validity include heterogeneous definitions of hypnosis and imprecision in the way hypnosis is conducted.

Strength. The Montgomery et al. (2000) meta-analysis found a moderate to large effect size (d = 0.74) for the effect of hypnosis on pain. The hypnosis literature still lacks any tendency to report outcome data in a manner that will allow the combination of data across studies (L'Abbé plots, odds ratios, effect sizes, and numbers needed to treat).

CONCLUSIONS

There is sufficient clinical evidence, of sufficient quality, for several high-quality reviews to have concluded that hypnosis has demonstrable efficacy in the treatment of pain. Because high-quality studies and high-quality reviews justify greater confidence in their findings, it is hoped that dissemination of information about the assessment of quality, in both primary clinical trials and literature reviews, may help to promote greater rigor in both types of studies in the future.

RUSSELL HAWKINS

REFERENCES

Baram DA. Hypnosis in reproductive health care: a review and case reports. *Birth* 1995; 22:37–42.

Barber J, Adrian C. *Psychological Approaches to the Management of Pain.* New York: Brunner/Mazel, 1982.

Bowers KS. Hypnotizability, creativity, and the role of effortless experiencing. *Int J Clin Exp Hyp* 1978; 26:184–202.

Edelson J, Fitzpatrick JL. A comparison of cognitive-behavioral and hypnotic treatments of chronic pain. *J Clin Psychol* 1989; 45:316–323.

Elton D, Burrows GD, Stanley GV. Hypnosis and chronic pain. *Aust J Clin Exp Hypn* 1980; 8:63–90.

Everett JJ, Patterson DR, Burns GL, Montgomery B, Heimbach D. Adjunctive interventions for burn pain control: comparison of hypnosis and Ativan: the 1993 Clinical Research Award. *J Burn Care Rehabil* 1993; 14:676–683.

Forbes A, MacAuley S, Chiotakakou-Faliakou E. Hypnotherapy and therapeutic audiotape: effective in previously unsuccessfully treated irritable bowel syndrome? *Int J Colorectal Dis* 2000; 15:328–334.

Freeman RM, Macaulay AJ, Eve L, Chamberlain GVP, Bhat AV. Randomised trial of self hypnosis for analgesia in labour. *BMJ* 1986; 292:657–658.

Galovski TE, Blanchard EB. The treatment of irritable bowel syndrome with hypnotherapy. *Appl Psychophysiol Biofeedback* 1998; 23:219–232.

Gay MC, Philippot P, Luminet O. Differential effectiveness of psychological interventions for reducing osteoarthritic pain. *Eur J Pain* 2002; 6:1–16.

Haanen HCM, Hoenderdos HTW, van Romunde LKJ, et al. Controlled trial of hypnotherapy in the treatment of refractory fibromyalgia. *J Rheumatol* 1991; 18:72–75.

Harmon TM, Hynan MT, Tyre TE. Improved obstetric outcomes using hypnotic analgesia and skill mastery combined with childbirth education. *J Consult Clin Psychol* 1990; 58:525–530.

Hawkins RMF. A systemic meta-review of hypnosis as an empirically supported treatment for pain. *Pain Rev* 2001; 8:47–73.

Hilgard ER. *Divided Consciousness: Multiple Controls in Human Thought and Action.* New York: John Wiley and Sons, 1977.

Hofbauer RK, Rainville P, Duncan GH, Bushnell MC. Cognitive modulation of pain sensation alters activity in human cerebral cortex. *Neurophysiologia* 2001; 86:402–411.

Houghton LA, Heyman DJ, Whorwell PJ. Symptomatology, quality of life and economic features if irritable bowel syndrome—the effect of hypnotherapy. *Aliment Pharmacol Ther* 1996; 10:91–95.

James FR, Large RG, Beale IL. Self-hypnosis in chronic pain: a multiple baseline study of five highly hypnotizable subjects. *Clin J Pain* 1989; 5:161–168.

Kiernan BD, Dane JR, Phillips LH, Price DD. Hypnotic analgesia reduces R-III nociceptive reflex: further evidence concerning the multifactorial nature of hypnotic analgesia. *Pain* 1995; 60:39–47.

Langenfeld MC, Cipani E, Borckardt JJ. Hypnosis for the control of HIV/AIDS related pain. *Int J Clin Exp Hypn* 2002; 50:170–188.

Liossi C. Clinical hypnosis in paediatric oncology: a critical review of the literature. *Sleep and Hypnosis* 2000; 2:125–131.

Lu DP, Lu GP, Kleinman L. Acupuncture and clinical hypnosis for facial and head and neck pain: a single crossover comparison. *Am J Clin Hypn* 2001; 44:141–148.

McCauley JD, Thelen MH, Frank RG, Willard RR, Callen KE. Hypnosis compared to relaxation in the outpatient management of chronic low back pain. *Arch Phys Med Rehabil* 1983; 64:548–552.

McQuay HJ, Moore RA. *An Evidence-Based Resource for Pain Relief.* Oxford: Oxford University Press, 1998.

Melzack R, Perry C. Self-regulation of pain: the use of alpha-feedback and hypnotic training for the control of chronic pain. *Exp Neurol* 1975; 46:452–469.

Montgomery GH, DuHamel KN, Redd WH. A meta-analysis of hypnotically induced analgesia: how effective is hypnosis? *Int J Clin Exp Hypn* 2000; 48:138–153.

National Health and Medical Research Council. *A Guide to the Development, Implementation and Evaluation of Clinical Practice Guidelines.* Canberra: National Health and Medical Research Council, 1998.

Olness K, MacDonald JT, Uden DL. Comparison of self-hypnosis and propranolol in the treatment of juvenile classic migraine. *Pediatrics* 1987; 79:593–597.

Oxman AD, Guyatt GH. Validation of an index of the quality of review articles. *J Clin Epidemiol* 1991; 44:1271–1278.

Pan CX, Morrison RS, Ness J, Fugh-Berman A, Leipzig RM. Complementary and alternative medicine in the management of pain, dyspnea and nausea and vomiting near the end of life: a systematic review. *J Pain Symptom Manage* 2000; 20:374–387.

Patterson DR, Ptacek JT. Baseline pain as a moderator of hypnotic analgesia for burn injury treatment. *J Consult Clin Psychol* 1997; 65:60–67.

Patterson DR, Adcock RJ, Bombardier CH. Factors predicting hypnotic analgesia in clinical burn pain. *Int J Clin Exp Hypn* 1997; 45:377–395.

Pekula RJ, Kumar VK. Predicting hypnotic susceptibility by a self-report phenomenological instrument. *Am J Clin Hypn* 1984; 27:114–121.

Porro CA, Balraldi P, Pagnoni G, et al. Does anticipation of pain affect cortical nociceptive systems? *J Neurosci Res* 2002; 22:3206–3214.

Price DD. The neurological mechanisms of hypnotic analgesia. In: Joseph Barber WW (Ed). *Hypnosis and Suggestion in the Treatment of Pain.* New York: Norton, 1996, pp 117–136.

Price DD, Barrell JJ. The structure of the hypnotic state: a self-directed experiential study. In: Barrell JJ (Ed). *The Experiential Method: Exploring the Human Experience.* Massachusetts: Copely, 1990, pp 85–97.

Prior A, Colgan SM, Whorwell PJ. Changes in rectal sensitivity after hypnotherapy in patients with irritable bowel syndrome. *Gut* 1990; 31:896–898.

Rainville P, Hofbauer RK, Paus T, et al. Cerebral mechanisms of hypnotic induction and suggestion. *J Cogn Neurosci* 1999; 11:110–125.

Rainville P, Hofbauer RK, Bushnell MC, et al. Hypnosis modulates activity in brain structures involved in the regulation of consciousness. *J Cogn Neurosci* 2002; 14:887–901.

Sellick SM, Zaza C. Critical review of 5 nonpharmacologic strategies for managing cancer pain. *Cancer Prev Control* 1998; 2:7–14.

Spinhoven P. Similarities and dissimilarities in hypnotic and nonhypnotic procedures for headache control: a review. *Am J Clin Hypn* 1988; 30:183–194.

Spinhoven P, Linssen AC. Education and self-hypnosis in the management of low back pain: a component analysis. *Br J Clin Psychol* 1989; 28:145–153.

Spinhoven P, Linssen AC, van Dyck R, Zitman FG. Autogenic training and self-hypnosis in the control of tension headache. *Gen Hosp Psychiatry* 1992; 14:408–415.

Talley N, Owen BK, Boyce P, Paterson K. Psychological treatments for irritable bowel syndrome: a critique of controlled treatment trials. *Am J Gastroenterol* 1996; 91:277–286.

ter Kuile MM, Spinhoven P, Linssen AC, et al. Autogenic training and cognitive self-hypnosis for the treatment of recurrent headaches in three different subject groups. *Pain* 1994; 58:331–340.

ter Kuile MM, Spinhoven P, Linssen AC, van Houwelingen HC. Cognitive coping and appraisal processes in the treatment of chronic headaches. *Pain* 1996; 64:257–264.

Turner JA, Chapman CR. Psychological interventions for chronic pain: a critical review. II. Operant conditioning, hypnosis, and cognitive-behavioral therapy. *Pain* 1982; 12:23–46.

van Dyck R, Zitman FG, Linssen AC, Spinhoven P. Autogenic training and future oriented imagery in the treatment of tension headache: outcome and process. *Int J Clin Exp Hypn* 1991; 39:6–23.

Whorwell PJ, Prior A, Faragher EB. Controlled trial of hypnotherapy in the treatment of severe refractory irritable-bowel syndrome. *Lancet* 1984; ii:1232–1234.

Correspondence to: Robert G. Large, MBChB, PhD, The Auckland Regional Pain Service, Auckland District Health Board, Auckland Hospital, Building 7, Private Bag 92024, Auckland, New Zealand. Email: boblarge@actrix.co.nz.

Correspondence regarding database search to: Russell Hawkins, PhD, Psychological Studies, National Institute of Education, Nanyang Technological University, 1 Nanyang Walk, Singapore 637616. Email: rhawkins@nie.edu.sg.

Proceedings of the 10th World Congress on Pain,
Progress in Pain Research and Management, Vol. 24,
edited by Jonathan O. Dostrovsky, Daniel B. Carr, and
Martin Koltzenburg, IASP Press, Seattle, © 2003.

66

Translating Evidence for Psychological Interventions to Manage Recurrent Pain and Chronic Pain in Children and Adolescents: Three Trials[1]

Christopher Eccleston,[a,b] Vivian P.B.M. Merlijn,[c]
Joke A.M. Hunfeld,[c] and Gary A. Walco[d,e]

[a]Pain Management Unit, University of Bath, Bath, United Kingdom; [b]Royal National Hospital for Rheumatic Diseases, Bath, United Kingdom; [c]Department of Medical Psychology and Psychotherapy, Erasmus University, Rotterdam, The Netherlands; [d]David Center for Children's Pain and Palliative Care, Joseph M. Sanzari Children's Hospital at Hackensack University Medical Center, Hackensack, New Jersey, USA; [e]Department of Pediatrics, University of Medicine and Dentistry of New Jersey, Newark, New Jersey, USA

The medical community has matured to the point where it is now acceptable to openly acknowledge and discuss the fact that children and adolescents experience pain on a regular basis (Fearon et al. 1996; Perquin et al. 2000). From this acknowledgment follows the responsibility to recognize that there are subpopulations of adolescents and children with pain who require pain management. In this chapter we report on three studies that share the goal of successful translation of clinical research findings to populations of children with disabling pain. All three evaluate cognitive behavioral therapy (CBT) for the management of pain. Walco and colleagues conducted the first study in the United States. This study enrolled children with cancer, for whom repeated exposure to procedures is a common and necessary part of treatment, and for whom these interventions are typically painful and distressing. Merlijn and Hunfeld conducted the second study in the

[1] Based on a Congress workshop.

Netherlands. This study assessed a pilot educational program delivered in the community for adolescents with chronic and recurrent pain. Eccleston and colleagues conducted the third study in the United Kingdom. This study employed an interdisciplinary residential program for adolescents with chronic pain (Eccleston et al., in press).

THE EVIDENCE BASE

Before focusing on individual studies it is instructive to assess the evidence for psychological interventions for chronic and recurrent pain in children and adolescents. There are many randomized controlled trials and effectiveness studies of CBT for pediatric chronic pain. Recent systematic reviews and meta-analyses have found that the strongest evidence for effectiveness lies with relaxation and biofeedback training for chronic headache (Herman et al. 1995; Holden et al. 1999; Eccleston et al. 2002). Fewer published trials describe psychological interventions for children and adolescents with chronic nonheadache pain (Janicke et al. 1999; Kibby et al. 1999; Walco et al. 1999). Significant problems that hamper the design and delivery of randomized controlled trials of CBT in children and adolescents are discussed at length in the evidence reviews and elsewhere (e.g., Durlak et al. 1995; Kazdin and Weisz 1998). Table I summarizes the main challenges.

These challenges are difficult, but not impossible, to overcome. International efforts are needed to allow psychosocial researchers to pilot interventions, develop study protocols, refine measurement technologies, and to enhance methods for evaluation other than randomized controlled trials. In time, the evidence base will be become stronger. The three studies we report herein are part of the foundation work to strengthen and broaden the evidence base.

PROCEDURE-RELATED PAIN

In all trials, but particularly in pediatric pain studies, it is essential to define specific outcomes. Pain, distress, and responses to intervention may be assessed in three major dimensions, as summarized in Table II.

The first study was designed to compare systematically a number of indicators of procedure-related distress in children with cancer undergoing lumbar puncture. A secondary aim was to assess the impact of three different treatment modalities on these outcomes: deep sedation (propofol),

Table I
Barriers to successful randomized controlled trials of psychosocial interventions for pediatric chronic pain (after Eccleston et al. 2002; Walco et al. 1999)

1) Small numbers of patients and other participants in any one study site
2) Difficulty with participants adhering to study protocols
3) Lack of clarity over what is an acceptable or desirable outcome
4) Lack of age- and developmentally appropriate measurement tools
5) Lack of clear guidance on therapy content

conscious sedation (midazolam plus an opioid), and CBT strategies plus topical anesthetic.

Forty-eight participants between the ages of 3.1 and 17.7 years (mean = 8.9, SD = 4.46) were receiving treatment at a large suburban medical center in the United States. Most were diagnosed with acute lymphocytic leukemia. Time elapsed since initial diagnosis ranged from 2 weeks to 4.25 years.

In order to assess the child's subjective experience, levels of anxiety, anticipated pain, self-efficacy, expectancy, and coping self-efficacy prior to the procedure were taken using visual analogue scales (VAS). Parents rated their own anxiety as well as their child's level of anxiety using a similar VAS. Behavioral distress was assessed with the Procedure Behavior Checklist (LeBaron and Zeltzer 1984) before, during, and after the procedure, focusing on muscle tension, screaming, crying, restraint used, pain verbalized, anxiety verbalized, verbal stalling, physical resistance, flinching, and groaning. Physiological parameters were assessed using a cardiac vagal tone monitor (Porges 1995). Mean cardiac vagal tone and mean heart rate were calculated over 10-second epochs, with a primary focus on the three epochs prior to initial needle insertion, the epoch that included initial needle insertion, and the three epochs immediately after needle insertion. A second index of physical reactivity to stress was the change in salivary cortisol

Table II
Three-systems approach to measurement of pain and distress in children and adolescents undergoing painful medical procedures (after Morison et al. 2001)

Subjective Experience
Self-report of the child's subjective experience, typically focused on pain, anxiety, or other aspects of emotional arousal using various means, such as intensity ratings or visual analogue scales

Behavior
Behavioral indicators are often assessed through observation of their frequency, intensity, or duration

Physiology
Physiological parameters that indicate increased arousal, such as heart rate variability or increases in salivary cortisol

concentration from before procedure to 20 minutes afterward. Physicians rated the difficulty of the procedure. Finally, the duration of the procedure and physician stress during the procedure were also recorded.

The choice of pain management strategy was made independent of the study, typically reflecting physician or family preference. For those children receiving propofol, an anesthesiologist administered the drug through a central venous catheter, after which the lumbar puncture was performed by a pediatric oncologist. Other children were administered conscious sedation, a combination of midazolam and an opioid, by the oncologist. Children using CBT were coached by a child life specialist who was trained with a semi-standardized protocol for self-regulatory strategies to be used during invasive procedures (Solomon et al. 1998). A topical anesthetic consisting of 2.5% lidocaine and 2.5% prilocaine (EMLA Cream, Astra Pharmaceuticals) was also placed over the site of the lumbar puncture at least 90 minutes prior to the procedure. Regardless of the method of sedation or coping, local infiltration of buffered lidocaine was used prior to the lumbar puncture.

Both behavioral and self-report measures indicated low levels of distress overall. In contrast, physiological parameters indicated that regardless of treatment strategy, stress was still significant for children undergoing lumbar punctures. Cardiac vagal tone and heart rate measures were significantly negatively correlated within and across time frames (pre-, during, and postprocedure). This finding is expected in that these systems generally operate in an antagonistic fashion. Intriguingly, there was a very strong correlation between cardiac vagal tone during the epoch immediately prior to needle insertion and the subsequent epoch that included the insertion itself. This correlation implies that although many participants were consciously or deeply sedated, they had an anticipatory response to a nociceptive stimulus. Across epochs, heart rate was relatively stable while cardiac vagal tone was more erratic. Beginning in the epoch immediately prior to needle insertion, the autonomic system appears to consolidate as heart rate increases while vagal tone concomitantly decreases. Once the acute threat subsides, the parasympathetic nervous system reactivates to restore homeostasis.

Postprocedure salivary cortisol levels were significantly higher than preprocedure levels. The average 300% increase is substantial, as a 10% increase from pre-stress levels is deemed significant (Klimes-Dougan et al. 2001). It is also important to note that neither propofol nor midazolam are expected to increase cortisol levels; if anything they suppress production of stress hormones (Aitkenhead et al. 1989).

As for relationships across physiological and behavioral dimensions, those individuals with higher levels of behavioral distress prior to the procedure had higher heart rates at the time of needle insertion. In this case, the behavioral response preceded the increase in heart rate at the time of needle insertion. It may be the case that certain individuals, perhaps through temperament, react with increased levels of arousal in both behavioral and physiological dimensions. Future studies should explore this possibility.

Self-report and behavioral measures indicated that children were fairly comfortable undergoing the observed lumbar punctures with all three treatment modalities. In addition, ratings of technical difficulty and times needed to complete the procedure were nearly identical across the three groups. Thus, even in the absence of protocolized assessments of patients' needs, current strategies appear to address the subjective experience and behavioral indicators of procedure-related distress among children with cancer.

Physiological parameters, however, differed between the groups. First, children who relied on CBT strategies and topical anesthesia had significantly lower heart rates, especially at the time of needle insertion, than did those who received conscious or deep sedation. Second, changes in salivary cortisol before and after the procedure were more marked in children receiving conscious or deep sedation than in those using CBT strategies and topical anesthesia. The differences were dramatic and appeared to be clinically significant, but barely failed to reach levels of statistical significance. There also appears to be a high level of within-subject variability for changes in cortisol levels as a function of stress, as indicated by a near-zero correlation of pre- and post-procedure salivary cortisol levels.

In sum, a desirable goal in managing procedural distress in children is to implement systematic decision-making processes to match patients to appropriate interventions, which maximize clinical efficacy and minimize deleterious effects and cost. The present data show that during ongoing research one must be extraordinarily careful in defining outcome measures and that a combination of self-report, behavioral, and physiological indicators of distress must be addressed.

COMMUNITY-BASED ADOLESCENT CHRONIC PAIN MANAGEMENT

Recent studies on the potential determinants and maintenance factors of chronic pain and disability have shown that adolescents with chronic pain have higher levels of negative affect and fear of failure, greater use of emotion-focused avoidance coping strategies, and less strong perceptions of themselves as socially accepted. In addition, adolescents with chronic pain report receiving less attention for their pain behavior from peers and parents and are exposed to a higher number of adults with pain behavior (Merlijn et al. 2003). The identification of psychosocial variables that help maintain pain has led to the development of psychosocial therapies for children and adolescents with chronic pain and associated distress and disability. Most programs make use of relaxation techniques, biofeedback, and cognitive techniques for pain control (e.g., Osterhaus et al. 1993). A self-management program using a printed manual and telephone contacts, although less expensive than a clinic-based program guided by a therapist, may be equally effective (e.g., Griffith and Martin 1996). Programs involving the guidance of parents also have positive effects on the pain of their children (Sanders et al. 1994; Allen and Shriver 1998).

Much of the evidence base is, as previously stated, focused on headache. Few trials have included adolescents suffering from nonheadache pain or have specifically focused on parental or peer involvement with nonheadache pain. We now report an outpatient, educationally based program for adolescents in The Netherlands with chronic pain in which parents and peers are invited to participate. This pilot study includes an evaluation of the feasibility of an education-based program, as well as preliminary indications of its potential effectiveness. The program included a number of components of CBT, including cognitive reframing, techniques of relaxation, and attention to and advice for increasing physical activity. The ideas of reinforcement and modeling of pain behavior were discussed in separate meetings with parents. These meetings emphasized the value of taking pain seriously and not ignoring pain behavior. Prior research indicates that parents often report a belief that their children complain of pain in order to avoid aversive or non-preferred activity (Hunfeld et al. 2002). Doubting the credibility of another's pain experience may shape adolescent pain complaints and associated disability. Equally unwanted may be overattentiveness, which reinforces pain complaint and disability. General guidelines on how to deal with pain and pain behavior are offered to the parents (based on Allen and Shriver 1998). Inviting parents and the children's peers to the training provided support for the participating adolescent with pain. To enhance understanding and support from parents for mechanisms behind coping with pain, attention was paid to this process. Thus, the ways in which parents experienced their own pain and managed their own distress were discussed and compared with the coping strategies of their children.

The program was 9 weeks long and comprised five group meetings and four telephone contacts. During the latter, a psychologist and assistant psychologist discussed the material the adolescents had studied at home and the homework assignments completed without therapist contact. At the beginning and end of the education program, the parents attended parent-only education sessions. Self-management was promoted by trainer reinforcement and directed problem-solving. During week five of the program telephone contact was made with parents to discuss their experiences with the guidelines and the program. In the same week, peers were invited to an adolescent group meeting. General information on pain in adolescence and pain behavior was provided. The peers were asked to perform an "obstacle course" in order to experience possible interference by pain with daily activities.

For this pilot study, eight adolescents with headache and nonheadache pain were interviewed about their training experience and asked whether this type of program was worth pursuing. Brief biographical and pain-related information is reported in Table III.

Adolescents completed a pain diary consisting of pain intensity VAS scores and questionnaires on psychosocial determinants (vulnerability, reinforcement, modeling, and coping) and quality of life. They did so 2 weeks before the program commenced and immediately after treatment. Details of the instruments are available on request from the authors (Merlijn and Hunfeld; merlijn@mpp.fqq.eur.nl).

Because of the small number of participants, preliminary statistical data are not reported. Qualitative data from the interviews showed that although adolescents found the group meetings relatively challenging at first, they came to enjoy the experience. A common comment after treatment was a wish for more time to practice coping skills under trainer direction. Parents judged the information they received to be useful and described their involvement as an important element in the program. Recruitment to the program from a community population was a significant problem in this study,

Table III
Pain characteristics from the first eight patients in a community-based adolescent chronic pain management program

Age (years)	Primary Type of Pain	Pain Frequency	Severity*	Problem*	Disability*
14	Limb pain	At least twice a week	38	62	56
14	Limb pain	At least twice a week	12	39	25
16	Headache	Every day	33	55	56
16	Abdominal pain	Every day	66	85	59
16	Headache	At least twice a week	66	62	59
16	Abdominal pain	At least twice a week	55	80	59
17	Headache	At least twice a week	–	–	–
18	Limb pain	Once a week	77	70	56

* Measured with visual analogue scales of 0–100 anchored by the phrases "no pain" and "the worst pain you can imagine," "no problem" and "the biggest problem you can imagine," and "no disability" and "the most disability you can imagine."

as was adherence to training and to the research protocol. In summary, although there was a strong theoretical basis to the training program and those attending were generally satisfied with their experience, the research team had difficulty in recruiting and retaining participants. Continuation and expansion of the study will incorporate means to increase motivation and adherence to the education-based training program.

RESIDENTIAL ADOLESCENT CHRONIC PAIN MANAGEMENT

Malleson et al. (2001) recently argued that the optimal treatment regime for adolescents with severe chronic pain is an interdisciplinary cognitive behavioral treatment (ICBT) program that focuses on pain management and rehabilitation to normal activity, and involves family members in treatment. In the Bath Pain Management Unit in the United Kingdom 57 patients (41 girls) were entered into a residential ICBT pain management program with a parent. Both the adolescents and their accompanying parent or guardian were required to be resident for the 3-week duration of the program. The mean age of the patients was 14 years, and the mean duration of chronic pain was 4.02 years. The most common diagnosis was of complex regional pain syndrome (CRPS) type I (26.4%). The mean length of time away from full-time education was 17 months, with a median of 12 months. Multiple assessments were made in a number of areas for both the adolescents and their primary accompanying adult. Included were the VAS for pain intensity, the Spence Children's Anxiety Scale (Spence 1998), the internalizing subscale of the Pain Coping Questionnaire (Reid et al. 1998), the Functional Disability Index (Walker and Green 1991), the Child Depression Inventory (Kovaks 1981), physical performance measures of a timed walk over 10 meters, and the maximum number of sit to stand movements possible in 60 seconds. Also included was a measure of school performance. Adults were also asked to complete measures of their child's pain and functional disability. Adults also reported on their own anxiety and depression with the Hospital Anxiety and Depression Scale (Zigmund and Snaith 1983), and rated the stress they experienced as parents using the Parenting Stress Index (Abidin 1995).

Operant and cognitive behavioral principles were incorporated in all aspects of the treatment. Primary themes of the program were the promotion of positive change despite pain, encouragement to achieve independence from medical and social care, and a return to normal everyday adolescent activity. The treatment was organized over 3 weeks. The day was structured like a school day to facilitate the development of skills to manage a return to full-time education. Many sessions required evening or weekend homework.

A rationale for therapy was introduced before each component. Emphasis was placed on normalization, home practice, and the maintenance and promotion of change at home. Patients received written information about all aspects of the program and compiled a patient manual. The clinical psychologist managed the therapy process, ensuring coherence and consistency. Regular team meetings were scheduled and monitored. Changes in therapeutic direction were decided and agreed upon in team meetings. Notes were taken after each session and routinely audited. The treatment program consisted of three main themes running across the delivery of all coping strategies: education, activity, and cognitive therapy.

Immediately following treatment the adolescents reported no significant changes on any self-report measure. However, they had significant improvement on the timed measures of physical function, with an average improvement on the timed walk of 2.61 seconds (95% confidence interval [CI], –1.02 to –4.2) and for sit to stand of 3.22 movements per patient per minute (CI +0.79 to +5.65). Three months following treatment the adolescents had maintained these physical improvements and also had statistically significant improvements in the self-report measures of anxiety, disability, and somatic awareness. Immediately following treatment the adults reported significant improvement in their adolescents' disability and in their own depression and parental stress. Three months following treatment all significant improvements were maintained. Of the 42 patients whose category of schooling could have improved, 27 improved at least one category of schooling (chi square 17.71, $P < 0.001$). An example of a category shift is from less than half the week to more than half the week spent in class. Twelve patients remained in the same category and three worsened by one category. The number of half-day sessions of school attended increased significantly from a mean of 3.28 to 5.69 (range 0–10) with a mean difference score of 2.41 (CI 1.13 to 3.69). The more conservative test of the effect of treatment overall for all 56 patients was also significant, with a mean difference score of 1.97 (CI 1.0 to 3.0).

By using measurement instruments in a range of domains of chronic pain experience it was possible to explore differential improvement at different time points after treatment. Immediate treatment gains were evident for children only in physical performance, and this improvement increased in the long term. There were more treatment gains for parents of adolescents immediately after treatment, raising the question of a relationship between positive changes in parents (reduced anxiety and parenting stress) and longer-term positive changes in adolescents. These results provide evidence for the effectiveness of ICBT in the improvement of psychological status, physical performance, and return to normal daily activity. Our findings offer a foundation for building future studies to translate the evidence base into clinical practice and that incorporate nontreatment or alternative treatment control groups.

CONCLUSION

Evidence exists for the effectiveness of psychological treatments to manage chronic pain in children and adolescents. In some areas this evidence base is excellent and the story is a positive report of achievements and successes (e.g., in headache). In other areas (e.g., chronic musculoskeletal pain) the evidence base is poor and the story resembles more a plan of action, or an adventure one is contemplating. However, there is guidance for this adventure. We have reported on three very different studies from three different parts of the world that exemplify the promise in this field of work. All show the importance of defining the domains of outcome and the tools for measuring effectiveness. All show the importance of involving significant other people, and in particular parents, in treatment. Finally, all show that clinical research with distressed children and adolescents is challenging but can produce interesting and worthwhile results from which to build. We look forward to the next generation of studies.

REFERENCES

Abidin RR. *Parenting Stress Index*. Odessa, FL: Psychological Assessment Resources, 1995.

Aitkenhead AR, Pepperman ML, Willatts SM, et al. Comparison of propofol and midazolam for sedation in critically ill patients. *Lancet* 1989; 2:704–709.

Allen KD, Shriver MD. Role of the parent-mediated pain behaviour management strategies in biofeedback treatment of childhood migraine. *Behav Ther* 1998; 29:477–490.

Durlak JA, Wells AM, Cotton JK, et al. Analysis of selected methodological issues in child psychotherapy research. *J Clin Child Psychol* 1995; 24:141–148.

Eccleston C, Morley S, Williams A, et al. Systematic review of randomised controlled trials of psychological therapy for chronic pain in children and adolescents, with a subset meta-analysis of pain relief. *Pain* 2002; 99:157–165.

Eccleston C, Malleson PN, Clinch J, et al. Chronic pain in adolescents: evaluation of a programme of inter-disciplinary cognitive behaviour therapy. *Arch Dis Child;* in press.

Fearon I, McGrath PJ, Achat H. Booboos: the study of everyday pain among young children. *Pain* 1996; 68:55–62.

Griffiths, JD, Martin PR. Clinical- versus home-based treatment formats for children with chronic headache. *Br J Health Psychol* 1997; 1:151–166.

Hermann C, Kim M, Blanchard EB. Behavioral and prophylactic pharmacological intervention studies of pediatric migraine: an exploratory meta-analysis. *Pain* 1995; 60:239–256.

Holden EW, Deichmann, MM, Levy J. Empirically supported treatments in pediatric psychology: recurrent pediatric headache. *J Pediatr Psychol* 1999; 24:91–109.

Hunfeld JAM, Perquin CW, Hazebroek-Kampschreur AAJM, et al. Physically unexplained chronic pain and its impact on children and their families: their mother's perception. *Psychol Psychother Theory Res Pract* 2002; 75:251–260.

Janicke DM, Finney JQ. Empirically supported treatments in pediatric psychology: recurrent abdominal pain. *J Pediatr Psychol* 1999; 24:115–127.

Kazdin AE, Weisz JR. Identifying and developing empirically supported child and adolescent treatments. *J Consult Clin Psychol* 1998; 66:19–36.

Kibby MY, Tyc VL, Mulhern RK. Effectiveness of psychological intervention for children and adolescents with chronic medical illness: a meta-analysis. *Clin Psychol Rev* 1998; 18:103–117.

Klimes-Dougan B, Hastings PD, Granger DA, Usher B, Zahn-Waxler C. Adrenocortical activity in at risk and normally developing adolescents: individual differences in salivary cortisol basal levels, diurnal variation and responses to social challenges. *Dev Psychopathol* 2001; 13:695–719.

Kovaks M. Rating scales to assess depression in school aged children. *Acta Paedopsychiatr* 1981; 46:305–315.

LeBaron S, Zeltzer L. Assessment of acute pain and anxiety in children and adolescents by self-report, observer reports, and a behavior checklist. *J Consult Clin Psychol* 1984; 52:729–738.

Malleson PN, Connell H, Bennett SM, et al. Chronic musculoskeletal and other idiopathic pain syndromes. *Arch Dis Child* 2001; 84:189–192.

Merlijn VPBM, Hunfeld JAM, van der Wouden JC, et al. Psychosocial factors associated with chronic pain in adolescents. *Pain* 2003; 101:33–43.

Morison SJ, Grunau RE, Oberlander TF, Whitfield MF. Relations between behavioral and cardiac autonomic reactivity to acute pain in preterm neonates. *Clin J Pain* 2001; 17:350–358.

Osterhaus SO, Passchier J, van der Helm-Hylkema H, et al. Effects of behavioral psychophysiological treatment on schoolchildren with migraine in a non-clinical setting: predictors and process variables. *J Pediatr Psychol* 1993; 18:697–715.

Perquin CW, Hazebroek-Kampscheur AAJM, Hunfeld JAM, et al. Pain in children and adolescents: a common experience. *Pain* 2000; 87:51–58.

Porges SW. Cardiac vagal tone: a physiological index of stress. *Neurosci Biobehav Rev* 1995; 19:225–233.

Reid GJ, Gilbert CA, McGrath PJ. The Pain Coping Questionnaire: a preliminary validation. *Pain* 1998; 76:83–96.

Sanders MR, Shepherd RW, Cleghorn G, et al. The treatment of recurrent abdominal pain in children: a controlled comparison of cognitive behavioral family intervention and standard pediatric care. *J Consult Clin Psychol* 1994; 62:306–314.

Solomon R, Walco GA, Robinson MR, Dampier CD. Pediatric pain management: program description and preliminary evaluation results of a professional course. *J Dev Behav Pediatr* 1998; 19:193–195.

Spence SH. A measure of anxiety symptoms among children. *Behav Res Ther* 1998; 36:545–566.

Walco GA, Sterling CM, Conte PM, Engel RG. Empirically supported treatments in pediatric psychology: disease related pain. *J Pediatr Psychol* 1999; 24:155–167.

Walker LS, Greene JW. The Functional Disability Inventory: measuring a neglected dimension of child health status. *J Pediatr Psychol* 1991; 16:39–58.

Zigmund AS, Snaith RP. The Hospital Anxiety and Depression Scale. *Acta Psychiatr Scand* 1983; 67:361–370.

Correspondence to: Christopher Eccleston, PhD, Director, Pain Management Unit, Department of Psychology, University of Bath, Claverton Down, Bath BA2 7AY, United Kingdom. Email: hssce@bath.ac.uk.

Proceedings of the 10th World Congress on Pain,
Progress in Pain Research and Management, Vol. 24,
edited by Jonathan O. Dostrovsky, Daniel B. Carr, and
Martin Koltzenburg, IASP Press, Seattle, © 2003.

67

A Biopsychosocial Approach to Fibromyalgia and Chronic Fatigue Syndrome[1]

Laurence A. Bradley,[a] Milton L. Cohen,[b] and Egil A. Fors[c]

[a]Division of Clinical Immunology and Rheumatology, University of Alabama at Birmingham, Birmingham, Alabama, USA; [b]Darlinghurst Arthritis and Pain Research Clinic, St Vincent's Medical Centre, Sydney, New South Wales, Australia; [c]Multidisciplinary Pain Center, Norwegian University of Science and Technology, Trondheim, Norway

Fibromyalgia (FM) and chronic fatigue syndrome (CFS) are perplexing syndromes characterized by musculoskeletal pain, fatigue, and high levels of health care utilization. In addition, few pharmacological or behavioral therapies have produced better outcomes than those evoked by appropriate placebo interventions. There is considerable debate regarding the mechanisms underlying these disorders and the extent to which basic and clinical research will lead to improved treatment outcomes.

This chapter critically examines these issues, beginning with Dr. Cohen's contribution, "The Failure of Fibromyalgia." Dr. Cohen identifies several weaknesses associated with the classification criteria for FM and with its conceptualization as a construct that is distinct from other chronic pain syndromes. This is followed by Dr. Bradley's section, "Current Models of Fibromyalgia and Chronic Fatigue Syndrome," which reviews recent findings concerning physiological and psychosocial factors that influence pain sensitivity in persons with FM or CFS. The chapter concludes with Dr. Fors' survey of "Guided Imagery, Attention to Pain, and Antidepressants in Fibromyalgia," which examines the effects of training FM patients to use mental imagery techniques to reduce pain.

---

[1] Based on a Congress workshop.

THE FAILURE OF FIBROMYALGIA

The American College of Rheumatology (ACR) formed a committee of investigators to perform a multi-site empirical study to establish reliable and valid classification criteria for FM (Wolfe et al. 1990). Those classification criteria are (a) widespread pain that has persisted for at least 3 months and (b) abnormal pain sensitivity at 11 or more of 18 specific anatomic sites termed "tender points." Although previous investigators had differentiated FM that occurs in the absence of other medical disorders (i.e., primary FM) from that which occurs after the development of other conditions (i.e., secondary FM), the ACR committee concluded that this distinction was no longer necessary.

The study performed by the ACR committee was characterized by several methodological and semantic weaknesses. For example, the criteria used by each investigator to identify patients as having FM were idiosyncratic. This approach was understandable in the absence of a gold standard, but it was likely to produce heterogeneity in case identification across study sites.

In addition, the definition of "widespread pain" led to a high level of heterogeneity within the FM construct. This definition required pain to be present on the left and right sides of the body, above and below the waist, plus axial pain. Shoulder and buttock pain were each defined as "involved side" pain whereas low back pain was defined as "below waist" pain. Thus, pain in one shoulder, the contralateral buttock and the anterior chest would fit the definition of "widespread pain." How this might differ from "pain all over" was not clear.

Finally, major problems were involved in the quantification of tenderness given that ordinal categories (grades of tenderness) were subjected to statistical tests appropriate for continuous variables (Cohen and Quintner 1998). The absence of reliable measures of mechanical allodynia that could act as a gold standard for the diagnosis of FM clearly influenced the deliberations of the ACR committee which, on the basis of receiver-operator plots, "reduced the number of tender points required for examination from 24 to 18" before determining that any 11 of these 18 provided the best diagnostic criteria. The end result of the exercise was this diagnostic equation: FIBROMYALGIA = WIDESPREAD PAIN + TENDER POINTS.

DOES THE "TENDER POINT" CRITERION DISTINGUISH FIBROMYALGIA FROM OTHER PAINFUL CONDITIONS?

The construct of FM asserts that its tender point criterion allows it to be differentiated from other conditions associated with persistent pain. Table I

Table I
Performance of ACR classification criteria for fibromyalgia

Criterion	Sensitivity (%)	Specificity (%)	False Positive (%)
Widespread pain	98	31	69
Pain "all over"	67	81	19
11 of 18 tender points	90	78	22
12 of 14 tender points*	65	89	11
Widespread pain and 11 of 18 tender points†	88	81	19

* Smythe and Moldofsky (1977).
† ACR criteria (Wolfe et al. 1990).

extends the published data on sensitivity and specificity from the ACR study by adding the false positive rate (the proportion of those meeting the specified diagnostic criteria who are considered not to have the condition). Despite the fact that tender points were the basis for provisionally labeling patients with widespread pain as having FM, the ACR criteria had sensitivity of only 88%. With regard to specificity, 19% of patients fulfilled the diagnostic criteria but were considered not to have FM.

The problems of sensitivity and specificity associated with the classification criteria raised three challenges to this construct of FM. First, it was not possible to determine the medical conditions responsible for the pain experienced by the 19% of the patients who were false positives. Indeed, it will never be possible to meet this challenge so long as FM is allowed to coexist with any other painful condition.

The second challenge was to diagnose the false-negative patients, i.e., those with widespread pain but fewer than 11 tender points. This challenge was solved by the decision to award such patients the diagnosis of FM, provided that their pain was "widespread", and that they suffered many of the symptoms considered to be characteristic of the syndrome such as fatigue, sleep disturbance, irritable bowel syndrome, paresthesiae, and psychological disturbance (Wolfe et al. 1996). This moving of the goal posts was a blatant violation of methodological integrity.

The third challenge was to interpret the significance of high tender point counts in individuals who do not report widespread pain. In other words, can tender point counts be used as a pathognomonic diagnostic criterion if a high count (≥11 tender points) can occur independently of widespread pain? This challenge has been met by a community-based study that found that tender points are associated with psychological and general distress, independently of the pain status of the individual (Croft et al. 1994).

Thus, the diagnostic validity of the tender point count has been refuted, reducing the defining equation to: FIBROMYALGIA = WIDESPREAD PAIN. That is, the name became a synonym for the presenting complaint although widespread pain is neither a syndrome nor a diagnosis.

Nevertheless, it is still asserted that FM is a "recognizable clinical entity," although simultaneously it is conceded that the construct is a "clinical invention," that there is no discrete boundary between it and non-FM, and that there are no uniformly accepted tests that can differentiate FM from other common pain disorders (e.g., Wolfe 1997a,b).

ERRORS IN ARGUMENT

In essence the FM label has been attached to an unbounded combination of recognizable clinical phenomena. As it admits all possibilities, this label constitutes a tautology, thus depriving it of any clinical or scientific meaning. What were the errors in argument that led to this situation, which threatens to withdraw legitimacy from those who suffer?

First, the use of the most prominent clinical feature of FM, the tender points, as the gold standard for a putative disease process represented a fallacious circular argument. This concentration on nosology—and the rush to diagnostic application—obscured any proper discussion of the clinical phenomena, repeating unlearned lessons from the history of "occupation neurosis," "railway spine," and "neurasthenia."

The second error was the attempt to group together disparate clinical features to create an apparently homogenous entity without a unifying theory. It would have been more appropriate to use the FM construct as a working hypothesis in order to test hypotheses of causation.

Finally, the tender point phenomenon itself—more correctly, mechanical allodynia—was all but ignored by the proponents of FM. It was asserted that "tender points" are central to the diagnosis but are mostly unknown to the patient and in any case are epiphenomenal to the pain (Littlejohn 1996). The number of tender points became the focus of concern; the nature or interpretation of the tenderness was considered irrelevant. This assertion of diagnostic utility over pathophysiological understanding constituted a logical and scientific contradiction.

CAN THE FIBROMYALGIA CONSTRUCT SURVIVE?

Clearly, the construct of FM does not survive critical analysis. However, the failure of this construct does not detract from the clinical problem it attempted to address. The key to understanding that problem is to dissect the clinical feature of mechanical allodynia. Only relatively recently has evidence appeared that the clinical phenomena of widespread pain and mechanical allodynia may represent disturbances of nociception at a central level (e.g., Kosek et al. 1995). Nevertheless, it remains difficult to distinguish between altered nociceptive function and increased propensity to pay attention to bodily events. Evolving insights from the neurobiology of pain and nociception will help in this respect. When conceptualized as the outcome of a complex interaction between nociceptive and psychosocial influences, FM is no different from other chronic pain entities: the clinical challenge it has bequeathed us is to understand the mechanisms underlying allodynia.

MILTON L. COHEN

CURRENT MODELS OF FIBROMYALGIA AND CHRONIC FATIGUE SYNDROME

Fibromyalgia and CFS are characterized by similar symptoms and by the absence of biological diagnostic markers that might be used to distinguish them from one another and from other disorders. The primary symptoms of FM are widespread, persistent, musculoskeletal pain and abnormal pain sensitivity at multiple anatomical sites in response to mechanical pressure and electrocutaneous and thermal stimulation (Wolfe et al. 1990).

Chronic fatigue syndrome is characterized by persistent, debilitating fatigue and secondary symptoms such as myalgias, sleep disturbance, and postexertional malaise. Persons with CFS or FM frequently report that they experience similar comorbidities such as irritable bowel syndrome (Aaron et al. 2000). It is not surprising, then, that among patients with CFS, between 35% and 70% meet criteria for FM and that 64% of patients with FM also meet criteria for CFS (Aaron et al. 2000). Nevertheless, individuals with CFS do not display abnormal pain sensitivity unless they also fulfill the classification criteria for FM (Buchwald 1996).

The following discussion examines two recent models of the pathogenesis of FM and CFS. It then describes the results of several investigations that have tested hypotheses derived from these models regarding abnormal pain sensitivity in persons with these disorders.

THEORETICAL MODELS

The development of classification criteria for FM and CFS (Wolfe et al. 1990; Fukuda et al. 1994) was followed by a substantial increase in research concerning the factors that contribute to pain in persons with these disorders.

Only recently, however, have investigators begun to develop models of the pathogenesis of FM and CFS and to test hypotheses derived from these models (e.g., Weigent et al. 1998). These models posit that among genetically predisposed individuals, interactions between one or more inciting events (e.g., physical trauma, environmental stressors, infection) and dysregulated central nervous system (CNS) functions (e.g., sleep, hypothalamic-pituitary-adrenal axis activity) can evoke or exacerbate abnormalities in pain transmission or inhibition that produce abnormal pain sensitivity and illness behaviors characteristic of FM. These models also suggest that environmental stressors or psychiatric illness may heighten affective distress and pain affect.

TESTS OF THE MODELS

Gracely and colleagues (2002) recently tested the hypothesis that cortical or subcortical augmentation of pain processing occurs in individuals with FM. Using functional magnetic resonance imaging (fMRI), the investigators compared changes in brain activation among patients with FM and healthy individuals in response to phasic, mechanical pressure stimulation of the left thumbnail bed under two conditions. In one condition, both patients and controls received stimulation at intensity levels (approximately 2.4 kg/cm^2) that evoked mean ratings of moderate pain intensity (11.3 on a 20-point scale) among the patients but evoked relatively low mean pain ratings among the controls (3.1). In the second condition, the controls received pressure stimulation at an intensity level (4.2 kg/cm^2) that evoked a mean pain rating (11.9) that was nearly identical to that produced by the patients in response to the lower stimulus.

When FM patients and controls received similar low levels of stimulation, patients exhibited significant increases in fMRI signal in 12 brain regions while the controls showed significant activation in only 2 regions. In contrast, when all subjects experienced similar levels of pain intensity, the controls displayed significant activation in a larger number of brain regions than the FM patients (i.e., 19 vs. 12), but there were 7 brain regions in which both the patient and control groups exhibited significant increases in fMRI signal. Together, these findings suggest that the abnormal pain sensitivity shown by patients with FM may be attributed to central augmentation of pain sensitivity rather than a generalized tendency of the patients to label stimulation as highly painful.

My colleagues and I have begun to test several hypotheses derived from Weigent's model regarding pain sensitivity in patients with FM, healthy controls, and in comparison groups such as patients with CFS or major depressive disorder (MDD). This model posits that interactions among multiple endogenous and exogenous factors (e.g., genetic influences, physical trauma) may produce symptoms such as pain and fatigue that are common to FM, CFS, and related disorders such as MDD. Nevertheless, the factors that distinguish persons with FM from those with similar disorders are the alterations in CNS function related to central sensitization that produce abnormal pain sensitivity at multiple anatomical sites. As noted earlier, the model also posits that environmental stressors and psychological distress may influence verbal and behaviorial displays of pain, but these factors are neither necessary nor sufficient to produce abnormal pain sensitivity. Therefore, the first hypothesis is that, although patients with FM, CFS, and MDD report similar symptoms, only patients who meet criteria for FM have verbal and physiological responses consistent with abnormal pain sensitivity.

We have found that, consistent with our first hypothesis, FM patients exhibit significantly lower pain thresholds in response to mechanical pressure stimulation than do patients with CFS or MDD and healthy controls (Cianfrini et al. 2001). We also have used single photon emission computed tomography (SPECT) to assess changes among these groups in brain regional cerebral blood flow (rCBF) in response to phasic pressure stimulation of three right-sided tender points (lower cervical, trapezius, and second rib). The stimulus intensity was calibrated so as to span each subject's respective pain threshold level (Cianfrini et al. 2001). The intensity of the pressure stimulation was about twice that used by Gracely et al. (2002) and produced relatively high mean pain intensity ratings of approximately 8.5 on a 10-cm visual analogue scale (VAS) among all subject groups. SPECT imaging revealed that the pressure stimulation evoked significant increases in brain rCBF in three brain regions (thalamus, somatosensory cortex, and anterior cingulate) in each group. The patients with FM displayed significant, bilateral (left and right hemisphere) increases in rCBF in the three regions. The CFS patients exhibited significant activation in the left and right somatosensory cortex and thalamus as well as in the contralateral anterior cingulate cortex. In contrast, the MDD patients and the controls showed significant activation in these brain regions primarily in the contralateral hemisphere.

Our finding that pressure stimulation evoked similar levels of pain intensity and activation of the same brain structures across all four subject groups is consistent with the results reported by Gracely et al. (2002). In addition, the activation of brain regions in both the left and right hemispheres among patients with FM or CFS suggests that pressure stimulation tended to evoke augmented neural input in these individuals. However, in accord with our hypotheses, the finding that FM patients displayed these responses to relatively low levels of pressure stimulation suggests that FM is

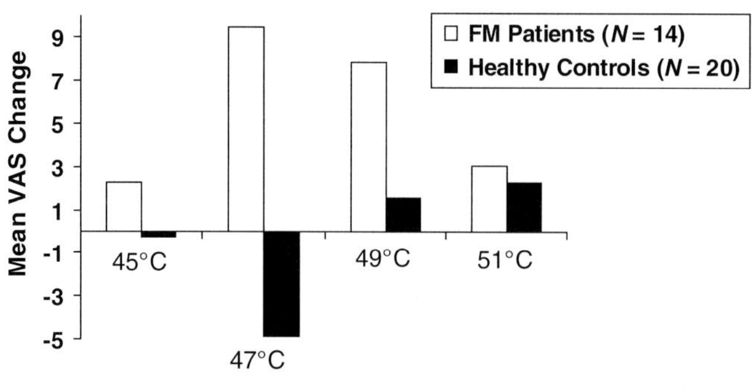

Fig. 1. Mean changes in visual analogue scale (VAS) ratings of pain unpleasantness evoked by thermal (heat) stimulation as a function of subject group and stimulus intensity. Patients with fibromyalgia showed significantly greater increases in VAS ratings than healthy controls ($P = 0.04$).

characterized by physiological alterations in pain processing that are distinct from the mechanisms underlying the symptoms of CFS or MDD.

We also have evaluated the effect of personally relevant, stressful imagery on magnitude estimates of pain evoked by thermal (heat) stimulation among patients with FM and healthy controls (McKendree-Smith et al. 2002). Our initial findings indicate that stressful imagery tends to produce modest increases in pain intensity ratings among patients and controls. However, Fig. 1 shows that stressful imagery produced significantly greater increases in ratings of pain unpleasantness among the patients with FM. The mechanisms underlying the patients' altered pain unpleasantness ratings remain to be determined in future studies.

In summary, publication of classification criteria for FM and CFS was gradually followed by the development of models of the pathogenesis of these disorders. Initial tests of hypotheses derived from these models suggest that, although FM and CFS are characterized by similar symptoms, only patients with FM exhibit abnormal pain sensitivity and augmented neural input in response to relatively low levels of pressure stimulation. In addition, personally relevant stressors produce greater increases in pain affect among FM patients relative to controls. Future tests of the models described above should lead to better understanding of the mechanisms underlying the symptoms of FM and CFS.

Laurence A. Bradley

GUIDED IMAGERY, ATTENTION TO PAIN, AND ANTIDEPRESSANTS IN FIBROMYALGIA

Cognition, emotion, and behavior influence individuals' pain perceptions. For example, focusing attention on painful symptoms through imagery or in consultation with a health professional may amplify the intensity of pain and other bodily sensations (Fors and Götestam 2000). In contrast, the use of guided imagery to divert attention from symptoms may reduce pain (Eller 1999). However, clinicians often provide both cognitive interventions and psychotropic medications to patients with FM (e.g., Arnold et al. 2000), which makes it difficult to assess the independent effects of these interventions and the extent to which changes in patients' pain reports covary with changes in mood. It is thus necessary to perform systematic, well-controlled trials to determine the independent effects of or interactions between cognitive and psychotropic therapies on FM patients' reports of pain and psychological distress. Therefore, my colleagues and I recently examined the effects of two cognitive interventions and amitriptyline versus those produced by appropriate placebos on VAS pain intensity ratings and self-reports of psychological function among patients with FM (Fors et al. 2002).

METHODS AND PROCEDURE

The patients consisted of 55 women previously diagnosed with FM with a mean age of 45.7 years (range 21–68 years); the mean time from onset of symptoms was 15.6 years. After providing informed consent, patients were randomly assigned to one of three cognitive and one of two pharmacological conditions. The cognitive interventions were (a) pleasant guided imagery; (b) attention imagery; and (c) a standard care control condition. Patients assigned the pleasant guided imagery condition used a 30-minute audiotape on a daily basis that instructed them to visualize beautiful natural settings on pleasant summer days. Patients in the attention imagery condition used a 30-minute audiotape on a daily basis that described how endorphins and inhibitory neurons act to modulate pain and instructed them to visualize the workings of their body's internal pain control systems. Patients in the control condition had an initial consultation with a supportive therapist who listened to their pain-related problems; following this consultation, the patients received their usual medical treatment without any other adjunct interventions.

The pharmacological interventions consisted of amitriptyline at a dose of 50 mg/day or a placebo that were prepared in identical capsules. The patients were instructed to take their medication once daily. Dosages were increased from 1 capsule (10 mg) the first day to 2 capsules (20 mg) the second day; dosages were then increased 10 mg every three days until 50 mg was reached on day 11. The first administration of both the cognitive and pharmacological interventions took place in our laboratory. The patients then managed their interventions at home for the next 28 days.

Outcome measures included a pain diary and three standardized measures of psychological function. The pain diary consisted of 28 pages with a 100-mm VAS with endpoints of "no pain" (0) to "severe pain" (100). The psychological measures included the Trait Anxiety Inventory, the Beck Depression Inventory, and the Automatic Negative Thoughts Questionnaire.

Patients completed the psychological measures and a pain VAS immediately prior to randomization to the treatment interventions. Following the first administration of their respective cognitive interventions, the patients completed a second pain VAS. They were instructed that, after returning home, they should complete their first pain diary VAS at 2 pm that day as well as on each subsequent day of the study. The patients returned to the laboratory on the final day of the study to deliver their pain diaries and again complete the psychological measures.

RESULTS

There were no baseline differences among the patient groups in age, education, time since symptom onset, baseline pain ratings, and psychological measures. However, there were significant group differences in pain outcomes. We found that the first exposure to pleasant guided imagery, compared to the control condition, produced a significantly greater reduction in patients' VAS pain ratings. There also was a positive effect of pleasant guided imagery on the pain diary ratings. Fig. 2 shows the results of a growth curve analysis of patients' pain diary ratings over the 28-day study period. Patients assigned to the pleasant guided imagery condition produced significantly greater reductions in pain diary ratings than did those assigned to the attention imagery and standard care control conditions. There was no effect of amitriptyline on patients' pain diary ratings, nor was there an interaction between the pharmacological and imagery conditions. In addition, all patient groups showed significant improvements in their self-reports of anxiety, depression, and automatic negative thoughts during the course of the study. Therefore, the positive effects of pleasant guided imagery were independent of both the pharmacological interventions and improvements in psychological function.

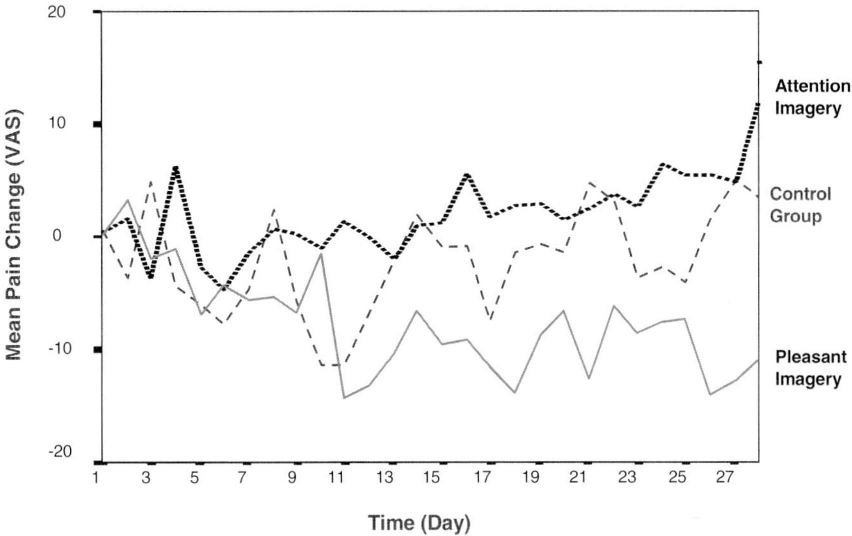

Fig. 2. Mean VAS ratings of pain intensity as a function of subject group and day of study. Guided pleasant imagery, compared to attention imagery and the standard care control condition, produced significantly greater reductions in pain intensity ratings over the 28-day study period.

DISCUSSION

Our findings suggest that it is beneficial to teach FM patients to divert attention from their pain both in a consultation setting and over a 28-day period. This finding is in accord with previous evidence that distractive coping strategies reduce subjective pain ratings (e.g., Petrovic et al. 2000). In contrast, the attention imagery condition tended to increase patients' pain diary ratings. This effect is consistent with evidence that intense monitoring of somatic symptoms or cues may serve to heighten subjective pain (Miller et al. 1988).

The lack of efficacy of amitriptyline is not surprising given that approximately two-thirds of patients with FM do *not* respond to this medication (Lautenschläger 2000). One might suggest that our 28-day study period may have been too short. However, previous placebo-controlled trials have shown that positive effects of amitriptyline begin to decline after 4 to 5 weeks of treatment (e.g., Carette et al. 1994). Nevertheless, some patients with FM respond to amitriptyline. Future studies should attempt to identify the characteristics that differentiate responders from nonresponders to this agent.

In summary, our findings suggest that audiotape-based instruction in guided pleasant imagery is a useful adjunct treatment for patients with FM. The positive effects of this intervention occur independently of changes in psychological function. It is necessary to determine whether our results may be replicated in other patient samples and whether the effects of guided pleasant imagery are maintained for more than 28 days.

EGIL A. FORS

ACKNOWLEDGMENTS

Preparation of this paper was supported by NIH grants 1-R01-AR-43136 and P60-AR-20164 from the National Institute of Arthritis and Musculoskeletal and Skin Diseases and by grant 5M0100032 from the National Center for Research Resources.

REFERENCES

Aaron LA, Burke MM, Buchwald D. Overlapping conditions among patients with chronic fatigue syndrome, fibromyalgia, and temporomandibular disorder. *Arch Intern Med* 2000; 160:221–227.

Arnold LM, Keck PE Jr, Welge JA. Antidepressant treatment of fibromyalgia: a meta-analysis and review. *Psychosomatics* 2000; 41:104–113.

Buchwald D. Fibromyalgia and chronic fatigue syndrome: similarities and differences. *Rheum Dis Clin North Am* 1996; 22:219–243.

Carette S, Bell MJ, Reynolds WJ, et al. Comparison of amitriptyline, cyclobenzaprine, and placebo in the treatment of fibromyalgia: a randomized, double-blind clinical trial. *Arthritis Rheum* 1994; 37:32–40.

Cianfrini LR, Bradley LA, Sotolongo A, et al. Abnormal pain sensitivity and chemical intolerance are not common to fibromyalgia and chronic fatigue syndrome. *J Pain* 2001; 2:12.

Cohen ML, Quintner JL. Fibromyalgia syndrome and disability: a failed construct fails those in pain. *Med J Aust* 1998; 168:402–404.

Croft P, Schollum J, Silman A. Population study of tender point counts and pain as evidence of fibromyalgia. *BMJ* 1994; 309:696–699.

Eller L. Guided imagery interventions for symptom management. *Annu Rev Nurs Res* 1999; 17:57–84.

Fors EA, Götestam KG. Patient education, guided imagery and pain related talk in fibromyalgia coping. *Eur J Psychiatry* 2000; 14:233–240.

Fors A, Sexton H, Götestam KG. The effect of guided imageries and amitriptyline on daily fibromyalgic pain: a prospective, randomized, controlled trial. *J Psychiatr Res* 2002; 36:179–187.

Fukuda K, Straus SE, Hickie I, et al. The chronic fatigue syndrome: a comprehensive approach to its definition and study. *Ann Intern Med* 1994; 21:953–959.

Gracely RH, Petzke F, Wolf JM, Clauw DJ. Functional magnetic resonance imaging evidence of augmented pain processing in fibromyalgia. *Arthritis Rheum* 2002; 46:1333–1343.

Kosek E, Ekholm J, Hanson P. Increased pressure pain sensibility in fibromyalgia patients is located deep to the skin but not restricted to muscle tissue. *Pain* 1995; 63:335–339.

Lautenschläger J. Present state of medication therapy in fibromyalgia syndrome. *Scand J Rheumatol* 2000; 113 (Suppl):32–36.

Littlejohn GO. Fibromyalgia syndrome. *Med J Aust* 1996; 165:387–391.

McKendree-Smith NL, Bradley LA, Alarcón GS, et al. Thermal pain sensitivity in fibromyalgia: patients exhibit greater stress-related increases in pain unpleasantness than healthy controls. *Arthritis Rheum* 2002; 46(Suppl):S108.

Miller S, Brody D, Summerton J. Styles of coping with threat: implications for health. *J Pers Soc Psychol* 1988; 54:142–148.

Petrovic P, Petersson KM, Ghatan PH, et al. Pain-related cerebral activation is altered by a distracting cognitive task. *Pain* 2000; 85:19–30.

Smythe HA, Moldofsky H. Two contributions to the understanding of the 'fibrositis' syndrome. *Bull Rheum Dis* 1977; 28:928–931.

Weigent DA, Bradley LA, Blalock JE, Alarcón GS. Current concepts in the pathophysiology of abnormal pain perception in fibromyalgia. *Am J Med Sci* 1998; 315:405–412.

Wolfe F. The fibromyalgia problem. *J Rheumatol* 1997a; 24:1247–1249.

Wolfe F. The relationship between tender points and fibromyalgia symptom variables: evidence that fibromyalgia is not a discrete disorder in the clinic. *Ann Rheum Dis* 1997b; 56:268–271.

Wolfe F, Smythe HA, Yunus MB, et al. The American College of Rheumatology 1990 criteria for the classification of fibromyalgia. *Arthritis Rheum* 1990; 33:160–172.

Wolfe F, Allen M, Bennett RM, et al. The Fibromyalgia Syndrome: a consensus report on fibromyalgia and disability. *J Rheumatol* 1996; 23:534–539.

Correspondence to: Laurence A. Bradley, PhD, Division of Clinical Immunology and Rheumatology, University of Alabama at Birmingham, 805 Faculty Office Tower, 510 20th Street South, Birmingham, AL 35294, USA. Email: Larry.Bradley@ccc.uab.edu.

Proceedings of the 10th World Congress on Pain,
Progress in Pain Research and Management, Vol. 24,
edited by Jonathan O. Dostrovsky, Daniel B. Carr,
and Martin Koltzenburg, IASP Press, Seattle, © 2003.

68

Rehabilitation of the Injured Worker: Measurement, Management, and Evidence[1]

Margareta Nordin,[a] Jenny Strong,[b]
Maurits van Tulder,[c,d] and Harriët Wittink[e]

[a]*Occupational and Industrial Orthopaedic Center, Hospital for Joint Diseases, Mount Sinai New York University, New York, New York, USA;* [b]*Academic Board, The University of Queensland, Brisbane, Queensland, Australia;* [c]*Department of Clinical Epidemiology and Biostatistics, and Institute for Research in Extramural Medicine, Free University of Amsterdam, Amsterdam, The Netherlands;* [d]*Institute for Work and Health, Toronto, Ontario, Canada;* [e]*Department of Physical Therapy, Free University Medical Center, Amsterdam, The Netherlands*

Work-related pain, disability, and the rehabilitation of injured workers continue to be of enormous cost to Western societies. The concepts of *work* (in the sense of industrialized paid employment) and *unemployment* originate from the 18th century (Garraty 1978). In etymological analysis of European languages, *work* means trouble, worry, or toil. The French word *travailler,* for example, is derived from the Latin word *tripotium,* meaning a feared instrument of torture (Janlert 1997). The diverse linguistic origins of the word *work* may in part account for local and international cultural differences in patients' and clinicians' attitudes toward work-related back injuries. Kafka created the concept of *disability* in the early 1900s in Bohemia (Hadler 1993). The most common definition for disability used today by clinicians is that of the International Classification of Functioning, Disability and Health (ICF) (World Health Organization 2001). This definition includes the criteria of being unable to perform paid work, to perform unpaid work, to perform leisure tasks, and/or to lead a healthy life. These components are translated to activity and participation in society by the World Health Organization (2001)

[1] Based on a Congress workshop.

standards. This chapter employs the first component of the definition, "not able to perform paid work," because this is a common outcome measure for studies of low back pain.

Biological, social, and psychological factors contribute to the development of chronic pain in the injured worker. Measurement and management of the injured worker should therefore occur within a biopsychosocial framework. Studies of mixed methodological quality report poor to excellent rates for return to work (RTW) in patients with occupational low back problems. Few studies have examined work retention and early predictors of the transition from acute to chronic pain. One challenge for the future is to rapidly identify the individual at risk for extended or permanent disability, so as to intervene with an active multidisciplinary program with a focus on ability to work. At present, patients with work-related pain and incapacity must undergo testing to determine their need for rehabilitation and their current level of work-related disability. Clinical and claims decisions based on the results of these evaluations have serious short- and long-term implications for the worker, the rehabilitation practitioner, the employer, and the insurer.

This chapter examines the issues and evidence for assessment and management strategies used in rehabilitating injured workers. Different assessment methods used in the context of occupational rehabilitation and prediction of RTW will be surveyed. In addition, the evidence underlying the effectiveness of specific rehabilitation approaches and occupational outcomes will be reviewed.

CLASSIFICATION OF LOW BACK PAIN

The classification of low back pain as specific versus nonspecific has been adopted in several guidelines. (Spitzer et al. 1987; Bigos et al. 1994; Waddell and Burton 2001). The primary purpose for this crude classification is to encourage practitioners to seek medical history responses or physical examination findings that may identify a serious underlying spinal condition. The specific spinal conditions are fracture, tumor, infection, or cauda equina syndrome. Findings on the history or physical examination that carry increased risk for such conditions are referred to as "red flags." Specific nonspinal conditions are vascular, abdominal, urinary, and pelvic pathology causing referred low back symptoms. Nonspecific low back pain (NSLBP) is the absence of any of these specific conditions. Once a clinician has failed to identify "red flags" and nonspinal pathology, the patient's symptoms can be categorized as either sciatica or NSLBP.

The above crude classification of NSLBP was revisited and refined by Abenhaim et al. (2000), in the report of the International Paris Task Force. It was clear to the task force that clinicians require a more refined classification for NSLBP. The revised classification was derived from 1,141 articles published between 1966 and 1997, and by task force consensus discussion. The task force suggests two classifications for NSLBP, one based on signs and symptoms and the other on duration of an episode. There are many other classifications. The International Paris Task Force classifications extended the work of previous task forces' from Canada (Spitzer et al. 1987), the United Kingdom (Waddell et al. 1996), and New Zealand (Accident Compensation Corporation and National Health Committee 1997). Using the same or similar classifications for NSLBP facilitates communication between different stakeholders in the aim of preventing disability from NSLBP. A strong recommendation (Abenhaim et al. 2000) is to use a classification of low back pain rather than to omit one.

NATURAL HISTORY OF NONSPECIFIC LOW BACK PAIN

Studies examining recovery from NSLBP do not in general include patients with sciatica. Patients with NSLBP, once correctly diagnosed, will recover spontaneously from their activity limitations within 1 month. This aggregate course of recovery or nonrecovery may be termed the natural history of NSLBP (Fig. 1). About 80% of patients diagnosed with their first episode of NSLBP will recover within a month and an additional 10% within 3 months, while up to 10% will be left with chronic pain.

Recurrence rates, however, are high in patients with NSLBP and vary from 5% to 45% in different studies (Rossignol et al. 1992; Garcy et al.

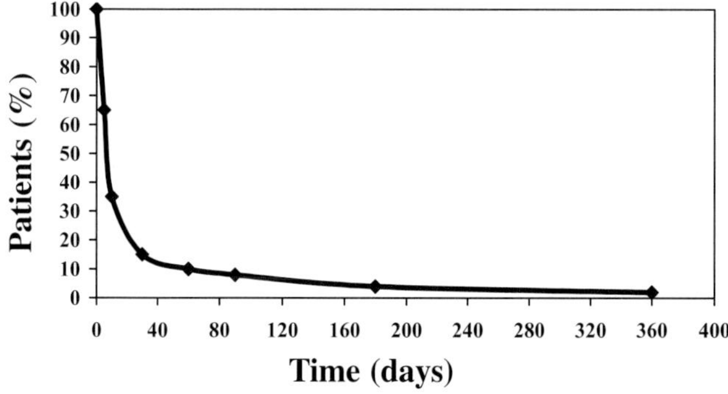

Fig. 1. The natural history of the first episode of low back pain: the percentage of patients with disabling pain as a function of time (in days) from the onset of symptoms.

1996). In a recent literature review, Campello (2002) showed recurrence rates to be associated with negative beliefs, fear-avoidance, depression, job dissatisfaction, pain intensity, previous history of low back pain, and physical work demands. Campello cautions about the difficulty in comparing and evaluating the literature on recurrence of NSLBP because most studies use different definitions of recurrence.

MODEL FOR TREATMENT OF NONSPECIFIC LOW BACK PAIN

Treatment of uncomplicated low back pain should focus on the early identification of pain behavior, impairment, and loss of function in the social environment, and on preventing permanent disability from NSLBP. The best model to embrace biological, social and psychological factors in the prevention of chronicity is the biopsychosocial model put forward by Fordyce and later adapted by Waddell (1992) for patients with NSLPB. This model provides an effective framework for management of NSLBP. A number of studies have operationalized this model to investigate the association between biopsychosocial factors and different outcomes of NSLBP, such as report of low back pain, incidence of NSLBP, success of a treatment program, sick leave, and disability (Bigos et al. 1991; Hazard et al. 1991; Lindstrom et al. 1992; Garcy et al. 1996; Hildebrandt et al. 1997).

PREDICTORS OF DELAYED RECOVERY FROM NONSPECIFIC LOW BACK PAIN

Early identification (within 4 weeks) of factors delaying recovery from NSLBP is helpful to identify patients at risk for extended or permanent work disability. Few studies have initially measured factors predictive of delayed recovery in patients with new, acute NSLBP. However, the following factors are moderately to strongly associated with delayed recovery and work disability in patients with acute NSLBP: previous disability from a back pain episode, depression, pain intensity, perception of disability, job demands/job controls, level of fitness and physical function, use of medication, use of medical services, and comorbidity (Bongers et al. 1993; Klenerman et al. 1995; Dionne et al. 1997; Nordin et al. 1997, 2002; Linton and Hallden 1998). Psychosocial factors are better predictors for chronicity and disability than are clinical or physical factors. These findings indicate that early screening and documentation for psychosocial factors are useful, as is screening for comorbidity. They also indicate the necessity for a broader approach to care that includes coping strategies, problem solving, relaxation, work intervention, and possibly individualized education about the condition itself. The Accident Compensation Corporation and National Health Committee of New Zealand (1997) incorporated some of these factors in the "yellow flags" to identify psychosocial aspects after 2–4 weeks of NSLBP. This prognostic tool is currently being tested.

A MULTIDISCIPLINARY TREATMENT

Evidence from the literature suggests that careful evaluation, cognitive behavioral therapy, education, and progressive physical activity are successful components of treatment for a patient experiencing delayed recovery from an episode of NSLBP. The literature also suggests that work problems need to be addressed early. The evidence suggests that optimal treatment requires a multidisciplinary team with expertise in the above areas. A key randomized controlled study (n = 103) performed at the Volvo Company in Sweden, discussed later in this chapter, was published by Lindström et al (1992). The authors obtained a 96% RTW rate. The success rate of this study is attributed to early management; patients were identified within 6 weeks of onset. The team (management, union, clinicians, and researchers) had extensive training and gave the patient an unambiguous message that returning to work is healthy. The program was based on the operant-conditioning behavioral approach. The content of the intervention included four parts: (1) functional capacity evaluation (FCE); (2) workplace visit; (3) back school education; and (4) an individual, submaximal, gradually progressive exercise program based on the functional capacity evaluation and the demands of the individual's job. The control group received regular care. The average durations of sick leave attributed to low back pain at 2-year follow-up were 12.1 (SD = 18.4) weeks and 19.6 (SD = 20.7) weeks for the intervention group and the control group, respectively (P = 0.05). Another important finding was that four patients in the control group received permanent disability compared with only one patient in the active intervention group. This study was repeated in New York City, and the first pilot study (n = 62) showed a 92% RTW rate (Campello et al. 1998) with a recurrence rate of 25%. A major difference between the two studies was their design (Lindström et al. used a randomized controlled study design, whereas Compello et al. used a prospective outcome design). Also, the duration of prior sick leave was 6.3 months (range 1–21 months) in the New York study, significantly longer than in the Swedish study. It proved very difficult in New York to have patients referred to a multidisciplinary program within 4–6 weeks. Furthermore, New York State legislation prohibits company physicians from referring patients directly to a particular center.

MEASUREMENT

Return to work, an important goal for the injured worker, can pose difficulties for the person with chronic pain (Strong 1996). Because chronic pain from work disability causes high personal and economic costs, considerable interest exists in early intervention to return injured workers to work (Gibson et al. 2002). With appropriate assessment and intervention directed at both the individual and the workplace, it is possible for a person with chronic pain to return to productive employment (Johns et al. 1994; Schmidt et al. 1995). An RTW program must be based on an individualized assessment of the person's functional capacities in conjunction with a thorough assessment of the demands of the job (Innes 1997; Shrey and Hursh 1999). Such assessment is needed to determine the most appropriate RTW goal. Whenever possible, the demands of the person's job should be assessed, or at least considered, *before* assessment of the person's capacity to return to work (Gibson et al. 2002). Doing so allows criteria to be set against which the person's capacity can be measured (Gibson and Strong 1997). The person's capacity to meet these specific demands is then established through work assessment.

Functional capacity evaluation (FCE) is a work assessment tool that evaluates the person's capacity to perform the physical demands of the job, or when there is no job available, the person's performance of physical demands of work in general. A trained therapist observes the person performing physical tasks such as sitting, standing, walking, crouching, kneeling, lifting, and carrying, and notes the person's abilities and limitations. The physical tasks observed during FCE are usually based on the physical demands defined in the *Revised Handbook of Analyzing Jobs* (United States Department of Labor 1991a), a companion publication of the *Dictionary of Occupational Titles* (United States Department of Labor 1991b). The latter publication is widely used to evaluate the match between a worker's functional capacity and the physical demands of the job (Lechner et al. 1994; Randolph 1996; Wickstrom 1996; King et al. 1998).

Based on the person's performance in the FCE, the therapist extrapolates whether the person could perform these demands in the workplace at the frequency required by the job. The therapist comments on the physical level of work the person can perform and recommends any limitations in performance, or restrictions, that may be required for safe performance in the workplace (Gibson et al. 2002). FCE provides a more objective measure of the person's functional capacity for RTW than self-report from interview and questionnaires and is "much better than 'clinical impression'" (Waddell 1998, p. 41). It is also a valuable baseline follow-up treatment outcome measure.

Another benefit of FCE is its focus on function (Gibson and Strong, in press, a), specifically on evaluation of the functional abilities of the person to perform the physical demands of work (Fishbain et al. 1995; King et al. 1998). For the person with pain wanting to return to work, an evaluation based on impairment alone may provide a distorted understanding of functional abilities. The person's diagnosis is a poor indication of his or her actual function (World Health Organization 2001) and is poorly correlated with function during work activities. Impairment refers to the loss or abnormality of body structure or of physiological or psychological function (World Health Organization 2001). Measurement of impairment provides information about the potential impact of the injury or condition upon functional activities. For example, the therapist may need to evaluate the person's impairment level before FCE to screen for potential underlying problems, precautions, or contraindications for testing. The therapist, however, is most interested in function during the activities the person would normally perform at work. Measures of impairment, such as range of motion, will not show what the person with pain can or cannot do in the workplace, and so the focus of the FCE should be on meeting the physical demands of work and potential to return to work (Gibson et al. 2002).

There are many approaches to FCE, ranging from commercial and standardized to nonstandardized. Research to date comparing these approaches has been limited. Innes and Straker (1999a,b) provided reviews of the reliability and validity of many different commercial approaches. These reviews, along with a three-part clinician's guide to work-related assessments (Innes and Straker 1998a,b,c), are valuable resources for therapists working in this area.

A recent survey of work practice by occupational therapists in the United States (Jundt and King 1999) confirmed that FCE was a frequently offered service. With such widespread use of FCEs by workers' compensation authorities and legal, employment, and welfare systems, FCEs incur considerable costs each year. Nevertheless, this use occurs in the absence of solid scientific research on the psychometric properties of FCEs (King et al. 1998; Innes and Straker 1999a,b). In addition to limited research, particularly regarding their reliability and validity, FCEs have other limitations. One such limitation of FCEs, and of work evaluations in general, has been their focus on biomechanical factors. Purely biomechanical factors are of limited predictive value for RTW. Many constructs operating in a complex and dynamic interaction are relevant to the RTW of a person with chronic back pain. These include demographic, physical or medical, psychosocial, behavioral, and ergonomic factors (Feuerstein et al. 1999; Carter and Birrell 2000; Turk and Gatchel 2000). Increasing evidence shows that psychosocial factors have greater value than medical or physical factors in predicting RTW (Haldorsen et al. 1998; Truchon 2001). Evidence has also been increasing of the contribution of psychosocial factors on physical performance, such as during an FCE (Rudy et al. 1996).

Gibson (2002) has developed an evidence-based, integrated, and comprehensive approach to FCE: the Gibson APProach to FCE (or GAPP FCE). This tool considers the various aspects of performance of the physical demands of work and incorporates measurement of variables shown to be relevant to the RTW of injured workers with back pain. The research and development of the GAPP FCE has followed standardized processes, from planning of the purpose and content of the items, to construction of the items and adjunct questionnaires, to quantitative evaluation of its psychometric properties (Dunn 1989; Hambleton 1991; Hambleton and Rogers 1991; Popham 1993). The GAPP has detailed and standard procedures and score sheets and an accompanying Users' Manual. The score sheets provide the therapist with a framework for using the three main models of FCE—biomechanical, physiological, and psychophysical—in observing the person's performance of the physical demands (Matheson 1988).

Four studies examining the feasibility, reliability, and expert validity of the GAPP FCE have been conducted (Gibson and Strong, in press, b). Participants were 7 healthy subjects (with an average age of 20.6 years, SD = 1.67 years) and 19 back pain clients (with an average age of 39.95 years, SD = 11.7 years) who were assessed using the GAPP FCE. Client assessments took an average of 3.25 hours to complete. Thirteen therapists were trained in the approach, procedural reliability was established prior to use with clients, and the therapists were silently observed conducting the evaluations by one other trained therapist and the senior investigator. A pilot study with healthy individuals indicated that the GAPP FCE was a feasible approach with good utility. A study with two trained therapists assessing five back pain clients revealed excellent inter-rater reliability, with an intraclass correlation (ICC) value of 0.96 for the total scores, and 0.80 for the recommended physical level of work. An expert review with five occupational therapists found support for GAPP FCE. A further study of inter-rater reliability of the GAPP FCE found ICC values of 0.80 (2,1) (n = 9) for the recommended physical level of work between the expert and therapist. In summary, the GAPP FCE appears to be a useful FCE tool in the work rehabilitation process for workers with back injury.

REHABILITATION OF WORKERS WITH SUBACUTE AND CHRONIC LOW BACK PAIN: THE EVIDENCE

Low back pain is a major medical and socioeconomic problem. It is one of the most frequent reasons for absence from paid or unpaid work and temporary or permanent disability, and is associated with high losses of productivity (van Tulder et al. 1995; Frank et al. 1996). Considering the socioeconomic impact of low back pain there is an obvious need for effective interventions, especially in occupational health care. The ultimate goal of such interventions for workers with low back pain is to return to work, either at the pre-injury level or with modified duties. Given the favorable natural course in the acute phase, the challenge is to return people to work later in the subacute and chronic phases.

Many interventions are used to treat workers with low back pain. This overview is limited to recently published systematic reviews of rehabilitation interventions for subacute and chronic low back pain (Frank et al. 1996; van Tulder et al. 2000a,b; Guzman et al. 2001; Karjalainen et al. 2001; Philadelphia Panel 2001).

Systematic reviews conclude that exercise therapy reduces pain and improves function in workers with subacute low back pain, but does not speed up RTW. Graded activity leads to earlier RTW and reduced long-term sick leave in workers with subacute low back pain. Lindström et al (1992) have described the graded activity approach. The goal of this approach (described above) is to return the worker to the previous, nonmodified workplace. Positive reinforcement is an important aspect of graded activity, as is continuous encouragement to return to work. No ergonomic or other changes in the work situation are included (Lindström et al. 1992). Other rehabilitation interventions for subacute low back pain (e.g., heat, cold, ultrasound) are not supported by evidence from randomized trials, although this does not necessarily mean that they are ineffective.

Systematic reviews have found that exercise therapy, behavioral therapy, and intensive multidisciplinary rehabilitation with functional restoration reduce pain and improve function, but do not have a clear benefit on RTW. Mitchell and Carmen (1994) have described the functional restoration approach. The goal is to restore function, which consequently leads to decrease and control of pain. The functional restoration program combines exercise with functional simulation and behavioral support. The exercise program uses a sports exercise approach that emphasizes mobility, strengthening, endurance, and flexibility. The functional simulation program is conducted in a specially developed occupational gymnasium and includes tasks that are commonly required in the workplace. The behavioral support consists of cognitive-behavioral treatment, relaxation, education, biofeedback, and individual and group counseling. The workers are treated in groups of 10–12 individuals. Other interventions for chronic low back pain have no or insufficient evidence.

In summary, multifactorial or multidisciplinary treatment consisting of a combination of exercises, education, and a behavioral approach seems the most effective intervention. Graded activity (Lindström et al. 1992) for workers with subacute low back pain, and functional restoration (Mitchell and Carmen 1994) for workers with chronic low back pain are the most promising concepts on which these interventions are based. However, optimal multidisciplinary treatment is still an open question as it is unclear what the most effective components are. Also, comprehensive economic evaluations examining the cost-effectiveness and cost-utility of multidisciplinary treatment programs are lacking.

Scientific evidence from clinical trials, systematic reviews, and meta-analyses of the effectiveness of interventions form a sound basis for clinical guidelines. Guidelines are an attractive means to close the gap between research and practice. Good clinical guidelines, however, also consider other aspects such as side effects, costs, and availability of various treatments, as well as preferences of injured workers and clinicians (Shekelle et al. 1999). At present, several guidelines have been published dealing with the specific issues of management of low back pain in an occupational health care setting: (1) Quebec Task Force, Canada (Spitzer et al. 1987); (2) Victoria Workcover Authority, Australia (1996); (3) American College of Occupational and Environmental Medicine, USA (Harris 1997); (4) Dutch Association of Occupational Medicine, The Netherlands (Nederlandse Vereniging voor Arbeids- en Bedrijfsgeneeskunde 1999); (5) Accident Compensation Corporation and National Health Committee, New Zealand (2000); and (6) Faculty of Occupational Medicine, United Kingdom (Carter et al. 2000). These guidelines agree on numerous issues fundamental to occupational management of low back pain. The assessment recommendations consisted of diagnostic triage, screening for "red flags" and neurological symptoms, and identification of potential psychosocial and workplace barriers to recovery. Their recommendations for treatment of workers with low back pain include:

(1) Reassure the worker and provide adequate information about the self-limiting nature and good prognosis of low back pain. (2) Advise the worker to continue ordinary activities and work, or to return to normal activity and work as soon as possible, even if there is still some pain. (3) Most workers with low back pain manage to return to more or less normal duties quite rapidly. Consider temporary adaptations of work duties

(hours/tasks) only when necessary. (4) When a worker fails to return to work within 2–12 weeks (there is considerable variation in the time scale in different guidelines), refer him or her to a gradually increasing exercise program, or multidisciplinary rehabilitation (exercises, education, reassurance, and pain management according to behavioral principles). These rehabilitation programs should be offered in an occupational setting.

The guidelines also agree on providing support and encouragement to patients that low back pain is a self-limiting condition and, importantly, that remaining at work or an early (gradual) return to work, with modified duties if necessary, is the best approach.

The management of low back pain in an occupational health setting should aim at a safe and timely return to work. Current occupational guidelines are consistent regarding their recommendations to reassure the worker with low back pain, and to encourage and support return to work even with some persisting symptoms. Evidence on the effectiveness of ergonomic and workplace adaptations is lacking, and guidelines do not specifically recommend this type of intervention. "Participatory ergonomics" interventions that propose consultations with the worker, the employer, and an ergonomist might be effective because the potential value of "getting all the players onside" has been stressed (Frank et al. 1998). Further evaluation of this approach and its implementation is needed.

REFERENCES

Abenhaim L, Rossignol M, Valat JP, et al. The role of activity in the therapeutic management of back pain. Report of the International Paris Task Force on Back Pain. *Spine* 2000; 25(4 Suppl):1S–33S.

Accident Compensation Corporation and National Health Committee. *New Zealand Acute Low Back Pain Guide.* Wellington, New Zealand, 1997.

Accident Compensation Corporation and National Health Committee. *Active and Working! Managing Acute Low Back Pain in the Workplace.* Wellington, New Zealand, 2000.

Bigos SJ, Battie MC, Spengler DM, et al. A prospective study of work perceptions and psychosocial factors affecting the report of back injury. *Spine* 1991; 16(1):1–6.

Bigos SJ, Bowyer O, Braen G, et al. *Acute Low Back Problems in Adults.* Clinical Guideline No. 14. AHCPR Publication No. 95-0642. Rockville, MD: U.S. Department of Health and Human Services, Agency for Health Care Policy and Research, 1994.

Bongers PM, de Winter CR, Kompier MA, Hildebrandt VH. Psychosocial factors at work and musculoskeletal disease. *Scand J Work Environ Health* 1993; 19(5):297–312.

Campello M. Physical and psychosocial predictors of work retention after a multidisciplinary rehabilitation program for non-specific low back pain patients. Dissertation. New York: New York University, 2002.

Campello M, Weiser S, van Doorn, JW, Nordin, M. Approaches to improve the outcome of patients with delayed recovery. In: Nordin M, Vischer TL, Cedraschi C (Eds). *Bailliere's Clinical Rheumatology: New Approaches to the Low Back Pain Patient.* London: Bailliere Tindall, 1998, pp 93–113.

Carter JT, Birrell LN. *Occupational Health Guidelines for the Management of Low Back Pain at Work—Principal Recommendations*. London: Faculty of Occupational Medicine, 2000.

Dionne CE, Koepsell TD, Von Korff M, et al. Predicting long-term functional limitations among back pain patients in primary care settings. *J Clin Epidemiol* 1997; 50(1):31–43.

Dunn G. *Design and Analysis of Reliability Studies*. New York: Oxford University Press, 1989.

Feuerstein M, Berkowitz SM, Huang GD. Predictors of occupational low back disability: implications for secondary prevention. *J Occup Environ Med* 1999; 41(12):1024–1031.

Fishbain DA, Khalil TM, Abdel-Moty E, et al. Physician limitations when assessing work capacity. A review. *J Back Musculoskeletal Rehabil* 1995; 5:107–113.

Frank JW, Brooker AS, DeMaio SE, et al. Disability resulting from occupational low back pain. Part II: What do we know about secondary prevention? A review of the scientific evidence on prevention after disability begins. *Spine* 1996; 21(24):2918–2929.

Frank J, Sinclair S, Hogg-Johnson S, et al. Preventing disability from work-related low-back pain. New evidence gives new hope—if we can just get all the players onside. *CMAJ* 1998; 158:1625–1631.

Garcy P, Mayer T, Gatchel RJ. Recurrent or new injury outcomes after return to work in chronic disabling spinal disorders. Tertiary prevention efficacy of functional restoration treatment. *Spine* 1996; 21(8):952–959.

Garraty JT. *Unemployment in History: Economic Thoughts and Public Policy*. New York: Harper and Row, 1978.

Gibson E. The research and development of a new approach to functional capacity evaluation for rehabilitation clients with chronic back pain. Dissertation. University of Queensland, Department of Occupational Therapy, 2002.

Gibson L, Allen M, Strong J. Re-integration into work. In: Strong J, Unruh AM, Wright A, Baxter GD (Eds). *Pain: a Textbook for Therapists*. Edinburgh: Churchill Livingstone, 2002, pp 267–287.

Gibson L, Strong J. A review of functional capacity evaluation practice. *Work* 1997; 9:3–11.

Gibson L, Strong J. A conceptual framework of functional capacity evaluation for occupational therapy in work rehabilitation. *Aust Occup Ther J;* in press (a).

Gibson L, Strong J. Expert review of an approach to functional capacity evaluation. *Work;* in press (b).

Guzman J, Esmail R, Karjalainen K, et al. Multidisciplinary rehabilitation for chronic low back pain: systematic review. *BMJ* 2001; 322(7301):1511–1516.

Hadler NM. *Occupational Musculoskeletal Disorders*. New York: Raven Press, 1993.

Haldorsen EMH, Indahl A, Ursin H. Patients with low back pain not returning to work. A 12 month follow-up study. *Spine* 1998; 23(11):1202–1208.

Hambleton RK. Validating the test scores. In: Berk RA (Ed). *A Guide to Criterion-Referenced Test Construction*. Baltimore, MD: John Hopkins University Press, 1991, pp 199–230.

Hambleton RK, Rogers HJ. Advances in criterion-referenced measurement. In: Hambleton RK, Zaal JN (Eds). *Advances in Educational and Psychological Testing*. Boston: Kluwer Academic, 1991, pp 3–43.

Harris JS. *Occupational Medicine Practice Guidelines*. Beverly, MA: OEM Press, 1997.

Hazard RG, Bendix A, Fenwick JW. Disability exaggeration as a predictor of functional restoration outcomes for patients with chronic low-back pain. *Spine* 1991; 16(9):1062–1067.

Hildebrandt J, Pfingsten M, Saur P, Jansen J. Prediction of success from a multidisciplinary treatment program for chronic low back pain. *Spine* 1997; 22(9):990–1001.

Innes E. Work assessment options and the selection of suitable duties: an Australian perspective. *N Z J Occup Ther* 1997; 48(1):14–20.

Innes E, Straker L. A clinician's guide to work-related assessments. 2. Design problems. *Work* 1998a; 11:191–206.

Innes E, Straker L. A clinician's guide to work-related assessments. 3. Administration and interpretation problems. *Work* 1998b; 11:207–219.

Innes E, Straker L. A clinician's guide to work-related assessments: 1. Purposes and problems. *Work* 1998c; 11:183–189.

Innes E, Straker L. Reliability of work-related assessments. *Work* 1999a; 13(2):107–124.

Innes E, Straker L. Validity of work-related assessments. *Work* 1999b; 13(2):125–152.

Janlert U. Unemployment as a disease and diseases of the unemployed. *Scan J Work Environ Health* 1997; 23(Suppl):379–383.

Johns REJ, Bloswick DS, Elegante JM, Colledge AL. Chronic, recurrent low back pain. A methodology for analyzing fitness for duty and managing risk under the Americans with Disabilities Act. *J Occup Med* 1994; 36(5):537–547.

Jundt J, King PM. Work rehabilitation programs. A 1997 survey. *Work* 1999; 12:139–144.

Karjalainen K, Malmivaara A, van Tulder M, et al. Multidisciplinary biopsychosocial rehabilitation for subacute low back pain in working-age adults: a systematic review within the framework of the Cochrane Collaboration Back Review Group. *Spine* 2001; 26(3):262–269.

King PM, Tuckwell N, Barrett TE. A critical review of functional capacity evaluations. *Phys Ther* 1998; 78(8):852–866.

Klenerman L, Slade PD, Stanley IM, et al. The prediction of chronicity in patients with an acute attack of low back pain in a general practice setting. *Spine* 1995; 20(4):478–484.

Lechner DE, Jackson JR, Roth DL, Straaton KV. Reliability and validity of a newly developed test of physical work performance. *J Occup Med* 1994; 36:997–1004.

Lindström I, Ohlund C, Eek C, et al. The effect of graded activity on patients with subacute low back pain: a randomized prospective clinical study with an operant-conditioning behavioral approach. *Phys Ther* 1992; 72(4):279–290.

Linton SJ, Hallden K. Can we screen for problematic back pain? A screening questionnaire for predicting outcome in acute and subacute back pain. *Clin J Pain* 1998; 14(3):209–215.

Matheson LN. Integrated work hardening in vocational rehabilitation: an emerging model. *Vocational Evaluation Work Adjustment Bull* 1988;22.

Mitchell RI, Carmen GM. The functional restoration approach to the treatment of chronic pain in patients with soft tissue and back injuries. *Spine* 1994; 19(6):633–642.

Nederlandse Vereniging voor Arbeids- en Bedrijfsgeneeskunde (NVAB). Handelen van de bedrijfsarts bij werknemers met lage-rugklachten. Richtlijnen voor Bedrijfsartsen. [Dutch Association of Occupational Medicine (NVAB). Dutch guideline for the management of occupational physicians of employees with low back pain.] April 1999.

Nordin M, Skovron ML, Hiebert R, et al. Early predictors of delayed return to work in patients with low back pain. *J Musculoskeletal Pain* 1997; 5:5–27.

Nordin M, Hiebert R, Pietrek M, et al. Associations of comorbidity and outcome in episodes of nonspecific low back pain in occupational problems. *J Occup Environ Med* 2002; 44(7):677–684.

Philadelphia Panel. Philadelphia Panel evidence-based clinical practice guidelines on selected rehabilitation interventions for low back pain. *Phys Ther* 2001; 81(10):1641–1674.

Popham JW. *Educational Evaluation.* Needham Heights, MA: Allyn and Bacon, 1993.

Randolph DC. Functional capacity evaluation and disability management. *J Back Musculoskeletal Rehabil* 1996; 7:181–186.

Rossignol M, Suissa S, Abenhaim L. The evolution of compensated occupational spinal injuries. A three-year follow-up study. *Spine* 1992; 17(9):1043–1047.

Rudy TE, Lieber SJ, Boston JR. Functional capacity assessment: Influence of behavioural and environmental factors. *J Back Musculoskeletal Rehabil* 1996; 6:277–288.

Schmidt SH, Oort-Marburger D, Meijman TF. Employment after rehabilitation for musculoskeletal impairments: the impact of vocational rehabilitation and working on a trial basis. *Arch Phys Med Rehabil* 1995; 76(10):950–954.

Shekelle PG, Woolf SH, Eccles M, Grimshaw J. Clinical guidelines: developing guidelines. *BMJ* 1999; 318(7183):593–596.

Shrey DE, Hursh NC. Workplace disability management: International trends and perspectives. *J Occup Rehabil* 1999; 9(1):45–59.

Spitzer WO, LeBlanc FE, Dupuis M, et al. Scientific approach to the assessment and management of activity-related spinal disorders. A monograph for clinicians. Report of the Quebec Task Force on Spinal Disorders. *Spine* 1987; 12(Suppl 7):S1–59.

Strong J. *Chronic Pain: The Occupational Therapist's Perspective.* New York: Churchill Livingstone, 1996.

Truchon M. Determinants of chronic disability related to low back pain: towards an integrative biopsychosocial model. *Disabil Rehabil* 2001; 23(17):758–767.

Turk DC, Gatchel RJ. Psychosocial assessment of chronic occupational musculoskeletal disorders. In: Mayer TG, Gatchel, RJ, Polatin PB (Eds). *Occupational Musculoskeletal Disorders.* Philadelphia: Lippincott Williams & Wilkins, 2000, pp 587–608.

United States Department of Labor. *The Revised Handbook of Analyzing Jobs.* Washington, DC: U.S. Department of Labor, Employment and Training Administration, 1991a.

United States Department of Labor. *Dictionary of Occupational Titles,* 4th ed. Washington, DC: U.S. Government Printing Office, 1991b.

van Tulder M, Koes B, Bouter LM. A cost-of-illness study of back pain in the Netherlands. *Pain* 1995; 62(2):233–240.

van Tulder MW, Malmivaara A, Esmail R, Koes BW. Exercise therapy for low back pain. *Cochrane Database of Systematic Reviews* 2000a; (2):CD000335.

van Tulder MW, Esmail R, Bombardier C, Koes BW. Back schools for non-specific low back pain. *Cochrane Database of Systematic Reviews* 2000b; (2):CD000261.

Victorian WorkCover Authority. Guidelines for the management of employees with compensable low back pain. Melbourne: Victorian WorkCover Authority, 1996.

Waddell G. Biopsychosocial analysis of low back pain. In: Nordin M, Vischer TL (Eds). *Bailliere's Clinical Rheumatology: Common Low Back Pain: Prevention of Chronicity.* London: Bailliere Tindall, 1992, pp 523–557.

Waddell G. *The Back Pain Revolution.* Edinburgh: Churchill Livingstone, 1998.

Waddell G, Burton AK. Occupational health guidelines for the management of low back pain at work: evidence review. *Occup Med (Lond)* 2001; 51(2):124–135.

Waddell G, Feder G, McIntosh A, et al. *Low Back Pain: Evidence Review.* London: Royal College of General Practitioners, 1996.

Wickstrom RJ. Evaluation physical qualifications of workers and jobs. In: Bhattacharya A, McGlothin JJ (Eds). *Occupational Ergonomics: Theory and Application.* New York: Marcel Dekker, 1996, pp 367–386.

World Health Organization. *ICF: International Classification of Functioning, Disability and Health.* Geneva: World Health Organization, 2001.

Correspondence to: Harriët Wittink, PhD, PT, Department of Physical Therapy, Vrije Universiteit Medical Center, De Boelelaan 1117, P.O. Box 7057, 1007 MB Amsterdam, The Netherlands. Tel: 31 20 4440461; Fax: 31 20 4440469; email: h.wittink@vumc.nl.

Proceedings of the 10th World Congress on Pain,
Progress in Pain Research and Management, Vol. 24,
edited by Jonathan O. Dostrovsky, Daniel B. Carr, and
Martin Koltzenburg, IASP Press, Seattle, © 2003.

69

Rehabilitation: Assessing the Outcome[1]

Alice Kvåle,[a] A. Elisabeth Ljunggren,[a] Liv I. Strand,[a]
Thomas E. Rudy,[b] and Dennis L. Hart[c]

[a]*Section of Physiotherapy Science, Department of Public Health and Primary Health Care, Faculty of Medicine, University of Bergen, Bergen, Norway;* [b]*Departments of Anesthesiology, Psychiatry, and Biostatistics and Pain Evaluation and Treatment Institute, University of Pittsburgh, Pittsburgh, Pennsylvania, USA;* [c]*Consulting and Research, Focus on Therapeutic Outcomes, White Stone, Virginia, USA*

Rehabilitation may be defined as a planned program in which a patient progresses toward, or maintains, the highest possible level of physical and psychological function, with illness and disease taken into account. Patients with persistent pain commonly have biopsychosocial problems. Selection of outcome instruments and choice of treatment should therefore be based on multi-method assessment batteries (Rudy et al. 1990; Turk et al. 1993; Turk and Rudy 1994). Test data can be prescriptive of treatment and predictive of outcome. Data can also discriminate between different groups of subjects and evaluate outcome after treatment. Whether each test included within a testing array is equally useful for every purpose can be questioned. While all assessment tools should be reliable, valid, and feasible, outcome measures also should be sufficiently sensitive to discern important changes (Beattie and Maher 1997; Simmonds et al. 2000).

Evaluation of the effectiveness of rehabilitation programs depends most often on outcome measures that are repeated before and after treatment (Deyo et al. 1991, 1994; Guyatt et al. 1987). Selected outcome measures must fit the patient, as well as the type and aim of treatment, and should address the following types of questions: Has treatment been clinically efficient and the program cost-effective? Which biopsychosocial dimensions are included? For whom are the outcome measures made: patient, health

[1] Based on a Congress workshop.

care provider, employer, health care system, or society? Increased emphasis on treatment outcome and cost-effectiveness in rehabilitation of persistent pain has placed additional pressure on clinicians and researchers to accurately report treatment effectiveness. The need to validate the utility of specific treatments requires not only the development of new assessment tools, but also additional validation of existing instruments to determine the degree to which they can accurately detect treatment effects.

This chapter will briefly suggest major domains of outcome assessment, followed by description and discussion of factors influencing the responsiveness of outcomes instruments to clinically important change. Because evaluation of treatment changes presents several important psychometric challenges, new methods to evaluate the validity of existing instruments will also be discussed. Additionally, recent psychometric advances permit the combination of multiple outcome instruments into a single item bank. Developments in these methods for functional health questionnaires (Hart and Wright 2002) will be discussed.

MAIN DOMAINS OF OUTCOME ASSESSMENT

Pain. Pain experience is regularly examined in various ways at baseline. Several subdimensions may be assessed, such as pain intensity (Jensen et al. 1986); sensory, affective, and evaluative components (Melzack 1975); anatomical location (Werneke et al. 1999); interference with activities (Ware et al. 1992, 1993); fear and avoidance (Waddell et al. 1993); and bothersomeness (Patrick and Deyo 1995). Degree of change along each dimension is measured, often at discharge, and if possible, at follow-up from rehabilitation, to evaluate how long treatment effects are maintained (Main and Burton 1995; Strong et al. 2002).

Function. Function can be measured on different levels according to the World Health Organization's *International Classification of Functioning, Disability and Health* (2001). According to this classification, the first level of outcome concerns losses or abnormalities of body function or structure, and comprises measures of impairment, i.e., joint range of motion or muscle strength. The second level focuses on limitations of activities, and comprises measures of activities of daily living. The third level relates to restrictions in participation, and comprises measures of life situations, i.e., work or obtaining a driving license (Dionne et al. 1999). Function may focus on physical aspects, and can be measured by self-reports as well as by different functional capacity and performance tests. Several studies have shown that although there is a correlation between scores on questionnaires and performance tests, the shared variance between these methods is so low that both should be included in outcome assessment (Grönblad et al. 1997; Simmonds et al. 1998; Waddell 1998).

Emotional distress. This domain focuses on psychosocial aspects, but may also comprise such questions as: What were the patient's mood and general well-being before treatment, and what was he/she thinking about his/her situation? Different types of psychological and quality of life questionnaires can be used to assess this dimension and to evaluate changes that occur during rehabilitation (Spilker 1996; Vlaeyen and Crombez 1999; Main and Spanswick 2000; Vlaeyen and Linton 2000).

Patient satisfaction. The patient's perception of the treatment can be evaluated, most commonly through questionnaires, but sometimes through interviews (Osborn 1998).

Health care utilization. The amount and type of medication taken before and after treatment is often used as an outcome measure when treating patients with persistent pain. Type and number of contacts with the health care system are other variables that may be reported (Andersson et al. 1994; Robertson and Colborn 1997).

ASPECTS TO CONSIDER WHEN DEVELOPING A TOOL FOR ASSESSING CLINICALLY IMPORTANT OUTCOME

GENERIC VERSUS CONDITION-SPECIFIC MEASURES

Quality of life is considered important to patients, and generic health-related quality of life measures are often used to assess important outcomes in rehabilitation studies. However, condition-specific measures should also be used to better capture key problems addressed in treatment of a particular group of patients. Heald et al. (1997) demonstrated that more than 60% of patients with shoulder pain had no problem identified by the generic Sickness Impact Profile (SIP). A wide range of scores was, however, demonstrated when the condition-specific Shoulder Pain and Disability Index (SPDI) was used, and only 2% reported no problem (Roach et al. 1991). This finding suggests that the SPDI is a better measure to detect treatment effects in this patient group than the SIP.

The Back Performance Scale (BPS) was recently developed as a condition-specific measure to assess clinically important outcomes in rehabilitation studies of patients with back pain (Strand 2001). Performances of five daily activities requiring mobility of the trunk were assessed on a 4-point ordinal scale. The test scores were found to be correlated and internal consistency was demonstrated ($\alpha = 0.73$, representing the average of the correlations among all the items in the measure). Accordingly, the five test scores could be summarized, providing a broad measure of sagittal trunk mobility (scores ranging from 0–15). The BPS sum scores were higher (worse) in patients with back pain than for other musculoskeletal pain, and discriminated between patients who did or did not return to work after rehabilitation.

RESPONSIVENESS AND CLINICALLY IMPORTANT CHANGE

Responsiveness connotes the ability of the measure to assess and quantify clinically important change (Cole et al. 1994). Test-retest variability of a responsive measure should be low when the condition is stable and high when the condition changes. High test-retest variability in a stable condition may be due to factors such as (a) learning effects among patients performing a test, or (b) inconsistency in scoring by the tester (i.e., low intra- or intertester reliability). Change in scores by a measure examined for responsiveness should be related to external indicators of whether or not an important change has occurred. No "gold standard" for important change exists, and so different indicators are used. Farrar et al. (2001) used the Patient Global Impression of Change to examine the responsiveness of the Numeric Pain Rating Scale. Patients who reported their condition to have changed for the better were expected to have improved considerably on the pain scale, while little or no improvement was expected of those who reported their condition to be the same or worse.

Return to work was used as an external indicator of responsiveness of the BPS (Strand et al. 2002). Because the patients in our study were all on long-term sick leave at the beginning of the study, full return to work at the 1-year follow-up was considered an important change for the patient, as well as for society. Physical performance, however, is only one of many factors (socioeconomic, psychological, and demographic factors, job characteristics) that influence whether or not patients return to work after long-term sick leave.

METHODS TO EXAMINE RESPONSIVENESS TO IMPORTANT CHANGE

Deyo and Centor (1986) suggested that outcome measures might be viewed as diagnostic tests to discriminate between improved and unimproved patients, and so their sensitivity and specificity in detecting improvement could be calculated on the basis of external criteria of important change. Thus, sensitivity is defined as the number of patients correctly identified as having improved by a particular change in scores on the assessment tool, divided by the number who had in fact improved, and specificity as the number of patients correctly identified by the assessment tool as not having improved, divided by the number who had not improved. Sensitivity is plotted against one minus specificity to generate a receiver operating characteristic (ROC) curve for each possible change in scores from baseline to follow-up. If the ROC curve is a diagonal straight line with area under the curve = 0.50, then the change in scores by the measure is no better than chance in discriminating improved from unimproved patients. The larger the area under the ROC curve (maximum = 1.00), the better the responsiveness of the measure.

The ability of the BPS to discriminate between improved and unimproved patients as defined by the dichotomous return to work variable (yes/no) was examined by constructing a ROC curve. The area under this ROC curve was 0.77. Assuming equal importance of sensitivity and specificity, the best cut-off point of change for discriminating improved and unimproved patients was 2.5 on the 0–15 BPS sum score (sensitivity 67% and specificity 70%).

Effect size, another commonly used method to examine responsiveness of assessment tools, is defined as the mean change of a variable (from baseline to follow-up) divided by the standard deviation of that variable (Kazis et al. 1989). A value of responsiveness can thus be derived of an assessment tool and compared to that of others, regardless of units of measurement (percentage, centimeters, degrees). Effect sizes, unlike *P* values in *t* tests, are less dependent on the number of subjects included, but still are affected by differences in standard deviation due to number. As suggested by Cohen (1988), an effect size of 0.20 is small, 0.50 moderate, and 0.80 large. A responsive measure should demonstrate a marked difference in effect size between improved and unimproved patients, defined by an external standard. The responsiveness of the BPS in terms of effect size statistics is shown in Table I (Strand et al. 2002).

Table I
Effect size of the Back Performance Scale sum scores in improved and unimproved patients; data are means (standard deviations)

Patient Group	*n*	Baseline	Follow-up	Change	Effect Size*
Improved	57	7.7 (3.4)	3.7 (3.3)	4.0 (3.0)	1.33
Not improved	57	7.1 (3.1)	6.3 (3.7)	0.9 (2.9)	0.31

* Calculated as the mean change divided by the standard deviation of the change.

PSYCHOMETRIC ISSUES IN EVALUATING TREATMENT OUTCOME

Numerous internal and external factors may affect rehabilitation and distort true changes, making it unclear whether observed change or lack of change is due to the intervention under study or some other effect that was not controlled for in the experimental design. For example, apparent changes may be due to unique events that occur during intervention (e.g., maturation, history), poor study controls, experimental bias, and treatment diffusion, to name a few (Cook and Campbell 1979).

Far less attention, however, has been devoted to psychometric issues, particularly measurement error, that may confound the interpretation of treatment outcome. Hebert et al. (1997, p. 1305) state that "it is vital to distinguish the signal (true change) from the noise caused by the unreliability of the instrument." When study participants are measured on multiple occasions using observational and self-report instruments, as commonly occurs in chronic pain outcome studies, additional confounders may be introduced into the evaluation process. It then may become difficult to determine which dimensions of the measurement system have changed and which have not (Wright 1996). If the intervention is successful, we might expect the indicators used to measure this change (e.g., test items) to alter their relative positions on the underlying scale or latent construct being measured (e.g., pain intensity, depression level). It may also be expected that study participants change the ways that they conceptualize the construct being measured. Only when items and scales demonstrate invariance across testing occasions can differences between multiple measures of participants be validly interpreted. Unfortunately, the classical test theory models that are most commonly used in outcomes research on persistent pain conditions do not disentangle changes in individuals, rating scales, and test items over different periods of assessment.

Recently, Wright (1996) proposed a Rasch-based algorithm for disentangling rating scale and item changes over repeated assessment, and Wolfe and Chiu (1999) demonstrated how this algorithm could be applied to evaluation settings involving measurement over two or more occasions. The Rasch Rating Scale Model (RSM) is part of a family of single-parameter Item Response Theory (IRT) models, which offer considerable advantages over more traditional classical test theory approaches that have been used by most test developers in pain research. The RSM is an additive linear model that describes the probability that a specific person (n) will respond to a specific Likert-type item (i) with a specific rating scale category (x) (Andrich 1978). The mathematical model for this probability (Eq. 1) contains three parameters: the person's ability-, disability-, or severity index (θ_n), according to the type or purpose of scale being evaluated, the item's difficulty or severity (β_I), and the rating category threshold (i.e., the threshold between two adjacent rating scale levels) (τ_x). In this model, it is assumed that the items are equally discriminating, response categories are ordered, and distance between each category threshold is constant across all items in the scale. Calibration of questionnaire data to this model results in a separate parameter estimate and a standard error for that estimate for each person, item, and rating category threshold:

$$P(X_{ni} = x) = \frac{\exp\sum_{j=0}^{k}[\theta_n - (\beta_i + \tau_j)]}{\sum_{k=0}^{m_j}\exp\sum_{j=0}^{k}[\theta_n - (\beta_i + \tau_j)]}, x = 0,1,\ldots,m \qquad (1)$$

where $P(X_{ni} = x)$ is the probability that a person n responds with rating scale category x to item i, which has $(m + 1)$ response options.

AN EXAMPLE USING THE INTERFERENCE SCALE OF THE MULTIDIMENSIONAL PAIN INVENTORY

The Multidimensional Pain Inventory (MPI) (Kerns et al. 1985) has been established as a valid and reliable measure in the field of chronic pain rehabilitation. However, in all previous studies of the MPI, classical test theory was used, which assumes that the underlying psychometric properties are stable or invariant with repeated assessments over time. This assumption may be a false and should be tested explicitly.

To evaluate the potential utility of the Rasch RSM in outcome assessment, a pilot study was conducted to investigate the Interference Scale of the MPI. Subjects included 212 patients with temporomandibular disorders who completed the MPI on three occasions: at the pretreatment assessment, 6 weeks later after participating in a standardized treatment intervention, and at 6-month follow-up. Specific aims study were to: (a) verify that the Interference Scale is unidimensional in nature, (b) test whether the items and the rating scale thresholds are invariant, (c) correct the measurement error associated with lack of invariance, and (d) determine whether these correction procedures result in the Interference Scale of the MPI being a more precise measurement tool for detecting treatment effects.

Summarized results will be reported for most analyses, with the exception of the rating scale test, which will be described in more detail to highlight several of the potential strengths of this methodology. Unidimensionality, an important requirement for IRT models, assumes that only a single component or factor influences subjects' performances along a particular scale. Conducting a factor analysis on the residuals following the fitting of the Rasch RSM to the data did support unidimensionality of the Interference Scale.

Tests for the rating scale threshold parameter estimates (the τ parameters in Eq. 1) revealed a lack of invariance over repeated testing. Linacre (1999) suggests several guidelines for evaluating the utility of a rating scale, specifically: (a) a minimum of 10 observations per category, (b) a unimodal distribution, (c) monotonically increasing parameter estimates (τ), (d) monotonically increasing step calibrations, and (e) an acceptable mean-square outfit statistic (0.60 to 1.40). (Outfit is a standardized outlier-sensitive mean square fit statistic that detects grossly unexpected responses that deviate from the Rasch Measurement Model.) Analyses of the Interference Scale across the three periods of testing disclosed some significant rating scale problems.

The MPI uses a 7-point rating scale (0 to 6) to collect subjects' ratings of the amount of interference that pain causes in different activity domains. An inspection of the average rating scale characteristics for the Interference Scale (Table II) indicated that the data had the minimum number of observations per category, had a unimodal distribution, and had monotonically increasing parameter (τ) estimates. However, the rating scale did not meet the criteria of having monotonically increasing step calibrations and acceptable outfit statistics. The step calibrations for categories 4 and 5 at the post-treatment and the 6-month follow-up were disordered, that is, not increasing monotonically. The outfit statistics indicated that category 6 did not fit the RSM at each of the three testing occasions, whereas, category 5 did not fit the RSM at the post-treatment follow-up. Additionally, the standardized differences (*t* tests) reported in Table II indicated that no rating scale thresholds, with the exception of category 1, were invariant across testing occasions. These findings indicated that the rating scale threshold parameter estimates were unstable across testing occasions, and thus potentially introduced measurement error into subjects' outcome scores. In order to create an invariant rating scale that functioned comparably across testing occasions, it was necessary to combine rating categories 4 and 5 to yield a six-point rating scale.

Additional lack of invariance across testing occasions was found for two of the 11 items that comprise the MPI Interference Scale. Specifically, the items concerning pain-related interference with day-to-day activities and the amount of change in ability to work due to pain were not invariant across the three testing occasions. The lack of invariance in these items presents a problem in score interpretation because these items' instability over time could result in decreased precision and validity.

In general, the Rasch RSM procedures for correcting lack of invariance over repeated assessments, as developed by Wolfe and Chiu (1999), were useful in adjusting the unwanted measurement error in the MPI Interference Scale. The ability of the uncorrected and corrected parameter estimates to accurately detect change was evaluated using a two-way ANOVA (correction vs. time). A significant interaction was found to exist in the Interference Scale between the correction factor and time ($P < 0.001$). Inspection of this interaction revealed that the effect sizes for the post-treatment and 6-month follow-up periods were significantly larger when corrected scale scores were used. These findings are relevant for the evaluation of treatment effectiveness in chronic pain rehabilitation. Even a well-established measure such as the MPI may under-report the magnitude of the treatment effect if measurement rating scale and item measurement error are not corrected during repeated assessments with the same instrument.

CAN COMPUTERIZED ADAPTIVE TESTING OF FUNCTIONAL HEALTH STATUS IMPROVE CLINICAL MANAGEMENT OF PATIENTS?

As noted above, the selection of outcome instruments for patients with painful syndromes is complex and can be affected by many factors. The number and variety of self-report outcome instruments can make it difficult to select the most appropriate one. Evolving mathematical models may improve the efficiency of outcome data collection by gathering and cocalibrating items from existing pain instruments in a single questionnaire. Equating is a mathematical procedure to allow different items or instruments to be meaningfully related, even if administered to different patients (Feuer et al. 1999; Cella and Chang 2000; McHorney and Cohen 2000; Ware et al. 2000; Hart and Wright 2002). Equating places scores from different instruments on a common metric, facilitating score comparisons.

Items from several outcome surveys describing physical functioning have been equated into one item bank for physical functional health status (Hart and Wright 2002). Item banks also exist for activities of daily living for the elderly (McHorney and Cohen 2000) and patients with headaches (Ware et al. 2000). However, for outcomes assessment in pain rehabilitation there are no studies demonstrating that dimensions can or should be assembled and cocalibrated within a single item bank.

Experts in assessment of generic health status (McHorney 1997) support the use of item response theory (IRT) (Hambleton et al. 1991) for equating items from validated outcome instruments into a common metric (McHorney

Table II
Calibrations, standard errors, fit statistics, and standardized differences for the Interference Scale of the Multidimensional Pain Inventory

Rating	Percentage (Counts)			τ			Step Calibration* (SE)			Outfit†			Standardized Differences‡	
Category	Pre	Post	6 Mo	Pre	Post	6 Mo	Pre	Post	6 Mo	Pre	Post	6 Mo	$\tau_1-\tau_2$	$\tau_1-\tau_3$
0	29 (662)	40 (859)	46 (828)	–2.37	–2.63	–2.86	–	–	–	1.03	1.08	1.08	–	–
1	18 (398)	25 (527)	26 (479)	–1.60	–1.56	–1.75	–1.47 (0.06)	–1.62 (0.06)	–1.73 (0.06)	0.91	0.74	0.74	1.77	*3.06*
2	15 (341)	13 (273)	11 (205)	–1.00	–0.92	–0.88	–1.17 (0.06)	–0.62 (0.06)	–0.51 (0.07)	0.82	0.89	0.74	*–6.48*	*–7.16*
3	14 (327)	10 (205)	8 (149)	–0.36	–0.36	–0.32	–0.67 (0.07)	–0.37 (0.08)	–0.38 (0.09)	0.88	1.19	0.99	*–2.82*	*–2.54*
4	11 (239)	4 (95)	3 (51)	0.29	0.00	0.12	0.22 (0.08)	**0.58** 0.10	**0.94** (0.13)	0.94	1.31	1.40	*–2.81*	*–4.70*
5	7 (159)	3 (71)	2 (36)	0.85	0.20	0.51	0.97 (0.09)	**0.49** (0.13)	**0.61** (0.16)	1.25	<u>1.47</u>	1.10	*3.04*	*1.96*
6	3 (77)	1 (25)	1 (22)	1.78	0.38	–0.28	2.11 (0.14)	1.53 (0.22)	1.07 (0.24)	<u>1.54</u>	<u>1.56</u>	<u>5.48</u>	2.22	*3.00*

* Step calibrations in boldface type do not increase monotonically.
† Outfit statistics that are underlined indicate a misfit.
‡ Standardized differences in italics indicate a lack of invariance.

and Cohen 2000). When items on a common metric are maintained in a single list (i.e., item bank), they may be selected and presented to patients via computerized adaptive testing (CAT) (Revicki and Cella 1997; Sands et al. 1997; Hays et al. 2000; Ware et al. 2000) in order to estimate a latent trait related to the pain dimension being assessed. The foundation of CAT applications is an IRT model.

ITEM RESPONSE THEORY

IRT models (Hambleton 2000; Hays et al. 2000) are mathematical equations describing the association between patient ability or severity on a latent trait or construct, in this case a pain dimension, and the probability of a particular item response (Hambleton et al. 1991). IRT models transform ordinal responses from items describing pain into linear measures, which are used to estimate item difficulty (i.e., item calibrations) along a measurement continuum or hierarchical scale. Models place items along a single, continuous dimension according to the proportion of persons who have limitations in that dimension. Patients with chronic pain are placed on the same scale according to the number of items in which they have limitations due to pain (Wright and Masters 1982). Item difficulty and patient ability are estimated with nonlinear regression-type models (Hambleton et al. 1991) that allow items from different scales to be cocalibrated to a common metric. In this way, the item difficulty on one scale can be directly compared to the difficulty or severity of an otherwise unrelated item on another scale, provided that the items fit the specific IRT model selected to calibrate the items.

One CAT process uses the following steps. The computer selects an item from the bank, and a patient answers the item (Ware et al. 2000). If the patient perceives that he/she has no difficulty with the activity, i.e., no limitation secondary to pain, the computer asks about a more difficult item. If the patient has problems with the activity, i.e., limitation secondary to pain, the computer asks about an easier item. After each response, an estimate of the latent pain dimension and its standard error is calculated (Hambleton et al. 1991), allowing assessment of measure precision in real time. The CAT stops when a predetermined level of precision is obtained producing an estimate of the pain dimension with an estimate of error per patient (Sands et al. 1997; Hays et al. 2000). CAT reduces administrative and respondent burdens by presenting pertinent items according to the patient's ability level while providing a precise estimate of the pain dimension.

IRT AND PHYSICAL FUNCTIONING

Several IRT models exist (Hambleton et al. 1991). Discussion of the assumptions, strengths, and weaknesses of different models is beyond the scope of this chapter. However, in a recent paper (Hart and Wright 2002), items describing physical functioning were equated using RSM (Eq. 1) (Andrich 1978). Some physical functioning items were queried in conjunction with pain interference (Fairbank et al. 1980; Vernon and Mior 1991), but pain dimensions were not analyzed separately.

Preliminary results support the reliability of item calibrations, as well as the construct and content validity of the physical function item bank hierarchical scale (Hart and Wright 2002). The CAT reduced the number of items required to estimate measures of physical functioning with a preselected level of precision, making CAT more efficient than the original outcome instruments. Correlational coefficients of estimates of physical functioning, using the CAT subset of items with the estimates of physical functioning calculated from all items answered by the patients, were greater than 0.95, suggesting test-retest reliability of the CAT process. Although preliminary results are promising, tests of different IRT models are warranted along with further tests of IRT model fit, unidimensionality, invariance, and validity.

Whether a physical functional health status CAT should include items representing pain dimensions should be investigated. We recommend that items representing the many pain dimensions be evaluated to determine if they can be arrayed into a unidimensional or multidimensional computer item bank. We hypothesize that many pain items will be multidimensional, and that the evolving CAT will require multiple scales or a complex multidimensional mathematical model. How pain dimensions interact with test scales is also of considerable clinical and research interest.

REFERENCES

Andersson GB, Bombardier C, Cherkin DC, et al. An introduction to therapeutic trials for low back pain. *Spine* 1994; 19:2066S–2067S.

Andrich D. A rating formulation for ordered response categories. *Psychometrika* 1978; 43:561–573.

Beattie P, Maher C. The role of functional status questionnaires for low back pain. *Aust J Physiother* 1997; 43:29–38.

Cella D, Chang CH. A discussion of Item Response Theory and its applications in health status assessment. *Med Care* 2000; 38(Suppl II):66–72.

Cohen J. *Statistical Power Analysis for the Behavioral Sciences*. New Jersey: Lawrence Erlbaum, 1988.

Cole B, Finch E, Gowland C, Mayo N. *Physical Rehabilitation Outcome Measures*. Toronto: Canadian Physiotherapy Association, 1994.

Cook TD, Campbell DT. *Quasi-Experimentation: Design and Analysis Issues for Field Settings*. Chicago: Rand McNally, 1979.

Deyo RA, Centor RM. Assessing the responsiveness of functional scales to clinical change: an analogy to diagnostic test performance. *J Chron Dis* 1986; 39:897–906.

Deyo RA, Diehr P, Patrick DL. Reproducibility and responsiveness of health status measures—statistics and strategies for evaluation. *Control Clin Trials* 1991; 12:142S–158S.

Deyo RA, Andersson G, Bombardier C, et al. Outcome measures for studying patients with low back pain. *Spine* 1994; 19:2032S–2036S.

Dionne CE, Von Korff M, Koepsell TD, et al. A comparison of pain, functional limitations, and work status indices as outcome measures in back pain research. *Spine* 1999; 24:2339–2345.

Fairbank JCT, Couper J, Davies JB, O'Brien JP. The Oswestry low back pain disability questionnaire. *Physiotherapy* 1980; 66(8):271–273.

Farrar JT, Young JP, LaMoreaux L, Werth JL, Poole RM. Clinical importance of changes in chronic pain intensity measured on an 11-point numerical pain rating scale. *Pain* 2001; 94:149–158.

Feuer MJ, Holland PW, Green BF, Bertenthal MW, Hemphill FC (Eds). *Uncommon Measures: Equivalence and Linkage among Educational Tests*. Washington, DC: National Academy Press, 1999.

Grönblad M, Hurri H, Kouri JP. Relationships between spinal mobility, physical performance tests, pain intensity and disability assessments in chronic low back pain patients. *Scand J Rehabil Med* 1997; 29:17–24.

Guyatt G, Walter S, Norman G. Measuring change over time: assessing the usefulness of evaluative instruments. *J Chron Dis* 1987; 40:171–178.

Hambleton RK. Emergence of item response modeling in instrument development and data analysis. *Med Care* 2000; 38(Suppl II):60–65.

Hambleton RK, Swaminathan H, Rogers HJ. *Fundamentals of Item Response Theory*. Newbury Park: Sage Publications, 1991.

Hart DL, Wright BD. Development of an index of physical functional health status in rehabilitation. *Arch Phys Med Rehabil* 2002; 83(5):655–665.

Hays RD, Morales LS, Reise SP. Item response theory and health outcomes measurement in the 21st century. *Med Care* 2000; 38(Suppl II):28–42.

Heald SL, Riddle DL, Lamb RL. The shoulder pain and disability index: the construct validity and responsiveness of a region-specific disability measure. *Phys Ther* 1997; 77:1079–1089.

Hebert R, Spiegelhalter DJ, Brayne C. Setting the minimal metrically detectable change on disability rating scales. *Arch Phys Med Rehabil* 1997; 78:1305–1308.

Jensen MP, Karoly P, Braver S. The measurement of clinical pain intensity: a comparison of six methods. *Pain* 1986; 27:117–126.

Kazis LE, Anderson JJ, Meenan RF. Effect sizes for interpreting changes in health status. *Med Care* 1989; 27:S178–S189.

Kerns RD, Turk DC, Rudy TE. The West Haven-Yale Multidimensional Pain Inventory (WHYMPI). *Pain* 1985; 23:345–356.

Linacre JM. Investigating rating scale category utility. *J Outcome Meas* 1999; 3:103–122.

Main CJ, Burton AK. The patient with low back pain: who or what are we assessing? An experimental investigation of a clinical puzzle. *Pain Rev* 1995; 2:203–209.

Main CJ, Spanswick CC. *Pain Management. An Interdisciplinary Approach*. Edinburgh: Churchill Livingstone, 2000.

McHorney CA. Generic health measurement: past accomplishments and a measurement paradigm for the 21st century. *Ann Intern Med* 1997; 127:743–750.

McHorney CA, Cohen AS. Equating health status measures with Item Response Theory. Illustrations with functional status items. *Med Care* 2000; 38(Suppl II):43–59.

Melzack R. The McGill Pain Questionnaire: major properties and scoring methods. *Pain* 1975; 1:277–299.

Osborn CE. Developing instruments for assessment of patient outcomes. *J Rehabil Outcome Meas* 1998; 2:18–25.

Patrick DL, Deyo RA, Atlas SJ, et al. Assessing health-related quality of life in patients with sciatica. *Spine* 1995; 20(17):1899–1909.

Revicki DA, Cella DF. Health status assessment for the twenty-first century: item response theory, item banking and computer adaptive testing. *Qual Life Res* 1997; 6:595–600.

Roach KE, Budiman-Mak E, Songsiridej N, Lertratanakul Y. Development of a shoulder pain and disability index. *Arthritis Care Res* 1991; 4(4):143–149.

Robertson SC, Colborn AP. Outcomes research for rehabilitation: issues and solutions. *J Rehabil Outcome Meas* 1997; 1:15–23.

Rogers WH, Wittink HM, Wagner A, Cynn D, Carr DB: Assessing individual outcomes during outpatient, multidisciplinary chronic pain treatment by means of an augmented SF-36. *Pain Med* 2000;1:44–54.

Rudy TE, Turk DC, Brena SF, Stieg RL, Brody MC. Quantification of biomedical findings of chronic pain patients: development of an index of pathology. *Pain* 1990; 42:167–182.

Sands WA, Waters BK, McBride JR (Eds). *Computerized Adaptive Testing: From Inquiry to Operation*. Washington, DC: American Psychological Association, 1997.

Simmonds MJ, Olson SL, Jones S, et al. Psychometric characteristics and clinical usefulness of physical performance tests in patients with low back pain. *Spine* 1998; 23:2412–2421.

Simmonds MJ, Harding V, Watson PJ, Claveau Y. Physical therapy assessment: expanding the model. In: Devor M, Rowbotham MC, Wiesenfeld-Hallin Z (Eds). *Proceedings of the 9th World Congress on Pain,* Progress in Pain Research and Management, Vol. 16. Seattle: IASP Press, 2000, pp 1013–1030.

Spilker B. *Quality of Life and Pharmacoeconomics in Clinical Trials,* 2nd ed. New York: Lippincott-Raven, 1996.

Strand LI. Assessment tools of pain and activity limitations in musculoskeletal conditions. Thesis. University of Bergen, 2001.

Strand LI, Moe-Nilssen R, Ljunggren AE. Back Performance Scale (BPS) for the assessment of mobility-related activities in people with back pain. *Phys Ther* 2002; 82(12):1213–1223.

Strong J, Sturgess J, Unruh AM, Vincenzino B. Pain assessment and measurement. In: Strong J, Unruh AM, Wright A, Baxter GD (Eds). *Pain: A Textbook for Therapists*. Edinburgh: Churchill Livingstone, 2002, pp 123–147.

Turk DC, Rudy TE. A cognitive-behavioral perspective on chronic pain: beyond the scalpel and syringe. In: Tollison DT, Satterthwaite JR, Tollison JW (Eds). *Handbook of Pain Management,* 2nd ed. Baltimore: Williams & Wilkins, 1994, pp 136–151.

Turk DC, Rudy TE, Sorkin BA. Neglected topics in chronic pain treatment outcome studies: determination of success. *Pain* 1993; 53:3–16.

Vernon H, Mior S. The Neck Disability Index: a study of reliability and validity. *J Manipulative Physiol Ther* 1991; 14(7):409–415.

Vlaeyen JW, Crombez G. Fear of movement/(re)injury, avoidance and pain disability in chronic low back pain patients. *Man Ther* 1999; 4:187–195.

Vlaeyen JW, Linton SJ. Fear-avoidance and its consequences in chronic musculoskeletal pain: a state of the art. *Pain* 2000; 85:317–332.

Waddell G. *The Back Pain Revolution*. Edinburgh: Churchill Livingstone, 1998.

Waddell G, Newton M, Henderson I, et al. A Fear-Avoidance Beliefs Questionnaire (FABQ) and the role of fear-avoidance beliefs in chronic low-back pain and disability. *Pain* 1993; 52:157–168.

Ware JE, Sherbourne CD. The MOS 36-item short-form health survey (SF-36) I. Conceptual framework and item selection. *Med Care* 1992; 30:473–483.

Ware JE, Snow KK, Kosinski M, Gandek B. *SF-36 Health Survey Manual and Interpretation Guide*. Boston: The Health Institute, New England Medical Center, 1993.

Ware JE, Bjorner JB, Kosinski M. Practical implications of Item Response Theory and computerized adaptive testing. A brief summary of ongoing studies of widely used headache impact scales. *Med Care* 2000; 38(Suppl II):73–82.

Werneke M, Hart DL, Cook D. A descriptive study of the centralization phenomenon: a prospective analysis. *Spine* 1999; 24(7):676–683.

Wolfe EW, Chiu CW. Measuring change across multiple occasions using the Rasch rating scale model. *J Outcome Meas* 1999; 3:360–381.

World Health Organization. *International Classification of Functioning, Disability and Health: ICF*. Geneva: World Health Organization, 2001.

Wright BD. Time 1 to time 2 comparison. *Rasch Meas Trans* 1996; 10:478–479.

Wright BD, Masters GN. *Rating Scale Analysis*. Chicago: MESA Press, 1982.

Correspondence to: Alice Kvåle, PT, MS, Section of Physiotherapy Science, Department of Public Health and Primary Health Care, Faculty of Medicine, University of Bergen, Ulriksdal 8c, 5009 Bergen, Norway. Email: alice.kvale@isf.uib.no.

Index

Locators in *italic* refer to figures.
Locators followed by t refer to tables.

D

Progress in Pain Research and Management Series

Proceedings of the 10th World Congress on Pain, edited by Jonathan O. Dostrovsky, Daniel B. Carr, and Martin Koltzenburg, 2003

Spinal Cord Injury Pain: Assessment, Mechanisms, Management, edited by Robert P. Yezierski and Kim J. Burchiel, 2002

Complex Regional Pain Syndrome, edited by R. Norman Harden, Ralf Baron, and Wilfrid Jänig, 2002

Neuropathic Pain: Pathophysiology and Treatment, edited by Per T. Hansson, Howard L. Fields, Raymond G. Hill, and Paolo Marchettini, 2001

Acute and Procedure Pain in Infants and Children, edited by G. Allen Finley and Patrick J. McGrath, 2001

The Child with Headache: Diagnosis and Treatment, edited by Patricia A. McGrath and Loretta M. Hillier, 2001

Pain Imaging, edited by Kenneth L. Casey and M. Catherine Bushnell, 2000

Sex, Gender, and Pain, edited by Roger B. Fillingim, 2000

Proceedings of the 9th World Congress on Pain, edited by Marshall Devor, Michael C. Rowbotham, and Zsuzsanna Wiesenfeld-Hallin, 2000

Psychological Mechanisms of Pain and Analgesia, by Donald D. Price, 1999

Opioid Sensitivity of Chronic Noncancer Pain, edited by Eija Kalso, Henry J. McQuay, and Zsuzsanna Wiesenfeld-Hallin, 1999

Chronic and Recurrent Pain in Children and Adolescents, edited by Patrick J. McGrath and G. Allen Finley, 1999

Assessment and Treatment of Cancer Pain, edited by Richard Payne, Richard B. Patt, and C. Stratton Hill, 1998

Sickle Cell Pain, by Samir K. Ballas, 1998

Measurement of Pain in Infants and Children, edited by G. Allen Finley and Patrick J. McGrath, 1998

Molecular Neurobiology of Pain, edited by David Borsook, 1997

Proceedings of the 8th World Congress on Pain, edited by Troels S. Jensen, Judith A. Turner, and Zsuzsanna Wiesenfeld-Hallin, 1997

Pain Treatment Centers at a Crossroads: A Practical and Conceptual Reappraisal, edited by Mitchell J.M. Cohen and James N. Campbell, 1996

Reflex Sympathetic Dystrophy: A Reappraisal, edited by Wilfrid Jänig and Michael Stanton-Hicks, 1996

Visceral Pain, edited by Gerald F. Gebhart, 1995

Temporomandibular Disorders and Related Pain Conditions, edited by Barry J. Sessle, Patricia S. Bryant, and Raymond A. Dionne, 1995

Touch, Temperature, and Pain in Health and Disease: Mechanisms and Assessments, edited by Jörgen Boivie, Per Hansson, and Ulf Lindblom, 1994

Proceedings of the 7th World Congress on Pain, edited by Gerald F. Gebhart, Donna L. Hammond, and Troels S. Jensen, 1994

Pharmacological Approaches to the Treatment of Chronic Pain: New Concepts and Critical Issues, edited by Howard L. Fields and John C. Liebeskind, 1994